SPINAL CORD MEDICINE

SPINAL CORD MEDICINE

Editors

STEVEN KIRSHBLUM, M.D.

Associate Professor
Department of Physical Medicine and Rehabilitation
University of Medicine and Dentistry–New Jersey Medical School
Newark, New Jersey
Director, Spinal Cord Injury Services and Ventilator Dependent Program
Associate Medical Director
Kessler Institute for Rehabilitation
West Orange, New Jersey

DENISE I. CAMPAGNOLO, M.D.

Associate Professor
Department of Physical Medicine and Rehabilitation
University of Medicine and Dentistry–New Jersey Medical School
Clinical Director
Spinal Cord Injury Program
University of Medicine and Dentistry–The University Hospital
Newark, New Jersey

JOEL A. DeLISA, M.D.

Professor and Chairman
Department of Physical Medicine and Rehabilitation
University of Medicine and Dentistry–New Jersey Medical School
Newark, New Jersey
President and Chief Executive Officer
Kessler Medical Rehabilitation Research and Education Corporation
West Orange, New Jersey

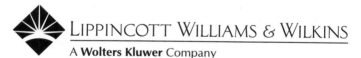

LIPPINCOTT WILLIAMS & WILKINS
A **Wolters Kluwer** Company
Philadelphia · Baltimore · New York · London
Buenos Aires · Hong Kong · Sydney · Tokyo

Acquisitions Editor: Robert Hurley
Developmental Editor: Stacey L. Baze
Production Editor: Thomas J. Foley
Manufacturing Manager: Colin J. Warnock
Cover Designer: Mark Lerner
Compositor: Maryland Composition Co., Inc.
Printer: The Maple Press Company

© 2002 by LIPPINCOTT WILLIAMS & WILKINS
530 Walnut Street
Philadelphia, PA 19106 USA
LWW.com

Printed in the USA

Library of Congress Cataloging-in-Publication Data

Spinal cord medicine / [edited by] Steven Kirshblum, Denise I. Campagnolo, Joel A. DeLisa.
   p. ; cm.
  Includes bibliographical references and index.
  ISBN 0-7817-2869-X (alk. paper)
  1. Spinal cord—Wounds and injuries. I. Kirshblum, Steven. II. Campagnolo, Denise I.
III. DeLisa, Joel A.
  [DNLM: 1. Spinal Cord Injuries. 2. Spinal Cord Diseases. WL 400 S757766 2001]
RD594.3 .S6695 2001
617.4'82044—dc21

2001038563

---

10 9 8 7 6 5 4 3 2 1

CONTENTS

CONTRIBUTING AUTHORS

James C. Agre, M.D., Ph.D. Staff Physiatrist, Department of Physical Medicine and Rehabilitation, Howard Young Medical Center, Woodruff, Wisconsin

Beth E. Anderson, OTR/L, CDRS Certified Driver Rehabilitation Specialist, Assistive Technology Center, Shepherd Center, Atlanta, Georgia

Filip Banovac, M.D. Department of Radiology, Georgetown University School of Medicine, Washington, D.C.

Kresimir Banovac, M.D., Ph.D. Professor, Department of Orthopedics and Rehabilitation, University of Miami School of Medicine; and Director, Spinal Cord Rehabilitation, Jackson Memorial Medical Center, Miami, Florida

William A. Bauman, M.D. Professor, Departments of Medicine and Rehabilitation Medicine, Mount Sinai School of Medicine, New York, New York; Director, Spinal Cord Damage Research Center, Spinal Cord Injury Service, Veterans Affairs Medical Center, Bronx, New York; and Senior Investigator, Rehabilitation Research and Training Center on Aging with Spinal Cord Injury, Rancho Los Amigos National Rehabilitation Center, Downey, California

Randal R. Betz, M.D. Professor of Orthopedic Surgery, Temple University School of Medicine; and Chief of Staff and Medical Director, Spinal Cord Injury Unit, Shriners Hospital for Children, Philadelphia, Pennsylvania

William L. Bockenek, M.D. Clinical Associate Professor, Department of Medicine, University of North Carolina, Chapel Hill, North Carolina; and Director of Spinal Cord Injury Program, Department of Physical Medicine and Rehabilitation, Charlotte Institute of Rehabilitation, Charlotte, North Carolina

Stephen P. Burns, M.D. Assistant Professor, Department of Rehabilitation Medicine, University of Washington; and Staff Physician, Spinal Cord Injury Service, Veterans Affairs Puget Sound Health Care System, Seattle, Washington

Denise I. Campagnolo, M.D. Associate Professor, Department of Physical Medicine and Rehabilitation, University of Medicine and Dentistry of New Jersey–New Jersey Medical School; and Clinical Director, Spinal Cord Injury Program, University of Medicine and Dentistry of New Jersey–The University Hospital, Newark, New Jersey

Gregory T. Carter, M.D. Clinical Associate Professor, Department of Rehabilitation Medicine, University of Washington School of Medicine, Seattle, Washington; and Regional Medical Director of Rehabilitation Services, Providence Health System, Southwest Washington Medical Center, Centralia, Washington

John Chae, M.D., M.E. Assistant Professor of Physical Medicine and Rehabilitation and Biomedical Engineering, Case Western Reserve University; and Attending Physician, Department of Physical Medicine and Rehabilitation, MetroHealth Medical Center, Cleveland, Ohio

Susan W. Charlifue, M.A. Research Supervisor, Department of Research, Craig Hospital, Englewood, Colorado

David Chen, M.D. Assistant Professor, Department of Physical Medicine and Rehabilitation, Northwestern University Medical School; and George M. Eisenberg Chair in Spinal Cord Injury Rehabilitation and Director, Spinal Cord Injury Program, Rehabilitation Institute of Chicago, Chicago, Illinois

Stuart D. Cook, M.D. Professor of Neurosciences, University of Medicine and Dentistry of New Jersey–New Jersey Medical School; and President, University of Medicine and Dentistry of New Jersey, Newark, New Jersey

Graham H. Creasey, M.D., F.R.C.S.Ed. Associate Professor, Department of Medicine, Case Western Reserve University; and Research Physician, Department of Spinal Cord Injury, Veterans Affairs Medical Center, Cleveland, Ohio

Joel A. DeLisa, M.D. Professor and Chairman, Department of Physical Medicine and Rehabilitation, University of Medicine and Dentistry of New Jersey–New Jersey Medical School, Newark, New Jersey; and President and Chief Executive Officer, Kessler Medical Rehabilitation Research and Education Corporation, West Orange, New Jersey

Michael J. DeVivo, Dr. P.H. Professor, Department of Physical Medicine and Rehabilitation, University of Alabama at Birmingham; and Director, National Spinal Cord Injury Statistical Center, Spain Rehabilitation Center, Birmingham, Alabama

Anthony F. DiMarco, M.D.   Professor, Department of Medicine, Case Western Reserve University; and Staff Physician, Department of Medicine, University Hospital, Cleveland, Ohio

John F. Ditunno, M.D.   Professor of Rehabilitation Medicine, Jefferson Medical College; and Project Director, The Regional Spinal Cord Injury Center for Delaware Valley, Thomas Jefferson University, Philadelphia, Pennsylvania

William H. Donovan, M.D.   Professor and Chairman, Department of Physical Medicine and Rehabilitation, University of Texas Health Science Center-Houston; and Medical Director, The Institute for Rehabilitation and Research, Houston, Texas

Susan Drastal, OT   Occupational Therapist, Kessler Institute for Rehabilitation, West Orange, New Jersey

Erica Druin, P.T.   Director of Rehabilitation Services, Kessler–Adventist Rehabilitation Hospital, Rockville, Maryland

Elie Elovic, M.D.   Co-Director TBI Research, Kessler Medical Rehabilitation Research Education Corporation, West Orange, New Jersey

Joyce Fichtenbaum, Ph.D.   Former Assistant Director, Department of Psychology and Neuropsychology, Kessler Institute of Rehabilitation, West Orange, New Jersey; Currently Stay-At-Home Mom, Montville, New Jersey

Rosemarie Filart, M.D., M.P.H.   Spinal Cord Injury Medicine Fellow, Kessler Institute for Rehabilitation, West Orange, New Jersey

Adam E. Flanders, M.D.   Professor, Department of Radiology, Thomas Jefferson University Hospital, Philadelphia, Pennsylvania

Susan V. Garstang, M.D.   Assistant Professor, Department of Physical Medicine and Rehabilitation, University of Texas Southwestern Medical Center at Dallas, Dallas, Texas

Lance L. Goetz, M.D.   Department of Physical Medicine and Rehabilitation, University of Texas-Southwestern Medical Center at Dallas; and Veterans Affairs North Texas Health Care System, Spinal Cord Injury Service, Dallas, Texas

Virginia Graziani, M.D.   Assistant Professor, Department of Rehabilitation Medicine, Philadelphia, Pennsylvania; and Director, Spinal Cord Injury Program, Bacharach Institute for Rehabilitation, Pomona, New Jersey

Andrew J. Haig, M.D.   Assistant Professor, Department of Physical Medicine and Rehabilitation and Surgery, University of Michigan; and Director, The Spine Program, University of Michigan Health Systems, Ann Arbor, Michigan

Margaret C. Hammond, M.D.   Associate Professor, Department of Rehabilitation Medicine, University of Washington School of Medicine; Chief Consultant, Spinal Cord Injury Disorders, Strategic Health Care Group; and Chief, Spinal Cord Injury Service, Veterans Affairs Puget Sound Health Care System, Seattle, Washington

Robert F. Heary, M.D.   Associate Professor of Neurological Surgery, Department of Neurosurgery, University of Medicine and Dentistry of New Jersey–New Jersey Medical School, Newark, New Jersey

Chester H. Ho, M.D.   Senior Instructor, Division of General Medicine Sciences Center for Physical Medicine and Rehabilitation, Case Western Reserve University School of Medicine; and Department of Spinal Cord Injury/Disorder, Cleveland Veterans Affairs Medical Center, Cleveland, Ohio

John A. Horton III., M.D.   Assistant Professor, Department of Physical Medicine and Rehabilitation, University of Pittsburgh; and Director, Department of Spinal Cord Injury, University of Pennsylvania Medical Center, Rehabilitation Hospital, Pittsburgh, Pennsylvania

Jamie G. House, M.D.   Former Spinal Cord Injury Fellow, Department of Physical Medicine and Rehabilitation, University of Medicine and Dentistry of New Jersey, Kessler Institute for Rehabilitation, Newark, New Jersey; and Attending Physician, Department of Physical Medicine and Rehabilitation, Penrose Hospital, Colorado Springs, Colorado

Stephen S. Kamin, M.D.   Associate Professor, Department of Neurosciences, University of Medicine and Dentistry of New Jersey–New Jersey Medical School; and Department of Neurology, University Hospital, Newark, New Jersey

Kevin L. Kilgore, Ph.D.   Adjunct Assistant Professor, Department of Biomedical Engineering, Case Western Reserve University; Program Manager, Department of Orthopedics, MetroHealth Medical Center, Cleveland, Ohio

Steven Kirshblum, M.D.   Director of Spinal Cord Injury Services and Ventilator Dependent Program, Associate Medical Director, Kessler Institute for Rehabilitation, West Orange, New Jersey; and Associate Professor, Department of Physical Medicine and Rehabilitation, University of Medicine and Dentistry of New Jersey–New Jersey Medical School, Newark, New Jersey

James S. Krause, Ph.D.   Adjunct Professor, Department of Behavioral Science, Health Education, Rollins School of Public Health, Emory University; and Behavioral Scientist, Crawford Research Institute, Shepherd Center, Atlanta, Georgia

Lisa S. Krivickas, M.D. Assistant Professor, Department of Physical Medicine and Rehabilitation, Harvard Medical School; and Director of Electrodiagnostic Medicine, Department of Physical Medicine and Rehabilitation, Spaulding Rehabilitation Hospital, Boston, Massachusetts

Daniel P. Lammertse, M.D. Assistant Clinical Professor, Department of Rehabilitation Medicine, University of Colorado, Denver, Colorado; and Medical Director, Craig Hospital, Englewood, Colorado

Todd A. Linsenmeyer, M.D. Associate Professor, Departments of Surgery (Urology) and Physical Medicine and Rehabilitation, University of Medicine and Dentistry of New Jersey–New Jersey Medical School, Newark, New Jersey; and Director of Urology, Kessler Institute for Rehabilitation, West Orange, New Jersey

James W. Little, M.D., Ph.D. Professor, Department of Rehabilitation Medicine, University of Washington; and Spinal Cord Injury Service, Veterans Affairs Puget Sound Health Care System, Seattle, Washington

William O. McKinley, M.D. Associate Professor, Department of Physical Medicine and Rehabilitation; and Director, Spinal Cord Injury Rehabilitation Medicine, Medical College of Virginia, Virginia Commonwealth University, Richmond, Virginia

Geno J. Merli, M.D., F.A.C.P., C.A.C.P. Ludwig A. Kind Professor of Medicine; and Acting Chairman, Department of Medicine, Jefferson Medical College, Thomas Jefferson University Hospital, Philadelphia, Pennsylvania

Jay M. Meythaler, M.D., J.D. Professor, Department of Physical Medicine and Rehabilitation, University of Alabama School of Medicine; and Medical Director, UAB Model TBI System, Department of Physical Medicine and Rehabilitation, Spain Rehabilitation Center, Birmingham, Alabama

Linda Marie Muccitelli, OTR Occupational Therapist, Department of Occupational Therapy, Rancho Los Amigos National Rehabilitation Center, Downey, California

Mary Jane Mulcahey, MS, OTR/L Associate Professor, School of Allied Health, Temple University; and Director of Rehabilitation and Clinical Research, Shriners Hospital for Children, Philadelphia, Pennsylvania

Mark S. Nash, Ph.D. Associate Professor, Department of Orthopaedics & Rehabilitation, University of Miami School of Medicine, Coral Gables, Florida

Cindy Nead, COTA Senior COTA, Specialty in Assisted Technology and SCI, Kessler Institute for Rehabilitation, West Orange, New Jersey

Steven B. Nussbaum, M.D. Assistant Professor, Department of Physical Medicine and Rehabilitation, Northwestern University Medical School; and Associate Medical Director, Spinal Cord Injury Unit, Department of Medicine and Rehabilitation, Rehabilitation Institute of Chicago, Chicago, Illinois

Kevin C. O'Connor, M.D. Chief, Spinal Cord Injury, Veterans Affairs San Diego Healthcare System, San Diego, California; and Department of Orthopedics, University of California, San Diego, LaJolla, California

W. Peter Peterson, M.D. Former Medical Director (Retired), Department of Respiratory Care, Craig Hospital, Englewood, Colorado

Mary Ann Picone, M.D. Medical Director, The Bernard W. Gimbel Multiple Sclerosis Comprehensive Care Center, Teaneck, New Jersey

Michael M. Priebe, M.D. Associate Professor, Department of Physical Medicine and Rehabilitation, University of Texas–Southwestern Medical Center at Dallas; and Chief, Spinal Cord Injury Service, Veterans Affairs North Texas Health Care System, Dallas, Texas

Arthur A. Rodriquez, M.D. Associate Professor, Department of Rehabilitation Medicine, University of Washington School of Medicine; and Director, Rehabilitation Care Services, Veterans Affairs Puget Sound Health Care System, Seattle, Washington

Sandra Salerno, OT/ATP Manager, Clinical Affairs, Independence Technology, Warren, New Jersey

Richard Salcido, M.D. The William Erdman Professor and Chair of Rehabilitation Medicine; Director of Rehabilitation Services; Senior Fellow, Institute on Aging; and Associate, Institute for Medical Bioengineering, University of Pennsylvania Health System, Philadelphia, Pennsylvania

Hreday N. Sapru, Ph.D. Professor, Department of Neurosurgery, University of Medicine and Dentistry of New Jersey–New Jersey Medical School, Newark, New Jersey

Carson D. Schneck, M.D., Ph.D. Professor, Department of Anatomy and Diagnostic Imaging, Temple University School of Medicine, Philadelphia, Pennsylvania

Ann M. Spungen, Ed.D. Research Associate Professor, Departments of Medicine and Rehabilitation Medicine, Mount Sinai School of Medicine, New York, New York; and Associate Director, Spinal Cord Damage Research Center, Veterans Affairs Medical Center, Bronx, New York

Paula J. B. Stewart, M.D. Physiatrist, Department of Physical Medicine and Rehabilitation, Charlotte Institute of Rehabilitation, Charlotte, North Carolina

Denise G. Tate, Ph.D., ABPP Associate Professor, Department of Physical Medicine and Rehabilitation, University of Michigan School of Medicine; and Chief Psychologist, Spinal Cord Injury Service, Department of Physical Medicine and Rehabilitation, University Hospital, Ann Arbor, Michigan

Alan Tessler, M.D.   Professor, Department of Neurobiology and Anatomy, MCP/Hahnemann University; and Department of Neurology, Philadelphia Veterans Affairs Hospital, Philadelphia, Pennsylvania

Ronald J. Triolo, Ph.D.   Assistant Professor, Department of Orthopedics, Case Western Reserve University; and Director of the Motion Study Laboratory, Louis Stokes Cleveland Department of Veterans Affairs Medical Center, Cleveland, Ohio

Lawrence C. Vogel, M.D.   Associate Professor, Department of Pediatrics, Rush Medical College; and Chief, Department of Pediatrics, Shriners Hospital for Children, Chicago, Illinois

Robert L. Waters, M.D.   Clinical Professor, Department of Orthopedic Surgery, University of Southern California, Los Angeles, California; and Chief Medical Officer, Rancho Los Amigos Rehabilitation Center, Downey, California

Lisa-Ann Wuermser, M.D.   Assistant Professor, Department of Physical Medicine and Rehabilitation, University of Texas-Southwestern Medical Center; and Chief, Department of Physical Medicine and Rehabilitation, Parkland Health and Hospital System, Dallas, Texas

Wise Young, M.D., Ph.D.   Professor and Director, Department of Cell Biology and Neuroscience, Rutgers University, The State University of New Jersey, Piscataway, New Jersey

Ross D. Zafonte, D.O.   Professor and Chairman, Department of Physical Medicine and Rehabilitation, University of Pittsburgh; and Vice President, Clinical Rehabilitation Services, UPMC Health System, Pittsburgh, Pennsylvania

PREFACE

The field of spinal cord injury (SCI) medicine has grown at an unprecedented pace. In the last decade, advances have been seen in the areas of acute and chronic medical care, in rehabilitation techniques and technology, and in basic science research.

This text is intended as a comprehensive resource of spinal cord injury medicine for clinicians and clinical investigators. SCI medicine encompasses both traumatic as well as nontraumatic disorders affecting the spinal cord. The topics covered in this text follow the blueprint of the subspecialty examination for board certification in SCI medicine.

The text begins with an overview of the subspecialty of SCI medicine, followed by the important aspects of spinal cord anatomy (Chapter 2), bony anatomy and radiology (Chapter 3), and epidemiology of traumatic SCI (Chapter 4). The next section includes the evaluation, examination, and classification (Chapter 5), treatment (Chapter 6), and prognostication after injury (Chapter 7) of SCI. Medical complications by organ system are then discussed, encompassing acute and chronic issues (Chapters 8–17), issues regarding dual disability (traumatic brain injury with SCI) (Chapter 18). Comprehen-

sive rehabilitation topics are also discussed, including adjustment, vocational, sexuality and fertility, recreational, driving, functional neuromuscular stimulation, and pain management issues (Chapters 19–26). Aging with SCI (Chapter 27) is followed by surgery for the upper extremity after injury (Chapter 28) and pediatric SCI (Chapter 29). Topics in nontraumatic disorders of the spinal cord are covered, including tumors, infections, vascular and nutritional diseases, multiple sclerosis, motor neuron disorders, and post–polio syndrome (Chapters 30–36). Acute and chronic demyelinating polyneuropathies are also covered since they are a part of the subspecialty examination (Chapter 37). The text then concludes with an in-depth review of wheelchairs (Chapter 38) and a review of research in the field of SCI (Chapter 39).

Well respected experts of varied specialties which include basic science research, physiatry, neurology, neurosurgery, and radiology have contributed to this book. The text is designed to give a view of the past, concentrate on the pulse of the present, and touch on the advances and opportunities for the future.

Steven Kirshblum, M.D.

DEDICATION

To my parents, Beverly and Judah, who taught me that without compassion, knowledge was not efficient or effective. To my grandfather, Rabbi Max Kirshblum, who taught me the importance of caring for those who were not otherwise being cared for. To all my past, present, and future patients and families, whose strength, desire, and motivation to achieve have served as an inspiration. To my professional mentors, Dr.'s Jerry Weissman and Joel DeLisa, who taught me that the continuous pursuit of knowledge was crucial for patient care and should be enjoyable. Most of all, to my wife Anna and three children Aryeh, Rena, and Max whose love, understanding, and support have allowed me to accomplish anything that I have.

I would like to thank Kessler Institute for Rehabilitation; and my colleagues, professional staff, and administration for allowing patient care to remain the main focus of what we do despite the changes in healthcare.

We thank all the fellows and residents that we have had the pleasure of being involved in their training. Your motivation to learn serves as our energy to teach. We would also like to recognize two organizations that have been so instrumental in furthering research and clinical care in the field of spinal cord injury, the American Paraplegia Society and the Spinal Cord Injury Model System Program sponsored by NIDRR. These along with the many other organizations dedicated to SCI help improve the knowledge base for which to treat persons with SCI, as well as to enhance their quality of life.

—S.K.

To my loving husband Tom who is my strength; to my children Thomas and Emily who are the lights of my life; and to my parents Rosalie and Carmine, who have always believed in me.

—D.I.C.

To my friend and colleague, Dr. Joseph W. Cheu, a dedicated physician researcher who lost his battle with hepatocellular carcinoma on September 22, 2001. Joe inspires all of us, through his writings, to view adversity, no matter how devastating, as an opportunity for personal growth. He reminds us to consider the spiritual and psychosocial needs of the individuals we care for, and that the pathway to providing compassionate, holistic care lies in finding our own inner peace.

—J.A.D.

SPINAL CORD MEDICINE

1

THE HISTORY OF THE SUBSPECIALTY OF SPINAL CORD INJURY MEDICINE

JOEL A. DeLISA

MARGARET C. HAMMOND

The approval in 1995 of spinal cord injury (SCI) medicine as a subspecialty of the American Board of Medical Specialties (ABMS) represented the culmination of concerted efforts by many dedicated individuals over the course of decades. Formal recognition of SCI medicine has promoted more focused research efforts and improved training for physicians who care for patients with injuries and diseases of the spinal cord. As a result of this milestone, there is better cooperation and communication among the various specialties that contribute to the complex care of the SCI population. With the growing number of board-certified specialists in SCI medicine, we are likely to see more rapid application of research findings to clinical practice. Our challenge for the future is to sustain this new subspecialty by expanding the opportunities for fellowship training and recruiting clinicians dedicated to improving the care of individuals with SCI.

The steps that led to the creation of this new subspecialty were detailed by Dr. Joel DeLisa in his sixteenth annual Donald Munro Lecture, "Subspecialty Certification in Spinal Cord Injury Medicine: Past, Present, and Future," presented at the forty-fifth annual conference of the American Paraplegia Society (APS) in September 1999 (1). The groundwork for this specialty was laid by the Veterans Administration (VA) during the period following World War II. Beginning in 1943, the VA developed multidisciplinary centers devoted solely to the care of veterans with SCI. The VA currently operates 23 of these specialized facilities throughout the nation (2). Based on this model, similar centers were established in Europe, the United Kingdom, and Australia.

A comparable initiative in the private sector, the Model Spinal Cord Injury Systems (MSCIS), was implemented in the United States in 1970 to coordinate research efforts and improve the management of individuals with SCI. The MSCIS is federally funded by the Department of Education, through the National Institute on Disability and Rehabilitation Research (NIDRR). The current system includes 16 centers that are funded for the 2000 to 2005 project period (3). The APS played a pivotal role in the development of the subspecialty of SCI medicine. Formed in 1954 by physicians involved primarily in the care of patients with SCI, most of the original members were working in the VA health care system. The APS was the outcome of a movement among professionals to improve the treatment of patients with SCI and to recognize the dedication and expertise of physicians who cared for "myelopathy cases" (4).

In its early days, the APS focused exclusively on scientific, charitable, and educational endeavors. The established goals of the APS were as follows (4):

- To advance, foster, encourage, promote, and improve the care and rehabilitation of individuals with SCI
- To develop and promote research and education initiatives related to SCI
- To recognize physicians who devote their careers to SCI
- To promote the exchange of ideas among SCI professionals

The dawn of the twenty-first century finds the APS making great strides toward its targeted goals.

By the late 1970s, significant advances had been made toward understanding the physiologic changes in major organ systems that commonly occur after SCI. Moreover, promising strategies had been developed for managing post-SCI pain and for addressing the myriad psychosocial issues associated with long-term care. With this foundation in place, the APS decided to pursue the establishment of a specialty board for certification in SCI medicine, to be called the American Board of Spinal Cord Injury (ABSCI). Organized medicine, however, remained unconvinced of the need for a new, separate certification board (1). In the early 1990s, renewed efforts by the community of SCI professionals met with greater success. In 1991, a new initiative was developed to support SCI medicine as a subspecialty certificate of the American Board of Physical Medicine and Rehabilitation (ABPMR). At a conference sponsored by the Eastern Paralyzed Veterans Association (EPVA), draft proposals detailing the professional and educational requirements for this new subspecialty were prepared for both the ABMS and the Accreditation Council for Graduate Medical Education (ACGME). After extensive review and critique, these proposals were submitted to the ABMS and the ACGME. Table 1.1 lists the required documentation for the ABMS proposal. This time, the efforts were fruitful—the proposal to issue a certificate in the subspecialty of SCI medicine was approved by the ABMS in March 1995. The approval stipulated that applicants for subspecialty certification in SCI medicine must be current diplomates of a member board of ABMS, and specified additional training and/or practice

TABLE 1.1. AMERICAN BOARD OF MEDICAL SPECIALISTS COMPONENTS FOR A NEW SUBSPECIALITY

1. Name of proposed new special qualifications
2. Purpose of proposed special qualifications
3. Documentation of the professional and scientific status of this special field
   a. History
   b. The existence of a body of scientific medical knowledge underlying the area, which is in large part distinct from, or more detailed than, that of the other areas in which certification is offered
   c. The existence of a group of physicians concentrating their practice in the proposed area, the number of such physicians and the annual rate of increase in the past decade, and their geographic distribution at present
   d. The existing national societies, the principal interest of which is in the proposed area, with an indication of the distribution of academic degrees held by their members and of the association of the membership with the specialties of medicine
   e. Numerical and geographic identification of medical school and hospital departments, divisions, or other units in which the principal educational effort is devoted to the area proposed for special certification
4. The number and names of institutions providing residency and other acceptable educational programs in the specialty, the total number of positions available, and the number of trainees completing training annually
5. The duration and curriculum of existing programs
6. The number and type of additional educational programs that can be developed
7. The cost of the required special training
8. Outline of the qualifications required of applicants for certification
9. Outline of proposed scope of the evaluation for candidates and a description of the method of evaluation
10. Copy of the proposed application form for candidates for certification
11. A written statement indicating concurrence or specific grounds for objection from each
12. A statement projecting the needs for, and the effect of, the new certification on the existing patterns of speculate practice, including the effect on the quality as well as the cost of providing such specialty care

From By Laws of the American Board of Medical Specialities. Chicago: 1991, with permission.

experience requirements (5). In recognition of the new subspecialty, the ACGME subsequently approved the program requirements for SCI medicine training programs in February 1996.

In June 1995, the EPVA awarded a 2-year grant to the ABPMR for the development of the SCI medicine certification examination, support that was crucial to the success of this new venture. Over a period of 2 years, contributing writers were trained through a series of item-writing workshops held at professional meetings of the APS, the American Spinal Injury Association, the American Academy of Physical Medicine and Rehabilitation, and the American Academy of Neurology. More than 80 physicians participated in the workshop series and submitted test items for consideration by the ABPMR.

In addition to the considerable efforts devoted to generating the item bank, essential supporting documents were developed. The first edition of the *Subspecialty Certification in Spinal Cord Injury Medicine, Booklet of Information* for prospective candidates was developed in April 1997 (5). Another key document, the examination question topic outline (blueprint), was completed in January 1998 (Table 1.2).

The first "Examination in Spinal Cord Injury Medicine" was administered to 92 candidates in October 1998. Of the 80 physicians who achieved a passing score, 70 were diplomates of the ABPMR, and 10 were diplomates in other disciplines, including internal medicine, orthopedic surgery, pediatrics, psychiatry and neurology, and urology. The second certification examination was given in October 1999, with 87 of 101 candidates receiving passing scores.

Today, there are 16 approved training sites for SCI fellowship programs. The "grandfather" period for certification extends to 2002 for candidates who are eligible based on clinical experience alone. After 2002, completion of a 1-year fellowship in an ACGME-approved SCI medicine training program will be a prerequisite for the SCI medicine certification examination. Fellows in these programs must devote a minimum of two thirds of their time to patient care, including the inpatient and outpatient settings.

It is evident that our colleagues endorse the purpose set forth for this certification (5). The subspecialty certification in SCI medicine offered through the ABPMR enhances the quality of care available to individuals with spinal cord dysfunction. As a result of formal specialty training in SCI medicine, we have a growing community of expert clinicians, teachers, and investigators who are equipped to achieve the following:

- Demonstrate special expertise in clinical knowledge and skill in SCI medicine
- Improve the rehabilitation and care of individuals with SCI
- Provide expert primary diagnostic and management services for complex and severe clinical problems related to SCI that require interspecialty management in SCI centers
- Support principal care providers of patients with SCI who practice in non-SCI centers, by rendering follow-up care to prevent and manage complications related to SCI

From the standpoint of future development of the profession, this new subspecialty credentials accomplish the following:

- Improve the quality of teaching of SCI medicine in residency programs of related primary specialties by increasing the number of subspecialists with additional knowledge and skills in SCI medicine
- Stimulate research that addresses the problems of individuals with spinal cord dysfunction while developing potential faculty members with special interests in SCI medicine
- Improve interspecialty and interdisciplinary communication and cooperation among specialists caring for patients with SCI
- Provide access to certification in SCI medicine to diplomates of all ABMS member boards, particularly those in specialties directly related to the care of patients with SCI

The 235 physicians board certified in SCI medicine constitute the nucleus for achieving our long-term goals: improving the quality of care and stimulating research into improved diagnosis and treatment of SCI. The 16 fellowship training programs are educating the next generation of leaders in this important subspecialty.

TABLE 1.2. AMERICAN BOARD OF PHYSICAL MEDICINE AND REHABILITATION EXAMINATION OUTLINE FOR SPINAL CORD INJURY MEDICINE

I. Types of Myelopathy
  A. Traumatic (fractures, dislocations, contusions)
    1. Cervical (C1–C8)
    2. Thoracic (T1–T12)
    3. Lumbar (L1–L5)
    4. Sacral
    5. Multiple
    6. Nonspecified
  B. Nontraumatic
    1. Motor neuron diseases
      a. Amyotrophic lateral sclerosis
      b. Spinal muscular atrophy
      c. Other motor neuron diseases
    2. Spondylotic myelopathies
      a. Spondylolysis; spondylolisthesis
      b. Spinal stenosis
      c. Disk herniation; ruptures
      d. Atlantoaxial instability
      e. Other spondylotic myelopathies
    3. Infectious and inflammatory diseases
      a. Multiple sclerosis
      b. Epidural abscesses
      c. Transverse myelitis
      d. Poliomyelitis; postpoliomyelitis
      e. Osteomyelitis
      f. Arachnoiditis
      g. Human immunodeficiency virus
      h. Chronic inflammatory demyelinating polyradiculoneuropathy; acute inflammatory demyelinating polyradiculoneuropathy
      i. Other infectious and inflammatory diseases
    4. Neoplastic diseases
      a. Malignant and metastatic tumors
      b. Nonmalignant tumors
      c. Other neoplastic diseases
    5. Vascular disorders
      a. Ischemic myelopathy
      b. Arteriovenous malformations
      c. Other vascular disorders
    6. Toxic and metabolic conditions
      a. Radiation-induced myelopathy
      b. Subacute combined degeneration
      c. Other toxic and metabolic conditions
    7. Congenital and developmental disorders
      a. Myelodysplasia
      b. Developmental syringomyelia
      c. Other congenital and developmental disorders
  C. Nonspecified and Other Spinal Cord Injury Myelopathies

II. Physiologic Complications Due to Spinal Cord Injury
  A. Cardiovascular
    1. Arrhythmias
    2. Ischemic heart disease
    3. Autonomic dysfunction
    4. Peripheral arterial disease
    5. Venous disease
    6. Deep vein thrombosis
    7. Edema
    8. Hypertension
    9. Orthostatic hypotension
    10. Applied sciences
    11. Other cardiovascular complications
  B. Pulmonary
    1. Restrictive pulmonary syndrome
    2. Pneumonia
    3. Hypoventilation and respiratory failure
    4. Pulmonary embolism
    5. Applied sciences
    6. Other pulmonary complications

  C. Genitourinary
    1. Neurogenic bladder
    2. Renal impairment
    3. Urinary tract infection
    4. Sexuality and reproductive issues
    5. Applied sciences
    6. Other genitourinary complications
  D. Gastrointestinal
    1. Neurogenic bowel
    2. Upper gastrointestinal problems
    3. Liver dysfunction
    4. Applied sciences
    5. Other gastrointestinal complications (e.g., pancreatitis)
  E. Musculoskeletal
    1. Joint complications (e.g., neuropathic, Charcot)
    2. Soft tissue complications (e.g., bursitis, contracture)
    3. Arthritis; arthritides
    4. Heterotopic ossification
    5. Demineralization (e.g., osteoporosis)
    6. Fractures (nonvertebral)
    7. Scoliosis
    8. Deconditioning
    9. Overuse and repetitive use (e.g., rotator cuff)
    10. Spine fractures (vertebral) and dislocations
    11. Applied sciences
    12. Other musculoskeletal complications
  F. Neurologic and Neuromuscular
    1. Spasticity
    2. Seizures
    3. Peripheral nerve dysfunction
    4. Dysphagia
    5. Hydrocephalus
    6. Syringomyelia
    7. Autonomic dysreflexia
    8. Applied sciences
    9. Other neuro complications (e.g., coma, stroke)
  G. Integumentary
    1. Sacral ulcers
    2. Trochanteric ulcers
    3. Ischial ulcers
    4. Other and combined ulcers
  H. Systemic
    1. Infectious disease
    2. Immunosuppression
    3. Metabolic disorders (e.g., hypercalcemia; thermoregulation)
    4. Endocrine disorders
    5. Diabetes
    6. Nutrition deficiency
    7. Applied sciences
    8. Other systemic complications (e.g., fatigue)
  I. Cognitive and Psychological
    1. Sleep disorders
    2. Communication disorders
    3. Depression and affective disorders
    4. Maladaptive behavior
    5. Substance abuse
    6. Applied sciences
    7. Other cognitive or psychological complications (including traumatic brain injury)
  J. Pain
    1. Peripheral nerve pain
    2. Central spinal cord pain
    3. Visceral pain
    4. Muscle and mechanical pain
    5. Psychogenic pain
    6. Other pain
  K. Nonspecified and Multiple Complications (including comorbidities)

(continued)

TABLE 1.2. Continued.

III. Clinical Decision Making
  A. Patient Evaluation and Diagnosis
    1. Diagnostic and clinical sciences
      a. Epidemiology
      b. Risk factors
      c. Etiology
      d. Classification, other
    2. Physical exam, signs, symptoms
    3. Specific diagnostic procedures
      a. Cardiopulmonary assessment
      b. Urodynamics
      c. Gait analysis
      d. Lab studies (e.g., blood gases)
      e. Medical imaging (e.g., x-ray, computed tomography, magnetic resonance imaging)
      f. Psychosocial evaluation
      g. Other diagnostic procedures
    4. Functional evaluation
      a. By level
      b. Energy expenditure analysis
    5. Spinal cord injury classification (ASIA)
    6. Prognosis
      a. Probable complications
      b. Life expectancy
      c. Outcomes
  B. Electrodiagnosis
    1. Nerve conduction
    2. Electromyography
    3. Somatosensory evoked potential
    4. Special studies
  C. Patient Management
    1. Emergency care (e.g., initial care, patient transport)
    2. Physical agents
      a. Heat and cryotherapy
      b. Ultrasound
      c. Multiple and other physical agents
    3. Therapeutic exercise and manipulation
      a. Reeducation; motor control
      b. Mobility and range of motion
      c. Strength and endurance
      d. Manipulation and massage
      e. Multiple and other therapeutic exercise and manipulation
    4. Pharmacologic interventions
      a. Analgesics
      b. Antispasticity medications
      c. Antiinflammatory agents
      d. Antibiotics
      e. Antidepressants
      f. Antihypertensives
      g. Anticoagulants
      h. Immunomodulatory agents
      i. Bowel and bladder medications (e.g., anticholinergics, receptor blockers, colonic stimulants)
      j. Multiple and other pharmacologic interventions
    5. Procedural and interventional
      a. Surgery
      b. Nerve blocks (e.g., phenol, botulinum toxin)
      c. Anesthetic injections
      d. Serial casting
      e. Traction and immobilization
      f. Multiple and other procedural and interventional
    6. Functional training
      a. Mobility and ambulation
      b. Activities of daily living
      c. Bladder function
      d. Bowel function
      e. Sexual function
      f. Multiple and other functional training
    7. Rehabilitation technology
      a. Orthotics
      b. Functional electrical stimulation
      c. Transcutaneous electrical nerve stimulation
      d. Ventilation
      e. Wheelchair and seating
      f. Communication devices
      g. Multiple and other assistive devices
    8. Psychosocial Issues
      a. Relaxation therapy
      b. Behavior modification
      c. Psychotherapy and counseling
      d. Patient and family education
      e. Vocational rehabilitation
      f. Multiple and other psychosocial issues
    9. Nutrition therapy
    10. Health care teams
    11. Ethics
  D. Basic and Clinical Sciences
    1. Anatomy
    2. Physiology
    3. Pathology; pathophysiology
    4. Genetics
    5. Kinesiology; biomechanics
    6. Neuroregeneration
    7. Research and statistics
    8. Other basic and clinical sciences
  E. Nonspecified and Multiple Clinical Decision Making

Looking back on the past 50 years in SCI medicine, the outcome of hard work, persistence, and cooperation is evident. By adhering to this approach, we can build on the solid framework we have established, resulting in improvements in care that will ease the burdens of living with SCI for patients and their families.

REFERENCES

1. DeLisa JA. Subspecialty certification in spinal cord injury medicine: past, present and future. *J Spinal Cord Med* 1999;22(3):218–225.

2. Veterans Affairs Spinal Cord Injury and Disorders (SCI&D) Centers. Available from SCI&D Strategic Healthcare groups, 1660 S. Columbian Way (128 NAT), Seattle, WA 98108.

3. National Center for the Dissemination of Disability Research (NCDDR) web site. Available at http://www.ncdrr.org/rpp/hf/webres_spinal.html. Accessed October 16, 2000.

4. *Historical information re: American Board of Spinal Cord Injury.* (n.d.) Unpublished work. (Available from American Paraplegia Society, 75-20 Astoria Blvd, Jackson Heights, NY 11370.)

5. *Subspecialty certification in spinal cord injury medicine, booklet of information.* American Board of Physical Medicine and Rehabilitation. (Available from ABPM&R, 21 First Street SW Suite 674, Rochester, MN, 55902-3092.)

SPINAL CORD: ANATOMY, PHYSIOLOGY, AND PATHOPHYSIOLOGY

HREDAY N. SAPRU

The spinal cord receives sensory information from somatic and visceral receptors through dorsal roots, transmits this information to higher brain structures through ascending tracts, receives signals from higher centers through descending tracts, and finally transmits these signals to somatic and visceral target sites through the ventral roots. The spinal cord, therefore, is a critical component for the transmission of sensory information to the brain and for the subsequent regulation of motor and autonomic functions. In this chapter, a brief review is presented of the important anatomic features of the spinal cord, including its ascending and descending tracts (1–3). Descriptions of several animal models of spinal cord injury (SCI) and pathophysiologic correlates derived from them are also included (4).

COVERINGS OF THE SPINAL CORD

The coverings (meninges) of the spinal cord include the dura, arachnoid, and pia mater. Although the spinal coverings are generally similar to those of the brain, there are some differences, which are subsequently listed. The spinal dura is single-layered and lacks the periosteal layer of the cranial dura. The spinal epidural space is an actual space in which venous plexuses are located and is used clinically for the administration of epidural anesthesia to produce a paravertebral nerve block. On the other hand, the cranial epidural space is a potential space that becomes filled with a fluid only in pathologic conditions; normally, there is no space between the dura and the cranium. The spinal epidural space is located between the meningeal layer of the dura (there is no periosteal layer) and the periosteum of the vertebra, whereas the cranial epidural space (when present) is located between the periosteal layer of the dura and the cranium (Fig. 2.1).

Dura Mater

As stated earlier, the spinal dura consists of the meningeal layer only and lacks the periosteal layer of the cranial dura. Rostrally, the spinal dura joins the meningeal layer of the cranial dura at the margins of the foramen magnum. The spinal epidural space separates the spinal dura from the periosteum of the vertebra and is filled with fatty connective tissue and plexuses of veins. Caudally, the spinal dura ends at the level of the second sacral vertebra (Fig. 2.2). At this level, the spinal dura becomes a thin extension (the coccygeal ligament or filum terminale externum) and serves to anchor the spinal dura to the base of the vertebral canal.

Arachnoid

The arachnoid membrane loosely invests the spinal cord and is connected to the dura by connective tissue trabeculae. Rostrally, it passes through the foramen magnum to join the cranial arachnoid; caudally, it surrounds the cauda equina (a bundle of nerve roots of all the spinal nerves caudal to the second lumbar vertebra) (Fig. 2.2). The subarachnoid space contains cerebrospinal fluid (CSF).

Pia Mater

The spinal pia is thicker than the cranial pia. It is a vascular membrane and projects into the ventral fissure of the spinal cord. At intervals, toothed ligaments of pial tissue, called *dentate ligaments*, extend from the lateral surfaces of the spinal cord; these ligaments serve to anchor the spinal cord to the arachnoid and through it to the dura. As mentioned earlier, at caudal levels, spinal pia continues along the filum terminale, which then anchors the spinal cord to the dura at the level of the second sacral vertebra. Rostrally, the spinal pia joins the cranial pia.

GROSS ANATOMY

The spinal cord is a long, cylindrical structure that is continuous with the medulla rostrally and ends at the rostral border of the second lumbar vertebra. At the caudal end, the spinal cord is conical in shape and is known as the *conus medullaris* (Fig. 2.2). A filament extending from the conus medullaris is called the filum terminale. This filament is enclosed in pia and consists of glial cells, ependymal cells, and astrocytes. As stated earlier, the

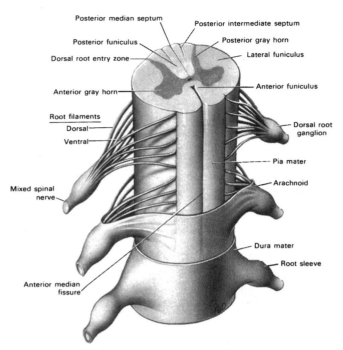

FIGURE 2.1. Coverings of the spinal cord. (From Parent A, ed. *Human neuroanatomy*. 9th ed. Baltimore: Lippincott Williams & Wilkins, 1996: 327, with permission.)

composition of the CSF in disorders such as meningitis. As noted previously, the caudal end of the spinal cord in the normal adult is located at the second lumbar vertebra. A puncture is usually made between the third and fourth lumbar vertebrae, and 5 to 15 mL of the CSF is removed to perform the cell count, protein analysis, and microbiologic studies. The patient is placed in a lateral recumbent position, and the CSF pressure is measured by a manometer. Normally, the CSF pressure should be less than 200 mm H_2O. If the intracranial pressure is high, withdrawal of CSF is contraindicated because brain tissue may herniate through the foramen magnum.

caudal thin extension of spinal dura is called the *coccygeal ligament*. This ligament surrounds the filum terminale internum of the spinal cord and attaches to the coccyx in order to anchor the spinal cord.

Up through the third month of fetal life, the spinal cord occupies the whole length of the vertebral canal. After the third month, the rate of lengthening of the spinal cord is slower than the lengthening of the vertebral column. In an adult, therefore, the spinal cord occupies only the upper two thirds of the vertebral column, with its caudal end located at the level of the second lumbar vertebra. For this reason, it is necessary for the lumbar and sacral nerve roots to descend some distance within the vertebral canal in order to exit from their respective intervertebral foramina. The filum terminale is surrounded by lumbosacral nerve roots to form a cluster, which resembles the tail of a horse and is called the *cauda equina* (Fig. 2.2).

Lumbar Cistern and Lumbar Puncture

The lumbar cistern extends from the caudal end of the spinal cord located at the second lumbar vertebra to the second sacral vertebra. The subarachnoid space is widest at this site and contains the filum terminale internum and nerve roots of the cauda equina. Because of the large size of the subarachnoid space and relative absence of neural structures, this space is most suitable for the withdrawal of CSF by lumbar puncture. This procedure is used to gain specific information about the cellular and chemical

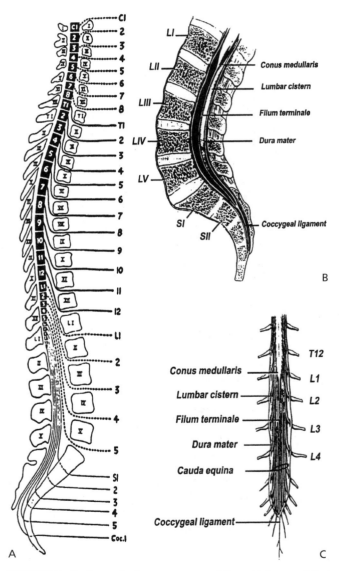

FIGURE 2.2. Bodies and spinous processes of the vertebrae and their position with reference to the spinal cord segments (**A**). Caudal part of the vertebral column showing the conus medullaris, filum terminale, cauda equina and coccygeal ligament (**B,C**). (From Carpenter MB, Sutin J. *Human neuroanatomy*. 8th ed. Baltimore: Lippincott Williams & Wilkins, 1983;8:235, with permission.)

Lesions of the Conus Medullaris and Cauda Equina

Usually, tumors are responsible for the lesions of the conus medullaris. The symptoms of such lesions include early sphincter dysfunction, urinary incontinence, difficulty or loss of voluntary bladder emptying, enhancement of residual urine volume, lack of urge to urinate, constipation, impaired penile erection and ejaculation in males, and lack of sacral sensation (saddle anesthesia). The symptoms of lesions in the cauda equina are related to the nerve roots involved. For example, lesions involving right L2 through L4 nerves cause ipsilateral wasting, weakness of quadriceps and adductor thigh muscles, absence of knee jerk, and sensory loss in L2 through L4 dermatomes (3).

SPINAL NERVES

Thirty-one pairs of spinal nerves emerge from the spinal cord. At each level of the spinal cord, spinal nerves exit through the intervertebral foramina. In the thoracic, lumbar, and sacral regions of the cord, spinal nerves exit through the intervertebral foramina just caudal to the vertebra of the same name. In the cervical region, however, these nerves exit through the intervertebral foramina just rostral to the vertebra of the same name. Because there are eight cervical nerve roots and only seven cervical vertebrae, the eighth cervical spinal nerve exits through the intervertebral foramen just rostral to the first thoracic vertebra (Fig. 2.2).

Each spinal nerve consists of a dorsal root containing afferent fibers and a ventral root containing efferent fibers. The dorsal root is absent in the first cervical and coccygeal nerves. The dorsal and ventral roots travel within the dural sac surrounding the spinal cord, penetrate the dura, and then enter the intervertebral foramen. Because of the length difference between the spinal cord and vertebral column, cervical and upper thoracic rootlets run at right angles to the spinal cord, whereas lower thoracic, lumbar, and sacral rootlets are increasingly oblique. The neurons that give rise to afferent fibers entering the spinal cord are located in the spinal ganglion (dorsal root ganglion), which resides within the intervertebral foramen.

The dorsal and ventral roots join together at a site distal to the spinal ganglion to form the common spinal nerve trunk. Usually, the following four branches (rami) arise from the common spinal nerve trunk: (a) the dorsal ramus, which innervates the muscles and skin of the back; (b) the ventral ramus, which innervates the ventrolateral part of the body wall and all extremities; (c) the meningeal branch, formed by several small branches arising from the common nerve trunk and the ramus communicans, which reenters the intervertebral foramen and innervates the meninges, blood vessels, and vertebral column; and (d) the ramus communicans, which consists of the white and gray portions. The white ramus communicans carries myelinated preganglionic fibers from the spinal cord to the sympathetic ganglion, whereas the gray ramus communicans contains the unmyelinated postganglionic fibers.

The spinal cord has two enlargements, one in the cervical region that is relatively larger than the one in the lumbar region. The cervical enlargement includes four lower cervical segments and the first thoracic segments. The nerve roots emerging from this enlargement form the brachial plexus, which innervates the upper extremities. The lumbar plexus (consisting of nerve roots from L1 through L4) and the lumbosacral plexus (consisting of nerve roots from L4 through S2) emerge from the lumbar enlargement. The lumbar plexus innervates the lower extremities. The sacral spinal nerves emerge from the conus medullaris and contain parasympathetic and somatic motor fibers innervating the smooth muscle of the bladder wall and external urethral sphincter, respectively.

INTERNAL STRUCTURE

A transverse section of the spinal cord reveals the presence of a butterfly-shaped central gray matter, which contains cell columns oriented along the rostrocaudal axis of the spinal cord (Fig. 2.3). The central gray area is surrounded by white matter, consisting of ascending and descending bundles of myelinated and unmyelinated axons (tracts or fasciculi). A bundle containing one or more tracts or fasciculi is called a *funiculus*. In each half of the spinal cord, there are three funiculi: the posterior (dorsal) funiculus (located between the dorsal horn and a midline structure called the *dorsal* or *posterior median septum*), the lateral funiculus (located between the sites where the dorsal roots enter and ventral roots exit from the spinal cord), and the anterior (ventral) funiculus (located between a ventral midline structure called the *anterior median fissure* and the site where the ventral roots exit). The two sides of the gray matter are connected by the gray commissure. The white commissure is located ventral to the gray commissure and contains decussating axons of nerve cells. The central canal is located in the gray commissure and is well defined in the spinal cord of the fetus and the newborn. In the adult spinal cord, the lumen of the central canal may be filled with debris consisting of macrophages and neuroglial processes.

The gray matter of the spinal cord contains primarily neurons, dendrites, and myelinated and unmyelinated axons, which are either exiting from the gray matter to the white matter or projecting from the white matter to innervate neurons located in the gray matter. The ascending and descending tracts of myelinated and unmyelinated fibers constitute the white matter.

SPINAL SEGMENTS

The spinal cord has been divided into 31 segments (8 cervical, 12 thoracic, 5 lumbar, 5 sacral, and 1 coccygeal) based on the existence of 31 pairs of spinal nerves. Each segment receives dorsal and ventral root filaments on each side.

Cervical Segments

As stated earlier, the cervical segments are the largest segments because the amount of nerve fibers in the ascending and descend-

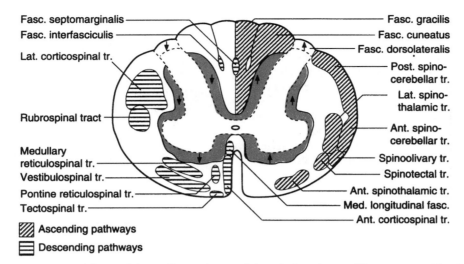

FIGURE 2.3. Ascending and descending pathways of the spinal cord. Two different types of *hatched areas* are used to differentiate ascending from descending pathways. The fasciculus proprius system (*shaded areas*) and dorsolateral fasciculus contain both ascending and descending nerve fibers. (From Parent A, ed. *Human neuroanatomy.* 9th ed. Baltimore: Lippincott Williams & Wilkins, 1996:401, with permission.)

ing spinal tracts is greatest at this level. The anteroposterior diameter is smaller than the transverse diameter, giving these segments their characteristic oval shape. Cervical segments below C5 (i.e., C5 through T1) are related to the brachial plexus and provide motor innervation of the upper extremities. These segments have well-developed posterior and anterior horns; the latter extend into the lateral funiculi.

Thoracic Segments

The thoracic segments are smaller than the cervical segments. All thoracic segments contain a lateral horn, which includes the intermediolateral cell column where the preganglionic sympathetic neurons are located. In all thoracic segments, a prominent structure, called the *dorsal nucleus of Clarke*, is located medially at the base of the dorsal horn and contains large cells. At rostral levels of the thoracic cord (T1 through T6), both the fasciculi gracilis and cuneatus are present, whereas at caudal levels, only the fasciculus gracilis is present. The spinal nerves providing motor innervation to the back and intercostal muscles (axial muscles) emerge from the rostral levels of the thoracic cord (except T1). The spinal nerves providing innervation to the abdominal muscles in addition to the axial muscles emerge from the caudal thoracic levels.

Lumbar Segments

Nerve roots emerging from the segments at L1 through L4 form the lumbar plexus, whereas those emerging from L4 through S2 form the lumbosacral plexus. The segments at L1 and L2 contain the dorsal nucleus of Clarke as well as the intermediolateral cell column and resemble lower thoracic spinal segments. The lumbar segments provide the motor innervation to the large muscles in the lower extremities.

Sacral Segments

These segments are relatively small and contain small amounts of white matter and abundant quantities of gray matter. The dorsal gray column is thicker due to the presence of a well-developed substantia gelatinosa. Preganglionic parasympathetic neurons innervating pelvic viscera are located along the lateral surface of the base of anterior gray horn in S2 through S4 sacral segments.

Coccygeal Segments

The coccygeal segment resembles the sacral segments in that the gray matter of this segment is much more developed than the white matter. It is smaller than the sacral segments.

CYTOARCHITECTURAL ORGANIZATION

The cytoarchitectural lamination of the cat spinal cord was described in detail by Rexed (5,6). A similar lamination is believed to be present in the spinal cord of all mammals (Fig. 2.4). A brief description of Rexed laminae is presented below (see also Table 2.1).

The zone of Lissauer (Fasciculos dorso-Lateralis) consists of fine myelinated and unmyelinated dorsal root fibers, which enter the medial portion of this zone. A large number of propriospinal fibers, which interconnect different levels of the substantia gelatinosa, are also present in this zone (Fig. 2.3).

Laminae I through IV are located in the dorsal horn of the spinal cord. The cells situated in these laminae receive primarily exteroceptive (i.e., pain, temperature, and tactile) inputs from the periphery. Lamina I contains terminals of dorsal root fibers mediating pain and temperature sensations, which synapse, in part, on cells called the posteromarginal nucleus. The axons of

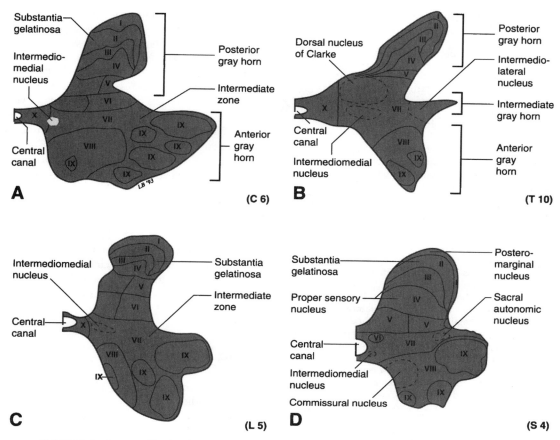

FIGURE 2.4. Structural lamination of human spinal cord segments at C6 (**A**), T10 (**B**), L5 (**C**), and S4 (**D**). (From Parent A, ed. *Human neuroanatomy.* 9th ed. Baltimore: Lippincott Williams & Wilkins, 1996:334, with permission.)

the cells in the posteromarginal nucleus cross to the opposite side and ascend as the lateral spinothalamic tract. Immediately below lamina I lies lamina II, which contains the substantia gelatinosa. The neurons in the substantia gelatinosa modulate the activity of pain and temperature afferent fibers. Activation of peripheral pain receptors results in the release of substance P and glutamate in the substantia gelatinosa. Laminae III and IV, both of which contain the proper sensory nucleus, are located in the lower aspect of the dorsal horn. The proper sensory nucleus receives inputs from the substantia gelatinosa and contributes to the spinothalamic tracts, mediating pain, temperature, and crude touch. Lamina V neurons, which are located at the neck of the dorsal horn, receive descending fibers from the corticospinal and rubrospinal tracts and give rise to axons, which contribute to the spinothalamic tracts. Lamina VI is present only in cervical and lumbar segments. It contains a medial segment, which receives muscle spindle and joint afferents, and also a lateral segment, which receives fibers from descending corticospinal and rubrospinal pathways. Neurons in this region are involved in the integration of somatic motor processes. Lamina VII, located in an intermediate region of the spinal gray matter, contains the nucleus dorsalis of Clarke, which extends from C8 through L3. This nucleus receives muscle and tendon afferents.

Axons of this nucleus form the dorsal spinocerebellar tract, which relays this information to the ipsilateral cerebellum. Other important neurons located in lamina VII include the sympathetic preganglionic neurons, which constitute the intermediolateral cell column in the thoracolumbar cord (T1 through L3), parasympathetic neurons located in the lateral aspect of sacral cord (S2 through S4), and numerous interneurons, such as Renshaw cells.

The output of alpha motor neurons is regulated by Renshaw cells through a mechanism called *recurrent inhibition.* Renshaw cells are interneurons that make inhibitory (glycinergic) synapses on the alpha motor neurons and receive excitatory (cholinergic) collaterals from the same neurons. When an alpha motor neuron is excited, it activates Renshaw cells through the excitatory (cholinergic) collaterals. Renshaw cells, in turn, inhibit through glycinergic synapses, the activity of the same alpha motor neuron.

Laminae VIII and IX are located in the ventral horn of the gray matter of the spinal cord. Neurons in this region, which receive inputs from the descending motor tracts from the cerebral cortex and brain stem, give rise to both alpha and gamma motor neurons that innervate skeletal muscles. Neurons in these laminae are somatotopically arranged; neurons situated in the medial aspect of the ventral horn receive afferents from the ves-

TABLE 2.1. IMPORTANT STRUCTURES IN SPINAL REXED LAMINAE

Laminae	Important Structures
I	Dorsal root fibers mediating pain, temperature, touch sensations; posteromarginal nucleus
II	Substantia gelatinosa neurons mediating pain transmission
III, IV	Proper sensory nucleus that receives inputs from substantia gelatinosa and contributes to spinothalamic tracts, mediating pain, temperature, and touch sensations
V	Neurons receiving descending fibers from corticospinal and rubrospinal tracts; neurons that contribute to ascending spinothalamic tracts
VI	Present only in cervical and lumbar segments; lateral segment receives descending corticospinal and rubrospinal fibers; medial segment receives afferents from muscle spindles and joint afferents
VII	Nucleus dorsalis of Clarke extending from C8 through L1, receives muscle and tendon afferents; axons from this nucleus form spinocerebellar tract; intermediolateral cell column containing sympathetic preganglionic neurons from T1 through L3; parasympathetic neurons located in S2 through S4 segments; Renshaw cells
VIII, IX	Located in the ventral horn; alpha and gamma motor neurons innervating skeletal muscles; neurons in medial aspect receive inputs from vestibulospinal and reticulospinal tracts and innervate axial musculature for posture and balance; neurons in lateral aspect receive inputs from corticospinal and rubrospinal tracts and innervate distal musculature; phrenic motoneurons (C3–C5); thoracic respiratory neurons (thoracic levels)
X	Gray matter surrounding central canal

tibulospinal and reticulospinal systems, and, in turn, innervate the axial musculature. This anatomic arrangement allows descending pathways to regulate the axial musculature (i.e., posture and balance). In contrast, neurons situated in the lateral aspect of the ventral horn receive afferents from the corticospinal and rubrospinal pathways. Axons of these neurons mainly innervate the distal musculature. This arrangement provides a basis by which these descending pathways can have a preferential influence on the activity of the distal musculature. In the ventral horn, motor neurons are located according to the muscle that they innervate. Neurons providing innervation to the extensor muscles are located ventral to those innervating the flexors. Neurons providing innervation to the axial and limb girdle musculature are medial to those innervating muscles in the distal parts of the extremity (Fig. 2.5). In the cervical part of the spinal cord (segments C3, C4, and C5), lamina IX contains phrenic motor neurons that provide innervation to the diaphragm. Thoracic respiratory motor neurons, which innervate intercostal and other rib cage and back muscles, are located in lamina IX of the thoracic segments. The gray matter surrounding the central canal constitutes lamina X.

SPINAL CORD TRACTS

In the white matter of the spinal cord, different tracts are grouped together and are referred to as *dorsal, ventral,* and *lateral funiculi.* A description of these different tracts follows.

Long Ascending Tracts

Dorsal (Posterior) Column

The fasciculi gracilis and cuneatus are also referred to as the *posterior (dorsal) columns.* Damage to these tracts results in symptoms that appear ipsilateral to the affected dorsal columns in the dermatomes at and below the level of the spinal cord lesion.

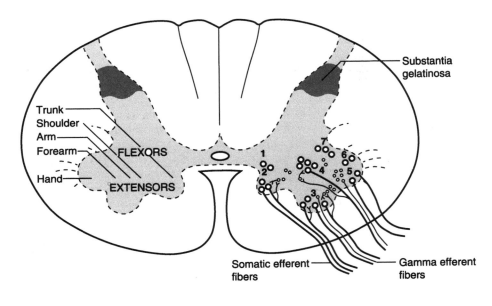

FIGURE 2.5. A diagrammatic representation of motor nuclei in anterior gray horn of a lower cervical spinal segment. **Left**; Location of anterior horn cells, which send motor axons to different muscle groups in the upper extremity. **Right**; Different motor nuclei: (1) posteromedial, (2) anteromedial, (3) anterior, (4) central, (5) anterolateral, (6) posterolateral, (7) retroposterolateral. Neurons in the *dotted area* represent internuncial neurons. Smaller anterior horn neurons send gamma efferents to small muscle fibers of neuromuscular spindle. Somatic efferent fibers emerging from neurons located in regions 2, 3, and 4 send collaterals, which synapse on Renshaw cells located in the gray matter. (From Parent A, ed. *Human neuroanatomy.* 9th ed. Baltimore: Lippincott Williams & Wilkins, 1996:334, with permission.)

A *dermatome* is defined as the area of skin innervated by a single dorsal root. The sensations transmitted in these tracts include tactile (vibration, deep touch, and two-point discrimination) and kinesthetic (position and movement) senses. The patient with a lesion affecting the cervical cord cannot identify an object placed in the hand ipsilateral to the lesion. If the lesion is located at the level of the lumbar cord, then the loss of these forms of sensation is restricted to the ipsilateral lower limbs. The patient can perceive passive movements such as touch or pressure, and the patient's movements will be poorly coordinated and clumsy because of the loss of conscious proprioception.

Fasciculus Gracilis

This tract contains long ascending fibers from the lower limbs (i.e., sacral, lumbar, and the caudal six thoracic segments) and exists at all levels of the spinal cord. Myelinated afferents, from the ipsilateral dorsal root ganglion, enter the dorsal funiculus (medial to the dorsal horn) and the ascending fibers occupy a medial position in the posterior (dorsal) funiculus (Fig. 2.6). Fibers from the lumbosacral regions mediating sensations from the lower limbs ascend medially, and those from higher regions ascend progressively in a more lateral direction, so that fibers from the upper limbs that enter at upper thoracic and lower cervical levels can ascend in the lateral position. The neurons located in the dorsal root ganglion represent the first-order neuron. The peripheral processes of the first-order neuron innervate the pacinian (sensing tactile and vibratory stimuli) and Meissner corpuscles (sensing touch) in the skin and the proprioceptors in the joints that are involved in kinesthesia (sense of position and movement). The central processes of the first-order neuron ascend ipsilaterally in the spinal cord (i.e., the ascending fibers of the first-order neuron are uncrossed) and terminate somatotopically on the second-order neuron in the ipsilateral nucleus gracilis in the medulla. Axons of the second-order neuron travel ventromedially as the internal arcuate fibers and cross in the midline to form the medial lemniscus. This crossed tract ascends through the medulla, pons, and midbrain and then terminates on the third-order neuron located in the contralateral ventral posterolateral nucleus of thalamus. Axons of the third-order neuron travel in the internal capsule and terminate in the sensorimotor cortex. The fasciculus gracilis is involved in mediating conscious proprioception, which includes kinesthesia and discriminative touch.

Fasciculus Cuneatus

The fasciculus cuneatus tract exists in cervical segments and in thoracic segments above T6. It contains long ascending fibers from the upper limbs. Myelinated afferents from the dorsal root ganglion enter the dorsal funiculus medial to the dorsal horn, and the fibers ascend to occupy a lateral position in the posterior (dorsal) funiculus (Fig. 2.6). The peripheral processes of the first-order neuron innervate pacinian and Meissner corpuscles in the skin and the proprioceptors in joints. Its central processes ascend ipsilaterally to terminate on second-order neurons located in the ipsilateral nucleus cuneatus of the medulla. Axons of these second-order neurons travel as internal arcuate fibers, cross the midline to form the medial lemniscus, and terminate on third-

order neurons located in the contralateral ventral posterolateral nucleus of thalamus. The axons of these third-order neurons then terminate in the sensorimotor cortex. The fasciculus cuneatus is involved in mediating conscious proprioception.

Spinocerebellar Tracts

Dorsal (Posterior) Spinocerebellar Tract

The dorsal spinocerebellar tract, located in the dorsal half of the lateral aspect of the lateral funiculus of spinal cord, arises from neurons located in the nucleus dorsalis of Clarke, which extends from L3 to C8. Afferent fibers arising from muscle spindles, and to a lesser extent Golgi tendon organs, reach the nucleus dorsalis of Clarke through dorsal roots. Axons of neurons located in the nucleus dorsalis of Clarke ascend ipsilaterally (i.e., the tract is uncrossed) and reach the cerebellum by way of the inferior cerebellar peduncle, where they terminate primarily in the cerebellar vermis of the anterior lobe. The tract first appears at L3 and increases in size until it reaches C8. Afferent fibers in segments caudal to L2 ascend in the fasciculus gracilis and synapse with the nucleus dorsalis of Clarke at the level of L2. The nucleus dorsalis of Clarke transmits information about muscle spindle and tendon afferents from the ipsilateral caudal aspect of the body and hind limb. The dorsal (posterior) spinocerebellar tract provides the cerebellum with information about the status of individual as well as groups of muscles, therefore enabling this region to coordinate and integrate neural signals controlling movement of individual lower limb muscles and posture.

Ventral (Anterior) Spinocerebellar Tract

The ventral spinocerebellar tract is located immediately below the dorsal spinocerebellar tract in the lateral aspect of the lateral funiculus. Neurons giving rise to this tract (second-order neurons) are located in the lateral part of the base and neck of the dorsal horn (laminae V, VI, and VII). Afferent fibers from the Golgi tendon organ reach the second-order neurons through the dorsal roots. The first-order neurons are located in the dorsal root ganglion. The axons of the second-order neurons cross in the spinal cord and ascend through the medulla to the pons. The fibers then join the superior cerebellar peduncle at the pontine level. Many of these fibers then recross and enter the cerebellum, where they terminate in the vermal region of the anterior lobe. This tract conveys information about whole limb movements and postural adjustments to the cerebellum.

Cuneocerebellar Tract

The nucleus dorsalis of Clarke does not extend to spinal segments rostral to C8. Therefore, afferent fibers entering the spinal cord rostral to this level ascend ipsilaterally in the fasciculus cuneatus and project to neurons located in the accessory cuneate nucleus located in the dorsolateral part of the medulla. Neurons located in this nucleus then give rise to the cuneocerebellar tract, which is functionally related to the upper limbs. The fibers in this tract terminate in the cerebellar cortex. Thus, the cuneocerebellar tract is the upper limb equivalent of the dorsal (posterior) spinocerebellar tract.

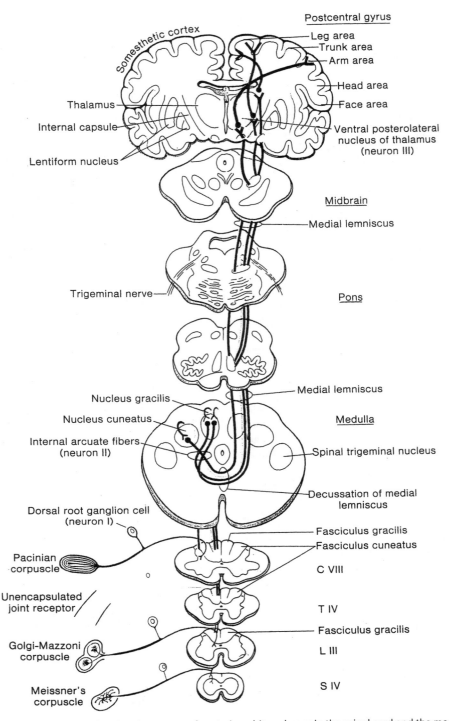

FIGURE 2.6. Diagram showing the courses of posterior white columns in the spinal cord and the medial lemniscus in the brain stem. (From Parent A, ed. *Human neuroanatomy*. 9th ed. Baltimore: Lippincott Williams & Wilkins, 1996:369, with permission.)

Anterolateral System of Ascending Tracts

Conventionally, the lateral spinothalamic tract is believed to transmit pain and temperature sensations, whereas the anterior spinothalamic tract transmits the sensation of nondiscriminative touch to the primary sensory cortex. Currently, it is believed

that all components of the anterolateral ascending spinal system carry all sensory modalities (i.e., pain, temperature, and simple tactile sensations) but that the pathways carrying them are different. The direct pathway, consisting of the neospinothalamic tract, mediates pain, temperature, and simple tactile sensations, whereas several indirect pathways mediate the affective and arousal components of these sensations. The revised concepts and new terminology for various tracts transmitting these sensations are presented subsequently.

Direct Pathway

Neospinothalamic Tract

The neurons that give rise to the neospinothalamic tract arise mainly from the nucleus proprius (the dorsal proper sensory nucleus), which is located in laminae III and IV. The axons of these neurons cross obliquely through the anterior white com-

missure to enter the contralateral white matter, where they ascend in the lateral funiculus. This tract has a somatotopic organization throughout its course. Fibers arising from the lowest part of the body associated with the sacral and lumbar levels of spinal cord ascend dorsolaterally, whereas those arising from the upper extremities and neck in association with the cervical cord ascend ventromedially. The ascending axons synapse on third-order neurons located primarily in the ventral posterolateral nucleus of the thalamus which, in turn, project to the primary sensory cortex in the postcentral gyrus (Fig. 2.7).

Deficits following damage to the direct neospinothalamic

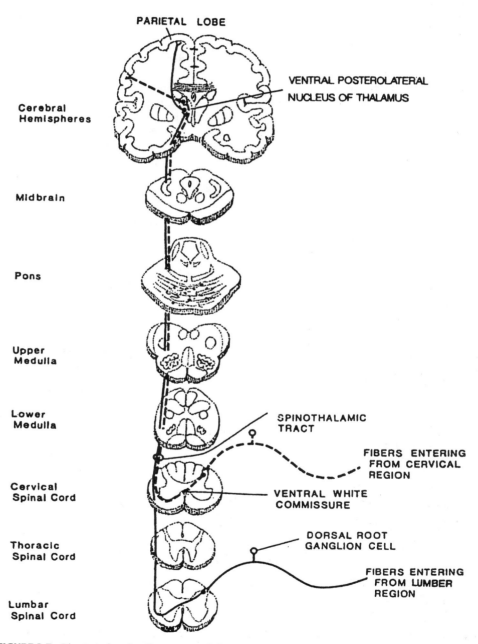

FIGURE 2.7. Diagram showing the courses of the spinothalamic tract. (From Benarroch EE, Westmoreland BF, Daube JR, et al. *Medical neurosciences.* 4th ed. New York: Lippincott Williams & Wilkins, 1999: 165, with permission.)

pathway on one side result in complete loss of pain (anesthesia), thermal (thermoanesthesia), and simple tactile sensations on the contralateral side of the body at and below the level of the lesion.

Loss of pain, temperature, and tactile sensations can also occur at a specific segment after damage to the area around the central spinal canal. This occurs in a condition called *syringomyelia*, in which a lesion (e.g., cavitation) occurs in or around the central canal and affects the crossing fibers from the neospinothalamic tracts on either side but only in or around the segment in which the lesion is present. Accordingly, such a disorder results in bilateral loss of pain, temperature, and simple tactile sensations at the affected segment.

The neospinothalamic tract is somatotopically organized; sacral and lumbar fibers lie dorsolateral to those of the thoracic and cervical fibers. Accordingly, a lesion within the spinal cord is likely to affect the thoracic and cervical fibers early, whereas the sacral and lumbar fibers are affected late or not at all.

When the dorsal columns and anterolateral spinothalamic tracts on one side are damaged, the following phenomenon is observed. On the ipsilateral side below the level of the lesion, there is a loss of conscious proprioception, but the sensations of pain, temperature, and simple touch are preserved. On the contralateral side below the level of the lesion, the reverse is true. There is a loss of pain, temperature, and simple tactile sensations, but conscious proprioception is preserved. This is observed in Brown-Séquard syndrome.

Indirect Pathways

The indirect pathways mediate the autonomic, endocrine, motor, and arousal components of pain, temperature, and simple tactile sensations. In addition, these indirect pathways are involved in the activation of pain-inhibiting mechanisms. The axons of these neurons ascend in the spinal cord bilaterally, show poor somatotopic organization, and make multiple synapses in the reticular formation, hypothalamus, and limbic system. The following pathways are included in this system.

Paleospinothalamic Tract

The neurons of this pathway are located deep in the dorsal horn and the intermediate gray matter. Their axons ascend contralaterally as well as ipsilaterally in the ventrolateral quadrant of the spinal cord. The axons make several synapses in the reticular formation, and project to the midline and intralaminar thalamic nuclei. These, in turn, project in a diffuse manner to the cerebral cortex, especially the limbic regions, such as the cingulate gyrus (Fig. 2.8A).

Spinoreticular Tract

The neurons of this pathway are also located deep in the dorsal horn and intermediate gray matter. The axons of these neurons project to different regions of the lower brain stem. One group of fibers terminates in the medullary reticular formation, and another ascends to the pontine reticular formation. Details concerning the origins and distributions of these pathways are not known. However, it is believed that the projections from the spinal cord to the brain stem are both crossed and uncrossed (Fig. 2.8B). A key feature of these pathways is that ascending spinoreticular fibers are believed to transmit sensory information to the reticular formation which, in turn, activate the cerebral cortex through secondary and tertiary projections through the

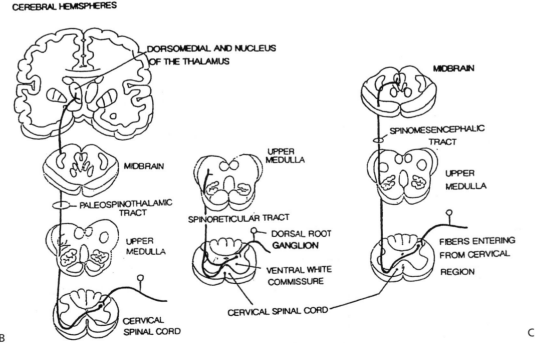

FIGURE 2.8. Diagram showing the course of the paleospinothalamic tract (**A**), the spinoreticular tract (**B**), and the spinomesencephalic tract (**C**). (From Benarroch EE, Westmoreland BF, Daube JR, et al. *Medical neurosciences.* 4th ed. New York: Lippincott Williams & Wilkins, 1999:173, with permission.)

midline and intralaminar thalamic nuclei. The thalamocortical projections are highly diffuse and influence wide areas of the cerebral cortex. The spinoreticular fibers constitute a part of a polysynaptic system, which is involved in the maintenance of the state of consciousness and awareness. Accordingly, a lesion of these fibers is likely to affect these functions.

Spinomesencephalic Tract

The neurons of this pathway are also located deep in the dorsal horn and intermediate gray matter. The axons of these neurons ascend to the midbrain, where they terminate in periaqueductal gray, a region surrounding the cerebral aqueduct (Fig. 2.8C). Similar to spinoreticular fibers, details regarding the distribution of these fibers have not been clearly established. It is believed that sensory information associated with this tract is transmitted to the cerebral cortex through secondary and tertiary projections through midline and intralaminar thalamic nuclei.

Long Descending Tracts

These tracts mediate motor functions, such as voluntary and involuntary movement, regulation of muscle tone, modulation of spinal segmental reflexes, and regulation of visceral functions. The corticospinal tract arises from the cerebral cortex, and the tectospinal and rubrospinal tracts arise from the midbrain. The remaining tracts arise from different nuclear groups within the lower brain stem. These include lateral and medial vestibulospinal tracts and one reticulospinal tract, which arise from the pons and medulla. In addition, other descending pathways arising from medullary nuclei modulate autonomic functions. The corticospinal and rubrospinal pathways are mainly concerned with control over the flexor motor system and fine movements of the limbs, whereas the vestibulospinal and reticulospinal systems principally regulate antigravity muscles, posture, and balance.

Corticospinal Tract

The corticospinal tract arises from the cerebral cortex. The axons arising from the cortex converge in the corona radiata; descend through the internal capsule, crus cerebri, pons, and medullary pyramids, and terminate in the spinal cord (Fig. 2.9). Within the cortex, the sites from which the fibers in this tract arise are the precentral area (area 4; deeper part of lamina V), the premotor and supplementary motor areas (area 6), and the postcentral gyrus (areas 3, 1, and 2). The corticospinal tract is somatotopically organized throughout its entire projection (1). The cells of origin functionally associated with the arm are located in the lateral convexity of the cortex, whereas the cells of origin functionally associated with the leg are located along the medial wall the hemisphere. This somatotopic organization is called *cortical homunculus*. Many of these axons control fine movements of the distal parts of the extremities. At the juncture of the medulla and spinal cord, about 90% the fibers cross to the contralateral side, forming the lateral corticospinal tract. About 8% of the fibers are uncrossed as they descend through the cord, and this pathway is called the *anterior corticospinal tract*. This tract ultimately crosses over at different segmental levels of the cord to

synapse with anterior horn cells on the contralateral side. A scant 2% of the corticospinal tract remains uncrossed throughout its entire trajectory and is called the *uncrossed lateral corticospinal tract* (Fig. 2.10A,B).

This tract controls voluntary movements of both the contralateral upper and lower limbs. Depending on the extent of the lesion, these functions are lost when the corticospinal tract is damaged. After an SCI, the first event to occur is for the affected muscles to lose their tone. After several days or weeks, the muscles become spastic (i.e., they resist passive movement in one direction), and hyperreflexia occurs (i.e., the force and amplitude of the deep tendon, myotatic reflexes are increased, particularly in the legs). The superficial reflexes (abdominal, cremasteric, and normal plantar) are either lost or diminished. A Babinski sign, which usually indicates damage to the corticospinal tract, is also present. This sign is characterized by an abnormal plantar response (extension of great toe while the other toes fan out) when the sole of a foot is stroked by a blunt instrument. The normal plantar response consists of a brisk flexion of all toes when the sole of a foot is stroked by a blunt instrument.

A lower motor neuron (LMN) is one whose cell body lies in the central nervous system (CNS) but whose axon innervates muscles or glands. An upper motor neuron (UMN) is one that descends from the cerebral cortex to the brain stem or spinal cord or that descends from the brain stem to the spinal cord and synapses with an LMN. In general, an LMN is usually thought of as a spinal cord motor horn cell or cranial nerve motor neuron, whereas UMNs are thought of as corticospinal or corticobulbar (projecting from cerebral cortex to the brainstem nuclei) neurons.

The symptoms of damage to the corticospinal tract (i.e., loss of voluntary movement, spasticity, increased deep tendon reflexes, loss of superficial reflexes, and Babinski sign) constitute a UMN paralysis. Thus, the pyramidal cells and their axons are designated as UMNs. The neurons located in the ventral horn of the spinal cord are designated as LMNs. The symptoms of LMN paralysis include the loss of muscle tone, atrophy of muscles, and the loss of all reflex as well as voluntary movement. After an SCI, there is often LMN injury at the level of injury, with UMN injury to levels below the injury.

Rubrospinal Tract

The rubrospinal tract arises from neurons called the *red nucleus*, which are located in the rostral half of the midbrain tegmentum. The axons of these neurons cross the midline in the ventral midbrain (called the *ventral tegmental decussation*) and descend to the contralateral spinal cord. Fibers in the rubrospinal tract are somatotopically arranged; the cervical spinal segments receive fibers from the dorsal part of the red nucleus, which in turn receives input from the upper limb region of the sensorimotor cortex; the lumbosacral spinal segments receive fibers from the ventral half of the red nucleus, which in turn receives input from the leg region of sensorimotor cortex. The fibers of the rubrospinal tract enter laminae V, VI, and VII of the spinal cord. They end on interneurons that, in turn, project to the dorsal aspect of ventral (motor) horn cells. The neurons in the red nucleus receive projections from ipsilateral cerebral cortex

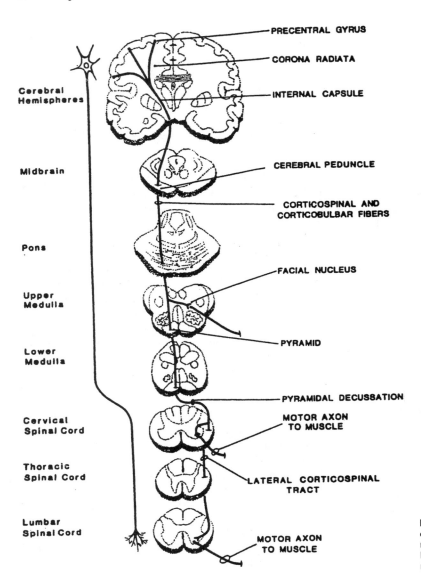

PRECENTRAL GYRUS

CORONA RADIATA

INTERNAL CAPSULE

Cerebral Hemispheres

Midbrain

CEREBRAL PEDUNCLE

CORTICOSPINAL AND CORTICOBULBAR FIBERS

Pons

FACIAL NUCLEUS

Upper Medulla

PYRAMID

Lower Medulla

PYRAMIDAL DECUSSATION

MOTOR AXON TO MUSCLE

Cervical Spinal Cord

Thoracic Spinal Cord

LATERAL CORTICOSPINAL TRACT

Lumbar Spinal Cord

MOTOR AXON TO MUSCLE

FIGURE 2.9. Diagram showing the origin and course of corticospinal and corticobulbar fibers (From Benarroch EE, Westmoreland BF, Daube JR, et al. *Medical neurosciences.* 4th ed. New York: Lippincott Williams & Wilkins, 1999:211, with permission.)

and contralateral deep cerebellar nuclei. Thus, the cerebral cortex and cerebellum can influence the activity of the alpha and gamma motor neurons of the spinal cord through the rubrospinal tract, which facilitates the activity of the flexor muscles and inhibits the activity of the extensor muscles. Damage to this tract is likely to compromise precise and well-controlled movements of the distal limb musculature. However, in the human nervous system, the rubrospinal tract may be of little clinical significance because it does not extend below cervical levels (7).

Tectospinal Tract

The neurons giving rise to the tectospinal tract are located in the superior colliculus. The axons of these neurons descend around the periaqueductal gray, cross the midline in the dorsal tegmental decussation, join the medial longitudinal fasciculus in the medulla, and descend in the anterior funiculus of the spinal cord. They terminate in laminae VI, VII, and VIII in upper cervical segments. Because this tract is believed to aid in directing head movements in response to visual and auditory stimuli, damage to this tract is likely to affect the aforementioned head movements.

Lateral Vestibulospinal Tract

The lateral vestibulospinal tract is an uncrossed tract that arises from neurons of the lateral vestibular nucleus, which is located at the border of the pons and medulla. It descends the entire length of the spinal cord. The descending fibers enter laminae VII and VIII and terminate directly on motor neurons mainly in cervical and lumbar levels. The lateral vestibular nucleus receives inhibitory inputs from the cerebellum and excitatory inputs from the vestibular apparatus. Impulses transmitted to the spinal cord by the lateral vestibular nucleus powerfully facilitate ipsilateral extensor motor neurons, thereby increasing extensor motor tone.

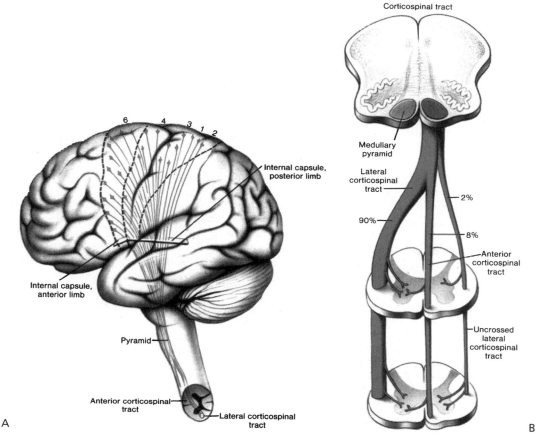

FIGURE 2.10. A,B; Diagram showing the divisions of the corticospinal tract. (From Parent A, ed. *Human neuroanatomy*. 9th ed. Baltimore: Lippincott Williams & Wilkins, 1996:384–385, with permission.)

Main functions of this tract are to control the muscles that maintain upright posture and balance. Therefore, maintenance of upright posture and balance is compromised by a lesion of this tract.

Medial Vestibulospinal Tract

The medial vestibulospinal tract arises from ipsilateral and contralateral medial vestibular nuclei, descends in the ventral funiculus of the cervical spinal cord, and terminates in the ipsilateral ventral horn. Because the main function of this tract is to control the head position in association with vestibular stimulation, this function is affected by a lesion of this tract.

Reticulospinal Tracts

The reticular formation gives rise to three functionally different fiber systems. One component of this system mediates motor functions, a second mediates autonomic functions, and a third modulates pain impulses.

Fibers arising from the medulla issue from a group of large cells located medially called the *nucleus gigantocellularis*. These cells project bilaterally to all levels of the spinal cord, and this pathway is referred to as the *lateral reticulospinal tract*. A key function of this pathway is that it powerfully suppresses extensor spinal reflex activity. In contrast, a separate reticulospinal pathway arises from two distinct nuclear groups in the medial aspect of the pons called the *nucleus reticularis pontis caudalis* and *nucleus reticularis pontis oralis*. These neurons project ipsilaterally to the entire extent of the spinal cord, but their principal function is to facilitate extensor spinal reflexes. This fiber bundle is called the *medial reticulospinal tract*.

A second group of descending reticulospinal fibers mediates autonomic functions. They arise largely from the ventrolateral medulla and project to the intermediolateral cell column of the thoracolumbar cord. This fiber system excites sympathetic preganglionic neurons in the intermediolateral cell column, which provide sympathetic innervation to visceral organs.

A third group of descending fibers modulates pain and is multisynaptic. The first limb of this pathway consists of enkephalinergic neurons, which arise from the midbrain periaqueductal gray and project to serotoninergic neurons located in the nucleus raphe magnus of the medulla. These serotoninergic neurons then project to the dorsal horn of the spinal cord, making synapse with a second group of enkephalinergic interneurons, which, in turn, synapse on primary afferent pain fibers. Therefore, a key function of this descending fiber system is to modulate the activity of pain impulses that ascend in the spinothalamic system.

Medial Longitudinal Fasciculus

The fibers in the medial longitudinal fasciculus bundle are mainly ascending, but this bundle also contains some descending fibers. Both ascending and descending fibers arise from different vestibular nuclei (lateral, superior, medial, inferior vestibular nuclei) located in the pons. Descending fibers of the medial longitudinal fasciculus are situated in the dorsal part of the ventral funiculus and project principally to upper cervical segments of the spinal cord. These fibers monosynaptically inhibit motor neurons located in the upper cervical cord. By virtue of its connections with motor neurons in the cervical cord, this pathway controls the position of the head in response to excitation by the labyrinth.

Fasciculi Proprii

The fasciculi proprii consist of ascending and descending, crossed or uncrossed fibers that arise and end in the spinal cord. They connect different segments of the spinal cord. These fibers mediate intrinsic reflex mechanisms of the spinal cord, such as the coordination of upper and lower limb movements. Signals entering the spinal cord at any segment are thus conveyed to upper or lower segments and finally transmitted to the ventral horn cells either directly or through interneurons.

SPINAL CORD AND THE AUTONOMIC NERVOUS SYSTEM

The function of the autonomic nervous system is to maintain the internal environment of the body constant (homeostasis). This system regulates involuntary functions, such as blood pressure, heart rate, respiration, digestion, glandular secretion, reproduction, and body temperature. Currently, the autonomic nervous system is divided into three divisions: sympathetic, parasympathetic, and enteric.

Sympathetic Division

The neurons from which the outflow of the sympathetic division originates (preganglionic neurons) are located in the intermediolateral cell column of the first thoracic to second lumbar vertebrae. For this reason, the sympathetic nervous system is sometimes called the thoracolumbar division. Generally, the axons of these preganglionic neurons exit the spinal cord through the ventral roots and enter the main trunk of the spinal nerve (Fig. 2.11). After traveling in the spinal nerve, the axons of the sympathetic preganglionic neurons exit through the white ramus and reach one of the sympathetic ganglia. The axon of the preganglionic neuron follows one or more of the following pathways:

1. The sympathetic preganglionic axon synapses on one of the neurons (called a *postganglionic neuron*) in the paravertebral sympathetic ganglion. The axon of this postganglionic neuron (postganglionic fibers) exits through the gray ramus com-

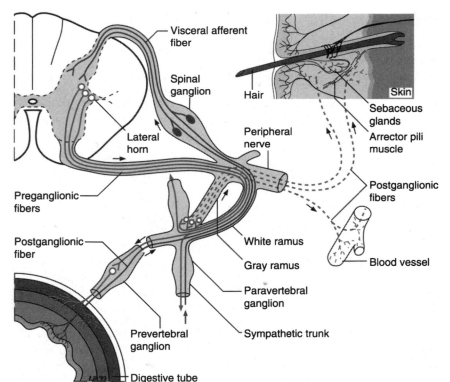

FIGURE 2.11. Diagram showing the reflex arcs of the sympathetic nervous system. (From Parent A, ed. *Human neuroanatomy.* 9th ed. Baltimore: Lippincott Williams & Wilkins, 1996:295, with permission.)

municantes and returns to the spinal nerve. The sympathetic postganglionic fibers then innervate the target organ (e.g., a blood vessel or sweat gland).

2. The sympathetic preganglionic axon does not synapse on any neuron in the paravertebral ganglion; it passes through the ganglion, exits through a nerve (e.g., the greater splanchnic nerve), and synapses on a neuron in one of the prevertebral ganglia. The sympathetic postganglionic fiber exiting from the neuron in the prevertebral ganglion then innervates the target organ (e.g., a segment of the gastrointestinal tract).

3. The sympathetic preganglionic axon branches: one of these branches synapses on a neuron in a particular paravertebral ganglion; others ascend or descend in the paravertebral sympathetic chain and synapse on neurons located in several ganglia. In this manner, one preganglionic neuron located in the intermediolateral column of the thoracolumbar cord innervates as many as 30 postganglionic neurons located in several paravertebral ganglia.

Sympathetic Ganglia

There are two types of sympathetic ganglia: paravertebral and prevertebral. The paravertebral ganglia (22 pairs) are located on either side of the vertebral column. They are connected together by a sympathetic nerve trunk, thus forming a sympathetic chain on either side (Fig. 2.12). The prevertebral ganglia (e.g., celiac and mesenteric ganglia) are located in different places in the thorax, abdomen, and pelvis. In addition, a few terminal ganglia, with short postganglionic fibers, are located in the urinary bladder and the rectum.

The sympathetic division of the autonomic nervous system is activated in stressful situations. Thus, activation of sympathetic nervous system results in pupillary dilatation and an increase in heart rate, blood pressure, blood flow in the skeletal muscles, and blood sugar. These effects are widespread because one preganglionic sympathetic axon innervates several postganglionic neurons. All of these responses prepare the individual for fight or flight. For example, increase in blood flow in the skeletal muscles helps in running away from the site of danger (flight), increase in heart rate and blood pressure helps in better perfusion of different organs, increase in blood sugar provides energy, and pupillary dilatation provides for better vision under these circumstances. The effects of simultaneous activation of the parasympathetic division of the autonomic nervous system complements these actions.

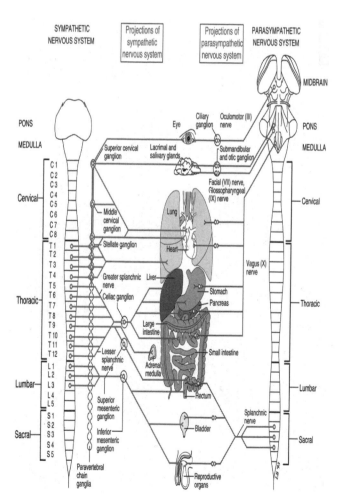

FIGURE 2.12. Diagram showing the sympathetic and parasympathetic components of the autonomic nervous system. Preganglionic fibers (*solid lines*) and postganglionic fibers (*broken lines*). (From Carpenter MB, Sutin J. *Human neuroanatomy.* 8th ed. Baltimore: Lippincott Williams & Wilkins, 1983:211, with permission.)

Parasympathetic Division

The preganglionic neurons from which the parasympathetic outflow arises are located in the brain stem (midbrain, pons, and medulla oblongata) and the sacral region of the spinal cord. For this reason, this division is sometimes referred to as *craniosacral division* (Fig. 2.12).

The parasympathetic preganglionic neurons are located in the brain stem and the spinal cord. In the spinal cord, the preganglionic parasympathetic neurons are located in the intermediolateral column of the sacral spinal cord at the S2 through S4 level. Their axons exit through the ventral roots, travel through pelvic nerves, and synapse on postganglionic neurons, which are located close to or within the organs being innervated. The postganglionic parasympathetic nerve fibers are, therefore, very short compared with the sympathetic postganglionic nerve fibers.

Activation of the parasympathetic division of the autonomic nervous system results in conservation and restoration of body energy. For example, decrease in heart rate brought about by the activation of parasympathetic nervous system also decreases the demand for energy, whereas the increased activity of the gastrointestinal system promotes restoration of body energy. The effects of parasympathetic activation are localized and last for a short time.

Enteric Nervous System

The enteric division consists of neurons in the wall of the gut (intrinsic innervation) that regulate gastrointestinal motility and secretion. The gastrointestinal system is also controlled by sympathetic and parasympathetic innervation (extrinsic innervation). The extrinsic system can override the intrinsic system under certain situations.

Autonomic Innervation of Selected Organs

Many organs are innervated by sympathetic as well as parasympathetic divisions (Fig. 2.12). As a rule, in most of the organs with dual innervation, the parasympathetic and sympathetic divisions have antagonistic actions. Exceptions to this rule are the salivary glands, for which activation of either system results in an increase in the secretion of saliva: sympathetic stimulation produces viscous saliva, whereas parasympathetic stimulation produces watery saliva. The autonomic innervation of some selected organs, often affected by SCI, are described in chapters 10, 12, and 22.

Neurotransmitters in the Autonomic Nervous System

Preganglionic Terminals

Within the autonomic ganglia, acetylcholine is the transmitter released at the terminals of the sympathetic as well as parasympathetic preganglionic fibers. The terminal branches of the preganglionic fibers contain vesicles (membrane-bound saclike structures) enclosing the neurotransmitter. The terminals make synaptic contacts with the postganglionic neurons located in the ganglia.

Postganglionic Terminals

The terminals of the sympathetic and parasympathetic postganglionic neurons innervate the effector cells in the target organs. At the terminals of most sympathetic postganglionic neurons, norepinephrine is the transmitter liberated, with the exception of those innervating sweat glands and blood vessels of the skeletal muscles for which acetylcholine is the neurotransmitter. At the terminals of all the parasympathetic postganglionic neurons, acetylcholine is the neurotransmitter liberated.

BLOOD SUPPLY OF THE SPINAL CORD

Arteries

The following major arteries supply the spinal cord (Fig. 2.13).

Posterior Spinal Arteries

The posterior spinal arteries, one on each side, are given off by the vertebral arteries as they ascend on the anterolateral surface of the medulla. They descend on the posterolateral surface of the spinal cord slightly medial to the dorsal roots.

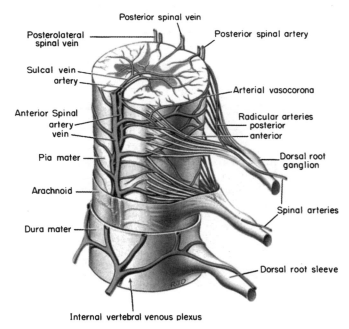

FIGURE 2.13. Diagram showing the blood supply of the spinal cord. (From Parent A, ed. *Human neuroanatomy.* 9th ed. Baltimore: Lippincott Williams & Wilkins, 1996:95, with permission.)

Anterior Spinal Arteries

The anterior spinal arteries also arise from the vertebral arteries as they ascend on the anterolateral surface of the medulla. They unite to form one single artery that courses along the midline of the spinal cord.

Radicular Arteries

The radicular arteries arise from segmental levels, including the ascending cervical, deep cervical, intercostal, lumbar, and sacral arteries, which, in turn, arise from the thoracic and abdominal aorta. The radicular arteries pass through the intervertebral foramina and then bifurcate into anterior and posterior radicular arteries. These arteries provide blood supply to the thoracic, lumbar, sacral, and coccygeal regions of the spinal cord. Radicular arteries travel along the ventral roots and enter the subarachnoid space. The radicular artery present at T12 through L2 supplies blood to the caudal two thirds of the spinal cord. In the lumbar region of the spinal cord, one anterior radicular artery (artery of Adamkiewicz) is larger than others.

The cervical segments of the spinal cord are supplied by branches of the vertebral and ascending cervical arteries. Because of the dual source of blood supply, these segments are usually less vulnerable to ischemia. On the other hand, upper thoracic segments depend on radicular branches of the intercostal arteries. If one or more branches of the intercostal arteries are injured, the spinal segments from T1 through T4 are not adequately perfused and are vulnerable to spinal cord infarction. Similarly, the L1 spinal segment is vulnerable to spinal infarction.

Veins

Six longitudinal veins drain the spinal cord; three are located on the ventral side and three on the dorsal side (Fig. 2.13). On the ventral side, one of the three veins is located in the midline (anteromedian vein), and two others (anterolateral veins) are located along the line of attachment of the ventral roots. Branches of the sulcal veins drain both sides of the spinal cord and then join and enter the anteromedian vein. The anteromedian and anterolateral veins empty into the anterior radicular veins, which, in turn, empty into the anterior epidural venous plexus. On the dorsal side, one of the veins (the posteromedian vein) is located in the midline, and the two posterolateral veins are located along the line of attachment of the dorsal roots. The posteromedian and posterolateral veins are drained by the posterior radicular veins, which, in turn, empty into the posterior epidural venous plexus.

ANIMAL MODELS OF SPINAL CORD INJURY

Human spinal cord injuries are multifactorial; therefore, it is difficult to design experimental models in which such injuries can be replicated precisely. Nevertheless, some useful data regarding the pathophysiology of SCI have derived from animal models (4). For example, in the weight-drop model, SCI has been experimentally induced by dropping a weight on the surface of the spinal cord (8). Recently, a more sophisticated electromechanical impacter has been developed based on the same principle (9). In the experimental weight-drop model, some of the features of SCI resemble those observed in human SCI. For example, weight-drop injury in both experimental animals and humans causes hemorrhage and tissue necrosis, which later develops into a cyst (4). The main disadvantages of the weight-drop model are that the results obtained are variable (4) and that the sites of injury do not simulate those observed in human SCI. For example, injury in the weight-drop model involves posterior cord compression, whereas in humans, anterior compression of the cord due to burst fractures or circumferential cord compression due to fracture dislocation is more common (4). In another model, balloon inflation in the spinal epidural space is used to induce SCI (10). In a novel approach, spinal cord vascular endothelium has been injured photochemically by injecting an organic photosensitive dye into the bloodstream (11). The spinal cord is then irradiated with a light beam of appropriate wavelength. The vascular endothelium is damaged, and the subsequent thrombosis results in ischemic lesions and vasogenic edema (11). Because the vertebral dorsal surface is adequately translucent, a laminectomy is not necessary in the model using photosensitive dyes. Microsurgical procedures have also been used to produce lesions in specific spinal pathways (12).

PATHOPHYSIOLOGY OF SPINAL CORD INJURY

A summary of the pathophysiologic changes that occur in a time-dependent manner secondary to SCI follows (4).

Ischemia

Hypoperfusion of the gray matter is a consistent feature of SCI (13). Diverse metabolites, such as serotonin, thromboxanes, platelet-activating factor, peptidoleukotrienes, and opioid peptides, have been reported to be released after SCI (4). These agents are believed to induce vasoconstriction of the vessels supplying the spinal cord and to cause ischemia of the gray matter (14). This decrease in blood flow results in a decrease in oxygen tension at the site of injury (15). The contributions of ischemia to the neurologic deficits that follow SCI remain unclear (16).

Edema

In experimental models of SCI, it has been observed that edema first occurs in the central part of the spinal cord, then spreads centrifugally to the white matter. The maximum formation of edema occurs during the initial stages of SCI (17).

Changes in Ionic Composition at the Site of Injury

The calcium ion concentration at the site of injury has been reported to increase within minutes after SCI, to peak at about

8 hours, and then to remain elevated for at least 1 week after the injury (18–21). This increase in intraaxonal calcium has been attributed to the calcium ion entry through voltage-gated calcium channels, voltage-dependent N-methyl-D-aspartate (NMDA) receptor channels, release of calcium from intracellular storage sites such as smooth endoplasmic reticulum, and the failure of the extrusion of calcium ions through the Ca^{2+}-ATPase exchange pump. Increased concentrations of calcium results in the activation of phospholipase C and A_2. Arachidonic acid is one of the products generated in these reactions (21). Metabolites of arachidonic acid, such as free radicals, thromboxanes, and peptidoleukotrienes, are known to cause tissue injury (22). Another ion that is known to play a role in SCI is the potassium ion (K^+) (23). Immediately after SCI, there is an increase in extracellular K^+, which results in the depolarization of cells, leading to a conduction block. Eventually, there is a loss of K^+ in the injured spinal cord tissue due to damaged cell membranes (23).

Hydrolysis of Phospholipids and Generation of Free Radicals

Activation of phospholipases by increased calcium concentrations results in hydrolysis of phospholipids and generation of free fatty acids, which, in turn, cause irreversible tissue damage (24). Activation of phospholipase A_2 results in an increase in the levels of platelet-activating factor, which is known to reduce blood flow and compromise the blood–CNS barrier. Phospholipid hydrolysis also results in the release of free radicals, which are very reactive. Free radical reactions damage the phospholipid and cholesterol components of cell membranes (25). Because spinal cord injuries are accompanied by hemorrhage, the iron contained in hemoglobin catalyzes the oxygen radical and lipid peroxidase reactions, which mediate further cell injury (4).

Role of Excitatory Amino Acids

Excitatory amino acids serve as transmitters in several different spinal pathways (26–30). The levels of excitatory amino acids, such as glutamate and aspartate, have been reported to be increased in response to SCI (31). Activation of glutamate receptors results in an increase in intracellular levels of Ca^{2+}, which, as previously noted, has been implicated in cell death (32). This phenomenon is known as *excitotoxicity*. NMDA, as well as DL-[α]-amino-3-hydroxy-5-methylisoxazole-propionic acid (AMPA) receptors have been implicated in this type of cell injury (33). Specific blockers for these receptors have been tested with variable success for their neuroprotective effects (34).

DIFFERENT PHASES OF TRAUMA

Acute Phase

Changes in the microvasculature of the central gray matter appear at the site of injury within minutes of the trauma and increase progressively within the first few hours (4). These changes are characterized by the appearance of multifocal hemorrhages, distention of postcapillary venules with erythrocytes, and the appearance of red blood cells in perivascular spaces through damaged vascular endothelium. The endothelial cells of capillaries and postcapillary venules appear vacuolated and swollen. This damage is believed to be induced by free radicals because pretreatment with antioxidants in experimental SCI prevented these endothelial cell abnormalities. Aneurysms and ruptured arteries appear in the lateral columns within 4 to 8 hours, and microthrombi appear in capillary size vessels within 24 hours. Some of the necrotic alterations are characterized by the presence of shrunken neurons with indistinct nuclei, loss of Nissl bodies, and swelling of rough endoplasmic reticulum. Necrotic changes occur in both glia and neurons. The neurons and glia in the anterior horn are affected earlier than those in the posterior horn. These changes occur in the gray matter within the first hours of injury. In the white matter, vacuoles appear in the myelin sheaths, and axons dilate or split, giving it a spongy appearance under a light microscope (4,35).

Subacute Phase

The phase of hemorrhagic necrosis is followed by the subacute phase, which is characterized by the presence of several different cell populations at the site of injury (4). Activated microglia at the site of injury exhibit an increased number of processes and an upregulation of cell surface molecules, such as the histocompatibility complex class I and II antigens, the complement C3 receptor, and the macrophage activation marker ED1. This activation process, regulated by special signals such as cytokines, leads to the transformation of microglia into large phagocytic brain macrophages. At the site of injury, the astrocytes hypertrophy and proliferate and contain an increased number of filaments consisting of glial fibrillary acidic protein. These astrocytes also exhibit increased activity of different oxidative and lysosomal enzymes. Another feature of this phase is the appearance of inflammatory cells at the site of the lesion. Within a few hours of SCI, polymorphonuclear granulocytes (neutrophils) infiltrate the lesion and adjacent sites. Their main function is to destroy any bacteria causing infection at the injury site. These neutrophil cells have also been reported to exert cytotoxic effects on neurons; however, this view is not universally accepted. Neutrophils are attracted to the site of injury by the degradation products of hemoglobin, thrombin, and bradykinin. Other peripheral cells that appear at the site of injury include monocytes and macrophages, which are involved in phagocytosis of cell debris (36). Additional cell types found at the site of SCI include Schwann cells and fibroblasts. Schwann cells have the ability to modify their myelin sheaths and generate neurotrophic factors. Therefore, they may be involved in axonal regeneration, thus providing a basis for the physiologic recovery of neurons after some types of experimental SCI (37). Fibroblasts produce basic fibroblast growth factor, a powerful angiogenic factor (38) that has been implicated in neovascularization in such injuries (39).

Late Phase

The late phase, which extends over a period of weeks to months after spinal injury, follows the acute and subacute phases (4).

Within a few days after the injury, phagocytic macrophages in the injured region disappear, and fluid-filled cysts (cavities surrounded by extensive scar tissue) appear. These cysts are connected to the central canal and are filled with CSF. In humans, elongated cavities are formed rostral to the injury after several months. This leads to syringomyelia (40). About 1 week after the spinal injury, a scar consisting of a dense network of processes is formed between the intact and the damaged tissue. This scar formation has been attributed to the accumulation of astrocytes at the margins of the lesion. Meningeal cells may also contribute to scar formation (41). The cavities formed at the site of injury are partly surrounded by white-matter tissue consisting of demyelinated fibers that are incapable of conducting sensory or motor information. Demyelination is an important feature of SCI (42, 43). This abnormality is responsible for impaired conduction in ascending and descending axons. Demyelination begins within 24 hours of the injury and increases progressively. Within 3 weeks, many fibers undergo wallerian degeneration. However, there is evidence of some remyelination after experimental SCI during the late phase, although the internodes of these remyelinated axons are abnormally short and the myelination is thin. In smaller lesions, oligodendrocytes and Schwann cells may be involved in the process of remyelination, although evidence of this is scanty (44). This feature may explain the limited spontaneous recovery of function in some cases of SCI.

INFLAMMATORY PROCESSES

As noted earlier, the first cells to infiltrate the site of injury after spinal cord trauma are polymorphonuclear granulocytes (neutrophils) (4). The primary function of these neutrophils at the site of injury is to combat bacterial infection. However, other properties of these cells may contribute to further cellular injury. For example, neutrophils produce lysosomal enzymes and oxygen radicals that degrade the connective tissue matrix and cause tissue destruction. The reperfusion of blood into ischemic tissue has been observed to cause further tissue damage. This "reperfusion injury" is believed to be due to the mechanical obstruction caused by the reentry of neutrophils into the blood vessels in the ischemic tissue, the subsequent cytotoxic effects of neutrophils, and the infiltration of neutrophils into the parenchyma. The adhesion of leukocytes is mediated by a glycoprotein complex (β_2-integrin subunit, CD18) on their membranes. Treatment of experimentally induced SCI with an antibody to this glycoprotein reduced tissue damage, most likely by preventing the aggregation of leukocytes in the blood vessels (45).

The appearance of neutrophils at the site of SCI is followed by the appearance of phagocytic macrophages. Macrophages play a dual role at the site of injury, one involving tissue destruction and the other involving tissue repair. Their primary role is to remove cellular debris. Axonal injury results in wallerian degeneration (i.e., degeneration of the distal nerve stump). Macrophages at the site of injury are believed to mediate the degradation of myelin by secreting neutral proteases. However, macrophages are also implicated in initiating the mitosis of Schwann cells and the proliferation of fibroblasts, which results in enhancement of the production of nerve growth factor by

non-neural tissue. Macrophages also alter the glial cell surfaces by producing a substance that permits elongation of neurites. These observations suggest that macrophages are also involved in tissue repair after spinal injury.

RECOVERY PROCESSES
Observations in Animal Studies

Based on experimental evidence in animals and humans, it is well established that pattern generators for rhythmic movements, such as walking and swimming, are located in the spinal cord (4, 46). These central pattern generators are independent of sensory input and retain their independence even after complete deafferentation. It has been reported that in rats with experimentally induced injuries to the lower thoracic spinal cord, relatively few intact descending fibers (1% to 10%) are necessary to initiate functions such as postural control and locomotion. Similarly, in adult cats with spinal cord injuries at the C5 level, capabilities for reaching and retrieving food were initially completely lost, but these behaviors reappeared later.

Observations in Human Studies

Success in the recovery of some spinal cord function in experimental animals has prompted new approaches to provide rehabilitation therapy to patients with SCI (47). It has been reported that in incomplete or complete paraplegic patients, the spinal pattern generator for locomotion can be initiated and trained (48). Impairment of motility depends on the extent of SCI. For example, it has been observed that lesions in ventral and ventrolateral funiculi do not impair motility in humans (49). On the other hand, lesions in the dorsolateral funiculi (which contain corticospinal and rubrospinal tracts) on one side, combined with 90% transection on the contralateral side, result in complete lower limb paralysis. However, functional recovery, such as walking, was even observed in these patients within 2 months (49). In other studies, when patients with partial spinal cord injuries with residual small sensory or motor innervation and patients with neurologically complete spinal cord lesions (50,51) were trained on treadmills, substantial improvement in functional recovery was observed. Some of these recovered patients showed electromyograms with typical rhythmic alternating patterns in flexor and extensor muscles. In other patients, the need for weight support on the treadmill decreased gradually, and spinal walking with the aid of crutches was achieved. The following explanation has been provided for the functional improvement observed in these patients in response to the treadmill training. The functional integrity of neuronal circuits is dependent on their activity. The loss of activity is likely to result in the loss of uninjured neural connections in the spinal cord. Therefore, training on a treadmill may have prevented the loss of the uninjured spinal connections in these patients. In addition, spared descending fibers after the SCI may have, to some extent, sprouted and made functionally useful connections. Treadmill training may have also reinforced this process.

TREATMENT STRATEGY

In SCI, the tissue damage and the related loss of function are usually irreversible. Irrespective of the nature of the injury, whether it is a closed contusion, open contusion, or partial transection, cell death occurs within hours, whereas the secondary pathologic changes take place within days and weeks of injury. Therefore, early intervention is of crucial importance for a better clinical outcome. In acute SCI, the first aim should be to arrest the cascade of secondary injury processes, in order to limit the tissue damage and interrupt or reverse sensorimotor dysfunction. The second aim is focused on the rehabilitation and stabilization of the consequences of injury and activation of residual neuronal circuits by training. This will improve the condition of living for the patient. The third aim is still in an experimental stage and involves the enhancement of axonal regeneration by different interventions.

Steroids have also been used extensively in the treatment of SCI in animals and humans (52). In the National Acute Spinal Cord Injury Study (NASCIS-I) (53), two groups were randomized, and both groups received 1,000-mg bolus within 48 hours after injury. The high-dose and the low-dose groups received maintenance doses of 1,000 mg and 100 mg of methylprednisolone (MP), respectively, administered for 10 days. No statistical difference was found between the two regimens at 6 months or at 1 year; however, there was a trend for the patients with the higher doses of MP to have better scores than the lower-dose group (53).

Criticisms of NASCIS-I included that the dose of MP (even the high dose) used was below the theoretic therapeutic threshold believed to be about 30 mg/kg of body weight from animal models; there was no placebo arm; all types of injury were grouped together; and the doses of MP were not based on body weight. It was also thought that the MP treatment was started too late (within 48 hours) after injury.

NASCIS-II, initiated in 1985, was a multicenter, double-blinded, placebo-controlled study in which 487 patients were randomized (54). The inclusion criterion was a SCI diagnosis within 12 hours of injury. Exclusion criteria included nerve root or cauda equina injury only; gunshot wounds; life-threatening morbidity; pregnancy; addiction to narcotics; use of maintenance steroid for any reason; age under 13 years; administration of more than 100 mg of MP or its equivalent or 1 mg of naloxone before admission to the study center; and difficult-to-follow cases.

Sensation and motor status were measured at admission, after 6 weeks, and after 6 months. Sensation was studied using 29 dermatomal segments from C2 through S5 and tabulating the sum of 14 myotomes using the standard six-point (0 through 5) Medical Research Council scale, which assessed motor score. Subjects received one of the following three regimens: MP and placebo naloxone, active naloxone and placebo MP, or placebo MP and placebo naloxone.

Results of the study revealed that patients, both neurologically complete and incomplete, who received MP within 8 hours after injury at a dosage of 30 mg/kg, maintained at 5.4 mg/kg/hr for a total of 23 hours, had significantly improved neurologic (motor and sensory) recovery 6 weeks, 6 months, and 1 year after injury. Patients treated with MP initiated more than 8 hours after injury had no beneficial effect, and in fact did marginally worse than the placebo group. Naloxone did not have a significant effect on recovery at the dose used. The wound infection rate was 7.1% in those receiving MP as compared to 3.6% in the placebo group, and the gastrointestinal bleeding rate was 4.5% in MP group as compared with 3.0% in the placebo group. Both of these potentially life-threatening complications, although higher in the MP group, did not reach statistical significance. One of the keys to NASCIS-II was the evidence that medication can improve neural recovery, thus indicating that secondary injury (injury occurring after the initial trauma to the cord) occurs.

The third study (NASCIS-III), initiated in 1991, was a double blind, randomized study with three treatment regimens (55). This included MP 24 hours (30 mg/kg bolus within 8 hours followed by MP 5.4 mg/kg/hr for 24 hours); MP 48 hours (30 mg/kg bolus followed by MP 5.4 mg/kg/hr for 48 hours); and tirilazad mesylate (TM) (30 mg/kg bolus MP followed by TM 2.5 mg/kg every 6 hours for 48 hours). Tirilazad mesylate (Upjohn U-74006F) is a 21-aminosteroid and potent antioxidant with no glucocorticoid receptor activity that has been shown to be neuroprotective in animal SCI models. Motor scores and Functional Independence Measure (FIM) scores were measured at 6 weeks and 6 months. There was no true placebo group included.

Results from 499 patients recruited from 16 centers revealed a significant improvement in motor scores in those who received 48 hours of MP when started in the 3- to 8-hour window at 6 weeks and 6 months of follow-up. There were no differences in sensory scores at any time between the groups. In NASCIS-III, there was a twofold higher incidence of pneumonia, and a four-fold higher incidence of sepsis, and sixfold higher incidence of death due to respiratory complications in the 48-hour group as compared with the 24-hour group, although these differences did not reach statistical significance. Although corticosteroids are known to possess antiinflammatory properties, their beneficial effects have been ascribed to their free radical scavenger properties (56,57) and their ability to inhibit lipid peroxidation (52).

Lazaroids (21-aminosteroids) are known to inhibit lipid peroxidation and are devoid of glucocorticoid activity (52,58). It was concluded from NASCIS-III that tirilazad was as effective as MP in treating acute SCI when administered for a 24-hour duration. In addition, the incidence of sepsis, pneumonia, and cardiovascular side effects was lower when tirilazad was used.

Although the previously mentioned recent trials support the use of MP in acute SCI, there have been some reports that question the effectiveness and use of steroids (see chapter 6) (59–61).

Gangliosides, which are glycolipids present in cell membranes, are also undergoing clinical trials for treatment of acute SCI (62). Administration of a ganglioside (GM-1; 100 mg, i.v. within 72 hours of injury) in patients with acute SCI has resulted in a significant improvement in neurologic function. Gangliosides have been reported to promote neurite outgrowth, regeneration, and neuronal sprouting (63–65). It is not clear yet whether these properties of gangliosides are responsible for their beneficial effect in treating SCI.

In experimental animals, opiate receptor antagonists have also been shown to exert neuroprotective effects after SCI (52). Initial clinical trials indicated that naloxone, a nonselective opiate receptor antagonist, did not elicit a significant neuroprotective effect in patients with acute SCI (54). However, a 1-year follow-up study indicated that naloxone did elicit a significant neuroprotective effect in acute SCI in humans (57,66). The neuroprotective effects of selective opiate receptor antagonists remain to be investigated.

As stated earlier, the accumulation of excess glutamate at the site of injury has been demonstrated in patients with spinal cord trauma. Administration of competitive and noncompetitive NMDA receptor antagonists has been reported to influence the pathologic process in SCI (67–69). However, these antagonists have many adverse side effects; therefore, none of the competitive or noncompetitive NMDA receptor antagonists is considered a potential therapeutic agent for treating SCI in humans.

Currently, the only medication being studied for chronic SCI patients is 4-aminopyridine (4-AP). This drug blocks fast voltage-dependent potassium channels in nerve membranes and, therefore, delays the repolarization of the membrane following an action potential. This effect results in an increase in the excitability of nerve cells and axons. 4-AP has been reported to restore conduction in demyelinated nerve fibers. Multiple studies with 4-AP in multiple sclerosis and some preliminary work in SCI have shown a trend toward increased motor function in incomplete injuries and decreased pain and spasticity (70–72). Newer studies are underway.

ACKNOWLEDGMENTS

This work was supported by a grant (HL 24347) from the National Heart, Lung and Blood Institute (NHLBI) awarded to Dr. H. N. Sapru.

REFERENCES

1. Benarroch EE, Westmoreland BF, Daube JR, et al. *Medical neurosciences.* 4th ed. New York: Lippincott Williams & Wilkins, 1999: 151–223.
2. Carpenter MB, Sutin J. *Human neuroanatomy.* 8th ed. Baltimore: Williams & Wilkins, 1983:232–262.
3. Afifi AK, Bergman RA. *Functional neuroanatomy.* New York: McGraw-Hill, 1998:102–103.
4. Schwab ME, Bartholdi D. Degeneration and regeneration of axons in the lesioned spinal cord. *Physiol Rev* 996;76:319–370.
5. Rexed B. The cytoarchitectonic organization of the spinal cord in the cat. *J Comp Neurol* 1952;96:415–494.
6. Rexed B. A cytoarchitectonic atlas of the spinal cord in the cat. *J Comp Neurol* 1954;100:297–379.
7. Burt AM. *Textbook of neuroanatomy.* Philadelphia: WB Saunders, 1993: 318.
8. Noble LJ, Wrathall R. Correlative analyses of lesion development and functional status after graded spinal cord contusive injuries. *Exp Neurol* 1989;103:34–40.
9. Bresnahan JC, Beattie MS, Todd FD, et al. A behavioral and anatomical analysis of spinal cord injury produced by a feedback-controlled impaction device. *Exp Neurol* 1987;95:548–570.
10. Tarlov IM, Klinger H. Spinal cord compression studies. *Am Med Assoc Arch Neurol Psychiatry* 1954;71:272–290.
11. Bartlett Bunge M, Holets VR, Bates ML, et al. Characterization of photochemically induced spinal cord injury in the rat by light and electron microscopy. *Exp Neurol* 994;127;76–93.
12. Theriault E, Tator CH. Persistence of rubrospinal projections following spinal cord injury in the rat. *J Comp Neurol* 1994;342:249–258.
13. Holtz A, Nyström B, Gerdin B. Spinal cord blood flow measured by ¹⁴C-iodoantipyrine autoradiography during and after graded spinal cord compression in rats. *Surg Neurol* 1989;31:350–360.
14. Olsson Y, Sharma HS, Pettersson A, et al. Release of endogenous neurochemicals may increase vascular permeability, induce edema and influence cell changes in trauma to the spinal cord. *Prog Brain Res* 1992; 91:197–203.
15. Stokes BT, Garwood M, Walters P. Oxygen fields in specific spinal loci of the canine spinal cord. *Am J Physiol* 1981;240:H761–766.
16. Tator CH. Hemodynamic issues and vascular factors in acute experimental spinal cord injury. *J Neurotrauma* 1992;9:139–141.
17. Nobel LJ, Wrathall JR. Distribution and time course of protein extravasation in the rat spinal cord after contusive injury. *Brain Res* 1989; 482:57–66.
18. Young W, Flamm ES. Effect of high-dose corticosteroid therapy on blood flow, evoked potentials, and extracellular calcium in experimental spinal cord injury. *J Neurosurg* 1982;57:667–673.
19. Moriya T, Hassan AZ, Young W, et al. Dynamics of extracellular calcium activity following contusion of the rat spinal cord. *J Neurotrauma* 1994;11:255–263.
20. Siesjö BK. Historical overview: calcium, ischemia, and death of brain cells. *Ann N Y Acad Sci* 1988;522:638–661.
21. Rasmussen H. The calcium messenger system (first of two parts). *N Engl J Med* 1986;314:1094–1101.
22. Xu J, Hsu CY, Junker H, et al. Kininogen and kinin in experimental spinal cord injury. *J Neurochem* 1991;57:975–980.
23. Young W, Koreh I. Potassium and calcium changes in injured spinal cords. *Brain Res* 1986;365:42–53.
24. Faden AI, Chan PH, Longar S. Alterations in lipid metabolism, (Na⁺, K⁺)-ATPase activity, and tissue water content of spinal cord following experimental traumatic injury. *J Neurochem* 1987;48:1809–1816.
25. Braughler JM, Hall ED. Central nervous system trauma and stroke. I. Biochemical considerations for oxygen radical formation and lipid peroxidation. *Free Radical Biol Med* 1989;6:289–301.
26. Chitravanshi VC, Sapru HN. NMDA as well as non-NMDA receptors mediate the neurotransmission of inspiratory drive to phrenic motoneurons in the adult rat. *Brain Res* 1996;715:104–112.
27. Chitravanshi VC, Sapru HN. NMDA as well as non-NMDA receptors in the phrenic motonucleus mediate respiratory effects of carotid chemoreflex. *Am J Physiol* 1997;272:R322–333.
28. Sundaram K, Murugaian J, Sapru HN. Cardiac responses to the microinjections of excitatory amino acids into the intermediolateral cell column of the rat spinal cord. *Brain Res* 1989;482:12–22.
29. Sundaram K, Sapru HN. NMDA receptors in the intermediolateral column of the spinal cord mediate sympathoexcitatory responses elicited from the ventrolateral medullary pressor area. *Brain Res* 1991;544: 33–41.
30. Murugaian J, Sundaram K, Krieger AJ, et al. Relative effects of different spinal autonomic nuclei on cardiac sympathoexcitatory function. *Brain Res Bull* 1990;24:537–542.
31. Liu D, Thangnipon W, McAdoo DJ. Excitatory amino acids rise to toxic levels upon impact injury to the rat spinal cord. *Brain Res* 1991; 547:344–348.
32. Choi DW. Excitotoxic cell death. *J Neurobiol* 1992;23:1261–1276.
33. Wrathall JR, Choiniere D, Teng YD. Dose-dependent reduction of tissue loss and functional impairment after spinal cord trauma with AMPA/kainate antagonist NBQX. *J Neurosci* 1994;14:6598–6607.
34. Sun FY, Faden AI. High- and low-affinity NMDA receptor-binding sites in rat spinal cord: effects of traumatic injury. *Brain Res* 1994;666: 88–92.
35. Dusart I, Schwab ME. Secondary cell death and the inflammatory reaction after dorsal hemisection of the rat spinal cord. *Eur J Neurosci* 1994;6:712–724.
36. Perry VH, Anderson PB, Gordon S. Macrophages and inflammation in the central nervous system. *Trends Neurosci* 1993;16:268–273.

37. Li Y, Raisman G. Schwann cells induce sprouting in motor and sensory axons in the adult rat spinal cord. *J Neurosci* 1994;14:4050–4063.

38. Folkman J, Klagsbrun M. Angiogenic factors. *Science* 1987;235:442–447.

39. Blight AR. Morphometric analysis of blood vessels in chronic experimental spinal cord injury: hypervascularity and recovery of function. *J Neurol Sci* 1991;106:158–174.

40. Madsen PW, Yezierski RP, Holets VR. Syringomyelia: clinical observations and experimental studies. *J Neurotrauma* 1994;11:241–254.

41. Sievers J, Pehlemann FW, Gude S, et al. Meningeal cells organize the superficial glia limitans of the cerebellum and produce components of both the interstitial matrix and the basement membrane. *J Neurocytol* 1994;23:135–149.

42. Blight AR, Young W. Central axons in injured cat spinal cord recover electrophysiological function following remyelination by Schwann cells. *J Neurol Sci* 1989;91:15–34.

43. Waxman SG. Demyelination in spinal cord injury. *J Neurol Sci* 1989;91:1–14.

44. Tator CH. The relationship among the severity of spinal cord injury, residual neurological function, axon counts, and counts of retrogradely labeled neurons after experimental spinal cord injury. *Exp Neurol* 1995;132:220–228.

45. Clark WM, Madden KP, Rothlein R, et al. Reduction of central nervous system ischemic injury in rabbits using leukocyte adhesion antibody treatment. *Stroke* 1991;22:877–883.

46. Rossignol S, Dubuc R. Spinal pattern regeneration. *Curr Opin Neurobiol* 1994;4:894–902.

47. Barbeau H, Rossignol S. Enhancement of locomotor recovery following spinal cord injury. *Curr Opin Neurol* 1994;7:517–524.

48. Wernig A, Muller S, Nanassy A, et al. Laufband therapy based on "rules of spinal locomotion" is effective in spinal cord injured persons. *Eur J Neurosci* 1995;7:823–829.

49. Nathan PW. Effects on movement of surgical incisions into the human spinal cord. *Brain* 1994;117:337–346.

50. Dietz V, Colombo G, Jensen L, et al. Locomotor capacity of spinal cord in paraplegic patients. *Ann Neurol* 1995;37:574–582.

51. Dietz V, Colombo G, Jensen L, et al. Locomotor capacity of spinal man. *Lancet* 1994;344:1260–1263.

52. Seidl EC. Promising pharmacological agents in the management of acute spinal cord injury. *Crit Care Nurs Q* 1999;22:44–50.

53. Bracken MB, Collins WF, Freeman DF, et al. Efficacy of methylprednisolone in acute spinal cord injury. *JAMA* 1984;251:45–52.

54. Bracken MB, Shepard MJ, Collins WF, et al. A randomized, controlled trial of methylprednisolone or naloxone in the treatment of acute spinal cord injury. *N Engl J Med* 1990;322:1405–1411.

55. Bracken MB, Shepard MJ, Holoford TR, et al. Administration of methylprednisolone for 24 or 48 hours or tirilazad mesylate for 48 hours in the treatment of acute spinal cord injury. Results of the Third National Acute Spinal Cord Injury Randomized Controlled Trial. *JAMA* 1997;277:1597–1604.

56. Faden AI, Salzman S. Pharmacological strategies in CNS trauma. *Trends Pharmacol Sci* 1992;13:29–35.

57. Bracken MB, Shepard MJ, Collins WF, et al. Methylprednisolone or naloxone treatment after acute spinal cord injury: 1-year-follow-up data. *J Neurosurg* 1992;76:23–31.

58. Clark WM, Hazel S, Coull BM. Lazaroids: CNS pharmacology and current research. *Drugs* 1995;50:971–983.

59. Nesathurai S. Steroids and spinal cord injury: revisiting the NASCIS 2 and 3 trials. *J Trauma* 1998;45:1088–1093.

60. Short DJ. High dose methylprednisolone in the management of acute spinal cord injury: a systematic review from a clinical perspective. *Spinal Cord* 2000;38:278–286.

61. Hurlbert RJ. Methylprednisolone for acute spinal cord injury: an inappropriate standard of care. *J Neurosurg* 2000;93(Suppl 1):1–7.

62. Geisler FH, Dorsey FC, Coleman WP. Recovery of motor function after spinal cord injury: a randomized, placebo-controlled trial with GM-1 ganglioside. *N Engl J Med* 1991;324:1829–1838.

63. Gorio AG, Fusco M, Janigro D, et al. Gangliosides and their effects on rearranging peripheral and central neural pathways. *Cent Nerv Syst Trauma* 1984;1:29–37.

64. Sabel BA, Slavin MD, Stein DG. GM-1 ganglioside treatment facilitates behavioral recovery from brain damage. *Science* 1984;225:340–342.

65. Geisler FH, Dorsey FC, Coleman WP. Past and current clinical studies with GM-1 ganglioside in acute spinal cord injury. *Ann Emerg Med* 1993;22:1041–1047.

66. Bracken MB, Holford TR. Effects of timing of methylprednisolone or naloxone administration on recovery of segmental and long-tract neurological function in NASCIS 2. *J Neurosurg* 1993;79:500–507.

67. Faden AI, Demediuk P, Panter SS, et al. The role of excitatory amino acids and NMDA receptors in traumatic brain injury. *Science* 1989;244:798–800.

68. Hao JX, Watson BD, Xu XJ, et al. Protective effect of NMDA antagonist MK-801 on photochemically induced spinal lesions in the rat. *Exp Neurol* 1992;118:143–152.

69. Kochhar A, Zivin JA, Mazzarella V. Pharmacologic studies of the neuroprotective actions of a glutamate antagonist in ischemia. *J Neurotrauma* 1991;8:175–186.

70. Segal JL, Brunnemann SR. 4-Aminopyridine alters gait characteristics and enhances locomotion in spinal cord injured humans. *J Spinal Cord Med* 1998;21:200–204.

71. Davis FA, Stefoski D, Rush J. Orally administered 4-AP improves clinical signs in multiple sclerosis. *Ann Neurol* 1990;27:186–192.

72. Segal JL, Brunnemann SR. 4-Aminopyridine improves pulmonary function in quadriplegic humans with longstanding spinal cord injury. *Pharmacotherapy* 1997;17:415–423.

ANATOMY, MECHANICS, AND IMAGING OF SPINAL INJURY

CARSON D. SCHNECK

GENERAL ANATOMIC, MECHANICAL, AND IMAGING FEATURES OF THE SPINE RELEVANT TO SPINE AND SPINAL CORD INJURY

Each level of the spine has some unique structural and functional attributes; however, an overview of general anatomic, mechanical, and imaging features of the spine can provide insights into many of the common mechanisms of spine and spinal cord injury. The unique morphologic, functional, and imaging characteristics of specific spine levels are described with their regional injuries.

General Bony Features

The typical vertebra is composed of a body and a vertebral or neural arch (Fig. 3.1A). The vertebral body is the major load-bearing element of most vertebrae. The progressive increase in cross-sectional area of the vertebral bodies from cervical through lumbar levels of the spine is a structural adaptation to the progressively increasing superincumbent loads (1). This tends to maintain intervertebral pressures within safe physiologic limits. The neural arch protects the contents of the spinal canal and transmits both muscular and gravitational forces. It is composed of paired pedicles and laminae. Transverse processes usually arise at the pedicle–lamina junction, and spinous processes attach at the mid-sagittal junction of the laminae. These processes serve as elongated moment arms for muscular attachment, thereby increasing the torque the muscles can generate. Spinous processes can suffer compression fractures in hyperextension injuries and distractive fractures by hyperflexion injuries (e.g., Chance fractures) and occasionally can be avulsed by violent muscular contraction. Transverse processes can be fractured by direct or indirect trauma or by muscular avulsion.

Paired superior and inferior articular processes project from the pedicle–lamina junction. The inferior articular processes of one vertebra articulate with the superior articular processes of the next lower vertebra to form the hyaline cartilage–covered synovial facet (zygapophyseal) joints. The facing direction of facet joints helps determine the kind and amount of motion normally present at each vertebral level. At cervical levels, the facet joints are oriented at about a 45-degree angle midway between the coronal and transverse planes (2). As the facet joints with the most horizontal orientation, they can permit unilateral or bilateral facet dislocation without fracture. The more coronal orientation of thoracic facet joints and the relatively sagittal ori-

entation of lumbar facet joints predispose them to fracture with dislocation.

From the axis to the sacrum, the vertebral column is a tripod load transmission system and a trijoint motion mechanism. It is an asymmetric tripod load transmission system that in the upright neutral position generally transmits 80% to 90% of the superincumbent loads through the vertebral bodies and 5% to 10% of the loads through each of the facet joints. However, in some regions, like the cervical level and lumbosacral junction, where the facet joints are most horizontally oriented, they bear a greater proportion of the loads, whereas at thoracic and lumbar levels, their more vertical orientation implies reduced load transmission in the upright position. With flexion, vertebral bodies bear greater loads, whereas in extension, facet joints bear increased loads. Pedicles and laminae serve as tie-rods or cross-braces between the legs of the tripod load-transmitting system. They can transmit externally applied compressive, distractive, and shearing stresses between the legs of the tripod as well as internally generated muscular torques applied to the transverse or spinous processes.

Intervertebral or neural foramina are located between the pedicles of adjacent vertebrae (Fig. 3.1B). They are bounded posteriorly by facet joints and anteriorly by the posterior aspect of the adjacent vertebral bodies and their intervening intervertebral disk. At cervical levels, the intervertebral disk is situated near the middle of the anterior wall of the intervertebral foramen, whereas at thoracic and lumbar levels, it is in the lower portion of the anterior wall. The location of the disk is an important determinant of the nerve likely to be encroached on by a traumatically acquired or degenerative disk protrusion, as described later.

General Ligamentous Supports of the Spine

The ligaments of the spine both stabilize the upright spine and limit excessive motion of the spine. The anterior longitudinal ligament extends from the foramen magnum to the sacrum (Fig. 3.2A). It is situated on both the anterior and lateral aspects of the vertebral bodies. It reinforces these aspects of the intervertebral disks and resists extension. It is most commonly injured by hyperextension trauma, but it can also be disrupted in compression burst fractures and flexion or extension teardrop fractures.

The posterior longitudinal ligament extends from the foramen magnum to the sacrum (Fig. 3.2A,B). At thoracic and lumbar levels, it is narrow and attaches to the posteromedial aspect

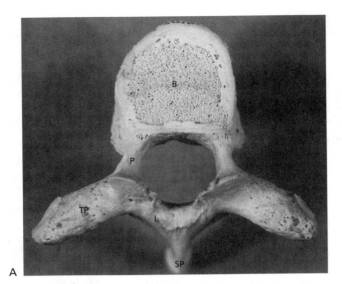

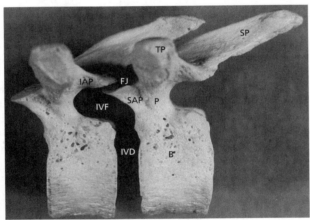

FIGURE 3.1. Typical (thoracic) vertebra. **A**; Superior view of a thoracic vertebra. **B**; Lateral view of two thoracic vertebrae in an articulated position demonstrating the body (*B*), pedicles (*P*), laminae (*L*), transverse processes (*TP*), spinous processes (*SP*), superior articular processes (*SAP*), inferior articular processes (*IAP*), intervertebral foramen (*IVF*), facet joint interval (*FJ*), and the position of intervertebral disk (*IVD*). (From Schneck CD. Functional and clinical anatomy of the spine. In: *Physical medicine and rehabilitation: state of the art reviews*, Vol. 9. Philadelphia: Hanley & Belfus, 1995:526, with permission.)

are continuous with the anterior capsule of the facet joints. The ligamenta flava resist spine flexion and can be ruptured by hyperflexion injuries. In acute hyperextension injury, approximation of the laminae can buckle the ligamenta flava into the spinal canal and contuse the cord. With degenerative disk disease, narrowing of the disk interval also causes an approximation of adjacent laminae, which can produce a permanent buckling of the ligamenta flava into the spinal canal and intervertebral foramen. This can contribute to progressive spinal or foraminal stenosis and predispose the patient to spinal cord or nerve injury during hyperextension trauma.

The capsule of the facet joints is sufficiently slack to permit motions in planes compatible with the facing direction of the facets. The capsules can be ruptured by hyperflexion trauma to cause facet subluxation or unilateral or bilateral facet dislocation. As previously noted, this can occur at cervical levels with or without fracture. Interspinous ligaments bridge the intervals between spinous processes. Supraspinous ligaments connect the tips of adjacent spinous processes. Both interspinous and supraspinous ligaments resist flexion and are commonly torn by hyperflexion injury because the posterior distracting forces act on a very long moment arm at this point.

The intervertebral disks form unique anatomic and functional joints between vertebral bodies. The periphery of the disk is composed of concentric layers of fibrocartilage called the *anulus fibrosus* and a more central gel-like *nucleus pulposus* (Fig. 3.3A–C). The collagen fibers in each layer of the anulus course at an oblique angle of about 30 degrees to the plane of the disk (5). They insert above and below into the hyaline cartilage plates and ring epiphyses that cover the upper and lower surfaces of the vertebral body. The fibers in adjacent layers spiral in opposite directions, so that, in one layer they spiral upward and clockwise and in the next layer upward and counterclockwise. The vertical vector component of these obliquely running collagen fibers resists the tensile stresses applied to the disk during flexion-extension and lateral bending movements of the spine. The horizontal component of these fibers resists rotational tensile stresses and also the shearing stresses of anteroposterior or mediolateral translational motions between vertebrae. In addition, when the spine is under vertical load, the fibers of the anulus resist the tensile stresses that cause the periphery of the disk to bulge. Hyperflexion injury most often ruptures the posterior anulus, whereas hyperextension injury most commonly ruptures the anterior anulus.

The young, healthy nucleus pulposus is a relatively fluid gel composed of glycosaminoglycans that bind large amounts of water and make up 90% of the young nucleus (6). Because the circumference of the nucleus is surrounded by the anulus and bounded above and below by the hyaline cartilage plates on the vertebral body ends, the young nucleus behaves like a fluid mass within a completely closed but somewhat distortable container (Fig. 3.3A,B). As such, it obeys Pascal's law, which says that given fluid in a completely closed container (e.g., water within a balloon), if the pressure is increased at one point on the surface of the container (e.g., press on the balloon with one finger), that local increase in pressure will be transmitted undiminished over the entire walls of the container (7). Hence, when the spine is bent in a particular direction (e.g., flexion), there is increased

of the vertebral body margins and the intervening intervertebral disk, but bridges across the concave mid-portion of each vertebral body. At cervical levels, it is wider and thicker (3,4). Because vertebral flexion-extension axes generally lie within the vertebral body (2), the posterior longitudinal ligament normally resists flexion and also reinforces the posteromedial aspect of the disk. It is disrupted in most unstable spine injuries. The posterior longitudinal ligament is also subject to degenerative ossification, which can contribute to spinal stenosis.

Ligamenta flava connect adjacent laminae (Fig. 3.2C). They attach to the anterior aspect of the lower border of the higher lamina and the posterior aspect of the upper border of the lower lamina. Therefore, the laminae and ligamenta flava overlap each other in a shingled arrangement. Laterally, the ligamentum flava

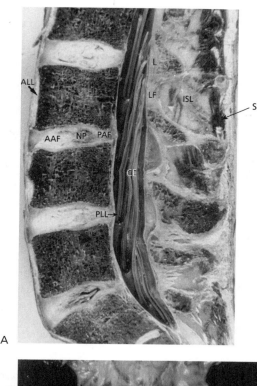

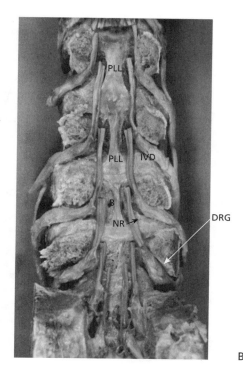

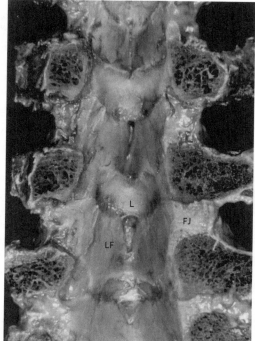

FIGURE 3.2. Major ligaments of the spine. **A**; Mid-sagittal section of the lumbosacral spine shows the anterior longitudinal ligament (*ALL*), anterior anulus fibrosus (*AAF*), nucleus pulposus (*NP*), posterior anulus fibrosus (*PAF*), posterior longitudinal ligament (*PLL*), cauda equina (*CE*), laminae (*L*), ligamenta flava (*LF*), interspinous ligament (*ISL*), and supraspinous ligament (*SSL*). **B**; Posterior view of the vertebral bodies with the neural arches removed by cutting the pedicles. The posterior longitudinal ligament has an hourglass shape (*PLL*), widening over the intervertebral disks (*IVD*) and narrowing over the vertebral bodies (*B*). Nerve roots (*NR*) and dorsal root ganglia (*DRG*) are also seen. **C**; Anterior view of the laminae (*L*) and ligamenta flava (*LF*) after the neural arch has been separated from the vertebral body by cutting the pedicles. The ligamenta flava make up most of the posterior wall of the spinal canal and are continuous laterally with the anterior capsule of the facet joints (*FJ*). (**A,C**, From Schneck CD. Functional and clinical anatomy of the spine. In: *Physical medicine and rehabilitation: state of the art reviews*, Vol. 9. Philadelphia: Hanley & Belfus, 1995:528, with permission.)

compressive load and stress on that side of the anulus and nucleus (Fig. 3.3C). Tensile stresses develop on the opposite side of the anulus and nucleus. The young, relatively fluid nucleus is able to distribute this load more evenly over a larger surface area of the vertebral body to prevent undue loading of the edge of the vertebral body toward which the spine is bent. If these flat interbody joints were synovial joints, which lack this pressure re-

ducing mechanism, the very high pressure produced on the vertebral body edges during motion would cause early hypertrophic degenerative changes. The young, healthy disk provides a hydraulic mechanism that permits motion, absorbs shock, and causes loads to be distributed over a larger surface area, thereby maintaining pressures within physiologically tolerable limits.

As intervertebral disks age, the amount of glycosaminoglycans

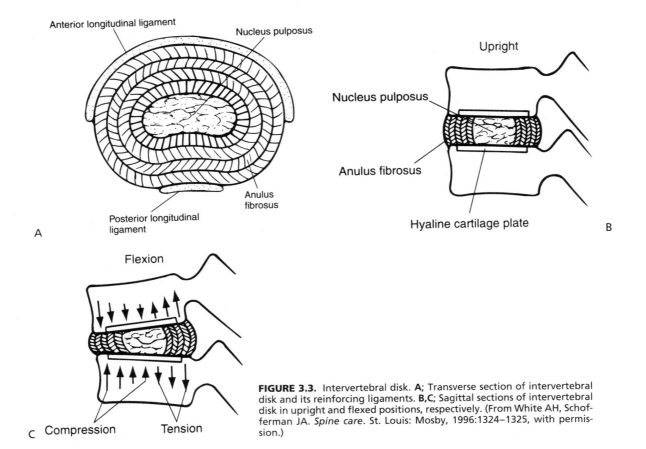

FIGURE 3.3. Intervertebral disk. **A**; Transverse section of intervertebral disk and its reinforcing ligaments. **B,C**; Sagittal sections of intervertebral disk in upright and flexed positions, respectively. (From White AH, Schofferman JA. *Spine care*. St. Louis: Mosby, 1996:1324–1325, with permission.)

in the nucleus is reduced, and the character of the disks changes. This reduces the water content and makes the nucleus a more viscous gel, which is less able to distribute loads over a larger surface area. As a result, increased loads are concentrated on the vertebral body edges toward which the spine is bent, with a resultant marginal osteophytosis that can cause either spinal canal stenosis or intervertebral foraminal stenosis (8). The loss in disk volume and vertebral body approximation can produce many other secondary degenerative or neural encroachment processes (9). These interrelated changes include the following:

1. A slackening of all longitudinally running ligaments, like the anterior and posterior longitudinal ligaments, ligamenta flava, and interspinous and supraspinous ligaments (10,11). This may increase mobility of the involved vertebral interval or even of adjacent vertebral segments and thereby hasten their degeneration.
2. Bulging of the peripheral anulus that can narrow both spinal canal and intervertebral foramen.
3. Pedicle approximation, which narrows the superoinferior dimension of the intervertebral foramen.
4. Laminar approximation, which can produce the previously described bulging of the ligamenta flava into the spinal canal or intervertebral foramina (12).
5. A superior and anterior subluxation of the superior articular process of the lower vertebra, which narrows the anteroposterior dimension of the intervertebral foramen.

6. An inferior and posterior subluxation of the inferior articular process of the higher vertebra, which can cause a retrolisthesis of the higher vertebral body to narrow the anteroposterior dimension of the spinal canal and intervertebral foramen.
7. Increased loading of the facet joints, which may cause hypertrophic degenerative facet disease that, in turn, can produce spinal or foraminal stenosis.

These various effects of chronic degenerative disk disease can by themselves produce myelopathy or radiculopathy. If they are preexisting at the time of spine injury, they can increase the probability of spinal cord or spinal nerve injury from traumatic incidents that might not otherwise cause neural injury.

General Neural Relationships of the Spine

Spinal nerves are named by the vertebrae adjacent to which they emerge from the spinal canal. The first seven cervical nerves emerge above the vertebra for which they are named (Fig. 3.4). The thoracic, lumbar, and sacral spinal nerves emerge below the vertebra for which they are named. This leaves the intervertebral foramen between C7 and T1 for the eighth cervical spinal nerve to emerge from the spinal canal. This occurs because during the embryonic splitting and fusion of the vertebral (sclerotomic) portions of the cervical somites, two half cervical somites are lost, leaving only seven cervical vertebrae but eight cervical spinal nerves (7). The spinal cord segments are, in turn, named by the

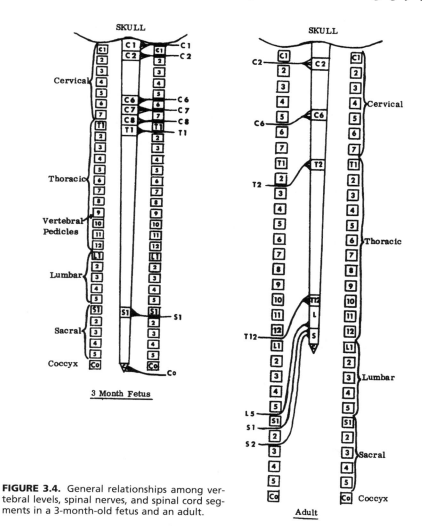

FIGURE 3.4. General relationships among vertebral levels, spinal nerves, and spinal cord segments in a 3-month-old fetus and an adult.

spinal nerve rootlets that emerge from a specific longitudinal segment of the spinal cord (Fig. 3.4).

Up to the third month of fetal development, the spinal cord and vertebral column are the same length, and each spinal cord segment is at the same level as its corresponding vertebra (Fig. 3.4). Therefore, the spinal nerve roots and nerves pursue a horizontal course to their intervertebral foramina. Beyond the first trimester, the vertebral column grows in length at a greater rate than the spinal cord, so that by birth, the spinal cord ends at the L2 to L3 vertebral level. By 5 years of age, the adult spinal cord relationships are established, with the spinal cord ending at the L1 to L2 vertebral level. In adults, only the upper cervical cord segments are at the same level as their vertebrae. At lower cervical and upper thoracic levels, the spinal cord segments are situated one vertebral level higher than their corresponding vertebrae. At mid-thoracic levels, the cord segments are two vertebral levels higher. The lumbar cord segments are situated at the T11 to T12 vertebral levels, and the sacral cord is located at the L1 vertebral level. Hence, below mid-cervical levels, the nerve roots course progressively more vertically, ultimately forming the cauda equina below the L1 vertebral level. Appreciation of the disparity between spinal cord and vertebral levels can be clinically significant. For example, in a burst fracture of the T11 vertebra that affects the spinal cord, the sensory and motor levels with which the patient presents at physical examination can be at upper lumbar levels rather than T11 because the upper lumbar cord levels are at the T11 vertebral level and the T11 cord level is at the T8 or T9 vertebral level. An awareness of this disparity allows reconciliation of the imaged vertebral level of injury with the neurologic findings.

At most levels, dorsal and ventral roots fuse to form a spinal nerve as they approach the intervertebral foramen. The spinal nerve and the dorsal root ganglia are located within the intervertebral foramen. The spinal nerve terminates as it emerges from the intervertebral foramen by dividing into dorsal and ventral rami. Dorsal rami perform only four functions. They innervate facet joints, interspinous and supraspinous ligaments, deep muscles of the back, and the skin of the medial two thirds of the back. Ventral rami innervate all other areas of the trunk and limbs that spinal nerves supply.

The major sensory innervation of the pain-sensitive walls and contents of the spinal canal is provided by the recurrent meningeal (sinuvertebral) nerve of Luschka. This nerve arises from the spinal nerve or its rami communicans and recurs through the intervertebral foramen. It supplies sensory innervation to the periosteal lining of the spinal canal, posterior longitudinal ligament, posterior anulus fibrosus, ligamenta flava, epidural fat and vessels, and the dura. The sensory innervation of the anterolateral anulus fibrosus and anterior longitudinal ligament is primarily from the rami communicans that connect the spinal nerve with the sympathetic trunk.

General Perispinal Soft Tissue Relationships

Rupture, edema, or hemorrhage involving the soft tissues that are closely related to the spine can serve as secondary or associated signs of spinal injury. These soft tissue injuries are typically best visualized by magnetic resonance imaging (MRI). From superficial to deep erector spinae, semispinalis, multifidus, and rotator muscles fill in the interval between the spinous processes medially and the laminae and transverse processes deeply. These are overlain by the splenius, levator scapulae, rhomboid, trapezius, and latissimus dorsi muscles (Fig. 3.5A). Hyperflexion or major fracture-dislocation injuries can involve these posteriorly situated muscles. The anterolaterally situated longus, scalene, sternocleidomastoid, and psoas muscles can be involved in hyperextension or major fracture-dislocation injuries (Fig. 3.5B). Closely related vessels like the vertebral vessels, aorta, and inferior vena cava can also be injured by vertebral trauma. The sympathetic trunk is closely related to the anterolateral aspect of spine throughout its length. Rupture of the cervical sympathetic trunk by hyperextension trauma can produce Horner syndrome.

Spine injury can also be associated with trauma to closely related visceral structures like the pharynx, esophagus, kidneys, and rectum.

General Biomechanics and Stability of the Spine

An appreciation of the normal mechanics of the spine provides the basis for understanding the pathomechanics of spine injury and the injury parameters that determine spine stability and instability. Basically, there are only two major kinds of motion that occur in the universe: translation and rotation. Translational motion occurs when all particles in a body move along parallel paths in the same direction with equal velocities (13). Rotational motion occurs when all particles in a body follow circular paths about a common axis with the same angular velocity. Because of the curved articular surfaces of most joints, rotational motion is the predominant motion in the human body. However, the flat ends of vertebral bodies make translational motions of the interbody joints feasible, although these may be normally limited at some levels by the facing direction of the facet joints or by local modifications of the vertebral body ends, such as uncinate processes at cervical levels. The combined constraints of the facing direction of the facet joints and the deformability of the intervertebral disk also permit rotational motions to occur about the trijoint intevertebral motion system. White and Panjabi applied a three-dimensional cartesian coordinate system to the spine to describe its complete mechanical behavior. They then described translational displacements acting along and rotational displacements acting around each of the three mutually perpen-

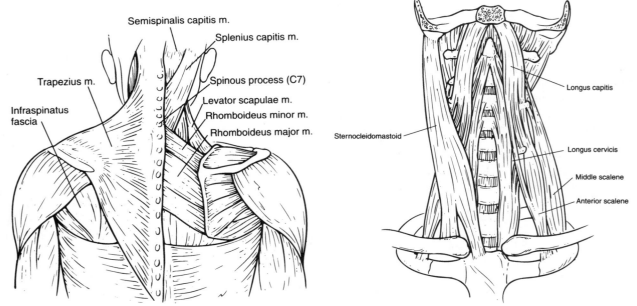

A

B

FIGURE 3.5. Musculature closely related to the spine. **A**; Some of the superficial back muscles, including the trapezius, rhomboids, and levator scapulae muscles. **B**; Anteriorly situated sternocleidomastoid, longus, and scalene muscles. (From White AH, Schofferman JA: *Spine care.* St. Louis: Mosby, 1995:1331, 1333, with permission.)

dicular axes (2). Injury forces can likewise be resolved along or around any of these axes.

The evaluation of spinal stability is critical to the management of the spine-injured patient. Yet the subject of stability or instability of the spine is a matter of controversy amongst biophysicists, orthopedic surgeons, neurosurgeons, and radiologists (14–17). There is even no agreement about the definition of spine stability or instability (18,19).

In 1977, Whitesides offered an early definition of the stable spine as one "that can withstand compressive force anteriorly through the vertebral bodies, tension forces posteriorly and rotational stresses . . . , thus being able to function to hold the body erect without progressive kyphosis and to protect the spinal contents from further injury" (20).

More recently in 1996, Daffner defined stability as "the ability of the vertebral column to maintain its normal alignment, to provide support for the head and torso and to protect the neural elements under physiologic stress" (14). He defined unstable injuries as "those that have the potential to cause progressive neurologic deterioration or skeletal deformity under normal physiologic motion or loading."

White and Panjabi, who have performed the most exhaustive studies of the biomechanics of the spine, defined clinical instability as "the loss of the ability of the spine under physiologic loads to maintain relationships between vertebrae in such a way that there is neither initial damage nor subsequent irritation to the spinal cord or nerve roots and, in addition there is no development of incapacitating deformity or pain due to structural changes" (2).

Some short simple definitions include those of Denis and Young. Denis said, "a stable spine is one that can withstand stress without progressive deformity or further neurologic damage" (21). He similarly defined an unstable spine as "one that can lead to an increased deformity or an increased neurologic defect." Young said an "unstable injury is one in which the spinal canal is unable to maintain its anatomic relationships under physiologic conditions" (22).

The attributes that are common to most of these definitions of stability and instability appear to be the spine's ability to resist immediate or progressive spinal deformity or neurologic damage under physiologic loads. This then raises the question, which of the potentially stabilizing features of the spine are most critical in delineating the stable from the unstable spine?

Kelly and Whitesides proposed an early model of spinal stability in 1968 (23). They proposed a two-column weight-bearing function of the spine made up anteriorly of a "solid column of vertebral bodies" and posteriorly of the "hollow column of the neural canal." They suggested that disruption of the anterior column without the posterior column will not create an unstable spine, whereas the additional failure of the posterior column will make the spine unstable. In 1977, Whitesides again divided the vertebral column into two major functional elements (20). But he then described the vertebral bodies as functioning to withstand compressive forces and the posterior elements as functioning to withstand tension. He claimed that failure of either of these elements would cause instability. Holdsworth also stressed the importance of the "posterior ligamentous complex," which he defined as the supraspinous ligament, interspinous ligament,

facet capsules, and ligamenta flava (24). He claimed that after injury, it is on the integrity of the posterior ligamentous complex that stability of the spine depends.

In 1983, Denis developed a three-column theory of spinal stability (21,25). He arrived at this concept because a number of well-designed investigations had demonstrated that complete rupture of the posterior ligamentous complex is insufficient to create spinal instability in flexion, extension, rotation, and shear (26–28). These studies revealed that when there is, in addition, also a disruption of the posterior longitudinal ligament and the posterior anulus fibrosus, spinal instability may be present, at least in flexion. Therefore, Denis described a third or middle column that has to be torn in addition to the posterior ligamentous complex to create acute instability. He said that the posterior longitudinal ligament, the posterior anulus fibrosus, and the posterior wall of the vertebral body form this middle column. Hence, Denis's three-column spine includes (a) an anterior column formed by the anterior longitudinal ligament and anterior part of the anulus fibrosus, (b) a middle column formed by the posterior longitudinal ligament, posterior anulus fibrosus, and posterior wall of the vertebral body, and (c) a posterior column formed by the posterior bony neural arch alternating with a posterior ligamentous complex made up of the supraspinous ligament, interspinous ligament, facet joint capsule, and ligamentum flavum. Denis cited the middle column as being crucial to spinal instability because the mode of its failure correlated well with both the type of spinal fracture and its neurologic injury.

Many authors have since embraced Denis's middle column as being an important determinant of spinal stability or instability. McAfee and associates claimed that the mode of failure of the middle osteoligamentous complex determined the pattern of spinal injury, the severity of neural deficit, the degree of instability, and the type of instrumentation required to stabilize the spine (29). They claimed that if the middle column has not failed, operative fixation is rarely indicated. They said the single exception to that generalization was multiple-level wedge compression fractures associated with progressive neural deficit. Ferguson and Allen modified Denis's three-column concept slightly by quantifying the limits of the middle column, or "element," as they preferred, as including the posterior one third of the vertebral body, posterior one third of the anulus fibrosus, and posterior longitudinal ligament (18). Thus, their anterior column came to be composed of the anterior two thirds of the vertebral body, anterior two thirds of the anulus fibrosus, and anterior longitudinal designation. Most subsequent authors have adopted the Ferguson and Allen modification of Denis's three-column concept (Fig. 3.6).

Young stressed the importance of the middle column by stating that the integrity of the middle column in the absence of displacement would indicate spinal stability (22). He further stressed that the importance of the middle column lies in its effect on surgical management of spine injuries. He emphasized that an intact middle element allows the positioning of posterior compression rods using the middle element as a fulcrum, whereas involvement of the middle element with fracture mandates the use of distracting rods.

Daffner interpreted Denis's three-column concept as imply-

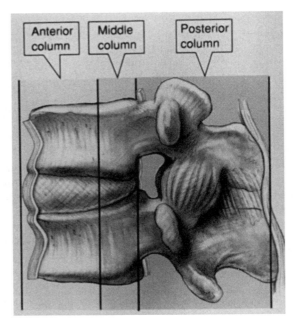

FIGURE 3.6. Denis's three-column concept of vertebral stability. (From Daffner NM. *Imaging of vertebral trauma*, 2nd ed. Philadelphia: Lippincott-Raven, 1996:224, with permission.)

TABLE 3.1. VERTEBRAL INSTABILITY

Radiographic Sign	Zones[a]		
Displacement	A	M	P
Wide interlaminar space		M	P
Wide facet joint		M	P
Wide vertebral canal	A	M	P
Disrupted posterior vertebral body line	A	M	

A, anterior; M, middle; P, posterior.
[a] The middle zone is disrupted in all of the signs.

ing that "instability would result only when disruption occurred in two contiguous zones, or more specifically when the middle zone was disrupted. This can only occur in conjunction with anterior or posterior disruption; middle zone disruption never occurs alone" (14,17).

Buitrago-Tellez and colleagues, writing as recently as 2000, supported the importance of the three-column concept and said that although it was conceived for the thoracolumbar spine, it could also be applied to the middle and lower cervical spine (19). They cited the middle column as the key to spinal instability, stating that lesions of the posterior column are unstable if one structure in the middle column is also affected and that lesions of both the anterior and middle column are unstable at least in flexion-compression. Further, they said lesions of just the anterior or posterior column are stable, and lesions of all three columns are unstable.

General Imaging Signs of Spinal Instability

In 1981, Gehwiler and associates analyzed 117 patients with thoracolumbar fractures and dislocations and concluded that all unstable lesions showed one or more of the following four signs: displaced vertebra, widened interspinous space, abnormal intervertebral disk or facet joints, and a widened vertebral canal (interpedicular distance) (30).

In 1987, Daffner and colleagues added to this list disruption of the posterior body line as a valid sign that a disruption has occurred within the middle column (31). By this, they meant disruption of the thin radiodense line normally observed along the posterior aspect of each individual vertebral body on lateral radiographs. They found that all 114 of their patients who had

computed tomography (CT)-confirmed pure burst fractures had either a posterior displacement of a portion of this line, a rotation of a portion of the line, or an obliteration of all or a portion of the line. By CT correlation, they found these findings to be consistent with retropulsion of one or more fragments from the posterior margin of the vertebral body into the vertebral canal.

Later, Daffner and colleagues more fully described these five findings of instability and related them to specific disruptions of Denis's three columns (14,17) (Table 3.1). They claimed that "the presence of only one of these signs is sufficient to establish a diagnosis of instability." First, they said vertebral displacement of more than 2 mm implies injury to the major ligamentous and articular structures. This could be anterior, posterior, or lateral dislocation of greater than 2 mm by all or a major portion of a vertebra. It implies that all three columns or zones are involved. Second, they claimed that widening of the interlaminar or interspinous spaces by greater than 2 mm can occur only when there is injury to the posterior ligamentous structures, the facet joints, and the posterior aspect of the anulus fibrosus, thus implying disruption of the posterior and middle zones. Third, they assert that facet joint disruption, indicated by an increase in the width of the facet joint interval, malalignment of the joints, or loss of contact between contiguous joints up to the level of naked facets involves posterior ligamentous damage that extends anteriorly to include the posterior longitudinal ligament and posterior anulus fibrosus. It thereby involves both the posterior and middle zones. Fourth, a widening of the vertebral canal, as indicated by an increase in interpedicle distance of more than 2 mm compared with contiguous levels, implies injury to the entire vertebra (both body and lamina) in the sagittal plane, thereby indicating disruption of all three zones. Fifth, they allege that disruption of the posterior vertebral body line is an indication of injury to the anterior bony structures and the posterior longitudinal ligament, thereby disrupting the anterior and middle zones (Table 3.1).

General Imaging Techniques for the Injured Spine

The techniques most commonly used to image a suspected spine injury include plain film radiography, CT, MRI, and occasionally conventional tomography.

Plain Film Radiography

For a patient suspected of having a cervical spine injury, most authors recommend as a minimum initial study a cross-table lateral, anteroposterior, and open-mouth atlantoaxial projection (14,19,32,33). The lateral should provide full visualization of the cervical spine from the base of the skull to the cervicothoracic junction. If the cervicothoracic junction is obscured by the superimposition of the shoulders, a "swimmer's view," with one limb fully abducted overhead and the other limb adducted, or a supine oblique view typically allows full visualization of this region. On the lateral film, five curved lines can be drawn that can be useful in detecting subtle vertebral malalignment (3) (Fig. 3.7). An anterior vertebral body line can be drawn along the anterior aspect of the vertebral bodies, approximating the position of the anterior longitudinal ligament. A posterior body line

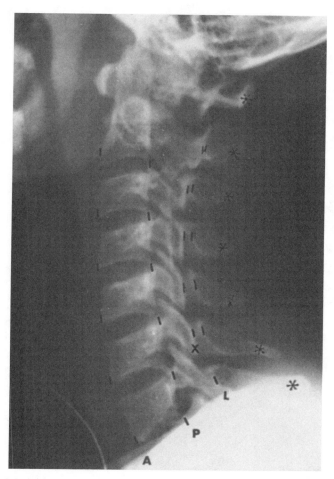

FIGURE 3.7. Lateral C-spine radiograph. Five "lines" should be drawn for reference: *A*; line of the anterior vertebral bodies; this outlines the position of the ALL; *P*; line of the posterior vertebral bodies; this outlines the line of the *PLL*; ***; line drawn through the tip of the spinous processes; this is most useful for assessing displacement of the posterior elements or fanning of the spinous processes; *L*; laminal line drawn between the posterior aspect of the spinal canal at each level, which is also helpful in determining displacement of the posterior elements; *X*; line drawn along the posterior margin of the contiguous articular pillars (using this line, displacement of articular pillars can be identified, and rotational anomaly of the spine can be judged by evaluating the distance between this line and the laminal line at each level) (see text). (From Mirvis SE, Young JWR. *Imaging in trauma and critical care*. Baltimore: Williams & Wilkins, 1992:293, with permission.)

along the posterior aspect of the vertebral body simulates the position of the posterior longitudinal ligament. A posterior pillar line can be constructed along the posterior margin of the articular pillars. A laminal or spinolaminar line can be drawn along the junction of the laminae and the spinous processes. An abrupt change in the space between the posterior pillar line and the spinolaminar line can be an accurate determinant of rotational disruption of the cervical spine, especially unilateral facet dislocation (34). A spinous process line can also be drawn along the tips of the spinous processes. The lateral view also permits evaluation of the uniformity of the interspinous and interlaminar distances, the orderly overlapping of the facet joints, any widening or luxation of the facet joint intervals or the intervertebral disk interval, the dens and the atlas–dens joint interval, the integrity of the pars interarticularis of the axis, and the integrity of the vertebral body ends, as well as the height of their anterior and posterior margins. Abrupt changes in the normal superimposition of the articular pillars of the two sides are another sign of rotation injury. Lateral views also permit an evaluation of the cervical prevertebral soft tissues. Changes in the contour of these soft tissues can be an indication of hemorrhage secondary to spinal trauma, but measurements of thickness tend to be unreliable, except anterior to the third cervical vertebra, where measurements of more than 10 mm are usually indicative of injury (33).

Anteroposterior cervical spine films permit an evaluation of the integrity of the uncinate processes, alignment of the lateral vertebral body margins, symmetry of alignment, integrity of spinous processes and pedicles, and uniformity of interspinous, interpedicle, and interbody distances (Fig. 3.8).

Open-mouth atlantoaxial views allow evaluation of the symmetry of the median and lateral atlantoaxial joints by examining the distance between the dens and the medial aspect of the lateral masses and the alignment of the lateral borders of the inferior articular facet of the atlas with the superior articular facet of the axis (Fig. 3.9). It also permits evaluation of the integrity of the dens, lateral masses, other parts of the vertebrae, and to some extent the atlantooccipital joint.

At thoracic and lumbar levels, supine anteroposterior and cross-table lateral projections allow evaluation of most of the same attributes of general vertebral integrity and symmetry that they provide at the C3 through C7 levels.

Functional radiographic examinations are used to detect segmental instability in patients with signs of localized spinal pain and tenderness, but without significant neurologic deficit, whose initial plain film examination revealed no osseous or ligamentous injuries. Most commonly, these are flexion-extension views of the cervical spine, but they can involve other spinal movements and levels. In normal flexion and extension views of the cervical spine, a fully alert and cooperative patient is instructed to flex and extend their spine only to the point of discomfort. In normal individuals, the cervical spine curves smoothly in both flexion and extension, with a relatively uniform mild (usually less than 2 mm) anterior or posterior subluxation of the vertebral bodies on the next lower vertebra. There is also a relatively uniform sliding forward, of each inferior articular process upon the next lower superior articular process, of about 5 mm in flexion (14, 33) (Fig. 3.10A,B). With hyperflexion subluxation, there is typically increased anterior subluxation at the level of injury, some-

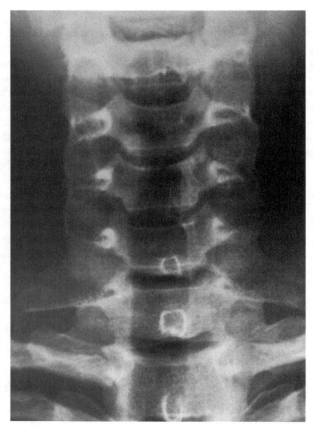

FIGURE 3.8. Normal anteroposterior cervical radiograph. Alignment at the lateral margins is normal. The pedicles are normally aligned, and the distances between them do not deviate more than 2 mm from level to level. The interspinous spaces are uniform. This patient has prominent transverse processes at C7. (From Daffner NM. *Imaging of vertebral trauma*, 2nd ed. Philadelphia: Lippincott-Raven, 1996:58, with permission.)

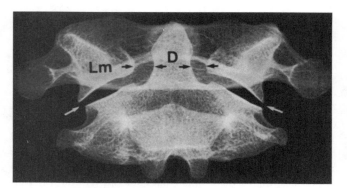

FIGURE 3.9. The atlantoaxial articulation, frontal view. Note the relation of the lateral masses of C1 and their articulations to the body of C2. Under normal circumstances, there should never be more than 2 mm of unilateral of bilateral atlantoaxial overlap at the point indicated by the *white arrows*. Similarly, there should never be more than 2 mm difference in the distance between the lateral margins of the dens and the medial margins of the lateral masses of C1 (*black arrows*). (From Daffner NM. *Imaging of vertebral trauma*, 2nd ed. Philadelphia: Lippincott-Raven, 1996:34, with permission.)

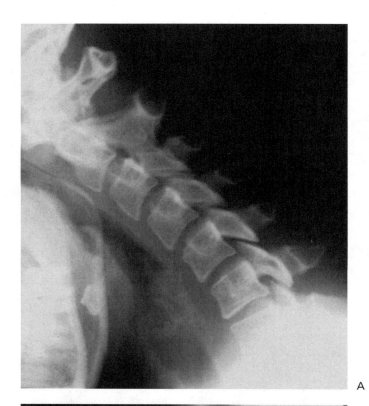

A

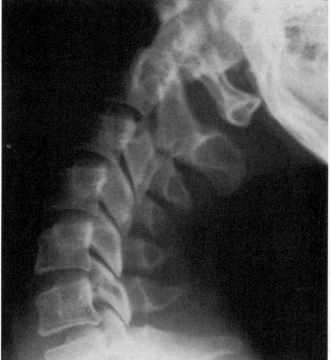

B

FIGURE 3.10. Normal flexion and extension. The cervical column curves smoothly in both flexion (**A**) and extension (**B**). There are minor degrees of subluxation at multiple levels, anteriorly in flexion and posteriorly in extension. This is normal, more so in younger patients. The articular surfaces are slightly asymmetric at some facet joints, which is also normal in young patients. (From Daffner NM. *Imaging of vertebral trauma*, 2nd ed. Philadelphia: Lippincott-Raven, 1996:200, with permission.)

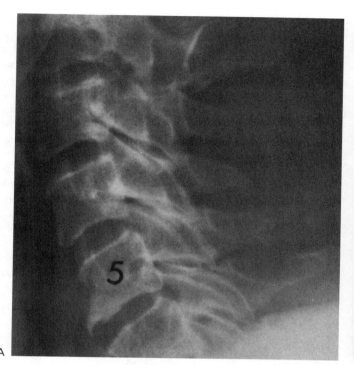

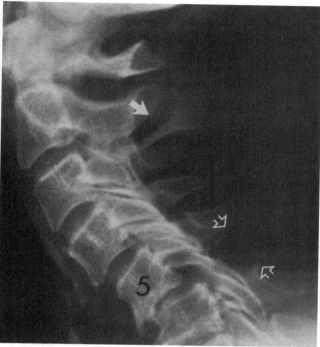

FIGURE 3.11. Occult instability. Flexion sprain of C5 in a 72-year-old patient involved in a rear-end automobile accident. **A**; Supine radiograph shows mild degenerative changes. **B**; Upright radiograph shows anterolisthesis of C5 on C6, narrowing of the C5 disk space, widening of the interlaminar (interspinous) space of C5-6 (*open arrows*), and fracture through the spinous process of C2 (*thick arrow*). Continuity is almost completely lost along the articular surfaces of the facet joints of C5 and C6. This case illustrates the need for erect radiographs before a patient is discharged from the hospital. (From Daffner NM. *Imaging of vertebral trauma*, 2nd ed. Philadelphia: Lippincott-Raven, 1996:3, with permission.)

times visualized only by assuming the upright position, with same-segment increases in facet luxation and in interspinous, interlaminar, and interpedicle dimension (Fig. 3.11A,B). With hyperextension subluxation, there can be increased posterior subluxation of the inferior articular process and widening of the intervertebral disk interval at the injured level.

Plain Film Tomography

The advent of fast spiral CT has replaced many of the indications for plain film tomography in the acute phase of spinal trauma. However, horizontal or axially oriented fractures parallel to the standard CT imaging plane, such as dens or Chance fractures, can be missed by the volume-averaging effect of CT. They can usually be well demonstrated by anteroposterior or lateral conventional tomograms.

Computed Tomography

Computed tomography has the technical advantages of eliminating the superimposition of plain films, enhancing contrast, and reformatting the images in sagittal, coronal, or oblique planes as well as three-dimensional reconstructions. It is especially useful for evaluating the middle and posterior columns of Denis, which form the walls of the spinal canal (19). Hence, it can be

invaluable in assessing spine instability, the presence and degree of spinal canal encroachment, or intervertebral foramen encroachment. It can assess the potential for spinal cord injury by detecting impingements on the thecal sac by bone fragments, epidural hematoma, or chronic degenerative processes. It is also useful in detecting fractures of laminae, pedicles, and articular pillars and for fully evaluating spine dislocations, fracture-dislocations, and complex vertebral body fractures. Important indications for CT include evaluation of (a) patients with equivocal plain film findings, (b) patients with focal spine pain or neurologic deficits unexplained by radiography, (c) patients with known spine injury to determine the extent of injury to help determine the best mode of therapy, and (d) patients with postoperative complications (33). CT myelography can be useful in further evaluating dural (thecal) sac or neural encroachment, identifying cervical nerve root avulsions or detecting posttraumatic cystic myelopathy (14). However, its value must be weighed against its invasive nature.

Magnetic Resonance Imaging

Some of the unique advantages of MRI are that (a) it can provide direct imaging of injury to spinal ligaments and the intervertebral disk; (b) it provides good contrast resolution of paraspinal soft tissues and detects edema or hemorrhage within these tissues as an associated sign of spinal injury; (c) it can provide a "myelographic effect" with T2-weighted images that will permit good visualization of spinal canal or spinal cord compromise by bone fragments, herniated disks, osteophytes, or epidural hematoma; (d) it permits differentiation of the type of spinal cord injury (contusion, hemorrhage, complete disruption), which can be of prognostic value for recovery of neurologic function; and (e) it is also invaluable for identifying the late sequelae of spinal cord trauma, including myelomalacia and posttraumatic spinal cord cysts or syringomyelia (32,35).

The typical MRI examination includes T1-, T2-, and proton density–weighted sequences in the sagittal and axial planes. On a T1-weighted image, fat within the vertebral marrow and epidural space has a high signal intensity (Fig. 3.12A). Cortical bone and the anterior and posterior longitudinal ligaments, ligamenta flava, interspinous and supraspinous ligaments, the anulus fibrosus, and the dura exhibit low signal intensity. Normal anterior and posterior longitudinal ligaments blend with the adjacent cortical bone and anulus fibrosus. The cerebrospinal fluid (CSF)

also has a low signal intensity, which makes it indistinguishable from its bounding dura and from the posterior longitudinal ligament and posterior vertebral body cortex. The central part of the intervertebral disk, spinal cord, and nerve roots demonstrate moderate signal intensity (Fig. 3.12A).

T2-weighted images provide a "myelographic effect" because of the high signal intensity of the CSF and moderate signal intensity of the spinal cord (Fig. 3.12B). Signal intensity of the marrow fat is decreased. The myelographic effect permits evaluation of the degree of encroachment of the dural sac or spinal cord by bone fragments, herniated disks, spinal stenosis or epidural hematoma. The signal intensity of the central disk is increased. Proton density images also show increased central disk intensity, and the signal intensity of the CSF is intermediate between that seen on T1- and T2-weighted images, thereby producing less contrast with the spinal cord (Fig. 3.12C).

The acutely injured spinal cord often enlarges to fill more of the spinal canal and to displace the epidural fat (35). This can

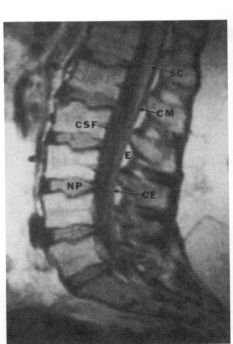 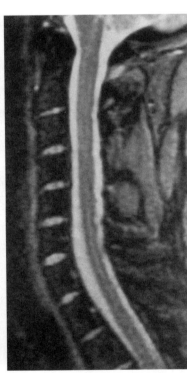 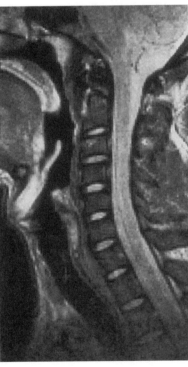

A,B   C

FIGURE 3.12. A; T1-weighted mid-sagittal magnetic resonance image (MRI) of the lumbosacral spine displays the nucleus pulposus (*NP*) of the intervertebral disks, spinal cord (*SC*), conus medullaris (*CM*), and nerve roots of the cauda equina (*CE*) as areas of moderate signal intensity. Cerebrospinal fluid (*CSF*) is of low signal intensity, and epidural fat (*E*) is hyperintense. **B**; Midline sagittal T2-weighted MRI. Image shows very dark bone marrow with bright intervertebral disks producing sharp contrast between bone and disk material. The ligaments remain very low in signal intensity, whereas the CSF is very bright. The cord is of intermediate signal intensity and markedly contrasted with surrounding CSF. Again, the anulus fibers and longitudinal ligaments cannot be distinguished. **C**; Midline sagittal proton density image obtained with TR = 2,500 and TE = 40 msec. One signal acquisition shows darkening of bone marrow signal and brightening of CSF signal. This has produced increased contrast between the relatively bright disk material as compared with adjacent cortical bone and ligaments. There is poor contrast between the CSF and spinal cord. The posterior anulus fibrosus and posterior or longitudinal ligament are well contrasted between the bright nuclear disk material and the CSF. (**A**, from DeLisa JA, Gans BM: *Rehabilitation medicine: principles and practice*, 3rd ed. Philadelphia: Lippincott-Raven, 1998:457, with permission. **B,C**, from Harris JH Jr, Mirvis SE. *The radiology of acute cervical spine trauma*, 3rd ed. Baltimore: Williams & Wilkins, 1996:143–141, with permission.)

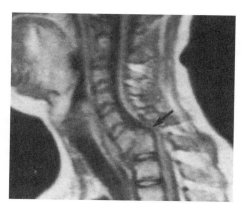

FIGURE 3.13. Fracture-dislocation of C6 to C7 with cord compression or transsection (*arrow*) as seen on a T1-weighted mid-sagittal magnetic resonance image. (From DeLisa JA, Gans BM. *Rehabilitation medicine: principles and practice*, 3rd ed. Philadelphia: Lippincott-Raven, 1998: 468, with permission.)

be visualized by both CT and MRI. However, MRI provides the best means of evaluating the type of spinal cord injury and its evolution. In the early stages of spinal cord injury, MRI can be valuable in determining the type of injury and the prognosis for recovery. It can identify the level and completeness of cord disruption by a direct visualization of the injury site (Fig. 3.13). In the early presentation of the nontransected spinal cord, it can differentiate spinal cord hemorrhage from contusion with edema. In the first 24 hours after injury, the edema of spinal cord contusion exhibits high signal intensity on T2-weighted images and a moderate signal intensity usually indistinguishable from normal cord on T1-weighted images (Fig. 3.14). The appearance of spinal cord hemorrhage depends on the state of the

hemoglobin in the hemorrhage (35,36). Within a few hours of a very early hemorrhage, the nonparamagnetic intracellular oxyhemoglobin is converted into paramagnetic intracellular deoxyhemoglobin. Hence, in the acute hemorrhage stage, lasting 1 to 3 days, intracellular deoxyhemoglobin causes the hemorrhage to appear very hypointense on T2-weighted images, slightly hypointense on T1-weighted images, and of intermediate hypointensity on proton density images (Fig. 3.15). Between the third and seventh day, intracellular deoxyhemoglobin is oxidized to methemoglobin as the clot enters its subacute phase. Although the subacute phase of hemorrhage has many substages in which the signal intensity of methemoglobin varies, in general, methemoglobin is hyperintense on T1-weighted images. Because the conversion to methemoglobin usually begins at the periphery of the clot, during the subacute phase, the clot can have a peripheral hyperintensity and a central hypointensity. Over several months, methemoglobin will be resorbed, and the clot will develop a rim of macrophages that contain hemosiderin, which is hypointense on both T1- and T2-weighted images. This is the chronic hemorrhage stage of the clot.

Kulkarni and colleagues found that the type of spinal cord injury visualized by MRI correlated with the patient's recovery of neurologic function (37). Patients with cord contusion and edema exhibited significant functional recovery, whereas those

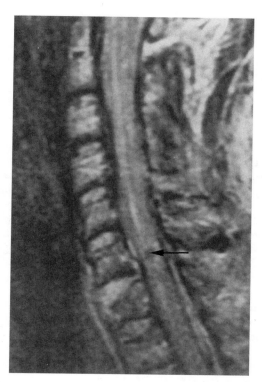

FIGURE 3.15. Sagittal proton density magnetic resonance image in a 45-year-old man sustaining severe hyperflexion injury shows a low-signal cord lesion at the C6 level representing intracellular deoxyhemoglobin or methemoglobin (*arrow*) with surrounding periphery of bright signal edema. (From Harris JH Jr, Mirvis SE. *The radiology of acute cervical spine trauma*, 3rd ed. Baltimore: Williams & Wilkins, 1996:168, with permission.)

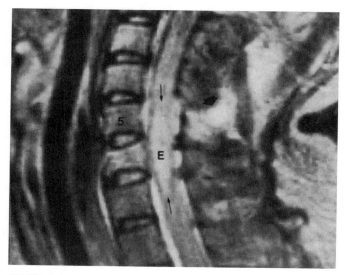

FIGURE 3.14. T2-weighted magnetic resonance image of central cord edema (*E*) after a C6 burst fracture. Note the extent of the edema (*thin arrows*). There is posterior soft tissue hemorrhage (*wide arrow*). (From Daffner NM. *Imaging of vertebral trauma*, 2nd ed. Philadelphia: Lippincott-Raven, 1996:88, with permission.)

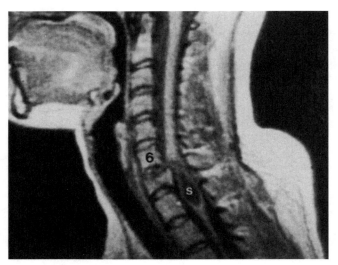

FIGURE 3.16. Posttraumatic syringomyelia. This patient suffered a burst fracture of C7. T1-weighted magnetic resonance image made 6 months after injury shows a localized low-signal area within the spinal cord representing a syrinx (s). (From Daffner NM. *Imaging of vertebral trauma*, 2nd ed. Philadelphia: Lippincott-Raven, 1996:84, with permission.)

with cord hemorrhage made little functional progress (see chapter 7 for details).

MRI is also useful for identifying the late sequelae of spinal cord injury. Myelomalacia is thought to develop within an injured cord segment either as a result of ischemia or because of enzymes released from autolyzed cells (35). The myelomalacic region is made up of the products of neural degeneration, scar tissue, and microcysts. It is hypothesized that the myelomalacic areas become larger intramedullary cysts either by virtue of coalescence of the microcysts or perhaps by CSF entering the cyst along the perivascular Virchow-Robin spaces that connect the subarachnoid space to the cyst.

On T1-weighted images, myelomalacia appears in the cord near the area of injury as a region of lower signal intensity than the cord but higher signal intensity than the CSF. It has indistinct margins with the surrounding cord. In contrast, intramedullary cysts (posttraumatic syringomyelia) have signal intensity like that of CSF and are sharply marginated from the surrounding cord or adjacent myelomalacic area (38) (Fig. 3.16). The development of an intramedullary cyst may cause a spinal cord patient whose clinical picture had stabilized to show progressive sensory and motor deficits. Although myelomalacia has no specific treatment, intramedullary cysts can be decompressed with a shunt, potentially to arrest the progression of neurologic signs. MRI can also be used postoperatively to ensure that the cyst is decompressed and that the shunt continues to function to prevent reaccumulation of fluid within the cysts.

ANATOMY, MECHANICS, AND IMAGING FEATURES OF OCCIPITOATLANTOAXIAL INJURIES

Atlas

Unlike the tripod load-transmitting mechanism of the rest of the spine, there is a dual load-transmitting system from the occipital

condyles to the axis. During embryologic development, the mesenchymal mass of the atlas body fuses with that of the axis to form the dens or odontoid process. Therefore, the atlas is formed of two load-bearing lateral masses joined by an anterior and posterior arch (Fig. 3.17A).

The superior aspect of the lateral masses bear concave ovoid articular surfaces with their major axis in the anteroposterior direction for articulation with the reciprocally convex occipital condyles (Fig. 3.17A,B). Because the superior articular surface faces superiorly and medially and the flat inferior articular surface for the axis faces inferiorly and medially, in a posterior or anterior view, the lateral masses are wedge shaped, with the apex of the wedge directed medially. This plays a major role in the pathomechanics of Jefferson fractures, as described later. On the medial aspect of each lateral mass, there is a tubercle for the attachment of the transverse atlantal ligament. The short straight anterior and the longer curved posterior arches of the atlas act as tie-rod stabilizers for the load-bearing lateral masses, as does the transverse atlantal ligament that is stretched between them. Both arches are thinnest where they attach to the lateral masses. The posterior arch is especially deeply grooved on its superior aspect by the vertebral arteries, which as they emerge from their foramina in the transverse processes, loop behind the lateral masses (Fig. 3.17B). These naturally narrowed portions of both arches are common sites of Jefferson fractures, described later. On its posterior aspect, the anterior arch has an articular facet for articulation with the dens of the axis (Fig. 3.17C).

Axis

The axis is also a unique vertebra that receives its name from the prominent dens or odontoid process that forms the axis of rotation of the atlantoaxial joint complex (Fig. 3.18A). It has an anterior articular surface on its head for articulation with the anterior arch of the atlas and a posterior articular surface on its neck for articulation with the transverse atlantal ligament. In an anterior view, the axis appears to have broad shoulders formed by its superior articular surfaces (Fig. 3.18A). The atlas functions as a load-splitting vertebra, which must convert the dual loads received from the inferior articular surface of the atlas into the tripod load-transmitting system of the rest of the spine. Most of the loads received from the inferiorly and medially directed inferior articular surfaces of the atlas are directed onto its vertebral body. However, in lateral view, it is clear that the inferior articular surface of the axis is offset posteriorly from the superior articular surfaces by a portion of the neural arch called the *pars interarticularis* (Fig. 3.18B). Hence, loads transmitted through the axis onto the facet joint it forms with the third cervical vertebra would tend to concentrate shearing stresses on the pars interarticularis, which is the usual site of failure in a traumatic spondylolisthesis of the axis (hangman's fracture).

Atlantooccipital Joints

The atlantooccipital joints are often described as "yes joints" because their freest motion is flexion and extension. They also permit some lateral bending, but rotation is limited. Many ligaments contribute to their stability. Anteriorly, a narrowed anterior longitudinal ligament and the anterior atlantooccipital

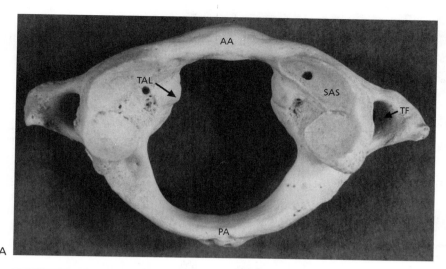

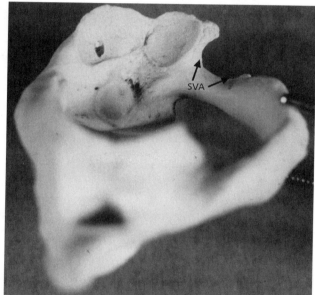

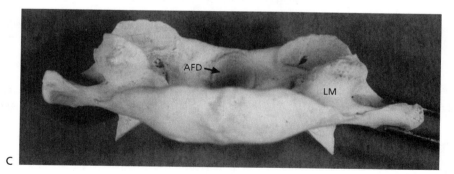

FIGURE 3.17. Atlas. **A**; Superior view displaying the anterior arch (*AA*), posterior arch (*PA*), superior articular surface of the lateral mass (*SAS*), tubercle for the transverse atlantal ligament (*TAL*), and transverse foramina for the transmission of the vertebral vessels (*TF*). **B**; Oblique superior and lateral view demonstrating the thinning of the posterior arch caused by the superiorly situated sulcus of the vertebral artery (*SVA*). **C**; Posterior view visualizing the ovoid articular facet for the dens (*AFD*) and the wedge shape of the lateral masses (*LM*). (From White AH, Schofferman JA. *Spine care*. St. Louis: Mosby, 1995:1312, 1313, with permission.)

membrane, which extends from the anterior margin of the foramen magnum to the anterior arch of the atlas, limit extension (Fig. 3.19A). A posterior atlantooccipital membrane extends from the posterior arch of the atlas and helps limit flexion (Fig. 3.19B). The upper end of the posterior longitudinal ligament broadens to become the tectorial membrane, which attaches to

the anterior aspect of the foramen magnum (Fig. 3.19C). The alar and apical ligaments are two joint ligaments extending from the tip of the dens to the foramen magnum. Because the flexion-extension axis of the atlantooccipital joint is situated just above the dens, it is thought that the closely related alar and apical ligaments, as well as the tectorial membrane, are little involved

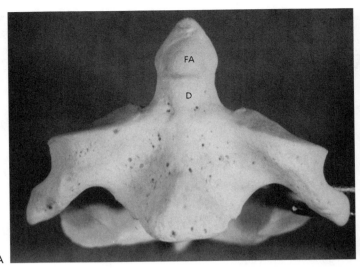
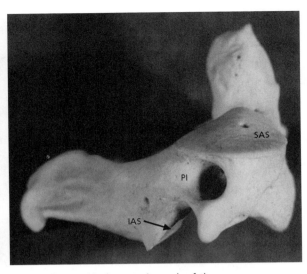

A

B

FIGURE 3.18. Axis. **A**; Anterior view showing the facet that articulates with the anterior arch of the atlas (*FA*) on the anterior aspect of the dens (*D*). **B**; Lateral view showing how the superior articular surface (*SAS*) is offset from the inferior articular surface (*IAS*) of the axis by the obliquely placed pars interarticularis (*PI*). (From White AH, Schofferman JA. *Spine care*. St. Louis: Mosby, 1995:1316, with permission.)

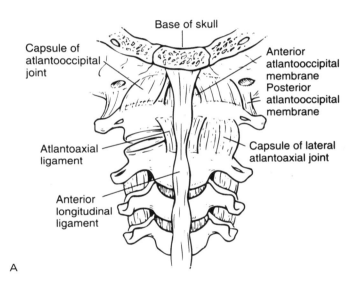

A

FIGURE 3.19. Ligaments of atlantooccipital joints and the lateral atlantoaxial joints. **A**; Anterior view. **B**; Posterior view. **C**; Posterior view with neural arches removed. (From White AH, Schofferman JA. *Spine care*. St. Louis: Mosby, 1995:1317, 1319, with permission.)

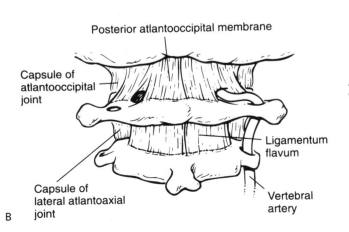

B

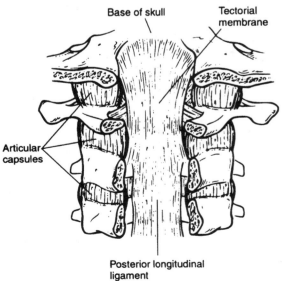

C

in resisting the physiologic range of flexion and extension (39, 40). However, all these ligaments must be disrupted in atlantooccipital dislocations secondary to hyperflexion, hyperextension, or distraction trauma.

Atlantoaxial Joints

The atlas and axis articulate at a median and two lateral atlantoaxial joints. The lateral atlantoaxial joints are formed between the inferior articular surfaces of the atlas and superior articular surfaces of the axis. The joint capsule is thin and loose and permits free motion. An extension-resisting anterior atlantoaxial ligament extends from the anterior arch of the atlas to the anterior body of the axis (Fig. 3.19A). A flexion-resisting posterior atlantoaxial ligament stretches from the posterior arch of the atlas to the lamina of the axis (Fig. 3.19B).

The median atlantoaxial joint is a pivot joint with two joint cavities. One joint is between the hyaline cartilage–covered artic-

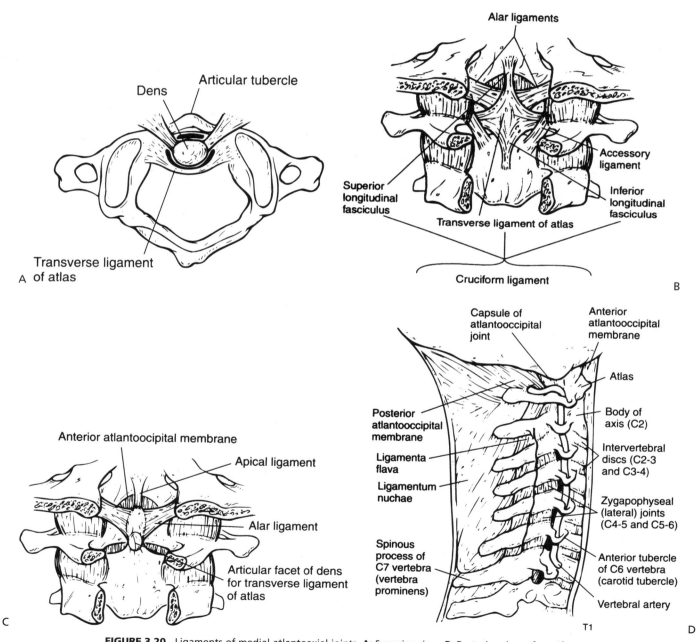

FIGURE 3.20. Ligaments of medial atlantoaxial joints. **A**; Superior view. **B**; Posterior view of cruciform ligament. **C**; Posterior view of alar and apical ligaments with cruciform ligament removed. **D**; Lateral view of cervical spine ligaments. (From White AH, Schofferman JA. *Spine care.* St. Louis: Mosby, 1995: 1319, with permission.)

ular facet on the anterior arch of the atlas and a similar facet on the head of the dens (Fig. 3.20A). The other is between the hyaline cartilage–covered facet on the back of the neck of the dens and the transverse atlantal ligament.

The strong, thick transverse atlantal ligament attaches to the tubercles on the medial aspect of the lateral masses (Fig. 3.20B). It has smaller superior and inferior longitudinal fasciculi attaching above to the anterior margin of the foramen magnum and below to the posterior body of the axis. The transverse atlantal ligament and the two longitudinal fasciculi are sometimes called the *cruciform ligament*. Just anterior to the superior longitudinal fasciculus, a narrow apical ligament extends from the apex of the dens to the anterior margin of the foramen magnum (Fig. 3.20C). Two broader but thinner alar ligaments extend from the superolateral margins of the dens to the medial aspect of the occipital condyles. Each alar ligament resists rotation and lateral bending of the head to the opposite side. Both the tectorial membrane and the ligamentum nuchae, which is a thin midline intermuscular septum between the posterior cervical muscles, resist flexion at the atlantoaxial joint and can be ruptured by hyperflexion injuries (Fig. 3.20D).

Atlantooccipital Dislocation

Dislocation or subluxation of the atlantooccipital joint can be caused by a number of diverse mechanisms, including flexion, extension, and distraction, most commonly by both flexion and distraction (32). This unstable fracture is frequently fatal because of injury to the closely related cardiovascular and respiratory centers of the medulla, but individuals have survived with major or even minor neurologic findings. On a lateral radiograph, the mastoid processes superimpose on this joint and may obscure some of the landmarks. Normally, the occipital condyles should occupy the superior articular surfaces (condylar fossae) of the atlas, with no intervening space; the posterior margin of the foramen magnum (opisthion) should lie along the upward continuation of the spinolaminar line of the atlas; the anterior margin of the foramen magnum (basion) should lie superior to the odontoid process; and a line constructed tangent to the posterior border of the clivus should pass close to the tip of the odontoid process (19,32,33) (Fig. 3.21A,B). In anterior atlantooccipital dislocations, the occipital condyles are distracted and anteriorly displaced, leaving an empty superior articular surface of the atlas; the opisthion is anterior to the spinolaminar junction of the atlas; and both the basion and clival line are anterior to the odontoid (Figs. 3.21A,B and 3.22). There can also be distortion and thickening of the soft tissues between the upper cervical spine and the nasopharynx caused by hemorrhage from injury to the ligaments bridging the atlantooccipital interval. A number of lines and ratios have been devised to assess this dislocation, but some of the bony landmarks are difficult to identify in many cases.

Jefferson Fracture

A Jefferson fracture is a burst fracture involving the arches of the atlas. It is caused by axial compression forces applied to the top of the head as, for example, when a football player spears

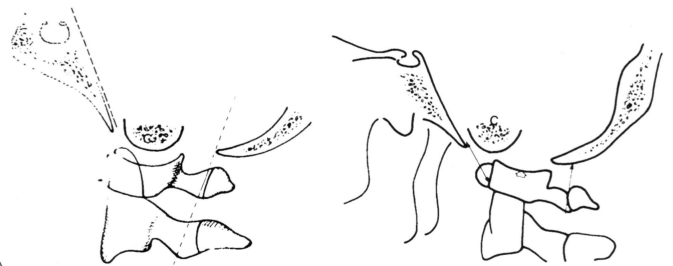

A   B

FIGURE 3.21. Atlantooccipital dislocation. **A**; Normal anatomic relationships of the skull base and atlas. A line drawn along the edge of the clivus should intersect the top of the odontoid process. The occipital condyle should occupy the condylar fossa of the atlas without an intervening gap. The posterior lip of the foramen magnum should align with the spinolaminar line of the atlas. **B**; Anterior displacement of the occiput in relation to the atlas. A line drawn along the posterior margin of the clivus intercepts the anterior aspect of the odontoid (*two-headed arrow*). The occipital condyle is displaced anterior to the condylar fossa of C1, leaving a "naked" condylar fossa (*open arrow*). A line drawn through the spinolaminar line of the atlas intercepts the occiput posterior to the posterior lip of the foramen magnum (*single-headed arrow*). (From Mirvis SE, Young JWR. *Imaging in trauma and critical care.* Baltimore: Williams & Wilkins, 1992:251, with permission.)

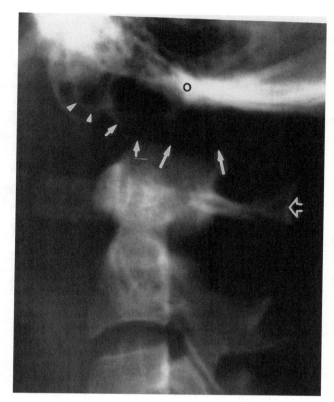

FIGURE 3.22. Anterior atlantooccipital dislocation. This lateral radiograph reveals empty condylar fossae (*long white arrows*) with the occipital condyles (*white arrowheads*) and the mastoid process (*short white arrows*) several centimeters anterior to the condylar fossae and the opisthion (*O*) several centimeters anterior to the spinolaminar line of the atlas (*open arrow*).

must be offset laterally at least 3 mm from the superior articular surface of the axis (14) (Fig. 3.23A). This typically indicates instability by virtue of rupture of the transverse atlantal ligament. The intervals between the dens and medial aspect of the lateral masses of the atlas may be abnormally wide or asymmetric, but asymmetry may also occur with normal physiologic rotation of the atlas on the axis or with rotary atlantoaxial dislocation (32, 42). On a lateral radiograph, the arch fractures may be visualized, and there may be widening or an abnormal contour of the cervicocranial prevertebral soft tissues. Axial CT routinely identifies all of the fracture sites and can identify rupture of the transverse atlantal ligament (Fig. 3.23B).

Traumatic Rotary Atlantoaxial Dislocation

In acute traumatic atlantoaxial dislocation, there is a rotational derangement of the lateral atlantoaxial joints secondary to an acute traumatic injury. It may involve some simultaneous rotation of the axis. It may be transient and resolve spontaneously in a few days or may persist (32). It typically produces no neural encroachment, but the resulting torticollis can be uncomfortable. In a right rotary dislocation (face deviated to the right), the left lateral mass moves forward and medially and therefore narrows the left lateral atlas dens interval and appears more rectangular. Whereas the right lateral mass moves posteriorly and the right lateral atlas dens interval appears wider (Fig. 3.24A). In a lateral radiograph, the lateral masses are unsuperimposed; the left lateral mass is anterior to the odontoid and appears narrow in its anteroposterior dimension, whereas the right lateral mass projects posterior to the odontoid with a greater anteroposterior dimension (Fig. 3.24B).

Atlantoaxial Instability

Atlantoaxial instability can cause an upper cervical myelopathy that presents with signs of compromised long ascending and descending tracts. It can be caused by disruption of the median atlantoaxial joint or by disruption of the odontoid. Disruption of the median atlantoaxial joint can be best visualized by a lateral cervical spine view with the neck flexed. The instability appears as a posterior displacement of the dens away from the anterior arch of the atlas (1). This brings the dens into the spinal canal, where it can encroach on the upper cervical spinal cord by narrowing the space between the dens and posterior arch of the atlas. On lateral cervical spine films, normal radiolucency is observed between the dens and the anterior arch of the atlas (Fig. 3.25A). This atlas–dens interval is produced by the hyaline cartilage on the posterior aspect of the anterior arch of the atlas and the anterior aspect of the dens. In normal adults, the atlas–dens interval (predental space) should not exceed 3 mm (43). In a child in whom ossification is incomplete, the upper limit of the normal atlas–dens interval is 5 mm (44). Atlantoaxial instability can be produced by simple disruption of the transverse atlantal ligament. This usually results from hyperflexion trauma, which may cause an avulsion or mid-substance tear of the transverse atlantal ligament and other ligaments of the dens (Fig. 3.25B,C).

an opposing player with his helmet. The pathomechanics of the injury is a function of the interaction between the wedge-shaped geometry of the lateral masses with the injuring forces. As compressive loads are transmitted from the occipital condyles onto the lateral masses, they are directed inferiorly and laterally onto its superior articular surface. As this load is transmitted through the lateral masses, it is directed inferiorly and medially onto the superior articular surface of the axis. By Newton's third law, the axis will exert a superiorly and laterally directed equal and opposite force onto the inferior articular surface of the atlas. Jefferson said the result of the inferior and lateral force acting on the superior articular surface of the atlas and of the superior and lateral force acting on its inferior articular surface is a laterally directed vector on each lateral mass (41). This produces a burst fracture of the ringlike atlas by placing the arches in tension. The arches most commonly fracture where they are thinnest, which is where each arch joins the lateral masses. Closed-ring structures like the atlas, pelvis, radius-ulna, and tibia-fibula are typically disrupted in at least two places. The arch fractures may be unilateral or bilateral. The transverse atlantal ligaments may be partially or completely disrupted. Stability depends on integrity of the transverse atlantal ligament (19).

To diagnose a Jefferson fracture on the open-mouth atlantoaxial view, the lateral margins of the lateral mass of the atlas

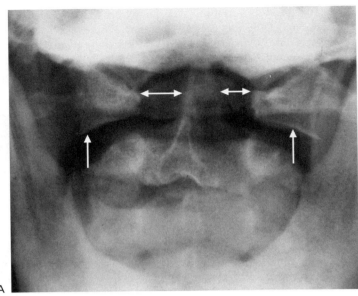

A

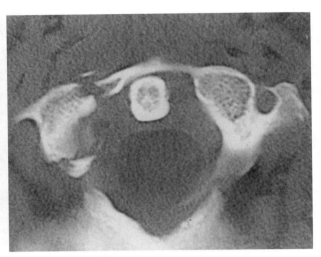

B

FIGURE 3.23. Jefferson's fracture. **A**; An open-mouth anteroposterior atlantoaxial view demonstrates that the lateral margins of both lateral masses are displaced laterally more than 5 mm from the lateral margins of the superior articular process of the axis (*vertical arrows*). The interval between the dens and the medial aspect of the right lateral mass is about twice as great as that of the left side (*double-headed horizontal arrows*). **B**; Bone window axial computed tomography scan visualizes comminuted fractures where the right anterior and posterior arches join the right lateral mass.

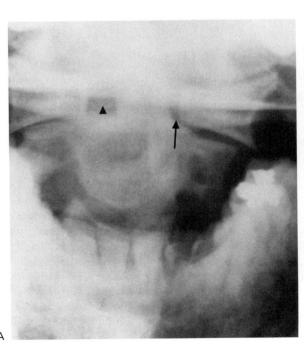

A

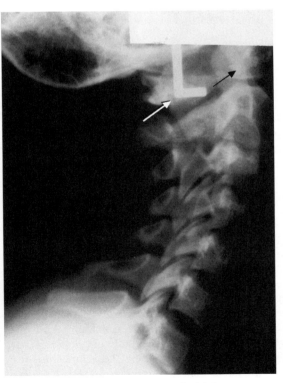

B

FIGURE 3.24. Traumatic rotary atlantoaxial dislocation. This 20-year-old woman presented with her head locked in rotation to the right after a sudden turn of her head after hair washing. **A**; Open-mouth anteroposterior atlantoaxial view reveals a narrowed left lateral atlas dens interval (*arrow*) and a widened right interval (*arrowhead*). **B**; Lateral radiograph shows substantially unsuperimposed lateral masses (*arrows*).

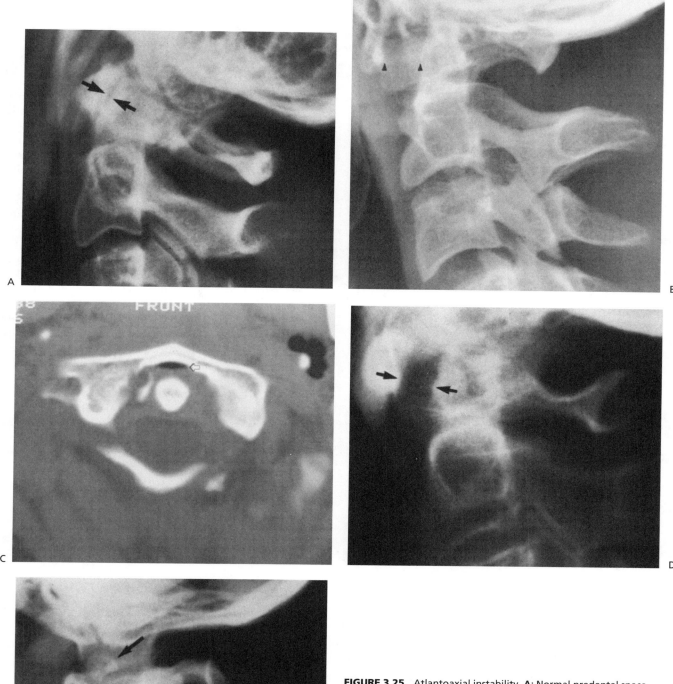

FIGURE 3.25. Atlantoaxial instability. **A**; Normal predental space in an adult (*arrows*). **B**; Lateral radiograph revealing marked anterior displacement of the anterior C1 arch relative to the odontoid with anterior displacement of the C1 spinolaminar line relative to that of C2 (*arrowheads*). Neither a C1 nor a C2 fracture was identified. **C**; Computed tomography image of a 40-year-old man after a motor vehicle accident shows widening of the atlantodental space with a vacuum joint (*open arrow*). There is an avulsion fracture of the medial aspect of the C1 lateral mass, probably secondary to the pull of the transverse alar ligament. **D**; Anterolisthesis of C1 on C2 with widened predental space (*arrows*) in a patient with rheumatoid arthritis. **E**; Atlantoaxial dislocation and wide predental space in a patient with os odontoideum (*arrow*). (**A,D,E**, from Daffner NM. *Imaging of vertebral trauma*, 2nd ed. Philadelphia: Lippincott-Raven, 1996:145, 180, with permission; **B,C**, from Mirvis SE, Young JWR: *Imaging in trauma and critical care*. Baltimore: Williams & Wilkins, 1992:356, with permission.)

47

However, it may be secondary to a Jefferson fracture. Ligament laxity from rheumatoid arthritis involving the atlantoaxial joints can also increase the atlas–dens interval in flexion (Fig. 3.25D). Os odontoideum, which involves either congenital failure of fusion of a dens ossification center with the rest of the dens or nonunion of a dens fracture, can also cause atlantoaxial instability, as can odontoid type 2 and 3 fractures, as described later. In these cases, the atlas–dens interval is intact, and the atlas and dens move forward on the axis in flexion and backward on the axis in extension. In flexion, the compromised spinal canal is the interval between the axis body and the posterior arch of the atlas (Fig. 3.25E), whereas in extension, the compromised interval is between the dens and lamina of the axis.

Odontoid Fracture

Fracture of the odontoid process or dens can be caused by hyperflexion, hyperextension, lateral bending, or some combination of these injury mechanisms. The traditional classification of dens fractures by Anderson and D'Alonzo divided these fractures into type I involving the dens tip, type II through the dens base, and type III extending into the axis body (45). Many investigators have failed to find examples of type I fractures that were not an os odontoideum (32). Hence, current authors have proposed dividing odontoid fractures into high (type II) and low (type III), although the low fractures might be better called *axis body fractures* (32,33). Both high and low fractures are typically unstable, and nonunion is common. High dens fractures appear as radiolucent intervals at the dens base on open-mouth films or conventional tomograms (Fig. 3.26A). Low dens fractures

can be similarly visualized (Fig. 3.26B) and are usually also well seen by sagittal or coronal reformatted CT.

Traumatic Spondylolisthesis of the Axis (Hangman's Fracture)

Traumatic spondylolisthesis of the axis most commonly involves bilateral fractures through the pars interarticularis (isthmus) of the axis. The most common mechanism of injury is hyperextension and axial compression of the cervical spine. This commonly occurs in deceleration injuries, like when the forehead strikes the car windshield. This causes axial loading of the neural arch, with concentration of shearing stresses on the pars interarticularis as previously described. It is not logical to call this a hangman's fracture because this differs from the usual judicial hanging with a submental knot, which produces hyperextension and distraction and rarely ever causes a pars interarticularis fracture (32). If there is minimal displacement of the pars interarticularis fracture and no disruption of the C2-3 intervertebral disk, the traumatic spondylolisthesis is classified as a type I fracture that is stable (46,47) (Fig. 3.27A,B). If there is also disruption of the intevertebral disk, it is classified as a type II fracture. Disruption of the intervertebral disk associated by a forward dislocation of the body of C2 on C3, possibly with bilateral interfacetal dislocation, is classified as a type III fracture (Fig. 3.27C). The type II and III fractures are thought to be complicated by a rebound hyperflexion following the hyperextension and are unstable. Many cases of traumatic spondylolisthesis show little neurologic deficit because the spinal cord occupies only about one third of the anteroposterior diameter of the spinal canal at axis

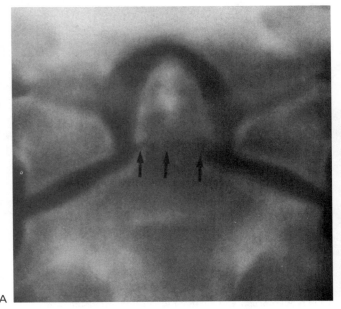

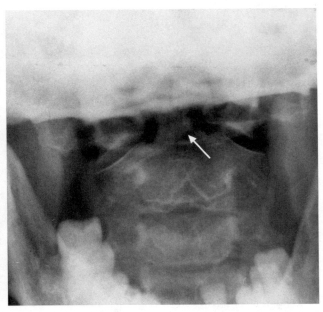

A　　　　　　　　　　　　　　　　　　　　　　　B

FIGURE 3.26. Odontoid fractures. **A**; Pleuridirectional tomogram of a high dens fracture (type II). The fracture line (*arrows*) involves only the dens. **B**, Open-mouth anteroposterior atlantoaxial view reveals a low (type III) fracture (*arrow*). (**A**, from Harris JH Jr, Mirvis SE. *The radiology of acute cervical spine trauma*, 3rd ed. Baltimore: Williams & Wilkins, 1996, with permission.)

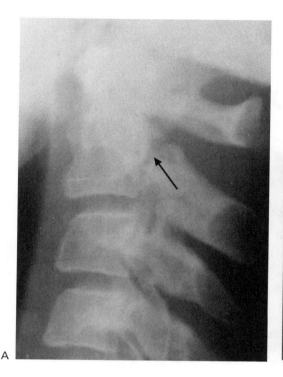

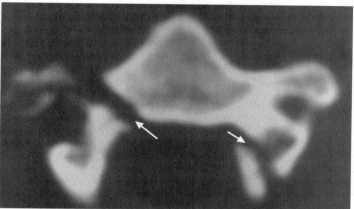

FIGURE 3.27. Traumatic spondylolisthesis of the axis. **A**; Lateral view of type I fracture with minimal displacement of the pars interarticularis fracture (*arrow*). **B**; Computed tomography scan of the bilateral pars fractures seen in **A** (*arrows*).

level and also because the pars interarticularis fracture tends to produce an autodecompression of the canal.

ANATOMY, MECHANICS, AND IMAGING FEATURES OF MIDDLE AND LOWER CERVICAL SPINE INJURIES

Anatomy and Mechanics of the Middle and Lower Cervical Spine

The lower five cervical vertebrae share many similar anatomic and mechanical features. One of their unique features are the prominent uncinate processes that protrude upward from the lateral border of the superior aspect of their vertebral bodies (Fig. 3.28A). They articulate with convexities on the lateral border of the lower aspect of the next higher vertebrae to form the uncovertebral or Luschka joints. However, it appears that Luschka joints are really degenerative clefts within the lateral aspect of the intervertebral disk rather than true joints because they do not appear until adolescence (48,49). Cervical disk degeneration probably occurs at this point because this is where cervical disks are thinnest in their superoinferior dimension and hence are subject to greatest strain (7). From a physics perspective, strain is the change in length of an object (deformation) under load divided by its original length. Hence, for the same displacement of the cervical spine in any direction (e.g., flexion, extension, lateral bending, or rotation), the part of the disk that is narrowest is subject to the greatest strain and is most likely to fail. Because Luschka joints are in the anterior wall of the intervertebral foramen, hypertrophic degenerative changes can cause foraminal stenosis (Fig. 3.28A).

The pedicles of the lower five cervical vertebrae are unique. First, they arise near the middle of the vertebral body. Hence, they are equally grooved on their upper and lower borders (Fig. 3.28B). This creates a symmetric intervertebral foramen with the intervertebral disk in the middle of its anterior wall. Second, the pedicles are directed posterolaterally, which causes the intervertebral foramina to face anterolaterally (Fig. 3.28B,C). Therefore, the best radiographic views of the foramina are the right and left anterior oblique views. The intervertebral foramina have Luschka joints in their anterior wall and facet joints in their posterior wall. Therefore, foraminal stenosis can be produced by hypertrophic degenerative changes in either joint.

The facet joints of the lower five cervical vertebrae are obliquely oriented on an angle of about 45 degrees to both the coronal and transverse planes. Because they are the most horizontally situated of any regional facet joints (Fig. 3.28B), they can be unilaterally or bilaterally dislocated without fracture. Their relatively horizontal orientation and the short stout cylindrical articular pillars that connect the inferior and superior articular surface of each vertebra imply that cervical facet joints probably bear more loads than those of other levels (Fig. 3.28B).

Cervical transverse processes also have many unique features. They are directed anterolaterally like the intervertebral foramina (Fig. 3.28B,C). They are composed of an anterior costal element that attaches to the vertebral body like a rib and a posterior transverse element that attaches to the pedicle–lamina junction like most transverse processes. It is the costal element that enlarges to form a cervical rib. Transverse foramina for the vertebral vessels are located between the costal and transverse elements. Hence, cervical fractures and dislocations can compromise vertebral artery blood supply to the cervical cord and brain

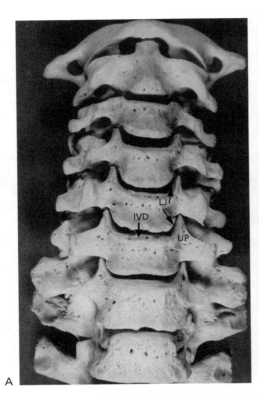
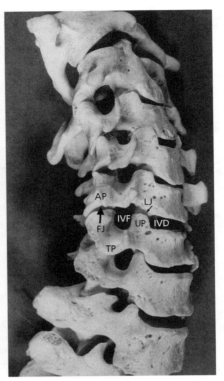

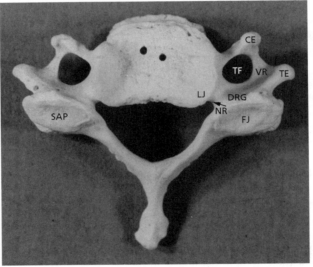

FIGURE 3.28. Lower cervical spine. **A**; Anterior view of the cervical spine. The uncinate processes (*UP*) protrude upward from the lateral margins of the superior surfaces of the lower five cervical vertebrae, and the Luschka joints (*LJ*) are positioned in the lateral portion of the intervertebral disk interval (*IVD*). **B**; Anterolateral view of the cervical spine displaying the anterolaterally facing direction of the intervertebral foramina (*IVF*) and the grooved transverse processes (*TP*). The uncinate processes (*UP*), Luschka joints (*LJ*), and intervertebral disks (*IVD*) are all in the anterior wall of the intervertebral foramina, whereas the facet joints (*FJ*) and their intervening articular pillars (*AP*) are in the posterior wall. **C**; Superior view of C5 demonstrating the costal (*CE*) and transverse (*TE*) elements of the deeply grooved transverse processes, the transverse foramina (*TF*), and the posterosuperior-facing direction of the superior articular processes (*SAP*). The positions of the nerve roots (*NR*) in the intervertebral foramen and of the dorsal root ganglion (*DRG*) and ventral rami (*VR*) within the grooved transverse process are indicated. Note the intimate relationship of the facet joints (*FJ*), Luschka joints (*LJ*), and intervertebral disks to these neural structures and to the vertebral arteries in the transverse foramina. (From Schneck CD. Functional and clinical anatomy of the spine. In: *Physical medicine and rehabilitation: state of the art reviews*, Vol. 9. Philadelphia: Hanley & Belfus, 1995:539, with permission.)

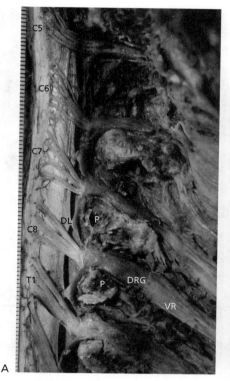

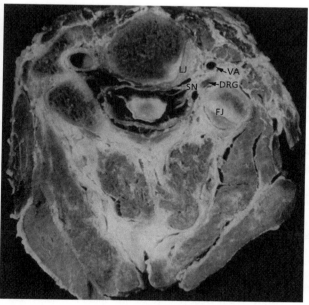

FIGURE 3.29. Neural relationships of the lower cervical spine. **A**; Posterior view of a dissection of the cervical spine where neural arches have been removed by sectioning the pedicles (*P*). Spinal cord segments C5 to T1 each give off multiple dorsal rootlets that converge as they penetrate the dural sac to enter the intervertebral foramina, which are delimited by the pedicles. The dorsal root ganglia (*DRG*), which are situated on the gross spinal nerve, extend extraforaminally into the trough of the transverse process, as do the ventral rami (*VR*). The dentations of the denticulate ligament (*DL*) attach to the dura between the rootlets of each emerging spinal nerve. **B**; Cross-section through C5 displaying the anterolateral course of the nerve roots and the intimate relationship of the spinal nerve (*SN*), dorsal root ganglion (*DRG*), and vertebral artery (*VA*) to both the Luschka joint (*LJ*) and the facet joint (*FJ*). (From Schneck CD. Functional and clinical anatomy of the spine. In: *Physical medicine and rehabilitation: state of the art reviews*, Vol. 9. Philadelphia: Hanley & Belfus, 1995:541, with permission.)

stem. Further, the vertebral vessels are within a few millimeters of the Luschka and facet joints and hence can be compromised by hypertrophic degenerative changes of these joints (Fig. 3.28C). The transverse processes are trough shaped, and the narrow interval between the vertebral vessels and the facet joints must accommodate the nerve roots, dorsal root ganglion, and ventral rami of the spinal nerve (Figs. 3.28C and 3.29A). All of these can be encroached by hypertrophic degenerative changes involving the Luschka or facet joints (Figs. 3.29B and 3.30A,B).

All of the joints between the lower five cervical vertebrae permit flexion-extension, lateral bending, and rotation. However, flexion-extension is freest at the C5-6 and C6-7 joints (5). This has been incriminated as a potential cause of the high incidence of degenerative changes and flexion-extension trauma at these levels. Lateral bending and rotation tends to be freest at the C3-4 and C4-5 levels.

The spinal cord is separated from the potentially injurious walls of the spinal canal by the meninges, subarachnoid space, and epidural fat (Fig. 3.29A). Both the cerebrospinal fluid and the epidural fat and its veins can help protect the cord from injury by providing a hydraulic cushion that can diminish cord

accelerations or decelerations relative to the walls of the spinal canal (1). The spinal cord is also somewhat stabilized by the denticulate ligaments, which are flangelike duplications of the pia on either side of the cord that attach to the dura between each emerging spinal nerve (Fig. 3.29A).

Because at lower cervical levels, the cord segments are one vertebral level above the vertebra of the same number, the nerve roots both descend and course anterolaterally to reach their intervertebral foramen (Fig. 3.29A). The spinal nerve and dorsal root ganglion occupy much of the foramen and are related anteriorly to the intervertebral disk, Luschka joint, and vertebral artery and posteriorly to the facet joint.

All of these bony and neural features of the cervical spine and its neural contents can be well visualized by bone or soft tissue window CT, metrizamide CT myelograms, and MRI (Fig. 3.31A–D).

Degenerative Cervical Spine Disease

Degenerative cervical spine disease can produce a chronic myelopathy or radiculopathy by encroaching on the spinal canal

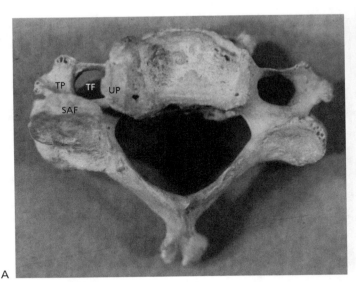

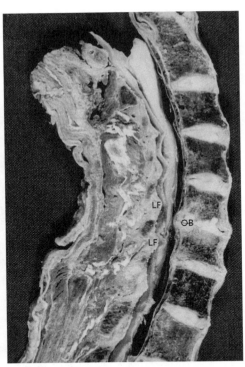

A

B

FIGURE 3.30. Degenerative cervical spine disease. **A**; Superior view of C6 demonstrating significant hypertrophic degenerative spurring of both the uncinate process (*UP*) of the Luschka joint and the superior articular facet (*SAF*) of the facet joint, which respectively encroached on the anteromedial and posterolateral aspects of the intervertebral foramen, the transverse foramen (*TF*) for the vertebral artery, and the sulcus of the transverse process (*TP*). **B**; Mid-sagittal section of a cervical spine with a substantial degeneration of the C5-6 intervertebral disk that has produced an osteophytic bar (*OB*) that intrudes into the anterior part of the spinal canal. The loss of disk height has caused a forward buckling of the ligamenta flava (*LF*) into the posterior part of the spinal canal. (From Schneck CD. Functional and clinical anatomy of the spine. In: *Physical medicine and rehabilitation: state of the art reviews*, Vol. 9. Philadelphia: Hanley & Belfus, 1995:542, with permission.)

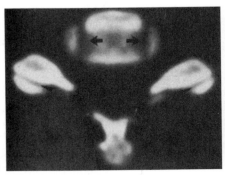

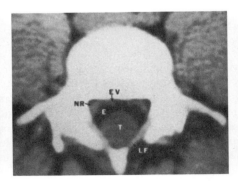

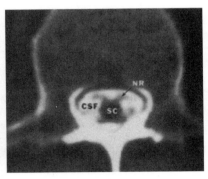

A,B

C

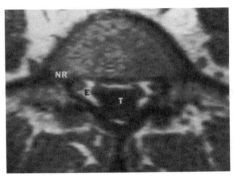

D

FIGURE 3.31. Computed tomography scan and magnetic resonance image of the normal cervical spine and spinal cord. **A**; Bone window computed tomography scan of the cervical spine displays normal facet joints (*arrowheads*) and Luschka joints (*arrows*). **B**; Soft tissue window computed tomography of L5 demonstrating thecal sac (*T*), nerve roots (*NR*) within the lateral recess, epidural fat (*E*), epidural veins (*EV*), and ligamentum flavum (*LF*). **C**; Metrizamide computed tomography myelogram at L1 level delimiting the spinal cord (*SC*), nerve roots (*NR*) arising from the cord, and contrast-enhanced cerebrospinal fluid. **D**; T1-weighted axial magnetic resonance image of L5 shows the thecal sac (*T*) as an area of low signal intensity, the nerve roots (*NR*) within their lateral recesses as areas of moderate signal intensity, and the epidural fat (*E*) as hyperintense. (From DeLisa JA, Gans MB. *Rehabilitation medicine: principles and practice*, 3rd ed. Philadelphia: Lippincott-Raven, 1998: 458, with permission.)

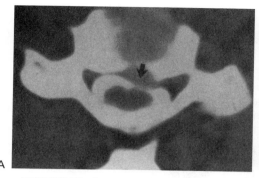
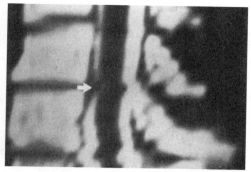

FIGURE 3.32. Computed tomography (CT) evaluation of a herniated C5 to C6 nucleus pulposus. **A;** An axial CT myelogram shows a radiodense protrusion of the C5 and C6 disks (*arrow*) that distorts the left anterior aspect of both the thecal sac and the spinal cord. **B;** Sagittal reconstruction shows the herniated C5 to C6 nucleus pulposus (*arrow*) indenting both the radiodense thecal sac and the radiolucent spinal cord. (From DeLisa JA, Gans MB. *Rehabilitation medicine: principles and practice,* 3rd ed. Philadelphia: Lippincott-Raven, 1998:458, with permission.)

or intervertebral foramen. By producing preexisting spinal or foraminal stenosis, it can also predispose the spine-injured patient to neural injury. The normal cervical lordosis is produced by wedge-shaped intervertebral disks that are narrower posteriorly than anteriorly (Fig. 3.30B). As previously described, the narrowness of the posterior anulus subjects it to increased strain, particularly with flexion movements. Soft intervertebral disk herniation is much less common at cervical than at lumbar levels.

This is probably because the wider and thicker posterior longitudinal ligaments of the cervical spine provide more support for the posterior disk and also because the uncinate processes help shield against posterolateral or lateral disk herniation. When present, soft tissue disk herniations are well visualized by CT or MRI (Figs. 3.32A,B and 3.33A–C). Disk degeneration at cervical levels more commonly produces osteophytes or hypertrophic bars, which can encroach on the spinal canal or intervertebral

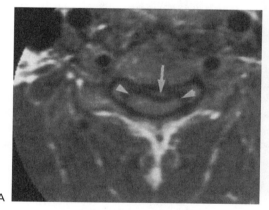
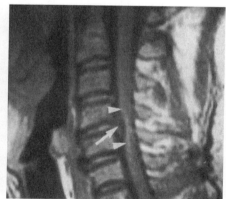

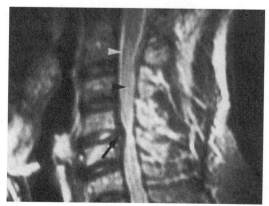

FIGURE 3.33. A; T1-weighted axial magnetic resonance image (MRI) shows a herniated C4 to C5 nucleus pulposus (*arrow*) indenting the thecal sac (*between arrowheads*). **B;** T1-weighted mid-sagittal MRI shows the herniated C4 to C5 disks (*arrow*) impinging on the moderately low signal intensity thecal sac (*arrowheads*). **C;** T2-weighted mid-sagittal MRI demonstrates that the herniated C4 to C5 disks (*arrow*) are compressing not only the high signal intensity dural sac (*white arrowhead*) but also the moderate signal intensity spinal cord (*black arrowhead*). (From DeLisa JA, Gans MB. *Rehabilitation medicine: principles and practice,* 3rd ed. Philadelphia: Lippincott-Raven, 1998:458, with permission.)

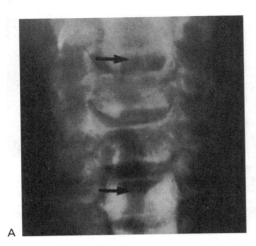

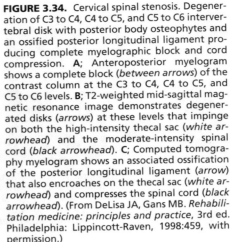

FIGURE 3.34. Cervical spinal stenosis. Degeneration of C3 to C4, C4 to C5, and C5 to C6 intervertebral disk with posterior body osteophytes and an ossified posterior longitudinal ligament producing complete myelographic block and cord compression. **A;** Anteroposterior myelogram shows a complete block (*between arrows*) of the contrast column at the C3 to C4, C4 to C5, and C5 to C6 levels. **B;** T2-weighted mid-sagittal magnetic resonance image demonstrates degenerated disks (*arrows*) at these levels that impinge on both the high-intensity thecal sac (*white arrowhead*) and the moderate-intensity spinal cord (*black arrowhead*). **C;** Computed tomography myelogram shows an associated ossification of the posterior longitudinal ligament (*arrow*) that also encroaches on the thecal sac (*white arrowhead*) and compresses the spinal cord (*black arrowhead*). (From DeLisa JA, Gans MB. *Rehabilitation medicine: principles and practice*, 3rd ed. Philadelphia: Lippincott-Raven, 1998:459, with permission.)

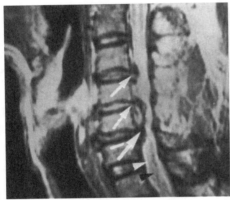

B

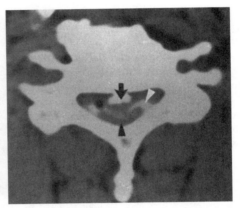

C

foramen (Fig. 3.30A,B). As the disks degenerate and lose height, approximation of the lamina can cause buckling of the ligamenta flava into the posterior spinal canal opposite the hypertrophic bars on the back of the disk (Fig. 3.30B). The resultant spinal and foraminal stenosis is well demonstrated by MRI or CT (Figs. 3.34A–C). All of these degenerative changes clearly predispose a spine-injured patient to spinal cord or nerve injury.

Classification of Middle and Lower Cervical Spine Injuries

Middle and lower cervical spine injuries can be classified mechanically into hyperflexion, hyperflexion with rotation, hyperextension, lateral bending, and vertical compression fractures (32). Hyperflexion injuries include hyperflexion sprain (anterior subluxation), simple wedge compression fracture, bilateral facet dislocation, flexion teardrop fracture, and clay shoveler's fracture. Hyperflexion with rotation injuries produce unilateral facet dislocation with or without fracture. Hyperextension injuries include hyperextension dislocation, extension teardrop fracture, and laminar fractures. Hyperextension with rotation produces pillar fractures or pedicolaminar fractures. Lateral flexion fractures can cause uncinate or transverse process fractures. Vertical compression produces burst fractures. Various combinations of

these mechanisms can also occur. Hyperextension with rotation and lateral bending injuries are discussed further because they are uncommon and rarely produce neurologic injury.

Hyperflexion Injuries

Hyperflexion injuries tend to apply compressive forces on the anterior column of the spine and distractive forces on the posterior spine. Hyperflexion sprain (anterior subluxation) involves varying degrees of disruption of the posterior ligaments of the spine, including the supraspinous, interspinous, ligamenta flava, facet joint capsules, posterior longitudinal, and posterior anulus fibrosus. Commonly, the anterior anulus and anterior longitudinal ligament are spared. Typically, this injury is initially stable, with no neurologic injury. However, there is a 30% to 50% incidence of delayed instability (32). The radiographic signs of hyperflexion sprain include a localized kyphotic angulation, widened interspinous and interlaminar spaces, forward displacement of the subluxed inferior articular facet on the lower superior facet, widening of the space between the subluxed vertebral body and the subjacent superior facet, posterior widening and anterior narrowing of the intervertebral disk space, and possible anterior displacement of the subluxed vertebral body (50) (Figs. 3.11 and

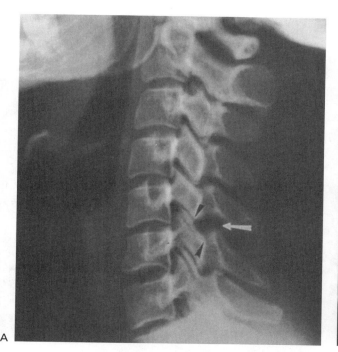
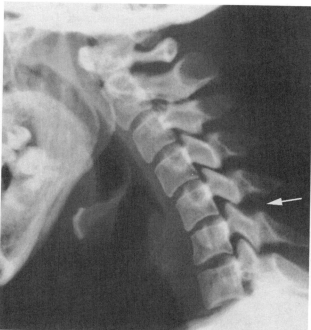

A

B

FIGURE 3.35. Subtle hyperflexion sprain. **A;** This supine lateral cervical radiograph of a young woman obtained after a vehicular accident demonstrates slight widening of the interspinous space between C5 and C6 (*white arrow*). There is diminished facet coverage at this level (*black arrowheads*) and slight narrowing of the intervertebral disk space as well. **B;** Lateral radiograph obtained in flexion confirms this injury (*white arrow*). (From Mirvis SE, Young JWR. *Imaging in trauma and critical care*, Baltimore: Williams & Wilkins, 1992:303, with permission.)

3.35A,B). These findings are usually exaggerated in supervised flexion films.

In a simple wedge compression fracture, there is decreased vertical height of the anterior aspect of the vertebral body, and there may be increased radiodensity along the superior endplate by trabecular buckling (Fig. 3.36). This is initially stable, but if there is accompanying posterior ligamentous injury that fails to heal, instability may occur.

Bilateral facet dislocations are unstable injuries caused by disruption of all posterior and anterior ligaments. They involve upward and forward dislocation of both inferior facets of the higher vertebra on the superior facets of the lower vertebra. In a complete facet dislocation, the higher inferior facet rests anterior to the lower superior facet and encroaches on the intervertebral foramen. This is often called *bilateral locked facets*, but the term "locked" implies stability, and this injury is not at all stable (Fig. 3.37). In an incomplete dislocation, the higher inferior facets come to rest on the superior margins of the lower superior facets and are often called "perched" facets (Fig. 3.38). In a complete dislocation, the dislocated vertebra is typically displaced forward more than half the anteroposterior diameter of the vertebral body; in an incomplete dislocation, the displacement is usually less than half that diameter. Neurologic injuries are common and can involve the spinal cord, the nerve in the involved intervertebral foramen, or the vertebral artery. This injury can be differentiated from unilateral facet dislocation because in this symmetric injury, the articular pillars of the two

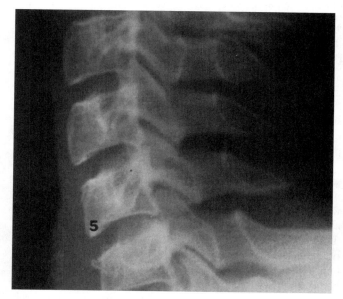

FIGURE 3.36. Simple wedge (compression) fracture of the bodies of C5 and C6 characterized by decreased anterior vertical height and disruption (C5) and buckling (C6) of the anterior cortex of the centrum. (From Harris JH Jr, Mirvis SE. *The radiology of acute cervical spine trauma*, 3rd ed. Baltimore: Williams & Wilkins, 1996:220, with permission.)

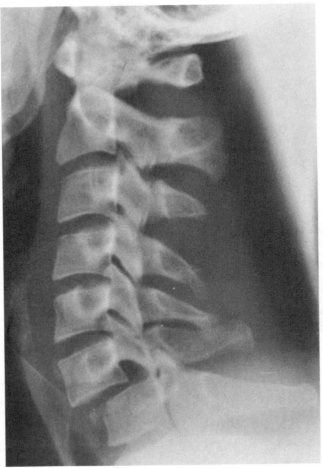

FIGURE 3.37. Bilateral locked facets. This lateral radiograph reveals a bilateral facet lock of C6 with respect to C7, with anterior dislocation of about 40% of the anteroposterior vertebral body length. Note the corner compression fracture of C7. (From Mirvis SE, Young JWR. *Imaging in trauma and critical care*, Baltimore: Williams & Wilkins, 1992:308, with permission.)

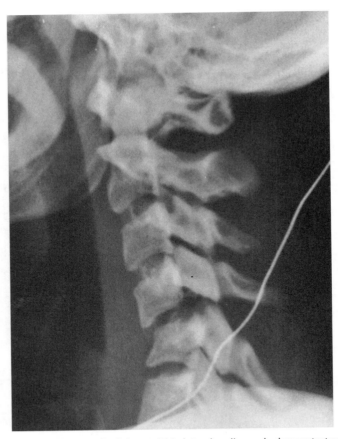

FIGURE 3.38. Perched facets. This lateral radiograph demonstrates perching of the facet tips between C4 and C5. Note the marked degree of spinous process fanning and focal kyphosis. There is mild swelling of the precervical soft tissue. (From Mirvis SE, Young JWR. *Imaging in trauma and critical care*, Baltimore: Williams & Wilkins, 1992:308, with permission.)

sides continue to superimpose on each other above the level of injury. This injury can be associated with vertebral body or posterior element fractures that may involve the vertebral artery.

Flexion teardrop fracture is generally considered the most serious cervical spine injury compatible with life because it almost invariably produces the anterior cervical cord syndrome with quadriplegia, loss of pain and temperature, and sparing of only the posterior white-column functions of proprioception, discriminative touch, and vibration. It is characterized by a large triangular fragment from the anteroinferior aspect of the vertebral body and retropulsion of the larger posterior part of the body into the vertebral canal (Fig. 3.39A,B). The triangular fragment has been analogized to a teardrop running down the cheek of the patient or the patient's family members (32). The facet joints are typically bilaterally dislocated or subluxed, and the posterior ligaments are disrupted. Hence, there is both bony and ligamentous instability.

Clay shoveler's fracture is an avulsion fracture of the spinous process of C7, C6, or T1, in that order, not typically associated with neurologic injury.

Hyperflexion and Rotation Injuries

Hyperflexion and rotation injuries are produced by combined flexion and rotation forces. They produce unilateral facet dislocation with or without associated fractures. The dislocated facet is on the side opposite that toward which the face was rotated. The dislocated inferior facet moves upward and forward on the lower superior facet around a vertical axis through the opposite intact facet. It comes to lie in the intervertebral foramen anterior to its subjacent superior facet. Above the level of injury, there is a loss of superimposition of the articular pillars of the two sides on lateral radiographs (Fig. 3.40). The dislocated pillar is superimposed on the vertebral body, and the offset pillars produce a bowtie or butterfly appearance. In anteroposterior radiographs, the spinous process above the dislocation is displaced toward the side of the displaced facet. These injuries are usually mechanically stable unless there is an associated major fracture of either of the articular processes involved in the dislocation.

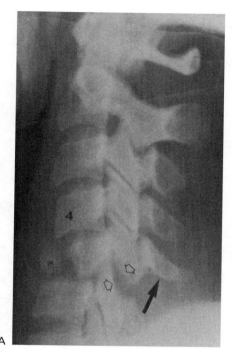

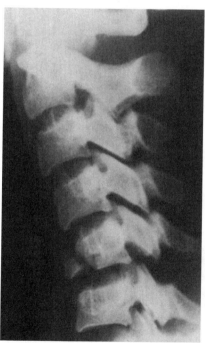

FIGURE 3.39. Flexion teardrop fracture of C5. The initial supine lateral radiograph demonstrates a severe kyphotic deformity at the C5 to C6 level. **A;** Compression of the anterior column of the spine has produced the characteristic large triangular fragment that constitutes the anteroinferior aspect of most of the body of C5 (*asterisk*). Concomitant and reciprocal distraction of the posterior column is evidenced by disruption of the interfacetal joints (*open arrows*) and the interlaminar and interspinous spaces ("fanning") (*long arrow*). Marked diffuse prevertebral soft tissue swelling in the lower cervical spine indicates hemorrhage and edema. **B;** A subsequent lateral radiograph demonstrates the characteristics of the teardrop fragment more clearly, as well as the flexion attitude of the upper cervical segment and total ligamentous disruption at the level of injury. (From Harris JH Jr, Mirvis SE. *The radiology of acute cervical spine trauma*, 3rd ed. Baltimore: Williams & Wilkins, 1996: 287, with permission.)

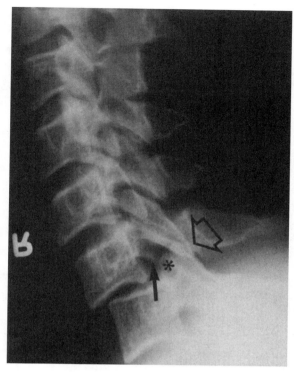

FIGURE 3.40. Unilateral facet dislocation with a fracture of the dislocated superior facet. Lateral radiograph shows that the amputated dislocated inferior articular process (*small arrow*) lies anterior to its next lower superior articular process. The contralateral inferior articular process (*open arrow*) has glided upward with respect to its next lower superior articular process but retains its normal position posterior to it. (From Mirvis SE. *The radiology of acute cervical spine trauma*, 3rd ed. Baltimore: Williams & Wilkins, 1996:263, with permission.)

Hyperextension Injuries

Hyperextension injuries are typically produced by an anteroposteriorly directed force to the face or mandible that distracts the spine anteriorly and compresses the posterior elements. The injuring force typically disrupts the anterior longitudinal ligament, intervertebral disk, and posterior longitudinal ligament and at least transiently displaces the vertebral body into the spinal canal. The approximation of the posterior elements causes buckling of the ligamenta flava into the posterior spinal canal. Hence, the spinal cord can be pinched between the vertebral body and the ligamenta flava, and the patient may present with neurologic findings that vary from transient to a central cord syndrome. However, after the injuring force is dissipated, the spine often returns to a near-normal alignment either as a result of rebound flexion or because of spine stabilization by emergency personnel. Hence, the lateral radiograph findings may belie the severity of the neurologic injury. Typically, there is anterior widening of the intervertebral disk space and marked prevertebral soft tissue swelling (Fig. 3.41). There may be an associated small avulsion fracture of the anteroinferior aspect of the higher vertebra, a vacuum effect causing increased radiolucency within the disk, or associated crush fractures of the articular pillars or laminae. Many of these injuries are stable unless there are fractures of the posterior elements. They are particularly devastating neurologi-

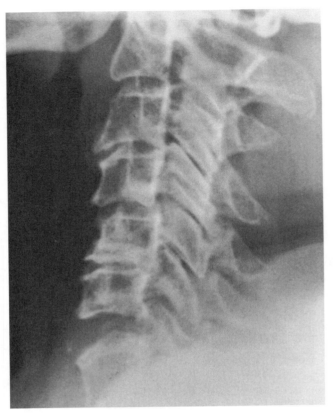

FIGURE 3.41. Hyperextension injury. This lateral radiograph shows marked widening of the C6-7 interspace and marked precervical soft tissue swelling consistent with hyperextension sprain. (From Mirvis SE, Young JWR. *Imaging in trauma and critical care*, Baltimore: Williams & Wilkins, 1992:323, with permission.)

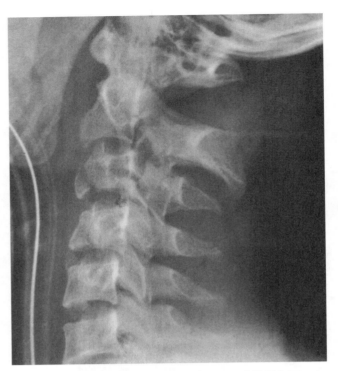

FIGURE 3.42. Hyperextension teardrop fracture of C3. This lateral radiograph demonstrates a triangular fracture off the anteroinferior corner of C3 consistent with a hyperextension teardrop fracture. (From Mirvis SE, Young JWR. *Imaging in trauma and critical care*. Baltimore: Williams & Wilkins, 1992:331, with permission.)

cally when there are preexisting degenerative changes of the cervical spine that chronically narrow the spinal canal, as previously described.

In hyperextension teardrop injuries, the anterior longitudinal ligament avulses a fragment from the anteroinferior border of the higher vertebral body (Fig. 3.42). It differs from flexion teardrop fractures by a lack of retropulsion of the larger vertebral body fragment into the spinal canal. These fractures are usually stable, with infrequent neurologic findings, unless there are associated posterior element fractures.

Hyperextension injuries can also cause laminar fractures, which are usually stable and produce no neurologic deficit unless the laminar fragments intrude into the spinal canal. They are best visualized by CT (Fig. 3.43).

Vertebral Compression (Burst Fracture) Injuries

Vertical loading of the vertebral column causes increased pressure in the nucleus pulposus that implodes the vertebral endplate. This increased intrabody pressure causes the vertebral body to explode, with comminuted fragments displaced in all direc-

tions. Retropulsion of fragments into the spinal canal can produce neurologic deficits ranging from transient findings to a complete cord syndrome. On lateral radiographs, both vertebral endplates are disrupted, and the retropulsed fragment can usually be visualized (Fig. 3.44A). Anteroposterior radiographs commonly show a vertical fracture of the vertebral body (Fig. 3.44B).

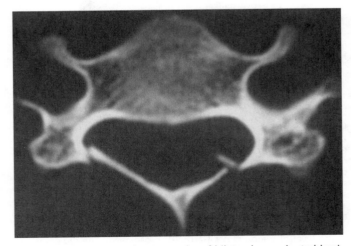

FIGURE 3.43. Computed tomography of bilateral comminuted laminar fractures caused by hyperextension injury.

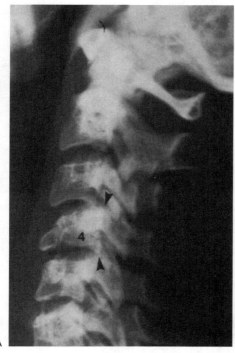

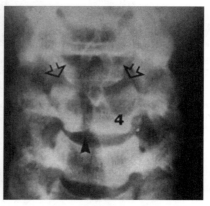

FIGURE 3.44. A; Lateral radiograph of a bursting fracture of C4 with severe comminution of the centrum and retropulsion of its posterior fragments (*arrowheads*) into the spinal canal. Note the essentially normal attitude of the cervical spine and the absence of signs of posterior column distraction that distinguished this injury from the flexion teardrop fracture. **B;** The projection demonstrates the characteristic vertical fracture of the vertebral body (*arrowhead*). Dispersion of the fragments is evidenced by lateral displacement of the major fragments and widening of the C3 to C4 Luschka joints (*open arrows*). (From Harris JH Jr, Mirvis SE. *The radiology of acute cervical spine trauma*, 3rd ed. Baltimore: Williams & Wilkins, 1996:353, 359, with permission.)

CT images typically reveal posterior element fractures, and MRI may reveal cord injury.

ANATOMY, MECHANICS, AND IMAGING FEATURES OF THORACOLUMBAR SPINE INJURIES

Anatomy and Mechanics of the Thoracic Spine

The normal kyphosis is produced by the slightly wedge-shaped vertebral bodies, which are 1.5 to 2 mm less in the superoinferior height of their anterior margins than their posterior margins. Although the coronal orientation of most thoracic facet joints (Fig. 3.1) would seem to permit very good flexion-extension, rotation, and lateral bending motions, a number of unique anatomic features limit these motions. First, the posterior attachments of the ribs to the vertebral bodies and transverse processes and the direct or indirect anterior attachments of most ribs to the sternum tend to limit all thoracic spine motions (1). Second, overlapping laminae and spinous processes limit extension. Third, the thin thoracic intervertebral disks also restrict deformation and limit all spine motions. Fourth, the general coronal facet joint orientation means that flexion and extension must occur by upward and downward motions that would be resisted by the longitudinally running ligaments of the spine.

The pedicles of thoracic vertebrae arise near the upper margin of the vertebral bodies. This creates an asymmetric intervertebral foramen with the intervertebral disk in the lower part of the anterior wall.

Anatomy and Mechanics of the Lumbar Spine

The shape of the spinal canal changes substantially from L1 to L5. At the L1 to L2 levels, it is oval, but by the L4 to S1 levels, it has developed prominent lateral recesses (1) (Fig. 3.45). These are created by a progressive shortening of the pedicles, which brings the superior articular process into the posterolateral part of the spinal canal. The lateral recesses are bounded laterally by the pedicle, anteriorly by the back of the vertebral body, and posteriorly at their upper end by the superior articular process and facet joint capsule. At lower levels, the lateral recesses are bounded posteriorly by the pars interarticularis of the lamina, which is the portion of the lamina between the superior and inferior articular processes. The anteroposterior dimension of the lateral recess is normally narrower at its upper end.

The lateral recesses are occupied by the nerve roots (surrounded by their dural sleeve) that will emerge from the next

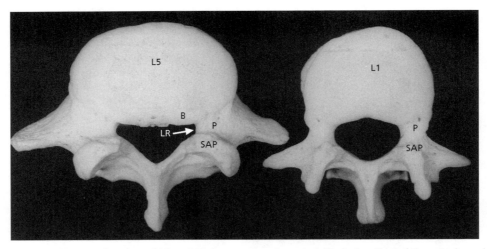

FIGURE 3.45. Superior view of L1 and L5 demonstrates how the elliptical outline of the spinal canal at L1 is converted into a trefoil outline with lateral recesses (*LR*) at L5 level by a shortening of the pedicles (*P*), which causes the superior articular processes (*SAP*) to encroach into the posterior aspect of the spinal canal. The superior part of each lateral recess is bounded posteriorly by the superior articular processes, laterally by the pedicle, and posteriorly by the body (*B*) of the vertebra. (From Schneck CD. Functional and clinical anatomy of the spine. In: *Physical medicine and rehabilitation: state of the art reviews*, Vol. 9. Philadelphia: Hanley & Belfus, 1995:544, with permission.)

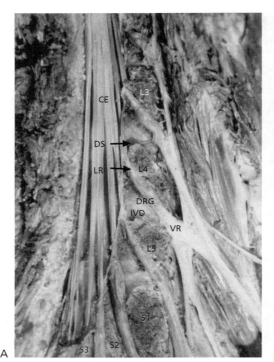

A

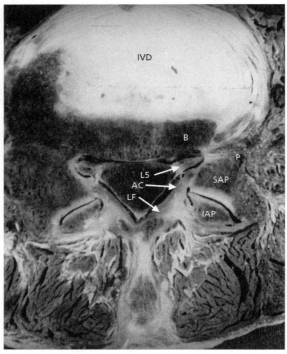

B

FIGURE 3.46. **A;** The neural relationships of the lumbar spine as seen in a posterior view of the lumbosacral spine with the right half of the neural arches removed by sectioning the right pedicles of L3 to S3. The posterior part of the dural sac (*DS*) has been removed to visualize the intradural course of the rootlets of the cauda equina (*CE*). Also displayed is the extradural course of the nerve roots as they descend the lateral recesses (*LR*) covered by a dural sleeve and then exit the intervertebral foramina between the pedicles to become continuous with the ventral rami (*VR*) of the lumbosacral plexus. The swellings on the nerves within the intervertebral foramina are the dorsal root ganglia (*DRG*). The nerves descend the lateral recesses in close apposition to the medial border of the pedicles. They then exit the upper part of the intervertebral foramen, whereas the intervertebral disks (*IVD*) occupy a lower portion of the foramen. **B;** Transverse section of the lower part of the L4 to L5 intervertebral disk (*IVD*) demonstrating the L5 nerve roots descending the upper part of their lateral recesses. Note the superior articular process of L5 (*SAP*) and anterior capsule of the L4 to L5 facet joint (*AC*) in the posterior wall of the lateral recess, the L5 pedicle (*P*) in the lateral wall of the recess, and the posterior body of L5 (*B*) in the anterior wall. Also note the more posteromedial position of the inferior articular process (*IAP*) of L4 and the continuity of the ligamenta flava (*LF*) with the anterior capsule of the facet joint. (From Schneck CD. Functional and clinical anatomy of the spine. In: *Physical medicine and rehabilitation: state of the art reviews*, Vol. 9. Philadelphia: Hanley & Belfus, 1995:544, with permission.)

and radial dimensions posteriorly, there are no posterolateral external reinforcing ligaments, and the predominant motion of flexion places increased tensile stress on the posterior anulus (Fig. 3.3C). When the disk herniates posterolaterally, it commonly spares the spinal nerve that exits through that foramen at a higher level and involves instead the next lower exiting nerve, either while it is still inside the dural sac or as it is about to enter its lateral recess (Fig. 3.48A,B).

Because the superior articular facet occupies the posterior wall of both the upper lateral recess and the intervertebral foramen, hypertrophic degenerative facet disease can cause both lateral and foraminal stenosis (Fig. 3.49). Lateral stenosis is typically defined as a narrowing of the anteroposterior dimension of the lateral recess to less than 3 mm. Because the predominant sagittal orientation of most lumbar facet joints places the inferior articular process relatively medial to the superior process, hypertrophic degenerative changes of the inferior process can encroach on a more central portion of the spinal canal to produce a central stenosis.

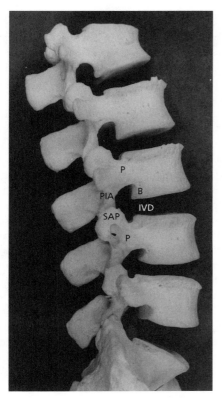

FIGURE 3.47. A lateral view of the lumbar spine demonstrates the relationships of lumbar intervertebral foramina. The pedicles (*P*) form the superior and inferior boundaries of each foramen. The upper anterior wall is formed by the posterior surface of the next higher vertebral body (*B*), whereas the lower anterior wall is formed by the interval for the intervertebral disk (*IVD*). Posteriorly, the upper foramen is bounded by the pars interarticularis (*PIA*) of the lamina, and the lower foramen is bounded by the superior articular process (*SAP*) of the facet joint. Note the lightbulb shape of the intervertebral foramen, the upper part of which has a wider anteroposterior dimension than the lower part. (From Schneck CD. Functional and clinical anatomy of the spine. In: *Physical medicine and rehabilitation: state of the art reviews*, Vol. 9. Philadelphia: Hanley & Belfus, 1995:544, with permission.)

lower intervertebral foramen (Fig. 3.46A,B). Because of their descending course, the nerve roots form the spinal nerve within the spacious upper part of their intervertebral foramen. Because the pedicles of lumbar vertebrae arise from the upper portion of their vertebral body, lumbar intervertebral foramina are asymmetric, with the intervertebral disk located in the lower part of the anterior wall of the foramen (Fig. 3.47). The intervertebral foramina have a more spacious anteroposterior diameter in their upper part than in their lower part.

Degenerative Thoracolumbar Spine Disease

Chronic degenerative thoracolumbar spine diseases, including herniated disks, central spinal stenosis, lateral stenosis, and foraminal stenosis, can produce chronic neurologic findings. They can also predispose the neural elements to injury in acute spinal trauma.

Thoracolumbar disk herniations most commonly occur posterolaterally because the anulus is thinnest in its anteroposterior

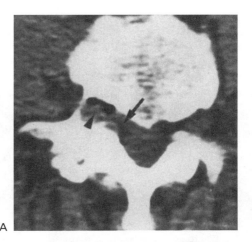

A

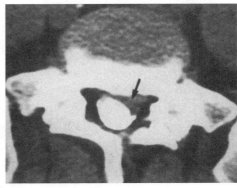

B

FIGURE 3.48. Computed tomography (CT) evaluation of herniated lumbar disks. **A**; A noncontrast CT image at the L4 to L5 level shows a dense mass (*arrow*) containing gas that displaces the right epidural fat and effaces the right L4 nerve roots within their neural foramen (*arrowhead*). Note the normal epidural fat on the left and the normal fat outlining the left L4 nerve roots. **B**; CT myelogram showing a left posterolateral herniation of the L5 to S1 disks (*arrow*) encroaching on the left anterior aspect of the contrast-enhanced thecal sac. (From DeLisa JA, Gans MB. *Rehabilitation medicine: principles and practice*, 3rd ed. Philadelphia: Lippincott-Raven, 1998:462, with permission.)

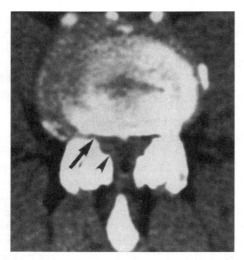

FIGURE 3.49. Computed tomography at the L4 to L5 level shows hypertrophic degenerative changes of the L5 superior articular process (*black arrow*), which produce lateral stenosis, and hypertrophic changes of the L4 inferior articular process (*black arrowhead*), which cause central stenosis. (From DeLisa JA, Gans MB. *Rehabilitation medicine: principles and practice*, 3rd ed. Philadelphia: Lippincott-Raven, 1998:465, with permission.)

Hyperflexion Injuries

Hyperflexion injuries of the thoracolumbar spine can be combined with other mechanisms of injury, such as compression, distraction, rotation, and shearing. They can produce simple anterior wedge fractures, burst fractures, distraction fractures, or facet dislocation.

Simple anterior wedge (anterior compression) fractures involve hyperflexion trauma that compresses only the anterior vertebral body. Typically, there is less than a 50% loss of anterior vertebral body height, and the posterior vertebral body height is normal (Fig. 3.50A,B). The posterior vertebral body is intact, and the posterior ligaments are intact. This is a stable injury that rarely produces neurologic deficits.

In thoracolumbar burst fractures, the mechanism commonly involves flexion and axial loading. This increases intrabody pressure to produce a comminuted fracture that disperses fragments radially in all directions, including posteriorly into the spinal canal. The loss of vertebral body height is typically greater than 50%, and both the anterior and posterior body margins are affected, although not necessarily equally (Fig. 3.51A–C). There is commonly involvement of the neural arch, and on anteroposterior films, interpedicle distance is increased. Typically, these fractures are unstable and produce neurologic deficits.

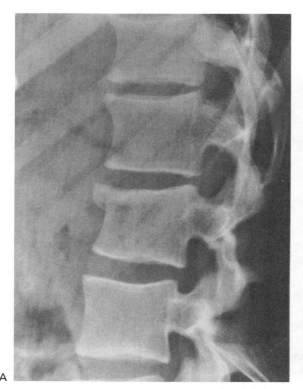

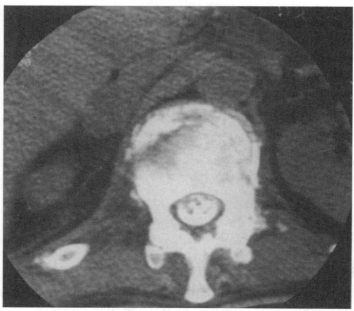

A   B

FIGURE 3.50. Wedge compression fracture of L1. **A**; Radiograph demonstrates loss of height of the anterior aspect of the vertebral body but not of the posterior aspect. **B**; Computed tomography scan after intrathecal contrast injection demonstrates disruption of the anterior body but an intact posterior cortex with no involvement of the spinal canal. (From Mirvis SE, Young JWR. *Imaging in trauma and critical care*, Baltimore: Williams & Wilkins, 1992:434, with permission.)

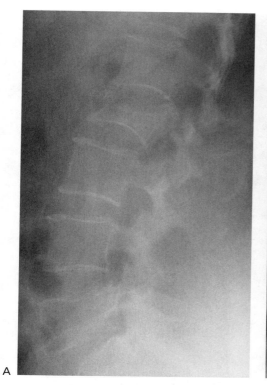

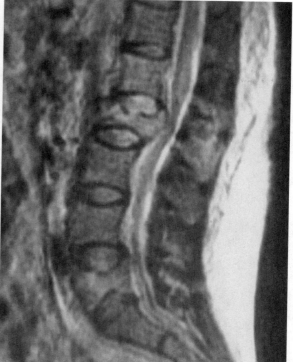

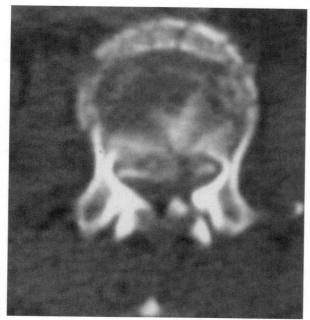

FIGURE 3.51. Flexion-compression burst fractures of L2 and L5 vertebrae. **A**; Lateral lumbar radiograph displays compression fractures of L2 and L5. **B**; Sagittal T2-weighted magnetic resonance image reveals that the L2 fracture compresses both the high signal intensity cerebrospinal fluid and the low signal intensity conus medullaris and cauda equina. **C**; Computed tomography scan of burst fracture of L2 showing radial dispersion of fragments, including retropulsion of fragments into the spinal canal.

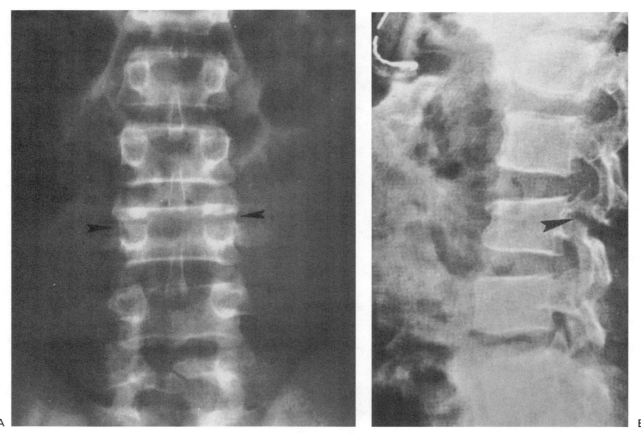

FIGURE 3.52. Chance or seat-belt fracture. **A**; Anteroposterior radiograph demonstrates horizontal fractures through the pedicles of L3 (*arrowheads*). **B**; On the lateral view, there is a horizontal fracture extending from the spinous process through the pedicles to the posterior margin of the vertebral body (*arrowhead*). The orientation of the fracture line indicates passage into the spinous process. (From Mirvis SE, Young JWR. *Imaging in trauma and critical care*, Baltimore: Williams & Wilkins, 1992:440, with permission.)

Flexion-distraction (seat-belt) fractures commonly involve the use of lap belts without a shoulder harness. In this type of injury, the seat belt against the anterior abdominal wall becomes the axis of rotation, and the spine is subjected to distraction forces that tend to rip it apart in the horizontal plane. If the fracture line passes horizontally through the spinous process and pedicles and into the vertebral body, it is called a Chance fracture (Fig. 3.52A,B). If it disrupts the posterior ligaments rather than the spinous process, with the fracture beginning at the lamina and extending into the vertebral body, it is a Smith fracture. The cleft spinous process and pedicles and the widened interlaminar and interspinous distances can be visualized on anteroposterior or lateral films. Lateral radiographs may also show lengthening and bowing of the posterior vertebral body. Axial CT may fail to visualize these fractures, although they can be seen on sagittal or coronal reconstructions. Because all columns are involved, these fractures are unstable, especially in flexion, and may cause neurologic injury.

Bilateral thoracolumbar facet dislocations are most commonly caused by hyperflexion with some distraction (Fig.

3.53A,B). This type of injury involves disruption of all posterior ligaments, facet capsule, intervertebral disk, and both longitudinal ligaments. On plain films, there is widening of the interspinous and interlaminar intervals, and the inferior articular facet of the higher vertebra rests in the narrow lower part of the intervertebral foramen just anterior to the subjacent superior articular process. Axial or sagittal CT and MRI images often visualize the locked facets, the disrupted ligaments, and the neural encroachment caused by this unstable fracture.

Hyperextension Injuries

Hyperextension injuries of the thoracolumbar spine are relatively rare. They may cause only a simple rupture of the anterior longitudinal ligament and disk space and remain stable with no neurologic deficits. Rarely, they can cause a hyperextension fracture-dislocation that disrupts both anterior and posterior elements to produce significant instability and neurologic injury (Fig. 3.54).

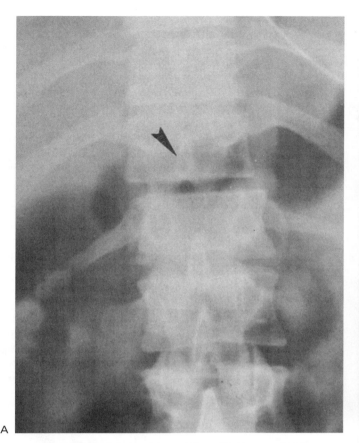

A

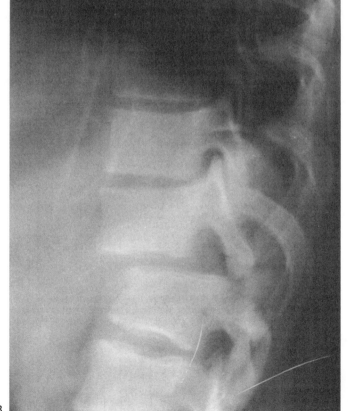

B

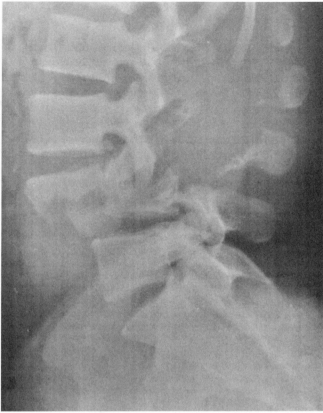

FIGURE 3.54. Lateral lumbar radiograph demonstrates a severe hyperextension fracture-dislocation. The L4 body has sheared off horizontally, with anterior displacement of the superior portion. The spinous processes of L1, L2, and L3 are fractured and markedly displaced posteriorly. The superior articular facets of L4 are fractured and anteriorly displaced. (From Mirvis SE, Young JWR. *Imaging in trauma and critical care*, Baltimore: Williams & Wilkins, 1992:451, with permission.)

FIGURE 3.53. Bilateral facet dislocation of T11 on T12. **A**; Anteroposterior radiograph demonstrates widening of the interspinous distance at T11 to T12, with superior displacement of the spinous process of T11 (*arrowheads*), giving rise to a vacant appearance to the superior aspect of the vertebral body of T12. **B**; Lateral view shows classical facet dislocation, much as is seen in the cervical spine. Of note is a mild wedge compression fracture of T12. (From Mirvis SE, Young JWR. *Imaging in trauma and critical care*, Baltimore: Williams & Wilkins, 1992:442, with permission.)

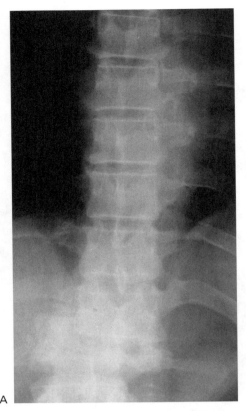

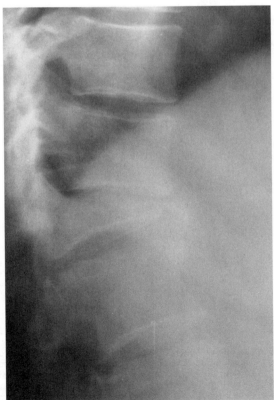

Rotation Injuries

Rotation injuries are frequently combined with other injury mechanisms, particularly flexion, axial loading, and shear. The vertebral body injury may be a horizontally oriented "slice" fracture of the superior part of the lower vertebra, or it may involve fragmentation of the body with radial dispersion of the fragments. The facet joints are typically asymmetrically disrupted as a result of the rotation, and facet fracture may be present. There may be associated rib or transverse process fractures. These highly unstable fractures typically cause severe neurologic deficits, with complete deficits in 50% to 70% of cases (22).

Shearing Injuries

Shearing injuries of the thoracolumbar spine may be caused by translatory shearing stress applied in sagittal, mediolateral, or oblique planes. They can cause significant anteroposterior, lateral, or oblique vertebral displacement (Fig. 3.55A,B). At times, the displaced vertebrae have a windswept appearance as a result of oblique shearing vectors (22) (Fig. 3.56). There are frequently fractures involving articular facets, ribs, and spinous or transverse processes.

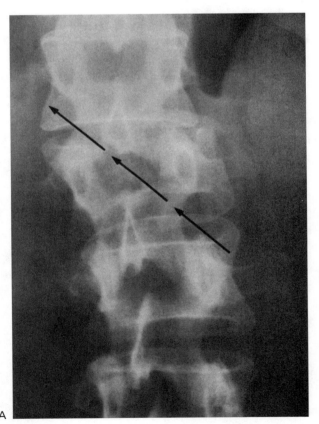

FIGURE 3.55. This paraplegic patient received a lateral shearing subluxation of T12 on L1 and a compression fracture of L1 by being pinned under a truck when a jack slipped. **A**; Anteroposterior thoracolumbar radiograph. **B**; Lateral thoracolumbar radiograph.

FIGURE 3.56. Typical shearing injury of L2. **A**; Frontal radiograph shows the windswept appearance of the vertebrae. The *arrows* indicate the force vector. *(Figure continues.)*

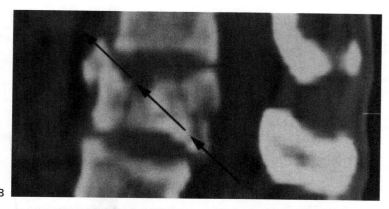

B

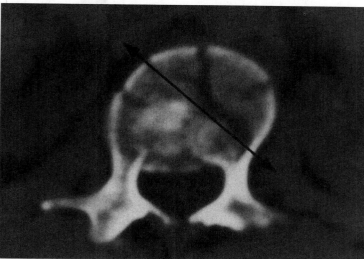

C

FIGURE 3.56. *Continued.* **B**; Sagittal computed tomography reconstruction also shows a windswept appearance. The *arrows* indicate the direction of the force vectors. **C**; Computed tomography section through L2 shows comminution, retropulsion of a bone fragment into the vertebral canal, and the windswept appearance. The *double arrow* indicates the force vector. (From Daffner NM. *Imaging of vertebral trauma*, 2nd ed. Philadelphia: Lippincott-Raven, 1996:140, with permission.)

REFERENCES

1. Schneck CD. Functional and clinical anatomy of the spine. In: Young MA, Lavin RA, eds. *Physical medicine and rehabilitation: state of the art reviews*, Vol. 9. 1995;9:571–604.
2. White AA III, Panjabi MM. *Clinical biomechanics of the spine*, 2nd ed. Philadelphia: JB Lippincott, 1990.
3. Bland JH, Boushey DR. Anatomy and physiology of the cervical spine. *Semin Arthritis Rheum* 1990;20:1–20.
4. Johnson RM, Orelin ES, White AA, et al. Some newer observations on the functional anatomy of the lower cervical spine. *Clin Orthop* 1978;111:192–200.
5. White AA, Panjabi MM. *Clinical biomechanics of the cervical spine*. Philadelphia: JB Lippincott, 1978.
6. Connell MD, Weisel SW. Natural history and pathogenesis of cervical disc disease. *Orthop Clin North Am* 1992;23:369–380.
7. Schneck CD. Clinical anatomy of the cervical spine. In: White AA, Schofferman JA, eds. *Spine care*. St. Louis: Mosby, 1995:1306–1334.
8. McNab I. *Backache*. Baltimore: Williams & Wilkins, 1977.
9. Schneck CD. The anatomical determinants of lumbar spondylosis. In: Ramani PS, ed. *Posterior lumbar interbody fusion*. Bombay: Associated Personnel Services, 1989:11–32.
10. Burton CV. High resolution CT scanning: the present and the future. *Orthop Clin North Am* 1983;14:539–551.
11. Sheldon JT, Serland T, Leborgne J. Computed tomography of the lower lumbar vertebral column. *Radiology* 1977;124:113–118.
12. Mikhael MA, Ciric I, Tarkington JA. Neurological evaluation of lateral recess syndrome. *Radiology* 1981;140:97–107.
13. Schneck CD, Jacob HA. Basic principles of functional biomechanics. In: Fortin JD, Falco FJE, Jacob HAC, eds. *Physical medicine and rehabilitation: state of the art reviews*, Vol. 11. 1997:731–751.
14. Daffner RH. *Imaging of vertebral trauma*, 2nd ed. Philadelphia: Lippincott-Raven Publishers, 1996:223–236.
15. Jacobs RE, Casey MP. Surgical management of thoracolumbar spinal injuries. *Clin Orthop* 1984;189:22–35.
16. Gaines RW, Humphreys WG. A plea for judgment in management of thoracolumbar fractures and fracture-dislocations. *Clin Orthop* 1984; 189:36–42.
17. Daffner RH, Deeb ZL, Goldberg AL, et al. The radiologic assessment of post-traumatic vertebral stability. *Skeletal Radiol* 1990;19:103–108.
18. Ferguson RL, Allen BL Jr. A mechanistic classification of thoracolumbar spine fractures. *Clin Orthop* 1984;189:77–88.
19. Buitrago-Tellez CH, Ferstl FJ, Langer M. Spine. In: Heller M, Fink A, eds. *Radiology of trauma*. Berlin: Springer, 2000:59–94.
20. Whitesides TE. Traumatic kyphosis of the thoracolumbar spine. *Clin Orthop* 1977;128:78–92.
21. Denis F. Spinal instability as defined by the three-column spine concept in acute spinal trauma. *Clin Orthop* 1984;189:65–76.
22. Young JWR. Fractures of the thoracic and lumbar spine. In: Mirvis SE, Young JWR, eds. *Imaging in trauma and critical care*. Baltimore: Williams & Wilkins, 1992:421–453.
23. Kelly RP, Whitesides TE Jr. Treatment of lumbodorsal fracture-dislocations. *Ann Surg* 1968;167:705–717.
24. Holdsworth F. Fractures, dislocations and fracture-dislocations of the spine. *J Bone Joint Surg Am* 1970;52:1534–1551.

25. Denis F. The three column spine and its significance in the classification of acute thoracolumbar spinal injuries. *Spine* 1983;8:817–831.

26. Panjabi MM, White AA III, Johnson RM. Cervical spine mechanics as a function of transsection of components. *J Biomechanics* 1975;8: 327–336.

27. Panjabi MM, Hausfeld JN, White AA III. A biomechanical study of the ligamentous stability of the thoracic spine in man. *Acta Orthop Scand* 1981;52:315–326.

28. Nagel DA, Koogle TA, Piziale RL, et al. Stability of the upper lumbar spine following progressive disruptions and the application of individual internal and external fixation devices. *J Bone Joint Surg Am* 1981; 63:62–70.

29. McAfee PC, Yuan HA, Fredrickson BE, et al. The value of computed tomography in thoracolumbar fractures. *J Bone Joint Surg Am* 1983; 65:461–473.

30. Gehwiler JA, Daffner RH, Osbourne RL Jr. Relevant signs of stable and unstable thoracolumbar vertebral column trauma. *Skeletal Radiol* 1981;7:179–183.

31. Daffner RH, Deeb ZL, Rothfus WE. The posterior vertebral body line: importance in the detection of burst fractures. *AJR Am J Roentgenol* 1987;148:93–96.

32. Harris JH Jr, Mirvis SE. *The radiology of acute cervical spine trauma*, 3rd ed. Baltimore: Williams & Wilkins, 1996.

33. Young JWR, Mirvis SE. Cervical spine trauma. In: Mirvis SE, Young JWR, eds. *Imaging in trauma and critical care*. Baltimore: Williams & Wilkins, 1992:291–379.

34. Young JWR, Resnik CS, DeCandido P, et al. The laminar space in the diagnosis of rotational flexion injuries of the cervical spine. *AJR Am J Roentgenol* 1989;152:103–107.

35. Schneck CD. Imaging techniques relative to rehabilitation. In DeLisa JA, Gans BM, eds. *Rehabilitation medicine: principles and practice*, 3rd ed. Philadelphia: Lippincott-Raven, 1998:433–479.

36. Grossman RI. Intracranial hemorrhage. In: Latchaw RE, ed. *MR and CT imaging of the head, neck and spine*. St. Louis: Mosby–Year Book, 1991:203–265.

37. Kulkarni MV, McArdle CB, Kopanicky D, et al. Acute spinal cord injury: MR imaging at 1.5 T. *Radiology*, 1987;164:837–843.

38. Quencer RM. Post-traumatic spinal cord cysts: characterization with CT, MRI and sonography. In: Latch RE, ed. *MR and CT imaging of the head, neck and spine*. St. Louis: Mosby–Year Book, 1991:1257–1267.

39. White AA, Panjabi MM. *Clinical biomechanics of the cervical spine*. Philadelphia: JB Lippincott, 1978.

40. White AA, Panjabi MM, Posner I, et al. Spinal stability: evaluation and treatment. In: Murray DG, ed. *Instructional course lectures*. St. Louis: Mosby, 1981:457–483.

41. Jefferson G. Fractures of the atlas vertebra: report of four cases, and a review of those previously recorded. *Br J Surg* 1920;7:407–422.

42. Helms CA. *Fundamentals of skeletal radiology*. Philadelphia: WB Saunders, 1995.

43. Dickman CA, Mamourian A, Sonntag VKH, et al. Magnetic resonance imaging of the transverse atlantal ligament for the evaluation of atlantoaxial instability. *J Neurosurg* 1991;75:221–227.

44. Fesmire FM, Luten FC. The pediatric cervical spine: developmental anatomy and clinical aspects. *J Emerg Med* 1989;7:133–142.

45. Anderson LD, D'Alonzo RT. Fractures of the odontoid process of the axis. *J Bone Joint Surg Am* 1974;56:1663–1672.

46. Effendi B, Roy D, Cornish B, et al. Fractures of the ring of the axis: a classification based on the analysis of 131 cases. *J Bone Joint Surg Br* 1981;63:319–327.

47. Levine AM, Edwards CC. The management of traumatic spondylolisthesis of the axis. *J Bone Joint Surg Am* 1985;67:217–226.

48. Bland JH, Boushey DR. Anatomy and physiology of the cervical spine. *Semin Arthritis Rheum* 1990;20:1–20.

49. Hayashi K, Yabuki T. Origin of the uncus and Luschka's joint in the cervical spine. *J Bone Joint Surg Am* 1985;67:788–791.

50. Green JD, Harle TS, Harris JH Jr. Anterior subluxation of the cervical spine: hyperflexion sprain. *AJNR Am J Neuroradiol* 1981;2:243–250.

4

EPIDEMIOLOGY OF TRAUMATIC SPINAL CORD INJURY

MICHAEL J. DeVIVO

Many studies of the epidemiology of traumatic spinal cord injury (SCI) in the United States have been undertaken since the 1970s. Initially, these studies were mostly descriptive, examining the demographic profile and other characteristics of patients treated at particular hospitals and rehabilitation centers (1,2). Local population-based studies of actual incidence of SCI were first conducted by Kraus and colleagues (3) for the northern California region and later by Griffin and associates (4) for one Minnesota county. National population-based epidemiologic investigations were first conducted by Kalsbeek and colleagues (5) and by Bracken and associates (6). However, other than immediate case fatality and hospital expenses, none of these investigations included patient follow-up or any measures of treatment outcome.

In the early 1970s, the model SCI care system program was initiated with funding from what is now the National Institute on Disability and Rehabilitation Research (NIDRR) in the U.S. Department of Education. As a part of this program, all funded model systems were required to contribute data on patients they treated to a national database. This database is now known as the National Spinal Cord Injury Statistical Center (NSCISC) Database and is located at the University of Alabama at Birmingham (7). This database has been used extensively to develop an epidemiologic profile of new SCIs that occur each year as well as changes in that profile that have occurred over time (8–11). It has been estimated that this database contains information on 15% of all new SCIs that occur in the United States each year (9). However, it is not population based, and as a result, it cannot be used to calculate incidence rates or directly assess risk factors for the occurrence of SCI. In general, when compared with population-based studies, it has been shown that patients in the NSCISC Database are representative of all SCIs, except that more severe injuries, injuries in nonwhites, and injuries due to acts of violence are slightly overrepresented (9). The strength of the NSCISC Database and of its unique contribution to the field of SCI epidemiology is that it was designed with a long-term follow-up component to track thousands of patients longitudinally over time for the purpose of assessing treatment outcomes.

Beginning in the 1980s, the Centers for Disease Control and Prevention began funding population-based SCI surveillance systems in many states (12–17). When combined with the more detailed information contained in the NSCISC Database, a rela-tively complete description of the epidemiology of SCI in the United States can be obtained.

OVERALL INCIDENCE

Published reports of the incidence of SCI vary from 25 new cases per million population per year in West Virginia to 59 new cases per million population per year in Mississippi (15, 17). Differences in SCI incidence rates among states are due to a combination of factors, including differences in population characteristics, such as age, gender, and race; differences in the definition of SCI; and differences in data collection methodology. Overall, when combining information from all the state SCI registries, the incidence rate appears to be about 40 new cases per million population, or just over 10,000 cases per year. This figure does not include patients who die at the scene of the accident. Interestingly, although there have been shifts in the underlying causes of these SCIs since the 1980s, the overall incidence appears to have remained relatively constant (18).

Incidence of fatal SCI before hospitalization was reported to be 21.2 cases per million population for northern California in 1970 to 1971, and 20.8 cases per million population in Olmsted County, Minnesota, from 1935 to 1981 (3,4). However, a more recent report from the SCI population-based registry in Utah suggests that the incidence rate of fatal SCI before hospitalization for 1989 to 1991 was only about 4 cases per million population, or about 1,000 cases per year if that figure were applied nationally (14). This decrease might be due to improved emergency medical services at the scene of the accident, but incomplete reporting of cases also cannot be ruled out.

Incidence of SCI in the rest of the world is consistently lower than in the United States and often does not exceed 20 new cases per million population per year (19–25). Much of this difference is due to the relatively high incidence of violence-related SCIs in the United States. Violence is a rare cause of SCI in other countries.

PREVALENCE

Prevalence can be estimated in one of two ways. Given that SCI is a relatively rare condition, initial attempts to assess prevalence were by using the epidemiologic formula linking prevalence to more established data on incidence and life expectancy. In 1980, using the best available data at the time, DeVivo and colleagues estimated SCI prevalence in the United States to be 906 patients per million population, or just under 200,000 existing cases (26). However, for this approach to be valid, both incidence and life expectancy would need to be relatively constant over time. Because life expectancy had been increasing and a current estimate was used, this approach resulted in a slight overestimate of prevalence.

The alternative approach of simply counting patients with SCI was eventually undertaken only when substantial funding was provided by the Paralyzed Veterans of America. Using a sophisticated probability sampling plan of small geographic areas and institutions, Berkowitz and associates conservatively estimated the prevalence of SCI in the United States to be 721 patients per million population, or about 176,965 patients in 1988 (27).

More recently, Lasfargues and coauthors combined the 1988 estimate of Berkowitz and associates with current estimates of age- and sex-specific incidence and mortality to project the growth in prevalence of SCI in the United States over time (28). Estimated prevalence of SCI from this mathematical model was 207,129 patients in 1994, 246,882 patients in 2004, and 276,281 patients in 2014. This growth results exclusively from improved life expectancies rather than an increase in incidence.

AGE

Several state registries have produced relatively comparable estimates of age-specific incidence rates. Typical is the state of Oklahoma, where the overall annual incidence rate of 40 cases per million population matches the national average. In Oklahoma, incidence rates are lowest for the pediatric age group (age less than 15 years, 6 cases per million population), are highest for those aged 15 to 19 years (94 per million population), and decline steadily after age 19 to 85 per million for ages 20 to 24 years, 71 per million for ages 25 to 29 years, 47 per million for ages 30 to 44 years, 32 per million for ages 45 to 59 years, and 26 per million patients at least 60 years of age (13). Looking at actual numbers of cases rather than rates, 3% of new cases in Oklahoma occurred among patients younger than 15 years of age, 47% occurred between the ages of 15 and 29 years, 27% occurred between the ages of 30 and 44 years, 12% occurred between the ages of 45 and 59 years, and 11% occurred at age 60 years or greater.

As seen in Fig. 4.1, the distribution of age at time of injury, for patients enrolled in the NSCISC Database, is strikingly similar to the population-based data from Oklahoma. The mean age at injury, for all patients in the NSCISC Database, is 31.8 years (±15.6 years), the median age at injury is 26.4 years, and the most common age at injury is 19 years (Table 4.1). Overall, 59.4% of all patients enrolled in the NSCISC Database were 30 years of age or younger at the time of injury. Interestingly, the percentage of new patients enrolled in the NSCISC Database

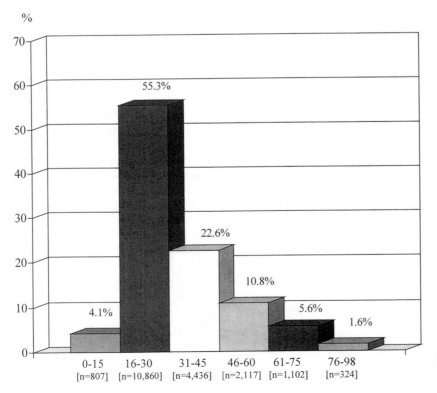

FIGURE 4.1. Age of patients enrolled in the National Spinal Cord Injury Statistical Center Database at time of injury (N = 19,646).

TABLE 4.1. CHARACTERISTICS OF PATIENTS ENROLLED IN THE NSCISC DATABASE, 1973–1999

Characteristic	
Age at injury (yr)	
Mean	31.8
Median	26.4
Mode	19.0
Male gender (%)	81.7
Race or ethnicity (%)	
White	66.4
African American	21.1
Native American	1.1
Asian	1.6
Hispanic	8.8
Other	1.0
Educational status at injury (%)	
Less than high school graduate	39.8
High school graduate	49.9
Associate degree	1.6
Bachelor's degree	5.9
Master's degree	1.3
Doctorate	0.8
Other degree	0.7
Marital status at injury (%)	
Single—never married	53.5
Married	30.4
Divorced	8.9
Separated	4.1
Widowed	2.4
Other/unknown	0.7

who were older than age 60 years at time of injury has increased steadily from 4.5% during 1973 to 1977 to 11.5% from 1994 to 1998 (11). This trend most likely reflects the advancing age of the general U.S. population, although shifts in referral patterns to model systems or changes in underlying age-specific incidence rates cannot be ruled out.

The distribution of ages at the time of injury (incident cases) is very different from the current ages of all patients who presently have a SCI (prevalent cases) because the latter is a function of both age at injury and long-term survival rates. Only the study by Berkowitz and colleagues has attempted to estimate the current ages of patients living with SCI in the United States (27). The median current age of all patients with SCI was estimated to be 41 years (15 years older than the median age of new cases), with only 5.4% younger than age 25 years, 54.2% between ages 25 and 44 years, 27.8% between ages 45 and 64 years, and 12.7% for those aged 65 years or greater (27). However, these estimates are now 12 years old, so that the median age of all patients with SCI alive today would likely be slightly higher than it was in 1988.

GENDER

The proportion of men in the NSCISC Database is 81.7% (Table 4.1). This is consistent with population-based registries,

such as in Oklahoma, where 80% of SCIs occurred among men (13). Underlying annual incidence rates in Oklahoma also reflect this 4:1 gender ratio, with men having an incidence rate of 65 and women having an incidence rate of 16 cases per million population per year (13). This 4:1 gender ratio has remained remarkably consistent over time despite significant trends in age at injury, ethnicity, and etiology of injury (11).

Because of differential survival rates between men and women, the percentage of patients with SCI who are alive today who are men is considerably lower than the percentage of new cases that occur among men. In 1988, Berkowitz and colleagues estimated that only 71% of prevalent cases of SCI in the United States were men (27). This figure should be slightly lower today than it was in 1988.

ETHNICITY

State registries consistently reveal higher incidence rates for African Americans than whites. Again, using Oklahoma as an example, the annual SCI incidence rate was 57 per million population for African Americans, 40 per million population for whites, and 29 per million for Native Americans (13). This difference between African Americans and whites is due entirely to injuries that result from acts of violence. Among African Americans, the cause-specific annual SCI incidence rate for acts of violence is 21 per million population, whereas the comparable figure for whites and Native Americans is only 3 per million population (13). Unfortunately, state registries have not yet published incidence rates for other racial and ethnic groups, such as Asians and Hispanics.

Since 1973, 66.4% of patients enrolled in the NSCISC Database have been white, 21.1% African American, 8.8% Hispanic, 1.6% Asian, 1.1% Native American, and 1% other race (11) (Table 4.1). However, a substantial trend has been observed in the racial distribution of patients enrolled in the NSCISC Database over time (11). During 1973 to 1977, 76.8% of new patients enrolled in the NSCISC Database were white, 14% were African American, 6.3% were Hispanic, 2.1% were Native American, and 0.8% were Asian. By comparison, between 1992 and 1999, only 58.9% of new patients enrolled in the NSCISC Database were white, whereas 28.1% were African American, 10.3% were Hispanic, 2.2% were Asian, and 0.5% were Native American. This trend is due in very small part to changes in the general U.S. population. Rather, it is related more to a combination of factors, including periodic changes in the identities and locations of participating model systems, changes in eligibility criteria for inclusion in the NSCISC Database, and changes in referral patterns to model systems. Given the substantial nature of this trend, some change in underlying race-specific incidence rates is also likely. However, the exact nature of any such change in race-specific incidence rates cannot be determined from the NSCISC Database.

ETIOLOGY OF INJURY

Eleven specific causes of traumatic SCI account for 93.4% of all new cases enrolled in the NSCISC Database each year. Automobile crashes rank first (34.3%), followed by falls (19%), gunshot wounds (17%), diving mishaps (7.3%), motorcycle crashes (5.6%), being hit by a falling object (3.3%), medical or surgical complications (2.1%), pedestrians being struck by motor vehicles (1.8%), and 1% each for stab wounds, bicycle mishaps, and violent personal contact. All other causes of SCI account for less than 1% each. Automobile crashes cause a lower percentage of cases among men than women (31.4% versus 51.0%). Conversely, a higher percentage of men, as compared to women, contract SCI from gunshot wounds (18.3% versus 11.3%), diving mishaps (8.0% versus 3.2%), and motorcycle crashes (6.1% versus 1.7%). Among men, diving mishaps have decreased over time as a cause of SCI from 10.6% during 1973 to 1977 to only 4.8% from 1994 to 1998. Automobile crashes have also caused a decreasing percentage of SCIs among men, ranging from 34.7% from 1978 to 1982 to 29.7% from 1994 to 1998; this is most likely due to the advent of air bags, passage of mandatory seat-belt laws, decreased speeding limits, and improvements in the design of newer-model cars. Conversely, the percentage of SCI caused by gunshot wounds increased from 12.7% among men during 1973 to 1977 to 24.1% from 1989 to 1993 before declining slightly to 22.4% from 1994 to 1998 (11).

Diving mishaps account for most SCIs due to recreational sports reported to the NSCISC Database between 1993 and 1996 (57.1%) (29). Snow skiing ranked second, at only 9.7%, followed by surfing at 4.1%, wrestling at 3.1%, and football at 2.8%. Interestingly, SCIs due to diving, football, and trampoline mishaps have declined markedly since the initiation of the NSCISC Database in the mid-1970s, whereas those due to snow skiing and surfing have increased in both raw numbers and percentages (29). The change of football rules in 1976 that banned deliberate "spearing" and the use of the top of the helmet as the initial point of contact in making tackles undoubtedly contributed to the decline in football-related SCIs. Similarly, removal of trampolines from schools in some states has undoubtedly contributed to the decline in trampoline-related SCIs.

It is important to keep in mind that those recreational sports activities that involve the most SCIs are not necessarily the most risky activities. To assess risk, one must know the underlying rate of exposure to that activity. For example, male gymnastics, which causes few SCIs but also has few participants, has an incidence rate of 14.3 per 100,000 athletes, whereas high school and college football, which causes more SCIs but also has more participants, has an incidence rate of only 1 per 100,000 athletes (30).

The NSCISC Database does not contain more specific information on the circumstances surrounding each SCI. However, a number of studies have been undertaken to examine the leading causes of SCI in more detail for the purpose of identifying possible preventive interventions that might be cost-effective. Specific causes of SCI that have been looked at include motor vehicle crashes, gunshot wounds, diving mishaps, and falls (31–36).

Individual causes of SCI are often grouped into five categories to facilitate analysis: vehicular crashes (any type of motor vehicle or bicycle), violence (gunshot wounds, stab wounds, personal contact, or explosion), recreational sports, falls, and all other

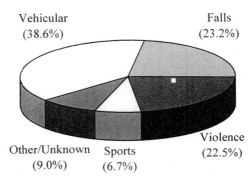

FIGURE 4.2. Grouped etiology for patients enrolled in the National Spinal Cord Injury Statistical Center Database between 1995 and 1999.

causes. Figure 4.2 reflects the distribution of grouped causes of SCI among all new patients enrolled in the NSCISC Database from 1995 to 1999. Overall, 38.7% of these injuries were due to vehicular crashes, 23.3% were due to falls, 22.5% were due to violence, 6.7% were due to sports, and 8.8% were due to all other causes.

A slightly different picture of grouped etiologies of SCI emerges from the population-based registries. In Oklahoma, 48% of SCIs are due to motor vehicle crashes, 20% are due to falls, 13% are due to recreational sports activities, 11% are due to violence, and 8% are due to other causes (13). Data from Utah are very similar to those from Oklahoma, with 49% of SCIs due to motor vehicle crashes, 21% due to falls, 16% due to recreational sports, 5% due to violence, and 9% due to other and unknown causes (14). Given the location of most model systems in large urban areas, it is not surprising that acts of violence are somewhat overrepresented in the NSCISC Database.

With the exception of injuries due to acts of violence, the most common causes of SCI in other countries are generally comparable to those observed in the United States. Typical is the case of Denmark, where 47% of SCIs are due to motor vehicle crashes, 26% are due to falls, 12% are due to recreational sports, 10% are due to acts of violence, and 5% are due to other causes (20). However, among the SCIs caused by acts of violence in Denmark, 80% result from failed suicide attempts, whereas in the United States, these injuries are usually either unintentionally inflicted (either by the individual or another person) or malicious. The pattern of causes of SCI in Taipei, Istanbul, and Spain is similar to that in Denmark (19,21,22). However, in Jordan, the distribution of causes of SCI looks more like that of the United States, with 29% due to acts of violence (almost all gunshot wounds) (24).

Grouped causes of SCI by age, at the time of injury, for all patients enrolled in the NSCISC Database appears in Table 4.2. Motor vehicle crashes are the leading cause of SCI until the age of 45 years old; however, falls represent the leading cause of SCI with the 46- to 60-year-old group. The percentage of SCIs due to falls increases steadily from only 8.4% among the pediatric age group to 59.0% in the oldest age group. Conversely, the percentages of SCIs due to recreational sports and acts of violence decrease with advancing age at time of injury. In the pediat-

TABLE 4.2. GROUPED ETIOLOGY FOR PATIENTS ENROLLED IN THE NSCISC DATABASE BY AGE AT INJURY

Age (yr)	Grouped Etiology (%)					Total (%)
	Vehicular	Violence	Sports	Falls	Other	
0–15	36.2	24.4	24.0	8.4	6.9	100.0
16–30	46.1	22.7	15.0	10.6	5.6	100.0
31–45	41.9	18.6	6.9	22.9	9.7	100.0
46–60	35.8	9.9	2.7	37.4	14.1	100.0
61–75	31.3	3.7	1.4	46.9	16.7	100.0
76–98	28.7	1.9	0.3	59.0	10.2	100.0

ric age group, recreational sports account for 24.0% and acts of violence for 24.4% of SCIs; whereas in the oldest age group, the comparable figures are 0.3% and 1.9%, respectively.

There are also significant differences in causes of SCI by racial and ethnic group. Among patients enrolled in the NSCISC Database, 87.9% of SCIs due to recreational sports, 77.5% due to motor vehicle crashes, 69.6% due to falls, and only 26.0% due to acts of violence occur among whites.

Closer inspection of the interaction of age, gender, race, year of injury, and cause of injury reveals the rather striking pattern depicted in Fig. 4.3. Among African American and Hispanic males aged 16 to 21 years at injury, enrolled in either the NSCISC Database or the comparable Shriners Hospital for Chil-

dren Spinal Cord Injury Database, the percentage of patients whose SCI was due to an act of violence increased dramatically from 34.9% between 1973 and 1979 to 73.6% between 1990 and 1994, before declining slightly to 68.5% since 1995. The comparable figures for white males aged 16 to 21 years were 4.7%, 9.3%, and 7.8%, respectively. Moreover, among adult (22 years of age or older) African American and Hispanic males enrolled in the NSCISC Database, the percentage of new injuries due to acts of violence only ranged from 33.5% between 1973 and 1979 to a peak of 44.5% between 1990 and 1994. Therefore, the epidemic of increased violence-induced SCIs has been limited almost entirely to African American and Hispanic males aged 16 to 21 years.

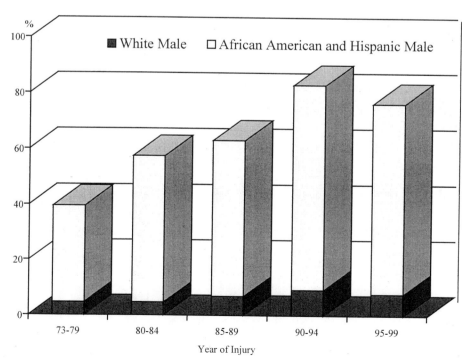

FIGURE 4.3. Percentage of 16- to 21-year-old men treated at a model system or Shriners Hospital whose spinal cord injury was due to an act of violence by a racial or ethnic group and year of injury.

ASSOCIATED INJURIES

SCIs are often accompanied by other significant injuries. Among patients enrolled in the NSCISC Database between 1986 and 1992, 29.3% had other broken bones, 28.2% experienced loss of consciousness at least briefly after the injury, 17.8% had a traumatic pneumothorax, and 11.5% had a head injury sufficient to affect cognitive or emotional functioning (9).

The nature and frequency of these other injuries is significantly associated with the etiology of SCI. Among patients injured in motor vehicle crashes, 42.5% experienced loss of consciousness, 39.7% had broken bones, 18.4% had a head injury, and 16.6% had traumatic pneumothorax (9). Conversely, among patients injured in recreational sports mishaps, 22.4% had loss of consciousness, but no other associated injury occurred in more than 5% of cases (9). Not surprisingly, traumatic pneumothorax is most common among patients injured by acts of violence (35.9% of cases), but other associated injuries are relatively rare among these patients (9).

TIME OF INJURY

Traumatic SCI occurs with greater frequency on weekends than other days of the week, with 19.3% of patients enrolled in the NSCISC Database since 1994 being injured on Saturday and another 17.2% being injured on Sunday (11). The least common injury days are Tuesday (11.3%) and Wednesday (11.4%). This pattern is typical of other types of injuries as well.

Substantial seasonal variation also exists in the incidence of SCI, with peak incidence occurring in July (9.8% of patients enrolled in the NSCISC Database since 1994), followed closely by August and June (11). The lowest incidence of SCI occurs in February (6.7%) (11). This seasonal pattern in SCI incidence is much more pronounced in the northern part of the United States, where seasonal variation in climate is greater. The increased incidence of SCI in the summer months is due mostly to higher frequencies of diving and other sports and recreational mishaps, and increased motor vehicle–related injuries secondary to greater summertime vehicular use. Interestingly, with the proportional decrease in SCIs due to sports and recreational activities described earlier, seasonal variation in overall SCI incidence has also declined in recent years (11).

NEUROLOGIC LEVEL AND EXTENT OF LESION

In the NSCISC Database, *neurologic level of injury* is defined as the lowest level of the spinal cord with both intact sensory and motor function bilaterally. Figure 4.4 reflects the distribution of neurologic levels of lesion at time of discharge from model system inpatient rehabilitation programs. Overall, 50.7% of patients in the NSCISC Database have cervical lesions, 35.1% have thoracic lesions, and 11.0% have lumbosacral lesions. The fifth cervical segment is the most common lesion level (14.7%), followed by C4 (13.2%), C6 (11.3%), T12 (7.2%), C7 (5.7%), and L1 (5.0%).

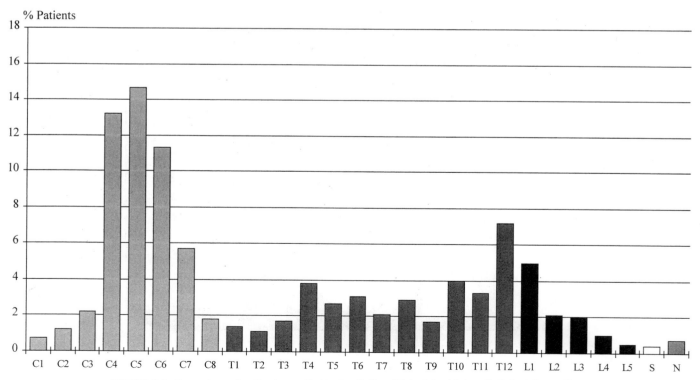

FIGURE 4.4. Percentage of patients enrolled in the National Spinal Cord Injury Statistical Center Database, by neurologic level of lesion at discharge.

Extent of injury is typically assessed using the five-category American Spinal Injury Association (ASIA) Impairment Scale (37). At time of discharge from inpatient rehabilitation, 48.6% of patients enrolled in the NSCISC Database had neurologically complete injuries (ASIA Classification A), 10.3% had incomplete injuries with sensory sparing (ASIA Classification B), 11.2% had incomplete injuries with nonfunctional motor capabilities below the lesion level (ASIA Classification C), 29.1% had incomplete injuries with functional motor capabilities below the lesion level (ASIA Classification D), and 0.8% had essentially complete neurologic recovery (ASIA Classification E). Thoracic injuries are the most likely to be neurologically complete (75.8% of T1 through T6 lesions and 65.4% of T7 through T12 lesions), whereas most lower level lesions are ASIA D injuries (52.9% of lumbar lesions and 85.1% of sacral lesions). Cervical injuries are usually classified as either ASIA A (43.2% for C1 through C4, 39.9% for C5 through C8) or ASIA D (33.1% for both high and low level cervical injuries).

Based on logistic regression analysis of the NSCISC Database, the odds of having a cervical injury relative to a lower injury level increase significantly with advancing age at time of injury, with male gender, and when the injury is due to sports or recreational activities. There has also been a trend toward increased likelihood of cervical injury since 1994 (11). Neurologically complete (ASIA A) injuries are more likely to occur as a result of acts of violence and among younger age groups. However, the proportion of incomplete injuries has not decreased significantly since the mid 1970s when the NSCISC Database was initiated (11).

Because severity of injury is a function of both neurologic level and extent of lesion, these two measures are often grouped together. Excluding ASIA E, one common method of grouping neurologic level and extent of lesion is to create four categories as follows: complete tetraplegia (C1 through C8 ASIA A), incomplete tetraplegia (C1 through C8 ASIA B–D), complete paraplegia (T1 through S5 ASIA A), and incomplete paraplegia (T1 through S5 ASIA B–D). Using this grouping approach, the most frequent combination at discharge from inpatient rehabilitation among patients enrolled in the NSCISC Database is incomplete tetraplegia (31.1%), followed by complete paraplegia (27.0%), complete tetraplegia (21.4%), and incomplete paraplegia (20.5%).

Etiology of injury is strongly associated with neurologic group. About half of motor vehicle crashes (54.6%) result in tetraplegia (32.5% incomplete and 22.1% complete). A somewhat similar pattern emerges for falls, with 52.2% resulting in tetraplegia (36.3% incomplete and 15.9% complete). However, acts of violence usually result in paraplegia (43.4% complete and 26.6% incomplete), whereas recreational sports–related SCIs almost always result in tetraplegia (47.1% incomplete and 42.1% complete).

MARITAL STATUS

It is not surprising given the relatively young age at which most SCIs occur that 53.5% of patients enrolled in the NSCISC Database had never been married at the time of their injury (Table 4.1). Moreover, only 30.4% had intact marriages at the time of injury, with the remainder being either separated, divorced, or widowed. Among those who were at least 15 years of age at the time of injury, 32.1% of patients in the NSCISC Database had still never married 20 years after SCI. The annual marriage rate after SCI is 59% below that of the general population of comparable age, gender, and marital status (never married versus previously married) (38). The annual divorce rate during the first 3 years after SCI is 2.3 times normal, and for those marriages that occur after injury, the divorce rate is still 1.7 times normal (39, 40).

Factors associated with increased likelihood of marriage after SCI include being a college graduate, having been previously divorced, having paraplegia rather than tetraplegia, being ambulatory, being independent in activities of daily living, and living in a private residence. There has been no trend in marriage rates among patients with SCI over the nearly 30-year existence of the NSCISC Database (38). Factors associated with divorce among patients with SCI who were married at the time of injury are younger age, female gender, being African-American, having no children, having a prior marriage ending in divorce, and being nonambulatory (39). Factors associated with divorce among marriages that occur after SCI include male gender, having less than a college education, having a previous marriage end in divorce, and having a thoracic injury level (40).

LEVEL OF EDUCATION

In general, the SCI population is not well educated. Among patients enrolled in the NSCISC Database, only 60.2% have at least completed high school (Table 4.1), whereas 83.5% are at least 19 years of age at the time of their injury. Moreover, very few have degrees beyond high school (1.6% associate's degree, 5.9% bachelor's degree, 1.3% master's degree, 0.8% doctorate, and 0.7% other degree). Among patients enrolled in the NSCISC Database who were in the ninth to eleventh grade at the time of their injury, 46.9% completed a high school diploma within 5 years of injury. However, among those who had a high school diploma at the time of their injury, only 11.6% completed a post–high school degree within 5 years. These low levels of educational attainment can magnify the difficulty in adjusting to one's disability and obtaining subsequent employment.

OCCUPATIONAL STATUS

Most patients enrolled in the NSCISC Database who are between the ages of 16 and 59 years are employed in the competitive labor market at the time of injury (60.5%). Another 18.6% of new SCIs occur among students. However, 17.1% of new SCIs occur among the unemployed, a figure that is substantially above the typical unemployment rate of the United States general population since the 1970s. Many of the model systems are located in large urban areas where unemployment is typically more common. Nonetheless, high rates of unemployment before injury are problematic because of the strong correlation between preinjury and postinjury employment status (41,42).

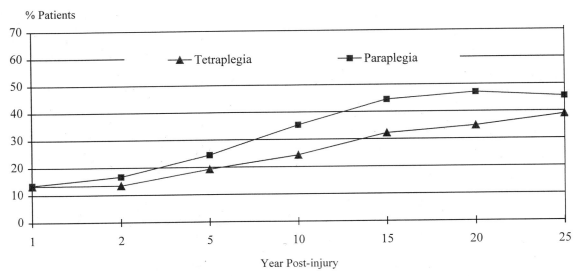

FIGURE 4.5. Percentage of patients enrolled in the National Spinal Cord Injury Statistical Center Database who are employed, by neurologic level of lesion and years after injury.

Virtually all studies of employment after SCI have focused on either obtaining employment or current employment status rather than maintaining employment over time. Figure 4.5 depicts occupational status by time after injury and neurologic level of injury in patients currently aged 16 to 59 years who are enrolled in the NSCISC Database. The percentage of patients with tetraplegia who are employed in the competitive labor market increases steadily with time from 13.4% at the first anniversary of injury to 38.9% at the twenty-fifth anniversary of injury. Among patients with paraplegia, the percentage employed in the competitive labor market is only slightly higher, ranging from 13.6% 1 year after injury to 47.1% 20 years after injury. Most of those who are employed have full-time rather than part-time jobs (41–43).

Predictors of increased likelihood of postinjury employment include younger age, male gender, white race, higher level of formal education, higher reported intelligence quotient (IQ), greater functional capability, less severe injury, being employed at the time of injury, having greater motivation to return to work, having a nonviolent injury etiology, being able to drive, and greater elapsed time after injury (41–47). Patients who return to work within the first year of injury usually return to the same job with the same employer, whereas those who return to work after more than 1 year has elapsed usually acquire a different job with a different employer, often after retraining (48). The most common types of jobs that patients with SCI obtain are professional/technical jobs and clerical/sales jobs (43,48).

Estimates of prevalence of current employment for patients enrolled in the NSCISC Database have also been produced. At the time of their most recent evaluation, 27% of patients with SCI were presently employed, but this varied substantially by neurologic level and extent of injury (41). Among patients with ASIA Impairment Scale A, B, or C injuries, 13.7% of patients with C1 to C4 injury levels, 22.7% of patients with C5 to C8 injury levels, and 28.5% of patients with thoracic, lumbar, or

sacral injuries were presently employed (41). Among patients with neurologically incomplete ASIA D injuries at any level, 38.7% were presently employed (41).

DISCHARGE PLACEMENT

Among all patients enrolled in the NSCISC Database, 88.6% are discharged to a private residence, and an additional 1.7% are discharged to a group living situation within the community. Only 1.3% are discharged to another acute care hospital, with 4.6% being discharged to a nursing home, 0.8% discharged to other environments, and the remaining 3% dying during hospitalization. Overall, among those who are actually discharged alive, 93.3% have historically been discharged back into the community, either in a private residence or group living situation.

Discharge back into the community is one patient outcome measure on which model systems differ from other hospitals and rehabilitation centers. Among 4,337 patients treated in 1996 at facilities participating in the Uniform Data System for Medical Rehabilitation program, only 81% were discharged back into the community, with 10% being discharged to long-term care facilities and another 5% being discharged to acute care hospitals upon completion of rehabilitation (49).

Significant predictors of nursing home discharge include having a cervical injury without useful motor functional capability below the injury level (ASIA Impairment Scale A, B, or C), being ventilator dependent, older age, being unmarried, being unemployed, being from a region of the United States other than the southeast, having an indwelling urethral catheter or external catheter bladder drainage, having either Medicaid or health maintenance organization (HMO) insurance, being dependent in performing activities of daily living, and being nonambulatory (50). There has also been a significant trend toward an increasing percentage of patients being discharged to nursing homes since 1995 with the advent of shorter inpatient rehabilitation lengths of stay (50,51). In 1997 and 1998, almost 9% of patients enrolled in the NSCISC Database were discharged to a nursing home (51). Of those who are initially discharged to a nursing home, about one third eventually move to a community residence (52).

Ten years after injury, about 98% of patients enrolled in the NSCISC Database who are still alive are still residing in private residences within the community (53). Age is the most significant predictor of long-term nursing home residence, with 12.4% of patients aged 61 to 75 years and 22.2% of patients who are at least 76 years of age residing in a nursing home at the time of their most recent anniversary of injury (54). During the first few years after injury, most patients who spend time in a nursing home eventually return to the community rather than spend the entire year in that institution; however, after the third anniversary of injury, full-year stays become more common (52).

LIFE EXPECTANCY

Life expectancy of patients with SCI has improved significantly during the past few decades but remains below normal. Among patients admitted to a model system within 24 hours of injury, the mortality rate during the first year after injury has been conservatively estimated at 6.3% (55). Mortality during postinjury year 2 has been estimated at only 1.7%, with a further decline to about 1.2% per year thereafter (55). Significant predictors of mortality during the first year after injury include advanced age, being male, being injured by an act of violence, having a higher injury level (particularly C4 or above), having

a neurologically complete injury, being ventilator dependent, and having either Medicare or Medicaid third-party sponsorship of care (56). There has also been a substantial decline in first-year mortality rates over time, such that after adjusting for other differences in patient characteristics, the odds of dying for patients injured between 1993 and 1998 were 67% lower than for patients injured between 1973 and 1977 (56).

The same factors that predict mortality during the first year after injury also predict increased likelihood of dying during subsequent years, albeit with somewhat reduced impact (56). Additional predictors of higher mortality rates in later years after SCI include lower satisfaction with life, poor health, emotional distress, being more dependent, and poor self-rated adjustment to disability (57). Interestingly, the substantial declines observed in mortality rates during the first year after injury have not been observed in subsequent years (56).

Using a variety of analytic techniques and the NSCISC Database, life expectancy estimates for patients with SCI have been developed and periodically updated (58–60). These estimates are typically based on neurologic level of injury, degree of injury completeness, age at injury, and ventilator dependency. Separate tables have been developed beginning at either the time of injury or the first anniversary of injury, with the latter reflecting higher life expectancies due to removing the higher mortality rate during the first year after injury. The similarity of results using these different analytic techniques serves to enhance the validity of these life expectancy estimates.

The latest life expectancy estimates from the NSCISC Database beginning at the first anniversary of injury appear in Table 4.3. An abridged version of this table is updated annually on the NSCISC website at *www.spinalcord.uab.edu*. These estimates are not adjusted for gender, race, presence of preexisting

TABLE 4.3. LIFE EXPECTANCY OF PATIENTS WITH SPINAL CORD INJURY TREATED AT MODEL SYSTEMS WHO SURVIVE AT LEAST 1 YEAR POSTINJURY

Current Age (yr)	Life Expectancy (yr)					
		Not Ventilator Dependent				Ventilator Dependent, Any Injury Level
	No SCI[a]	Motor Functional, Any Injury Level	Paraplegia	Tetraplegia		
				C5–C8	C1–C4	
10	66.9	62.0	55.5	50.3	46.0	34.9
15	61.9	57.1	50.7	45.6	41.3	30.4
20	57.2	52.5	46.2	41.2	37.1	26.8
25	52.4	47.9	41.8	37.0	33.1	23.5
30	47.7	43.3	37.3	32.7	29.0	20.1
35	43.0	38.7	33.0	28.5	25.0	16.8
40	38.4	34.3	28.7	24.5	21.2	13.7
45	33.9	29.9	24.6	20.6	17.6	10.8
50	29.5	25.7	20.6	16.9	14.1	8.2
55	25.2	21.8	17.0	13.6	11.1	5.9
60	21.2	18.1	13.7	10.6	8.4	4.0
65	17.5	14.9	10.9	8.1	6.3	2.7
70	14.1	12.1	8.4	6.0	4.4	1.6
75	11.1	9.8	6.5	4.4	3.1	0.9
80	8.4	8.0	5.1	3.2	2.0	0.2

[a] Values for patients with no spinal cord injury are taken from the 1996 U.S. Life Tables for the general population.

medical conditions, or other factors that significantly affect long-term survival. Therefore, Table 4.3 should only be used as a rough guide for estimating the life expectancy of any individual. It can also be used to track progress in prognosis after SCI by comparison to previous life-expectancy estimates.

As seen in Table 4.3, life expectancy is almost normal for patients with incomplete motor functional injuries but declines steadily as injury severity increases. Interestingly, in general, as age increases within each neurologic category, the percentage reduction in life expectancy also increases. For example, among patients with high-level (C1 to C4) tetraplegia who survive the first year after injury, life expectancy is 68.8% of normal for a 10-year-old patient, 60.8% of normal for a 30-year-old patient, 47.8% of normal for a 50-year-old patient, and 31.2% of normal for a 70-year-old patient.

Similar life-expectancy tables have recently been produced for patients with SCI in Great Britain, Denmark, Australia, and Canada (61–64). Life expectancies following SCI appear to be quite comparable in those countries to the experience in the United States. The Canadian study is of particular interest because it also assesses health expectancy, revealing that for patients aged 25 to 34 years at injury, on average, 79.3% of the remaining life expectancy should be accompanied by overall good health, with declining health presumably occurring during the last few years of life expectancy (64).

CAUSES OF DEATH

Primary (underlying) causes of death for all patients enrolled in the NSCISC Database who subsequently died of a known cause appear in Table 4.4. Diseases of the respiratory system are the leading cause of death after SCI, accounting for 20.8% of all deaths. Of deaths due to respiratory diseases, 72.3% are specifically due to pneumonia. Heart disease ranks second at 20.6%, with 7.3% being hypertensive or ischemic in nature and 13.3% being attributed to other types of heart disease. However, heart disease is somewhat overestimated as a cause of death because more than half of the "other heart diseases" reflect heart attacks that occur in young patients with no apparent underlying heart or vascular disease. Therefore, this probably reflects poor quality of cause of death data and reporting practices on many death certificates of patients with SCI rather than true underlying heart disease.

Infective and parasitic diseases (8.8%) are the next leading cause of death behind respiratory and heart disease. These are virtually always cases of septicemia (90.4%) and are usually associated with pressure ulcers, urinary tract infections, or respiratory infections. Often, the source of septicemia is not identified on death certificates.

The next most common cause of death is cancer (6.5%). The most common location of cancer is the lung (29% of fatal cancer

TABLE 4.4. PRIMARY (UNDERLYING) CAUSE OF DEATH IN PATIENTS WITH SPINAL CORD INJURY TREATED AT MODEL SYSTEMS (n = 2,476)

ICD9CM Codes	Primary Cause of Death	Percentage
460–519	Diseases of the respiratory system	20.8
420–429	Other heart disease	13.3
000–139	Infective and parasitic diseases	8.8
400–414	Hypertensive and ischemic heart disease	7.3
140–239	Neoplasms	6.5
415–417	Disease of pulmonary circulation	6.2
780–799	Symptoms and ill-defined conditions	5.3
E800–E949	Unintentional injuries	5.0
520–579	Diseases of the digestive system	5.0
E950–E959	Suicides	4.4
580–629	Diseases of the genitourinary system	3.6
E980–E989	Subsequent trauma of uncertain nature (unintentional, suicide, homicide)	3.4
430–438	Cerebrovascular disease	3.3
320–389	Diseases of the nervous system and sense organs	2.0
440–448	Diseases of the arteries, arterioles, and capillaries	1.5
240–279	Endocrine, nutritional, metabolic, and immunity disorders (includes acquired immunodeficiency syndrome)	1.4
E960–E969	Homicides	0.8
451–459	Diseases of veins, lymphatics, and other diseases of the circulatory system	0.3
290–319	Mental disorders	0.3
710–739	Diseases of the musculoskeletal system and connective tissue	0.3
Residual	All others	0.2
740–759	Congenital anomalies	0.1
280–289	Diseases of blood and blood-forming organs	0.1
E970–E979	Legal intervention	0.1
	Total known causes of death	100.0

cases), followed by bladder (8%), prostate (6.8%), and colon or rectum (6.8%). Diseases of pulmonary circulation (98% of which are cases of pulmonary emboli) rank next behind cancer. Deaths due to pulmonary emboli usually occur before discharge from acute care and rehabilitation and decline sharply with the passage of time after injury.

External causes of death such as unintentional injuries, suicide, homicide, and legal intervention account for a combined 13.7% of deaths after SCI. Among these deaths, unintentional injuries are slightly more common than suicides and considerably more common than other external causes.

Other causes of death after SCI include symptoms and ill-defined conditions (5.3%), diseases of the digestive system (5.0%), diseases of the genitourinary (GU) system (3.6%), and cerebrovascular disease (3.3%). The decline in deaths due to genitourinary system diseases is particularly striking because this was the leading cause of death in patients with SCI 30 years ago.

In addition to considering the most common causes of death, it is also important to consider the frequency of these causes of death in relation to the general population of comparable age, gender, and race but without SCI. Overall, it has been conservatively estimated that deaths due to septicemia among patients with SCI occur at 64.2 times the normal rate, whereas deaths due to diseases of pulmonary circulation occur at 47.1 times the normal rate, and deaths due to pneumonia and influenza occur at 35.6 times the normal rate (58). Conversely, the mortality rates for ischemic heart disease and cancer in patients with SCI are similar to those of the general population, although some specific cancer mortality rates, such as that of bladder cancer, are elevated (58,65).

During the first month after injury, most deaths are due to either pneumonia (300 times the normal rate), pulmonary embolism (500 times the normal rate), symptoms and ill-defined conditions (275 times the normal rate), or septicemia (500 times the normal rate) (66). However, these extraordinarily high cause-specific mortality multiples decline rapidly after the first month after injury. For example, after the fifth postinjury year, the mortality rate for pneumonia is reduced to 19 times normal, whereas the septicemia mortality rate is 46.7 times normal, and the pulmonary embolism mortality rate is 8.9 times normal (58).

Pneumonia is by far the leading cause of death for patients with tetraplegia (24.7% of deaths for C1 through C4 injuries and 19.7% of deaths for C5 through C8 injuries), whereas heart disease (16.1%), septicemia (13.2%), and suicide (11.5%) are more common among patients with paraplegia (58). Among patients with incomplete motor functional (ASIA D) injuries at any neurologic level, heart disease again ranks as the leading cause of death (24.1%), followed by pneumonia (11.0%) (58).

LIFETIME COSTS

Managed care and other cost-containment pressures have had a dramatic effect on the way in which patients with SCI are initially treated. Average length of stay in acute care for patients enrolled in the NSCISC Database has decreased from a peak of 33 days in 1976 to 16.8 days in 1997, whereas average length of stay in inpatient rehabilitation has decreased from a peak of 127.3 days in 1974 to 51 days in 1997 (51). Conversely, in Europe, lengths of hospital stay after SCI remain high. For example, in Denmark, acute care length of stay averages about 2 months, and average rehabilitation length of stay ranges from 5 months for patients with motor incomplete paraplegia to 9.5 months for patients with motor complete tetraplegia (20).

Among patients enrolled in the NSCISC Database in 1997, average acute care charges were $89,615, and average inpatient rehabilitation charges were an additional $97,487 (51). By comparison, average charges for patients enrolled in the NSCISC Database in 1973 (in 1997 dollars) were $34,072 for acute care and $96,798 for inpatient rehabilitation (51). Average charges per day in constant 1997 dollars rose during that same period from $836 in 1973 to $2,791 in 1997, reflecting increased intensity of service (51).

Table 4.5 depicts average first-year and annual expenses in 1999 dollars for patients with SCI over their remaining lifetime by neurologic level and extent of injury. These estimates are derived from a study of model system patients performed between 1988 and 1990 and updated for inflation by using the Medical Care Component of the Consumer Price Index (67). These charges include only items that are directly related to the SCI; other medical expenses that would be encountered in the absence of SCI were not counted. Moreover, items that might have been needed or at least desirable but that were not acquired were not counted. However, an appropriate value was assigned to items that were received free of charge, and those items were

TABLE 4.5. AVERAGE ANNUAL EXPENSES AND PRESENT VALUE OF LIFETIME DIRECT COSTS OF CARE FOR PATIENTS WITH SPINAL CORD INJURY TREATED AT MODEL SYSTEMS[a]

Injury	Average Annual Expenses		Estimated Lifetime Costs	
	First Year	Each Subsequent Year	25 Years Old	50 Years Old
C1–C4	$549,800	$98,483	$2,100,185	$1,236,390
C5–C8	$355,037	$40,341	$1,187,507	$752,019
T1–S5	$200,897	$20,442	$701,716	$478,614
ASIA D	$162,032	$11,355	$468,097	$399,239

[a] In 1999 dollars discounted at 2%.

counted. Lost wages, fringe benefits, and other indirect costs are not included in these estimates. These indirect costs frequently exceed the direct costs seen in Table 4.5 (43,67).

Average first-year charges range from $549,800 for patients with C1 through C4 injury levels (excluding incomplete motor functional injuries) down to $162,032 for patients with incomplete motor functional injuries at any level, whereas average annual charges for the remainder of life are estimated to range from $98,483 to $11,355 for those same two groups of patients, respectively. More detailed predictive models reveal that patients who are ventilator dependent will experience even higher average charges in 1999 dollars of $742,765 in the first year after injury and $291,434 per year for the remainder of their life (67). These estimates of first-year and annual charges are relatively consistent with results obtained from population-based studies after conversion of those results to 1999 dollars (43,68).

A detailed categorization of these charges has been reported previously (67). During the first year, most charges result from inpatient acute care and rehabilitation, although significant charges are also often incurred for attendant care after discharge, durable equipment, and environmental modifications, particularly for patients with cervical injuries. Recurrent annual charges are mostly for attendant care and rehospitalizations, although other items, such as durable equipment, outpatient services, medications, supplies, and in some instances, substantial nursing home charges, are also incurred (67,69).

The estimated present value of average lifetime direct costs of SCI in 1999 dollars using a real discount rate of 2% for patients injured at ages 25 and 50 years by neurologic level and extent of injury also appears in Table 4.5. At age 25 years, the present value of lifetime direct costs of care is estimated to be $2,100,185 for patients with C1 through C4 injury levels and $468,097 for patients with incomplete motor functional injuries at any level. Estimates of present value of lifetime costs at age 50 years are lower because of the lower life expectancy of these patients.

Estimates of average first-year and annual charges for SCIs of different etiologies have also been reported (70). First-year and annual recurring charges are highest for SCI resulting from sports mishaps because they almost always result in cervical injuries and for motor vehicle crashes that often involve other injuries in addition to the SCI that require more intensive acute care and may delay rehabilitation. Based on a 2% real discount rate, estimated present value of total annual aggregate direct costs in the United States that could be avoided if all new SCIs could be prevented was reported to be $7.7 billion in 1995 dollars or $8.8 billion if adjusted to 1999 dollars (70). Because they are the most frequent cause of injury, motor vehicle crashes accounted for just under half of that total aggregate cost, followed by acts of violence, falls, sports, and all other causes. These estimates of SCI costs by etiology are more useful when considered from a public health or primary prevention perspective than are estimates based on injury severity.

CONCLUSION

A broad understanding of the epidemiology of SCI has emerged from a variety of sources, including the NSCISC Database, the state population-based registries, and other studies conducted both within and outside the United States. Future efforts should be directed toward attempts to standardize data collection and combine these data sources in ways that take full advantage of the unique strengths of each available database.

REFERENCES

1. Wilcox NE, Stauffer ES, Nickel VL. A statistical analysis of 423 consecutive patients admitted to the spinal cord injury center, Rancho Los Amigos Hospital, 1 January 1964, through 31 December 1967. *Paraplegia* 1970;8:27–35.
2. Fine PR, Kuhlemeier KV, DeVivo MJ, et al. Spinal cord injury: an epidemiologic perspective. *Paraplegia* 1979;17:237–250.
3. Kraus JF, Franti CE, Riggins RS, et al. Incidence of traumatic spinal cord lesions. *J Chron Dis* 1975;28:471–492.
4. Griffin MR, Opitz JL, Kurland LT, et al. Traumatic spinal cord injury in Olmsted County, Minnesota, 1935-1981. *Am J Epidemiol* 1985; 121:884–895.
5. Kalsbeek WD, McLaurin RL, Harris BSH, et al. The national head and spinal cord injury survey: major findings. *J Neurosurg* 1980;Suppl: S19-31.
6. Bracken MB, Freeman DH, Hellenbrand K. Incidence of acute traumatic hospitalized spinal cord injury in the United States, 1970–1977. *Am J Epidemiol* 1981;113:615–622.
7. Stover SL, DeVivo MJ, Go BK. History, implementation, and current status of the national spinal cord injury database. *Arch Phys Med Rehabil* 1999;80:1365–1371.
8. DeVivo MJ, Rutt RD, Black KJ, et al. Trends in spinal cord injury demographics and treatment outcomes between 1973 and 1986. *Arch Phys Med Rehabil* 1992;73:424–430.
9. Go BK, DeVivo MJ, Richards JS. The epidemiology of spinal cord injury. In: Stover SL, DeLisa JA, Whiteneck GG, eds. *Spinal cord injury: clinical outcomes from the model systems.* Gaithersburg, MD: Aspen, 1995:21–55.
10. Vogel LC, DeVivo MJ. Pediatric spinal cord injury issues: etiology, demographics and pathophysiology. *Top Spinal Cord Inj Rehabil* 1997; 3(2):1–8.
11. Nobunaga AI, Go BK, Karunas RB. Recent demographic and injury trends in people served by the model spinal cord injury care systems. *Arch Phys Med Rehabil* 1999;80:1372–1382.
12. Acton PA, Farley T, Freni LW, et al. Traumatic spinal cord injury in Arkansas, 1980–1989. *Arch Phys Med Rehabil* 1993;74:1035–1040.
13. Price C, Makintubee S, Herndon W, et al. Epidemiology of traumatic spinal cord injury and acute hospitalization and rehabilitation charges for spinal cord injuries in Oklahoma, 1988–1990. *Am J Epidemiol* 1994;139:37–47.
14. Thurman DJ, Burnett CL, Jeppson L, et al. Surveillance of spinal cord injuries in Utah, USA. *Paraplegia* 1994;32:665–669.
15. Woodruff BA, Baron RC. A description of nonfatal spinal cord injury using a hospital-based registry. *Am J Prev Med* 1994;10:10–14.
16. Johnson RL, Gabella BA, Gerhart KA, et al. Evaluating sources of traumatic spinal cord injury surveillance data in Colorado. *Am J Epidemiol* 1997;146:266–272.
17. Surkin J. Spinal cord injury: *Mississippi's facts and figures.* Mississippi State Department of Health, Jackson, MS 1995.
18. Glick T. Spinal cord injury surveillance: is there a decrease in incidence? *J Spinal Cord Med* 2000;23[Suppl]:61(abst).
19. Chen CF, Lien IN. Spinal cord injuries in Taipei, Taiwan, 1978–1981. *Paraplegia* 1985;23:364–370.
20. Biering-Sorensen F, Pedersen V, Clausen S. Epidemiology of spinal cord lesions in Denmark. *Paraplegia* 1990;28:105–118.
21. Garcia-Reneses J, Herruzo-Cabrera R, Martinez-Moreno M. Epidemiological study of spinal cord injury in Spain 1984-1985. *Paraplegia* 1991;28:180–190.
22. Karamehmetoglu SS, Unal S, Karacan I, et al. Traumatic spinal cord injuries in Istanbul, Turkey: an epidemiological study. *Paraplegia* 1995; 33:469–471.

23. Schonherr MC, Groothoff JW, Mulder GA, et al. Rehabilitation of patients with spinal cord lesions in The Netherlands: an epidemiological study. *Spinal Cord* 1996;34:679–683.

24. Otom AS, Doughan AM, Kawar JS, et al. Traumatic spinal cord injuries in Jordan: an epidemiological study. *Spinal Cord* 1997;35:253–255.

25. Martins F, Freitas F, Martins L, et al. Spinal cord injuries: epidemiology in Portugal's central region. *Spinal Cord* 1998;36:574–578.

26. DeVivo MJ, Fine PR, Maetz HM, et al. Prevalence of spinal cord injury: a reestimation employing life table techniques. *Arch Neurol* 1980;37:707–708.

27. Berkowitz M, Harvey C, Greene CG, et al. *The economic consequences of traumatic spinal cord injury.* New York: Demos, 1992.

28. Lasfargues JE, Custis D, Morrone F, et al. A model for estimating spinal cord injury prevalence in the United States. *Paraplegia* 1995;33:62–68.

29. DeVivo MJ. Head and neck injuries in industries and sports. In: Yoganandan N, Pintar FA, Larson SJ, et al., eds. *Frontiers in head and neck trauma: clinical and biomechanical.* Amsterdam: IOS Press, 1998:92–100.

30. Clarke KS. Spinal cord injuries in organized sports. *Model Systems SCI Digest* 1980;2:9–17.

31. Kraus JF, Franti CE, Riggins RS. Neurologic outcome and vehicle and crash factors in motor vehicle related spinal cord injuries. *Neuroepidemiology* 1982;1:223–238.

32. Wigglesworth EC. Motor vehicle crashes and spinal cord injury. *Paraplegia* 1992;30:543–549.

33. Fine PR, Stafford MA, Miller JM, et al. Gunshot wounds of the spinal cord: a survey of literature and epidemiologic study of 48 lesions in Alabama. *Ala J Med Sci* 1976;13:173–180.

34. Weingarden SI, Graham PM. Falls resulting in spinal cord injury: patterns and outcomes in an older population. *Paraplegia* 1989;27:423–427.

35. DeVivo MJ. Prevention of spinal cord injuries resulting from falls. *J Spinal Cord Med* 2000;23[Suppl]:15–16.

36. DeVivo MJ, Sekar P. Prevention of spinal cord injuries that occur in swimming pools. *Spinal Cord* 1997;35:509–515.

37. American Spinal Injury Association. *International standards for neurological and functional classification of spinal cord injury, revised 1996.* Chicago: American Spinal Injury Association, 1996.

38. DeVivo MJ, Richards JS. Marriage rates among persons with spinal cord injury. *Rehabil Psychol* 1996;41:321–339.

39. DeVivo MJ, Fine PR. Spinal cord injury: its short-term impact on marital status. *Arch Phys Med Rehabil* 1985;66:501–504.

40. DeVivo MJ, Hawkins LN, Richards JS, et al. Outcomes of post-spinal cord injury marriages [published erratum appears in *Arch Phys Med Rehabil* 1995;76:397]. *Arch Phys Med Rehabil* 1995;76:130–138.

41. Krause JS, Kewman D, DeVivo MJ, et al. Employment after spinal cord injury: an analysis of cases from the model spinal cord injury systems. *Arch Phys Med Rehabil* 1999;80:1492–1500.

42. DeVivo MJ, Rutt RD, Stover SL, et al. Employment after spinal cord injury. *Arch Phys Med Rehabil* 1987;68:494–498.

43. Berkowitz M, O'Leary PK, Kruse DL, et al. *Spinal cord injury: an analysis of medical and social costs.* New York: Demos, 1998.

44. James M, DeVivo MJ, Richards JS. Postinjury employment outcomes among African-American and white persons with spinal cord injury. *Rehabil Psychol* 1993;38:151–164.

45. Krause JS, Anson CA. Employment after spinal cord injury: relation to selected participant characteristics. *Arch Phys Med Rehabil* 1996;77:737–743.

46. McShane SL, Karp J. Employment following spinal cord injury: a covariance structure analysis. *Rehabil Psychol* 1993;38:27–40.

47. Hess DW, Ripley DL, McKinley WO, et al. Predictors for return to work after spinal cord injury: a 3-year multicenter analysis. *Arch Phys Med Rehabil* 2000;81:359–363.

48. Young JS, Burns PE, Bowen AM, et al. *Spinal cord injury statistics: experience of the regional spinal cord injury systems.* Phoenix: Good Samaritan Medical Center, 1982.

49. Fiedler RC, Granger CV. Uniform data system for medical rehabilitation: report of first admissions for 1996. *Am J Phys Med Rehabil* 1998;77:69–75.

50. DeVivo MJ. Discharge disposition from model spinal cord injury care system rehabilitation programs. *Arch Phys Med Rehabil* 1999;80:785–790.

51. Fiedler IG, Laud PW, Maiman DJ, et al. Economics of managed care in spinal cord injury. *Arch Phys Med Rehabil* 1999;80:1441–1449.

52. Dijkers MP, Abela MB, Gans BM. The aftermath of spinal cord injury. In: Stover SL, DeLisa JA, Whiteneck GG, eds. *Spinal cord injury: clinical outcomes from the model systems.* Gaithersburg, MD: Aspen, 1995:185–212.

53. DeVivo MJ, Richards JS, Stover SL, et al. Spinal cord injury: rehabilitation adds life to years. *West J Med* 1991;154:602–606.

54. DeVivo MJ, Shewchuk RM, Stover SL, et al. A cross-sectional study of the relationship between age and current health status for persons with spinal cord injuries. *Paraplegia* 1992;30:820–827.

55. DeVivo MJ, Stover SL, Black KJ. Prognostic factors for 12-year survival after spinal cord injury. *Arch Phys Med Rehabil* 1992;73:156–162.

56. DeVivo MJ, Krause JS, Lammertse DP. Recent trends in mortality and causes of death among persons with spinal cord injury. *Arch Phys Med Rehabil* 1999;80:1411–1419.

57. Krause JS, Sternberg M, Lottes S, et al. Mortality after spinal cord injury: an 11-year prospective study. *Arch Phys Med Rehabil* 1997;78:815–821.

58. DeVivo MJ, Stover SL. Long-term survival and causes of death. In: Stover SL, DeLisa JA, Whiteneck GG, eds. *Spinal cord injury: clinical outcomes from the model systems.* Gaithersburg, MD: Aspen, 1995:289–316.

59. DeVivo MJ, Ivie CS. Life expectancy of ventilator-dependent persons with spinal cord injuries. *Chest* 1995;108:226–232.

60. Strauss DJ, DeVivo MJ, Shavelle RM. Long-term mortality risk after spinal cord injury. *J Insurance Med* 2000;32:11–16.

61. Frankel HL, Coll JR, Charlifue SW, et al. Long-term survival in spinal cord injury: a fifty year investigation. *Spinal Cord* 1998;36:266–274.

62. Hartkopp A, Bronnum-Hansen H, Seidenschnur AM, et al. Survival and cause of death after traumatic spinal cord injury: a long-term epidemiological survey from Denmark. *Spinal Cord* 1997;35:76–85.

63. Yeo JD, Walsh J, Rutkowski S, et al. Mortality following spinal cord injury. *Spinal Cord* 1998;36:329–336.

64. McColl MA, Walker J, Stirling P, et al. Expectations of life and health among spinal cord injured adults. *Spinal Cord* 1997;35:818–828.

65. Stonehill WH, Dmochowski RR, Patterson AL, et al. Risk factors for bladder tumors in spinal cord injury patients. *J Urol* 1996;155:1248–1250.

66. DeVivo MJ, Kartus PL, Stover SL, et al. Cause of death for patients with spinal cord injuries. *Arch Intern Med* 1989;149:1761–1766.

67. DeVivo MJ, Whiteneck GG, Charles ED. The economic impact of spinal cord injury. In: Stover SL, DeLisa JA, Whiteneck GG, eds. *Spinal cord injury: clinical outcomes from the model systems.* Gaithersburg, MD: Aspen, 1995:234–271.

68. Johnson RL, Brooks CA, Whiteneck GG. Cost of traumatic spinal cord injury in a population-based registry. *Spinal Cord* 1996;34:470–480.

69. Ivie CS, DeVivo MJ. Predicting unplanned hospitalizations in persons with spinal cord injury. *Arch Phys Med Rehabil* 1994;75:1182–1188.

70. DeVivo MJ. Causes and costs of spinal cord injury in the United States. *Spinal Cord* 1997;35:809–813.

NEUROLOGIC ASSESSMENT AND CLASSIFICATION OF TRAUMATIC SPINAL CORD INJURY

STEVEN KIRSHBLUM
WILLIAM H. DONOVAN

ASSESSMENT OF SPINAL CORD INJURY

A comprehensive examination of the patient with acute spinal cord injury (SCI) is of great clinical importance and should include a general assessment of all organ systems to discover associated injuries and preexisting conditions. This is detailed in chapter 6 and may influence treatment strategies as well as outcomes. Diagnostic evaluation of patients with spinal injury using different imaging and electrodiagnostic studies and the role of these studies in predicting neurologic recovery are discussed in chapter 7.

The most accurate way to assess a patient who has sustained a SCI is by performing a standardized physical examination as endorsed by the International Standards for Neurological and Functional Classification of Spinal Cord Injury Patients, also commonly called the American Spinal Injury Association (ASIA) guidelines (1). These standards provide basic definitions of the most common terms used by clinicians in the assessment of SCI and describe the neurologic examination. Key terms used in traumatic SCI are defined in Table 5.1.

The neurologic examination of the patient with SCI has two main components, sensory and motor, with certain required and optional elements. The required elements allow the determination of the sensory, motor, and neurologic levels; generation of sensory and motor index scores; determination of the completeness of the injury; and classification of the impairment. The rectal examination, which tests for voluntary anal contraction and deep anal sensation, is part of the required components of the examination. The information from this neurologic examination can be recorded on a standardized flow sheet that should be included in the medical records (Fig. 5.1). Optional elements (described later) include aspects of the neurologic examination that may better describe the patients' clinical condition but are not used for numeric scoring. To learn how to use the International Standards correctly, an instructional manual and three videotapes have been produced and can be obtained through the ASIA office in Atlanta.

Sensory Examination

There are 28 key dermatomes, each separately tested for pinprick/dull (with a safety pin) and light touch (with a cotton-tip applicator) on both sides of the body (Fig. 5.1). These points were adapted from Austin and received consensus among experienced spinal cord physicians (2). A three-point scale (0 to 2) is used, with the face as the normal control point. For the pinprick examination, the patient must be able to distinguish between the pin (sharp edge) and the dull edge of a disposable safety pin. Absent sensation, which includes the inability to distinguish between the sharp and dull edge of the pin, yields a score of 0. A score of 1 (impaired) for pinprick testing is given when the patient can distinguish between the sharp and dull edge of the pin, but the pin is not felt as sharp as on the face. The impaired score is also given if the patient reports altered sensation, including hyperesthesia. If there is a question about whether the patient can definitively discriminate between the pin and dull edges, 8 of 10 correct answers is considered accurate (3). The score of 2 (normal or intact) is given only if the pin is felt as sharp, in the tested dermatome, as when tested on the face.

For light touch, a cotton-tip applicator is used, with 2 (intact) being the same touch sensation as on the face and 1 (impaired) if less than on the face. The cotton-tip swab should be stroked across the skin moving over a distance not to exceed 1 cm (3). When testing the digits for dermatomes C6 through C8, the dorsal surface of the proximal phalanx should be tested. When testing the chest and abdomen, sensory testing should be performed at the mid-clavicular line.

It is extremely important to test the S4-5 dermatome (one area tested for the S4-5 dermatome) for both pinprick and light touch because this represents the most caudal aspect of the sacral spinal cord. To test for deep anal sensation, a rectal digital examination is performed. The patient is asked to report any sensory awareness, touch, or pressure, with firm pressure of the examiner's digit on the rectal walls. Deep anal sensation is recorded as either present or absent.

The *sensory level* is the most caudal dermatome to have intact (2/2) sensation for both pinprick and light touch on both sides of the body. *Sensory index scoring* is calculated by adding the scores for each dermatome, for a total score possible of 112 (56 on each side) for pinprick and for light touch.

An important feature regarding sensory testing is to recognize that the C4 dermatome comes down low on the upper part of the chest, even as far as the T3 interspace in some people. Therefore, when sensory loss begins at or just above the nipple line (T4 dermatome), careful sensory testing at key points on the

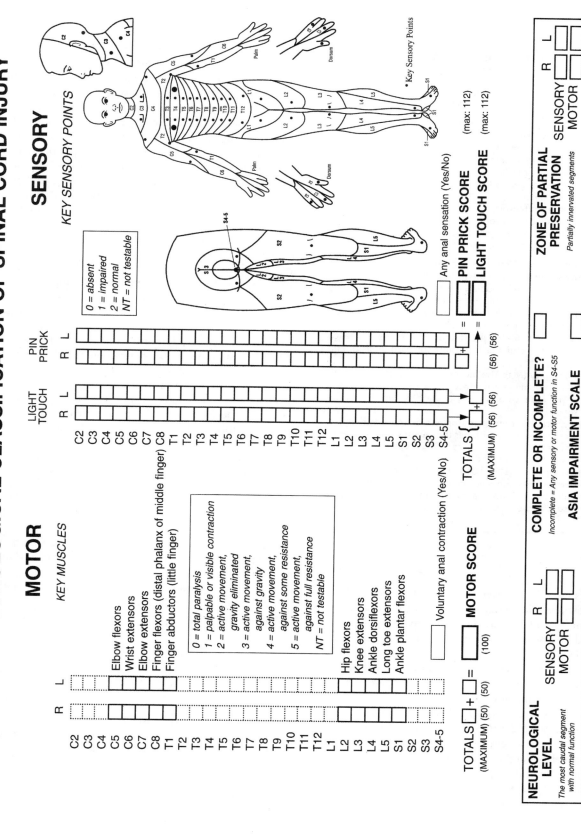

FIGURE 5.1. American Spinal Injury Association flow sheet. From American Spinal Injury Association/International Medical Society of Paraplegia. *International standards for neurological and functional classification of spinal cord injury patients.* Chicago: 2000, with permission.

TABLE 5.1. GLOSSARY OF KEY TERMS

Key muscle groups: Ten muscle groups that are tested as part of the standardized spinal cord examination.

Root Level	Muscle Group
C5	Elbow flexors
C6	Wrist extensors
C7	Elbow extensors
C8	Long finger flexors
T1	Small finger abductors
L2	Hip flexors
L3	Knee extensors
L4	Ankle dorsiflexors
L5	Long toe extensor
S1	Ankle plantarflexors

Motor level: The most caudal key muscle group that is graded 3/5 or greater with the segments cephalad graded normal (5/5) strength.

Motor index score: Calculated by adding the muscle scores of each key muscle group; a total score of 100 is possible.

Sensory level: The most caudal dermatome to have normal sensation for both pinprick/dull and light touch on both sides.

Sensory index score: Calculated by adding the scores for each dermatome; a total score of 112 is possible for each pinprick and light touch.

Neurologic level of injury (NLI): The most caudal level at which both motor and sensory modalities are intact.

Complete injury: The absence of sensory and motor function in the lowest sacral segments.

Incomplete injury: Preservation of motor and/or sensory function below the neurologic level that includes the lowest sacral segments.

Skeletal level: The level at which, by radiologic examination, the greatest vertebral damage is found.

Zone of partial preservation (ZPP): Used only with complete injuries, refers to the dermatomes and myotomes caudal to the neurologic level that remain partially innervated. The most caudal segment with some sensory and/or motor function defines the extent of the ZPP.

upper limbs is essential to determine properly a sensory level, rather than just assuming a T3 sensory level (3). In a patient who has absent T1 and T2 sensation with apparently preserved T3, T3 should be scored as absent if there is no sensation at the nipple level (T4).

If accurate sensory testing in any dermatome cannot be performed, NT (not tested) should be recorded, or an alternate location within the dermatome can be tested with notation that an alternate site was used. If NT has been documented at any level, then a sensory score cannot be calculated. Optional elements of the ASIA sensory examination are also important and strongly recommended and include proprioception (joint position and vibration) and deep-pressure sensations. These can be graded as absent, impaired, or normal. Only one joint is tested for each extremity; the index finger and the great toe are recommended (1).

Motor Examination

The required elements of the ASIA motor examination consists of testing 10 key muscles: 5 in the upper limb and 5 in the lower limb on each side of the body (Table 5.1). Other muscles are also clinically important but are viewed as optional in that they do not contribute to the motor scores or levels (4). The muscles should be examined in a rostral to caudal sequence, starting with the elbow flexors (C5 tested muscle) and finishing with the ankle plantar flexors (S1 muscle). Testing of all key muscles during the initial and the follow-up examinations are performed with the patient in the supine position and graded and recorded on the standard form, on a six-point scale from 0 to 5 (5). Testing in the supine position, although different from classic teaching for manual muscle testing (MMT), is recommended for SCI evaluations to allow for a valid comparison of a patient's scores obtained during the acute period (i.e., because of an unstable spine) to those obtained during the rehabilitation and follow-up phases of care. For purposes of inter-rater reliability, it has been recommended that only whole numbers (rather than pluses and minuses) be used when comparing data from one institution to another. To be confident that a true change in strength has occurred, muscle grades should change more than one full grade (6).

Although there is a clear distinction for each root level during sensory testing (one site per dermatome tested), the myotomes are not as clearly delineated. Although each of the key muscles has one root listed, more than one root segment and usually two segments innervate most muscles. The key muscles tested have been chosen because of their consistency for being innervated primarily by the segments indicated and for their ease of testing in the supine position. If a particular muscle has a grade of 3/5, it is considered to have full innervation by at least the more cephalad nerve root segment. In addition, a muscle with a grade of at least 3/5 has antigravity strength and is considered useful for functional activities (7,8). A muscle initially graded 5/5 (normal) would be considered to be fully innervated by both spinal root segments.

Voluntary anal contraction is tested as part of the motor examination by sensing contraction of the external anal sphincter around the examiner's finger and graded as either present or absent. It is important not to confuse a reflex contraction of the anal sphincter with voluntary contraction. During the rectal examination, one should also document the presence or absence of anal sensation, as previously described.

Placing the joints in the proper position during MMT, by stabilizing above and below the joint tested, to ensure proper biomechanics for the muscle being tested is important, especially if the muscles do not have antigravity strength. This will also help prevent confusion with vicarious movements that may occur. For example, when testing the flexor digitorum profundus, the wrist must be stabilized so that passive movement caused by extension of the wrist is not misinterpreted as voluntary movement of the distal phalanx.

An important aspect to remember when muscle testing a newly injured individual with a lesion below T8 is that the hip should not be flexed passively or actively beyond 90 degrees because this may place too great a kyphotic stress on the lumbar spine (4). In a patient who may have an unstable spine or be in too much pain to lift up their leg, MMT should be tested isometrically by placing a hand on the patient's thigh just above the knee and asking the patient to lift while the examiner offers resistance to movement. The examiner can grade the force between the grades of 2 and 5 (4). If the patient has only minimal movement, the examiner should palpate over the more superficial hip flexors (i.e., sartorius, rectus femoris) rather than the iliopsoas because the iliopsoas is too deep to palpate (4).

The *motor level* is the lowest normal motor segment, which may differ by side of the body. It is defined as the lowest key muscle that has a grade of at least 3, providing the key muscles represented by segments above that level are graded as 5 (1).

Often, the patients' clinical condition may prevent the completion of an accurate examination. Limiting factors, such as pain and deconditioning, may be present such that the patient only grades a 4/5. In these situations, the muscle should be graded as a 5 with an asterisk (*) to indicate that inhibiting factors were present (4). When the patient is not fully testable for any reason, including spasticity that prevents accurate stabilization of the joint, uncontrolled clonus, severe pain, or a fracture that limits the examination, the examiner should record NT instead of a numeric score. If a contracture limits less than 50% of the normal range, then the muscle is graded through its available range subject to the same criteria of the 0 to 5 scale. If the contracture limits more than 50% of the normal range, then the muscle should be graded NT (4). Other examples of when NT should be recorded include when a patient is comatose from an associated traumatic brain injury, has an injury to the brachial or lumbosacral plexi, or has a limb immobilized because of a fracture. If NT is used, and this muscle is required for determination of the motor level, the designation of the motor level for that side should be deferred.

Handheld instruments for objective muscle testing have been developed and have proved reliable and valid to assess strength (9,10). Herbison and colleagues found that the handheld myometer detected changes in muscle strength not detected by MMT, especially in muscles with strength graded higher than 3/5 (10). However, MMT remains the most common tool used by clinicians and researchers to assess individuals with SCI (10).

Motor index scoring is calculated by adding the muscle scores of each key muscle group (1). The total score possible is 100, 25 for each extremity. If NT has been documented, then a motor index score cannot be calculated. Pluses and minuses are not considered for motor index scoring (4).

A number of optional muscles (diaphragm, deltoids, abdominal muscles, medial hamstrings, and hip adductors) may also be tested, which may be helpful in determining involvement of certain regions of the spinal cord, but are not used to obtain a motor index score (4). The strength of the muscles is described as absent, weak, or normal (1). The diaphragm can be tested by measurement of the vital capacity but may also be tested under fluoroscopy to determine the extent of involvement. Movement of the hemidiaphragm two or more interspaces generally indicates normal function on that side. The deltoid, although important with respect to function because it provides a major contribution for reach of the upper extremity, is not used for motor scoring because it cannot properly be tested in the supine position. Looking for the Beevor sign can test the abdominal muscles (innervated by T6 through T12). With the patient flexing the head and neck (a half sit-up), if the patient has a lesion between T9 and T11, the umbilicus will move rostrally because the upper abdominal muscles are innervated at and above T10. This test should not be performed during the acute stages of thoracic and lumbar injuries. The hip adductor muscle, although not used as part of the motor score, is an important muscle to monitor because it is often the first muscle to recover in the lower extremities.

The *neurologic level of injury* (NLI) is the most caudal level at which both motor and sensory modalities are intact on both sides of the body. If the motor level is C7 and the sensory level is C8, the overall NLI is C7. The motor or sensory level may be different from side to side; therefore, up to four different levels are possible. It is strongly recommended that each level be recorded separately and that a single level not be used (i.e., right C6 motor, C7 sensory; left C7 motor, C6 sensory) because it presents a clearer picture of the patient's status. Motor and sensory levels are the same in less than 50% of complete injuries, and the motor level may be multiple levels below the sensory level 1 year after injury (11,12).

The motor level and upper extremity motor index score better reflect the degree of function and the severity of impairment and disability, relative to the NLI, after motor complete tetraplegia (11). This is because the sensory level may place the neurologic level more cephalad, thereby incorrectly implying poorer function. In addition, there is variability in dermatomes and dermatomal maps, which can lead to inconsistencies when using the sensory level in classifying individuals with SCI.

In cases in which there is no key muscle for a segment that has sensory dermatomes intact (these include C2 through C4, T2 through L1, and S2 through S5), the sensory level, and therefore the neurologic level, is the one that defines the motor level. In a case in which the elbow flexors graded 3/5 on both sides and the wrist extensors were 1 or 2/5, with a sensory level on the left at C4 and on the right C3, the motor level on the left would be C5 and on the right C3 (13). On the right side, because the C4 dermatome is abnormal, it is assumed that the C4 myotome is also impaired; therefore, the motor level is C3. On the left side, the C4 dermatome tests normal, so that the C4 myotome is considered normal. As a result, the left motor level is C5 because the C5 key muscle—elbow flexion—is at least 3, with the segments above being normal (13).

The *skeletal level of injury* is defined as the spinal level at which, by radiographic examination, the greatest vertebral damage is found.

CLASSIFICATION OF SPINAL CORD INJURY

Until recent years, there was confusion regarding the definitions of the neurologic and functional deficits of SCI. It was therefore difficult to measure clinically and scientifically the outcome of different treatments. Using a standard method of neurologic assessment is important to help determine the course of recovery and the effect of interventions in the treatment of SCI, including regeneration (14).

To address this issue, leading physicians in the field of SCI from 15 different countries responded to a questionnaire in 1969, to establish international agreement on neurologic terminology for SCI and to compare their opinions on the best time to make an accurate prognosis following SCI. Their recommendations were published, but there was no agreement on the overall classification of SCI (15). Below is described a historical per-

TABLE 5.2. FRANKEL SCALE

A—Complete: Motor and sensory function below the segmental level was absent.

B—Sensory only: Implies some sensation present below the lesion but that the motor paralysis was complete below that level. This does not apply when there is a slight discrepancy between the motor and sensory level but does apply to sacral sparing.

C—Motor useless: Some motor power present below the lesion but of no practical use to the patient.

D—Motor useful: Implies that there was some useful motor power below the level of the lesion, that is, some patients could move the lower limbs, and many could walk, with or without aids.

E—Recovery: Free of neurologic symptoms, that is, no weakness, no sensory loss, no sphincter disturbances. Abnormal reflexes may be present.

From Frankel HL, Hancock DO, Hyslop G, et al. The value of postural reduction in initial management of closed injuries of the spine with paraplegia and tetraplegia, *Paraplegia* 1969–70; 7:179–192, with permission.

spective on the development and changes in the ASIA standards over the years, leading to the current classification.

Many systems have since been developed for the classification of SCI. These have included those based on bony patterns of injury, mechanism of injury, neurologic function, and functional outcome (16–22). In 1969, Frankel and associates described a five-grade system of classifying traumatic SCI, with a division into complete and incomplete injuries (23) (Table 5.2). The amount of preserved sensory or motor function determined the specific Frankel classification. The purpose of this article was to describe results of postural reduction in the treatment of SCI, and they described their classification as "crude."

To improve accurate communication and consistency among clinicians and researchers, in 1982, ASIA first developed and published a booklet, *Standards for Neurological Classification of Spinal Injured Patients* (24). The 1982 standards incorporated the Frankel grades A through E and the classification of Lucas and Ducker who first introduced motor scores (25). Sensory testing was recommended in 29 dermatomes as adapted from Austin (2). Motor testing was recommended with scoring of 10 key muscle groups, with the deltoid or biceps used for testing the C5 myotome. Bracken and colleagues introduced the sensory scores on a three-point scale, testing each side of the body for light touch and pinprick (19). The 1982 standards defined the neurologic level of injury, quadriplegia and quadraparesis, paraplegia and paraparesis, and complete and incomplete injury. It provided sensory dermatomes for sensory classification and key muscles for motor classification; it also defined the "zone of injury" as up to three neurologic segments at the point of damage to the spinal cord, where there is frequently some preservation of motor or sensory function. The standards also described a number of anatomic incomplete clinical syndromes.

Chehrazi and associates presented the Yale Scale in 1981 that tested 10 muscles on each side of the body, using the six-point muscle grading system (21). Lucas and Drucker suggested testing 14 muscles (25), whereas Bracken initially chose 15 muscles on each side of the body using a modified grading system (26). Bracken and colleagues in the National Acute Spinal Cord Injury

Study I (NASCIS-I) and NASCIS-II used 14 muscles on each side of the body (27,28). The Frankel Classification and the subsequent ASIA Impairment Scale have used the 10 key muscle groups (1,24). El Masry and coauthors found the ASIA and NASCIS motor scoring systems comparable in representing motor deficits and recovery (29). Because the ASIA motor scoring system offers the smaller amount of muscles to be tested and is reliable in representing the conventional motor score, they suggested that it be used to assess muscle strength in individuals with SCI (29).

The motor level in the 1982 classification was defined as the level that graded 3 (fair) with the level above it grading 4 (good) or 5 (normal) (24). A complete injury was defined as "no preservation of any motor and/or sensory function below the zone of injury" and an incomplete injury as "preservation of any motor and/or sensory function below the zone of injury." Frankel A was defined as a complete injury. Frankel B was defined as the preservation of sensation below the level of injury, excluding phantom sensations, with absent voluntary motor function. Frankel C was initially described as nonfunctional motor sparing below the zone of injury, whereby there was "preservation of voluntary motor function which performs no useful purpose except psychologically," and Frankel D (functional) as "preservation of voluntary motor function which is useful functionally." Frankel E represented complete recovery, which included return of all motor and sensory function, but possibly with abnormal reflexes (24).

These standards were refined over the next 10 years, involving input from SCI clinicians and researchers (30). Tator and associates recommended changing the terminology of Frankel classifications C and D (31). Donovan and coauthors showed that considerable discrepancies existed, even among experienced clinicians, in the use of the 1982 standards to classify SCI patients (32). In 1989, Donovan led an ASIA ad hoc committee that further defined key muscles and sensory points and clarified Frankel grades and the *zone of partial preservation* (ZPP) (33). Changes included the use of specific key areas with anatomic landmarks to define the sensory level, combining the S4 and S5 dermatomes into a single S4-5 dermatome (perianal area), and redefining the zone of injury as the ZPP of sensory or motor function. Other changes included having only the elbow flexors examined to test the C5 myotome, clarifying muscle grading in the determination of motor levels, and clarifying the Frankel classification in terms of the degree of incompleteness. Frankel C was changed to be defined as the majority of key muscles below the level of injury graded less than 3/5, and Frankel D as the majority of key muscles below the NLI graded at least 3/5, as previously recommended by Tator and associates (31). Use of the terms quadraparesis and paraparesis was discouraged because they imprecisely described incomplete lesions. In 1989, ASIA adopted these changes (33).

Priebe and Waring found that the interobserver reliability of patient classification based on these revised (1989) standards, although improved from the 1982 standards, continued to be less than optimal (34). They recommended that a number of changes be made to improve interobserver reliability, including clearly identifying the inguinal ligament to better delineate the T12 and L1 dermatomes, clarifying the motor score needed to

TABLE 5.3. ASIA IMPAIRMENT SCALE

A—Complete: No sensory or motor function preserved in the lowest sacral segments, S4–S5.
B—Incomplete: Sensory but no motor function preserved below the neurologic level, including the sacral segments S4–S5.
C—Incomplete: Motor function is preserved below the neurologic level, and most key muscles below the neurologic level have a muscle grade less than 3.
D—Incomplete: Motor function is preserved below the neurologic level, and most key muscles below the neurologic level have a muscle grade greater than or equal to 3.
E—Normal: Sensory and motor functions are normal.

From American Spinal Injury Association/International Medical Society of Paraplegia. *International standards for neurological and functional classification of spinal cord injury patients.* Chicago: 1992, with permission.

identify the motor level with incomplete injuries, and instituting training methods to highlight the changes made (34).

The Frankel classification was replaced in 1992 by the *ASIA Impairment Scale* (Table 5.3). This scale was revised in 1996 and again in the year 2000 (1,35,36) (Table 5.4). The 1992 standards included additional features, such as the assessment of disability by incorporating the functional independence measure (FIM), and modification of the definitions of complete and incomplete injuries (requiring that "sacral sparing" be used to define the incompleteness of injury). Modifications were also made in some of the key sensory points, testing pinprick and light touch separately on a three-point scale, developing a new sensory scoring system (sensory index scoring), and modifying the definition of the ZPP. The name of the Frankel classification was officially changed, in 1992, to the ASIA Impairment Scale, and optional tests (position sense, vibration, and additional muscles to localize better the level of the lesion) were added. These standards were endorsed by the International Medical Society of Paraplegia and thereafter became known as the *International Standards for Neurological and Functional Classification of Spinal Cord Injury Patients* (36).

TABLE 5.4. ASIA IMPAIRMENT SCALE[a]

A—Complete: No motor or sensory function is preserved in the sacral segments S4–S5.
B—Incomplete: Sensory but not motor function preserved below the neurologic level and includes the sacral segments S4–S5.
C—Motor function is preserved below the neurologic level, and more than half of the key muscles below the neurologic level have a muscle grade less than 3.
D—Incomplete: Motor function is preserved below the neurologic level, and at least half of key muscles below the neurologic level have a muscle grade of 3 or more.
E—Normal: Motor and sensory function are normal.

[a]Revised 1996 (36) and 2000 (1) standards.
Note: For an individual to receive a grade of C or D, he or she must be incomplete, that is, have sensory or motor function in the sacral segments S4–S5. In addition, the individual must have either (a) voluntary anal sphincter contraction or (b) sparing of motor function more than three levels below the motor level (1).

The definition of the motor level was changed in 1992 to the lowest key muscle group that has a grade of at least 3, provided that the muscles innervated by segments above that level were graded 5 (normal). Grade 4 was not to be considered normal, as it was previously, unless the examiner judged that certain inhibiting factors, such as pain, positioning of the patient, hypertonicity, or disuse, inhibited full effort.

The 1992 standards further defined many key terms. *Tetraplegia*, preferred to the term quadriplegia, is defined as impairment or loss of motor or sensory function in the cervical segments of the spinal cord due to damage of neural elements within the spinal cord. It does not include brachial plexus lesions or injury to the peripheral nerves outside the neural canal (35). Tetraplegia results in impairment of function in the arms as well as the trunk, legs and pelvic organs. *Paraplegia* refers to impairment of motor or sensory function in the thoracic, lumbar, or sacral segments of the spinal cord secondary to damage of neural elements within the spinal canal. With paraplegia, neurologic function in the upper extremities is spared, but depending on the level of injury, the trunk, legs, and pelvic organs may be involved. Paraplegia can also refer to cauda equina and conus medullaris injuries, but not lumbosacral plexus lesions or injuries to peripheral nerves outside the neural canal (35). The terms quadriparesis (tetraparesis) and paraparesis are discouraged because they describe incomplete lesions imprecisely. Rather, a more precise description should be applied for incomplete lesions.

Since 1992, *complete* injury is defined as the absence of sensory or motor function in the lowest sacral segments, and *incomplete* injury is defined as preservation of motor function or sensation below the NLI that includes the lowest sacral segments (*sacral sparing*). Sacral sparing is tested by light touch and pinprick at the anal mucocutaneous junction (S4-5 dermatome), on both sides, as well as by testing voluntary anal contraction and deep anal sensation as part of the rectal examination. If any of these is present (sacral sparing), intact or impaired, the individual has an incomplete injury. According to this definition, a patient with cervical SCI can have sensory and motor function in the trunk or even the legs, but unless sacral sparing is present, the injury must be classified as complete (ASIA A), with a large ZPP (see later). When sacral sparing is used to define incompleteness, motor recovery is significantly more likely to occur than when it is not (37). The sacral sparing definition of the completeness of the injury is a more stable definition because fewer patients convert from incomplete to complete status over time after injury, which is the basis for changing the definitions (37). The ASIA Impairment Scale, similar to the Frankel classification, describes five different levels of SCI severity.

The ZPP, in 1992, was defined as all segments below the NLI with preservation of sensory function and used only in complete (ASIA A) injuries (1,35,36). When some impaired sensory or motor function was found below the lowest normal segment, the exact number of segments was to be recorded on the classification form for sensory and motor function bilaterally (35). Cohen and Bartko tested both the interrater and intrarater reliability of the skills of the examination and classification using the 1992 standards (38). The 1992 changes were thought to result in excellent reliability for the examination procedure but revealed that discrepancies still existed in the classification of injury (38,39). Clifton and colleagues tested the intrarater reliability of the 1992 standards and found the motor score to be very reliable but the sensory score less so (40). At the 1994 ASIA conference, the 1992 standards were tested after an instructional course (41). Results showed that further revisions were required to ensure accurate classification of SCI. Some of the areas of confusion noted were later clarified by the 1996 revision of the standards. Donovan and associates tested the 1992 standards, by having SCI specialists review two case reports (42). They also found that further revisions were needed to clarify the determination of sensory levels and how to score muscles whose strength is inhibited by pain.

The 1996 revision clarified how to score muscles whose strength may be affected by inhibiting factors, such that if any of the previously mentioned inhibiting factors impede muscle testing and grading, the muscle should be graded NT (36) (Table 5.4). However, if it is the examiner's judgment that the muscle would test grade 5 (normal), rather than grade 4, were it not for these inhibiting factors, the muscle may be graded as 5/5 (normal). To clarify the distinction between ASIA C and D, the term "majority" was replaced by the phrase of "at least half of the key muscles" for the classification of ASIA D and "more than half the key muscles" for the classification of ASIA C. The 1996 standards also included instructions regarding when the sensory level falls into a region where the muscles cannot be clinically tested (C1 through C4, T2 through L1, and S3 through S5), whereby the motor level is designated as being the same as the sensory level.

The revisions to the standards in 2000 clarified a few issues (1). First, for an individual to receive an ASIA classification of motor incomplete (ASIA C or D), they must have either (a) voluntary anal sphincter contraction, or (b) sensory sacral sparing with sparing of motor function more than 3 levels below the motor level (1). Previously, the patient needed only to have sparing more than two levels below the motor level (4,35). Another major change in the 2000 revisions is the elimination of the FIM from the standards.

Finally, there was a change in the way the ZPP is to be documented. Now, only the most caudal segment with some sensory or motor function should be recorded on the form for sensory and motor function bilaterally. For example, if the right sensory level is C5 and some sensation extends to C8, then C8 is recorded in the right sensory ZPP block on the classification form (1).

Utilizing the American Spinal Injury Association 2000 Standards

Below is a summary of the steps in classifying an individual with a SCI.

1. Perform sensory examination in 28 dermatomes bilaterally for pinprick and light touch, including the S4-5 dermatome, and test for anal sensation on rectal examination.
2. Determine sensory level (right and left) and total sensory score.

3. Perform motor examination in the 10 key muscle groups, including voluntary anal contraction on rectal examination.
4. Determine motor level (right and left) and motor index score.
5. Determine the NLI.
6. Classify injury as complete or incomplete.
7. Categorize ASIA Impairment Scale (A through E).
8. Determine ZPP if ASIA A.

If a patient has a sensory incomplete lesion and absence of all the key muscle groups below the NLI, but has voluntary sphincter contraction, the injury is classified as ASIA C. In a case like this, however, the examiner should be careful that he or she is feeling the anal sphincter rather than contracting gluteal muscles or a reflex sphincter contraction, as in a bulbocavernosus reflex. When in doubt, the patient should be scored as not having voluntary power of the anal sphincter (13).

Having a well-defined classification of SCI allows clinicians and researchers to study the effect of drug and rehabilitation interventions and to determine prognosis. The International Standards are the most valid and reliable classification to assess SCI and are used by the Model System Spinal Cord Injury database (43).

CLINICAL SYNDROMES OF SPINAL CORD INJURY

Different clinical syndromes of SCI are frequently referred to by clinicians and in the literature, and include central cord, Brown-Séquard, anterior cord, posterior cord, conus medullaris, and cauda equina syndromes. In general, these syndromes do not accurately describe the extent of the neurologic deficit; however, they are important to define (Table 5.5).

Bing reported on the Brown-Séquard, anterior cord, posterior cord, conus medullaris, and cauda equina syndromes (44), and Schneider and colleagues on the central cord syndrome (45). These original definitions have remained for the most part unchanged, except that central cord syndrome may be a predominately white-matter lesion in some instances (46,47). However, when this syndrome is accompanied by lower motor neuron findings in the arms, gray-matter involvement can be assumed (48).

Central Cord Syndrome

The most common of the incomplete syndromes is central cord syndrome. This applies almost exclusively to cervical injuries and is characterized by motor weakness in the upper extremities greater than the lower extremities, in association with sacral sparing (45). In addition to the motor weakness, other features include bladder dysfunction and varying sensory loss below the level of the lesion. Although central cord syndrome most frequently occurs in older patients with cervical spondylosis and hyperextension injury, the syndrome may occur in patients of any age and is associated with other etiologies, predisposing factors, and injury mechanisms. The postulated mechanism of injury involves compression of the cord both anteriorly and poste-

TABLE 5.5. INCOMPLETE CLINICAL SYNDROMES

Syndrome	Main Symptoms	Prognosis for Recovery
Central cord	• Greater weakness in the upper limbs than in the lower limbs • Occurs almost exclusively in the cervical region • Frequently seen in elderly patients and those with cervical stenosis	• Favorable prognosis for walking and activities of daily living based on age (<50 yr old greater improvement than >50) • Recovery occurs earliest in legs, followed by bladder, then proximal upper extremity muscles and intrinsics last
Brown-Séquard	• Greater ipsilateral proprioceptive and motor loss and contralateral loss of sensitivity to pain and temperature	• Best prognosis for ambulation • Recovery starts in ipsilateral proximal extensors, then the distal flexors
Posterior cord	• Loss of propioception • Maintains pain and temperature as well as varying degree of motor function	• Difficulty with ambulation secondary to proprioceptive losses
Anterior cord	• Variable loss of motor function and pain and temperature while preserving propioception	• Poor prognosis for recovery of lower extremity function and ambulation

riorly, with inward bulging of the ligamentum flavum during hyperextension in an already narrowed spinal canal (49).

Central cord syndrome usually has a favorable prognosis (50–53). The typical pattern of recovery usually occurs earliest and to the greatest extent in the lower extremities, followed by bowel and bladder function, upper extremity (proximal) function, and then intrinsic (distal) hand function. Penrod and others have noted that the prognosis for functional recovery of ambulation, activities of daily living, and bowel and bladder function is dependent on the patient's age, with a less optimistic prognosis in older patients relative to younger patients (50–53). Specifically, patients younger than 50 years of age were much more successful in becoming independent in ambulation than older patients (87% to 97% versus 31% to 41%) (50–52). Similar differences were seen between the younger and older patients in independent bladder function (83% versus 29%), independent bowel function (63% versus 24%), and dressing independently (77% versus 12%) (53). However, in patients with initial neurologic examinations (within 72 hours) with a classification of ASIA D tetraplegia, prognosis for recovery of independent ambulation is excellent, even for those older than 50 years of age (54).

Cruciate Paralysis

A syndrome with similar clinical features of upper extremity paresis or paralysis, with minimal to no lower extremity involvement, is cruciate paralysis, first described by Bell (55). This may occur with fractures of C1 and C2, with neurologic compromise at the cervicomedullary junction (56). In central cord syndrome, the injury is usually localized in the middle to lower segments of the cervical spinal cord, whereas in cruciate paralysis, the damage is higher, with respiratory insufficiency occurring in roughly 25% of patients (56). A number of reports have appeared in the literature of cases in which this diagnosis is sus-

pected (57–60). The prognosis for cruciate paralysis is good, with most patients demonstrating complete recovery.

Wallenberg proposed an anatomic explanation for this clinical syndrome (61). He suggested that the decussation of the fibers to the upper limb lay in a more rostral, medial, and ventral location in the cervicomedullary junction, as compared with a more lateral and caudal location of the lower limb decussating fibers. Therefore, injury to the canal where the upper extremity fibers travel alone after decussation causes preferential injury to the upper limbs. Neuroanatomic evidence to support this hypothesis, however, has not been found (62–64).

Brown-Séquard Syndrome

Brown-Séquard syndrome involves a hemisection of the spinal cord, consisting of asymmetric paresis with hypalgesia more marked on the less paretic side. It accounts for 2% to 4% of all traumatic spinal cord injuries (65–67). In the classic presentation, there is (a) ipsilateral loss of all sensory modalities at the level of the lesion; (b) ipsilateral flaccid paralysis at the level of the lesion; (c) ipsilateral loss of position sense and vibration below the lesion; (d) contralateral loss of pain and temperature below the lesion; and (e) ipsilateral motor loss below the level of the lesion. Neuroanatomically, this is explained by the crossing of the spinothalamic tracts in the spinal cord, as opposed to the corticospinal and dorsal columns, which decussate in the brain stem.

Only a limited number of patients have the pure form of Brown-Séquard syndrome; much more common is Brown-Séquard plus syndrome, which refers to a relative ipsilateral hemiplegia with a relative contralateral hemianalgesia (68). Although Brown-Séquard syndrome has traditionally been associated with knife injuries, a variety of etiologies, including those that result in closed spinal injuries with or without vertebral fractures, may be the cause (68–70). In addition, neoplastic causes, as well as intramedullary inflammatory lesions, such as in multiple sclerosis, can result in partial or complete Brown-Séquard syndrome (69).

Despite the variation in presentation, considerable consistency is found in the prognosis of Brown-Séquard syndrome. Recovery takes place in the ipsilateral proximal extensors and then the distal flexors (71,72). Motor recovery of any extremity having a pain or temperature sensory deficit occurs before the opposite extremity, and these patients may expect functional gait recovery by 6 months. Overall, patients with Brown-Séquard syndrome have the greatest prognosis for functional outcome and potential for ambulation. Seventy-five to 90% of patients ambulate independently at discharge from rehabilitation, and nearly 70% perform functional skills and activities of daily living independently (66,68). The most important predictor of function is whether the upper or lower limb is the predominant site of weakness: when the upper limb is weaker than the lower limb, patients are more likely to ambulate at discharge. Recovery of bowel and bladder function is also favorable, with continent bladder and bowel function achieved in 89% and 82% of patients, respectively, in one study (68).

Anterior Cord Syndrome

The anterior cord syndrome involves a lesion affecting the anterior two thirds of the spinal cord while preserving the posterior columns. It may occur with retropulsed disk or bone fragments, direct injury to the anterior spinal cord, or lesions of the anterior spinal artery, which provides the blood supply to the anterior spinal cord (73,74). There is a variable loss of motor and pinprick sensation, with a relative preservation of light touch, proprioception, and deep-pressure sensation. Usually, patients with anterior cord syndrome have only a 10% to 20% chance of muscle recovery, and even in those with some recovery, there is poor muscle power and coordination (75).

Posterior Cord Syndrome

The posterior cord syndrome is the least common of the incomplete SCI syndromes and has been omitted from recent versions of the International Standards (1,36). It is characterized by preservation of pain, temperature, and touch appreciation with varying degrees of motor preservation and an absence of all dorsal column function. Prognosis for ambulation is poor, secondary to the propioceptive deficits.

Conus Medullaris and Cauda Equina Injuries

The conus medullaris, which is the terminal segment of the adult spinal cord, lies at the inferior aspect of the L1 vertebra (see chapter 2 for details). The segment above the conus medullaris is termed the *epiconus* and consists of spinal cord segments L4 through S1. Nerve roots then travel, from the conus medullaris caudally, as the cauda equina. Lesions of the epiconus affect the lower lumbar roots supplying muscles of the lower part of the leg and foot, with sparing of reflex function of sacral segments. The bulbocavernosus reflex and micturition reflexes are pre-

served, representing an upper motor neuron or suprasacral lesion. Spasticity most likely develops in sacral innervated segments (toe flexors, ankle plantar flexors, and hamstring muscles). Recovery is similar to that of other upper motor neuron spinal cord injuries.

Conus medullaris lesions affecting neural segments S2 and below present with lower motor neuron deficits of the anal sphincter and bladder due to damage of the anterior horn cells of S2 through S4. Bladder and rectal reflexes are diminished or absent, depending on the exact level and extent of the lesion. There is paralysis of the bladder detrusor muscle due to destruction of the preganglionic parasympathetic fibers, with retention of urine and overflow incontinence. In men, there is failure of penile erections and ejaculation due to the destruction of the preganglionic parasympathetic neurons and the somatic motor ventral horn cells, respectively. Emission of semen can still occur because the motor fibers to the ductus deferens and seminal vesicles have sympathetic innervation. Motor strength in the legs and feet may remain intact if the nerve roots (L3 through S2) are not affected. The lumbar nerve roots may be spared partially or totally in the conus medullaris. This is referred to as *root escape*. If the roots are affected as they travel with the sacral cord in the spinal column, this will result in lower motor neuron damage, with diminished or absent reflexes. In low conus lesions, the S1 segment is not involved; therefore, the ankle jerks are normal, a finding accounting for most instances of failure to make the diagnosis. Because of the small size of the conus medullaris, lesions are more likely to be bilateral than are those of the cauda equina. With conus medullaris lesions, recovery is limited.

Injuries below the L1 vertebral level do not cause injury to the spinal cord, but rather injure the cauda equina or nerve rootlets supplying the lumbar and sacral segments of the skin and muscle groups. This usually produces motor weakness and atrophy of the lower extremities (L2 through S2) with bowel and bladder involvement (S2 through S4) and areflexia of the ankle and plantar reflexes. Often, the patient has spared sensation in the perineum or lower extremities but complete paralysis. In cauda injuries, there is loss of anal and bulbocavernosus reflexes as well as impotence. Cauda equina injuries are usually asymmetric, possibly because the rootlets are more mobile than the cord.

Cauda equina injuries have a better prognosis for recovery than spinal cord injuries. This is most likely because the nerve roots are more resilient to injury and because many of the biochemical processes that occur in the spinal cord and produce secondary damage occur to a much less extent in the nerve roots. Cauda equina injuries may represent a neuropraxia or axonotomesis and demonstrate progressive recovery over a course of weeks to months. Because the cauda equina rootlets are histologically peripheral nerves, regeneration can occur.

Separation of cauda equina and conus lesions in clinical practice is difficult because the clinical features of these lesions overlap. Isolated conus lesions are rare because the roots forming the cauda equina are wrapped around the conus. Traumatic SCI will likely produce a combination syndrome or a pure cauda equina lesion. The conus may be affected by a fracture of L1, whereas a fracture of L2 or lower impinges solely on the cauda equina. Sacral fractures and fractures of the pelvic ring also dam-

TABLE 5.6. COMPARISON OF DIFFERENT LEVEL OF LESIONS

Symptom	Epiconus	Conus Medullaris	Cauda Equina
Pain	Uncommon	Uncommon	Very common and may be severe
Bowel and bladder reflexes	Present	Absent	Absent
Anal and bulbocavernosus reflexes	Present	Absent[a]	Absent
Muscle tone	Increased	Depends[b]	Decreased
Muscle stretch reflexes	Increased[c]	Depends[b]	Decreased
Symmetry of weakness	Yes	Yes	No
Sensation	In dermatomal distribution	Absent in saddle distribution and may be dissociated	In root distribution
Recovery prognosis	Limited	Limited	Possible

[a] Unless a high conus lesion.
[b] Depends if nerve roots are affected. If so, then is decreased.
[c] Ankle plantarflexors and hamstrings, not knee jerks.

age the cauda equina as well as the sacral plexus. Bullet wounds can penetrate the bony structures to traumatize the cauda and conus. Intrinsic tumors of the conus medullaris can selectively damage the conus. Some differences between these lesions are noted in Table 5.6.

Pain is uncommon in conus lesions but is a frequent complaint in cauda equina lesions. Sensory abnormalities occur in a saddle distribution in conus lesions, and if there is sparing, there is usually dissociated loss with a greater loss of pain and temperature sensation but with spared touch sensation. In cauda equina lesions, sensory loss occurs in a more root-like distribution and is not dissociated.

Cauda equina lesions are multiple radiculopathies. Electrodiagnostic studies can be helpful in the diagnosis. Sensory nerve action potentials in lesions that are proximal to the dorsal root ganglia should remain normal, whereas in cauda equina lesions, they are affected. The electromyographic abnormalities in cauda lesions would be widespread and bilateral (but asymmetric). Other methods of studying root or nerve function (H reflexes, F waves, root stimulation, somatosensory evoked potentials) may be used to aid in diagnosis. Conus medullaris lesions should cause electrical abnormalities only where the lower motor neurons are affected. In that case, abnormalities may be present in muscles supplied by S2 through S4 levels (such as the anal sphincter).

THE FUNCTIONAL EVALUATION

To describe accurately the impact of the SCI on an individual and to monitor functional progress, it is necessary to use descriptive terms and a standard measure of activities of daily living. The World Health Organization has defined terms that are frequently used when functional deficits are discussed; losses or abnormalities of bodily function and structure (impairments), limitations of activities (previously referred to as *disabilities*), and restriction in participation (previously referred to as *handicap*) (76). *Impairment* is any loss or abnormality of bodily structure or of a physiologic or psychological function, such as paralysis.

Restriction or lack of ability to perform an activity in the nature and extent of functioning within the range considered normal (resulting from an impairment) may refer to the inability to walk from the paralysis. *Restriction in participation* (handicap) refers to a disadvantage for a given individual, resulting from an impairment and limitation of activity, that prevents the fulfillment of a role that is normal (depending on age, gender, and social and cultural factors) for that individual, such as being unable to walk and, therefore, unable to return to one's previous work.

There have been numerous articles attempting to correlate impairment with disability in SCI (8,9,77,78). The most commonly used disability measures in SCI are the FIM, the Modified Barthel Index (MBI), and the Quadriplegia Index of Function (QIF). A review of the reliability and validity of these scales is given elsewhere (79). The Craig Handicap and Reporting Technique (CHART) is an excellent measure of handicap (limitation of activity) in individuals with SCI (80).

Functional Independence Measure

The FIM was initially developed in 1983 to 1984 for the disabled population in general, not specifically for patients with SCI (81) (Fig. 5.2). The FIM is reliable and valid as an instrument and is sensitive to changes in functioning during rehabilitation. It is the most widely used functional assessment instrument in the United States and was used in NASCIS-III to attempt to measure functional change (82). Although the FIM was added to the International Standards in 1992, it was removed in the 2000 revisions (1). The FIM consists of 18 items (13 motor and 5 cognitive) clustered into six areas: self-care; sphincter control of bladder and bowel; mobility (transfers); locomotion; communication; and social recognition (83,84). Each of these 18 functions is evaluated using a seven-point scale with respect to independence. The scale used assigns to each subscore a value of 1 to 7, which describes the "burden of care" associated with the individual engaging in each activity (1 is the highest burden, 7 the lowest). Burden of care refers to the amount of time and energy provided by another person, or the use of an assistive device when the individual with a disability engages in each target activ-

L **E** **V** **E** **L** **S**	7 6	Complete independence (timely, safely) Modified independence (device)	**NO HELPER**
		Modified Dependence	**HELPER**
	5	Supervision (Subject = 100%+)	
	4	Minimal Assist (Subject = 76%+)	
	3	Moderate Assist (Subject = 50%+)	
		Complete Dependence	
	2	Maximal Assist (Subject +25%+)	
	1	Total Assist (Subject = less than 25%)	

Self-Care
A. Eating
B. Grooming
C. Bathing
D. Dressing – Upper Body
E. Dressing – Lower Body
F. Toileting

Sphincter Control
G. Bladder Management
H. Bowel Management

Transfer
I. Bed, Chair, Wheelchair
J. Toilet
K. Tub, Shower

Locomotion
L. Walk/Wheelchair
M. Stairs

Motor Subtotal Score:

Communication
N. Comprehension
O. Expression

Social Cognition
P. Social interaction
Q. Problem Solving
R. Memory

Cognitive Subtotal Score:

FIGURE 5.2. The Functional Independence Measure (FIM) instrument. (From Uniform data system for medical rehabilitation; a division of UB Foundation Activities, Inc. © 2001, all rights reserved, with permission.)

ity. An assistive device, for example, a brace or adapted telephone, is viewed as adding an additional potential burden of care; that is, if the device were not available, assistance from another person would be needed. The sum of all items represents the total FIM score, ranging from 18 (least independent) to 126 (most independent), which projects the cost of the disability in terms of safety and a person's dependence on others or technologic devices to achieve and maintain a certain quality of life.

Evidence has shown that reliability of assessments by trained users has reached highly acceptable levels, especially the reliability of the total score (85,86). Reliability of the individual items has been shown to be more variable and typically lower than reliability of the total scores (86). Analysis of FIM data has also shown that the cognitive domain may be inappropriate for use in SCI (87,88). The FIM is highly predictive of hours of assistance received by the individuals after discharge from inpatient rehabilitation. Data from the Model Spinal Cord Injury Systems indicate that for motor FIM items, differences exist at each neurological level from C4 through C8 between Frankel A to C and Frankel D (87).

The maximum gain in FIM occurs between rehabilitation admission and discharge, with little change beyond discharge (88). This is consistent with the practice of patients remaining in acute rehabilitation until maximum functional goals are reached. As length of stay in rehabilitation decreases, however, there may be larger increases in postdischarge FIM score changes. Modest gains in function continue to be made, however, as measured by the FIM in some individuals up to 5 years after injury (88).

Dijkers and Yavuzer evaluated a short telephone version of the motor FIM and found good correlation between a seven-item short version and the total motor FIM (89). This approach would allow data collection to be more time- and cost-efficient. Further study is underway.

Modified Barthel Index

The original Barthel Index consists of 10 self-care and mobility skills, with a scale range of 0 to 100 (90). Additions were made creating a modified 15-item scale, the MBI, still with the maximum score possible of 100 (91). Further modifications were made by researchers at the Midwest Regional Spinal Cord Injury Care System, by expanding the levels of certain items from two to three, adding the level of "assistance" to drinking, eating, grooming, and bathing, and adding a "limited independence" level for bowel and bladder continence (92). There are two main subscores: the self-care (drinking from a cup, eating, dressing upper and lower body, donning a brace or prosthesis, grooming, washing and bathing, and bladder and bowel continence) and the mobility (transfers to a chair, toilet, and tub or shower; walking 50 yards on level surfaces; ascending and descending one flight of stairs; and wheelchair propulsion 50 yards) subscores. Granger and associates have shown the MBI to be valid, reliable, and sensitive for describing functional abilities and change over time in patients with SCI (91). This scale has been used occasionally in the SCI studies (92–95). The MBI may not be sensitive in detecting small changes of functional ability in those with paraplegia because they can perform many of the criteria independently (96).

Quadriplegia Index of Function

The QIF was developed to help detect clinically relevant small changes in function in individuals with tetraplegia (97). The QIF consists of 10 categories of function with subdivisions: wheelchair mobility, transfers, bed activities, grooming, bathing, feeding, dressing, bladder and bowel programs, and understanding personal care. Weights are assigned for each category in the QIF for a total score, after calculation, of up to 100. A difference between this scale and the FIM and MBI is that credit is given in the QIF for completing even part of a task. There are also many more subdivisions to each task. For example, the range of score on the QIF for feeding is 0 to 28, compared with 1 to 7 on the FIM and 0 to 10 on the MBI (98). The QIF concentrates more on tasks that higher-level SCI patients can perform. For example, the task of feeding contributes to 8% of the total score in the FIM, 10% in the MBI, and 12% in the QIF, whereas transfers accounts for 23% in the FIM, 22% for the MBI, and only 8% in the QIF.

Compared with the FIM, the QIF feeding score shows a higher correlation to the degree of motor impairment in tetraplegia (98). The QIF has been found to be a better indicator of motor recovery than the FIM and is a more sensitive evaluation because it can reflect small gains in function that parallel small strength gains (99). In addition, the item scores differ for individuals with different levels of tetraplegia, that is, improved scores for patients with lower levels of injury (100). The QIF, however, has not been adopted by most rehabilitation centers, possibly because it is time-consuming to complete (roughly 30 minutes) or because of its complex weighted scoring system. In addition, some tasks are not easily tested in the hospital, such as meal preparation.

Because of redundancy within the QIF, a short-form QIF consisting of six items was developed for nonambulatory patients with tetraplegia (101). The six items are wash and dry hair, turn side to side in bed, put on lower extremity clothing, open carton or jar (feeding), transfer from bed to chair, and lock wheelchair. For the short-form QIF, no weighting system is used. This scale however, was not able to differentiate between C7 and C8 tetraplegia (101). Further work needs to be completed before the short-form QIF can be recommended as an assessment of disability.

Benzel Classification

Benzel and Larson described a slightly more detailed classification than the ASIA standards, in which functional motor individuals (Frankel D) were divided into three categories (102). The categories include the inability to walk independently, walking limited to 25 feet, and unlimited walking. Therefore, there are seven, rather than five, categories. This may more clearly classify the ability to ambulate with a motor incomplete injury. This scale was used in the recent Sygen (GM–1) trial (103).

Capabilities of Upper Extremity Instrument

The Capabilities of Upper Extremity Instrument (CUE) was recently designed to measure upper extremity functional limitations in patients with tetraplegia (104). This instrument is a 32-item questionnaire that assesses the difficulty in performing certain actions with the upper extremities (with one or both hands), including reaching and lifting, pulling and pushing, and so forth. CUE was found to be able to distinguish between different levels of tetraplegia more than one level apart and was correlated with ASIA motor scores and the FIM. Further work is needed to determine its sensitivity to change in function.

Walking Index for Spinal Cord Injury

The Walking Index for Spinal Cord Injury (WISCI) was developed to measure more precisely gradations of physical assistance and devices required for walking after SCI in clinical studies (105). In a pilot study, the WISCI showed good validity and reliability. Further clinical studies are underway to determine the responsiveness of the scale.

REFERENCES

1. American Spinal Injury Association/International Medical Society of Paraplegia. *International standards for neurological and functional classification of spinal cord injury patients.* Chicago: 2000.
2. Austin GM. The spinal cord: *Basic aspects and surgical consideration,* 2nd ed. Springfield, I: Thomas; 1972:762.
3. Neurological assessment: the sensory examination. In: Ditunno JF, Donovan WH, Maynard FM, eds. *Reference manual for the international standards for neurological and functional classification of spinal cord injury.* Chicago: American Spinal Injury Association, 1994.
4. Neurological assessment: the motor examination. In: Ditunno JF, Donovan WH, Maynard FM, eds. *Reference manual for the international standards for neurological and functional classification of spinal cord injury.* Chicago: American Spinal Injury Association, 1994.
5. Daniels L, Worthingham C. *Muscle testing techniques of manual examination,* 5th ed. Philadelphia: WB Saunders, 1986.
6. Hinderer KA, Hinderer SR. Muscle strength development and assessment in children and adolescents. In: Ringdal K, ed. *International perspectives in physical therapy,* Vol. on muscle strength. Edinburgh: Churchill Livingstone, 1992:20.
7. Long CII, Lawton EB. Functional significance of spinal cord lesion level. *Arch Phys Med Rehabil* 1955;36:249–255.
8. Welch RO, Lubley SJ, O'Sullivan SB, et al. Functional independence in quadriplegia critical levels. *Arch Phys Med Rehabil* 1986;67:235–240.
9. Marciello M, Herbison GJ, Ditunno JF Jr., et al. Wrist strength measured by myometry as an indicator of functional independence. *J Neurotrauma* 1994;12:99–105.

10. Herbison GJ, Isaac Z, Cohen ME, et al. Strength post-spinal cord injury: myometer vs manual muscle test. *Spinal Cord* 1996;34: 543–548.

11. Marino RJ, Rider-Foster D, Maissel G, et al. Superiority of motor level over single neurological level in categorizing patients. *Paraplegia* 1995;33:510–513.

12. Waters RL, Adkins R, Yakura J, et al. Motor and sensory recovery following complete tetraplegia. *Arch Phys Med Rehabil* 1993;74: 242–247.

13. Scoring, scaling and classification. In: Ditunno JF, Donovan WH, Maynard FM, eds. *Reference manual for the international standards for neurological and functional classification of spinal cord injury.* Chicago: American Spinal Injury Association, 1994:43–52.

14. Ditunno JF, Graziani V, Tessler A. Neurological assessment in Spinal Cord Injury. *Adv Neurol* 1997;72:325–333.

15. Michaelis LS. International inquiry on neurological terminology and prognosis in paraplegia and tetraplegia. *Paraplegia* 1969;7:1–5.

16. Cheshire DJE. A classification of the functional end-results of injury to the cervical spinal coed. *Paraplegia* 1970;8:70–73.

17. Maroon JC, Alba AA. Classification of acute spinal cord injury, neurological evaluation, and neurosurgical considerations. *Crit Care Clin* 1987;3:655–677.

18. Allen BL, Ferguson RL, Lehman TR, et al. A mechanistic classification of the lower cervical spine. *Spine* 1982;7:1–27.

19. Bracken MB, Webb SB, Wagner FC. Classification of the severity of acute spinal cord injury: implications for management. *Paraplegia.* 1977–78;15:319–326.

20. Roaf R. International classification of spinal injuries. *Paraplegia* 1972; 10:78–84.

21. Chehrazi B, Wagner FC, Collins WF, et al. A scale for evaluation of spinal cord injury. *J Neurosurg* 1981;54:310–315.

22. Jochheim KA. Problems of classification in traumatic paraplegia and tetraplegia. *Paraplegia* 1970;8:80–82.

23. Frankel HL, Hancock DO, Hyslop G, et al. The value of postural reduction in initial management of closed injuries of the spine with paraplegia and tetraplegia. *Paraplegia* 1969–70;7:179–192.

24. American Spinal Injury Association. *Standard for neurological classification of spinal injured patients.* Chicago: 1982.

25. Lucas JT, Ducker TB. Motor classification of spinal cord injuries with mobility, morbidity and recovery indices. *Am J Surg* 1979;45: 151–158.

26. Bracken MB, Hildreth N, Freeman DH, et al. Relationship between neurological and functional status after acute spinal cord injury: an epidemiological study. *J Chron Dis* 1980;33:115–125.

27. Bracken MB, Collins WF, Freeman DF, et al. Efficacy of methylprednisolone in acute spinal cord injury. *JAMA* 1984;251:45–52.

28. Bracken MB, Shephard MJ, Collins WF, et al. A randomized controlled trial of methylprednisolone or naloxone in the treatment of acute spinal cord injury: results of the second national acute spinal cord injury study. *N Engl J Med* 1990;332:1405–1411.

29. El Masry WS, Tsubo M, Katoh S, et al. Validation of the American Spinal Injury Association (ASIA) motor score and the National Acute Spinal Cord Injury Study (NASCIS) motor score. *Spine* 1996;21: 614–619.

30. Ditunno JF. American spinal injury standards for neurological classification of spinal cord injury: past, present and future. *J Am Paraplegia Soc* 1993;17:7–11.

31. Tator CH, Rowed DW, Schwartz ML. Sunnybrook cord injury scales for assessing neurological injury and neurological recovery in early management of acute spinal cord injury. In: Tator CH, ed. *Early management of acute spinal cord injury.* New York: Raven, 1982:7–24.

32. Donovan WH, Wilkerson MA, Rossi D, et al. A test of the ASIA guidelines for classification of spinal cord injury. *J Neurol Rehabil* 1990;4:39–53.

33. Standards for neurological classification of spinal cord injury patients. American Spinal Injury Association. Chicago, 1989.

34. Priebe MM, Waring WP. The interobserver reliability of the revised American Spinal Injury Association standards for the neurological classification of spinal injury patients. *Am J Phys Med Rehabil* 1991; 70:268–271.

35. American Spinal Injury Association/International Medical Society of Paraplegia (ASIA/IMSOP). *International standards for neurological and functional classification of spinal cord injury patients (revised).* Chicago: 1992.

36. American Spinal Injury Association/International Medical Society of Paraplegia. *International standards for neurological and functional classification of spinal cord injury patients.* Chicago:1996.

37. Waters RL, Adkins RH, Yakura JS. Definition of complete spinal cord injury. *Paraplegia* 1991;29:573–581.

38. Cohen ME, Bartko JJ. Reliability of the ISCSCI-92. International standards for neurological and functional classification of spinal cord injury patients. Chicago: 1994.

39. Cohen ME, Sheehan TP, Herbison GJ. Content validity and reliability of the international standards for neurological and functional classification of spinal cord injury. *Top Spinal Cord Injury Rehabil* 1996; 4:15–31.

40. Clifton GL, Donovan WH, Dimitrijevic MM, et al. Omental transposition in chronic spinal cord injury. *Paraplegia* 1996;4:193–203.

41. Cohen ME, Ditunno JF, Donovan WH, et al. A test of the 1992 international standards for neurological and functional classification of spinal cord injury. *Spinal Cord* 1998;36:554–560.

42. Donovan WH, Brown DJ, Ditunno JF, et al. Clinical case of the month: neurological issues. *Spinal Cord* 1997;35:275–281.

43. Stover S, DeLisa JA, Whiteneck GG, eds. *Spinal cord injury: clinical outcomes from the model systems.* Gaithersburg, MD: Aspen, 1995.

44. Bing R. *Compendium of regional diagnosis in affection of the brain and spinal cord,* 2nd ed. New York: Rebman, 1921.

45. Schneider RC, Cherry GR, Patek H. Syndrome of acute central cervical spinal cord injury with special reference to mechanisms involved in hyper-extension injuries of cervical spine. *J Neurosurg* 1954;11: 546–577.

46. Quencer RM, Bunge RP, Egnor M, et al. Acute traumatic central cord syndrome: MRI pathological correlations. *Neuroradiology* 1992; 34:85–94.

47. Bunge RP, Puckett WR, Becerra JL, et al. Observation on the pathology of human spinal cord injury: a review and classification of 22 new cases with details from a case of chronic cord compression with extensive focal demyelination. *Adv Neurol* 1993;59:75–89.

48. Kahulos BA, Bedbrook GM. Pathology of injuries of the vertebral column. In: Vinken PJ, Bruyn GW, eds. *Handbook of clinical neurology,* Vol. 25. Amsterdam: N. Holland, 1976:27–42.

49. Taylor AR. The mechanism of injury to the spinal cord in the neck without damage to the vertebral column. *J Bone Joint Surg Br* 1951; 33:543–547.

50. Foo D, Subrahamyan TS, Rossier AS. Post-traumatic acute anterior spinal cord syndrome. *Paraplegia* 1981;19:201–205.

51. Merriam WF, Taylor TKF, Ruff SJ, et al. A reappraisal of acute traumatic central cord syndrome. *J Bone Joint Surg Br* 1986;68: 708–713.

52. Penrod LE, Hegde SK, Ditunno JF. Age effect on prognosis for functional recovery in acute, traumatic central cord syndrome. *Arch Phys Med Rehabil* 1990;71:963–968.

53. Roth EJ, Lawler MH, Yarkony GM. Traumatic central cord syndrome: clinical features and functional outcomes. *Arch Phys Med Rehabil* 1990;71:18–23.

54. Burns SP, Golding DG, Rolle WA, et al. Recovery of ambulation in motor incomplete tetraplegia. *Arch Phys Med Rehabil* 1997;78: 1169–1172.

55. Bell HS. Paralysis of both arms from injury of the upper portion of the pyramidal decussation with "cruciate paralysis." *J Neurosurg* 1970; 33:376–380.

56. Dickmen CA, Hadley MN, Pappas CTE, et al. Cruciate paralysis: a clinical and radiographic analysis of injuries to the cervicomedullary junction. *J Neurosurg* 1990;73:850–858.

57. Erlich V, Snow R, Heier L. Confirmation by magnetic resonance imaging of Bells' cruciate paralysis in a young child with Chiari type I malformation and minor head trauma. *Neurosurgery* 1989;25: 102–105.

58. Marano SR, Calica AB, Sonntag VKH. Bilateral upper extremity pa-

ralysis (Bells cruciate paralysis) from a gunshot wound to the cervicomedullary junction. *Neurosurgery* 1986;18:642–644.

59. Schneider RC, Crosby EC, Russo RH, et al. Traumatic spinal cord syndromes and their management. *Clin Neurosurg* 1973;20:424–492.

60. Hatzakis M, Bryce N, Marino R. Case report: cruciate paralysis, hypothesis for injury and recovery. *Spinal Cord* 2000;38:120–125.

61. Wallenberg A. Anatomischer Befund in einem als "acute bulbaraffection (embolie der cerebellar post inf sinista?)" beschreiben falle. *Arch Phychiatr* 1901;34:923–959.

62. Pappas CTE, Gibson AR, Sonntag VKH. Decussation of hind-limb and fore-limb fibers in monkey corticospinal tract: relevance to cruciate paralysis. *J Neurosurg* 1991;75:935–940.

63. Coxe WS, Landau WM. Patterns of Marchi degeneration in the monkey pyramidal tract following small discrete cortical lesions. *Neurology* 1970;20:89–100.

64. Barnard JW, Woolsey CN. A study of localization in the corticospinal tracts of monkey and rat. *J Comp Neurol* 1956;105:25–50.

65. Bohlman HH. Acute fractures and dislocations of the cervical spine: an analysis of three hundred hospitalized patients and review of the literature. *J Bone Joint Surg Am* 1979;61:1119–1142.

66. Bosch A, Stauffer ES, Nickel VL. Incomplete traumatic quadraplegia: a ten year review. *JAMA* 1971;216:473–478.

67. Brown-Sequard CE. Lectures on the physiology and pathology of the central nervous system and the treatment of organic nervous affections. *Lancet* 1868;2:593–595,659–662,755–757,821–823.

68. Roth EJ, Park T, Pang T, et al. Traumatic cervical Brown-Sequard and Brown-Sequard plus syndromes: the spectrum of presentations and outcomes. *Paraplegia* 1991;29:582–589.

69. Tttersall R, Turner B. Brown-Sequard and his syndrome. *Lancet* 2000; 356:61–63.

70. Koehler PJ, Endtz LJ. The Brown Sequard syndrome: true or false? *Arch Neurol* 1986;43:921–924.

71. Graziani V, Tessler A, Ditunno JF. Incomplete tetraplegia: sequence of lower extremity motor recovery. *J Neurotrauma* 1995;12:121.

72. Little JW, Halar E. Temporal course of motor recovery after Brown-Sequard spinal cord injuries. *Paraplegia* 1985;23:39–46.

73. Bauer RD, Errico TJ. Cervical spine injuries. In: Errico TJ, Bauer RD, Waugh T, eds. *Spinal trauma*. Philadelphia: JB Lippincott, 1991: 71–121.

74. Cheshire WP, Santos CC, Massey EW, et al. Spinal cord infarction: etiology and outcome. *Neurology* 1996;47:321–330.

75. Bohlman HH, Ducker TB. Spine and spinal cord injuries. In: Rothman RH, ed. *The spine*, 3rd ed. Philadelphia: WB Saunders, 1992: 973–1011.

76. World Health Organization. *International classification of impairments, activities and participation*. Geneva: World Health Organization, 1998.

77. Rogers JC, Figne JJ. Traumatic quadriplegia: follow up study of self-care skills. *Arch Phys Med Rehabil* 1980;61:316–321.

78. Woolsey RM. Rehabilitation outcome following spinal cord injury. *Arch Neurol* 1985;42:116–119.

79. Marino RJ, Stineman MG. Functional assessment in spinal cord injury. *Top Spinal Cord Injury Rehabil* 1996;14:32–45.

80. Whiteneck GG, Charlifue SW, Gerhart KA, et al. Quantifying handicap: a new measure of long-term rehabilitation outcomes. *Arch Phys Med Rehabil* 1992;73:519–526.

81. Hamilton BB, Granger CV, Sherwin FS. A uniform national data system for medical rehabilitation. In: Fuhrer MJ, ed. *Rehabilitation outcomes: analysis and measurement*. Baltimore: Brooks, 1987: 137–147.

82. Bracken MB, Shephard MJ, Holford TR, et al. Administration of methylprednisolone for 24 or 48 hours or tirilizad mesylate for 48 hours in the treatment of acute spinal cord injury: results of the third national acute spinal cord injury randomized controlled trial. *JAMA* 1997;277:1597–1604.

83. *Guide for the uniform data set for medical rehabilitation (adult FIM)*, Version 5.1. Buffalo, NY: State University of New York at Buffalo, 1997.

84. Functional independence measure. In: Ditunno JF, Donovan WH, Maynard FM, eds. *Reference manual for the international standards for neurological and functional classification of spinal cord injury*. Chicago: American Spinal Injury Association, 1994:53–57.

85. Hamilton BP, et al. Intraagreement of the seven level functional independence measure (FIM). *Arch Phys Med Rehabil* 1991;31:790.

86. Segal ME, Ditunno JF, Stass WE. Institutional agreement of individual functional independence measure (FIM) items measured at two sites on one sample of SCI patients. *Paraplegia* 1993;31:622–631.

87. Ditunno JF, Cohen ME, Formal CS, et al. Functional outcomes in spinal cord injury. In: Stover SL, DeLisa J, Whiteneck GG, eds. *Spinal cord injury: clinical outcomes from the model system*. Gaithersburg, MD: Aspen, 1995:170–184.

88. Hall KM, Werner P. Characteristics of the functional independence measure in traumatic spinal cord injury. *Arch Phys Med Rehabil* 1999; 80:1471–1476.

89. Dijkers MPJM, Yavuzer G. Short version of the telephone motor functional independence measure for use with persons with spinal cord injury. *Arch Phys Med Rehabil* 1999;80:1477–1484.

90. Mahoney FI, Barthel DW. Functional evaluation: the Barthel index. *MD State Med J* 1965;14:61–65.

91. Granger CV, Albrecht GL, Hamilton BB. Outcomes of comprehensive medical rehabilitation: measurement by PULSES profile and the Barthel index. *Arch Phys Med Rehabil* 1979;60:145–154.

92. Yarkony GM, Roth EJ, Heinemann AW, et al. Benefits of rehabilitation for traumatic spinal cord injury: multivariate analysis in 711 patients. *Arch Neurol* 1987;44:93–96.

93. Yarkony GM, Roth EJ, Heinemann AW, et al. Rehabilitation outcomes in C6 tetraplegia. *Paraplegia* 1988;26:177–185.

94. Tow AMPE, Kong K. Central cord syndrome: functional outcome after rehabilitation. *Spinal Cord* 1998;36:156–160.

95. Dzidic I, Moslavac S. Functional skills after the rehabilitation of spinal cord injury patients: observation period after 3 years. *Spinal Cord* 1997;35:620–623.

96. Curtis KA, McClanahan S, Hall KM, et al. Health, vocational and functional status in spinal cord injured athletes and non-athletes. *Arch Phys Med Rehabil* 1986;67:862–865.

97. Gresham GE, Labi MLC, Dittmar SS, et al. The quadriplegia index of function (QIF): sensitivity and reliability demonstrated in a study of thirty quadriplegic patients. *Paraplegia* 1986;24:38–44.

98. Marino RJ, Huang M, Knight P, et al. Assessing self care status in quadriplegia: comparison of the quadriplegia index of function (QIF) and the functional independence measure (FIM). *Paraplegia* 1993; 31:225–233.

99. Yavus N, Tezyurck M, Akyuz M. A comparison of the functional tests in quadriplegia: the quadriplegia index of function and the functional independence measure. *Spinal Cord* 1998;36:832–837.

100. Zafonte RD, Demangone DA, Herbison GJ, et al. Daily self-care in quadriplegic subjects. *Neurorehabilitation* 1991;1:17–24.

101. Marino RJ, Goin JE. Development of a short form Quadriplegia Index of Function Scale. *Spinal Cord* 1999;37:289–296.

102. Benzel EC, Larson SJ. Functional recovery after decompressive spine operation for cervical spine fractures. *Neurosurgery* 1987;20:742–746.

103. Geisler FH. Personal communication, 2000.

104. Marino RJ, Shea JA, Steinman MG. The Capabilities of Upper Extremity Instrument: reliability and validity of a measure of functional limitation in tetraplegia. *Arch Phys Med Rehabil* 1998;79:1512–1521.

105. Ditunno JF, Ditunno PL, Graziani V, et al. Walking index for spinal cord injury (WISCI): an international multicenter validity and reliability study. *Spinal Cord* 2000;38:234–243.

ACUTE MEDICAL AND SURGICAL MANAGEMENT OF SPINAL CORD INJURY

DENISE I. CAMPAGNOLO
ROBERT F. HEARY

The acute management of a spinal cord injury (SCI) patient may make the difference between recovery and lifelong disability. Acute SCI is a complex, multifaceted process. Mechanical trauma causes direct neuronal damage; however, a large number of axons are lost as a result of secondary pathophysiologic events. It has been estimated that salvaging as little as 10% of adult axons makes walking a potential goal (1). Therefore, the most critical factors in recovery remain early prehospital recognition of injury, prompt resuscitation, stabilization of the injury, and avoidance of additional neurologic injury and medical complications (2,3). The principals of in-field resuscitation, medical stabilization, and emergency department care, along with surgical strategies, are reviewed in this chapter.

PRE-HOSPITAL (IN-FIELD) CARE

Successful in-field care is dependent on the recognition of the SCI. The first responders at any accident scene are typically personnel trained to deliver basic medical care, the emergency medical technicians (EMT-Basics). They provide basic life support; are trained in extrication, patient immobilization, and transport; and can administer oxygen (4). The second-level responders are the EMT-Paramedics. These technicians provide advanced life support, perform intravenous line insertion, and administer intravenous fluids and medications (4,5). The in-field responders not only provide immediate attention to the patient but also take a quick survey of the security and safety of the surroundings. For example, hostile crowds may need to be contained, traffic may need to be stopped, or fire may need to be controlled. Once the surroundings are secured, the primary survey of the patient is undertaken.

The primary survey ensures adequate airway, breathing, and circulation. Establishment of a secure airway is of highest priority. Adequately ventilating the patient and preventing hypoxemia also prevent potential secondary ischemia of the spinal cord in the initial critical period of minutes to hours after injury. While securing the airway, the responders must avoid cervical spine extension; therefore, the jaw-thrust maneuver is preferred over neck hyperextension. Proper airway control includes log-

rolling the patient secured on a long board and suctioning of the airway. In the unconscious patient, blind nasotracheal intubation is performed with in-line manual cervical immobilization (6). Supplemental oxygen is administered, as is manual ventilation, if needed.

Bleeding is handled with direct pressure. Foreign objects should not be removed until the patient is in the hospital because removal can cause potential exsanguination. Venous access is obtained with two large-bore peripheral venous catheters (7). The use of pneumatic antishock garments or military antishock trousers is not recommended because of the potential for peripheral tissue ischemia with lactic acid buildup and for further neurologic injury with the manipulation of the thoracolumbar spine needed to apply the garments (7).

Extrication from a motor vehicle can be prolonged and is especially risky in the unconscious patient. Five to 10% of unconscious people in this situation have a cervical spine injury; therefore, in the unconscious victim, a SCI is assumed to exist until proved otherwise (6). When a car crash victim is found sitting in the vehicle, the responder should perform a quick survey to assess for the size of the cervical collar needed. Most brands of cervical collars provide guidelines for quick assessment using fingerbreadth designations. In addition, there should be an opening in the front of the collar for assessment of tracheal deviation and to provide access for emergent cricothyroidotomy. One responder applies manual cervical traction while the other applies the collar, which must fit snugly. Once the cervical spine is secured, the use of the Kendrick extrication device (KED) is preferred over the short backboard. The KED has vertical battens for stability during the transfer out of the vehicle onto a spine board. Other techniques for transfer include the four-man lift or scoop stretcher (8). If the patient is found supine, the safest means of immobilization to secure the patient is to logroll the patient onto a rigid spine board. This board should extend from the top of the head to the feet. The patient should be strapped to the board at the forehead, thorax, and extremities. The ideal positioning of the spine on the backboard is to have the head in neutral alignment with the spine. To achieve this in adults, an occipital pad may need to be applied; in children younger than 6 years of age, however, because of the disproportionately large size of the head in relation to the torso, an occipital recess may be necessary (9). Cervical and head supports attached to the spine board should be used.

In a case in which the victim of a diving accident is still in the water, the patient should be floated on the back with the rescuers hands supporting the head, neck, and spine. Once at the water's edge the patient is floated onto a spine board and secured, and the board and patient are lifted from the water. In football-related injuries, the helmet should not be removed unless the airway is compromised. The shoulder pads should also be left in place. If the facemask must be cut away to secure the airway, inline manual traction should be applied.

During the first seconds after a SCI, there is release of catecholamines, with an initial hypertensive phase. This phase is fleeting, however, and is followed rapidly by the state of spinal shock, defined as flaccid paralysis and extinction of muscle stretch reflexes below the injury level (10). The cardiovascular manifestation of spinal shock is neurogenic shock, consisting of hypotension, bradycardia, and hypothermia. Hypothermia is most prominent in extended extrication times. Hypotension is initially managed with intravenous fluids in the field.

The method of patient transport is determined by the distance to be traveled, the patient's stability, and traffic conditions in the area. The general rule of thumb is that for distances less than 50 miles, an ambulance is used; for 51 to 150 miles or during periods of traffic congestion, a helicopter is used; and for distances greater than 150 miles, a fixed-wing aircraft (2).

The multidisciplinary emergency department team evaluating the patient should include the traumatologist or general surgeon, the neurologic surgeon, the orthopedic surgeon, the physiatrist, the anesthesiologist, and trained nursing and respiratory personnel. The goals are to normalize the patient's vital signs, prevent hypoxemia and aspiration, establish normal spine alignment, and consider the use of pharmacologic agents thought to limit secondary neuronal cell death.

Hypotension is common in patients with a neurologic level of injury at or above T6. These cervical and high paraplegic levels of injury leave most of the sympathetic outflow levels from the cord in a state of depressed function (spinal shock). Therefore, there is loss of sympathetically mediated vascular tone and possibly an inability to accelerate heart rate (11). The hypotension from neurogenic shock can be differentiated from hypotension secondary to hypovolemic shock by the presence of bradycardia. The parasympathetic influences on heart rate go unopposed in patients with a level of injury above T1; thus, heart rates are typically less than 60 beats/min. In contrast, tachycardia is present in patients with hypovolemic shock, although both can exist together, and all sources of potential bleeding must be excluded. Treatment of hypotension from either source involves fluid resuscitation to produce adequate urine output (>30 mL/hr). However, in neurogenic shock, further fluid administration must proceed judiciously. Loss of sympathetically mediated vasoconstriction and thus expanded intravascular tree, as well as capillary leak syndrome, place the SCI patient at risk for neurogenic pulmonary edema. Trendelenburg positioning can be used for symptomatic hypotension. Further, the use of vasopressors is preferred in this population over continued fluid

administration. To guide this, pulmonary artery catheterization (Swan-Ganz catheter) has been recommended because pulmonary artery wedge pressures will normalize before central venous pressures, giving an accurate assessment of the patient's volume status and avoiding fluid overload (12). Arterial blood pressure catheters are needed because maintaining the mean arterial blood pressure at more than 85 mm Hg has been associated with enhanced neurologic outcome (12). Dopamine (2.5 to 5 μg/kg per minute) is the vasopressor of choice in the setting of hypotension with bradycardia because it is both an α- and a β_1-agonist, both of which directly increase heart rate. This can be followed by norepinephrine (Levophed) if needed (0.01 to 0.2 μg/kg per minute) to keep the mean arterial blood pressure higher than 85 mm Hg (12). Phenylephrine is a pure α-agonist, and its use is limited by the potential reflex slowing of the heart rate in the setting of an already present bradycardia. The bradycardia can be treated with intravenous atropine, and pretreatment with atropine is done before a maneuver that may cause further vagal stimulation (such as nasotracheal suctioning). Temporary cardiac pacing and permanent pacemakers, although reported, are rarely needed (6) (see chapter 8).

Ventilatory assessment is critical in acute SCI patients and should include arterial blood gases with target PaO_2 of 100 mm Hg and $PaCO_2$ of less than 45 mm Hg. Measurement of forced vital capacity (VC) in the emergency department provides the best assessment of inspiratory muscle strength. A VC of less than 1,000 mL indicates an extreme ventilatory defect with impending ventilatory failure and necessitates intubation and mechanical ventilation. A VC of 1,000 to 1,500 mL is borderline and necessitates careful serial assessment each shift. Once the VC is above 1,500 mL, there is usually no need for mechanical ventilatory assist. All patients with levels of injury above T12 will have varying degrees of secretion clearance deficiencies. The higher the level of injury is, the worse the deficiency will be. Patients with tetraplegia, who have no measurable cough, are at greater risk for mucous plugging.

A nasogastric tube should be inserted during the initial assessment period to prevent emesis and potential aspiration. A Foley catheter should be inserted for urinary drainage because the bladder demonstrates the same flaccid paralysis as limb muscles during the period of spinal shock. In addition, an indwelling urinary catheter will allow for an accurate assessment of output.

Once the initial resuscitative measures have been taken, attention is turned to spinal realignment. A history of central nervous system disorders and known spinal abnormalities (e.g., ankylosing spondylitis, diffuse idiopathic skeletal hyperostosis) is obtained from the patient or family. A full initial neurologic assessment as described in the American Spinal Injury Association *International Standards for Neurological and Functional Classification of Spinal Cord Injury Patients* (2000) should be documented (see chapter 5). This will provide a clear baseline on which changes in neurologic status can be gauged. Inspection and palpation of the spine in search of bruising or abrupt stepoff should be undertaken. Imaging of the spine is needed to guide correction of malalignments. The most commonly used imaging studies are listed in Table 6.1 along with the information they provide. A standard trauma series includes cross-table lateral and anteroposterior views of the cervical and thoracolumbar spine.

TABLE 6.1. MOST COMMON IMAGING TECHNIQUES FOR THE SPINE

Anteroposterior and lateral radiographs of the entire spine (cervical, thoracic, lumbar, and sacral)	To assess position of spinal elements
Open mouth view of the cervical spine	To assess odontoid process and lateral masses of C1 and C2
Swimmer's view of the cervical spine if needed	To assess cervicothoracic junction
Computed tomographic (CT) scan with sagittal reconstruction	To assess the part of the spine that cannot be adequately visualized on plain radiograph
Tomography of C1 and C2 if needed	To assess a transverse fracture of the odontoid or lateral mass fracture
Oblique views	To assess facet fracture
Flexion-extension views	To assess instability and ligamentous injury

There is a 12% incidence of noncontiguous fractures; therefore, once one fracture is identified, careful inspection of the rest of the spine is imperative (7). Forty-seven percent of patients with spine trauma and 64% of patients with SCI have concomitant injuries, including head, chest, and long-bone fractures (13).

Knowing the mechanism of injury with an understanding of the force vectors involved allows the treating physician to anticipate which spinal elements will be involved. Manifestations of various injuries on plain film are listed in Table 6.2. In any of theses mechanisms, there may or may not be evidence of vertebral subluxation or dislocation, or loss of vertebral body height with vertebral body fractures. Additionally, soft tissues need to be carefully inspected because soft tissue swelling may be the only sign of a subtle vertebral body fracture. Increases in diameter of the prevertebral soft tissues may indicate a ligamentous injury, fracture, or fracture-dislocation. In adults, the retropharyngeal (C1 through C4) soft tissue diameter should be no more than 10 mm at C1 and 7 mm at C2 through C4. At C5 and below, the retrotracheal soft tissue should be no more than 22 mm in diameter (14).

If a spinal injury is identified, the spine surgeon must decide whether to pursue further imaging, such as magnetic resonance imaging (MRI), or to attempt immediately to realign the spinal

TABLE 6.2. MANIFESTATIONS OF VARIOUS INJURIES ON PLAIN FILM

Flexion	Widening of interspinous, interlaminar, and facet joint spaces; loss of vertebral body height anteriorly on lateral film.
Extension	Widening of disk space anteriorly; anterior avulsion fracture; fractures of the posterior elements.
Rotation	Malalignment of the spinal column.
Shear	Horizontal displacement of spinal elements with disruption of bone and soft tissue.

elements through traction or open surgical reduction. For cervical spine injuries, MRI has been recommended before attempting closed reduction to identify disk herniation and its potential for neurologic worsening with manipulation (15). Eismont and colleagues presented data showing the frequency of acute disk herniation compressing the neural elements ventrally in acute SCI. These authors proposed that an MRI should be obtained before the use of traction for fear that cervical traction could cause ascending (worse) neurologic deficit if the bony subluxation was reduced against a ventrally located (herniated) disk (15). On the other hand, Cotler and associates, in 1993, published a study demonstrating the safety of immediate skeletal traction, in patients who were awake, using evoked potentials. In this study, 24 patients treated this way demonstrated no neurologic worsening resulting from the use of immediate cervical traction before obtaining an MRI (16). Other centers have reported little risk if the reduction is performed with the patient awake (17). However, in the obtunded patient, an MRI should be obtained first. In all cases, after closed reduction, MRI is obtained to exclude spinal cord compression from disk herniation (7).

Closed cervical reduction is accomplished with traction applied as quickly and as safely as possible. The patient is placed in either a Stryker frame (Stryker Corp., Kalamazoo, MI) or a Roto-Rest bed (Kinetic Concept, San Antonio, TX). Gardner-Wells (stainless steel or titanium) tongs (Zimmer Inc., Warsaw, IN) or the halo ring is applied using local anesthetic after proper preparation of the skin. For straight traction, pins are inserted 1 cm superior to the middle of the pinna of the ear. The pins are tightened until the pressure indicator pin protrudes 1 mm (7). For a flexion or extension moment, the pins can be placed slightly posterior or anterior, respectively. The initial weight applied is 10 pounds, with weight added in 10-pound increments until reduction is achieved. Immediately after each increment of weight, a neurologic examination is performed, and a cross-table (lateral) radiograph is obtained. Up to 140 pounds of weight can be used to reduce dislocations in awake and cooperative patients (7). Once reduction is confirmed, 10 to 15 pounds of weight is used to maintain reduction. The patient is then brought to the operating room for open stabilization.

MEDICAL INTERVENTIONS

An ancient Egyptian physician wrote in the *Edwin Smith Surgical Papyrus* that SCIs were hopeless and recommended withholding water from spinal cord–injured soldiers (18). Improvement in emergency medical procedures, critical care medicine, and the development of model centers for the treatment of acute SCI have improved survival in this population (2,19,20). With improved survival, strategies to maximize neurologic recovery are of paramount importance. Several newly developed pharmacologic agents have shown promise in improving neurologic recovery in SCI survivors (21–26). Details regarding the National Acute Spinal Cord Injury Studies (NASCIS-I to -III) (21–23) and ganglioside (GM-1) are discussed in chapter 2.

Since the publication of the NASCIS-II results (22), methylprednisolone (bolus dose of 30 mg/kg followed by 5.4 mg/kg/hr maintenance dose for 23 hours) has been considered the standard of care. However, the scientific integrity of these studies has recently been reevaluated based on the quality of evidence needed to change pattern of practice (27). Hurlbert expressed in a recent review that both NASCIS-II and NASCIS-III were well designed and executed trials but that the data from NASCIS-III was weak and noncompelling (27). The conclusions of three recent systematic reviews are that the use of 24-hour methylprednisolone remains experimental and that the use of 48-hour methylprednisolone is potentially harmful (27–29). Because the evidence indicates that the use of methylprednisolone is still experimental, clinicians should keep within strict inclusion and exclusion criteria described in NASCIS-II and NASCIS-III when considering the use of methylprednisolone.

Inclusion criteria for steroids include a traumatic SCI diagnosis within 8 hours of injury. Exclusion criteria include age under 13 years, nerve root or cauda equina injury only, SCI secondary to gunshot wounds (GSWs), life-threatening morbidity, pregnancy, and addiction to narcotics. Unfortunately, the use of methylprednisolone has been extended to subgroups not included in NASCIS studies, such as those with penetrating SCI (i.e., from GSWs). Two retrospective nonrandomized studies have shown that the use of methylprednisolone in penetrating injuries is not supported (30,31). Currently, many clinicians use this experimental protocol because of medicolegal concerns (28), which may not be in the best interest of the patient.

Tirilazad mesylate, a lazaroid that was assessed in NASCIS-III (23), holds promise in limiting membrane lipid peroxidation, and thus limiting secondary neuronal loss after SCI. In a preliminary study, GM-1, a ganglioside that has shown some improved functional recovery in cats (32) and humans (26), is not available for routine clinical use after injury. Local hypothermia has been recognized as a method to protect neurons from secondary mechanisms of injury but is not practical (33). None of these treatments are a panacea, however. Prehospital recognition of injury, prompt medical resuscitation, stabilization of the injury, and avoidance of additional neurologic injury and medical complications are the factors that most significantly affect neurologic recovery.

PENETRATING INJURIES

Most of the published medical literature on the treatment of penetrating injures was generated from experience in the military with high-velocity missile wounds (30). Significant differences exist between the injuries that occur from high-velocity missiles and those from handguns in the civilian population. This section addresses only civilian GSWs, which are the third leading cause of SCI in the United States. Stab wounds account for only 8% to 10% of all penetrating spinal injuries in most North American series (34). Stab wounds and GSWs generally do not produce spinal instability and therefore generally do not require surgical stabilization or orthotic immobilization. Entrance and exit wounds should be examined to determine whether cerebrospinal fluid (CSF) leakage is present, suggesting dural incompetence and the presence of a CSF fistula (35). These wounds can be dressed with a sterile dressing. Plain films and computed tomography are used not only to assess extent of bony injury but also

to provide information regarding the location and path of bullet and bone fragments and the extent of soft tissue and vascular damage, in which case angiography would be required also. As a general rule, it is safe to perform an MRI after a GSW with the bullet retained because nonjacketed bullets do not pose a problem. If the bullet has a jacket, it may heat up and necessitate aborting the study. There are no reported cases of a bullet moving during the MRI and causing subsequent neurologic damage.

Knives or other sharp objects that are embedded around the spinal canal should be left in place until their exact location is known as well as the extent of pleural or abdominal injury (35). Removal is best done in the operating room under direct visualization of the spinal canal. Bullets that pass through the abdominal viscera hold a greater risk for infection for the central nervous system and should be treated with broad-spectrum antibiotics for 7 days (35,36). Tetanus prophylaxis is routinely administered in the emergency department. Indications for operative intervention are to close a CSF fistula or to decompress the spinal cord in cases in which bullet fragments, bone, or hematoma is causing neurologic deterioration (30,35). Bullets do not have to be removed during the course of a laminectomy to close a dural leak; only if the bullet is surgically accessible will it be removed (36). There is a generally poor outcome as far as neurologic recovery in civilian cases after GSWs; in one large series, the most common neurologic deficit was complete paraplegia (31). Complete injuries can result from bullets that do not actually enter the spinal canal. Steroids should not be used with penetrating injuries because they showed no benefit and their use is associated with a higher incidence of spinal and extraspinal infection (30,31,36).

SURGICAL MANAGEMENT OF ACUTE SPINAL CORD INJURY

The timing of surgical treatment for patients with acute SCI is controversial. Conflicting reports exist in the medical literature detailing whether surgery should be performed acutely or whether it is more appropriate to perform surgery after a delay to allow the neural elements to "cool off." In a large, widely quoted study by Marshall and colleagues in 1987, the rate of neurologic complications following spinal surgery was higher in patients who underwent surgery within the first 5 days than in a group who underwent surgery more than 6 days after the initial traumatic event (37). In 1997, Vaccaro and associates performed a prospective landmark study on survivors of acute cervical spinal cord trauma (38). These authors were unable to demonstrate a significant difference in neurologic outcome between patients operated on early (within 72 hours) versus late (5 days or later). Both of these studies have been criticized for substantial flaws in design or technique. In the study by Marshall and colleagues, decompressive laminectomy, through a dorsal approach, was frequently performed. Although this type of surgical procedure was reasonable and widely used in the 1980s, decompressive laminectomy alone is rarely performed in the surgical treatment of traumatic SCI in present times. The Vaccaro study has been criticized for the timing of the "early" population definition. In this study, early surgery was defined as surgery within 72 hours of the traumatic event. Many investigators have considered this to be an excessively long time interval to be categorized as early surgery. Critics of this review contend that early surgery would be performed within 24 hours or less from the time of the initial injury.

There is a common sentiment among many spine surgeons that early surgery offers an advantage to patients with an acute SCI. This concept has never been proved in a randomized, prospective study because there has never been a study that has been of proven benefit to early surgery. Tator and coworkers performed a multicenter retrospective review of 36 North American centers evaluating the timing of surgery on acute SCI patients. They determined that there was very little agreement on the optimum timing of surgical treatment (39). Likewise, Fehlings and Tator performed an evidenced-based review of the literature, in 1999, to evaluate the rationale and indications for the timing of decompressive surgery in the treatment of acute nonpenetrating SCI (40). Although they determined that evidence from experimental animal studies showed benefit to early decompressive surgery after acute SCI, they concluded that the relevant interventional timing in humans remains unclear. Both of these studies concluded that there is a need for a randomized controlled trial to assess the optimal timing of decompressive surgery in SCI (39,40).

The only uniformly agreed upon principle in the management of the acute SCI patient is that early surgery is indicated when a patient presents with a progressive neurologic deficit. This situation rarely occurs in clinical practice. However, if a patient with an adequate, documented neurologic examination is noted to demonstrate progressive loss of neurologic function, immediate surgical intervention is indicated. In all other cases, the choices of emergent, urgent, and elective surgery all appear to be supportable.

The timing of the diagnostic radiographic imaging studies depends on the neurologic status of the patient at the time of admission to the hospital. Patients who are neurologically intact should undergo plain film radiographs as well as advanced imaging studies. These advanced imaging studies usually include MRI and CT scans. Myelography may be indicated in patients unable to undergo MRI. In patients with a neurologic, incomplete SCI (America Spinal Injury Association [ASIA] classes B through D) with a stable neurologic examination, the workup should be identical to that in a patient with an intact neurologic examination and should include plain films as well as an advanced imaging study. In the relatively rare patient with an incomplete injury and an unstable or progressive examination consistent with neurologic deterioration, emergent treatment is necessary and may cause the diagnostic workup to be abbreviated. In patients presenting with a complete SCI (ASIA A), the routine evaluation should include plain film radiographs. As discussed earlier, there is further controversy involving whether to place a patient with a neurologic, complete SCI in traction immediately after plain film radiographs or to obtain advanced imaging studies.

SPINAL STABILITY

Any discussion of the surgical management of acute SCI requires an understanding of spinal stability. Numerous theories involving spine stability or instability have been postulated. White and

Panjabi have proposed the most widely accepted theory on spinal instability. They defined clinical instability as "the loss of the ability of the spine, under physiologic loads, to maintain its pattern of displacement so that there is no initial or additional neurological deficit, no major deformity, and no incapacitating pain" (41). This definition of spinal instability is applicable at all levels of the axial spine.

Radiographic criteria have been established for the diagnosis of clinical instability of the spine. In 1983, Denis published the widely accepted three-column theory for thoracolumbar fractures. In this theory, the spine is divided into three columns (Fig. 6.1). The anterior column is composed of the anterior vertebral body, the anterior longitudinal ligament, and the anterior half of the annulus fibrosus. The middle column consists of the posterior vertebral body, the posterior longitudinal ligament, and the posterior half of the annulus fibrosus. The posterior column includes all the posterior elements (including the pedicles). In this three-column theory of Denis, spinal instability is present if any two of the three columns are violated. In these situations, the spine is determined to be unstable (42).

In the cervical spine, plain film definitions of stability vary depending on the level involved. In the occipital–atlantoaxial regions, spinal instability is difficult to determine. Specific points related to instability are described in the treatment of these occipitocervical region injuries. In the subaxial cervical spine (C3 through C7), spinal instability is generally accepted as present on plain film radiographs in a lateral projection if a sagittal displacement of greater then 3.5 mm occurs or if relative sagittal plane angulation of greater than 11 degrees is present (41).

Benzel introduced the concept of the instantaneous axis of rotation (IAR). In work published from Benzel's biomechanics laboratory in 1997 by Resnick and colleagues, the biomechanical principles affecting the thoracolumbar spine are described (43). Specifically, forces on the spine act through vectors, and depending on the direction of the force and the relative location of the

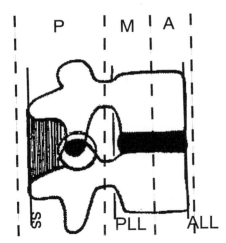

FIGURE 6.1. The three-column spine. P, posterior column; M, middle column; A, anterior column; SS, supraspinous ligament; PLL, posterior longitudinal ligament; ALL, anterior longitudinal ligament. (From, Denis F. The three-column spine and its significance in the classification of acute thoracolumbar spinal injuries. *Spine* 1983;8:817–831, with permission.)

IAR, different failure modes of the spine occur (9). An understanding of the location of the IAR and its importance to spinal stabilization procedures will help guide the spine surgeon to choose the most biomechanically advantageous form of stabilization procedure to be performed.

PRINCIPLES OF SPINAL STABILIZATION

Injuries to the spine or spinal cord are the result of failure of the bony elements, the ligamentous supporting structures, and the supporting musculature. Surgical treatments depend on an understanding of some basic principles. Injuries that are primarily ligamentous, such as facet dislocations, require internal stabilization procedures. As a general rule, ligamentous injuries have high failure rates when external orthoses alone are attempted as the sole treatment. The most common external orthoses currently used in the cervical spine are halo vest immobilization and hard cervical collar S (e.g., Philadelphia Collar, Westville, N.J.; Miami J Collar, Jerome Medical, Moorestown, N.J.). In the thoracolumbar spine regions, the commonly used external orthoses include a thoracolumbosacral orthosis (TLSO) or a body cast. Bony fractures may heal with external orthoses alone if the ligamentous structures are not badly disrupted. When fractures of the bone lead to spinal instability, open surgical intervention with internal surgical stabilization is necessary. This is frequently the case in significant spine injuries that result in a SCI.

The primary goal of surgical intervention in acute SCI is to decompress the neural elements. Either an anterior or a posterior approach may accomplish this. The approach chosen depends on the comfort and expertise of the operating surgeon as well as the specific pathophysiology of the injury. The most common etiology of SCI occurs from retropulsion of bone or disk material from a ventral location into the spinal canal. This injury pattern favors an anterior approach to decompress the neural elements. In addition, biomechanical advantages, related to the IAR, are realized when the anterior column may be reconstructed after decompressive surgery. This is not always feasible at certain locations of the spine, including the occipitocervical complex, the upper thoracic region, and the lower lumbar regions. When posterior surgery is used, there is a biomechanical disadvantage in that most posterior stabilization procedures, after the decompression, secure only the posterior elements. This requires use of longer constructs to achieve spinal stability. The more recent use of pedicle screw instrumentation at multiple levels of the spinal canal allows for a potential advantage of being able to stabilize all three columns of the spine through a posterior approach, thereby allowing for shorter segment stabilizations to be performed.

After adequate neural decompression (corpectomy or discectomy) is accomplished, through an anterior or a posterior approach, the spine must be stabilized and fused. Fusion is typically performed by using autologous bone, which is most frequently harvested from the iliac crest in trauma cases. The fibula can also be used as donor site for autograft bone; however, this is usually reserved for cases that require more than one level of fusion, such as in spinal tumor or infection in which three or more disks and two or more vertebral bodies need to be resected.

This is typically not the case in traumatic injuries, which usually span one vertebral level, and thus the iliac crest provides sufficient bone for the autograft. With anterior stabilization procedures, allograft bone, or most recently cages, may be used to provide anterior column support; however, iliac autograft is the gold standard in trauma because it yields the highest fusion rates when compared with cages or allograft bone. Posterior onlay fusions have significant failure rates when allograft bone is used, and as such, iliac autograft is greatly preferred when surgery is performed from a dorsal approach.

Surgical instrumentation, or hardware, is used to help fixate bones to allow a fusion to occur. It is essential to understand that surgical hardware is a temporary fixation device that merely facilitates an eventual long-term bony fusion. If a fusion does not develop, the hardware will eventually fail, leading to the development of a pseudarthrosis. As such, although hardware is frequently used in the treatment of spinal trauma, the spinal fusion must be solid for a long-term beneficial effect to occur.

The use of an external orthosis, in addition to the internal stabilization, is dependent on the comfort of the operating surgeon with the stabilization procedure as well as the inherent instability of the initial injury. When an external orthosis is used, it is kept on for 3 months because that is the length of time that complete fusion can be proved radiographically. Postoperative films are taken at 6 weeks, 12 weeks, 6 months, 1 year, and 2 years. If the 3-month film demonstrates good bony fusion, the orthosis is removed. The type of spinal orthotic chosen depends on the level of spinal injury; generally, for the occipital to C2 levels, the halo vest is used, although some surgeons will use a hard cervical collar such as the Miami J. A hard cervical collar is used for the C3 through C7 levels; for the T1 through T3 levels, a cervicothoracic orthosis is used. From T4 through L2, a TLSO is used; however, at L3 and below, a lumbosacral orthotic (LSO) with the incorporation of one hip-thigh (spica attachment to a LSO or TLSO) will ensure satisfactory immobilization of the low lumbar and sacral spine.

SPECIFIC INJURIES TO THE SPINE
Occipital–Atlantoaxial Complex

Occipitocervical (O through C1) dissociation (Fig. 6.2) is usually a fatal event. Numerous lines of craniometry have been devised to define the normal anatomic locations of the occiput with respect to the upper cervical spine. A detailed review of these lines of craniometry is beyond the scope of this chapter. Powers and coworkers, in 1979, defined occipitocervical subluxations with a ratio commonly referred to as the *Powers ratio* (44). If an occipitocervical subluxation has occurred and the patient has survived this injury, the surgical treatment requires a posterior occipitocervical fusion procedure.

Fractures of the atlas were initially described by Sir Geoffrey Jefferson and, as such, are commonly referred to as *Jefferson burst fractures*. These are most frequently stable injuries that can be treated with a halo vest orthosis. Spence and associates have defined unstable Jefferson fractures as those with more than 7 mm of combined lateral translation of the lateral masses of the atlas on an open-mouth odontoid radiograph (45). Unstable Jefferson burst fractures require posterior surgical stabilization.

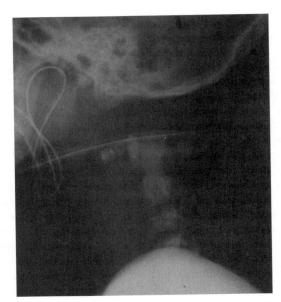

FIGURE 6.2. Lateral cervical spine radiographic demonstrating a severe occipitoatlantal subluxation.

Odontoid fractures are classified into three basic types. Type I odontoid fractures are very rare and involve fractures of the tip of the odontoid process. Type II odontoid fractures are much more common, particularly in the elderly population. They involve a fracture through the base of the odontoid process, or dens, at its junction with the C2 vertebral body (Fig. 6.3). Type III odontoid fractures are those injuries that extend from the base of the odontoid into the body of the C2 vertebra proper. Type I odontoid fractures typically require no specific surgical intervention. Type III odontoid fractures are typically treated with an external orthosis (either halo vest or hard cervical collar, depending on the surgeon's preference) for 3 months. Type II odontoid fractures may be treated with an external halo vest orthosis; however, there is a high failure rate with this treatment mode. As such, numerous internal stabilization procedures have been hypothesized for the treatment of type II odontoid fractures. Apfelbaum and colleagues have described the use of an anterior odontoid screw to fixate type II fractures (46). In anterior odontoid screw fixation, motion at the C1-2 joint is preserved, with fusion occurring between the vertebral body of C2 and the odontoid peg. This innovative procedure is feasible only with acute odontoid fractures (within 6 months) because the use of this procedure with chronic odontoid fractures has yielded unacceptably high failure rates. Additional accepted treatments for odontoid type II fractures include posterior C1 and C2 fusions. Numerous descriptions for C1 and C2 posterior stabilization have been described. In 1939, Gallie described a fusion between the posterior elements secured between the posterior ring of the atlas and the spinous process of the axis (47). Brooks and Jenkins described a modification in 1978 in which a C1 and C2 fusion is accomplished with two separate bone grafts placed between the posterior arch of the atlas and each lamina of C2 separately (48). Both the Gallie and the Brooks fusions require an intact C1 posterior arch. In a more recently described

procedure, Grob and Magerl, in 1987, described the use of C1 and C2 transarticular screws. These screws extend through the lateral mass of C2 into the lateral mass of C1 to immobilize effectively the C1 to C2 segment (49). In addition to the transarticular screws, augmentation of the fusion using a modification of the Gallie technique may also be performed. If the transverse atlantal ligament is disrupted, C1 and C2 instability is implied. This is best detected on lateral cervical spine radiographs where the distance between the anterior aspect of the odontoid process is measured with respect to the posterior aspect of the C1 anterior arch. This distance is referred as the *atlantodental interval.* If this interval is greater than 3 mm in an adult or 5 mm in a child, disruption of the transverse atlantal ligament is implied and surgery is indicated (41).

Fractures of the pedicles, or the isthmus region, of C2 are usually bilateral and are commonly referred to as *hangman's fractures.* These are most often stable injuries that are treated with external orthoses. When disruption is more significant, treatment with a halo vest orthosis, with slight extension, is used. In less severe injuries, a hard collar orthosis (Philadelphia or Miami J) may be used. In the rare unstable hangman's fracture, indicated by significant sagittal translation of the C2 vertebral body or significant angulation of the C2 vertebral body, an open surgical fusion may be necessary. The open treatment for hangman's fractures would include either an anterior C2 and C3 discectomy and fusion procedure or a posterior C1 and C2 fusion procedure.

The occipitocervical complex is responsible for a major degree (at least 50%) of neck rotational movement. Fractures in this region may be singular as previously described or may occur in combination. The surgical stabilization procedure necessary will depend on the overall stability of the various injuries, with the least stable segment dictating the mode of therapy.

Subaxial Cervical Spine (C3 through C7)

Fractures and subluxations of the subaxial cervical spine may be associated with SCI. Pure bony injuries without substantial neurologic compression may heal with an external orthosis alone. Most patients who have sustained an acute SCI secondary to fractures of vertebral column have ligamentous injuries that allow significant compression of the spinal cord. These patients require open surgical intervention to decompress or fuse the cervical spine.

The most common burst fracture in the cervical spine occurs at the C5 level. This typically leads to a retropulsion of bone into the spinal canal with compression of the spinal cord. These injuries are best treated surgically through an anterior approach. Skeletal traction is frequently applied, upon the initial evaluation, followed by a definitive surgical stabilization at a later time. The surgery typically involves a corpectomy (resection of the vertebral body) with a minimum width of bone resection of 15 mm. This allows for adequate decompression of the spinal cord in the lower cervical spine because the width of the cord is about 13 mm. After the corpectomy, a strut graft, usually autologous iliac crest, is positioned, and stabilization is accomplished with a screw plate device. Caspar and associates described stabilization with a screw plate device in 1989 (50). Since that description, numerous additional techniques have been used for anterior

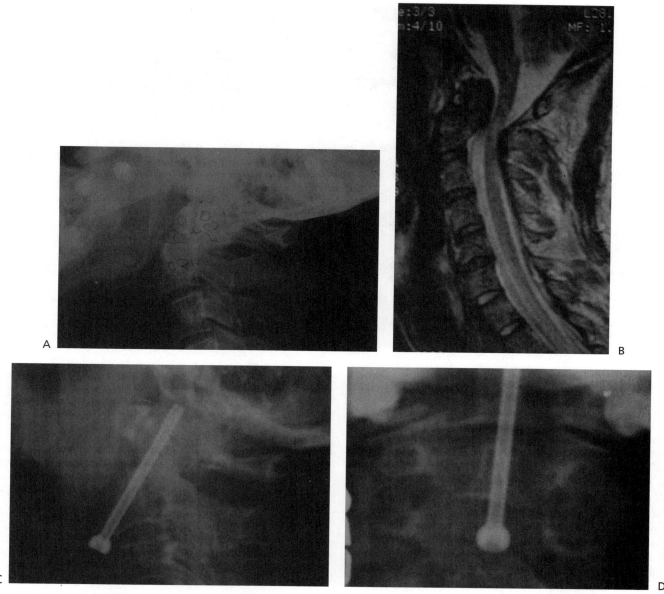

FIGURE 6.3. A; Lateral cervical radiograph demonstrating a type II dens fracture, with significant subluxation remaining and with the patient in a halo vest. **B;** T2-weighted magnetic resonance image of the same type II dens fracture with corresponding cervical cord edema. **C,D;** Treatment of the same fracture using an odontoid screw.

screw plate fixation in the cervical spine that allow for immediate stability of the region. As with upper cervical injuries, an external orthosis may, or may not, be applied in addition to the internal stabilization procedure. The use of an orthosis is determined by the comfort of the operating surgeon with the stabilization procedure, the inherent instability initially present, and often the patient's body habitus. Morbidly obese patients and patients with very short necks do not tolerate external orthoses well. In addition, halo vests are known to have higher failure rates in the lower cervical spine owing to a phenomenon referred to as "snaking." Snaking is defined by Johnson and colleagues as flex-

ion at one cervical level and compensatory extension at adjacent levels that allows substantial individual level motion with minimal total excursion of the entire cervical spine (51). In other words, there is excessive motion at the segments that need to be stabilized owing to the fixation points (head and thorax in the case of the halo and halo vest) being beyond these segments. This explains the nearly 10% incidence of lost reduction when the halo vest is used to attempt to control the middle to low cervical spine (52).

Subluxations of the cervical spine may involve unilateral or bilateral facet injuries (Fig. 6.4). The most common level af-

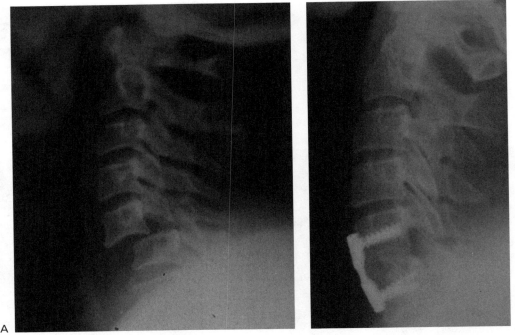

FIGURE 6.4. A; Lateral cervical radiograph demonstrating C5-on-C6 bilateral jumped facets. This patient sustained a complete injury. **B;** Postoperative lateral radiograph of the above-stated injury treated surgically with an anterior screw plate system.

fected by cervical spine subluxations is the C5 to C6 level. In a unilateral facet injury, the patient usually does not sustain a complete (ASIA A) SCI. More frequently, unilateral facet jumps are associated with a nerve root injury at the level of the facet subluxation. An incomplete injury may also be present, however. The usual treatments of facet subluxations involve urgent use of skeletal traction to realign the spinal elements. The timing of advanced imaging studies, with respect to the use of traction, has been previously discussed. Bilateral facet subluxations are typically associated with complete (ASIA A) SCI. These classically have a greater than 50% subluxation of the superior vertebral body with respect to the interior vertebral body.

After spinal realignment with skeletal traction, surgical stabilization is indicated for facet subluxations in the cervical spine. The surgical approach may be either anterior or posterior. If advanced imaging studies demonstrate the presence of a herniated disk or significant vertebral bony injury causing neural compression anteriorly, then an anterior decompressive procedure with fusion and screw plate fixation is indicated. In the absence of ongoing ventral neural compression, either an anterior or posterior approach may be used. From a posterior approach, techniques include use of interspinous wiring with bone grafting or placement of lateral mass plating with bone grafting.

Thoracic Spine Injuries

The most common thoracic spinal injury involves fractures of the T12 vertebra. This may, or may not, be associated with an acute SCI. Most T12 vertebral injuries do not have an associated

neurologic injury. Presumably as a result of increased stability afforded this region by the presence of stabilizing ribs, significant subluxations in the thoracic spine are uncommon. Recently, fractures involving the upper thoracic spine appear to be increasing in frequency. Fractures in the T5 vertebral body region may result from the use of shoulder harness belts, which place a moment of force in the upper thoracic region. This area is a vascular watershed area, with poor blood supply, and as such, if a SCI occurs in this region, it is more likely to be neurologically complete.

After determination of the stability of a thoracic spine fracture, unstable injuries are treated with stabilization and fusion procedures (Fig. 6.5). In addition, decompression may be necessary when retropulsion of bony elements into the spinal canal has occurred, or a significant ligamentous injury has accounted for a subluxation causing neural compression. In the lower thoracic spine region, either an anterior or posterior approach may be used. Anterior surgery is typically performed through a thoracotomy, or a thoracoabdominal approach, when a corpectomy is performed. This is followed by bone grafting and stabilization with either a screw plate or a screw and rod construct. These anterior surgical procedures allow for a short-segment stabilization to be accomplished. Anterior surgery in the upper thoracic spine is extremely difficult technically and is rarely performed. Posterior thoracic surgery may be performed in either the upper or lower thoracic spine. This classically involves the use of a hook and rod stabilization construct. Often, a laminectomy can be performed at the level of the injured segment, with hooks and rods placed at locations remote from the site of injury.

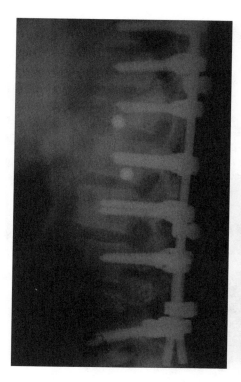

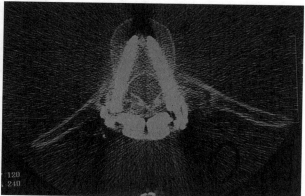

FIGURE 6.5. Two noncontiguous fractures (T10 and T6) treated with the same pedicle screw rod system during one surgical procedure.

Because of the biomechanical disadvantages of stabilizing merely the posterior elements, with an injury that may be prone to kyphotic deformity, long-segment stabilizations are necessary when posterior hook and rod constructs are used. Recently, pedicle screw implementation has been used in the thoracic spine, which may afford the advantage of stabilizing all three columns of the spine as well as allowing for shorter-segment stabilization.

Lumbar Spine Injuries

In the lumbar spine, L1 burst fractures are the most common cause of SCI (Fig. 6.6). These frequently result from a fall from a height and result in an injury that partially affects the conus medullaris and partially affects the cauda equina. Bowel and bladder function may be affected as well. Injuries to the lower lumbar sections are nerve root injuries alone because they affect the cauda equina. Of particular note is that the cauda equina, or peripheral nerve root injuries, should not be treated with steroid medications because there is no proven benefit to this treatment in the lower lumbar spine. The surgical treatment of upper lumbar injuries typically involves a corpectomy of either the L1 or L2 vertebral body followed by stabilization with a screw and rod or screw plate construct. On the other hand, posterior hook and rod constructs at the thoracolumbar junction may be used to treat upper lumbar injuries; however, these would require long-segment stabilization. In the lower lumbar region, posterior screw and rod stabilizations are typically performed. This involves placement of screws in the large pedicles of the lumbar spine, which provides excellent stabilization. Decompression can be accomplished through laminectomy, and

ventral compression may also be achieved from a posterior approach using this technique. Anterior surgery in the lower lumbar spine is extremely difficult because of the presence of the iliopsoas muscles and the great vessels. As such, anterior surgery below the level of L3 is rarely attempted. For L1 and L2 operations, the anterior approach is often used.

Miscellaneous

In certain instances of severe trauma, multiple spinal segments may be injured independently. In these circumstances, each injured segment must be treated appropriately while maintaining an understanding that major surgical procedures may need to be staggered, on different days, due to concerns of critical care or systemic medical concerns in the polytrauma patient. If possible, there are advantages to completing all stabilizations at the time of the initial procedure so that the patient may be mobilized more quickly after surgical stabilization (Fig. 6.5). In addition, some spinal disruptions causing SCI may be so severe that they necessitate a combined anterior and posterior approach in order to decompress and stabilize the spine adequately.

Laminectomy alone is rarely indicated in acute spine trauma causing SCI. If the predominant neural compression is from a dorsal direction with relative preservation of the anterior elements, laminectomy may be the procedure of choice. Practically, this occurs more commonly with penetrating trauma than with blunt trauma. Some surgeons who are uncomfortable with long anterior cervical surgeries perform cervical laminectomies for cervical spondylosis with central cord syndrome, but this is not the preferred method of decompression.

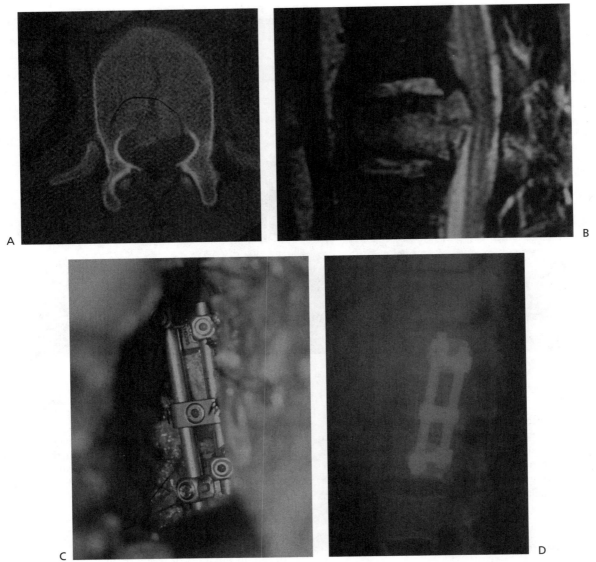

FIGURE 6.6. Computed tomography scan (**A**) and magnetic resonance image (**B**) demonstrating an L1 burst fracture. **C**; Intraoperative view of the treatment of the same fracture using a screw rod system. **D**; Postoperative lateral radiograph of the screw rod system in place.

SUMMARY REGARDING SURGERY

Conventional teaching states that the neurologic outcome after an acute SCI is frequently determined at the time of the injury or in the first 20 minutes after the injury. This means that the neurologic status is determined before the patient's arrival to the hospital. The time of the surgery and the use of traction have been described. At this time, there is no uniform consensus as to the timing; however, it is our belief that early traction and early surgical stabilization are advantageous to the patient with an acute SCI. Theories involving spinal stability have been explained, and surgical principles have been detailed. Specific segments and their treatments have been described. When surgery is planned to treat a patient with an acute SCI, the primary goal is neural decompression, with a secondary goal to stabilize and fuse the spine for long-term recovery. If a complete neurologic injury is present at the time of the initial evaluation, surgery may be performed to facilitate earlier rehabilitation, improve the ultimate posture obtainable, help with self-esteem issues, prevent the development of chronic pain, and possibly decrease the incidence of posttraumatic syringomyelia development. If an incomplete SCI or a neurologically intact state is present, surgery may then be performed to decompress the neural elements, prevent neurologic deterioration, prevent the development of chronic pain and deformity, and facilitate a more rapid entrance into the rehabilitation process.

REFERENCES

1. McDonald JW. Repairing the damaged spinal cord. *Sci Am* 1999;281: 64–73.
2. Slucky AV, Eismont FJ. Treatment of acute injury of the cervical spine. *J Bone Joint Surg Am* 1994;76:1882–1896.
3. Slucky AV, Eismont FJ. Treatment of acute injury of the cervical spine. *Instructional Course Lectures* 1995;44:67–80.
4. Ramzy AI, Parry JM, Greenberg J. Head and spinal injury: pre hospital care. In: Greenberg J, ed. *Handbook of head and spine trauma.* New York: Marcel Dekker, 1993:29–44.
5. Crosby LA, Lewallen DG, eds. *Emergency care and transportation of the sick and injured,* 6th ed. Rosemont, IL: American Academy of Orthopedic Surgery, 1995.
6. Cohen M. Initial resuscitation of the patient with spinal cord injury. *Trauma Q* 1993;9:38–43.
7. Vaccaro AR, An HS, Betz RR, et al. The management of acute spinal trauma: prehospital and in-hospital emergency care. *Instructional Course Lectures* 1997;46:113–125.
8. Sonntag VK, Douglas RA. Management of spinal cord trauma. *Neurosurg Clin North Am* 1990;1:729–750.
9. Fielding JW. Fractures of the spine. I. Injuries of the cervical spine. In: Rockwood CA Jr, Wilkins KE, King RE eds. *Fractures in children.* Philadelphia: JB Lippincott, 1984:683–705.
10. Atkinson PP, Atkinson JL. Spinal shock. *Mayo Clin Proc* 1996;71: 384–389.
11. Geisler FH. Acute management of cervical spinal cord injury. *MD Med J* 1998;37:525–530.
12. Vale FL, Burns J, Jackson AB, et al. Combined medical and surgical treatment after acute spinal cord injury: results of a prospective pilot study to assess the merits of aggressive medical resuscitation and blood pressure management. *J Neurosurg* 1997;87:239–246.
13. Savitsky E, Votey S. Emergency department approach to acute thoracolumbar spine trauma. *J Emerg Med* 1997;15:49–60.
14. Greenberg MS. *Handbook of neurosurgery,* 3rd ed. Lakeland FL: Greenberg Graphics, 1994.
15. Eismont FJ, Arena MJ, Green BA. Extrusion of an intervertebral disc associated with traumatic subluxation or dislocation of cervical facets: case report. *J Bone Joint Surg Am.* 1997;73:1555–1560.
16. Cotler JM, Herbison GJ, Nasuti JF, et al. Closed reduction of traumatic cervical spine dislocation using traction weights up to 140 pounds. *Spine* 1993;18:386–390.
17. Star AM, Jones AA, Cotler JM, et al. Immediate closed reduction of cervical spine dislocations using traction. *Spine* 1990;15:1068–1072.
18. Breasted JH. *Edwin Smith surgical papyrus.* Chicago: University of Chicago Press, 1930.
19. Nockels R, Young W. Pharmacologic strategies in the treatment of experimental spinal cord injury. *J Neurotrauma* 1992;9:S211–S217.
20. Young W. Medical treatment of spinal cord injury. *J Neurol Neurosurg Psychiatry* 1992;55:635–639.
21. Bracken MB, Collins WF, Freeman DF, et al. Efficacy of methylprednisolone in acute spinal cord injury. *JAMA* 1984;251:45–52.
22. Bracken MB, Shepard MJ, Collins WF, et al. A randomized controlled trial of methylprednisolone or naloxone in the treatment of acute spinal-cord injury: results of the Second National Acute Spinal Cord Injury Study. *N Engl J Med* 1990;322:1405–1411.
23. Bracken MB, Shepard MJ, Holford TR, et al. Administration of methylprednisolone for 24 or 48 hours or tirilazad mesylate for 48 hours in the treatment of acute spinal cord injury: results of the Third National Acute Spinal Cord Injury Randomized Controlled Trial. National Acute Spinal Cord Injury Study. *JAMA* 1997;277:1597–1604.
24. Bracken MB, Shepard MJ, Collins WF, et al. Methylprednisolone or naloxone in the treatment of acute spinal cord injury: 1 year follow up data. Results of the Second National Acute Spinal Cord Injury Study. *J Neurosurg* 1992;76:23–31.
25. Bracken MB, Shepard MJ, Holford TR, et al. Methylprednisolone or tirilazad mesylate administration after acute spinal cord injury: 1-year follow up. Results of the Third National Acute Spinal Cord Injury randomized controlled trial. *J Neurosurg* 1998;89:699–706.
26. Geisler FH, Dorsey FC, Coleman WP. Recovery of motor function after spinal cord injury: a randomized, placebo-controlled trial with GM-1 ganglioside. *N Engl J Med* 1991;324:1829–1838.
27. Hurlbert RJ. Methyprednisolone for acute spinal cord injury: an inappropriate standard of care. *J Neurosurg* 2000;93:1–7.
28. Nesathurai S. Steroids and spinal cord injury: revisiting the NASCIS 2 and NASCIS 3 trials. *J Trauma* 1998;45:1088–1093.
29. Short DJ, El Masry WS, Jones PW. High dose methylprednisolone in the management of acute spinal cord injury: a systematic review from a clinical perspective. *Spinal Cord* 2000;38:273–286.
30. Heary RF, Vaccaro AR, Mesa JJ, et al. Steroids and gunshot wounds to the spine. *Neurosurgery* 1997;41:576–583.
31. Levy ML, Gans W, Wijesinghe HS, et al. Use of methylprednisolone as an adjunct in the management of patients with penetrating spinal cord injury: outcome analysis. *Neurosurgery* 1996;39:1141–1148.
32. Constantini S, Young W. The effects of methylprednisolone and the ganglioside GM1 on acute spinal cord injury in rats. *J Neurosurg* 1994; 80:97–111.
33. Kuchner EF, Hansebout RR. Combined steroid and hypothermia treatment of experimental spinal cord injury. *Surg Neurol* 1976;6:371–376.
34. Kulkami A, Bhandari M, Stiver S, et al. Delayed presentation of spinal stab wound: case report and review of the literature. *J Emerg Med* 2000; 18:209–213.
35. Chiles BW III, Cooper PR. Acute spinal injury. *N Engl J Med* 1996; 334(8):514–520.
36. Heary RF, Vaccaro AR, Mesa JJ, et al. Thoracolumbar infections in penetrating injuries to the spine. *Orthop Clin North Am* 1996;27: 69–81.
37. Marshall LF, Knowlton S, Garfin SR, et al. Deterioration following spinal cord injury: a multicenter study. *J Neurosurg* 1987;66:400–404.
38. Vaccaro AR, Daugherty RJ, Sheehan TP, et al. Neurologic outcome of early versus late surgery for cervical spinal cord injury. *Spine* 1997; 22:2609–2613.
39. Tator CH, Fehlings MG, Thorpe K, et al. Current use and timing of spinal surgery for management of acute spinal surgery for management of acute spinal cord injury in North America: results of a retrospective multicenter study. *J Neurosurg* 1999;91:12–18.
40. Fehlings MG, Tator CH. An evidence-based review of decompressive surgery in acute spinal cord injury: rationale, indications, and timing based on experimental and clinical studies. *J Neurosurg* 1999;91:1–11.
41. White AA, Panjabi MM. *Clinical biomechanics of the spine,* 2nd ed. Philadelphia: Lippincott, 1990.
42. Denis F. The three column spine and its significance in the classification of acute thoracolumbar spinal injuries. *Spine* 1983;8:817–831.
43. Resnick DK, Weller SJ, Benzel EC. Biomechanics of the thoracolumbar spine. *Neurosurg Clin North Am* 1997;8:455–469.
44. Powers B, Miller MD, Kramer RS, et al. Traumatic anterior atlantooccipital dislocation. *Neurosurgery* 1979;4:12–17.
45. Spence KF Jr, Decker S, Sell KW. Bursting atlantal fracture associated with rupture of the transverse ligament. *J Bone Joint Surg Am* 1970; 52:543–549.
46. Apfelbaum RI, Lonser RR, Veres R, et al. Direct anterior screw fixation for recent and remote odontoid fractures. *J Neurosurg* 2000;93: 227–236.
47. Gallie WE. Fractures and dislocation of the cervical spine. *Am J Surg* 1939;46:495–499.
48. Brooks AL, Jenkins EB. Atlanto-axial arthrodesis by the wedge compression method. *J Bone Joint Surg Am* 1978;60:279–284.
49. Grob D, Magerl F. [Surgical stabilization of C1 and C2 fractures] (German). *Orthopade* 1987;16:46–54.
50. Caspar W, Barbier DD, Klara PM. Anterior cervical fusion and Caspar plate stabilization for cervical trauma. *Neurosurgery* 1989;25:491–502.
51. Johnson RM, Hart DL, Simmons EF, et al. Cervical orthoses: a study comparing their effectiveness in restricting cervical motion in normal subjects. *J Bone Joint Surg Am* 1977;59:332–339.
52. Glaser JA, Whitehill R, Stamp WG. Complications associated with the halo-vest. *J Neurosurg* 1986;65:762–769.

7

PREDICTING OUTCOME IN TRAUMATIC SPINAL CORD INJURY

JOHN F. DITUNNO
ADAM E. FLANDERS
STEVEN KIRSHBLUM
VIRGINIA GRAZIANI
ALAN TESSLER

Functional outcome in terms of capacity to walk and care for oneself are the most important issues for patients who have recently sustained a spinal cord injury (SCI) once they are aware that they will survive the immediate trauma. The prediction of this function is important to the family and loved ones of the injured patient and to the treatment team, in order to plan realistically for the future during rehabilitation in the hospital and after discharge. The insurance industry, under the best of circumstances, has made evidence-based justification of the rehabilitation treatment an *imperative* for those in need of care and those who wish to provide it (1).

In recent years, our knowledge of the course of neurologic recovery has increased to the point at which we can predict within a week of injury the recovery in strength of the arms and legs (1). This information, together with our understanding of the relationship of strength to function, allows us to predict functional capacity accurately for groups of patients. Fundamental to our ability to predict outcome in SCI is the knowledge and skill of performing an accurate neurologic examination based on the international neurologic standards, presented in chapter 5. Based on (a) an accurate neurologic assessment, (b) the knowledge of neurologic recovery after SCI, and (c) the relationship of function to recovery, we can prognosticate future functional capacity.

The purpose of this chapter is to review the evidence, which establishes the basis for predicting neurologic recovery after SCI. The initial sections examine the findings based on clinical examination alone, followed by discussions of the laboratory methods, including the electrodiagnostic evidence for recovery and the neuroradiologic findings correlated with neurologic outcome, which may supplement or at times substitute for a limited physical examination. Finally, an attempt to understand some of the underlying mechanisms responsible for the recovery is reviewed in an effort to pose potential strategies to enhance recovery in the future.

PREDICTION OF ARM AND LEG RECOVERY AND THE RELATIONSHIP OF NEUROLOGIC RECOVERY TO FUNCTIONAL CAPACITY

Long, in a provocative work based on clinical observation, set the stage for relating the final neurologic level following SCI with the self-care and mobility that was possible for those individuals (2). For close to 50 years, this has served the rehabilitation professional and patients with SCI, as a guide for estimating functional capacity or expectations based on the neurologic examination and level. Most textbooks over the years have used a similar outline with minor revisions of Long's original paper (3, 4). Stauffer, 25 years later, placed the actors on the stage set by Long, by introducing *prognosis of neurologic recovery* in cervical cord lesions and *walking* based on clinical syndromes (5). Although Stauffer's statement that all subjects with a cervical cord lesion would improve one neurologic level has been significantly qualified in recent years, it was the standard for prognosis of cervical injury for the latter part of the twentieth century. Based on improvement of one neurologic level, an individual admitted immediately after injury with a C5 level would improve to C6, thereby gaining independence in certain feeding and self-care tasks; and a patient with C6 injury, who would improve to C7, could possibly be independent in self-care and mobility in a wheelchair.

As a result of many studies from predominantly two authors, we can now predict the time course of reaching the final neurologic level and the functional capacity after injury that is possible. As stated by Kirshblum, the studies are not comparable because in Ditunno's reports, the prognosis is based on examination within 1 week, whereas in Water's studies, the initial examination is at 30 days (6–11). The use of the Frankel or American Spinal Injury Association (ASIA) classification makes little difference in change of motor scores and grades A, C, and D 1 year after injury (12). Although we understand the course of recovery much better than we did 25 years ago, the functional capacity measures have lagged behind the impairment measures of sensation, strength, and reflexes. Because the Functional Independence Measure (FIM) is a measure of burden of care, it has important implications in estimating costs and has become the standard for the rehabilitation industry since 1987 (13). The FIM is composed of motor items (self-care, sphincter control, and mobility) and cognitive items (communication and psychological adjustment) and is described in chapter 5. It fails, however, to portray accurately the full independence that individuals with SCI can achieve (14). The cognitive items are not informative for detecting changes over time, but the motor items appear to reflect changes in neurologic status (15). Improved measures of functional capacity, such as the Capacity for Upper Extremity function (CUE) and the Walking Index for Spinal Cord Injury (WISCI), may be more accurate for defining function, particularly for use in clinical trials (16,17).

The accuracy, frequency, thoroughness, and timing of the neurologic assessment during the first week after the injury is essential to predicting the motor recovery of individuals with SCI in order to relate this recovery to functional capacity (6). Multicenter studies, which show a more representative time course of recovery than single centers, enable the experienced clinician to prognosticate, provided individuals are examined by the methods of the ASIA standards. These standards include a *minimum* data set of key sensory points and key muscles, which are tested repeatedly in the supine position (18). The controversial testing technique of the gastrocnemius-soleus muscle group (plantar flexors) in the supine position of an acutely injured individual, because of spine instability, cannot be compared with the traditional testing of the same muscle group in the antigravity position after the patient can stand. Testing in the emergency room soon after injury is important, but testing over a period of days and by 72 hours after injury has been shown to be superior to a single early examination (19). The sensory examination is of greater value for predicting motor recovery in the lower extremities than for the upper extremities (20). The significance of reflexes in regard to functional recovery, which are currently optional in the ASIA minimum data set, are discussed later (21).

It is also important to appreciate that the skills mastered in the accurate performance of the neurologic assessment differ from the skills used in the classification of individuals by level and impairment, although the classification is derived from the neurologic assessment (18). Performance of functional tests, likewise, requires skill and understanding of differences in techniques (22). Thus, results of neurologic examination may vary based on the clinician or the time after injury and the functional assessment based on the use of observation or self-report (23). Finally, the prediction of functional recovery is valid only for groups of patients, up to a 95% confidence level (24).

NEUROLOGIC RECOVERY OF THE ARMS AND SELF-CARE FUNCTION IN INDIVIDUALS WITH TETRAPLEGIA

Stauffer's seminal work on prognosis for cervical lesions presumed the neurologic level was normal (defined as muscle grade 5) and not the 3/5 or better muscle grade used in the definition of the ASIA standards, with the next proximal level muscle grade 5, because it predated the standards (5). This should be kept in mind when comparing results of studies.

In a retrospective study of a group of motor complete tetraplegic subjects, it was concluded if motor strength was grade 2 to 5 at the zone of injury (ZOI) 1 week after injury, then there was an 80% chance that the patient would gain functional strength at the next neurologic level (7). The ZOI in this study refers to the most rostral neurologic levels that showed evidence of weakness due to spinal cord injury and may consist of one

to three levels immediately below the neurologically intact level rostrally. In 1992, the first multicenter study of recovery of arm strength in 150 subjects from four centers showed that 70% to 80% of motor complete tetraplegic patients with some motor strength (SMS, grade 1 to 2) at the ZOI 1 week after injury would recover to the next neurologic level within 3 to 6 months (8). In subjects, however, with no motor strength (NMS, grade 0/5), only 30% to 40% would gain a level during the same period. This study was unable to indicate, however, the prognosis for individual levels, such as C4, C5, or C6, because of the size of the sample and the method of analysis. Waters reported a similar recovery pattern at 1 year in 61 motor complete subjects with SMS at 30 days, but there was minimal significant recovery in subjects with NMS at 30 days (10).

In data presented during the past several years and recently published, we have reported on a mathematic model for very accurately prognosticating for groups of patients within the first week of injury (18,24). Using a generalized estimating equation and subjects from five centers, prognosis for complete versus incomplete tetraplegia patients in one study and 221 subjects with motor complete tetraplegia in a second study can be made with a 90% confidence level for groups at 1 week. These studies showed a significant difference between motor complete and incomplete patients at the C4 and C5 levels for those who would gain a motor level. This confirmed earlier reports, but no significant difference was found at C6, which was not expected.

Although individuals with complete lesions may improve one and sometimes two levels, those with incomplete lesions often have recovery at multiple levels below the injury site. In a 10-year, multicenter study of motor complete subjects, subjects with SMS compared with NMS at the C4 and C5 level showed a greater recovery ($p < 0.001$) than C6 subjects ($p < 0.014$), but all levels reached significance (9) (Fig. 7.1). Individuals with complete injuries show a plateau of recovery to the next level after 12 to 18 months (Fig. 7.1). Whereas individuals with incomplete injuries achieve a plateau of recovery to the next level more rapidly, in 9 to 12 months (9,24). Figure 7.1 portrays the recovery of the wrist extensors in C5 motor complete tetraplegic patients from no muscle strength (MS = 0/5) in the wrist extensors and from some strength (MS − 1 to 2.5/5) on initial examination to various points over a 2-year period.

Kirshblum has extensively reviewed the literature on neurologic recovery in tetraplegic subjects and these reviews are recommended for a more thorough discussion of nuances of recovery based on initial motor strength, sensory examination and timing of the examination (25). Caution is warranted in reaching conclusions from these studies, however, because in most studies, the sample is small (30 to 50 subjects) and from one center and therefore less representative than samples in larger multicenter studies (Table 7.1).

Several authors have shown a correlation of motor recovery with improved feeding or other self-care function (26–28). Patients with a C7 motor level may be independent in most self-care activities and were reported to be significantly more functional than those with a C6 motor level if motor strength was a grade 3 or higher (26). In fact, Zafonte and colleagues reported that patients with a C7 motor level on one side could be independent in feeding activities (27). These studies correlated motor

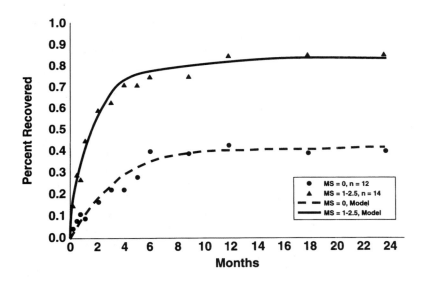

FIGURE 7.1. Pattern of recovery of wrist extensors to grade higher than 3 in C5 right motor complete tetraplegic subjects.

level with self-care, but Marino and associates also looked at upper extremity motor scores, in addition to motor levels, and showed a correlation with feeding activities (28). It is important to realize that the motor level is superior to the single neurologic or sensory level in correlating self-care activities such as feeding, but often in tables correlating level with function, the level is not specified as motor, sensory, or neurologic (29).

The Model Systems centers, in an analysis of more than 2,500 subjects, showed a good correlation of FIM scores and neurologic level, and the third National Acute Spinal Cord Injury Study (NASCIS-III) of almost 500 subjects showed a significant improvement in self-care that correlated with improved motor

function (30,31). The recent model systems report divided neurologic recovery and change based on the FIM into two separate studies (12,15). Changes in motor scores and Frankel or ASIA grade from 1 week of injury to discharge and 1 year follow-up in more than 3,500 subjects were comparable to data reported in 1995 (12). This study showed that the sensory level determines the neurologic level, and the sensory level was higher (more rostral) in more than 20% of cases (12). In about 4,000 subjects, the FIM showed that it was sensitive to change over time, but this was reflected only in the motor FIM scores, not to be confused with motor scores, which are summated scores of the key muscles (15). The study made reference to cervical neurologic levels and did not define detailed function but, rather, motor scores (FIM). Eating, grooming, and transfers of all types were highly correlated with the changes in FIM scores.

Based on these studies and the prediction model of motor recovery described previously, it is now possible to predict functional recovery for groups of patients after a careful neurologic assessment within 1 week of injury.

TABLE 7.1. SUMMARY OF RECOVERY FROM COMPLETE TETRAPLEGIA

A. Patients (30%–80%) regain one motor level from 1 week to 1 year.
B. At 72 hours to 1 week, recovery of the next motor level to at least 3/5 at 1 year depends on the motor level and initial strength:
   About 30%–40% of first 0/5 muscles
   70%–80% of muscles 1 or 2/5
   Presence of sensation at that level increases chances of recovery
C. At 1 month; recovery at 1 year:
   Greater than 95% of 1 or 2/5 muscles recover to 3/5
   50%–60% of first 0/5 muscles recovers to 1/5
   About 25% of first 0/5 muscles recover to 3/5
   Less than 10% of second 0/5 muscles recover to 1/5
   About 1% of second 0/5 muscles recover to 3/5
D. The initial strength of the muscle is a significant predictor of achieving antigravity strength and its rate of recovering strength.
E. The faster an initial 0/5 muscle starts to recover some strength, the greater the prognosis for recovery.
F. Most upper extremity recovery occurs during the first 6 months, with the greatest rate of change during the first 3 months.
G. Most patients with some initial power plateau at an earlier time and at a higher level than patients with no motor power. Motor recovery can continue, with lesser gains seen in the second year, especially in patients with initially 0/5 strength.

NEUROLOGIC RECOVERY OF THE LEGS AND WALKING IN SPINAL CORD INJURY PATIENTS

The first study on the prognosis for recovery of walking based on the pattern of the anatomic lesion was from Bosch and colleagues (32). They reported that 90% of patients with Brown-Séquard lesions would be able to walk, followed by 50% of those with central cord syndromes, whereas individuals with anterior cord lesions had an extremely poor prognosis. Maynard and coauthors reported that 72 hours after injury, 47% of sensory incomplete patients were walking, and 87% of motor incomplete subjects at 72 hours were walking at 1 year (33). They classified patients by Frankel grade and suggested walking levels be added to the Frankel grades to categorize further Frankel D (motor functional) subjects. Benzel and Larson added three walking categories to the Frankel grades, and this scale was used in the recent Sygen trial (34,35). Both the anatomic and Frankel classifications use the interpretation of a detailed neurologic examination and have been used to predict functional recovery. The Frankel grades have been modified to the ASIA Impairment Scale, and both the anatomic and ASIA Impairment Scale have been incorporated into the *International Standards for Neurological and Functional Classification of Spinal Cord Injury* (21).

Thirty-five hundred patients admitted to the Model Systems centers within 1 week of injury with clinically complete lesions (Frankel or ASIA A) show only 2% to 3% improvement to Frankel or ASIA D by 1 year (12). This improvement in patients with clinically complete injuries has not apparently changed since the 1990s (30). The data do not reveal how many of the 2% to 3% will be ambulatory, nor does it distinguish between tetraplegia and paraplegia. In several smaller studies, we found that community ambulation (150 feet or more) is not seen in complete tetraplegia (Frankel or ASIA A) nor at times in some Frankel or ASIA B or C patients classified within 1 week of injury (36,37). These studies did not include subjects who required bilateral long leg braces or functional electrical stimulation to ambulate. Waters reported on only 5% of complete paraplegic patients achieving community ambulation, and others showed that these individuals required pelvic control with at least one hip flexor and knee extensor at grade 3/5 muscle strength (38,39).

Frankel or ASIA B patients with complete motor paralysis but preserved sensation are not categorized by the presence or absence of pinprick sensation. Frankel or ASIA B subjects with preservation of pinprick sensation within the first few weeks after injury have a 70% to 90% chance of motor recovery sufficient to walk. Patients who are motor complete but have only light touch present with the absence of pinprick sensation do not have a favorable prognosis for walking (20). Patients with incomplete injuries manifested by some movement, however slight, have an excellent prognosis for walking if younger than 50 years of age. Older patients (50 years of age or older) with incomplete injuries similar to Brown-Séquard or central cord syndromes have only a 40% chance of walking, if motor strength is slight (ASIA C) within a week of injury, but an excellent chance if strength is classified as ASIA D (36). Waters has also reported that 46% of incomplete tetraplegic patients experience sufficient motor recovery to ambulate at 1 year (11). He used lower extremity motor scores and correlated them with community ambulation (40). In subjects with a lower extremity motor score of 20/50 or below at 1 month, the ambulation was poor, but with motor scores of 30/50 or above, subjects were able to achieve community ambulation. Although we lack population-based studies and multicenter studies on recovery of walking, there is consistency in patterns of neurologic recovery in the lower extremities from a number of centers and the Model Systems centers. Therefore, it is possible to correlate community walking in most patients with a final Frankel or ASIA D grade and in those with lower extremity motor scores of 30 or greater.

NEUROLOGIC RECOVERY IN THE LOWER EXTREMITIES IN PATIENTS WITH PARAPLEGIA

Recovery from injuries below the cervical spine (resulting in paraplegia) has not been studied to the degree of tetraplegia. In

thoracic level and high lumbar level injuries [neurologic level of injury (NLI) above L2], one can usually test only for sensory modality change to document an improvement in NLI because there are no corresponding key muscle groups between T1 and L2. Therefore, it is especially difficult to document the degree of neurologic improvement, especially for those with a complete injury.

For those with a complete injury, Waters and colleagues found that the NLI did not change in 73% of patients from 1 month to 1 year after injury, with 18% improving a single level, 7% two levels, and the remainder greater than two levels (5). For patients with a complete injury above T8, these investigators reported that no patients regained lower extremity motor strength. The potential for lower extremity motor strength recovery improves with lower initial neurologic levels of injury; 15% of patients with an NLI between T9 and T11 and 55% of those with an initial NLI below T12 recovered some function. Most of the volitional movement gained is in the proximal lower extremity musculature (41). This improvement of lower extremity strength may represent recovery of partially injured lumbar roots, or "root escape" as described by Holdsworth over 30 years ago (42).

Individuals with incomplete paraplegia have the best prognosis for ambulation (38,43). Between 1 month and 1 year, the average increase in motor index scoring is 12 points, with the greatest increase occurring in the first 3 months. Eighty percent of individuals with incomplete paraplegia regain hip flexors and knee extensors (strength greater than 3/5) at 1 year. Individuals with no lower extremity strength at 1 month may still show significant return by 1 year. The mechanism of recovery often includes recovery of the spinal roots and spinal cord and therefore differs from the mechanism of recovery of leg function in tetraplegic patients.

PROGNOSIS BASED ON REFLEX RECOVERY AND SPINAL SHOCK

Considerable confusion exists regarding the role of spinal shock and the ability to predict recovery at that time following injury (5,44). Stauffer is frequently cited as warning against prognosticating during spinal shock, and several authors suggest spinal shock is associated with a more serious prognosis (5). Spinal shock, however, has been poorly defined, and because the definitions are vague or misleading, it is not helpful to clinicians to make reference to it in predicting recovery, unless they are very precise in regard to reflexes. Stauffer and others define spinal shock as an absence of all reflexes, but this rarely is seen in completely injured individuals. Recovery of reflexes has also been described as caudal to cephalad with the bulbocavernosus reflex (S4 to S5) occurring first and then the ankle jerk (L5 to S1), followed by the knee jerk (L3 to L4). A recent report that carefully monitored 50 subjects from the initial day of injury failed to confirm these previous descriptions (44). The delayed plantar response (DPR) in this study was seen most often as the first reflex after injury, rather than the bulbocavernosus reflex, and the DPR had prognostic value for walking. The cremasteric reflex occurred in males often before the deep tendon reflexes (ankle jerk and knee jerk), from the L1 dermatome. Therefore, the DPR (L5 to S1) and the cremasteric reflex are often present on the day of injury and are followed by the deep tendon reflex. This is not consistent with previous descriptions of spinal shock, as stated earlier, in which the recovery of reflexes was stated to be from caudal to rostral, but typically referred only to the bulbocavernosus and deep tendon reflexes (45).

In two studies from the same center, the DPR, particularly if it persisted for several days after the injury, was associated with a poor prognosis for ambulation (44,46). This reflex is elicited by stroking the sole of the foot in the same area as for the Babinski sign but requires deep pressure rather than a light stimulus. The response is always delayed in comparison to a normal plantar response or Babinski sign, and the toes flex and then relax slowly. The DPR was always seen in severe injuries and less frequently and of shorter duration (usually 1 day) in ASIA D patients but was associated with a poor prognosis for walking when it persisted longer than 2 days in ASIA A, B, and C patients. It is probably unwise to predict future function based on only one examination on the day of injury for scientific and psychological reasons, particularly if the findings are consistent with a complete lesion. Occasionally, the patient cannot cooperate fully in an examination, and the eliciting of reflexes that do not require a cooperative patient may be the only clinical clue to the prognosis.

The presence of a bulbocavernosus reflex in a patient with an upper motor neuron (UMN) lesion has no prognostic significance because it is usually present in all UMN cases. Its persisting absence for more than several days is indicative of a lower motor neuron (LMN) lesion, and this has functional significance in bladder, bowel, and sexual function. Although LMN lesions usually occur at the T12 to S5 levels, a significant number of T9 to T11 injuries result in absence of bulbocavernosus or deep tendon reflexes (47).

In summary, persistence of reflexes such as the DPR has prognostic significance for walking, and the absence of reflexes such as the bulbocavernosus would define an LMN lesion associated with different bladder, bowel, and sexual function than an UMN lesion. The evolution of reflexes in the week following injury is probably of greater significance than the presence or absence of reflexes on one examination and references to the presence or absence of spinal shock.

CLINICAL SIGNIFICANCE OF SPINAL CORD MAGNETIC RESONANCE IMAGING FINDINGS

Magnetic resonance imaging (MRI) has revolutionized the diagnosis of diseases of the spine and spinal cord. In the setting of spinal cord injury, MRI has become an essential diagnostic tool in the initial period after injury and for long-term assessment when late neurologic deterioration occurs. MRI is the only noninvasive imaging tool that depicts the structure of the spinal cord. Since it was first applied in the setting of SCI, numerous experimental and clinical investigations have shown a direct correlation between the appearance of the damaged spinal cord on MRI and the degree of functional deficit at the time of injury and the capacity for neurologic recovery. The ultimate clinical value of MRI in SCI may be realized in the selection and monitoring of patients for novel forms of therapeutic intervention.

Three MRI features that characterize SCI are spinal cord hemorrhage, spinal cord edema, and spinal cord swelling. A typical SCI on MRI is spindle shaped and characterized by a central focus of hemorrhage and a peripheral margin of edema that may span a variable length of the spinal cord. Edema appears brighter (hyperintense) relative to normal spinal cord parenchyma on T2-weighted images, whereas subacute hemorrhage appears dark (hypointense). In some instances, no central focus of hemorrhage is identifiable on MRI, in which case, only edema is present. The damaged region of spinal cord is usually larger in caliber (swollen) than the normal adjacent parenchyma. The MRI features are often described in terms of presence or absence, location, and extent.

In one of the first studies that examined the relationship between MRI findings and neurologic injury. Kulkarni and associates proposed three MRI injury patterns for SCI and correlated these with the ASIA impairment scale and total motor scores (48). Intramedullary hemorrhage (type I pattern of injury) equated with a severe neurologic deficit and a poor prognosis. Cord edema alone (type II pattern of injury) was associated with mild to moderate initial neurologic deficits that subsequently improved. Similar findings were reported in other studies (49–52).

A subsequent study by Schaefer and colleagues refined the MRI patterns of SCI by including the size of the injured segment (53). Cord edema that extended for more than the span of one vertebral segment was associated with a more severe initial deficit than smaller areas of edema. Identification of spinal cord hemorrhage was also associated with the most severe neurologic abnormalities (53).

In a larger study, Flanders and coworkers found that the cervical MRI features of spinal cord hemorrhage were a strong predictor of a complete neurologic injury (54). The location of the hemorrhage corresponded anatomically to the level of neurologic injury. The location of spinal cord edema related imprecisely to the neurologic level; however, the proportion of spinal cord affected by edema was directly related to the severity of initial neurologic injury. Moreover, although vertebral body fracture, disk herniation, and ligamentous injury were not predictive of the initial neurologic deficit, the presence of residual spinal cord compression by disk, bone, or epidural hematoma was more frequently associated with a hemorrhagic spinal cord lesion than injuries without residual compression. This suggests that early decompressive surgery may minimize the severity of tissue damage to the spinal cord (54–56).

There is additional substantial evidence that suggests that the MRI changes of SCI offer prognostic information regarding neurologic recovery (48–52,57–66). In two original studies that demonstrated the prognostic correlate of MRI in SCI, the authors categorized MRI spinal cord injury patterns into five types (65,66). They showed that poor recovery from SCI was associated with severe cord compression, cord swelling, and abnormal signal on T1-weighted and T2-weighted images. Moreover, patients with persistent signal changes in the spinal cord on follow-up MRI examinations demonstrated little or no clinical improvement in ASIA grade, whereas prognosis was improved for patients who demonstrated resolution of signal abnormalities (65, 66). Signal patterns that correlated with the best prognosis included normal spinal cord signal or hyperintensity on T2-weighted images (intramedullary edema). Hypointensity or hyperintensity on T1-weighted images with hyperintense signal on T2-weighted images (indicative of tissue necrosis) was a poor prognostic indicator (5,51,58–60,66). In two very similar studies, Shimada and colleagues also showed that persistent signal changes in the spinal cord on serial MRI studies were associated with no significant clinical improvement, whereas marked improvement in neurologic status was found in the subset of patients whose MRI studies became normal (58,60).

Silberstein and associates confirmed that there is a direct relationship between spinal fractures, subluxation, ligamentous injury, prevertebral swelling, epidural hematoma and the initial clinical deficit, as well as an indirect relationship to prognosis (59). All these associated imaging features suggested that residual spinal cord compression might be an important factor in determining poor neurologic recovery. However, other investigations have been less conclusive (67).

Selden and associates identified four MRI characteristics that were significant negative prognosticators of neurologic recovery as measured by the ASIA grade and were independent from the initial clinical examination: presence of spinal cord hemorrhage, length of spinal cord hemorrhage, length of spinal cord edema, and spinal cord compression (66).

Although there is an apparent relationship between spinal cord compression and neurologic injury, there are no consistent methods for characterizing spinal cord compression or posttraumatic reduction in canal diameter. Rao and Fehlings recently provided a critical, evidence-based analysis of existing radiologic literature, which correlated the degree of posttraumatic spinal cord compression to neurologic deficit (68). The studies that were evaluated contained both quantitative and qualitative assessments of spinal canal and spinal cord dimensions. Preexisting mid-sagittal canal stenosis (developmental or congenital stenosis) was generally associated with more severe neurologic deficit after injury, notably when the mid-sagittal diameter of the spinal canal was 10 mm or less. Studies that assessed the capability of the Torg ratio to predict the degree of neurologic function after injury were found to be inconclusive (68).

In another study, 30% of patients with severe spinal cord compression (defined as a two-thirds reduction in spinal cord diameter) had a complete motor deficit at the time of injury, compared with 20% of patients with mild spinal cord compression (defined as less than one-third reduction in spinal cord diameter). Moreover, 90% of patients with mild spinal cord compression improved by one or more ASIA grade, compared with 30% of patients with severe spinal cord compression (57).

Fehlings and colleagues developed a standardized method for measuring mid-sagittal spinal canal compromise and spinal cord compression that is applicable to both computed tomography (CT) and MRI (69). The authors found excellent agreement with CT and T1-weighted MRI images in determining canal compromise after injury. T2-weighted sagittal MRI studies provided the most reliable assessment of spinal cord compression. CT alone was a relatively poor predictor of spinal cord compression (98% specificity and 72% sensitivity). Overestimation of

canal compromise occurred with MRI; however, agreement between CT and MRI in assessing canal narrowing in patients with preexisting spondylosis was excellent. Spinal canal compromise on CT by 25% or more was 100% specific for spinal cord compression on MRI. The authors also identified a statistically significant difference in neurologic deficit for patients with and without spinal cord compression or spinal canal compromise (69).

In the first study that analyzed the relationship between motor index scores and MRI, Schaefer and colleagues correlated the MRI appearance of the spinal cord on admission to changes in total motor index score in 57 patients (70). Patients with hemorrhagic spinal cord lesions showed no statistical improvement in motor index score at follow-up. The group of patients with small areas of edema (less than one vertebral segment in length) demonstrated the largest improvement in motor index score (72% recovery), whereas larger areas of edema showed intermediate recovery of motor index score (42%) (70).

A similar study by Marciello and colleagues compared the presence or absence of intramedullary hemorrhage to changes in individual motor scores for the upper and lower extremities in 24 subjects (61). For patients with documented spinal cord hemorrhage on MRI, only 16% of muscles in the upper extremities and 3% of muscles in the lower extremities improved to a useful grade (>3/5) at follow-up; only 7% improved one or more motor levels. For patients without MRI evidence of spinal cord hemorrhage, 73% of upper extremity and 74% of lower extremity muscles improved to useful grade, and 78% of subjects improved one or more motor levels (61). In a subsequent comprehensive study, the prognostic capabilities of MRI were assessed in forecasting motor recovery in 104 cervical SCI patients (71). Individual manual muscle test scores were compiled for the upper and lower extremities both at the time of admission and 12 months after injury. The motor recovery rate for the upper and lower extremities was also determined using the method of Lucas and Ducker (71). The injured spinal cord segment on MRI was quantified using a unique method that expressed spinal cord hemorrhage and edema by length and location relative to known anatomic landmarks. Lesion length was directly proportional to neurologic impairment at the time of injury ($p < 0.001$). In addition, spinal cord hemorrhage was associated with the most severe injuries ($p < 0.001$). Improvement in motor function after 1 year was observed in all patients; subjects with spinal cord hemorrhage on MRI had lower initial motor scores and had less improvement than those without hemorrhage. Nonhemorrhagic MRI lesions were associated with significantly higher motor recovery rates in the lower and upper extremities and had a higher proportion of useful muscle function. Multiple regression analysis was used to determine the contribution of MRI in predicting the outcomes parameters of motor function independent of the initial clinical evaluation. Initial motor scores, the presence of hemorrhage, and the length of edema were independent predictors of final motor score and the proportion of muscles with useful function at 1 year. A statistical model that used *both* the MRI parameters and the initial clinical information was 18% more effective in predicting motor recovery than a statistical model based on initial clinical data alone (72).

In a subsequent prognostic study using the FIM, changes in the four distinct motor scales were compared with the initial MRI findings at the time of injury (73). The clinical assessment was based on changes in the motor FIM subscales between rehabilitation admission and discharge. Patients without spinal cord hemorrhage on MRI had significant improvement in self-care and mobility scores compared with patients with hemorrhage. The upper limit of the lesion (edema) correlated with admission and discharge self-care, admission mobility, and locomotion scores. Edema length correlated negatively with all FIM scores at admission and discharge. At the time of admission to rehabilitation, all subjects were completely dependent on equipment or caregivers to perform the tasks, whereas at the time of discharge, only patients with nonhemorrhagic MRI lesions improved to a modified dependence category (73).

Similar results have been reproduced using serial MRI studies in experimental models of SCI. In one study, two types of paralysis were induced in rats using a weight-drop model (20 and 35 gm, respectively), resulting in a transient and persistent motor paralysis (74). The animals were imaged, and motor strength was tested 2 and 28 days after induction of the injury. The animals with the milder injury showed significant improvement in motor function after 28 days. Spinal cord edema was identified on the initial and final MRI studies corresponding histologically to edema and reactive gliosis. The subset of animals with the severe injuries featured a central focus of hemorrhage surrounded by edema on the T2-weighted images at initial MRI. Low signal was observed on the T1-weighted images on the subsequent MRI study, suggesting cavitation. Histopathology of the more severe injury featured hemorrhages, cavitation, and reactive gliosis (74). This supports the concept that identification of hemorrhage on MRI after SCI portends a poor neurologic recovery.

There is only one major study that minimized the value of MRI in predicting neurologic recovery after SCI (75). Shepard and Bracken compared the results of MRI studies in 191 cervical SCI patients from multiple institutions to motor and sensory evaluations obtained at admission and 6 weeks after injury. The authors reported no statistical difference in the presence of contusions or edema between complete and incomplete injuries. MRI studies that featured hemorrhage or contusion were more likely to be associated with lower initial motor, pinprick, and touch sensation scores. Motor function recovery parameters were found to be lower in patients showing hemorrhage, contusion, and edema on MRI; however, the differences were not statistically significant. After controlling for the results of the initial clinical assessment, the authors found no added value of the MRI findings (cord hemorrhage, contusion, and edema) in predicting neurologic recovery (75).

The validity of this ambitious study is questionable, especially in consideration of the number of other investigations that contradict their results. There are a number of critical flaws in Shepard and Bracken's study design that undoubtedly contribute to their conclusions. First, they neglected to provide central review of the MRI images by a panel of experts. Instead, interpretations of written reports and anecdotal information were primarily used to "assess" the MRI studies. Second, the authors failed to control, address, or discuss the imaging protocols that were used

at the participating institutions. Third, overall image quality, variability between different vendors, and static field strength were not controlled for or addressed in the discussion. Many published MRI studies have shown that an MRI instrument's sensitivity in depicting the characteristic features of SCI (hemorrhage and edema) are highly dependent on factors such as static field strength, choice of pulse sequences, and imaging protocol. Fourth, critical definitions or criteria of contusion, edema, and hemorrhage were inconsistent or omitted. Any one of these flaws could have serious consequences on the results of a study that purports to evaluate the accuracy of MRI. In principle, the authors failed to validate the prognostic utility of MRI because they neglected to evaluate the instrument itself.

The utility of MRI in the assessment, management, and treatment of SCI has matured significantly since the 1990s as a result of refinements in hardware and software design. Moreover, the dissemination of this technology worldwide has helped to move MRI into the routine clinical armamentarium of available diagnostic tools in SCI. The diagnostic power of MRI in the assessment of spinal cord disease is still in its infancy. Continued development in MRI spectroscopy, anisotropic diffusion, and functional MRI as applied to the spinal cord will unquestionably enhance the diagnostic power of this clinical tool.

ELECTROPHYSIOLOGIC TESTING IN PROGNOSTICATING NEUROLOGIC OUTCOME

There are a number of electrophysiologic tests that have been used in the acute period after SCI to assess the level and severity of the SCI as well as to prognosticate neurologic and functional outcome. Techniques include nerve conduction studies (NCS), late responses (H reflex and F wave), somatosensory evoked potentials (SSEPs), motor evoked potentials (MEPs), and sympathetic skin responses (SSRs), all of which can supplement clinical and neuroradiologic examinations. These tests, however, are most useful in differentiating lesions of the central and peripheral nervous system and in uncooperative or unconscious patients because they do not require the cooperation of the patient (76). They are not recommended as a routine part of the acute workup of a newly injured patient to offer prognosis for neurologic or functional outcome.

Nerve Conduction Studies

The most important information that can be obtained from NCS, motor and sensory, is whether the injury affects the LMN, that is, nerve root, plexus, or peripheral nerves. In a LMN injury, both motor and sensory conduction responses are impaired (77, 78). In an UMN lesion, NCS below the level of the injury is within normal limits for compound motor action potentials (CMAPs) and nerve conduction velocity (NCV) (79). If the nerve tested is at or just below the level of injury (e.g., median or ulnar nerves with cervical injury), the CMAP may be diminished but the NCV normal (77,80). Over the course of the first month, the CMAP may diminish, especially in paraplegic injuries, but then stabilize (79). Sensory nerve action potentials remain intact in UMN lesions.

Upper extremity recordings in patients with tetraplegia may help predict hand function (81,82). No patients with a loss of motor potentials of the median and ulnar nerves recovered active hand function because all patients had LMN weakness of the intrinsic hand muscles (81). NCS of the upper extremities can also help determine whether functional electrical stimulation can be used to improve hand function or as an indicator for tendon transfers.

In the lower extremities, Rutz and colleagues used NCS in acute patients with paraplegia and found that the CMAPs can be used to differentiate between conus or cauda equina and epiconal lesions (77). In contrast to patients with an epiconal injury, almost all patients with conus or cauda equina lesions presented with a severe axonal neuropathy of the tibial and peroneal nerves (loss of tibial CMAP in 71% and of peroneal CMAP in 68%), compared with patients with epiconal lesions (no loss of tibial CMAP and abolished peroneal CMAP in 14%). Pathologic CMAPs in these cases developed as early as 1 to 2 weeks after injury, whereas the motor NCV remained normal when elicited. The NCS, however, in contrast to the ASIA examination, was not of value in predicting the outcome of ambulatory capacity for ambulation (77). This is explained by the fact that ambulatory capacity requires at least proximal lower extremity musculature, whereas the NCS tests only the distal lower extremity nerves (e.g., tibial and peroneal nerves). However, recording of the tibial and peroneal nerves can help diagnose LMN injury to determine whether interventions such as functional electrical stimulation can be used.

Late Responses

The H reflex, an electrically induced monosynaptic reflex, although possibly depressed for the first 24 hours after SCI, can be elicited acutely (after 24 hours), even during spinal shock (79,83–85). While tendon reflexes are still absent, the H reflex has a normal latency and the H-to-M ratio is normal acutely as compared with normal subjects. The presence of an intact H reflex confirms that there is no associated peripheral nerve (LMN) injury. It is unclear whether an increase in the H-to-M ratio over time (weeks to months) suggests an increased incidence of developing increased hyperreflexia (79,84).

The F wave, an antidromic afferent motor and efferent motor response to supramaximal electrical stimulation, unlike the H reflex, is influenced by spinal shock and may take up to 6 months to return to normal in UMN lesions (79,80). This may reflect reduced alpha motor neuron excitability, possibly because of the sudden loss of tonic input or trophic support from supraspinal to spinal neuronal centers (79). F waves are initially absent, even in the presence of a normal CMAP. Once present (80% at 3 months, all by 6 months after injury), the mean F-wave latencies are within normal limits. Although the frequency of the F waves elicited progressively increases over time, it is reduced as compared with normal subjects. F-wave latencies are not related to the development of spasticity. Preserved responses relate to conduction through the peripheral nerve.

Somatosensory Evoked Potentials

A large number of studies have been performed to determine the value of SSEPs in the evaluation and prognostication of the SCI patient (86–98). Recordings of lower extremity SSEPs enables differentiation between complete and incomplete lesions, and the lack of cortical evoked responses elicited by stimulation of nerves below the lesion associated with a complete injury indicates a poor recovery (94–97,99). Although SSEP primarily evaluates the function of the dorsal columns, it also reflects the extent of lesions of peripheral nerves after acute SCI (92,96,97,100,101). The inability to pick up a peripheral response (e.g., at the popliteal fossa with tibial nerve stimulation) is associated with a probable LMN injury. SSEP recordings are not influenced by spinal shock or by the patient's level of consciousness, even if sedated (95,102–104). A return of the early SSEP components in the initial stage after SCI can proceed to clinically detectable improvements in motor and sensory function (96,99,105–108).

Different techniques for SSEP recordings, dermatomal versus mixed nerve, have been used. Some authors have suggested that dermatomal SSEPs of the upper extremity (ring electrodes on the thumb [C6]; forefinger [C7], and little finger [C8]) is a sensitive technique for detecting levels of injury (97,109). Recording is from the ipsilateral Erb point (N9) and over the contralateral somatosensory cortex. Other investigators have tested mixed nerves, such as the median, ulnar, pudendal, and tibial nerves, for prognostication purposes. Different grading systems for potential recording have been used in relation to amplitude or latency in different studies, which may account for some of the differences in their conclusions regarding prognostic capability.

Many studies have found that SSEPs are no more effective for prognosticating outcome than is a proper examination (ASIA protocol) for both complete and incomplete patients (89–92, 94–96,110). The presence of an SSEP recording is not always associated with motor recovery because the SSEP represents spared sensory fibers of the posterior columns, whereas motor activity depends on the functioning of the anterior and anterolateral spinal cord with a different blood supply. Other studies, however, have shown that SSEPs offer additional prognostication to the clinical examination (86,87,98). SSEPs are especially helpful in an unresponsive or uncooperative patient to determine whether the patients has a SCI because in these patients, a clinical examination, and consequently the use of the ASIA Impairment Scale, is limited. In addition, the differentiation between SCI and conversion reaction may be difficult, and SSEP may be helpful (105,107).

Curt and Dietz reported that SSEP recordings of the upper extremities correlate with the sensory impairment and have prognostic value for recovery of hand function (86). With combined recordings of median and ulnar SSEP, they were able to distinguish between lesions of the upper (C3 to C6) and lower (C6 or C7 to T1) cervical spine. With C3 to C6 lesions, the median SSEP was pathologic in 52% of cases, compared with only 20% in C6 to T1 lesions. Ulnar nerve SSEPs were pathologic in more than 80% of all cervical injuries. All patients with a loss of median and ulnar SSEPs did not achieve hand function. More than 90% of patients with normal median and ulnar SSEP latencies recovered active hand function, with correspondingly more independence in daily living in most cases. SSEP results showed sensitivity similar to ASIA scores in predicting the outcome of hand function (86). Jacobs and colleagues, however, did not find a correlation between median and superficial radial nerve SSEPs with recovery of extensor carpi radialis muscle function (89).

Curt and Dietz reported that recordings of the tibial and pudendal SSEP are related to the outcome of ambulatory capacity in acute SCI patients to a similar extent as the ASIA scores (87). This was consistent with other studies showing their value in predicting ambulation (20,90,98). Most patients (>80%) with normal tibial SSEP latency and amplitude progress to full ambulation capacity, whereas no patients with acute tetraplegia and absent responses up to 2 weeks after injury recovered to full independence (87). Of those subjects with no tibial SSEP elicited, only 20% achieved functional or therapeutic ambulation. Of the patients with a pathologic tibial SSEP (prolongation of latency), 10% regained full ambulation capacity, with 70% regaining functional or therapeutic ambulation capacity (87). In incomplete subjects, the SSEP was more strongly related to the outcome of ambulatory capacity than the clinical examination. This may reflect the fact the ambulation depends not only on anterior cord function (i.e., muscle strength) but also on the function of somatosensory tract fibers.

Iseli and coworkers found that tibial SSEP recordings were strongly indicative of the degree of ambulatory recovery in both traumatic and ischemic causes of paraplegia (98). Pudendal SSEP recordings were significantly related to ambulatory capacity, but only in trauma patients. They concluded that, in general, the SSEP recordings were of less prognostic value in the ischemia compared with the trauma injury patients. In addition, of all the clinical and electrophysiologic indices, the best prediction of outcome of ambulatory capacity was achieved by the combination of the motor score (on clinical examination) and tibial SSEP in both patient groups (98).

For prognosticating bladder function, SSEP recordings of pudendal and tibial nerves correlate with recovery of somatic nerve function (external urethral sphincter function) but not with autonomic nerve function (detrussor function) (88). Most patients with no pudendal SSEP elicited (90% paraplegia, about 70% tetraplegia) had complete loss of voluntary external urethral sphincter function 6 months after injury. Pudendal SSEP recordings have a value similar to the ASIA scores in predicting the outcome of bladder function. However, neither of these (SSEP nor ASIA scoring) can predict detrussor function (88,111).

It is important to recognize that SSEP recordings do not improve parallel to functional recovery. Although motor recovery takes place over time, the pathologic SSEP recordings do not show significant improvement (86,112).

Motor Evoked Potentials

In the acute phase after SCI, MEP recordings can provide a measure of functional integrity of the corticomotor neuronal connection (113). Whereas SSEPs reflects dorsal column function, cortical stimulation examines the corticospinal tract by recording from different peripheral muscles, allowing assessment of the level and extent of the lesion (114). MEP can be elicited by magnetic or electrical stimulation. Although magnetic cortical stimulation is preferable to electrical stimulation as a means of assessing central motor conduction in conscious patients because

it is more powerful and less painful, it is difficult to use in patients who have metal plates surgically implanted (97,115).

MEP can be used to document the level of injury in the upper extremities with electrodes on the deltoid (C5), biceps (C6), forearm extensors (C7), and first dorsal interosseous muscle (C8 to T1) (97). Thresholds to elicit compound MEPs are greater and latencies and duration of the potentials are longer or absent in SCI patients, and these measures correlates with function (116–119). Voluntary muscle contraction enhances the amplitude and shortens the onset latency of the MEP.

In neurologic complete injuries, MEP are absent in muscles below the level of injury, whereas in incomplete injuries, MEPs can usually be elicited (120–123). When MEPs are absent in the early stages after injury, a poor outcome is usually observed. Weakness of voluntary muscle contraction in patients with incomplete SCI correlates well with delayed (about 80%) or absent responses in the muscle. Of interest is that an enlarged MEP is seen in muscles above the level of injury with a shortened latency as well as an enlarged cortical map of motor output. This is seen in chronic SCI, as well as in acute SCI, as early as 6 days after injury (124–127). This suggests that early motor reorganization may occur after acute SCI.

MEP recordings of proximal upper limb muscles can help predict mobility and activities of daily living function. Patients with early MEP responses (within 4 days) have the best recovery of motor and ambulation capability (128). Curt and colleagues, studying 36 acute SCI patients, found MEP recordings to be related to the outcome of ambulatory and hand function, similar to ASIA scores on examination (123). All patients with an elicitable MEP initially recovered functional motor activity (>3/5) of that respective muscle. Those who lacked MEP of the abductor digiti minimi did not regain active hand function, and most patients (about 80%) who achieved full ambulatory capacity had normal MEP latencies of the tibialis anterior and quadriceps femoris muscles. All patients with a normal MEP in the tibialis anterior muscle recovered full ambulatory capacity, whereas only 11% who lacked a tibialis anterior MEP acutely recovered full ambulatory capacity. Less than 20% of acute patients with loss of lower limb SSEP progressed to full or functional ambulatory capacity (123).

As is the case for SSEP, MEP recordings do not parallel recovery of function over time because latency does not improve, whereas motor recovery and function may improve (123).

Sympathetic Skin Responses

The SSR can help examine the common efferent pathway of the sympathetic nervous system. The SSR can be recorded by surface disk electrodes applied to the skin (i.e., palm of the hands, plantar aspects of the feet) to assess lesions of the spinal and sympathetic nerve fibers supplying these areas (129).

In a study by Curt and associates, all patients with complete tetraplegia had abnormal SSR potentials in the hands and feet, whereas 73% of patients with incomplete tetraplegia had normal responses (130). No patient with preserved SSR potentials had symptoms of autonomic dysreflexia during urodynamics testing. By contrast, all patients with autonomic dysreflexia symptoms had pathologic SSRs. The loss of SSR in the hands was associated with the development of autonomic dysreflexia in 93% of the patients studied. In the incomplete injury subjects, only those with absent SSR had signs of autonomic dysreflexia during urodynamics testing. Therefore, SSR recordings can assess autonomic failure, even when not clinically evident, as in incomplete lesions.

MECHANISMS OF RECOVERY AFTER SPINAL CORD INJURY

Most patients with SCI demonstrate some degree of neurologic recovery after injury. The recovery of motor function involves the resolution of the injury-induced spinal cord pathology and plasticity of the central nervous system. Severity and extent of the injury are the primary determinants of the amount of recovery (119). The primary injury in spinal cord trauma is followed by two opposing sets of processes: one resulting in further tissue damage and functional loss (secondary injury or damage), and the other promoting tissue repair and behavioral recovery (131). Secondary injury processes include posttraumatic ischemia, neuronal electrolyte shifts, elaboration of oxygen free radicals and lipid peroxidation, glutamate excitotoxicity, and inflammation involving cytokines and other deleterious factors (132). To understand recovery of function after SCI, the overlapping variables associated with the primary injury, secondary damage, and repair processes must be considered (131). Using an adult guinea pig model of SCI in which a brief lateral compression of the thoracic spinal cord to a thickness of 1.2 mm is applied over a length of 5 mm, evaluation of several measurements can be used to demonstrate recovery of specific pathways over time. The cutaneous trunci muscle reflex represents function of a specific ventrolateral ascending pathway, and the toe spread response provides evaluation of a descending system (probably the reticulospinal system). In addition to these measures, other behaviors (motor responses to specific interventions or tasks) provide measurement of lumbar spinal cord function and less specific effects of descending input (133–135). These studies demonstrated that the time course and extent of change of the specific behavioral responses varies within an individual animal, indicating that the mechanisms of loss and recovery of function are localized to particular tracts within the spinal cord and cannot be attributed to generalized depression of activity in the cord (131). In addition, these studies suggested that long-term recovery of function approximates the degree of function spared in the first few hours after injury and that secondary deficits in the first week after injury can extend to both segmental and long-tract function (131).

Certain histopathologic features have been shown to correlate with functional outcome in the guinea pig model. In these studies, the central measurement was the cross-sectional area of the spinal cord lesion. This measurement was shown to correlate with the number of myelinated axons surviving in the outer rim of the tissue at the center of the lesion and a combined neurologic score. This finding supports the concept that the combined primary and secondary loss of tissue is proportional to the axon survival in the white matter, which is then proportional to the sparing of overall function (131). The combined neurologic

score correlated negatively with the density of blood vessels and with the proportion of surviving axons with thin myelin sheaths in the outer rim of the white matter at the site of the lesion. This indicates that at least two separate processes are involved in secondary loss and recovery of function (one represented by hypervascularity and the other by incomplete remyelination) and suggests that the overall survival of axons and the best neurologic score predominantly indicate the extent of primary mechanical damage, with perhaps a small contribution from secondary losses. The change in neurologic score, blood vessel density, and the proportion of thinly myelinated axons possibly represent the outcome of the counteracting influences of secondary damage and repair mechanisms. The cross-sectional area of the lesion, therefore, is related to the summation of the effects of primary damage, secondary degeneration, and repair processes (131).

An incomplete spinal cord injury that interrupts descending axons will partially denervate target neurons in the lumbar spinal cord. Partial denervation may result in receptor supersensitivity, which can enhance recovery by allowing target neurons to respond to diminished levels of neurotransmitter (136). Axonal sprouting, or reactive reinnervation, has been demonstrated after spinal hemisection in cats and rats (137,138). In the adult animal, sprouting is spatially limited and regulated, whereas in the neonate, the amount of sprouting is usually greater. In some animal models, the sprouting has been associated with recovery of postural reflexes and locomotion (136). In humans, it has also been demonstrated that there is lesser degree of functional recovery, specifically walking, after motor incomplete tetraplegia (ASIA C) in older patients, and it is suggested that this may be a result of a loss of potential for neural plasticity or remyelination with increasing age (36). Other studies have suggested that reduced cortical inhibition and reorganization at a cortical level after SCI may contribute to functional recovery (119).

Little and Halar postulated that recovery after incomplete spinal cord injury is based on central synaptic mechanisms that allow spared inputs to assume new function caudal to the lesion (139). They suggested a hypothetical model in which two neuronal mechanisms act sequentially to mediate an early and a late phase of recovery, reversing the hyperpolarization of spinal cord neurons responsible for spinal shock. The early-phase mechanisms are thought to act within hours to days after injury and to be mediated by receptor upregulation in hyperpolarized cord neurons, resulting in supersensitivity to neurotransmitter. The late phase occurs over weeks to months and is proposed to result from local synapse growth in preexisting pathways, both spared descending pathways and reflex pathways. There is competition between descending motor and reflex input recovery, and an inverse relationship between recovery of strength and development of spasticity has been demonstrated. In larger lesions, there is a longer delay in late-phase recovery, presumably because fewer supraspinal axons are spared, and each axon must generate many new synapses before a functioning pathway is reestablished (139). The pattern of recovery of lower extremity muscles may provide further insight into this mechanism of recovery. It has been shown, in primates, that contralateral descending pathways are preferentially distributed to ipsilateral proximal extensors rather than distal flexors. In motor incomplete SCI patients, proximal flexor muscles recover before distal extensor muscles, supporting the theory that motor recovery depends on the number of spared descending inputs (140,141).

Functional recovery after complete SCI is far more limited than that after incomplete SCI. Although 10% to 15% of SCI patients classified as ASIA A at time of injury convert to incomplete status, only about 2% regain functional strength below the level of the lesion (12). Most complete tetraplegia patients, however, recover strength in the first caudal myotome below the level of injury (25). The degree of recovery depends on the neurologic level of injury, the initial sensation, and the initial muscle strength (7,8,10,142–147). Less than 25% of complete patients have motor recovery below the first caudal level from the neurologic level of injury (10).

Recovery after complete SCI occurs as a result of recovery of nerve roots adjacent to the level of the lesion, recovery of the spinal cord (gray matter) at the level of the lesion, and peripheral mechanisms. This recovery seen in complete SCI may be based on the following processes: (a) resolution of acute injury events, (b) resolution of secondary injury processes, (c) peripheral mechanisms of axon sprouting and muscle fiber hypertrophy, and possibly (d) regrowth or regeneration of nervous tissue (7,132). Acute injury events, including cord compression and contusion, frequently begin to resolve within minutes of injury and can continue to resolve over several days. Conduction block resulting from potassium leakage into the extracellular space can resolve as normotension and sodium and potassium gradients are restored (132). Recovery from neurapraxia in peripheral nerve usually occurs within 6 weeks but may take longer, and it has been suggested that similar injury to the cervical root should follow the same course of recovery (148–150). In addition to resolution of conduction block and neurapraxia, early hemorrhage into the cord can cease within minutes depending on the severity of the injury. Clearing of the hemorrhagic tissue by macrophages proceeds in the succeeding days (132). These mechanisms of resolution of early injury events may be responsible for early recovery of neurologic function in the zone of injury in complete injury patients. Muscle fiber hypertrophy and peripheral sprouting of nerve fibers in partially innervated muscles may account for improvement of strength in the zone of injury between 2 and 8 months after injury (7,151). Further strength recovery seen after 12 months following injury may be due to regeneration of the axon at the zone of injury, although this has not been clearly demonstrated in the literature (7).

Most of the recovery following SCI is spontaneous, but it may be enhanced or limited by several factors. It has been demonstrated that active exercise can promote motor recovery, whereas immobilization has been shown to impede motor recovery, suggesting that synapse growth may be activity dependent (152–155). Using a body-weight support system and interactive locomotor training on a treadmill, ambulation recovery may be enhanced in incomplete SCI patients. It has been postulated that upregulation of neurotransmitters due to sensory input and training of a central pattern generator may be the mechanisms responsible for the improved function when using this training method (112,156–161). Serotoninergic and neuroadrenergic drugs may enhance locomotor recovery, whereas γ-aminobutyric acid (GABA)-ergic drugs may impede ambulation (162). Neural prostheses are currently in use to enhance upper extremity function but are less successful for improvement of ambulation (163, 164). Combinations of pharmacologic and rehabilitative therapies may be more effective in improving function than any of these interventions when used alone (165).

Another approach to improving function after SCI is to transplant cells or tissues into the damaged spinal cord. Several groups of investigators have already used transplants of fetal spinal cord to occlude posttraumatic cysts that cause late functional deterioration after spinal cord injury (166). These studies also serve as phase I clinical trials that test the safety of the grafts, which studies in experimental animals suggest may act in several different ways to contribute to functional recovery. They have, for example, been reported to reduce astrocytic scarring at the injury site; the scar is thought to present a mechanical or chemical barrier to local axon sprouting and long-distance regeneration (167). They have also been reported to reduce the number of neurons that die after spinal cord injury (168). Rescued neurons can contribute to both sparing and recovery of function. In addition, in newborn animals, supraspinal axons regenerate through the transplants and caudal host spinal cord and enhance the development of locomotor function (169). Fetal tissue transplants placed into adult hosts, however stimulate little regeneration, and most of the growth derives from neurons located very close to the grafts (170). Recovery in adult hosts has also been limited.

The available experimental evidence suggests that other types of cells provide more efficacious intraspinal transplants than fetal spinal cord, at the same time avoiding the complicated political, ethical, and logistical problems that encumber the use of fetal tissue. Cells genetically modified to express neurotrophic factors have received the most attention to date. For example, fibroblasts engineered to express the neurotrophic factor NT-3 have been shown to rescue axotomized Clarke nucleus neurons from retrograde cell death as efficiently as transplants of fetal spinal cord (171). Schwann cells engineered to express a different neurotrophic factor, BDNF, and grafted into adult hosts stimulated regeneration of supraspinal axons across the site of a complete spinal cord transection (172). Several instances have also been reported in which genetically modified fibroblasts promoted both long-distance regeneration and recovery of locomotor function. Transplants of fibroblasts expressing NT-3 enhanced regeneration of corticospinal axons and recovery on a grid-walking task, and fibroblasts expressing BDNF stimulated regeneration of rubrospinal axons and recovery of forelimb and hindlimb locomotor performance as measured by several quantitative assays (173,174). Neurotrophic factor production may also be one of the mechanisms by which activated macrophages promote regeneration and partial recovery following transplantation into a complete spinal cord transection site in adult rats (175). A phase I trial of activated macrophage transplants in patients with spinal cord injury is in progress in Israel (Proneuron Biotechnology, USA; Weizmann Institute of Science, Rehovot, Israel).

Neural stem cells, defined by their capacity to renew themselves and to differentiate into neurons, astrocytes, and oligodendrocytes, are particularly attractive types of cells to use as transplants. They have been isolated from the brain and spinal cord of mature as well as developing mammals, including humans, and are readily maintained in culture in an undifferentiated state.

In principle, therefore, stem cells can be derived from a patient with a spinal cord injury and used to replace lost neurons, astrocytes, and oligodendrocytes. They are also amenable to genetic modification. Several different types of stem cells, including those isolated from embryonic human forebrain, have been reported to integrate into the uninjured brain of adult rats and to express the phenotype of neurons present in the area into which they have been transplanted (176). Progenitor cells isolated from the postnatal rat brain, which have a more restricted range of differentiation than stem cells, have also been reported to differentiate into Schwann cells and oligodendrocytes that remyelinate experimentally denuded axons in adult rat spinal cord (177). Embryonic stem cells transplanted into an intraspinal contusion site have been observed to differentiate into oligodendrocytes that contribute to remyelination and recovery of locomotor function (178). Phase I clinical trials treating spinal cord injury with porcine fetal stem cells are expected to begin soon (Diacrin; ●www.diacrin.com).

REFERENCES

1. Ditunno JF Jr. The John Stanley Coulter Lecture. Predicting recovery after spinal cord injury: a rehabilitation imperative. *Arch Phys Med Rehabil* 1999;80(4):361–364.
2. Long C, Lawton EB. Functional significance of spinal cord lesion level. *Arch Phys Med Rehabil* 1955;36:249–255.
3. Freed MM. Traumatic and congenital lesions of the spinal cord. In: Kottke FJ, Leo-Summers L, eds. *Krusen's handbook of physical medicine and rehabilitation.* Philadelphia: WB Saunders, 1990:717–748.
4. Staas WE Jr, Formal CS, Gershkoff AM, et al. Rehabilitation of the spinal cord-injured patient. In: DeLisa JA, editor. *Rehabilitation medicine: principles and practice.* Philadelphia: JB Lippincott, 1988: 635–659.
5. Stauffer ES. Diagnosis and prognosis of acute cervical spinal cord injury. *Clin Orthop* 1975;112:9.
6. Kirshblum SC, O'Connor KC. Levels of spinal cord injury and predictors of neurologic recovery. *Phys Med Rehabil Clin North Am* 2000; 11(1):1–27, vii.
7. Ditunno JF Jr, Sipski ML, Posuniak EA, et al. Wrist extensor recovery in traumatic quadriplegia. *Arch Phys Med Rehabil* 1987;68:287–290.
8. Ditunno JF Jr, Stover SL, Freed MM, et al. Motor recovery of the upper extremities in traumatic quadriplegia: a multicenter study. *Arch Phys Med Rehabil* 1992;73(5):431–436.
9. Ditunno JF Jr, Cohen ME, Hauck W. Early prediction of upper extremity motor recovery in tetraplegia: results of a 10 year multicenter study. *J Spinal Cord Med* 1998;21(2):162.
10. Waters RL, Adkins RH, Yakura J, et al. Motor and sensory recovery following complete tetraplegia. *Arch Phys Med Rehabil* 1993;74: 242–247.
11. Waters RL, Adkins RH, Yakura JS, et al. Motor and sensory recovery following incomplete tetraplegia. *Arch Phys Med Rehabil* 1994;75(3): 306–311.
12. Marino RJ, Ditunno JF, Donovan WH, et al. Neurologic recovery after traumatic spinal cord injury: data from the Model Spinal Cord Injury Systems. *Arch Phys Med Rehabil* 1999;80(11):1391–1396.
13. Hamilton BB, Granger CV, Sherwin FS. A uniform national data system for medical rehabilitation. In: Fuhrer MJ, ed. *Rehabilitation outcomes: analysis and measurement.* Baltimore: Paul H. Brookes, 1987: 137–147.
14. Catz A, Itzkovich M, Agranov E, et al. SCIM—Spinal Cord Independence Measure—a new disability scale for patients with spinal cord lesions. *Spinal Cord* 1997;35(12):850–856.
15. Hall KM, Cohen ME, Wright J, et al. Characteristics of the Func-

16. Marino RJ, Shea JA, Stineman MG. The Capabilities of Upper Extremity instrument: reliability and validity of a measure of functional limitation in tetraplegia. *Arch Phys Med Rehabil* 1998;79(12): 1512–1521.
17. Ditunno JF, Ditunno PL, Graziani V, et al. Walking Index for Spinal Cord Injury (WISCI): an international multicenter validity and reliability study. *Spinal Cord* 2000;38(5):234–243.
18. Ditunno JFJ. Scoring, scaling and classification. In: Ditunno JF, Donovan WH, Maynard FM, eds. *Reference manual for the international standards for neurological and functional classification of spinal cord injury.* Atlanta: American Spinal Injury Association, 1994:19–42.
19. Brown PJ, Marino RJ, Herbison GJ, et al. The 72-hour examination as a predictor of recovery in motor complete quadriplegia. *Arch Phys Med Rehabil* 1991;72(8):546–548.
20. Crozier KS, Graziani V, Ditunno JF Jr, et al. Spinal cord injury: prognosis for ambulation based on sensory examination in patients who are initially motor complete. *Arch Phys Med Rehabil* 1991;72(2): 119–121.
21. Maynard FMJ, Bracken MB, Creasey G, et al. International Standards for Neurological and Functional Classification of Spinal Cord Injury. American Spinal Injury Association. *Spinal Cord* 1997;35(5): 266–274.
22. Marino RJ, Stineman MG. Functional assessment in spinal cord injury. *Top Spinal Cord Injury Rehabil* 1998;4(1):32–45.
23. Marino RJ, Cohen ME. Post discharge changes in self-report Functional Independence Measure in relationship to severity of injury. *J Spinal Cord Med* 2000;23(1):29.
24. Ditunno JF Jr, Cohen ME, Hauck WW, et al. Recovery of upper-extremity strength in complete and incomplete tetraplegia: a multicenter study. *Arch Phys Med Rehabil* 2000;81(4):389–393.
25. Kirshblum SC. Predicting neurologic recovery in traumatic cervical spinal cord injury. *Arch Phys Med Rehabil* 1998;79(11):1456–1466.
26. Welch RD, Lobley SJ, O'Sullivan SB, Freed MM. Functional independence in quadriplegia. *Arch Phys Med Rehabil* 1986;67(4): 235–240.
27. Zafonte RD, Demangone DA, Herbison GJ, et al. Daily self-care in quadriplegic subjects. *Neurol Rehabil* 1991;1(4):17–24.
28. Marino RJ, Huang M, Knight P, et al. Assessing selfcare status in quadriplegia: comparison of the quadriplegia index of function (QIF) and the functional independence measure (FIM). *Paraplegia* 1993; 31(4):225–233.
29. Marino RJ, Rider-Foster D, Maissel G, et al. Superiority of motor level over single neurological level in categorizing tetraplegia. *Paraplegia* 1995;33(9):510–513.
30. Ditunno JFJ, Cohen ME, Formal C, et al. Functional outcomes. In: Stover SL, Whiteneck GG, DeLisa JA, eds. *Spinal cord injury: clinical outcomes from the Model Systems.* Gaithersburg, MD: Aspen, 1995: 170–184.
31. Bracken MB, Shepard MJ, Holford TR, et al. Administration of methylprednisolone for 24 or 48 hours or tirilazad mesylate for 48 hours in the treatment of acute spinal cord injury: results of the Third National Acute Spinal Cord Injury Randomized Controlled Trial. National Acute Spinal Cord Injury Study. *JAMA* 1997;277(20): 1597–1604.
32. Bosch A, Stauffer ES, Nickel VL. Incomplete traumatic quadriplegia: a ten-year review. *JAMA* 1971;216(3):473–478.
33. Maynard FM, Reynolds GG, Fountain S, et al. Neurological prognosis after traumatic quadriplegia: three-year experience of California Regional Spinal Cord Injury Care System. *J Neurosurg* 1979;50(5): 611–616.
34. Benzel EC, Larson SJ. Functional recovery after decompressive spine operation for cervical spine fractures. *Neurosurgery* 1987;20(5): 742–746.
35. Geisler FH. Personal communication, 1999.
36. Burns SP, Golding DG, Rolle WA, et al. Recovery of ambulation in motor-incomplete tetraplegia. *Arch Phys Med Rehabil* 1997;78(11): 1169–1172.
37. Penrod LE, Hegde SK, Ditunno JF Jr. Age effect on prognosis for

functional recovery in acute, traumatic central cord syndrome. *Arch Phys Med Rehabil* 1990;71(12):963–968.

38. Waters RL. Donald Munro lecture: functional and neurologic recovery following acute SCI. *J Spinal Cord Med* 1998;21(3):195–199.

39. Hussey RW, Stauffer ES. Spinal cord injury: requirements for ambulation. *Arch Phys Med Rehabil* 1973;54(12):544–547.

40. Waters RL, Adkins R, Yakura J, et al. Prediction of ambulatory performance based on motor scores derived from standards of the American Spinal Injury Association. *Arch Phys Med Rehabil* 1994;75(7):756–760.

41. Waters RL, Yakura JS, Adkins RH, et al. Recovery following complete paraplegia. *Arch Phys Med Rehabil* 1992;73:784–789.

42. Holdsworth F. Fractures, dislocations, and fracture-dislocations of the spine. *J Bone Joint Surg Am* 1970;52:1534–1551.

43. Waters RL, Akins RH, Yakura JS, et al. Recovery following incomplete paraplegia. *Arch Phys Med Rehabil* 1994;75:67–72.

44. Ko HY. The pattern of reflex recovery during spinal shock. *Spinal Cord* 1999;37(6):402–409.

45. Guttmann L. Studies on reflex activity of the isolated cord in spinal man. *J Nerv Ment Dis* 1952;116:957–972.

46. Weinstein DE, Ko HY, Graziani V, et al. Prognostic significance of the delayed plantar reflex following spinal cord injury. *J Spinal Cord Med* 1997;20(2):207–211.

47. More-O'Ferrall D, Doherty J, Ditunno JFJ. Upper motor neuron lesion vs. lower motor neuron lesions in lower thoracic complete spinal cord injury. *J Spinal Cord Med* 1988;21:181(abst).

48. Kulkarni MV, McArdle CB, Kopanicky D, et al. Acute spinal cord injury: MRI imaging at 1.5T. *Radiology* 1987;164(3):837–843.

49. Bondurant FJ, Cotler HB, Kulkarni MV, et al. Acute spinal cord injury: a study using physical examination and magnetic resonance imaging. *Spine* 1990;15(3):161–168.

50. Kulkarni MV, Bondurant FJ, Rose SL, et al. 1.5 tesla Magnetic resonance imaging of acute spinal trauma. *Radiographics* 1988;8(6):1059–1082.

51. Ramon S, Dominguez R, Ramirez L, et al. Clinical and magnetic resonance imaging correlation in acute spinal cord injury. *Spinal Cord* 1997;35(10):664–673.

52. Cotler HB, Kulkarni MV, Bondurant FJ. Magnetic resonance imaging of acute spinal cord trauma: preliminary report. *J Orthop Trauma* 1988;2(1):1–4.

53. Schaefer DM, Flanders A, Northrup BE, et al. Magnetic resonance imaging of acute cervical spine trauma: correlation with severity of neurologic injury. *Spine* 1989;14:1090–1095.

54. Flanders AE, Schaefer DM, Doan HT, et al. Acute cervical spine trauma: correlation of MRI imaging findings with degree of neurologic deficit. *Radiology* 1990;177(1):25–33.

55. Beers GJ, Raque GH, Wagner GG, et al. MRI imaging in acute cervical spine trauma. *J Comput Assist Tomogr* 1988;12(5):755–761.

56. Harrington JF, Likavec MJ, Smith AS. Disc herniation in cervical fracture subluxation. *Neurosurgery* 1991;29:374–379.

57. Hayashi K, Yone K, Ito H, et al. MRI findings in patients with a cervical spinal cord injury who do not show radiographic evidence of a fracture or dislocation. *Paraplegia* 1995;33(4):212–215.

58. Shimada K, Takahashi C, Satoru A, et al. Sequential MRI studies in patients with cervical cord injury but without bony injury. *Paraplegia* 1995;33:573–578.

59. Silberstein M, Tress BM, Hennessy O. Prediction of neurologic outcome in acute spinal cord injury: the role of CT and MRI. *Am J Neuroradiol* 1992;13:1597–1608.

60. Shimada K, Tokioka T. Sequential MR studies of cervical cord injury: correlation with neurological damage and clinical outcome. *Spinal Cord* 1999;37(6):410–415.

61. Marciello M, Flanders AE, Herbison GJ, et al. Magnetic resonance imaging related to neurologic outcome in cervical spinal cord injury. *Arch Phys Med Rehabil* 1993;74:940–946.

62. Silberstein M, Tress BM, Hennessy O. Delayed neurologic deterioration in the patient with spinal trauma: role of MRI imaging. *Am J Neuroradiol* 1992;13:1373–1381.

63. Sato T, Kokubun S, Rijal KP, et al. Prognosis of cervical spinal cord

injury in correlation with magnetic resonance imaging. *Paraplegia* 1994;32:81–85.

64. Schneider, RC, Thompson JM, Bebin J. The syndrome of the acute central cervical spinal cord injury. *J Neurol Neurosurg Psychiatry* 1958;21:216–227.

65. Yamashita Y, Takahashi M, Matsuno Y, et al. Acute spinal cord injury: magnetic resonance imaging correlated with myelopathy. *Br J Radiol* 1991;64(759):201–209.

66. Selden NR, Quint DJ, Patel N, et al. Emergency magnetic resonance imaging of cervical spinal cord injuries: clinical correlation and prognosis. *Neurosurgery* 1999;44:785–792.

67. Dai L, Jia L. Central cord injury complicating acute cervical disc herniation in trauma. *Spine* 2000;25:331–335.

68. Rao SC, Fehlings MG. The optimal radiologic method for assessing spinal canal compromise and cord compression in patients with cervical spinal cord injury. I. An evidence-based analysis of the published literature. *Spine* 1999;15:598–604.

69. Fehlings MG, Rao SC, Tator CH, et al. The optimal radiologic method for assessing spinal canal compromise and cord compression in patients with cervical spinal cord injury. II. Results of a multicenter study. *Spine* 1999;24(6):605–613.

70. Schaefer DM, Flanders AE, Osterholm JL, et al. Prognostic significance of magnetic resonance imaging in the acute phase of cervical spine injury. *J Neurosurg* 1992;76(2):218–223.

71. Lucas JT, Ducker TB. Motor classification of spinal cord injuries with mobility, morbidity and recovery indices. *Am Surg* 1979;45:151–158.

72. Flanders AE, Spettell CM, Tartaglino LM, et al. Forecasting motor recovery after cervical spinal cord injury: value of MR imaging. *Radiology* 1996;201:649–655.

73. Flanders AE, Spettell CM, Friedman DP, et al. The relationship between the functional abilities of patients with cervical spinal cord injury and the severity of damage revealed by MR imaging. *AJNR Am J Neuroradiol* 1999;20:926–934.

74. Ohta K, Fujimura Y, Nakamura M, et al. Experimental study on MRI evaluation of the course of cervical spinal cord injury. *Spinal Cord* 1999;37:580–584.

75. Shepard MJ, Bracken MB. Magnetic resonance imaging and neurological recovery in acute spinal cord injury: observations from the National Acute Spinal Cord Injury Study 3. *Spinal Cord* 1999;37:833–837.

76. Houlden DA, Schwartz ML, Klettke KA. Neurophysiologic diagnosis in uncooperative trauma patients: confounding factors. *J Trauma* 1992;33:244–251.

77. Rutz S, Dietz V, Curt A. Diagnostic and prognostic value of compound motor action potentials of lower limbs in acute paraplegic patients. *Spinal Cord* 2000;38:203–210.

78. Krasilowsky G. Nerve conduction studies in patients with cervical spinal cord injuries. *Arch Phys Med Rehabil* 1980;61:204–208.

79. Hiersemenzel LP, Curt A, Dietz V. From spinal shock to spasticity: Neuronal adaptations to a spinal cord injury. *Neurology* 2000;54:1574–1582.

80. Curt A, Keck ME, Dietz V. Clinical value of f-wave recordings in traumatic cervical spinal cord injury. *Electroencephalogr Clin Neurophysiol* 1997;105:189–193.

81. Curt A, Dietz V. Nerve conduction study in cervical spinal cord injury: significance for hand function. *Neurorehabilitation* 1996;7:165–173.

82. Curt A, Dietz V. Neurographic assessment of intramedular motorneurone lesions in cervical spinal cord injury; consequences for hand function. *Spinal Cord* 1996;34:326–332.

83. Cadilhac J, Georgesco M, Benezech J, et al. Potential evoque cerebral somesthesique et d'Hoffmann dans les lesions medullaires aigues interet physiopathologique et prognostic. *Electroenceplalogr Clin Neurophysiol* 1977;43:160–167.

84. Little JW, Halar EW. H-reflex changes following spinal cord injury. *Arch Phys Med Rehabil* 1985;66:19–22.

85. Diamatopoulos E, Zander Olson P. Excitability of motor neurons in spinal shock in man. *J Neurol Neurosurg Psychiatry* 1967;30:427–431.

86. Curt A, Dietz V. Traumatic cervical spinal cord injury: relation be-

tween somatosensory evoked potentials, neurologic deficit, and hand function. *Arch Phys Med Rehabil* 1996;77:48–53.

87. Curt A, Dietz V. Ambulatory capacity in spinal cord injury: significance of somatosensory evoked potentials and ASIA protocol in predicting outcome. *Arch Phys Med Rehabil* 1997;78:39–43.

88. Curt A, Rodic B, Schurch B, et al. Recovery of bladder function in patients with acute spinal cord injury: significance of ASIA scores and somatosensory evoked potentials. *Spinal Cord* 1997;35:368–373.

89. Jacobs SR, Sarlo FB, Baran EM, et al. Extensor carpi radialis recovery predicted by qualitative SEP and clinical examination in quadriplegia. *Arch Phys Med Rehabil* 1992;73:790–793.

90. Jacobs SR, Yeaney NK, Herbison GJ, et al. Future ambulation prognosis as predicted by somatosensory evoked potentials in motor complete and incomplete quadriplegia. *Arch Phys Med Rehabil* 1995;76:635–641.

91. Kaplan PE, Rosen JS. Somatosensory evoked potentials in spinal cord injured patients. *Paraplegia* 1981;19:118–122.

92. Katz RT, Toleikio RJ, Knuth AE. Somatosensory-evoked and dermatomal-evoked potentials are not clinically useful in the prognostication of acute spinal cord injury. *Spine* 1991;16(7):730–735.

93. Louis AA, Gupta P, Perkash I. Localization of sensory levels in traumatic quadriplegia by segmental somatosensory evoked potentials. *Electroencephalogr Clin Neurophysiol* 1985;62:313–316.

94. Rowed DW. Value of somatosensory evoked potentials for prognosis in partial cord injuries. In: Tator CH, ed. *Early management of acute spinal cord injury.* New York: Raven, 1982:167–180.

95. York DH, Watts C, Raffensberger M, et al. Utilization of somatosensory evoked cortical potentials in spinal cord injury: prognostic limitations. *Spine* 1983;8:832–839.

96. Young W. Correlation of somatosensory evoked potentials and neurological findings in spinal cord injury. In: Tator CH, ed. *Early management of acute spinal cord injury.* New York: Raven, 1982:153–165.

97. Cheliout-Heraut F, Loubert G, Mastri-Zada T, et al. Evaluation of early motor and sensory evoked potentials in cervical spinal cord injury. *Neurophysiol Clin* 1998;28:39–55.

98. Iseli E, Cavigelli A, Dietz V, et al. Prognosis and recovery in ischaemic and traumatic spinal cord injury: Clinical and electrophysiological evaluation. *J Neurol Neurosurg Psychiatry* 199;67:567–571.

99. Gruninger W, Ricker K. Somatosensory cerebral evoked potentials in spinal cord diseases. *Paraplegia* 1991;9:206–215.

100. Jones SJ. Investigation of brachial plexus traction lesions by peripheral and spinal somatosensory evoked potentials. *J Neurol Neurosurg Psychiatry* 1979;42:107–116.

101. Beric A, Light JK. Function of the conus medularis in cauda equina in the early period for long spinal cord injury and the relationship to recovery of detrussor function. *J Urol* 1992;148:1845–1880.

102. Grundy BL, Friedman W. Electrical physiological evaluation of the patient with acute spinal cord injury. *Crit Care Clin* 1987;3:519–548.

103. Guttmann L. Spinal shock and reflex behavior in man. *Paraplegia* 1970;8:100–110.

104. Sedgwick EM, El-Negamy E, Frankel H. Spinal cord potentials in traumatic paraplegia and quadriplegia. *J Neurol Neurosurg Psychiatry* 1980;43:823–830.

105. Dickson H, Cole A, Engle S, et al. Conversion reaction presenting as acute spinal cord injury. *Med J Aust* 1984;141:427–429.

106. Dimitrijevic MR, Prevec TS, Sherwood AM. Somatosensory perception and cortical evoked potentials in established paraplegia. *J Neurol Sci* 1983;60:253–265.

107. Kaplan BJ, Friedman WA, Gavenstein D. Somatosensory evoked potential in hysterical paraplegia. *Surg Neurol* 1985;23:502–506.

108. Li C, Houlden DA, Rowed DQ. Somatosensory evoked potentials and neurological grades as predictors of outcome in acute spinal cord injury. *J Neurosurg* 1990;72:600–609.

109. Date ES, Ortega R, Hall K, et al. Somatosensory evoked responses to dermatomal stimulation in cervical spinal cord injured and normal subjects. *Clin Electroencephalogr* 1988;19:144–154.

110. Afls CM, Koelman JHTM, Meyjes FEP, et al. Posterior tibial and sural nerve somatosensory evoked potentials: a study in spastic paraparesis in spinal cord lesions. *Electroencephalogr Clin Neurophysiol* 1993;89:437–441.

111. Roussier AS, Ott R. Bladder and urethral recordings in acute and chronic spinal cord injury. *Urol Int* 1976;31:49–59.

112. Dietz V, Wirz M, Curt A, et al. Locomotor pattern in paraplegic patients: training effects and recovery of spinal cord function. *Spinal Cord* 1998;36:380–390.

113. Mckay WB, Stokic DS, Dimitrjevic MR. Assessment of corticospinal function in spinal cord injury. Using transcranial motor cortex stimulation: a review. *J Neurotrauma* 1997;14:539–548.

114. Curt A, Dietz V. Scientific Review. Electophysiological recordings in patients with spinal cord injury: significance for predicting outcome. *Spinal Cord* 1999;37:157–165.

115. Bordelli A, Inghillari M, Formisano R, et al. Stimulation of motor tracts in motor neuron disease. *J Neurol Neurosurg Psychiatry* 1987;50:732–737.

116. Cheng CW, Lien IN. Estimate of motor conduction in human spinal cord injury. *Muscle Nerve* 1991;14:990–996.

117. Davey NJ, Smith HC, Wells E, et al. Responses of thenar muscles to transcranial magnetic stimulation of the motor cortex in patients with incomplete spinal cord injury. *J Neurol Neurosurg Psychiatry* 1998;65:80–87.

118. Smith HC, Davey NJ, Savic G, et al. Modulation of single motor unit discharges using magnetic stimulation of the motor cortex in incomplete spinal cord injury. *J Neurol Neurosurg Psychiatry* 2000;68:516–520.

119. Smith HC, Savic G, Ellaway PH, et al. Corticospinal function studied over time following incomplete spinal cord injury. *Spinal Cord* 2000;38:292–300.

120. Clarke CE, Modarres-Sudeghi H, Twomey JA, et al. Prognostic value of cortical magnetic stimulation in spinal cord injury. *Paraplegia* 1994;32:554–560.

121. MacDonell RAL, Donnan GA. Magnetic cortical stimulation in acute spinal cord injury. *Neurology* 1995;45:303–306.

122. Bondurant CP, Haghighi SS. Experience with transcranial magnetic stimulation in evaluation of spinal cord injury. *Neurol Res* 1997;19:497–500.

123. Curt A, Keck ME, Dietz V. Functional outcome following spinal cord injury: significance motor evoked potentials and ASIA scores. *Arch Phys Med Rehabil* 1998;79:81–86.

124. Cohen LG, Bandinelli S, Topka HR, et al. Topographic maps of human motor cortex in normal humans, patients with congenital mirror movements, amputations, and spinal cord injuries. *Electroencephalogr Clin Neurophysiol* 1991(Suppl 43):36–50.

125. Levy WJ, Amassian VE, Traad M, et al. Focal magnetic coil stimulation reveals motor cortical system reorganized in humans after traumatic quadriplegia. *Brain Res* 1990;510:130–134.

126. Topka HR, Cole R, Hallet M, et al. Reorganization of corticospinal pathways following spinal cord injury. *Neurology* 1991;41:1276–1283.

127. Streletz LJ, Belevich JKS, Jones SM, et al. Transcranial magnetic stimulation: cortical motor maps in acute spinal cord injury. *Brain Topogr* 1995;7:245-250.

128. Hirayama T, Tsubokawa T, Maejima S, et al. Clinical assessment of the prognosis and severity of spinal cord injury using corticospinal motor evoked potentials. In: Shimoji K, Kurokawa T, Tamaki T, et al., eds. *Spinal cord monitoring and electrodiagnosis.* Heidelberg: Springer, 1991:503–510.

129. Yokota T, Matsunaga T, Okiyama R, et al. Sympathetic skin response in patients with multiple sclerosis compared with patients with spinal cord transections and normal controls. *Brain* 1991;114:1381–1394.

130. Curt A, Nitschie B, Rodic B, et al. Assessment of autonomic dysreflexia in patients with spinal cord injury. *J Neurol Neurosurg Psychiatry* 1997;62:473–477.

131. Blight AR. Remyelination, revascularization and recovery of function in experimental spinal cord injury. *Adv Neurol* 1993;59:91–104.

132. Tator CH. Biology of neurological recovery and functional restoration after spinal cord injury. *Neurosurgery* 1998;42(4):696–707.

133. Blight AR. Morphometric analysis of a model of spinal cord injury in guinea pigs, with behavioral evidence of delayed secondary pathology. *J Neurol Sci* 1991;103:156–171.

134. Blight AR, McGinnis ME, Borgens RB. Cutaneous truci muscle reflex of the guinea pig. *J Comp Neurol* 1990:296:614–633.

135. Gruner JA. Comparison of vestibular and auditory startle responses in the rat and cat. *J Neurosci Methods* 1989;27:13–23.

136. Goldberger MM, Murray M, Tessler A. Sprouting and regeneration in the spinal cord: their roles in recovery of function after spinal injury. In: Gorio A, ed. *Neuroregeneration*. New York: Raven Press, 1993:241–264.

137. Murray M, Goldberger ME. Restitution in function and collateral sprouting in the cat spinal cord: the partially hemisected animal. *J Comp Neurol* 1974;158:19–36.

138. Huselbosch CE, Coggeshall RE. A comparison of axonal numbers in dorsal roots following spinal cord hemisection in neonate and adult rats. *Brain Res* 1983;265:187–197.

139. Little JW, Halar E. Temporal course of motor recovery after Brown-Sequard spinal cord injuries. *Paraplegia* 1985;23:39–46.

140. Graziani V, Tessler A, Ditunno JF. Incomplete tetraplegia: sequence of lower extremity muscle recovery. *J Neurotrauma* 1995;12:121.

141. Little JW, Harris RM, Lerner SJ. Immobilization impairs recovery after spinal cord injury. *Arch Phys Med Rehabil* 1991;72:408–412.

142. Browne BJ, Jacobs SR, Herbison GJ, et al. Pin sensation as a predictor of extensor carpi radialis recovery in spinal cord injury. *Arch Phys Med Rehabil* 1993;74:14–18.

143. Eschbach KS, Herbison GJ, Ditunno JF. Sensory root level recovery in patients with Frankel A quadriplegia. *Arch Phys Med Rehabil* 1992; 73:618–621.

144. Kornsgold LN, Herbison GJ, Decena BF, et al. Biceps vs extensor carpi radialis recovery in Frankel A and B in spinal cord patients. *Paraplegia* 1994;32:340–348.

145. Mange KC, Marino RJ, Gregory PC, et al. The course of motor recovery at the zone of injury in complete spinal cord injury. *Arch Phys Med Rehabil* 1992;73:437–441.

146. Wu L, Marino RJ, Herbison GJ, et al. Recovery of zero grade muscles in the zone of partial preservation in motor complete quadriplegia. *Arch Phys Med Rehabil* 1992;73:40–43.

147. Young JS, Dexter SR. Neurological recovery distal to the zone of injury in 172 cases of closed, traumatic spinal cord injury. *Paraplegia* 1978;16:39–49.

148. Seddon H. *Surgical disorders of peripheral nerves*. Edinburgh and London: Churchill Livingstone, 1972:32–56.

149. Sunderland S. Avulsion of nerve roots. In Vinken PJ, Bruyn GW, eds. *Handbook of clinical neurology. Vol. 25, Injuries of spine and spinal cord: part I*. Amsterdam, North Holland Publishing: 1976:393–435.

150. Trojaberg W. Prolonged conduction block with axonal degeneration: electrophysiological study. *J Neurol Neurosurg Psychiatry* 1977;40: 50–57.

151. Marino RJ, Herbison GJ, Ditunno JF Jr. Peripheral sprouting as a mechanism for recovery in the zone of injury in acute quadriplegia: a single-fiber EMG study. *Muscle and Nerve* 1994;17:1466–1468.

152. Dietz V, Wirz M, Jensen L. Locomotion in patients with spinal cord injuries. *Phys Ther* 1997;77:508–516.

153. Barbeau H, Rossignol S. Recovery of locomotion after chronic spinalization in the adult cat. *Brain Res* 1987;412:84–95.

154. Little JW, Ditunno JF Jr, Stiens SA, et al. Incomplete spinal cord injury: neuronal mechanisms of motor recovery and hyperreflexia. *Arch Phys Med Rehabil* 1999;80:587–599.

155. Muir GD, Steeves JD. Sensorimotor stimulation to improve locomotor recovery after spinal cord injury. *Trends Neurosci* 1997;20:72–77.

156. Dobkin BH, Edgerton VR, Fowler E, et al. Training induces rhythmic locomotor EMG patterns in a subject with complete spinal cord injury. *Neurology* 1992;42(3 Suppl):207–208.

157. Edgerton VR, de Leon RD, Tillakartne N, et al. Use-dependent plasticity in spinal stepping and standing. *Adv Neurol* 1997;72:233–247.

158. de Leon RD, Hodgson JA, Roy RR, et al. Locomotor capacity attribut-

159. Ladouceur M, Pepin A, Norman KE, et al. Recovery of walking after spinal cord injury. *Adv Neurol* 1997;72:249–255.

160. Visintin M, Barbeau H. The effects of body weight support on the locomotor pattern of spastic paretic patients. *Can J Neurol Sci* 1989; 16::315–325.

161. Wernig A, Muller S, Nanassy A, et al. Laufband therapy based on rules of spinal locomotion is effective in spinal cord injured persons. *Eur J Neurosci* 1995;7:823–829.

162. Barbeau H, Ladouceur M, Norman KE, et al. Walking after spinal cord injury: evaluation, treatment and functional recovery. *Arch Phys Med Rehabil* 1999;80:225–235.

163. NIH Publication No. 97-4201. *Spinal cord injury: emerging concepts*. Proceedings of an NIH Workshop September 30-October 1, 1996. September 1997, NIH, Bethesda, Maryland.

164. Stein RB, Belanger M, Wheeler G, et al. Electrical systems for improving locomotion after incomplete spinal cord injury: an assessment. *Arch Phys Med Rehabil* 1993;74:954–959.

165. Fung J, Stewart JE, Barbeau H. The combined effects of clonidine and cyproheptadine with interactive training on the modulation of locomotion in spinal cord injured subjects. *J Neurol Sci* 1990;100: 85–93.

166. Falci S, Holtz A, Akesson E, et al. Obliteration of a posttraumatic spinal cord cyst with solid human embryonic spinal cord grafts: first clinical attempt. *J Neurotrauma* 1997;14:875–884.

167. Houle J. The structural integrity of glial scar tissue associated with a chronic spinal cord lesion can be altered by transplanted fetal spinal cord tissue. *J Neurosci Res* 1992;31:120–130.

168. Himes BT, Goldberger ME, Tessler A. Grafts of fetal central-nervous-system tissue rescue axotomized Clarke nucleus neurons in adult and neonatal operates. *J Comp Neurol* 1994;339:117–131.

169. Miya D, Giszter S, Mori F, et al. Fetal transplants alter the development of function after spinal cord transection in newborn rats. *J Neurosci* 1997;17:4856–4872.

170. Jakeman LB, Reier PJ. Axonal projections between fetal spinal cord transplants and the adult rat spinal cord: a neuroanatomical tracing study of local interactions. *J Comp Neurol* 1991;307:311–334.

171. Tessler A, Fischer I, Giszter S, et al. Embryonic spinal cord transplants enhance locomotor performance in spinalized newborn rats. *Adv Neurol* 1997;72:291–303.

172. Menei P, Montero-Menei C, Whittemore SR, et al. Schwann cells genetically modified to secrete human BDNF promote enhanced axonal regrowth across transected adult rat spinal cord. *Eur J Neurosci* 1998;10:607–621.

173. Grill R, Murai K, Blesch A, et al. Cellular delivery of neurotrophin-3 promotes corticospinal axonal growth and partial functional recovery after spinal cord injury. *J Neurosci* 1997;17:5560–5572.

174. Liu Y, Kim D, Himes BT, et al. Transplants of fibroblasts genetically modified to express BDNF promote regeneration of adult rat rubrospinal axons and recovery of forelimb function. *J Neurosci* 1999;19: 4370–4387.

175. Rapalino O, Lazarov-Spiegler O, Agranov E, et al. Implantation of stimulated homologous macrophages results in partial recovery of paraplegic rats. *Nat Med* 1998;4(7):814–821.

176. Fricker RA, Carpenter MK, Winkler C, et al. Site-specific migration and neuronal differentiation of human neural progenitor cells after transplantation in the adult rat brain. *J Neurosci* 1999;19:5990–6005.

177. Keirstead HS, Ben-Hur T, Rogister B, et al. Polysialylated neural cell adhesion molecule-positive CNS precursors generate both oligodendrocytes and Schwann cells to remyelinate the CNS after transplantation. *J Neurosci* 1999;19:7529–7536.

178. McDonald JW, Liu XZ, Qu Y, et al. Transplanted embryonic stem cells survive, differentiate and promote recovery in injured rat spinal cord. *Nat Med* 1999;5:1410–1412.

able to step training versus spontaneous recovery after spinalization in adult cats. *J Neurophysiol* 1998;79:1329–1346.

AUTONOMIC AND CARDIOVASCULAR COMPLICATIONS OF SPINAL CORD INJURY

DENISE I. CAMPAGNOLO
GENO J. MERLI

Understanding and being able to treat the medical complications that often follow spinal cord injury (SCI) is critical to improving quality of life and maximizing independence. This chapter discusses the acute and subacute cardiovascular complications after SCI.

Cardiovascular problems can be broadly categorized into direct and indirect complications. The direct sequelae result from the neurologic injury itself, owing to interruption and decentralization of the autonomic nervous system. Indirect complications are typically the result of immobilization and sedentary lifestyle. The most common direct cardiovascular complications include hypotension, bradycardia, and, once spinal shock has resolved, autonomic dysreflexia (AD). Fortunately, cardiopulmonary arrest is rare in the acute rehabilitation settings (1). The most significant indirect cardiovascular complications include thromboembolic disorders that occur acutely, such as deep venous thrombosis (DVT) and pulmonary embolism (PE). In the chronic phase, ischemic heart disease is one of the leading causes of death in patients with SCI.

Direct cardiovascular complications of spinal cord injury are due to injury to the spinal cord or nerves that interrupts communication between brain-stem centers and the effectors and receptors of the autonomic nervous system. A brief review of the autonomic nervous system is needed to understand the direct cardiovascular complications of SCI. The parasympathetic neurons have a cranial and sacral outflow from the central nervous system and orchestrate such "rest" state functions as digestion, gastrointestinal motility, slowing of the heart rate and respiration, and lowering of blood pressure. The sympathetic system has cell bodies in intermediolateral gray columns of the cord from the T1 to L2 level. Activation of the system increases heart rate, provides vasoconstriction, and increases arterial blood pressure; thus, it is predominantly activated in stressful ("fight-or-flight") situations, and its activity predominates during daytime hours.

The heart and blood vessels for the entire body are supplied by sympathetic outflow from levels T1 to T7 (2). The radial muscle of the iris causes dilation of the pupil (mydriasis) and receives its sympathetic innervation from the first thoracic segment of the spinal cord. Vasculature below the diaphragm, also called *splanchnic vasculature*, receives its innervation from the T5 through T7 levels. This becomes important in patients with high paraplegia and tetraplegia who suffer from the possible medical complication of AD, discussed later. The heart receives its sympathetic innervation from levels T1 through T4. The more severe the SCI, the more severe the cardiovascular problems because most preganglionic sympathetic neurons would no longer be under the control of suprasegmental input. Thus, in patients with enough damage to the lateral funiculus (corticospinal tract) to cause motor loss, it follows that the greatest autonomic derangement would be present (3).

HYPOTENSION

Cardiovascular derangements seen in acute spinal cord injury are typically hypotension and in cervical levels of injury, bradycardia. In the first few seconds to minutes after cord injury, however, there is a systemic pressor response due to the acute activation of sympathetic nervous system and the adrenal medulla. This is followed by hypotension due to loss of sympathetic tone (3). The classic triad of neurogenic shock includes hypotension, bradycardia, and hypothermia. The loss of sympathetic tone produces hypotension because of a decrease in systemic vascular resistance and dilatation of the venous vessels, thereby reducing preload to the heart. During spinal shock, the cardioaccelerator reflexes are also lost, resulting in bradycardia. Pulmonary edema is a known complication, and its association has been recognized since the 1800s (4).

The pathophysiology of neurogenic pulmonary edema includes the initial mechanical trauma to the cord, stimulating massive sympathetic discharge initially, with hypertension in the first seconds to minutes after SCI. This marked increase in afterload to the heart, as well as bradycardia, produces potential for left ventricular strain or failure and direct cardiac pulmonary edema. Also, β-endorphin release may depress the cardiorespiratory drive and thus decrease left ventricular function. Additionally, capillary leak syndrome is prominent in the acute minutes to hours after SCI, with disruption of pulmonary capillary endothelium resulting in a noncardiac component to the pulmonary edema.

Acute hypotension due to neurogenic shock is common. It is most prominent during the period the patient is neurologically in spinal shock. Bleeding sources must be excluded. Neurogenic hypotension is due to loss of vasomotor tone and the expanded vascular bed that results. Pulmonary artery catheterization (Swan-Ganz catheterization) is useful to guide fluid resuscitation in high tetraplegia patients and can provide information on central venous pressures, pulmonary capillary wedge pressures, and cardiac output (5,6). Judicious volume expansion with intravenous colloids to raise wedge pressures and produce optimal left ventricular function is recommended. General guidelines include administering enough intravenous fluids to maintain pulmonary capillary wedge pressures and adequate urine output (>30 mL/hr). Enhanced neurologic recovery was observed in a prospective study in subjects whose mean arterial blood pressure was maintained over 85 mm Hg (5). The Trendelenburg position can be used for symptomatic episodes. The use of vasopressors to treat further symptomatic hypotension is recommended, as opposed to increasing fluid administration. Typically, the vasopressors used are dopamine or phenylephrine. Dopamine is an α- more than β_1-agonist, which directly increases heart rate, and is the vasopressor of choice for hypotension and bradycardia as seen in neurogenic shock. Phenylephrine is a pure α-agonist and causes vasoconstriction of the venous and arterial trees, thus increasing preload and afterload. Caution must be used in the setting of bradycardia because use of phenylephrine may cause a reflex increase in vagal tone and slow the heart rate, with no ability to cardioaccelerate. Atropine is used for reflex bradycardia, which can be seen especially with phenylephrine.

BRADYCARDIA

The cardiovascular system is highly dependent on autonomic influences; therefore, it is logical that acute spinal cord trauma might interfere with complex mechanisms involved in cardiovascular homeostasis. Although bradyarrhythmias are common, occurring in up to 100% of tetraplegic patients, cardiac arrest is rare (7). Sympathetic innervation exits from T1 through T4. Parasympathetic control to the heart comes from the vagus nerve, which originates in the medulla. Bradycardia (and other cardiovascular abnormalities) resolves as spinal shock gradually resolves. The proposed mechanism of bradyarrhythmias, sinus slowing, and cardiac arrest is disruption of cardiac sympathetic influences during spinal shock. In addition to baseline sinus bradycardia, tracheal suctioning, defecation, and belching can cause sinus pauses and reflex vagal (parasympathetic) activity that is unopposed by sympathetics. Hypoxia may contribute to the bradycardia (7). Bradycardia is most pronounced 2 to 3 weeks after injury, and by 6 weeks, rhythm is usually normal.

Management of bradycardia includes prevention through pretreatment with atropine, 0.1 to 1 mg given intravenously 1 to 5 minutes before suctioning if needed. Careful monitoring of the patient during susceptible activities is extremely important. Transvenous pacing can be used if the above measures fail, but some patients may require a permanent demand pacemaker (8, 9).

THERMOREGULATION

Body temperature is normally regulated by the hypothalamus. When core temperature requires an adjustment, the hypothalamus can employ shivering and vasoconstriction to increase temperature. This serves to generate increased heat and also to decrease heat loss. Similarly, sweating and vasodilation decrease temperature through increased heat loss. SCI decreases the ability of the hypothalamus to direct the periphery. In patients with a complete SCI above T6, thermoregulation is significantly impaired as a result of interruption of efferent pathways (10). Spinal cord–injured patients are partially poikilothermic in that they usually have difficulty maintaining a normal core temperature in response to environmental change in temperature (10,11).

ORTHOSTATIC HYPOTENSION

Orthostatic hypotension can be defined as a decrease in blood pressure that results from a change in body position toward the upright posture. The symptoms include lightheadedness, dizziness, nausea, and even syncope. Associated symptoms may include numbness around the face and pallor. Orthostatic hypotension is more likely to occur in high levels of injury and is less likely in injuries below T6 and in incomplete injuries. The true incidence of orthostatic hypotension is not known (12). Symptoms decrease after the first few weeks of rehabilitation, helped by repeated postural challenges.

The mechanism of orthostatic hypotension involves pooling of blood in the lower extremities and viscera with change in posture. This, coupled with interruption of efferent sympathetic activity in the spinal cord, produces reflexive arterial vasoconstriction (12). In able-bodied patients during tilting, there is a decreased blood pressure that is sensed by the aortic and carotid baroreceptors, which would usually cause an increase in sympathetic outflow, resulting in tachycardia and vasoconstriction (13). However, in patients with SCI, the efferent pathway is interrupted; therefore, there is no increase in sympathetic outflow and no increase in norepinephrine and epinephrine (14, 15). The spinal cord–injured patient; therefore, has little or no increase in heart rate, which is not sufficient to counterbalance the decrease in blood pressure. The symptoms depend on cerebral blood flow rather than absolute arterial blood pressure (16). The venous pooling that occurs also limits venous return to the heart and thus limits cardiac output. The extent of the syndrome lessens with time. The reasons for this are not entirely understood but likely involve vascular wall receptor hypersensitivity, the development of spinal postural reflexes or spasticity causing vasoconstriction, improved autoregulation of cerebrovascular circulation in response to low perfusion pressures, and adaptation of the plasma renin-angiotensin system (12,13). Renin levels are elevated in patients with tetraplegia, especially in the head-up tilt position. This is dependent on intrinsic renal mechanisms and leads to production of angiotensin II, a vasoconstrictor.

This, in turn, leads to release of aldosterone, which causes volume expansion and vasoconstriction and limits drop in blood pressure.

The treatment of orthostatic hypotension involves daily tilting sessions with gradual change to the upright posture (this includes the use of the recliner wheelchair and tilt table). Elastic binders help with compression of the abdomen that limits blood accumulation in the abdominal vasculature. Elastic stockings likewise limit the accumulation of blood in the lower extremities. The patient needs to be adequately hydrated; therefore, initiating an intermittent catheterization program with a fluid restriction may best wait until this complication is resolved. Salt tablets, usually in a dose of 1 g four times daily, can be useful. Ephedrine sulfate, which stimulates norepinephrine release, is administered orally in doses of 20 to 30 mg one to four times daily (17,18). Mineral corticoid (fludrocortisone) is a salt-retaining steroid and can be started at a dose of 0.05 to 0.1 mg daily. Pitting edema is a common complication with the use of fludrocortisone. Midodrine hydrochloride, an α_1-adrenergic receptor agonist has been used as treatment at a dose of 2.5 mg twice to three times daily, titrating up to maximum of 10 mg twice to three times daily (19). A complication of these medications is supine hypertension. Also, in those patients with cardiac insufficiency, all volume-enhancing medications need to be used with caution. It is notable that patients who are susceptible to AD must be treated more cautiously with these medications because they can potentially increase the blood pressure response during an autonomic dysreflexic episode.

Functional electrical stimulation (FES) has been successfully used to increase blood pressure of recently injured subjects by as much as at least 20 mm Hg, allowing subjects to tolerate higher angles of tilt (20). Because blood pressure response was stimulus dependent and was independent of site stimulation (bone versus muscle), the investigators postulated that it was the noxious stimulus itself that augmented blood pressure by an AD–type sympathetic response (20). Future research is needed to clarify whether a small, unobtrusive FES device could be used clinically to control orthostatic hypotension.

AUTONOMIC DYSREFLEXIA

AD is a syndrome characterized by a sudden exaggerated reflex increase in blood pressure, sometimes accompanied by bradycardia, in response to a stimulus originating below the level of injury (12). This sympathetic discharge occurs in patients with SCI above most sympathetic outflow levels (T6 and above), although isolated cases of AD in patients with level of injury as low as T8 have been reported (21,22). AD goes by various names: autonomic hyperreflexia, paroxysmal hypertension, hypertensive autonomic crisis, visceroautonomic stress syndrome, autonomic spasticity, sympathetic hyperreflexia, and mass reflex. The incidence varies in the literature; however, it is generally reported to occur in 48% to 85% of all SCI patients with injury at T6 and above (23–25). The mechanism involves a strong stimulus that enters the spinal cord through intact peripheral nerves. The stimulus ascends through the spinothalamic tract and posterior

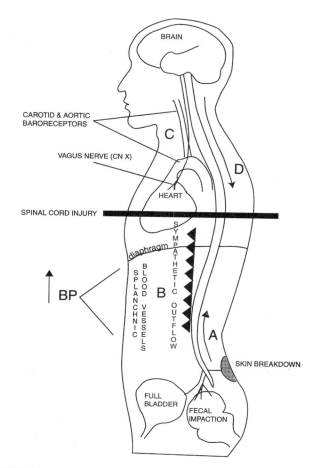

FIGURE 8.1. *A;* A strong sensory input (not necessarily noxious) is carried into the spinal cord through intact peripheral nerves. The most common origins are bladder and bowel. *B;* This strong sensory input travels up the spinal cord and evokes a massive reflex sympathetic surge from the thoracolumbar sympathetic nerves. This sympathetic surge causes widespread vasoconstriction, most significantly in the subdiaphragmatic (or splanchnic) vasculature. Thus, peripheral arterial hypertension occurs. *C:* The brain detects this hypertensive crisis through intact baroreceptors in the neck delivered to the brain through cranial nerves IX and X (vagus). *D:* The brain attempts two maneuvers to halt the progression of this hypertensive crisis. First, the brain attempts to shut down the sympathetic surge by sending descending inhibitory impulses. Unfortunately, these inhibitory impulses do not reach most sympathetic outflow levels because of the spinal cord injury at T6 or above. Therefore, inhibitory impulses are blocked in the injured spinal cord. The second maneuver orchestrated by the brain, in an attempt to bring down peripheral blood pressure, is heart rate slowing through an intact vagus (parasympathetic) nerve. This may result in a compensatory bradycardia but is inadequate, and hypertension continues. In summary, the sympathetic nerves prevail below the level of neurologic injury, and the parasympathetic nerves prevail above the level of injury. Once the inciting stimulus is removed, the reflex hypertension resolves.

columns below the level of lesion (Fig. 8.1). This stimulus incites a reflex release of sympathetic activity from the preganglionic sympathetic neurons in the intermediolateral cell column below the lesion level. This causes release of norepinephrine, dopamine-β-hydroxylase, and dopamine. The result is regional vasoconstriction, especially in the vasculature of the gastrointestinal tract (subdiaphragmatic or splanchnic vasculature). Peripheral vascular resistance and cardiac output increase, with a resultant marked rise in arterial blood pressure. A compensatory reflex bradycardia is seen as the brain-stem vasomotor centers attempt to reduce blood pressure. This maneuver is not effective because of Poiseuille's law—that pressure within a tube (blood vessel) is affected to the fourth power by change in radius (vasoconstriction) and only linearly by change in flow rate (slowed heart rate). The second attempt at correction of hypertension also fails because descending inhibitory tracts are unable to block this sympathetic surge owing to the spinal cord injury (Fig. 8.1). The patient, therefore, has a continued hypertensive crisis (21). The symptoms with which a patient usually presents include hypertension (defined as blood pressure of 20 to 40 mmHg above baseline for that patient), headache, sweating, and flushing above level of lesion. The headache is usually pounding in nature, found in the frontal and occipital areas. The pounding headache is caused by lack of sympathetic tone, which allows extensive vasodilation of pain sensitive intracranial arteries (12). Headaches are likely not caused by the hypertension directly because they have not been shown to correlate with the level of hypertension (12). Piloerection occurs below the injury level, owing to sympathetic stimulation of hair follicles below the level of injury. Pupillary changes are varied depending on whether the level of injury is above T1, the level from which the eye receives its sympathetic innervation. In that case, the circular or sphincter muscle of the iris responds to the sympathetic input causing mydriasis (2). This is not the case in lesions at T1, with interruption of fibers to the superior cervical ganglion and loss of sympathetic input to the eye, causing miosis, ptosis, and anhydrosis of the facial skin (Horner syndrome) (2). The patient can also experience nasal congestion and anxiety. These signs and symptoms categorized by their parasympathetic or sympathetic origin are listed in Table 8.1. The patient can also experience no symptoms at all, with silent elevation of blood pressure (26).

Possible complications of AD include retinal hemorrhage, subarachnoid hemorrhage, intracerebral hemorrhage, myocardial infarction, seizure, and potentially death (27). Hypertension is particularly important in elderly patients who have a baseline hypertensive nature. Pressure ulcer development, although not a direct complication of AD, has been considered to result from sympathetic denervation to the skin causing arteriovenous shunt and thus ischemia (28).

The single most common source of the stimulus to the cord is bladder distention. This can result from a blocked indwelling urinary catheter or a missed intermittent catheterization. In addition, a bladder infection or bladder stones can incite AD. The second most common cause is bowel distention due to fecal impaction. Other causes include pressure ulcers, ingrown toenails, abdominal emergencies, fractures, and body positioning. In women, AD is known to occur during labor and delivery. Ejaculation can also incite AD (Table 8.2).

Patients with SCI at T6 and above who are undergoing surgery are at particular risk for AD. AD occurs commonly during the induction phase of anesthesia regardless of the type of anesthetic technique used (27). Gastrointestinal, urologic, and plastic surgical procedures are the most common type to cause AD (27). This problem requires the full attention of anesthesiologists and surgeons. Spinal (intrathecal) anesthesia is ideal because it interrupts the autonomic reflex arc that produces AD (27). AD

TABLE 8.1. CLINICAL MANIFESTATIONS OF AUTONOMIC DYSREFLEIA

Signs and Symptoms	Autonomic Origin
General	
Systemic hypertension	Sympathetically mediated vasoconstriction in the peripheral blood vessels, especially the splanchnic vasculature
Bradycardia	Reflex compensatory parasympathetic influence through the intact vagus nerve
Anxiety	Nonspecific
Above and Around the Level of Injury	
Pounding headache	Inhibition of sympathetics allows extensive vasodilation of pain-sensitive intracranial arteries
Mydriasis (pupillary dilatation)	If the level of injury is above T1, sympathetic outflow from the first thoracic segment will cause pupillary dilation
Flushing	Inhibition of sympathetics allows extensive vasodilation of skin microcirculation
Sweating	Sympathetic cholinergic stimulation of sweat glands
Nasal congestion	Inhibition of sympathetics allows extensive vasodilation in mucosa of nasal passages
Below the Level of Injury	
Pallor, cool extremities	Sympathetically mediated vasoconstriction
Piloerection	Sympathetically mediated sudomotor activity at hair follicles
Bladder sphincter contraction	Sympathetically mediated through direct adrenergic receptors
Intestinal or stomach sphincter contraction	Sympathetically mediated through direct adrenergic receptors
Penile erection or seminal fluid emission	Sacral parasympathetic outflow is also stimulated, causing erection; sympathetically mediated seminal fluid emission

is intentionally self-induced by some to enhance athletic performance. This risky maneuver is termed "boosting" (28–30). A comprehensive listing of reported causes of AD is provided in Table 8.2. An intact spinal cord needs to be present for AD to occur; therefore, in the setting of cord infarction, AD is usually not seen.

AD generally occurs after the period of spinal shock and therefore is rarely detected earlier than 2 months after injury. There are rare cases reported of early AD occurring once sacral reflexes returned. These were attributed to rapid bladder filling with stimulation of the bladder neck where sympathetic receptors predominate (31). AD is usually present by 6 months to 1 year after injury. In one study, 92% of subjects exhibited their first autonomic dysreflexic episode by 1 year (24). The lack of occurrence of AD early after spinal cord injury suggests that AD develops over time and is produced mainly by peripheral or central receptor hypersensitivity rather than blockade of de-

TABLE 8.2. STIMULI AND CONDITIONS ASSOCIATED WITH THE DEVELOPMENT OF AUTONOMIC DYSREFLEXIA

Gastrointestinal system
  Bowel distention
  Anal fissures
  Esophageal reflux
  Enemas
  Gastric dilatation
  Gastric ulcer
  Cholecystisis or cholelithiasis

Urogenital system
  Penile stimulation, intercourse
  Urethral, bladder distention
  Vaginal dilatation
  Urinary tract infections
  Epididymitis
  Renal calculus
  Testicular torsion

Skin
  Cutaneous stimulation
  Sunburns
  Pressure sores

Extremities
  Deep venous thromboses
  Ingrown toenails
  Functional electrical stimulation
  Spasticity
  Bone fractures
  Range-of-motion exercises
  Position changes

Procedures and conditions
  Urodynamics and cystoscopy
  Surgical procedures
  Radiologic procedures
  Pulmonary emboli
  Electroejaculation
  Labor

Miscellaneous
  Medications
  Emergence in cold water
  Self-induced autonomic dysreflexia (intentional boosting)
  Sentinel event of another serious medical complication

Adapted from Teasell RW, Arnold JM, Krassioukov A. Cardiovascular consequences of loss of supraspinal control of the sympathetic nervous system after spinal cord injury. *Arch Phys Med Rehab* 2000;81(4):506–516, with permission.

scending inhibitory tracts (12). Another theory has suggested that AD results from decreased neuronal reuptake and increased synaptic levels of norepinephrine (12). The fact that level of SCI plays such a critical role in the appearance of AD has conventionally supported the blockade of inhibitory tract as the main pathophysiologic event leading to AD. However, it may just be that receptor hypersensitivity or synaptic overload of norepinephrine also occurs below that critical T6 level, but that simply not enough blood vessels are constricted below this level to cause any meaningful rise in systemic arterial pressure (12).

In 1997, under the auspices of the Paralyzed Veterans of America, a panel was convened of physicians, nurses, and a phar-macist with many years of experience in the care of patients with SCI. This group produced the clinical practice guideline entitled "Acute Management of Autonomic Dysreflexia: Adults with Spinal Cord Injury Presenting to Health Care Facilities" (32). The successful treatment of AD begins with the rapid recognition of the symptoms, followed by the prompt removal of precipitating stimuli (32). After checking the blood pressure, if it is elevated and the patient is supine, immediately sit the patient up, and loosen any clothing or constrictive devices. This could lead to pooling of blood in lower extremities, which may reduce blood pressure. Monitor blood pressure and pulse every 2 to 5 minutes until stabilized; blood pressures have the potential of fluctuating quickly during an AD episode as a result of impaired autonomic regulation. A rapid survey of the patient for instigating causes, beginning with the urinary system (most common cause of AD), should be performed. If an indwelling urinary catheter is not in place, catheterize the individual. If an indwelling urinary catheter is already in place, check the system along its entire length for kinks, folds, constrictions, or obstructions and for correct placement of the indwelling catheter; if the catheter appears to be blocked, gently irrigate the bladder with a small amount of fluid, such as normal saline at body temperature. Avoid manually compressing or tapping on the bladder if the catheter is draining. If the blood pressure remains elevated, suspect fecal impaction (second most common cause of AD), and check the rectum for stool. The use of lidocaine (Xylocaine) gel before rectal examination is recommended. If the blood pressure is at or above 150 mm Hg systolic, consider pharmacologic management to reduce systolic blood pressure before checking for fecal impaction. Use of antihypertensive agents with rapid onset and short duration should be considered while the causes of AD are being investigated. The most commonly used agents are nifedipine and nitrates (nitroglycerine paste). Nifedipine should be the immediate release form; bite-and-swallow is the preferred method of administration, rather than sublingual administration (33). Nifedipine should be used with extreme caution in elderly patients or patients with coronary artery disease. Other agents that have been used are hydralazine, mecamylamine, diazoxide, phenoxybenzamine, β-blockers, and terazosin (34–37).

One should monitor the individual's symptoms and blood pressure for at least 2 hours after resolution of the AD episode to ensure that AD does not recur. AD may resolve because of medication, not because of resolution of the underlying cause if there is poor response to treatment or if the cause of the AD has not been identified. If this is the case, the patient should be sent to the nearest emergency department for monitoring, maintenance of pharmacologic control of blood pressure, and investigation of other causes of the AD. The episode should be documented.

ANEMIA

Anemia is common after acute SCI and is usually normochromic and normocytic (38–41). Serum iron, TIBC, and transferrin are usually low. Although the exact cause is not known, bleeding may be a factor in some cases (38–41). By 1 year after injury, anemia improves in most patients with SCI. In the chronic stage, anemia may be associated with chronic inflammatory complications, such as pressure ulcers and frequent urinary tract infection.

ATHEROSCLEROTIC HEART DISEASE

Sedentary lifestyle and a high-fat diet place patients with SCI at high risk for atherosclerotic heart disease (42). The Model Systems database shows that for patients surviving longer than 30 years after SCI, heart disease is the leading cause of mortality (43). Hyperlipidemia is an independent risk factor for the development of atherosclerotic heart disease. In the general population, total cholesterol levels of greater than 200 mg/dL, low-density lipoprotein levels above 135 mg/dL, and high-density lipoprotein levels below 35 mg/dL are of concern (44). Decreased high-density lipoprotein levels are frequently observed in patients with chronic SCI (45–47) (see chapter 11).

THROMBOEMBOLIC DISORDERS IN ACUTE SPINAL CORD INJURY

DVT in acute SCI with Frankel classification of A, B, or C has been reported to occur in 47% to 100% of SCI patients (48, 49). The cause of this high incidence has been postulated to be increased platelet aggregation, increased factor VIII, and stasis (50,51). Modalities of prophylaxis were developed to change all or each of these factors individually. Adjusted dose heparin, external pneumatic compression, external pneumatic compression plus aspirin and dipyridamole, electrical calf stimulation plus low-dose heparin, and low-molecular-weight heparin (LMWH) have all demonstrated a reduction in the incidence of DVT in this population (48,52–57). The use of mechanical methods with pharmacologic agents appears to be safer and more effective than either modality alone during the acute phase of SCI. New forms of LMWH have been evaluated in other high-risk groups and may become effective modalities of prophylaxis in acute SCI patients.

Etiology

The high incidence of DVT and pulmonary embolism in patients with SCI is related to stasis, intimal injury, and hypercoagulability, which are all sequelae of acute neurologic impairment. These effects are referred to as Virchow's triad for the development of thrombosis (58). Stasis is the first risk factor to consider following injury to the spinal cord. Acute paralysis results in loss of the gastrocnemius-soleus pump as well as peripheral venous dilatation. Frieden and colleagues, using venous occlusive plethysmography in acute SCI patients, showed a decreased maximum venous outflow and venous capacitance (59). These two concomitant factors reduce the venous return from the lower extremities. Seifert and associates, using xenon-133 and chromium-51 EDTA documented the blood flow in the lower extremities of paraplegics (60). They demonstrated a reduction

in blood flow of paralyzed muscle compared to normal resting muscle. The flow could be increased in the paralyzed muscles by passive exercise, but the flow could not be sustained longer than 8 to 9 minutes after exercise. These two factors established the conditions for thrombus generation in the lower extremities of SCI patients.

Hypercoagulability is the second factor that has been assessed in SCI. Rossi and colleagues demonstrated a chronology of events in 13 of 18 patients who developed DVT after spinal cord injury (51). Preceding the thrombotic episodes, there was noted an increase in factor VIII:C and marked elevation in factor VIII:Ag (von Willebrand factor antigen) and factor VIII:RcoF (ristocetin cofactor). Factor VIII:C is a procoagulant glycoprotein synthesized in the liver, which is a measure of factor VIII activity. This is classically decreased in hemophiliacs. Factor VIII:Ag and factor VIII:RcoF are necessary for normal platelet adhesion and thrombus formation at sites of endothelial injury. Because these factors are produced by endothelial cells, their elevation reflects either endothelial cell damage or stasis of blood from the paralysis (61). Concomitantly, there was a hyperactive platelet aggregation response to collagen before the development of thrombosis (62). This suggests an alteration of platelet function, causing greater adhesion that predisposes to thrombus formation. After the development of DVT, the platelet aggregation ratio became normal. This indicated that circulating platelet aggregates are a result of thrombus formation, not the cause. This sequence of events was documented in 13 patients.

Erzos and colleagues documented in 10 paraplegic patients an increase in collagen-induced platelet aggregation compared with 10 age-matched healthy volunteers (63). This increase was observed 12 to 48 weeks after the acute trauma. This finding has been supported by four other studies in SCI. Myllynen and coworkers reevaluated these factors and supported these observations. They noted that the ratio of factor VIII:Ag to factor VIII:C was predictive of DVT in the eight spinal injured patients evaluated (50). Rossi and associates had also documented this elevated ratio (51). The clinical importance of this observation of an elevated ratio of endothelial cell–produced glycoprotein to liver-synthesized procoagulant as a predictor of DVT in acute SCI needs further investigation. Mammen and coworkers studied a series of 29 spinal injured patients who completed prothrombotic testing that included: fibrinopeptide A, platelet factor 4, β-thromboglobulin, D-dimer, antithrombin III, α_2-antiplasmin, thrombin antithrombin III complex, fibrinogen, factor VIII:C, factor VIII:RcoF, platelets, and mean platelet volume (64). These markers were measured every other day for 31 days after injury. These investigators found that the best correlation with DVT was the thrombin–antithrombin III complex. Boudaoud and colleagues (65) and Petaja and associates (66) reported the slow recovery response of the fibrinolytic system in patients following spinal cord injury. All of the above mechanisms for increasing thrombotic risk need to be addressed when designing prophylaxis strategies in this patient population.

Incidence

A number of autopsy studies documented the incidence of PE in spinal cord injury. Dietrick and Russi (67) and Nyquist and

Bors (68) documented the incidence of PE to be 2.3% to 3.6% in acute and chronically injured spinal cord patients. Their respective study sizes were 55 and 49 patients. Munro (69) and Tribe (70) reported PE as the major cause of death in 8.6% and 37.5% of patients studied, respectively. Their populations focused on acute spinal cord–injured patients less than 3 months after injury. The lower incidence of 8.6% reported by Munro is due to the mixed population of thoracic, lumbar, and conus injuries, the latter group of which has a lower incidence of DVT than the higher-level, complete lesions. Although their cohorts were 23 (Munro) and 16 (Tribe) patients, these two necropsy studies defined the mortality of PE in the 3-month period after acute SCI.

Six retrospective studies have attempted to identify the incidence of DVT in spinal cord–injured patients (71–76). Three of these studies had populations varying from 234 to 500 patients. The remaining three had smaller populations of 20 to 50 subjects. These trials have a number of limitations that do not allow a uniform assessment of the data. The patient postinjury time of entry into the studies varied from 4 days to 3 months. The objective assessment of DVT and PE was performed only when indicated by clinical signs and symptoms. Endpoint testing was performed with either impedance plethysmography, compression ultrasound, or lung scanning. Three of the studies did not describe a methodology for evaluating DVT and PE. Because of these study designs, accurate conclusions on the clinical course of thrombosis cannot be drawn from these trials. The overall incidence of DVT from these six retrospective studies was 12.5% to 17%, whereas the incidence of PE ranged from 3% to 15.3%.

In seven well-designed studies (Table 8.3), the incidence of DVT varied from 24% to 100% (48,49,51,77–80). Three studies had varied entry times into the protocols. Although these trials had an objective endpoint of iodine-125 (^{125}I) fibrinogen scanning or venography, an assessment of the time course of thrombosis development could not be ascertained. Four of the studies evaluated patients with motor complete or motor nonfunctional injuries within 72 hours of injury using ^{125}I fibrinogen scanning, impedance plethysmography (IPG), or venogra-

phy. One study performed bilateral lower extremity venography on all patients in addition to confirming any positive IPG or ^{125}I fibrinogen scan. The development of DVT was noted to occur most frequently during the first 2 weeks after spinal cord injury. Merli and colleagues reported a 54% incidence of DVT between days 3 and 7, and 33% on days 8 through 14 (48). Rossi and colleagues documented a 62% incidence on days 6 to 8 and a 23% incidence on days 9 through 14 (51). Geerts and colleagues evaluated an unprophylaxed multiple trauma population for DVT and PE by performing bilateral venography between days 7 and 21 after injury (81). Motor vehicle accidents accounted for the largest cause of severe multisystem injuries. The overall incidence of DVT was 58% (201 or 349 patients), with only 3 of the 201 patients with DVT (1.5%) having any clinical suspicion of the diagnosis (81). Because of the heterogeneity of the trauma group, subgroup analysis revealed that SCI patients had a 62% overall incidence of DVT with 27% of the thrombi in the proximal venous system.

This window of risk for DVT is important for designing interventions for the prevention of this complication as well as understanding the need to assess patients who have not received prophylaxis early in the course of injury or who are being transferred from trauma centers to rehabilitation units.

Prophylaxis

Prophylaxis for DVT and PE in acute SCI has had a variety of approaches, ranging from heparin in varied dosage regimens, oral anticoagulants, antiplatelet agents, and physical modalities. These forms of prophylaxis were directed at reducing stasis and hypercoagulability immediately after injury. A review of the literature since 1970 allows a detailed assessment of the studies and an evaluation of the validity of their outcomes.

Table 8.4 lists five reported trials using heparin in varied dosage regimens, oral anticoagulants, and physical modalities as prophylaxis for thrombosis after injury (82–86). Hachen compared 76 patients treated with Sintrom (oral anticoagulant) from 1969 through 1972 and 44 patients who received heparin 10,000 units subcutaneously every 12 hours between 1973 and 1974 (86). The incidence of DVT was 21% in the former and 6.8% in the latter. Bleeding was present in 5.3% of the Sintrom group and 4.5% of the heparin group. The methodology for assessing the results was not clear in the study and was assumed to be physical examination. A second study, with 100 patients, with oral anticoagulation was completed by Silver (84). Sixty-eight patients received prophylaxis with phenindione, and the remaining 32 patients, who were ineligible for anticoagulation, served as the controls. The efficacy of therapy was evaluated by physical examination and doppler when indicated. In the treatment group, 6% developed DVT, as compared with 25% in the controls. Casas and associates evaluated two doses of heparin, either 5,000 units or 7,500 units, every 12 hours in 21 patients (83). Three patients did not complete the protocol, and DVT was not observed clinically in the remaining 18 patients. This study did not indicate which dosage each subject received, and only physical examination was used to assess the efficacy of the therapy. Watson compared a group of unprophylaxed SCI patients from 1973 to 1974 (82). Physical examination and dopp-

TABLE 8.3. INCIDENCE OF DEEP VENOUS THROMBOSIS IN ACUTE SPINAL CORD INJURY

Reference	No. of Patients	Entry Time	Patients with DVT	Method
Todd (77)	20	<2 mo	20 (100%)	^{125}I, V#
Bors (78)	67	1–4 yr	36 (58%) @	V*
	32	Same	19 (59%) @	
Rossi (51)	18	<72 hr	13 (72%)	^{125}I, V#
Myllynen (49)	9	<72 hr	9 (100%)	^{125}I, V#
Brach (79)	10	<72 hr	7 (70%)	^{125}I, IPG, V#
Merli (48)	17	<72 hr	8 (47%)	^{125}I, IPG, V*
Philipps (80)	25	Variable	6 (24%)	V*

^{125}I, radiolabeled fibrinogen uptake test; V#, venogram performed for positive noninvasive test; V*, venogram performed on all patients; @, complete and incomplete spinal cord injury, respectively; IPG, impedance plethysmography.

TABLE 8.4. PROPHYLAXIS FOR DEEP VENOUS THROMBOSIS IN ACUTE SPINAL CORD INJURY

Reference	No. of Patients	Entry Time	Prophylaxis	Patients with DVT	Method
Watson (82)	181	Admission	No Rx	14/99 (14%)	PE, D
			Heparin	5/82 (6%)	
Casas (83)	21	Admission	Heparin	0/18 (0%)	PE
Silver (84)	100	2–7 days	No Rx	8/32 (25%)	PE, D
			Phenindione	4/68 (6%)	
Van Hove (85)	41	Day of injury	PROM	6/15 (40%)	PE
			M/S	0/26 (0%)	
Hachen (86)	120	<6–7 days	Sintrom	16/76 (21%)	PE
			Heparin	3/44 (6.8%)	

PE, physical examination; D, Doppler performed only if clinically indicated; PROM, passive range of motion; M/S, massage and stockings.

ler were used as the modalities for evaluating the endpoint of DVT prevent. The incidence rates of DVT were 0% in the treated group and 17% in the untreated control. The patients received passive mobilization of the extremities or massage plus elastic stockings. The incidence of DVT was 40% in the passive mobilization group and 0% in the massage plus stockings cohort, as assessed by physical examination and leg circumference.

All five studies have a number of serious problems with methodology, making their interpretation difficult. First, the studies were neither randomized nor controlled. Second, the time window for entry in the protocols varied from not designated to within 36 hours of the injury. The lack of adherence to a defined entry period in light of the previous information on the time of occurrence of DVT again makes this information difficult to assess critically. Third, there was no uniformity in dosage or scheduling of the prophylactic agents chosen. The oral warfarin-like agents differ in their potency, side effects, and lack of proven efficacy in prophylaxis trials. The heparin doses were not standard, except in one study. The duration of the prophylaxis

ranged from 4 weeks to whenever the patient was wheelchair mobile.

A second group of more recent studies was more directed toward preventing stasis and hypercoagulability in acute SCI (48,52,53,87,88) (Table 8.5). Frisbie and Sasahara evaluated 32 patients, comparing placebo with low-dose heparin (5,000 units given subcutaneously every 12 hours) (87). The patients were enrolled within 1 week of injury. Prophylaxis was maintained for 60 days, with IPG as the endpoint of the protocol. The results showed 6.4% in the placebo group and 7.7% in the heparin-treated patients. A problem with this study was the use of IPG, which has a low sensitivity and specificity for calf vein thrombosis as the sole assessment of therapy efficacy. Green and colleagues selected a prophylactic modality based on his previous work with Rossi and associates, which demonstrated increased platelet aggregation and factor VIII:Ag as the cause of DVT (53). Twenty-eight patients were randomized within 72 hours of injury to receive external pneumatic compression (EPC) alone or EPC plus acetylsalicylic acid and dipyridamole for 4 weeks. All patients underwent IPG and ^{125}I fibrinogen scanning with

TABLE 8.5. STUDIES DIRECTED TOWARD PREVENTING STASIS AND HYPERCOAGULABILITY IN ACUTE SPINAL CORD INJURY

Reference	No. of Patients	Entry Time	Therapy	Patients with DVT	Method
Frisbie (87)	17	<1 wk	Placebo	1 (5.8%)	IPG
	15	Same	Heparin	1 (6.6%)	Same
Green (53)	15	<72 hr	EPC	6 (40%)	[125]I, IPG, V
	12	Same	EPC, ASA, D	3 (25%)	Same
Becker (88)	5	<72 hr	Rotation P	4 (80%)	[125]I, IPG
	10	Same	Rotation C	4 (40%)	Same
Merli (48)	17	<72 hr	Placebo	8 (47%)	[125]I, IPG, V
	16	Same	Heparin	8 (50%)	Same
	16	Same	ES, heparin	1 (6.7%)	Same
Gunduz (89)	31	<15 d	Heparin	16 (53.3%)	V
Green (52)	29	<72 hr	Heparin	9 (31%)	[125]I, VU, V
	29	Same	Adj. heparin	2 (7%)	Same

EPC, external pneumatic compression; ASA, aspirin; D, dipyridamole; ES, electrical calf stimulation; IPG, impedance plethysmography; ^{125}I, radiolabeled fibrinogen; V, venography; VU, venous ultrasound.

venographic confirmation of positive studies. The mechanical plus antiplatelet therapy had a 25% incidence of DVT, whereas the mechanical modality alone had an incidence of 40%. This was compared with a historical placebo control group that had an incidence of 78%.

Becker and colleagues completed a study of 15 patients that assessed the use of rotating beds (88). All patients were randomized within 72 hours of injury to receive periodic rotation or continuous rotation for a 10-day period. IPG and ^{125}I fibrinogen scanning were selected to evaluate the efficacy of prophylaxis. The continuous-rotation group had a 10% incidence of DVT, whereas the periodic-rotation group had an 80% incidence. When ^{125}I fibrinogen scanning was used as the endpoint, the incidence of DVT in the continuous-rotation group was 40%, whereas the patient in the periodic-rotation group remained at 80%. The study population of this protocol was small and included a mix of complete and incomplete injuries.

The fourth study by Merli and colleagues was a randomized, placebo-controlled trial comparing low-dose heparin (5,000 units given subcutaneously every 8 hours) and electrical stimulation of the calf muscles plus low-dose heparin (5,000 units given subcutaneously every 8 hours) for 4 weeks (48). Daily ^{125}I fibrinogen scanning for 28 days and weekly IPGs were performed for thrombosis surveillance. Venography was performed for all positive noninvasive testing and bilaterally at the completion of the study. DVT was documented in 8 of 17 patients (47%) in the placebo group, in 8 of 16 patients (50%) in the low-dose heparin group, and in 1 of 15 patients (6.7%) in the electrical stimulation plus low-dose heparin group. A second study assessing mechanical and pharmacologic modalities by Merli and associates compared a group of 20 patients treated with external pneumatic compression sleeves plus gradient elastic stockings and low-dose heparin (5,000 units given subcutaneously every 12 hours) to a matched historical placebo-controlled group. All patients had ^{125}I fibrinogen scanning and IPG, with venography performed for positive study results (54). DVT was documented in 2 of 20 (10%) of the treated patients.

Gunduz and colleagues evaluated 31 SCI patients transferred to a rehabilitation center (89). All patients were give 5,000 units

of heparin every 12 hours for 12 weeks. Bilateral venography was performed in patients who had 2.5 cm or more leg swelling or increased warmth and in patients admitted more than 15 days from the time of injury. The incidence of DVT was 53.3%, and no major complications, including postvenographic phlebitis and allergic reactions, were observed.

Green and colleagues used an adjusted-dose subcutaneous heparin regimen over a 7-week period that demonstrated a reduction in the incidence of DVT from 31% to 7% (52). This study used duplex ultrasound for screening with venography for positive studies. Although this study using a single pharmacologic agent was effective, a 24% incidence of major bleeding necessitated the discontinuation of the adjusted heparin prophylaxis.

New Agents for Prophylaxis

Recently, fractionated portions of the heparin molecule have been evaluated for their antithrombotic effects (Table 8.6). These new forms of heparin (the LMWHs) have a more specific antithrombotic effect, a longer half-life, greater bioavailability, less thrombocytopenia, and a lower incidence of major bleeding. In addition, they have been shown to be more or as effective as standard heparin and as safe.

Two of these agents have been evaluated as DVT and PE prophylaxis in acute SCI. Green and colleagues randomized 41 motor complete acute SCI patients to standard heparin (5,000 units given subcutaneously every 8 hours) or LMWH (logiparin [now known as tinzaparin], 3,500 units given subcutaneously every day) (55). Surveillance with IPG, duplex ultrasound, and venography for positive noninvasive testing was performed weekly for 8 weeks. Five patients in the standard heparin group (23.8%) had thrombotic events. Three had DVT documented by noninvasive testing or venography (14.2%), and two patients died from PE. Two patients had bleeding requiring the discontinuation of heparin therapy. In the LMWH group, there were no documented thrombotic events or bleeding complications.

Merli and associates randomized 67 Frankel A, B, and C acute SCI patients into either group A (danaparoid, 750 units

TABLE 8.6. PROPHYLAXIS FOR DEEP VENOUS THROMBOSIS AND PULMONARY EMBOLISM IN ACUTE SPINAL CORD INJURY[a]

Reference	No. of Patients	Entry	Therapy[b]	Patients with DVT	Method
Green (55)	21	<72 hr	Heparin	5 (24%)	IPG, VU, V
	20	Same	Tinzaparin	0 (0%)	Same
Merli (56)	16	<72 hr	^Danaparoid and EPC	3 (18%)	^{125}I, VU, V
	26	Same	*Danaparoid and EPC	2 (7%)	Same
	15	Same	#Danaparoid and ES	0 (0%)	Same
Harris (57)	105	6-mo period	Enoxaparin	0 (0%)	Clinical and VU

[a] Daily clinical examination, venous ultrasound of neurologically impaired acute spinal cord injury.
[b] Tinzaparin, 3,500 U, s.c. q.d.; ^danaparoid, 750 U, s.c. q12h; *danaparoid, 1,250 U, s.c. q.d.; #danaparoid, 750 U, s.c. q12h.
IPG, impedance plethysmography; VU, venous ultrasound; V, venography; EPC, external pneumatic compression; ES, electrical calf stimulation.

given subcutaneously every 12 hours plus EPC), group B (1,250 units danaparoid given subcutaneously every day plus EPC), or group C (danaparoid, 750 units given subcutaneously every day plus electrical calf stimulation) (56). All patients were treated for 14 days, with DVT surveillance completed by daily ^{125}I fibrinogen scanning and duplex ultrasound on day 14. All positive studies were confirmed by venography. Nineteen patients were randomized into group A, with 16 completing. DVT developed in 3 of 16 (18%) patients. Twenty-six of 30 patients entered into group B completed the study, and DVT developed in 2 of the 26 (7%) patients. Group C had 15 of 18 patients complete the trial, and no evidence of DVT was detected in this group.

Harris and coworkers completed a prospective, single-cohort study of 105 patients treated prophylactically with enoxaparin (30 mg given subcutaneously every 12 hours) for 6 months (57). Forty of the 105 patients had complete motor paralysis, and the remainder were neurologically intact. All patients had daily clinical examinations, with only the neurologically impaired group undergoing venous ultrasound. There was no evidence of clinical DVT or PE. The incidence of major bleeding was 2.8% (3 of 105 patients).

Recommendations for Prevention of Thromboembolism

A consortium for the prevention of thromboembolism in spinal cord injury was developed under the auspices of the Paralyzed Veterans of America in 1997 (90). This guideline recommended that patients receive both a method of mechanical prophylaxis of DVT and anticoagulant prophylaxis. Pneumatic compressive hose or devices should be applied to the legs of all patients during the first 2 weeks after injury. If this measure has been delayed for more than 72 hours after injury, tests to exclude the presence of clots in the leg should be performed. The mechanism of action of EPC in reducing the rate of venous thrombosis in the lower limbs is hypothesized to be caused not only by direct expulsion of blood from the lower extremities but also by enhancement of fibrinolytic activity (91,92). In fact, intermittent compression of the arms was effective in reducing DVT in the legs and maintained fibrinolytic activity in postoperative patients (92).

Nursing personnel should inspect the skin underneath these pneumatic compressive devices routinely during the patient's care. Anticoagulant prophylaxis with either LMWH or adjusted-dose unfractionated heparin should be initiated within 72 hours after SCI provided that there is no active bleeding or evidence of head injury or a coagulopathy. For patients with motor incomplete injury, unfractionated heparin, 5,000 units given subcutaneously every 12 hours, can be used along with the compressive devices. For patients with motor complete SCI or high-risk factors for DVT, unfractionated heparin that is dose-adjusted to keep a high-normal aPPT,' or LMWH, should be used. Vena cava filter placement is recommended in SCI patients who have failed anticoagulant prophylaxis or who have a contraindication to anticoagulation. Filters should also be considered in patients with high-level motor complete tetraplegia (C2 or C3) with poor cardiopulmonary reserve or with thrombosis of the inferior vena cava despite anticoagulant prophylaxis. Filter placement is not

a substitute for thromboprophylaxis, which should be commenced as soon as feasible if there is no contraindication. The prophylactic insertion of filters is increasingly common in high-risk patients, with reported low insertion complication rates (93). Very few studies have specifically addressed the prophylactic use of filters in patients with SCI.

In a prospective study by Rogers and associates of high-risk trauma patients, the incidence of PE was significantly reduced in those who received a filter as compared with historical controls and controls using heparin or compressive devices (94). Two other studies have shown the benefits of prophylactic filter insertion (95,96). Problems with vena cava filters include cava thrombosis, filter migration, perforation of the vena cava, and complications at the skin insertion site. (97,98). A prospective randomized study designed to assess the benefits and risks of caval filters in the prevention of PE in high-risk patients with proximal DVT showed that the initial benefits of vena caval filters was counterbalanced by an excess of recurrent DVT, with no difference in mortality (93). Further inferior vena caval filters do not protect the patient with upper extremity paralysis from DVT in the upper extremities, both of which have been associated with PE (99–101). The appropriate use of filters in patients with SCI has yet to be determined.

Anticoagulant prophylaxis for patients with a motor incomplete lesion (ASIA C and D) should continue while the patients are in the hospital (including rehabilitation). For motor complete injuries (ASIA A and B), prophylaxis should continue for 8 to 12 weeks after injury depending on other risk factors. With a documented clot, mobilization and exercise of the lower extremities should be withheld for 48 to 72 hours after appropriate medical therapy has been implemented. Anticoagulant prophylaxis should be reinstituted in the chronic phases of SCI if the patient is readmitted for medical illness or surgical procedures (90).

Patients, family, significant others, and caregivers should be educated in the recognition and prevention of DVT. Recognition of calf circumference side-to-side differences (unilateral edema), increase in the pattern of collateral veins, pain or tenderness, and low-grade fever can all be indicators of DVT. Caregivers must be made aware of the clinical manifestations of PE: breathlessness, apprehension, fever, and cough. Thromboembolism can also be completely asymptomatic. Elastic stockings should be applied to augment venous return; however, tight bands should be avoided. These hose must be removed and the skin beneath inspected twice daily.

REFERENCES

1. Chen D, Apple DF Jr, Hudson LM. Medical complications during acute rehabilitation following spinal cord injury: current experience of the Model Systems. *Arch Phys Med Rehabil* 1999;80(11):1397–1401.
2. Barron KW, Blair RW. The autonomic nervous system. In: Cohen H, ed. *Neuroscience for Rehabilitation*, 2nd ed. Philadelphia: Lippincott Williams & Wilkins, 1999:277–302.
3. Piepmeier JM, Lehmann KB, Lane JG. Cardiovascular instability following acute cervical spinal cord trauma. *Cent Nerv Syst Trauma* 1985;2:153–160.
4. Gilbert J. Critical care management of patient with acute spinal cord injury. *Crit Care Clin* 1987;3:549–567.

5. Vale FL, Burns J, Jackson AB, et al. Combined medical and surgical treatment after acute spinal cord injury: results of a prospective pilot study to assess the merits of aggressive medical resuscitation and blood pressure management. *J Neurosurg* 1997;87:239–246.

6. Bernard GR, Sopko G, Cerra F, et al. Pulmonary artery catheterization and clinical outcomes. *JAMA* 2000;283:2568–2572.

7. Lehmann KG, Lane JG, Piepmeier JM, et al. Cardiovascular abnormalities accompanying acute spinal cord injury in humans: incidence, time course and severity. *J Am Coll Cardiol* 1987;10:46–52.

8. Kay MM. Kranz JM. External transcutaneous pacemaker for profound bradycardia associated with spinal cord trauma. *Surg Neurol* 1984; 22:344–346.

9. Gilgoff IS, Ward SLD, Hohn AR. Cardiac pacemaker in high spinal cord injury. *Arch Phys Med Rehabil* 1991;72:601–603.

10. Schmidt KD, Chan CW. Thermoregulation and fever in normal persons and in those with spinal cord injuries. *Mayo Clin Proc* 1992;67: 469–475.

11. Menard MR, Hahn G. Acute and chronic hypothermia in a man with spinal cord injury: environmental and pharmacologic causes. *Arch Phys Med Rehabil* 1991;72:421–424.

12. Teasell RW, Arnold JM, Krassioukov A. Cardiovascular consequences of loss of supraspinal control of the sympathetic nervous system after spinal cord injury. *Arch Phys Med Rehabil* 2000;81(4):506–516.

13. Corbett JL, Frankel HL, Harris PJ. Cardiovascular reflex responses to cutaneous and visceral stimuli in spinal man. *J Physiol* 1971;215: 395–409.

14. Mathias CJ, Christensen NJ, Corbett JL, et al. Plasma catecholamines, plasma renin activity and plasma aldosterone in tetraplegic man, horizontal and tilted. *Clin Sci Mol Med* 1975;49:291–299.

15. Mathias CJ, Christensen NJ, Frankel HL, et al. Renin release during head-up tilt occurs independently of sympathetic nervous activity in tetraplegic man. *Clin Sci* 1980;59:251–256.

16. Gonzalez F, Chang JY, Banovac K, et al. Autoregulation of cerebral blood flow in patients with orthostatic hypotension after spinal cord injury. *Paraplegia* 1991;29:1–7.

17. Groomes TE, Huang C. Orthostatic hypotension after spinal cord injury: treatment with fludrocortisone and ergotamine. *Arch Phys Med Rehabil* 1991;72:56–58.

18. Naso F. Cardiovascular problems in patients with spinal cord injury. *Phys Med Rehabil Clin North Am* 1992;3(4):741–749.

19. Barber DB, Rogers SJ, Fredrickson MD, et al. Midodrine hydrochloride and the treatment of orthostatic hypotension in tetraplegic: two cases and a review of the literature. *Spinal Cord* 2000;38:109–111.

20. Sampson EE, Burnham RS, Andrews BJ. Functional electrical stimulation effect on orthostatic hypotension after spinal cord injury. *Arch Phys Med Rehabil* 2000;81:139–143.

21. Erickson RP. Autonomic hyperreflexia: pathophysiology and medical management. *Arch Phys Med Rehabil* 1980;61:431–440.

22. Kurnick NB. Autonomic hyperreflexia and its control in patients with spinal cord lesions. *Ann Intern Med* 1956;44:678–686.

23. Frankel HL, Mathias CJ. Cardiovascular aspects of autonomic dysreflexia since Guttmann and Whitteridge. *Paraplegia* 1979;17:46–51.

24. Lindan R, Joiner E, Freehafer AA, et al. Incidence and clinical features of autonomic dysreflexia in patients with spinal cord injury. *Paraplegia* 1980;18:285–292.

25. Braddom RL, Rocco JF. Autonomic dysreflexia: a survey of current treatment. *Am J Phys Med Rehabil* 1991;70:234–241.

26. Linsenmeyer TA, Campagnolo DI, Chou IH. Silent autonomic dysreflexia during voiding in men with spinal cord injuries. *J Urol* 1996; 155:519–522.

27. Eltorai IM, Wong DH, Lacerna M. Surgical aspects of autonomic dysreflexia. *J Spinal Cord Med* 1997;20(3):361–364.

28. Boulton TB, Scott PV, Heggs CG, et al. Deaths and anaesthesia. *Br Med J* 1982;285:730–731.

29. Burnham R, Wheeler G, Bhambani Y, et al. Intentional induction of autonomic dysreflexia among quadriplegic athletes for performance enhancement: efficacy, safety and mechanisms of action. *Clin J Sports Med* 1994;4:1–10.

30. Webborn AD. "Boosting" performance in disability sport. *Br J Sports Med* 1999;33:74–75.

31. Silver JR. Early autonomic dysreflexia. *Spinal Cord* 2000;38:229–233.

32. Clinical Practice Guidelines: Acute management of autonomic dysreflexia. *J Spinal Cord Med* 1997;20:284–318.

33. Grossman E, Messerli FH, Grodzicki T, et al. Should a moratorium be placed on sublingual nifedipine capsules given for hypertensive emergencies and pseudoemergencies? *JAMA* 1996;276:1328–1331.

34. Naftchi NE, Richardson JS. Autonomic dysreflexia: pharmacological management of hypertensive crises in spinal cord injured patients. *J Spinal Cord Med* 1997;20:355–360.

35. Pasquina PF, Houston RM, Belandres PV. Beta blockade in the treatment of autonomic dysreflexia: a case report and review. *Arch Phys Med Rehabil* 1998;79:582–584.

36. Teichman JM, Barber DB, Rogenes VJ. Malone antegrade continence enemas for autonomic dysreflexia secondary to neurogenic bowel. *J Spinal Cord Med* 1998;21:245–247.

37. Vaidyanathan S, Soni BM, Sett P. Pathophysiology of autonomic dysreflexia: long-term treatment with terazosin in adult and paediatric spinal cord injury patients manifesting recurrent dysreflexic episodes. *Spinal Cord* 1998;36:761–770.

38. Claus-Walker J, Dunn CDR. Spinal cord injury and serum erythropoietin. *Arch Phys Med Rehabil* 1984;65:370–374.

39. Huang CT, DeVivo MJ, Stover SL. Anemia in acute phase of spinal cord injury. *Arch Phys Med Rehabil* 1990;71:3–7.

40. Hirsch GH, Menard MR, Anton HA. Anemia after traumatic spinal cord injury. *Arch Phys Med Rehabil* 1991;72:195–201.

41. Lipetz JS, Kirshblum SC, O'Connor KC, et al. Anemia and serum protein deficiencies in patients with traumatic spinal cord injury. *J Spinal Cord Med* 1997;20:335–340.

42. Szlachcic Y, Adkins RH, Adal T, et al. The effect of dietary intervention on lipid profile in individuals with spinal cord injury. *J Spinal Cord Med* 2001;24(1):26–29.

43. DeVivo MJ, Stover SL. Long-term survival and causes of death. In: Stover SL, DeLisa JA, Whiteneck GG, eds. *Spinal cord injury: clinical outcomes from the Model Systems.* Gaithersburg, MD: Aspen, 1995: 289–316.

44. Sempos CT, Cleeman JI, Carroll MD, et al. Prevalence of high blood cholesterol among U.S. adults: an update based on guidelines from the Second Report of the National Cholesterol Education Program Adult Treatment Panel. *JAMA* 1993;269:3009–3014.

45. Breanes G, Dearwater S, Shapera R, et al. High density lipoprotein cholesterol concentrations in physically active and sedentary spinal cord injured patients. *Arch Phys Med Rehabil* 1986;67:445–450.

46. Bauman WA, Spungen AM, Zhong YG, et al. Depressed serum high density lipoprotein cholesterol levels in veterans with spinal cord injury. *Paraplegia* 1992;30:697–703.

47. Kocina P. Body composition of spinal cord injured adults. *Sports Med* 1997;23(l):48–60.

48. Merli G, Herbison G, Ditunno J, et al. Deep vein thrombosis: prophylaxis in acute spinal cord injured subjects. *Arch Phys Med Rehabil* 1988;69:661–664.

49. Myllynen P, Kammonen M, Rokkanen P, et al. Deep vein thrombosis and pulmonary embolism in patients with acute spinal cord injury: a comparison with nonparalyzed patients immobilized due to spinal fractures. *J Trauma* 1985;25:541–543.

50. Myllynen P, Kammonen M, Rokkanen P, et al. The blood FVIII: Ag/FVIII:C ratio as an early indicator of DVT during post-traumatic immobilization. *J Trauma* 1987;27:287–290.

51. Rossi E, Green D, Rosen J, et al. Sequential changes in factor VIII and platelets preceding deep vein thrombosis in patients with spinal cord injury. *Br J Haematol* 1980;45:143–151.

52. Green D, Lee M, Ito V, et al. Fixed versus adjusted dose heparin in the prophylaxis of thromboembolism in spinal cord injury. *JAMA* 1988;260:1255–1258.

53. Green D, Rossi E, Yao J, et al. Deep vein thrombosis in spinal cord injury: effect of prophylaxis with calf compression, aspirin, and dipyridamole. *Paraplegia* 1982;20:227–234.

54. Merli G, Crabbe S, Doyle L, et al. Mechanical plus pharmacologic prophylaxis for deep vein thrombosi in acute spinal cord injury. *Paraplegia* 1992;30:558–562.

55. Green D, Lee M, Lin A, et al. Prevention of thromboembolism after

spinal cord injury using low molecular weight heparin. *Ann Intern Med* 1990;113:571–574.

56. Merli G, Doyle L, Crabbe S, et al. Prophylaxis for deep vein thrombosis in acute spinal cord injury comparing two doses of low molecular weight heparinoid (ORG 10172) in combination with either external pneumatic compression or electrical stimulation. *Am Spinal Injury Assoc Dig* 1990:8;(abst).

57. Harris S, Chen D, Green D. Enoxaparin for thromboembolism prophylaxis in spinal injury: preliminary report on experience with 105 patients. *Am J Phy Med Rehabil* 1996;75:326–327.

58. Vichow R. Neuer fall von todlichen: emboli der lungenaterie. *Arch Pathol Anat* 1856;10:225–228.

59. Frieden R, Jung A, Pineda H, et al. Venous plethysmography values in patients with spinal cord injury. *Arch Phys Med Rehabil* 1987;68:427–429.

60. Seifert J, Stoephasius E, Probst J, et al. Blood flow in muscles of paraplegic patients under various conditions measured by a double isotope technique. *Paraplegia* 1972;10:185–191.

61. Jaffe E, Hoyer L, Nachman R. Synthesis of antihemophilic factor antigen by cultured human endothelial cells. *J Clin Invest* 1973;52:2757–2764.

62. Winther K, Gleerup G, Snorranson K, et al. Platelet function and fibrinolytic activity in cervical spinal cord injured patients. *Thromb Res* 1992;65:469–474.

63. Ersoz G, Ficicilar H, Pasin M, et al. Platelet aggregation in traumatic spinal cord injury. *Spinal Cord* 1999;37:644–647.

64. Mammen E, Farag A, Fujii Y, et al. Newer laboratory tests in the diagnosis of patients with deep vein thrombosis. *Haemostasis* 1988;18(Suppl)2:53.

65. Boudaoud L, Roussi J, Lortat-Jacob S, et al. Endothelial fibrinolytic reactivity and the risk of deep venous thrombosis after spinal cord injury. *Spinal Cord* 1997;35:151–157.

66. Petaja J, Myllynen P, Rokkanen P, et al. Fibrinolysis and spinal injury-relationship to post-traumatic deep vein thrombosis. *Acta Chir Scand* 1989;155:241–246.

67. Dietrick R, Russi S. Tabulation and review of autopsy findings in 50 paraplegics. *JAMA* 1958;166:41–44.

68. Nyquist R, Bors E. Mortality and survival in traumatic myelopathy during 19 years, from 1946 to 1965. *Paraplegia* 1967;5:22–48.

69. Munro D. Thoracic and lumbosacral cord injuries. *JAMA* 1943;122:1055–1063.

70. Tribe C. Causes of death in the early and late stages of paraplegia. *Paraplegia* 1963;1:19–47.

71. Perkash A, Prakash V, Perkash I. Experience with the management of thromboembolism in patients with spinal cord injury. I. Incidence, diagnosis, and role of some risk factors. *Paraplegia* 1978;79:16:322–331.

72. Watson N. Anticoagulant therapy in the treatment of venous thrombosis and pulmonary embolism in acute spinal injury. *Paraplegia* 1974;12:197–201.

73. Naso F. Pulmonary embolism in acute spinal cord injury. *Arch Phys Med Rehabil* 1974;55:275–278.

74. Walsh J, Tribe C. Phlebo-thrombosis and pulmonary embolism in paraplegia. *Paraplegia* 1965;3:209–213.

75. Watson N. Venous thrombosis and pulmonary embolism in spinal cord injury. *Paraplegia* 1968;6:113–121.

76. Cheshire D. The complete and centralized treatment of paraplegia. *Paraplegia* 1968;6:59–73.

77. Todd J, Frisbie J, Rossier A, et al. Deep venous thrombosis in acute spinal cord injury: a comparison of 125 I fibrinogen leg scanning, impedance plethysmography, and venography. *Paraplegia* 1976;14:50–57.

78. Bors E, Conrad C, Massell T. Venous occlusion of the lower extremities in paraplegic patients. *Surg Gynecol Obstet* 1954;49:451–454.

79. Brach B, Moser K, Cedar L, et al. Venous thrombosis in acute spinal cord paralysis. *J Trauma* 1977;17:289–292.

80. Philipps R. The incidence of deep venous thrombosis in paraplegics. *Paraplegia* 1963;1:116–130.

81. Geerts W, Code K, Jay R, et al. A prospective study of venous thromboembolism after major trauma. *N Engl J Med* 1994;331:1601–1606.

82. Watson N. Anticoagulant therapy in the prevention of venous thrombosis and pulmonary embolism in spinal cord injury. *Paraplegia* 1978;16:265–269.

83. Casas E, Sanchez M, Arias C, et al. Prophylaxis of venous thrombosi and pulmonary embolism in patients with acute traumatic spinal cord lesions. *Paraplegia* 1977;15:209–214.

84. Silver J. The prophylactic use of anticoagulant therapy in the prevention of pulmonary emboli in one hundred consecutive spinal injury patients. *Paraplegia* 1974;12:188–196.

85. Van Hove E. Prevention of thrombophlebitis in spinal injury patients. *Paraplegia* 1978;16:332–335.

86. Hachen H. Anticoagulant therapy in patients with spinal cord injury. *Paraplegia* 1974;12:176–187.

87. Frisbie J, Sasahara A. Low dose heparin prophylaxis for DVT in acute spinal cord injured patients: a controlled study. *Paraplegia* 1981;191:343–346.

88. Becker D, Gonzalez M, Gentili A, et al. Prevention of deep vein thrombosis in patients with acute spinal cord injuries: use of rotating treatment tables. *Neurosurgery* 1987;20:675–677.

89. Gunduz S, Ogur E, Mohur H, et al. Deep vein thrombosis in spinal cord injured patients. *Paraplegia* 1993;31:606–610.

90. Consortium for Spinal Cord Medicine. Prevention of thromboembolism in spinal cord injury. *J Spin Cord Med* 1977;20:259–283.

91. Salzman EW, McManama GP, Shapiro AH, et al. Effect of optimization of hemodynamics on fibrinolytic activity and antithrombotic efficacy of external pneumatic calf compression. *Ann Surg* 1987;206:636–641.

92. Knight MTN, Dawson R. Effect of intermittent compression of the arms on deep venous thrombosis in the legs. *Lancet* 1976;2(7998):1265–1267.

93. Decousus H, Leizorovicz A, Parent F, et al. A clinical trial of vena caval filters in the prevention of pulmonary embolism in patients with proximal deep-vein thrombosis. *N Engl J Med* 1998;338:409–415.

94. Rogers FB, Shackford SR, Ricci MA et al. Routine prophylactic vena cava filter insertion in severely injured trauma patients decreases the incidence of pulmonary embolism. *J Am Coll Surg* 1995;180:641–647.

95. Wilson JT, Rogers FB, Wald SL, et al. Prophylactic vena cava filter insertion in patients with traumatic spinal cord injury: preliminary results. *Neurosurgery* 1994;35:234–239.

96. Khansarinia S, Dennis JW, Velden HC, et al. Prophylactic Greenfield filter placement in selected high-risk trauma patients. *J Vasc Surg* 1995;22:231–236.

97. Balshi JD, Cantelmo NL, Menzoian JO. Complications of caval interruption by Greenfield filter in quadriplegics. *J Vasc Surg* 1989;9:558–562.

98. Kinney TB, Rose SC, Valji K, et al. Does cervical spinal cord injury induce a higher incidence of complications after prophylactic Greenfield inferior vena cava filter use? *J Vasc Interv Radiol* 1996;7:907–915.

99. Monreal M, Lofoz E, Ruiz J, et al. Upper-extremity deep venous thrombosis and pulmonary embolism. *Chest* 1991;99:280–283.

100. Monreal M, Raventos A, Lerma R, et al. Pulmonary embolism in patients with upper extremity DVT associated to venous central lines: a prospective study. 1991;99:280–283.

101. Prandoni P, Polistena P, Bernardi E, et al. Upper-extremity deep vein thrombosis: risk factors, diagnosis and complications. *Arch Intern Med* 1997;157:57–62.

PULMONARY MANAGEMENT OF SPINAL CORD INJURY

W. PETER PETERSON
STEVEN KIRSHBLUM

Respiratory complications after spinal cord injury (SCI) are the leading cause of mortality in patients with tetraplegia and paraplegia (1–10). Pneumonia is the leading cause of death during all postinjury time periods, ranging from 18.9% during the first postinjury year to 12.7% after the first postinjury year (1,2, 6–10). In the acute stage, respiratory complications increase the length of hospitalization by as long as 27 days (11). Unfortunately, although much is known regarding pulmonary complications, there is little literature on the management of this important issue. A recent review of 1,887 English language articles regarding traumatic SCI and pulmonary issues from the Duke Evidence-based Practice Center concluded that the "quality of the literature is relatively low" because there are few studies with large sample sizes and comparison groups (12).

The problem for SCI patients in terms of pulmonary issues is threefold: secretion management, atelectasis, and hypoventilation. First, acute patients with tetraplegia and high paraplegia have loss of innervation of the muscles that are used in forceful exhalation required for an effective cough. Because of this reduced ability to cough, there is difficulty in clearing secretions. Second, patients with tetraplegia have loss of intercostal muscle innervation and therefore are dependent mostly on the diaphragm for inhalation. Because of this weakness, there is a tendency to develop atelectasis. Most of the respiratory complications that develop are secondary to these issues.

The goals of management are related to these problems. Caregivers need to help the patient mobilize his or her secretions. In addition, the alveoli need to be stabilized, compliance of the lungs and chest wall needs to be maintained, and the lungs need to be kept inflated. This chapter focuses on the potential for respiratory problems after SCI, their diagnosis, and treatment options.

ANATOMY AND PHYSIOLOGY OF VENTILATION

In able-bodied people, ventilation is achieved by the coordinated action of muscles on the rib cage, producing expansion and contraction of the thoracic volume. There are three main sets of muscles involved in inspiration: diaphragm, external intercostals, and accessory muscles, including the scalene, sternocleidomastoid, trapezius, and pectoralis muscles. These accessory muscles act as either prime movers of the rib cage or stabilizers that adjust the configuration and affect the efficiency of the diaphragm. The muscles of expiration include mainly the abdominal muscles: recti, obliques, and transversus abdominis.

The diaphragm is a dome-shaped muscle and is the major muscle of inspiration, whereas expiration is primarily a passive process. The diaphragm is innervated by the phrenic nerve, which originates from C3 through C5, with C4 being the main source of diaphragmatic innervation (13). As the diaphragm contracts, it becomes flattened, the abdominal contents are displaced downward, and air movement commences as the thoracic cavity is increased. The diaphragm contributes to 65% of the vital capacity (VC) in able-bodied individuals (14,15). Rib cage stabilization, degree of expansion, and the starting position of the diaphragm affect the efficiency of air movement because they determine the length and tension efficiency of the diaphragmatic contraction.

The intercostal nerves from the T1 through T11 levels innervate the intercostal muscles. It is thought that both layers of intercostal muscles act to produce inspiration at low lung volumes and expiration at large lung volumes (16). The trapezius and sternocleidomastoid muscles have innervation from cranial nerve XI, with their motor neurons from the upper cervical root levels. The scalene muscles are innervated from the C4 through C8 root levels.

The abdominal muscles, innervated segmentally from the T6 through L1 root levels, are mainly muscles of expiration. They produce increased intraabdominal pressure that moves the diaphragm superiorly during high-effort expirations and cough. The diaphragm also benefits from abdominal muscular tone, which places the diaphragm in an optimal position for length and tension efficiency. The clavicular portion of the pectoralis major muscle has been shown to be an expiratory muscle in tetraplegia. If strengthened, cough is improved, and expiratory volume is increased.

The central control of respiration is mainly from the medulla, which predominately controls the depth and rhythmicity of breathing. There is volitional control of breathing from the cortex, which also controls coordination of breathing to produce speech.

RESPIRATORY DYSFUNCTION AFTER SPINAL CORD INJURY

SCI patients whose level of injury is L1 or lower usually do not have significant respiratory dysfunction. From a T12 up to T5 neurologic level of injury (NLI), the abdominal muscles and intercostal muscles are weakened; therefore, there is impairment of forceful ventilation and cough. From T5 up to the T1 level, the intercostals are progressively weakened. Therefore, forceful ventilation and cough are severely impaired, and at these higher thoracic levels, even quiet respiration is affected in that the position of the diaphragm is no longer optimum owing to lack of abdominal musculature. With cervical level of injuries (C4 through C8), expiration consists of passive recoil of the rib cage. These individuals are highly vulnerable to respiratory complications and should be monitored closely. At the C4 level of injury, the diaphragm may have lost some innervation, further compromising even quiet respiratory effort, which is largely the product of diaphragmatic movement. At the C3 level, the diaphragm is typically weakened to the point at which ventilation cannot be sustained, resulting in the need for ventilatory assistance. The accessory muscles of respiration are still largely functioning at this level, providing a VC of 100 to 300 mL acutely. However, they usually cannot sustain the patient in the acute stage of injury. In the more chronic post-injury stages, the accessory muscles alone can sometimes produce tidal volumes adequate for long-term ventilation. Patients with a complete injury at the C2 level and above have no diaphragmatic function and may be apneic.

Three major categories of severity of cervical SCI, with the level of injury relating to respiratory problems, are as follows:

1. Patients with a complete NLI of C2 and above have no function of the diaphragm and therefore need some type of ventilatory assistance.
2. Patients with C3 or C4 as the last preserved neurologic level have the potential to wean from ventilatory assistance if it is initially required. A study of the outcome of patients with functional C3 and C4 levels of injury revealed that 83% of patients at these levels weaned completely from the ventilator (17). To wean successfully, these patients initially need to be ventilated and weaned with optimal skill and technique, preventing complications and optimizing weaning techniques (17,18). Wicks and Menter reported successfully weaning 51% of patients with C3 injury levels and 78% of patients with C4 injuries who were initially ventilator dependent (19).
3. Patients injured at the NLI of C5 and below are usually able to breathe without respiratory assistance. However, some of these patients initially require ventilatory support. Any pulmonary compromise due to secretions, atelectasis, or infection can result in ventilatory insufficiency and the need for assisted ventilation. Vigorous preventive measures are extremely important for these patients, with close monitoring and early intervention. All acute SCI patients should be considered at risk for progressive respiratory insufficiency.

RESTRICTIVE VENTILATORY DEFECT

SCI patients typically have a restrictive pulmonary syndrome, with a decrease in all lung volumes (total lung capacity, VC, expiratory reserve volume [ERV] and functional residual capacity [FRC]) except the residual volume, which increases, because the patient does not have the strength to exhale to the normal residual volume. These individuals have lost most of their ERV because of paralysis of their expiratory muscles. As a result, their forced vital capacity (FVC) approximates their inspiratory capacity. During spinal shock, when paralyzed muscles are flaccid, the paralyzed abdominal wall moves outward rather than contracting to augment chest wall expansion. Paralyzed intercostals are drawn inward with inspiration. These paradoxical movements of the intercostals and abdominal muscles result in a significant drop in the efficiency of breathing (20). The VC in the newly injured tetraplegic patient is reduced to 24% to 31% of the predicted normal (21,22). The VC does improve in the subacute and chronic period after SCI, owing to improved strength and the development of intercostal and abdominal tone that stabilizes the rib cage, allowing for a more mechanically effective diaphragmatic action (16,21,23). Ledsome and Sharp documented that a significant increase in VC occurred within 5 weeks of injury, with an approximate doubling of VC 3 months after injury in patients with complete injuries at C4 to C6 (21). In general, VC in these later stages in tetraplegia is reduced by 30% to 50% in high-level cervical injuries, FRC by about 25%, and ERV by as much as 75% (24). The VC and forced expiratory volume in 1 second (FEV_1) are decreased similarly with rising SCI levels, most marked in those with complete tetraplegia (25,26). The typical functional loss associated with complete motor lesions at C5 and above is roughly half for FVC and FEV_1; for C6 to C8, about one third; for T1 to T7, only slightly below the lower limits of normal; and for low paraplegia, only slightly below predicted norms (26). Halo vests may further restrict the VC by up to 8% in SCI patients (27,28).

Longer duration of injury is also associated with greater functional loss of VC in individuals with tetraplegia. This loss in tetraplegia is more than expected for aging alone and may be clinically important in later years, especially in those injured at a younger age (26).

INCIDENCE OF COMPLICATIONS

Various studies have attempted to quantify the complication rates of respiratory issues during the acute and rehabilitation admissions, and found those rates to be at least 20% for pneumonia and for atelectasis, these being the most common pulmonary complications (1,29–32). Jackson and Groomes, in a retrospective review, reported that overall 67% of acutely injured individuals experienced some respiratory complication during the initial hospitalization; these complications included atelectasis (36%), pneumonia (31%), and respiratory failure (22.6%) (30). All levels of injury were at risk; 84% of acute patients with an NLI between C1 and C4 had at least one respiratory complication, 60% of patients with an NLI between C5 and C8, and 65% of those with thoracic level injuries.

There is a greater incidence of pulmonary complications, during the acute and rehabilitation phases, with increasing age, high level of injury, and complete tetraplegia (1,7,32,33). In patients undergoing rehabilitation, respiratory issues are a frequent cause of death, especially in those with complete tetraplegia (8,34). Respiratory complications during the acute and initial rehabilitation hospitalizations are associated with increased likelihood of requiring mechanical ventilation, which in turn is associated with lower functional status, greater probability of nursing home placement, greater medical costs, and the potential for decrements in survival and perceived quality of life (35,36). DeVivo reported that about 16% of ventilator-dependent patients were discharged to a nursing home, in comparison to 4% of patients who were able to breath independently (35). Fuhrer and associates found that 1 year after injury, 89% of ventilator-independent patients were living at home, in comparison with 79% of those requiring a ventilator (36).

RESPIRATORY COMPLICATIONS AFTER SPINAL CORD INJURY

Atelectasis

The incidence of atelectasis in patients with SCI is extremely high and should be avoided because of the potential for a cascade of complications that may follow, including pneumonia, pleural effusion, and empyema. The most important treatment of atelectasis consists of attempts to expand the lungs. For patients requiring ventilation, high tidal volumes are extremely helpful. In one series, 60% of patients with an NLI of C3 and C4, admitted on a ventilator to a tertiary care facility, had atelectasis (18). Although not randomized into treatment groups, 23 of 42 patients in this series were subsequently ventilated with "low" tidal volumes (<20 mL/kg body weight), and 19 of 42 patients were subsequently ventilated with "high" tidal volumes (>20 mL/kg body weight). The two groups were on comparable tidal volumes at the time of discharge from the referring hospital; 950 mL for those who were subsequently ventilated with lower tidal volumes, compared with 920 mL for those subsequently ventilated with higher tidal volumes. At the time of admission, 9 of 23 patients in the subsequent low tidal volume group had atelectasis (39%), and 16 of 19 patients in the subsequent high tidal volume group had atelectasis (84%). At the end of 2 weeks, 52% of those subsequently ventilated with low tidal volumes had atelectasis, whereas 16% of those subsequently ventilated with high tidal volumes had atelectasis (18). Other treatment modalities for atelectasis include assisted cough techniques, proper positioning, noninvasive positive-pressure ventilation, and respiratory treatments (see later).

Pneumothorax and Chest Injury

Patients with SCI may have associated chest injury, especially with thoracic level injuries or penetrating injuries (e.g., gunshot wounds). They may have rib fractures, contusion of the lung, pneumothorax or hemothorax, or injury to the diaphragm, heart, or aorta. A pneumothorax may also occur as a result of ventilation of the patient with high pressure. An important concept to remember is that if patients require thoracic surgery or a chest tube, there is a high likelihood that they will form adhesions between the parietal and visceral pleura, or even a trapped lung. If the patient is on a ventilator and ventilated at low tidal volumes, there may be persistent atelectasis, or a lung that is trapped at a volume that may prevent the patient from weaning. Keeping the long-term and short-term risks of treatment in mind, it is recommended that the patient with a pneumothorax be treated with large tidal volumes, at least 1,000 mL. The larger tidal volumes may increase the risk for barotrauma but will decrease the risk for lung trapping and permanent atelectasis. If the larger tidal volumes can be given with a peak inspiratory pressure on the ventilator of 40 cm H_2O or less, then the risk for further lung damage will be small, with the benefit being an increased likelihood of weaning completely from the ventilator.

Pneumonia

In patients with SCI, and especially with atelectasis, the pneumonia occurs because the patient cannot cough effectively. As previously mentioned, high levels of injury and older age are significantly associated with an increased risk. If there is atelectasis, the pneumonia is most likely to develop in the atelectatic area of lung.

Pulmonary Embolism

Individuals with SCI should be monitored closely for pulmonary emboli because they are at increased risk from their injuries and immobility. Prompt treatment is imperative. For further discussion of pulmonary emboli, see chapter 8.

Pleural Effusion

With atelectasis, the mediastinum may shift to the side of the atelectasis, and the diaphragm on the side of the atelectasis may rise. These shifts occur to fill the space that is left by the collapse of the affected areas of lung. Multiple studies have found that lobar collapse is associated with lower pleural pressure around the collapsed lobe when compared with the pressure around lobes without collapse (37–39). When the SCI patient has atelectasis, it is most often in the lower lobes. The lower lobe may pull away from the diaphragm and the parietal pleura in such a way that there is a space that is not filled by the shift in the mediastinum or diaphragm (40). This leaves an empty space, with low pressure, which may be filled by fluid. In a study of 100 consecutive admissions to the intensive care unit, it was shown that 62% of the patients had pleural effusions, and of those, 14 patients (23% of those with effusions) had atelectasis as a cause of the effusion (41). These effusions secondary to atelectasis resulted from severe muscle weakness, airway obstruction, or patient immobility, all of which are seen in SCI patients. In this study, the effusions rapidly disappeared with resolution of the atelectasis.

The following case study illustrates some of these points.

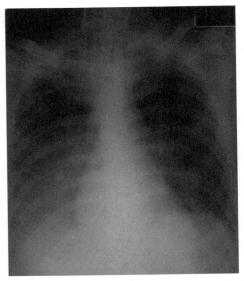

FIGURE 9.1. X-ray film. There is a pleural effusion on the right, with the patient on low ventilator tidal volumes.

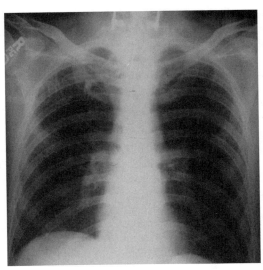

FIGURE 9.3. X-ray film. The pleural effusion is gone after institution of large ventilator tidal volumes.

Case study #1

GS is a 46-year-old man who suffered a C4 SCI and hypoxemic brain injury in a bodysurfing accident. He is 6′0″ tall. On arrival at a tertiary care institution, he was being ventilated at 1,000 mL, or 11.9 mL/kg ideal body weight (IBW). He had atelectasis of the right lower lobe, with shift of the mediastinum to the right, and elevation of the right hemidiaphragm (Fig. 9.1). There was also a large pleural effusion. Although the effusion was getting better with increases in the ventilator tidal volume, a thoracentesis was performed because of a body temperature of 104°F. At the time of the thoracentesis, GS was being ventilated with a tidal volume of 1,800 mL, or 21.4 mL/kg of IBW. The effusion was an exudate, with values of albumen of 3.3, specific gravity of 1.022, and cell count of 2,664 white blood cells and 9,590

red blood cells. The cultures were negative for routine culture, tuberculosis, and fungus; therefore, the effusion most likely represented a parapneumonic effusion. After 730 mL was removed by the thoracentesis, the patient still had a pleural effusion (Fig. 9.2). At the time of x-ray (Fig. 9.2), GS was being ventilated with 1,900 mL, or 22.6 mL/kg IBW. The patient was treated by increasing tidal volumes on the ventilator, with complete resolution of the effusion (Fig. 9.3). The choice not to treat with a chest tube was made because the effusion was not infected, and there is a risk for lung trapping secondary to the chest tube.

This case illustrates that pleural effusions occur in the presence of atelectasis and can be treated by filling the fluid-filled space with an inflated lung.

Empyema

The combination of atelectasis, pulmonary effusion, and pneumonia can lead to the development of empyema. This again points out the importance of avoiding atelectasis and pneumonia.

Trapped Lung

Atelectasis may lead to the development of a pleural effusion; if the effusion becomes infected, the patient has an empyema. A chest tube may be inserted to drain the empyema. With an empyema, or a chest tube, the patient runs the danger of having a trapped lung. The trapped lung occurs because of scarring and fusion of the parietal and visceral pleura. There may also be organization of the exudate in the pleural space, so that a "peel" is formed around the lung that prevents the lung from expanding, thereby trapping the lung. The patient may also have a chest injury associated with the initial SCI. If this injury requires a chest tube or surgery, there is the same risk for forming a pleural peel. If the patient with an infected pleural space is ventilated

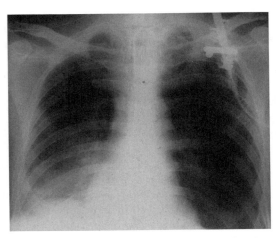

FIGURE 9.2. X-ray film. The pleural effusion is better after thoracentesis and increasing tidal volumes on the ventilator.

with a small tidal volume (e.g., 700 mL), then the patient forms a peel, or a type of "corset" around the lung set at 700-mL maximum VC.

Wicks and Menter showed that the SCI patient of average height will need a VC of 1,000 to 1,100 mL to be able to wean successfully from the ventilator (19). If the patient has a localized empyema and only a lobe is involved in the entrapment, that lobe will be trapped at a small volume, and atelectasis is inevitable. Therefore, the patient with an empyema or with chest tubes will need to be ventilated at a tidal volume of at least 1000 mL to wean from the ventilator. An article on chest tubes as a cause of failure to wean from the ventilator proposes ventilating the SCI patient at the highest possible ventilator tidal volume immediately after surgery or after insertion of a chest tube (42). The larger the tidal volume, the greater the potential VC when the time for weaning from the ventilator arrives. This management strategy also avoids permanent atelectasis.

Aspiration

Aspiration occurs in about 5% of all SCI patients, with a higher risk (about 13%) in patients older than 60 years of age (1). High-level SCI patients are also at a higher risk for aspiration, especially after anterior-approach surgery, in the older age group, or in the presence of a tracheostomy (43). This may also result from sedation and immobilization in the initial days after injury, in which case the patients may not be awake enough or able to turn their head to expectorate the fluid. A halo vest may also prevent turning of the head. The dangers of aspiration include pneumonia and acute respiratory distress syndrome (ARDS). The acute SCI patient is also at great risk for reflux or emesis because spinal shock may slow the emptying of the stomach; air from respiratory treatments or from the ventilator may distend the stomach; medications may slow the emptying of the stomach; the patient may have diabetes, in which case there may be slow gastric emptying; and the patient may have a tracheoesophageal fistula, or more commonly, an esophagolaryngeal fistula from hardware on the anterior surface of the spine.

One needs to be highly suspicious for the potential of aspiration in the acute high-level SCI patient. Any signs of aspiration should be quickly evaluated by a full workup, including a video-fluoroscopic swallowing study or ear, nose, and throat evaluation. Positioning may be used to reduce the chance of reflux, and some medications (i.e., metoclopramide) can help reduce the incidence of reflux and aspiration.

Abdominal Complications

Abdominal complications are common in SCI patients. Some of these are related to abdominal injury occurring at the time of the SCI. Patients may also develop ileus, with distended bowel pushing on the diaphragm and compromising the ability of the diaphragm to descend. This diminishes the ability of the patient to take a deep breath and may contribute to atelectasis.

DIAGNOSTIC OPTIONS

The importance of diagnosis is to assist in prevention of serious pulmonary complications. Options include plain x-ray, arterial blood gas (ABG) measurement, noninvasive oxygen saturation and end-tidal CO_2 monitoring, pulmonary function tests (PFTs), computed tomography (CT) scans, and fluoroscopy.

X-ray

Current practice is to follow the chest x-ray films (anteroposterior and lateral) of SCI patients, looking for atelectasis, pneumonia, and pneumothorax as the major complications, as well as diagnosing a paralyzed hemidiaphragm. Lateral decubitus films are helpful to exclude pleural effusions.

Arterial Blood Gas

It is important to perform an ABG on admission in high-level cervical SCI patients. If the patient is on a ventilator, obtaining the initial partial pressure of carbon dioxide in the blood (pCO_2) while simultaneously obtaining an end-tidal CO_2 level, allows the calculation of the alveolar-arterial CO_2 gradient. This may be important in adjusting the amount of dead space, or the respiratory rate, if the patient is on a ventilator. Blood gases, however, are expensive and invasive. Monitoring the end-tidal CO_2 level and oximetry (O_2 saturation) allows for the delivery of effective care, without drawing multiple ABG measurements. An ABG should subsequently be obtained if the clinical status of the patient changes and when changes are initially made in the ventilator settings. Usually, if the oximetry and end-tidal CO_2 are followed, only a few ABG measurements are needed during the care of the SCI patient on the ventilator.

Pulmonary Function Tests

It would be preferable to have PFTs in all patients, but this is not practical. A substitute for a formal PFT is to follow the spontaneous VC, the FEV_1, and the negative inspiratory force. Following these parameters is useful in assessing the status of the patient and monitoring the progress of the patient over time and can be performed at the bedside (21,44). Of these parameters, the VC is the most useful to measure and follow for an indication of the course of the patient (45,46). The VC can be used to determine the patient's ability to breathe deeply, to develop an effective cough, and to clear secretions (45,46). An easily transportable, handheld device can measure the VC. VC was found to be significantly correlated with FEV_1, inspiratory capacity, ERV, FRC, residual volume, and total lung capacity, although not with maximum positive expiratory pressure nor with maximum negative inspiratory pressure (24). The lack of correlation with these pressures may reflect that these are pressure measurements, whereas the VC and all other PFTs are volumetric in nature. Sometimes, the VC deteriorates because of secretions, or increasing atelectasis, which is a clue to the need for a chest x-ray or ventilatory assistance.

Computed Tomography

CT scans are not required as part of the initial pulmonary workup but may be helpful in clarifying areas of atelectasis or pleural effusions that occur behind the heart or diaphragm. CT scans have very little use in helping determine whether the patient has a trapped lung.

Fluoroscopy

Frequently, patients with C3 or C4 levels of injury have one lower lobe that is difficult to expand, or to keep expanded, when being weaned from the ventilator. This may be because one diaphragm is paralyzed. This works in effect like a flail chest, where the stronger diaphragm works well enough to keep one lung expanded, whereas the weaker diaphragm cannot keep the opposite lung expanded. Fluoroscopy of the diaphragm may be very useful in determining this situation.

Peak Expiratory Flow

Weakness of the abdominal muscles impairs the ability to cough. Peak cough flow is decreased (the average value in tetraplegic patients is 220 L/min, whereas in non-SCI subjects, it is 300 to 700 L/min), with the decrease varying with the level of injury (LOI) (47,48). This is an extremely important parameter to measure and has been correlated with the ability to decannulate a patient from the ventilator (49).

TREATMENT OPTIONS

Acute management in the initial hours after SCI is focused on securing an airway and providing adequate ventilatory support while preventing secretions and aspiration. Close monitoring (by measuring VC at least every 8 hours as well as oximetry) for ventilatory worsening is crucial. After the initial days of injury, close monitoring should be maintained because the immobilization of the SCI patient may predispose the patient to development of atelectasis.

The weakness of the SCI patient, as described previously, makes it difficult to keep the lungs inflated, with an inability to take a deep breath. This, in association with the difficulty in clearing secretions, makes them susceptible to atelectasis, accelerating a cascade of events that may lead to pneumonia. Many of the treatment options that follow are appropriate for the patient whether on or off the ventilator. Aggressive respiratory management has been shown to reduce pulmonary-related morbidity and mortality (49,50).

Postural Drainage and Beds

There is little information regarding the use of rotating beds as an intervention to prevent or treat pulmonary complications. Their use may decrease the risk for complications and the length of intensive care unit stay; however, their exact mechanism of action (i.e., improving mobilization of secretions or by decreasing atelectasis) is not known (51,52). Rotating beds, however, should be part of an aggressive prevention program for the acute SCI patient.

Chest Physiotherapy

Chest clapping, percussion, and vibration, either with a mechanical vibrator or by hand, may be used to loosen the secretions and may help drain lobes that have secretions in them. Positioning the patient so that the involved lung area is in a superior position allows gravity to help it drain. Frequently, however, in the acute SCI patient, the presence of a halo vest, the location of the patient's injury, pain, or blood pressure alterations limit the use of chest physiotherapy if the patient is placed in the Trendelenburg position. Some beds come with automatic turning and vibration settings that can be helpful in patients for whom positioning for treatments is a problem.

Suctioning

Suctioning may be a torturing procedure for the patient. However, it may be useful in the tetraplegic patient with a lot of secretions, if other types of secretion management are not used (i.e. mechanical insufflation-exsufflation [MI-E]). Several decisions related to suctioning need to be made, including the choice of a system—one that does not break the integrity of the ventilator tubing versus one that does break the integrity of the ventilator tubing system. Not breaking the integrity of the ventilator tubing system should lead to fewer infections. However, in this case, the suction catheters are stiff and potentially more damaging to the trachea. One may choose, however, to use red rubber catheters, which are softer and less damaging to the trachea, but these interrupt the integrity of the ventilator tubing system.

Another choice is whether to use sterile or clean technique. Sterile technique means a new suction catheter with every suctioning, whereas a clean technique involves storing a red rubber catheter in solution and using non-sterile (but clean) gloves. The choices depend on the situation of the patient. If the patient is being weaned from the ventilator, using a Passey-Muir valve, or a "trach talk," the ventilator tubing system is being interrupted for the weaning. If the patient is using this method of weaning, it makes sense to use clean suctioning with a red rubber catheter. It may also be helpful to use catheters with a curved tip, to direct the suction catheter into the affected lung, if there is atelectasis. However, clearing the lung of atelectasis and secretions depends more on delivering a deep breath than on the directing tip on the catheter.

Assisted Cough

Methods to assist the cough include manual pressure (*quad coughing*) applied to the abdomen timed with the patient's cough effort, positive-pressure insufflation, and electrical stimulation to the abdominal muscles.

The technique of quad coughing, a type of assisted cough, involves a forceful push on the upper abdomen at the end of a deep inspiration (Fig. 9.4). Quad coughing tries to mimic a true cough by helping to mobilize secretions from the lower portions of the lungs because these patients lack the strength of the abdominal and lower intercostal muscles to do so. The clinician's open hands are placed with the palms down below the patient's rib cage, between the xiphoid process and the umbilicus. After a deep breath is taken by the patient, or given through the

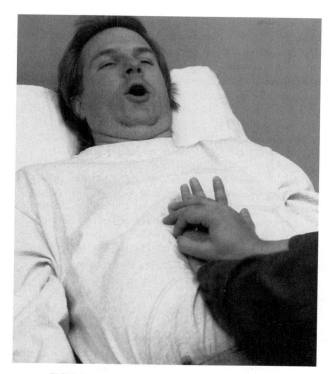

FIGURE 9.4. Picture of assisted cough technique.

ventilator or Ambu bag, the clinician pushes upward and inward as the patient coughs. This technique is similar to an abdominal thrust in the Heimlich maneuver. Contraindications include fractured ribs, chest trauma, and abdominal complications. There are reports in the literature of displacement of an inferior vena cava filter in the case of cardiac arrest, with cardiac compressions being used. It would probably be best not to use quad coughing in patients who have a new inferior vena cava filter placed.

Although the use of the abdominal binder or corset has shown little improvement (2% to 7%) in peak cough flow, manual assistive cough has shown a larger improvement (15% to 33%) (53–55). Electrical stimulation to the abdominal muscles may also help; however, all patients may not respond to or tolerate this (53,55). The use of oral positive pressure in combination with manual assistance improves peak cough flow as well (54).

Mechanical Insufflation-Exsufflation

The MI-E delivers a deep insufflation (positive pressure) to the airway that is immediately followed by an exsufflation (negative pressure). The rapid shift in pressure produces a high expiratory flow rate from the lungs, simulating a cough. Usual insufflation-exsufflation pressures are $+40$ to -40 cm H_2O, and these pressures generate about 10 L/sec of expiratory flow. An abdominal thrust may be applied during the mechanical exsufflation, increasing effective cough flows (56). This method can be used either through tracheostomy, facemask, or mouthpiece and has been shown to be effective in clearing secretions, while producing no macroscopic tissue damage (57).

MI-E is especially useful in patients using noninvasive ventilatory support because suctioning may be difficult without a tracheostomy tube. Bach observed an increase in VC, peak cough expiratory flow, and oxygen saturation after MI-E in patients with SCI, postpoliomyelitis, and muscular dystrophy (56). A survey of a group of SCI patients who had experience with both endotracheal suctioning and MI-E through tracheostomy found that MI-E was significantly less irritating, painful, tiring, and uncomfortable than endotracheal suctioning, with the patients overwhelmingly preferring MI-E to suctioning (58). MI-E has also been shown to have a high patient satisfaction rate in other populations (59–62).

The MI-E has a manual cycling feature that facilitates caregiver–patient coordination of inspiration and expiration with insufflation and exsufflation. One treatment consists of about 5 cycles of MI-E followed by a brief rest for assisted ventilation as needed for 20 to 30 seconds to avoid hyperventilation. Treatments may be repeated as needed to clear secretions. MI-E has effectively been used by patients to clear airways in chronic SCI during episodes of chest colds (56).

Indications for use include an inability to cough or clear secretions effectively because of a reduced peak cough expiratory flow (less than 5 to 6 L/sec). Contraindications include a history of bullous emphysema, susceptibility to pneumothorax or pneumomediastinum, and recent barotrauma. For the patient with acute high-level tetraplegia in spinal shock, severe bradyarrhythmias, including complete heart block, can occur, similar to suctioning.

The advantages of MI-E over other modalities include the ability to clear secretions better; MI-E can clear both lung fields and can clear out larger mucous plugs than can the suction catheter. Because the left main-stem bronchus branches off at an angle, the suction catheter has difficulty clearing secretions from this side. In addition, the limiting factor in suctioning large mucous plugs is the diameter of the suction catheter, whereas with MI-E, the limiting factor is the size of the tracheostomy, if present.

Intermittent Positive-pressure Breathing or Intermittent Positive-pressure Ventilation ''Stretch''

With this technique, an intermittent positive-pressure breathing (IPPB) machine is used to deliver large volumes to the patient. With IPPB "stretch," an IPPB treatment is started at a low pressure that the patient can tolerate, perhaps 15 cm H_2O of pressure, and as the treatment proceeds, the pressure is increased to as high a pressure as the patient can tolerate, up to 40 cm H_2O. An alternative to IPPB is nebulizer treatments. Inhaled medications, such as albuterol, cromolyn, and ipratropium, can be delivered to the patient with either nebulizer without pressure or with IPPB. Because the positive pressure is useful in expanding areas of atelectasis, using a nebulizer without positive pressure may not be as effective in expanding the patient's lungs as IPPB stretch.

Bilevel Positive Airway Pressure and Continuous Positive Airway Pressure

Bilevel positive airway pressure (BiPAP) and continuous positive airway pressure (CPAP) can be used with patients who do not have an endotracheal or tracheostomy tube or can be used with cuffed or uncuffed tracheostomy tubes. Patients can be placed on these machines, with settings starting at 5 to 8 cm H_2O for the CPAP and going as high as the patient can tolerate. When using BiPAP on a patient with a cuffed tracheostomy tube, the I-PAP can be set as high as tolerated, starting with lower pressures and working up to as high a pressure as 40 cm H_2O. The E-PAP can be set at 5 to 8 cm H_2O. The patient's chest x-ray film should be monitored to ascertain whether the desired effect of preventing or expanding atelectasis is being accomplished. Appropriate adjustments may need to be made in the pressures to accomplish the desired goals. Higher levels of pressure delivers higher volumes and helps with the prevention and treatment of atelectasis.

Intrapulmonary Percussive Ventilation

The intrapulmonary percussive ventilator delivers vibrations (200 cycles/min) inside the lungs with deep penetration of medications. A constant pressure is maintained to keep the airway open. The purpose is to help loosen secretions while the patient is receiving a deep breath. The procedure can be performed either through a tracheostomy tube, by mouth, or with a facemask. A variation on this is a flutter valve, which is used with an IPPB machine or a nebulizer.

Positioning of the Patient

Patients with cervical and high thoracic level SCI have a reduction in VC of about half (42% to 65%) in the sitting position as compared with the supine position (26,28,63,64). The VC improves in the supine position because of the relative placement of the diaphragm into the chest, resulting in improvement in the length-to-tension relation and in diaphragmatic function.

The reduction in VC associated with changing positions from supine to sitting is clinically important because it may lead to the inability to take a deep breath in the sitting position. This may result in a rapid shallow breathing pattern that can cause microatelectasis and decreased pulmonary compliance. Because of these factors, it is better for the patient who is initially weaning from the ventilator to do so in the supine position. This is in contrast to the desired position for most other patients who are weaning from a ventilator. Only after the patient has developed some tolerance for weaning should the weaning be performed in the wheelchair.

In patients with central cord syndrome, there may be preservation of the intercostal innervation but paralysis of the diaphragm. This can be determined by watching the patient breathe. If the chest is moving outward on inspiration, but the abdominal contents are not moving outward, that patient probably has intercostal innervation but paralysis of the diaphragm. This can be confirmed by fluoroscopy of the diaphragm. In these patients, there is a mechanical advantage for breathing when the head is elevated. This is because the air moves into the lungs when the ribs move up and out. A paralyzed diaphragm, which

is in a high position, will take up room that could be used for air. Therefore, these patients do better without a binder when in the wheelchair. When asleep in bed, it would be better for them to have the head of the bed elevated. Some patients with this problem have been observed to retain CO_2 when flat in bed but not when they have the head of the bed elevated.

Abdominal Binder

The loss of VC in the upright position may be partially corrected by the use of an abdominal binder or corset (64,65). When lying flat in bed, the abdominal contents tend to push up on the diaphragm. When this happens, the diaphragm starts in a position of mechanical advantage for the patient. The higher the diaphragm is at the end of expiration, the better the position for obtaining a deep breath. When the patient is up in the wheelchair, the abdominal contents are pulled caudally by gravity, and because of the lack of abdominal muscle tone in the acute tetraplegic patient, the tendency is for the abdominal contents to fall forward. This applies suction on the diaphragm, pulling it downward, and the patient thus starts an inhalation with the diaphragm already in a position of partial inhalation. Applying an abdominal binder forces the abdominal contents inward, pushing up on the diaphragm and thus allowing for a better position of the diaphragm for inhalation to proceed when sitting. Estenne and DeTroyer also found that the use of an abdominal binder eliminated the increase in residual volume that occurred when patients assume the seated position from the supine position (64).

Incentive Spirometry and Resistive Devices

Several training techniques may be used to improve respiratory function actively in tetraplegia. Exercises include inspiratory resistance muscle training, abdominal weights, and incentive spirometry and have been shown to improve pulmonary function by strengthening and improving the endurance of the diaphragm and accessory respiratory muscles (50,66–70).

Incentive spirometry is a technique that encourages the patient to inhale as deeply as possible. The purpose is to prevent or treat atelectasis. Using the spirometer also allows patients to see their progress. Resistive devices, through which the patient breathes, can be adjusted to make it harder for the patient to breathe in and are used to help strengthen the inspiratory muscles. Although the concept is for the patient to become stronger and better able to take a deep breath, there is question about the value of this device (68,71). Bach and Wang note that the VC of tetraplegic patients tends to improve without intervention and that the improvement seen in studies of resistive devices may actually reflect the normal healing process (72). Weights placed on the abdomen to help improve the strength of the muscles of respiration have a similar concept. Liaw and colleagues found that improvement in pulmonary parameters, including total lung capacity, VC, minute ventilation, FEV_1, and the resting Borg scale showed greater improvement with a resistive inspiratory muscle training program (73). Other studies have found similar results (74–77).

Glossopharyngeal Breathing

Glossopharyngeal breathing (GPB) is a technique that involves rapidly taking small gulps, six to nine gulps of 60 to 200 mL each, using the tongue and pharyngeal muscles to project the air past the glottis into the lungs. It is a useful technique even in patients who have no diaphragmatic strength; however, it requires an intact midbrain to be successful. Many patients can learn to use this technique to augment VC to assist with coughing or prolong ventilator-free time for patients with minimal spontaneous VC, if the patient does not have an inflated cuff on the tracheostomy tube (78). As an exercise, GPB can also increase the VC, which allows for assistance in cough, improvement in audibility of the patient's voice, and ventilator-free time in patients with otherwise minimal VC (79,80).

Bronchoscopy

Bronchoscopy can be helpful in removing secretions but should be performed in association with accompanying attempts to inflate the lung that contains the secretions. Without inflating the lung by using one of the previously listed techniques (or by using the ventilator), the secretions will reaccumulate, and the patient will have obstructing secretions that will require removal by bronchoscopy repeatedly. If repeated bronchoscopies are required, consideration should be given to using one of the treatment modalities outlined previously, or larger ventilator volumes if the patient is on a ventilator. If the lung is expanded, the tendency for secretions to form is reduced.

Types of Tracheostomy Tubes

The choice of tracheostomy tube is important. Although a comprehensive discussion is beyond the scope of this chapter, a few points should be noted. It is easier for the patient to wean from the ventilator the larger the inner diameter of the tracheostomy tube. It is often suggested that a tube with an inner cannula should be used, but that is probably not necessary, and the inner cannula reduces the inner diameter. It is better if the patient is weaned using a Passey-Muir valve or a trach talk, and if this method of weaning is used, the larger the inner diameter, the less the resistance to airflow. The less the resistance, the easier it will be to wean.

One decision will be whether to use a tracheostomy tube with fenestration and an inner cannula, which can be removed. A caution about this type of tube is that it can be a source of damage to the posterior portion of the trachea, if, on suctioning, there is mucosa suctioned into the lumen of the tracheostomy and the suction catheter damages that mucosa. A better choice would be to deflate the cuff on the tube and allow air to escape around the deflated cuff and out the patient's mouth. This will allow speech, without the danger of damage to the mucosa of the posterior trachea at the level of fenestration. There is a higher risk for aspiration if the patient is unable to swallow and the cuff is deflated. The air in the cuff can be gradually deflated. When the cuff can be deflated around the clock, a cuffless tube may be inserted.

There are choices between plastic and metal cuffless tracheostomy tubes. It is always desirable to have as few secretions as possible, and the metal tracheostomy tubes (Jackson tracheos-tomy tubes) appear to stimulate fewer secretions than the plastic tubes.

Medications

Because mobilizing secretions is a problem in the early post-injury stage, *mucolytics* are frequently indicated. Guaifenesin is commonly used and generally well tolerated. Saturated solution of potassium iodide (SSKI) may be helpful in patients who can tolerate it. The patient's ability to swallow and the need for a feeding tube may limit use of these.

Acetylcysteine (Mucomyst). This mucolytic can be nebulized into the lungs. If the patient has a tracheostomy or endotracheal tube, the acetylcysteine can be diluted with saline and shot down the tube from a syringe. Acetylcysteine breaks up the mucus, making it more liquid and therefore easier to be suctioned or coughed out. This is especially helpful in those patients who seem to form secretions that are very tenacious. A drawback of acetylcysteine is that it tastes like rotten eggs. It can be given in a nebulizer treatment, along with other medications (i.e., Proventil). Acetylcysteine may cause bronchospasm, especially if nebulized.

Theophylline. This agent relaxes smooth muscle and is therefore helpful in patients who have bronchospasm. In addition, it stimulates the medullary respiratory centers. Theophylline can improve diaphragmatic contractility, can reduce diaphragmatic fatigue, and is one of the few medications that stimulates the release of surfactant (81,82). However, theophylline medications have potentially deleterious effects, including arrhythmia, nausea, and seizures. Theophylline preparations should not be used in patients with the potential for arrhythmia, in patients with a history of seizures, or in patients who have a concomitant head injury.

Antibiotics. Appropriate antibiotics for identified respiratory infections are a frequent necessity. They need to be individualized for the patient. Prophylactic antibiotics are not recommended.

Inhaled medications. Patients with tetraplegia have unopposed parasympathetic innervation and, therefore, may benefit from the administration of both short acting and long acting β-agonist inhaled medications. Cromolyn and nedocromil may be beneficial antiinflammatory medications, but the benefit of these medications for SCI patients is not established. Inhaled steroids should be avoided, because of the propensity for these patients to develop respiratory infections. Many physicians use ipratropium because theoretically it would help block the effect of the parasympathetic stimulation. However, it is important to preserve the integrity of the surfactant in the patient's lungs, and atropine, which is similar to ipratropium, blocks the production of surfactant (82–84). As reported in the Duke Center study of the literature of respiratory issues in SCI, ipratropium may not be effective in blocking bronchospasm in SCI patients (12). More studies need to be done to determine whether ipratropium is beneficial or harmful in tetraplegic patients.

There is good reason to use both long acting (salmeterol) and short-acting β-agonists (albuterol and others). They act to offset the unopposed parasympathetic stimulation found in tetraplegic patients. They also reduce inflammation and stimulate the secretion of surfactant. One possible way to use these medications is to use salmeterol as 2 puffs twice daily, delivered through the ventilator tubing or using a spacer device in patients who are not on a ventilator. The short-acting β-agonists can be delivered as a nebulizer or by metered dose inhalers through the ventilator tubing or with a spacer device if the patient cannot coordinate with the puffs of a metered dose inhaler. This can be done every 4 hours as needed, around the clock, with gradual tapering as the patient improves. If needed, the short acting β-agonists can be delivered every hour, depending on the response of the patient's heart rate to this high dosage.

Asthma and Obstructive Lung Disease

Individuals with a premorbid history of obstructive airway disease present special problems. In concept, these patients may have hyperexpanded lungs, and the hyperexpansion should prevent atelectasis. The disadvantage with hyperexpanded lungs, however, is that the diaphragm will be lower because of air trapping, and the lungs will have high residual volumes. Thus, there is less lung volume available for exchange of air. Because high tetraplegic patients rely so much on the diaphragm, hyperexpanded lungs place the patient at a disadvantage.

The choices for treatment of bronchospasm or hyperexpanded lungs would include theophyllines, mucolytics, and leukotriene inhibitors. In selected patients, the leukotriene inhibitors can be helpful in relieving inflammation and reducing air trapping, thereby making it easier for the patient to breathe and wean from the ventilator. The decision to use inhaled steroids, to reduce the work of breathing, would need to be individualized for the patient. Because of the risk for respiratory infections in these patients, inhaled steroids should probably be avoided. Short-acting β-agonists can be helpful in patients with bronchospasm, and *in vitro*, they are also antiinflammatory (85). Long-acting β-agonists may be helpful for the same reasons.

Dairy Products

Some patients respond to dairy products by forming secretions. Therefore, in the patient with copious secretions, it may be helpful to limit dairy products until the patient is able to handle secretions easily.

RESPIRATORY FAILURE

Numerous studies suggest that higher-level cervical injuries (C5 and above) are almost twice as likely to require mechanical ventilator assistance as those are with lower cervical injuries (below C5) (1,32,86,87). Claxton and colleagues found that two thirds of patients with C5 or higher level of injury required mechanical ventilation, compared with only 39% with lower-level cervical injuries (86). Furthermore, patients with complete injuries are more likely than those with incomplete injuries to require mechanical ventilation. The amount of secretions and pneumonia is also associated with the need for mechanical ventilation. These findings reinforce the potential for treatments aimed at improving ventilation, cough, and secretion clearance to reduce the need for mechanical ventilation.

Criteria for intubation include the following: (a) intractable atelectasis that has not responded to conservative efforts to expand the lung; (b) hypoxemia or hypercapnia not responsive to conservative measures such as CPAP or BiPAP; (c) rapid shallow breathing, persistent tachycardia, fever related to unresponsive pneumonia, hypotension, or hypertension; and (d) noninvasive ventilation is not adequate or unavailable.

If the patient requires intubation, it is usually best to proceed with a tracheostomy if noninvasive means of ventilation are not an option. Advantages of the tracheostomy tube over the endotracheal tube include less chance of damage to the vocal cords; easier to clear secretions through a suction catheter or MI-E; ability to deflate the tracheostomy tube cuff to allow speech; and ability of the patient to eat, if swallowing problems do not prohibit this.

In the acute phase of injury, the patient may require fluid resuscitation to maintain the blood pressure. This, however, can lead to fluid overload of the lungs, reducing the oxygen transport from the alveoli to the pulmonary capillaries. The fluid will also reduce the lung compliance and the VC. Judicious use of fluid with pressor agents to maintain the blood pressure is important to diminish the chances of pulmonary edema. One of the most important aspects to caring for patients after SCI is to remember that unless they have premorbid lung disease, their lungs are healthy. One should not treat the oxygen saturation number on the pulse oximeter with oxygen alone, but rather should also treat the underlying cause.

Invasive versus Noninvasive Ventilation

It is better for the patient to avoid initial intubation and mechanical ventilation if this is possible. Patients with C2 levels of injury and higher are usually intubated, unless their first contact is with a medical center that has expertise in noninvasive ventilation. Without such expertise, it is more prudent to intubate these patients immediately. Patients with brain-stem injury usually do not have control of swallowing or tongue movement. These patients are especially prone to aspiration and should be intubated immediately.

A concern about noninvasive ventilation is the potential for emesis and aspiration. Aspiration increases the patient's chance for ARDS. The propensity for emesis may be aggravated if the noninvasive ventilation causes gastric distention. In addition, acutely after SCI, in the period of spinal shock, with the patient immobilized in bed, the stomach may empty slowly. If the patient is being fed while flat in bed, the risk for reflux or emesis and aspiration is increased. Older patients, as well as those with diabetic gastric atony, may be more prone to these problems. A cuffed endotracheal tube or tracheostomy tube may protect the patient from aspiration of gastric contents.

If these problems are considered and thought to be unlikely, then noninvasive ventilation is an option. The benefits of noninvasive ventilation include a decreased risk for infection as the presence of a foreign body in the patient's trachea is avoided, lower risk for hospital-associated pneumonia, and greater discharge to home. Bach and colleagues studied patients with tetraplegia on home ventilation and found that the incidence of pneumonia was lower in patients with noninvasive ventilation than in those with tracheostomy tubes (88). In addition, the hospitalization rate for patients receiving noninvasive ventilation was lower. This article suggested that noninvasive positive-pressure ventilation (NIPPV) may reduce the risk for pneumonia compared with tracheostomy for patients requiring chronic ventilatory support.

NIPPV can be delivered through oral, nasal, or oronasal interfaces. Oral interfaces can be attached to a wheelchair while the patient is sitting, or kept in the mouth, and can be used for full-time ventilation (89). Nasal interfaces can be used if the mouthpiece is not effective and at night (90).

Mechanical Ventilation

Patients requiring mechanical ventilation have a high mortality rate. The 1-year survival rate for patients identified on day of injury was about half of the 1-year survival for the total admissions to the Model Systems facility (25.4% versus 49.7%) (35). However, for patients who survived the first year on the ventilator, the 15-year survival rate was reported to be 61.4% (35). There has also been a marked improvement in survival since the 1970s, with patients injured since 1986 having a 91% lower mortality rate than patients injured between 1973 and 1979. Respiratory conditions, however, account for almost 50% of deaths among ventilator-dependent patients with SCI.

If the patient requires mechanical ventilation, perhaps the most important piece of information for the physician to know is the patient's height. Patients who are lying in bed may all appear to be 5'9″ tall, even if they are 6'5″. Therefore, very tall patients are apt to be ventilated with low tidal volumes, leading to atelectasis and carbon dioxide retention.

If ventilation is required, the patient should be started on the ventilator at a tidal volume of 12 to 15 mL/kg of IBW, with the volume adjusted upward according to the increasing tidal volume protocol included in Table 9.1. The plan, do, check (or study), and act (PDCA) cycle (Fig. 9.5) should be used to follow the progress of the patient. Sometimes, use of the PDCA cycle allows the physician to notice that the ventilator tidal volume is not adequate to keep the patient from developing atelectasis.

Protocol for Ventilation

In young patients affected by traumatic SCI, there is limited published data regarding ventilation and weaning techniques. The study that comes the closest to a matched controlled sample is a retrospective study of patients in which a protocol that gradually increased the tidal volume on the ventilator was compared with patients who were managed by conventional methods, within the same hospital setting (18). The higher tidal volume protocol resulted in faster clearing of atelectasis and in a 3-week shorter time on the ventilator for patients with C3 or C4 level injury.

If the patient develops atelectasis before going on the ventilator, this reflects the condition of weakness resulting from the SCI. Atelectasis, in many cases of tetraplegia, is an iatrogenic complication of ventilation (18,91). If the patient enters the hospital with clear lungs and, after being on the ventilator, develops atelectasis, this is because of the ventilator settings. Physi-

TABLE 9.1. RECOMMENDED PROTOCOL FOR VENTILATION OF PATIENTS WITH HIGH TETRAPLEGIA

I. Upon admission:
   1. Obtain patient's height and calculate ideal body weight (IBW)
      a. Male, 130 lb at 5 feet tall +5 lb per inch above 5 feet (change to kg) = kg IBW.
      b. Female, 115 lb at 5 feet +5 lb per inch above 5 feet (change to kg) = kg IBW.
   2. Place patient on ventilator.
      a. Mode—assist/control (A/C) or controlled mandatory ventilation (CMV)
      b. Tidal volume (TV)—set at 12–15 mL/kg IBW, or as per setting at previous hospital (if patient is transferred from another hospital)
      c. Respiratory rate, 12. Can decrease as TV is increased.
      d. Sigh—300–500 mL greater than the TV with rate of 8 times per hour, two sighs each sigh cycle.
      e. Flow rate—70 L/min
      f. Titrate oxygen to saturation greater than 92%.
      g. Positive end-expiratory pressure—zero, or same as previous hospital setting
      h. Dead space—heat and moisture exchanger (HME) of up to "14 inches"
      i. Obtain chest x-ray, patient's spontaneous vital capacity, and arterial blood gas after 1 hr on the ventilator.

II. Day 2 and thereafter:
   1. The patient is evaluated daily for the following steps in the protocol:
      a. If the peak pressure is under 40 cm H_2O, then tidal volume is increased by 100 mL/d. If the patient is less than 5 feet, 6 inches tall, the TV is increased by 50 mL/d.
      b. If the peak pressure is still less than 40 cm H_2O, after the increase in TV, then peak flow is increased by 10 L/min per day. Note that if the patient is less than 5 feet, 6 inches tall, the peak flow is increased by 5 L/min per day.
      c. Titrate fiO_2 to maintain oxygen saturation greater than 92%.
      d. Maintain end tidal pCO_2 (using capnograph) at 28–35 mm Hg, by adding or subtracting appropriate dead space.

III. Limits to be used with the ventilator protocol:
   1. Peak pressures not to exceed 40 cm H_2O.
      a. If peak pressure increases above 40 cm H_2O with a TV or peak flow change, return to previous settings.
      b. If the peak pressure measures more than 40 cm H_2O, decrease TV by 100 mL, then peak flow by 10 L/min until pressures remain below 40 cm H_2O. Then draw arterial blood gases.
   2. TV and flow rate limits:
      a. Increase TV until patient is afebrile and has minimal secretions, and chest x-ray film is clear.
      b. Maximum TV of 25 mL/kg IBW.
      c. Peak flow should not exceed 120 L/min.

cians tend to ventilate all patients with low tidal volumes, because of the literature regarding complications of large tidal volumes and high ventilation pressures. However, if the patient is given a deep breath on the ventilator, air will move past the mucus. The SCI patient is not able to generate an effective cough, especially if they are on a ventilator. If large ventilator tidal volumes are used, there will be air in the peripheral portions of the lung when the inspiration ends. With the end of inspiration, the abdominal contents, which have been pushed outward by the ventilator breath, fall back, pushing on the diaphragm and lower lung. The lower ribs also move in because of tissue

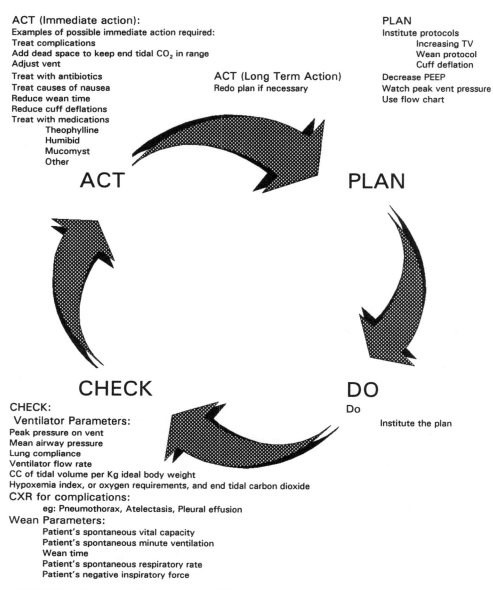

ACT (Immediate action):
Examples of possible immediate action required:
Treat complications
Add dead space to keep end tidal CO₂ in range
Adjust vent
Treat with antibiotics
Treat causes of nausea
Reduce wean time
Reduce cuff deflations
Treat with medications
   Theophylline
   Humibid
   Mucomyst
   Other

ACT (Long Term Action)
Redo plan if necessary

PLAN
Institute protocols
   Increasing TV
   Wean protocol
   Cuff deflation
Decrease PEEP
Watch peak vent pressure
Use flow chart

ACT

PLAN

CHECK

DO

CHECK:
  Ventilator Parameters:
Peak pressure on vent
Mean airway pressure
Lung compliance
Ventilator flow rate
CC of tidal volume per Kg ideal body weight
Hypoxemia index, or oxygen requirements, and end tidal carbon dioxide
  CXR for complications:
     eg: Pneumothorax, Atelectasis, Pleural effusion
Wean Parameters:
    Patient's spontaneous vital capacity
    Patient's spontaneous minute ventilation
    Wean time
    Patient's spontaneous respiratory rate
    Patient's negative inspiratory force

Do
Institute the plan

FIGURE 9.5. This chart is the plan, do, check (or study), and act (PDCA) cycle showing what items the caregivers should monitor as the plan is implemented. It is meant to be a rapid resource for the reference of the caregivers.

elasticity. The bronchi become smaller in diameter, and the air below the mucus exerts a force on the mucus, albeit lower than physiologic, pushing the mucus up toward the tracheostomy opening. If the problem is mucus and collapse of normal lungs, and if the lung tissue is not diseased, the lungs should be able to withstand pressures of up to 40 cm H_2O as measured at the tracheostomy. In the ventilated patient, there is a loss of about 5 to 10 cm H_2O pressure going through the tracheostomy tube and loss of still more pressure before the air gets to the visceral pleura. By the time the air–oxygen mixture gets to the visceral pleura, the pressure exerted is considerably lower than the pressure measured at the tracheostomy. With high flows and large ventilator tidal volumes, the pressure measured at the tracheostomy is higher for smaller tracheostomy tubes than for larger

tubes. There is more loss of pressure going through a small tracheostomy tube than through a large tube. The opening pressure at the alveolus (to open a closed alveolus) in patients with atelectasis is about 10 to 12 cm H_2O, and the pressure to keep the alveolus open is about 4 cm (91). In theory, to keep the lungs from developing atelectasis, the pressure measured at the tracheostomy needs to be high enough to generate these pressures at the alveolus. However, there are risk-to-benefit ratios that must be considered in the case of SCI patients, who either have atelectasis or have the risk for atelectasis. A consideration of the various risks and benefits of low ventilator tidal volumes, as compared with higher ventilator tidal volumes, is described in Table 9.2.

There are risks in expanding the atelectatic lung (92,93).

TABLE 9.2. COMPARISON OF HIGH AND LOW VENTILATOR TIDAL VOLUMES

Complication	Low Ventilator Tidal Volumes	High Ventilator Tidal Volumes
Atelectasis	Greater risk	Lower risk
Time to wean	Longer time	Shorter time
Pneumothorax	Less risk	More risk
Pneumonia	Greater risk	Less risk
Pleural effusion	Greater risk	Less risk
Empyema	Greater risk	Less risk
Trapped lung	Greater risk	Less risk
Decortication	Greater risk	Less risk

Frequently, the atelectatic lung is infected. Because the patient lacks the ability to cough, if the lung is expanded by the use of the ventilator, bacteria may be spread throughout the remaining lung, causing extensive pneumonia. There can also be reperfusion and reexpansion pulmonary edema with the sudden expansion of atelectatic lung. It is important to remember that atelectatic lung does not produce any surfactant (94). Without surfactant lining the alveoli, the lung may be more prone to injury. Therefore, a strategy needs to be devised that allows expansion of the lung, while trying to improve the presence of surfactant in the lung that has been atelectatic.

Factors to consider, therefore, include the following:

1. Is the atelectatic lung infected? If so, careful monitoring regarding the need for antibiotics should be undertaken.
2. Is the patient receiving adequate nutrition to make surfactant? Surfactant production decreases after just 3 days of starvation (95). Surfactant is a fat, and it may be that fats should be given to the patient, especially if the patient is malnourished. The desirability of this, however, is not established.
3. Because the only physiologic stimulus to the release of surfactant from the type II alveolar cells is stretching the cells, it is best to inflate the atelectatic areas slowly, rather than suddenly (83).

Case report #2

TJC, a 19-year-old man with a C4 level of injury, was injured as a result of a gunshot wound. His injury occurred on 7/28/94. At initial hospitalization, the patient was treated for 34 days. His chest x-ray film showed atelectasis at the left base, with a silhouette sign of the left hemidiaphragm (Fig. 9.6). During the initial hospitalization, he was treated with a ventilator tidal volume of 600 mL and was being weaned by SIMV and pressure support. His height is 5'7"; the IBW for that height is 73 kg. Therefore, he was being ventilated at 8.2 mL/kg IBW. The patient was transferred to a tertiary care facility on 8/30/94. The question that arises is whether the atelectasis and slow progress with weaning were caused by the low ventilator tidal volume and weaning with SIMV. On arrival at the tertiary hospital, TJC was treated with the increasing tidal volume protocol and weaned by progressive ventilator-free breathing (PVFB). The chest x-ray film showed no atelectasis with ventilator tidal volume slowly increased to 1,900 mL, or 26 mL/kg IBW (Fig. 9.7).

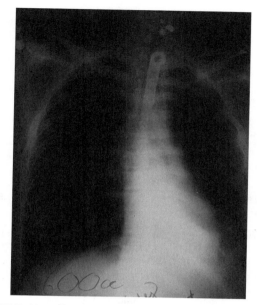

FIGURE 9.6. X-ray film. There is atelectasis, with retrocardiac density, and "sillouette" sign of the left hemidiaphragm, with low ventilator tidal volumes.

Figure 9.8 shows that as the tidal volume is increased, the peak inspiratory pressure on the ventilator rises very little. The lung compliance improved from 30 to 56 mL/cm. The patient's spontaneous VC improved from 550 mL on admission to 1,700 mL from day 1 to day 8. The patient was weaned from the ventilator in 18 days.

This patient represents a subject who serves as his own control. On low tidal volumes, he had atelectasis and was unable to wean from the ventilator. With larger tidal volumes, his lung compliance and spontaneous VC improved as the ventilator tidal

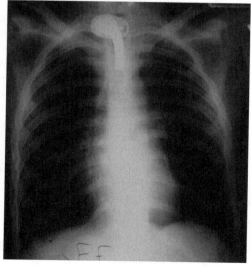

FIGURE 9.7. X-ray film. The lungs are clear, after slow increase in the ventilator tidal volumes.

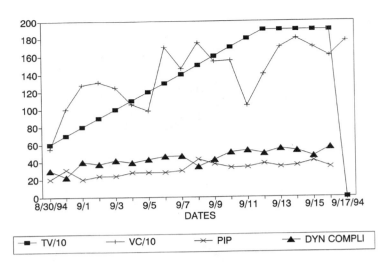

FIGURE 9.8. Chart showing the improvement in vital capacity (*VC*) of the patient as the ventilator tidal volume (*TV*) is increased. It also shows improvement in the dynamic compliance (*dyn compli*) of the lung. There is little increase in peak inspiratory pressure (*PIP*) as the tidal volume is gradually increased. The ventilator tidal volume and vital capacity have been divided by 10. This patient was subsequently removed from the ventilator.

volume was slowly increased. Figure 9.8 suggests that up to a certain point (depending on the spinal level of injury), the tidal volume used on the ventilator inflates the lung so that the patient has available a larger capacity for generating a VC. If the individual is provided with a more expanded lung with which to breathe, he uses that amount of lung to improve his VC. This patient was on the ventilator at low ventilator tidal volumes for 34 days, without weaning from the ventilator. With a ventilator tidal volume of 600 mL, his spontaneous VC was 550 mL. On larger ventilator tidal volumes, the atelectasis resolved, secretions diminished, and the positive inspiratory pressure increased very little because compliance improved, and the patient was totally weaned from the ventilator in 18 days. With a ventilator tidal volume of 1,900 mL, the patient's spontaneous VC improved to 1,700 mL.

Positive End-expiratory Pressure

Current practice is to almost always use positive end-expiratory pressure when ventilating patients. However, there are reasons for not using PEEP in patients with SCI. First, there is evidence that PEEP does not stimulate the release of surfactant (86). Second, PEEP increases the mean airway pressure and thereby may predispose the patient to barotrauma. To increase the level of PEEP to the point that it would open atelectatic areas of lung, the level would have to be very high, greatly increasing the mean airway pressure. In treating SCI patients, it is observed that the mean airway pressure is lower if patients are ventilated with large volumes, without PEEP. However, in a few patients, once the lung has been inflated, it may be difficult to keep the lung inflated, and PEEP may help keep an already inflated lung, inflated. As a general rule in SCI patients who are subject to atelectasis, it is better to stabilize the lungs by stimulating the release of surfactant by use of large volumes.

Surfactant

The surface tension of the alveoli is reduced and the compliance of the lungs is increased by the presence of surfactant. Massaro

and Massaro raised the "possibility that type 2 cells in collapsed . . . alveoli may not secrete until the alveoli in which they reside are opened" (94). Nicholas and Barr stated that "the only proven physiologic stimulus for surfactant release is an increase in tidal volume" (83). Atropine, propranolol, and indomethacin inhibit this release. Surfactant release is stimulated by cyclic adenosine monophosphate, β-adrenergic agonists, and theophylline, but not to the extent that it is stimulated by increasing the tidal volume (82–84,96).

The combination of β-adrenergic drugs (e.g., albuterol or salmeterol), theophylline, and larger tidal volumes should improve the release of surfactant and therefore the compliance of the lung. It would seem that although ipratropium would be a useful drug to offset bronchospasm caused by the unopposed parasympathetic system in the SCI patient, its use might be relatively contraindicated if it inhibited release of surfactant and it may also dry secretions (32). Whether ipratropium inhibits the release of surfactant, as atropine does, is not known. Further studies are needed in this area.

Weaning

Tetraplegic patients with lower cervical level of injury (C5 or below) are easier to wean than those with higher-level injuries. An initial VC of more than 1 liter on admission is a favorable prognostic factor for weaning of patients with high-level injuries. The decision about when to wean a patient is individualized. Several studies have given threshold values for VC, for example: attempts at weaning require a VC of at least 300 mL, more than 10 mL/kg body weight, or as little as 100 mL (97,98). Before initiating a weaning program, the procedure should be thoroughly explained to the patient and family. The protocol recommended for weaning is outlined in Table 9.3 (99).

Synchronized Intermittent Mandatory Ventilation versus Progressive Ventilator-free Breathing

In a study comparing success of synchronized intermittent mandatory ventilation (SIMV) and PVFB weaning, it was reported

TABLE 9.3. RECOMMENDED WEANING PROTOCOL IN SPINAL CORD INJURY

1. Criteria to begin or to increase weans:
   a. Patient's level of injury is such that part- or full-time weaning is a potential.
   b. Patient agrees and understands the procedure.
2. Each change should be closely monitored and may be increased under the following conditions:
   a. Patient agrees to increase the wean time.
   b. Oximetry on the wean is within acceptable limits.
3. Schedule for weans:
   a. Starting at 2–5 min t.i.d. and increasing slowly as tolerated. A schedule can be followed as follows: 10 min t.i.d., 20 min t.i.d., 30 min t.i.d., 1 hr t.i.d., 2 hr t.i.d., 3 hr t.i.d., 4 hr b.i.d., 5 hr b.i.d., 12 hr q.d., 14 hr q.d., 16 hr q.d., 18 hr q.d., 20 hr q.d., 22 hr q.d., 24 hr q.d.
   b. Based on the judgment of the physician or respiratory therapist, the patient may skip steps on the wean protocol schedule.
4. Weans should start in the bed, with the patient lying supine.
5. Weans are to be done with the cuff deflated and trach talk as tolerated.
6. Titrate oxygen to saturation of more than 92%.
7. Cuff should be inflated if the patient is nauseated or has reflux.
8. Once the patient can tolerate weaning for longer than 30 min, weans may be started in the wheelchair and then in therapy under supervision.
9. Weans can occur in the shower after able to wean for more than 1 hr, under supervision.
10. Weans may be discontinued or reduced in time if patient has persistent atelectasis.
11. Documented parameters for all weans:
    a. Forced vital capacity
    b. Respiratory rate
    c. Heart rate
    d. Oxygen saturation
    e. Negative inspiratory force
    f. Minute ventilation
12. Criteria to discontinue weaning:
    a. Respiratory rate increased to more than 30 breaths/min
    b. Heart rate increased by 20 beats/min from baseline or is more than 130 beats/min or less than 50 beats/min
    c. Blood pressure change of plus or minus 30 points from baseline or systolic pressure less than 70 mm Hg or diastolic more than 100 mm Hg
    d. Saturation less than 92% with an fiO_2 increase 20% higher than ordered.
    e. Forced vital capacity less than half of documented patient baseline
    f. Marked increase in spasms, diaphoresis, or change in mental status
    g. Marked increase of complaint of shortness of breath or fatigue
    h. Patient request

that although SIMV was used in most patients from referring hospitals across the country, it was a successful methodology in only 35% of the SIMV weaning attempts (17). On the other hand, PVFB weaning resulted in success in 68% of attempts. Thus, it would appear that although SIMV is used frequently for weaning other categories of patients, it is successful only sporadically when used with SCI patients.

If a T piece is used while the patient is being weaned with PVFB, humidified oxygen can be passed by the tracheostomy tube. This can be done with a trach talk in place. The trach talk has a one-way valve that allows the patient to talk and cough.

With the trach talk in place, the cuff on the tracheostomy tube must be deflated. This cannot be done if the patient is on SIMV or pressure support. The ability to talk improves the patient's mental outlook. The patient who is weaning with the cuff deflated can also benefit from the use of the one-way Passey-Muir valve. Humidified oxygen can be administered by use of a trach collar over the Passey-Muir valve. Another way of delivering oxygen is to use a cap, with a hole punched in it, and to administer oxygen through the cap. This method essentially gives the patient transtracheal oxygen.

SIMV may also cause additional complications in SCI patients. In order for SIMV to work, the patient has to have a drive to breathe. This drive to breathe comes from the lack of stretching of the stretch receptors in the lung by giving small tidal volumes on the ventilator, or from creating just enough hypoxemia, acidosis, or hypercapnia to cause the brain to have a stimulus to initiate a breath. To create these drives to breathe, the physician turns down the respiratory rate on the ventilator, or turns down the ventilator tidal volume. Therefore, in order for SIMV to work, the patient has to be on a low tidal volume. Low tidal volumes cause atelectasis in SCI patients and make it harder for the patient to breathe. SIMV does not allow for adequate rest for the weak SCI patient and will tire the patient. With PVFB, the patient has periods of total rest from the effort to breathe. In this way, patients can gradually build up their strength and utilize lung, which has been expanded and is compliant because of the bigger volumes used. Clearly, the compliance of the lung is adversely affected in SCI patients by SIMV, and it is favorably affected by increasing the ventilator tidal volumes and expanding areas of lung that have been atelectatic. One especially threatening problem results from the use of SIMV in patients who have a C3 or higher level of injury. These patients do not have the capacity to generate a minute ventilation that is adequate to keep the pCO_2 in a physiologic range, and the patient may develop respiratory acidosis, cardiac arrhythmia, and death.

Another approach to weaning an individual is by using noninvasive means of ventilation after extubating or decannulating the patient. This can be performed by having the patient wean themselves off by taking fewer mouthpiece-assisted breaths, as the need is felt (100) (see appendix 9).

Phrenic Nerve Pacing

Electrophrenic respiration (EPR), or phrenic nerve pacing, is enthusiastically supported by some centers; however, only a few studies reported on its success in patients with SCI. Full-time use of EPR ranged from 27% to 35% of patients attempted, failure occurred in 13% to 38%, and mortality in 3% to 39%, with follow-up ranging from 12 to 88.7 months (12). Weese-Mayer and associates reported that 15 of 25 patients were successfully paced and had no complications (101).

Sometimes, patients have recovery of diaphragmatic function over a period of several months. For this reason, EPR should not be performed until this recovery has had a chance to occur. Criteria for use of EPR include an injury at or above C2, with intact phrenic nerves as tested by percutaneous stimulation of the phrenic nerves by an individual trained and competent to perform this testing. Most patients injured at C3, C4, or C5 should be able to wean from the ventilator without EPR, and for patients injured at these levels, weaning attempts should be made for several months before EPR is attempted.

There is some risk involved with EPR because there can be electrical failure of the electrical transmitter. This event can be catastrophic for the patient; therefore, the patient will need to be monitored closely when alone and on EPR. Monitoring can be performed by a transducer, which would sense movement of the chest; an oximeter, which would indicate hypoxemia; by an end-tidal PCO_2 monitor placed at the nose or mouth; or by an electrocardiographic monitor.

One problem with EPR can be that the patient may not be able to develop a deep enough breath with this technique to prevent atelectasis. If this happens, the patient my develop pneumonia and other complications. Therefore, it is ideal for the patient to have no atelectasis before the EPR surgery is performed.

EPR is expensive and requires extensive training of the personnel who will care for the patients. EPR should be done by those experienced in the technique, with enthusiasm for use of EPR and a willingness to train caregivers, and patients should be followed closely. It would also seem that one criterion for EPR would be that the patient should live in proximity to the center performing the procedure and have adequate funding for caregivers in the home. Further detail regarding phrenic nerve pacing is given in chapter 25.

Pneumobelt

The pneumobelt is an inflatable "bladder" that fits around the abdomen and is attached to a ventilator. Like EPR, it allows for ventilation with the patient's tracheostomy cuff deflated, allowing speech. It is an alternative for ventilation, in selected patients, when the patient is up in the wheelchair, but it is not a good option for those in bed (102). Some patients find it difficult to use, including obese patients. Like EPR, it is best used in patients treated at centers with an enthusiasm for the device and with skill and experience in using it.

SLEEP DISORDERS AND SLEEP APNEA IN PATIENTS WITH SPINAL CORD INJURY

Sleep apnea is common in SCI patients. Incidences of sleep apnea and sleep disordered breathing are reported in a range between 15% and 60% (72,103–105). These reports of sleep apnea in SCI differ in their conclusions about whether there is a relationship between sleep apnea and obesity and neck circumference, higher level of injury, VC, the effect of certain medications (i.e. antispasticity medications), and length of time from the original injury. There may be a relationship between nasal stuffiness (possibly related to loss of thoracic sympathetic outflow), snoring, and medications given for pain and spasticity. Short and colleagues noted that these incidences of sleep apnea and sleep-disordered breathing in SCI patients compare to an

incidence of occult sleep apnea of 2% to 4% and an incidence of clinical sleep apnea of 0.3% in a survey of 1,001 nonparalyzed men between the ages of 35 and 65 years (103). The comparison data are from a study conducted in a large general practice (106). In SCI patients, the sleep apnea is primarily obstructive, with a small percentage of patients demonstrating central sleep apnea.

The complications of sleep apnea are hypertension, pulmonary hypertension and cor pulmonale, congestive heart failure, deterioration in mental function, daytime sleepiness, and cognitive changes, including poor judgment. In patients with previous normal sexual function, there may also be impotence.

Because of the high prevalence of sleep apnea in SCI patients and because of the severity of the side effects and complications of sleep-disturbed breathing, it is advisable to review questions about sleep disturbance, snoring, daytime somnolence, and nasal symptoms with the patient. In the SCI patient, the physician must have a high index of suspicion of sleep apnea. Optimal workup would include an overnight oximetry recording followed by a formal sleep study if the oximetry recording is abnormal. Treatment would include CPAP or BiPAP, depending on the situation, as well as possibly the use of tricyclic antidepressants, theophylline preparations, and medications directed toward relief of upper airway symptoms.

LONG-TERM RESPIRATORY MANAGEMENT

In caring for the patient with SCI, whether acutely or in the chronic phase, the goals remain the same: to stabilize the alveoli, clear secretions, and keep the patient free of atelectasis. There are certain items that should be periodically monitored. These include (a) the current level of injury, for improvement or deterioration; (b) the VC; (c) the chest X-ray film; (d) oxygenation; and (e) symptoms of sleep-disordered breathing, including sleep apnea.

Studies of life satisfaction issues in ventilator-dependent SCI patients have been undertaken. Most patients suggest that they would again receive mechanical ventilation (97). Bach and Tilton compared overall life satisfaction, well being, and level of distress in ventilator-dependent and ventilator-independent SCI patients (107). Long-term quality of life and well being were found to be similar and correlated with the degree of family and social interaction. Those requiring MV rated their distress over the loss of breathing lower than the independently breathing SCI subjects predicted that they would. In addition, the ratings of quality of life and well being reported by the ventilator-assisted patients were higher than ratings given by health care providers when asked to imagine themselves requiring ventilatory assistance. The study suggests that chronic ventilator support does not result in decrements in quality of life, as is often assumed (107).

Only a few studies have looked at what impact the respiratory system has on long-term medical morbidity and mortality during the subacute as well as chronic stages after injury (108–110). In a study of patients with complete tetraplegia during extended follow-up, pneumonia was the leading cause of death for each age group and all time periods (2). A recent report from Model Systems data, with follow-up extending through 1998, showed similar trends in respiratory diseases (111). The most comprehensive data on annual rates of respiratory complications were reported by McKinley and coworkers, who found that for patients with complete injuries, the probability of experiencing at least one episode of pneumonia or atelectasis during the preceding year was 9.9, 6.4, 4.9, 4.1, and 3.7% for 1, 5, 10, 15, and 20 years after injury, respectively (112). The gradual decrease in rates may be the result of those patients suffering respiratory complications being at higher risk for death. Meyers and colleagues found the annual rate of respiratory infections in an independent living facility, (e.g., including influenza and pneumonia, but not colds) to be in the range of 18% to 25% for SCI patients (113).

SCI patients with a history of ventilator usage at disease onset, a history of repeated atelectasis or pneumonia, a VC of less than 2 liters, nocturnal hypercapnia, and a mean SaO_2 of less than 95% are at risk for developing late-onset respiratory insufficiency. Close surveillance of inspiratory and expiratory muscle function should be undertaken. Patients with vital capacities below 2 liters are at risk for development of respiratory failure during upper respiratory infections or after surgical anesthesia. These individuals can be taught to monitor their oxygen saturation with a pulse oximeter and use assisted cough techniques (manual or mechanical) or assisted ventilation (NIPPV or BiPAP) until they improve.

Patients with tetraplegia should receive a yearly influenza vaccine. Patients who have had a splenectomy should also receive immunization for *Haemophilus influenzae* infection.

Thoughts on Chronic Hypocapnia

Often, in patients on chronic ventilation, ABG results reveal a low PCO_2 value. It may however, be helpful to keep the PCO_2 below 35. Experience has shown that if the PCO_2 is kept low, the kidneys compensate, and the pH remains between 7.40 and 7.45. In addition, it does not seem to be a problem if the patient has a mild alkalosis because the side effects, unless there is a history of seizures or heart disease, are minimal. Finally, mucus is more soluble in alkaline secretions than in acid secretions, and it is conceivable that if the blood pH is alkalotic, the secretions may be more soluble (also, dilute $NaHCO_3$ can be used to loosen secretions).

Continuous Quality Improvement Methods

Because there is a lack of prospective, blinded, paired, comparison trials for care of tetraplegic patients, the physician caring for these patients has little guidance from the literature. Dr. W. Edwards Deming promoted alternative methods to check on quality of performance in industry (114). Mary Walton writes about the use of charts in measuring quality (115). Many of these techniques and charts can be used in caring for SCI patients.

The accompanying PDCA chart (Fig. 9.5) demonstrates that the lung compliance and the ventilator peak inspiratory pressure, along with the trend for development or clearing of the atelectasis on chest x-ray films, are items to check when making changes on the ventilator. Using a trend chart in the acute phase of caring for a patient on a ventilator will tell the clinicians whether the

patient is achieving the goals of better VC, better compliance, and better oxygenation. If the ventilator TV is turned up 100 mL daily, the trend of the response in these parameters will become obvious. The goals for SCI patients would be a dynamic compliance of 60 to 100 mL/cm and a decreasing need for oxygen. As the tidal volume on the ventilator is increased gradually, the VC will also improve (see the trend chart for patient #2 in Fig. 9.8).

Benchmarking

Some benchmarks have been established for ventilation and weaning of quadriplegic patients (17,18). One benchmark is that 83% of C3 and C4 tetraplegic patients should wean from the ventilator. A second benchmark is that only 16% of patients should still have atelectasis at the end of 2 weeks on the ventilator. A third benchmark is that C3 and C4 tetraplegic patients should be weaned from the ventilator in an average of 35 to 40 days.

Protocols

Protocols offer a chance to "reduce variation" in the care of patients with SCI. The Institute for Healthcare Improvement has established reducing variation in care as a goal for improving health care (116). There are recommended protocols in this chapter for use in ventilation of patients with SCI. Using these protocols, keeping records of outcomes and individual patient checklists, and using the PDCA cycle will allow each institution to improve the care of its patients.

CONCLUSIONS AND SUMMARY

Patients with SCI have problems with secretions and atelectasis. Most of the respiratory complications can be attributed to these problems. The most important treatments to maintain alveolar stability involve delivery of deep breaths, both for patients who do and those who do not require mechanical ventilation. The height of the patient should be ascertained immediately to guide the caregiver in the noninvasive methods that can help the patient, and especially to guide the ventilator settings for those patients requiring invasive ventilation. Although small ventilator tidal volumes are very appropriate for patients with ARDS, they are not appropriate for patients with SCI. SIMV should not be used in SCI patients because it has a propensity to cause atelectasis in these patients, and the success rate for weaning with SIMV is not as great as the success rate for PVFB. The clinician should use continuous quality improvement methods to improve the care for the SCI patient. Benchmarks allow the caregiver to know how they compare with treatment delivered in other institutions.

There are many needed research projects in the area of respiratory management of SCI patients. These include comparison of weaning techniques, the rate of clearing of atelectasis at various ventilator tidal volumes (noninvasive and invasive), the incidence of sleep apnea, proper medications in the acute and chronic periods after SCI, and the long-term complication rates of ventilator-dependent patients.

APPENDIX: DO'S AND DON'TS

Do's

1. Ask patients how tall they are.
2. Use protocols.
3. Use the FOCUS (find a process to improve, organize a team, collect data, understand variation, and select a process for improvement) and PDCA (plan, do, check, and act) cycles.
4. Use large volumes and high flow rates, with a respiratory rate of 10-12. This will cause a lower mean airway pressure and lessen the chance of pneumothorax.
5. If using noninvasive methods for keeping the lungs clear, use methods that supply a deep breath.
6. Wean the patient while supine in bed initially. Sitting the patient up is a mechanical disadvantage for tetraplegic patients. The exception to this "do" is the patient with central cord syndrome with preserved intercostal muscles but paralysis of the diaphragm.
7. Use cromolyn—it is hydrophilic. It should help moisten the secretions.
8. Use theophylline (if no contraindications)—it stimulates the brain, is a bronchodilator, strengthens the diaphragms, liquefies secretions, and is one of the few pharmacologic stimulants to release surfactant from type II alveolar cells.
9. Rejoice, if after about 2-4 days into the increasing tidal volume protocol, the patient has increased secretions. Once the secretions are removed, the amount of secretions will diminish again. At large tidal volumes, the patient will require little suctioning.
10. Use β-agonists, both short and long acting, because they stimulate the release of surfactant and offset the parasympathetic effects that result from tetraplegia.
11. Stop what you are doing if it isn't working (Loeb's Laws of Medicine) (117).
12. If you are using synchronized intermittent mandatory ventilation (SIMV) without success, try the increasing tidal volume protocol and progressive ventilator free breath (PVFB) weaning.

Don'ts

1. Don't say that atelectasis in a ventilated, paralyzed patient is the fault of the patient or their disease; it is probably the fault of the way the ventilator is set up.
2. Don't use small volumes in a patient who is ventilator dependent and has had thoracotomy or chest tubes.
3. Don't let the paralyzed patient override the ventilator; adjust the ventilator.
4. Don't use SIMV. This will lead to atelectasis in the paralyzed patient. Using SIMV and overriding the ventilator encourage "flailing" of the weak diaphragm, which encourages the formation of atelectasis. Also, with SIMV, you can't let the cuff down so the patient can talk, but you can with assist/control.
5. Don't use high levels of positive end-expiratory pressure. This will cause more barotrauma than just increasing the tidal volumes cautiously. It may treat atelectasis if used very aggressively but will increase the mean airway pressure unnecessarily.
6. Don't increase the tidal volume to high volumes suddenly; this will result in expansion of atelectatic lung but can also cause acute respiratory distress syndrome and reperfusion-reexpansion pulmonary edema and will spread bacteria that had been trapped in the atelectatic area throughout the lungs.

REFERENCES

1. Ragnarsson KT, Hall KM, Wilmot CB, et al. Management of pulmonary, cardiovascular and metabolic conditions after spinal cord injury. In: Stover SL, DeLisa JA, Whiteneck GG, eds. *Spinal cord injury: clinical outcomes for the Model Systems.* Gaithersburg, MD: Aspen, 1995:79–99.
2. DeVivo MJ, Black KJ, Stover SL. Causes of death during the first 12 years after spinal cord injury. *Arch Phys Med Rehabil* 1993;74:248–254.
3. Silver JR, Gibbon NO. Prognosis in tetraplegia. Br Med J 1968;4(623):79–83.
4. Carter RE. Experiences with high tetraplegics. *Paraplegia* 1979;17(2):140–146.
5. Carter RE, Donovan WH, Halstead L, et al. Comparative study of electrophrenic nerve stimulation and mechanical ventilatory support in traumatic spinal cord injury. *Paraplegia* 1987;25(2):86–91.
6. Minaire P, Demolin P, Bourret J, et al. Life expectancy following spinal cord injury: a ten-years survey in the Rhon-Alpes Region, France, 1969–1980. *Paraplegia* 1983;21(1):11–15.
7. Reines HD, Harris RC. Pulmonary complications of acute spinal cord injuries. *Neurosurgery* 1987;21(2):193–196.
8. Kiwerski J. Respiratory problems in patients with high lesion quadriplegia. *Int J Rehabil Res* 1992;15(1):49–52.
9. Chen CF, Lien IN. Spinal cord injuries in Taipei, Taiwan, 1978–1981. Paraplegia 1985;23(6):364–370.
10. Nyquist RH, Bors E. Mortality and survival in traumatic myelopathy during nineteen years, from 1946 to 1965. Paraplegia 1967;5(1):22–48.
11. Tator CH, Duncan EG, Edmonds VE, et al. Complications and costs of management of acute spinal cord injury. Paraplegia 1993;31(11):700–714.
12. McCrory DC, Samsa GP, Hamilton BP, et al. *Draft evidence report: treatment of pulmonary disease following spinal cord injury.* Duke Evidence-based Practice Center, Center for Clinical Health Policy Research, Prepared for the Agency for Healthcare Research and Quality. Durham, NC, May 31, 2001.
13. Williams PL, Warwick R, Dyson M, et al., eds. *Gray's anatomy,* 37th ed. Edinburgh: Churchill Livingstone, 1989:1128.
14. Derenne J, Macklem PT, Roussos CH. The respiratory muscles: mechanisms, control and pathophysiology. *Am Rev Respir Dis* 1978;118:119–133, 373–390, 581–601.
15. Sharp JT. Respiratory muscles: a review of older and newer concepts. *Lung* 1980;157:185–199.
16. DeTroyer A, Heilporn A. Respiratory mechanics in quadriplegia: the respiratory function of the intercostal muscles. *Am Rev Respir Dis* 1980;122:591–600.
17. Peterson W, Charlifue W, Gerhart A, et al. Two methods of weaning persons with quadriplegia from mechanical ventilators. Paraplegia, 1994;32:98–103.
18. Peterson WP, Barbalata L, Brooks CA, et al. The effect of tidal volumes on the time to wean persons with high tetraplegia from ventilators. *Spinal Cord* 1999;37:284–288.
19. Wicks AB, Menter RR. Long-term outlook in quadriplegic patients with initial ventilator dependency. *Chest* 1986;90:406–410.
20. Mansel JK, Norman JR. Respiratory complications and management of spinal cord injuries. *Chest* 1990;97:1446–1452.

21. Ledsome JR, Sharp JM. Pulmonary function in acute cervical cord injury. *Am Rev Respir Dis* 1981;124:41–44.

22. McMichan JC, Michel L, Westbrook PR. Pulmonary dysfunction following traumatic quadriplegia: recognition, prevention, and treatment. *JAMA* 1980;243(6):528–531.

23. Morgan MD, Gourly AR, Silver JR, et al. The contribution of the rib cage to breathing in tetraplegia. *Thorax* 1985;40:613–617.

24. Roth EJ, Nussbaum SB, Berkowitz M, et al. Pulmonary function testing in spinal cord injury: correlation with vital capacity. *Paraplegia* 1995;33:454–457.

25. Almenoff PL, Spungen AM, Lesser M, et al. Pulmonary function survey in spinal cord injury: influence of smoking and level and completeness of injury. *Lung* 1995;173:297–306.

26. Linn WS, Adkins RH, Gong H Jr, et al. Pulmonary function in chronic spinal cord injury: a cross-sectional survey of 222 southern California adult outpatients. *Arch Phys Med Rehabil* 2000;81:757–763.

27. Lind B, Bake B, Lundqvist C, et al. Influence of halo vest treatment on vital capacity. *Spine* 1987;12(5):449–452.

28. Maeda CJ, Baydur A, Waters RL, et al. The effect of the halovest and body position on pulmonary function in quadriplegia. *J Spinal Disord* 1990;3(1):47–51.

29. Kendall RJ, Lafuente J, Hosie KB. Central pontine myelinolysis after an operation. *J R Soc Med* 1997;90(8):445–446.

30. Jackson AB, Groomes TE. Incidence of respiratory complications following spinal cord injury. *Arch Phys Med Rehabil* 1994;75(3):270–275.

31. Waters RL, Meyer PR, Adkins RH, et al. Emergency, acute, and surgical management of spine trauma. *Arch Phys Med Rehabil* 1999;80:1383–1390.

32. Branscomb BV, Stover SL, DeVivo MJ, et al. Final report: the pathophysiology of respiratory complications in spinal cord injury patients (unpublished). Birmingham, AL: Department of Rehabilitation Medicine and the Division of Pulmonary and Critical Care Medicine, University of Alabama School of Medicine, 1984.

33. Chen D, Apple DF, Hudson LM, et al. Medical complications during acute rehabilitation following spinal cord injury: current experience of the Model Systems. *Arch Phys Med Rehabil* 1999;80:1397–1401.

34. Fishburn MJ, Marino RJ, Ditunno JF Jr. Atelectasis and pneumonia in acute spinal cord injury. *Arch Phys Med Rehabil* 1990;71(3):197–200.

35. DeVivo MJ, Ivie CS. Life expectancy of ventilator-dependent persons with spinal cord injuries. *Chest* 1995;108(1):226–232.

36. Fuhrer MJ, Carter RE, Donovan WH, et al. Postdischarge outcomes for ventilator-dependent quadriplegics. *Arch Phys Med Rehabil* 1987;68(6):353–356.

37. Rigby M, Zylak CJ, Wood LD. The effect of lobar atelectasis on pleural fluid distribution in dogs. *Radiology* 1980;136:603–607.

38. Zidulka A, Nadler S, Anthonisen NR. Pleural pressure with lobar obstruction in dogs. *Respir Physiol* 1976;26:239–248.

39. D'Angelo E, Miserocchi G, Michelini S, et al. Local transpulmonary pressure after lobar occlusion. *Respir Physiol* 1973;18:328–337.

40. Fraser RS, Muller, NL, Colman N, et al. *Fraser and Pare's diagnosis of diseases of the chest*, 4th ed. Philadelphia: WB Saunders, 1999.

41. Mattison LE, Coppage L, Alderman DF, et al. Pleural effusions in the medical ICU: prevalence, causes and clinical implications. *Chest* 1997;111(4):1018–1023.

42. Peterson WP, Whiteneck GG, Gerhart KA. Chest tubes, lung entrapment, and failure to wean from the ventilator. *Chest* 1994;105:1292–1294.

43. Kirshblum S, Johnston MV, Brown J, et al. Predictors of dysphagia after spinal cord injury. *Arch Phys Med Rehabil* 1999;80:1101–1106.

44. Bluechardt MH, Weins M, Thomas SG, et al. Repeated measurements of pulmonary function following spinal cord injury. *Paraplegia* 1992;30:768–774.

45. Shapiro BA, Harrison RA, Trout CA. *Clinical application of respiratory care*, 2nd ed. Chicago: Year Book Medical, 1979.

46. Petty TL. *Intensive and rehabilitation respiratory care*. Philadelphia: Lea & Febiger, 1971.

47. Braun SR, Giovannoni R, O'Connor M. Improving the cough in patients with spinal cord injury. *Am J Phys Med Rehabil* 1984;63:1–10.

48. Wang AY, Jaeger RJ, Yarkony GM, et al. Cough in spinal cord injured patients: the relationship between motor level and peak expiratory flow. *Spinal Cord* 1997;35:299–302.

49. Niranjan V, Bach JR. Noninvasive management of pediatric neuromuscular ventilatory failure. *Crit Care Med* 1998;26:2061–2065.

50. Cheshire DJ, Flack WJ. The use of operant conditioning techniques in the respiratory rehabilitation of the tetraplegic. *Paraplegia* 1978;16:162–174.

51. Green BA, Green KL, Klose KJ. Kinetic nursing for acute spinal cord injury patients. *Paraplegia* 1980;18(3):181–186.

52. Lemons VR, Wagner FC Jr. Respiratory complications after cervical spinal cord injury. *Spine* 1994;19(20):2315–2320.

53. Lin KH, Lai YL, Wu HD, et al. Effects of an abdominal binder and electrical stimulation on cough in patients with spinal cord injury. *J Formos Med Assoc* 1998;97(4):292–295.

54. Kirby NA, Barneiras MJ, Siebens AA. An evaluation of assisted cough in quadriplegic patients. *Arch Phys Med Rehabil* 1966;47(11):705–710.

55. Jaeger RJ, Turba RM, Yarkony GM, et al. Cough in spinal cord injured patients: comparison of three methods to produce cough. *Arch Phys Med Rehabil* 1993;74(12):1358–1361.

56. Bach JR. Mechanical insufflation-exsufflation: comparison of peak expiratory flows with manually assisted and unassisted coughing techniques. *Chest* 1993;104(5):1553–1562.

57. Colebatch HJH. Artificial coughing for patients with respiratory paralysis. *Aust J Med* 1961;10:201–212.

58. Garstang SV, Kirshblum SC, Wood KE. Patient preference for inexsufflation for secretion management in spinal cord injury. *J Spinal Cord Med* 2000;23:80–85.

59. Bach JR. A comparison of long-term ventilatory support alternatives from the perspective of the patient and care giver. *Chest* 1993;104:1702–1706.

60. Barach AL, Beck GJ. Exsufflation with negative pressure: physiologic and clinical studies in poliomyelitis, bronchial asthma, pulmonary emphysema and bronchiectasis. *Arch Intern Med* 1954;93:825–841.

61. Barach AL, Beck GJ, Smith RH. Mechanical production of expiratory flow rates surpassing the capacity of human coughing. *Am J Med Sci* 1953;226:241–248.

62. Beck GJ, Scarrone LA. Physiological effects of exsufflation with negative pressure. *Dis Chest* 1956;29:1–16.

63. Fugl-Myer AR. Effects of respiratory muscle paralysis in tetraplegic and paraplegic patients. *Scand J Rehabil Med* 1971;3(4):141–150.

64. Estenne M, DeTroyer A. Mechanism of the postural dependence of vital capacity in tetraplegic subjects. *Am Rev Respir Dis* 1987;135(2):367–371.

65. Maloney FP. Pulmonary function in quadriplegia: effects of a corset. *Arch Phys Med Rehabil* 1979;60:261–265.

66. Derrickson J, Ciesla N, Simpson N, et al. A comparison of two breathing exercise programs for patients with quadriplegia. *Phys Ther* 1992;72(11):763–769.

67. Huldtgren AC, Fugl-Myer AR, Jonasson E, et al. Ventilatory dysfunction and respiratory rehabilitation in post-traumatic quadriplegia. *Eur J Respir Dis* 1980;61(6):347–356.

68. Loveridge B, Badour M, Dubo H. Ventilatory muscle endurance training in quadriplegia: effects on breathing pattern. *Paraplegia* 1989;27(5):329–339.

69. Lane CS. Inspiratory muscle weight training and its effect on the vital capacity of patients with quadriplegia. *Cardiopulmonary Q* 1982;5(10):13.

70. Walker J, Cooney M. Improved respiratory function in quadriplegics after pulmonary therapy and arm ergometry [Letter]. *N Engl J Med* 1987;316(8):486–487.

71. Gross D, Ladd HW, Riley EJ, et al. The effect of training on strength and endurance of the diaphragm in quadriplegia. *Am J Med* 1980;68:27–35.

72. Bach JR, Wang TG. Pulmonary function and sleep disordered breathing in patients with traumatic tetraplegia: a longitudinal study. *Arch Phys Med Rehabil* 1994;75:279–284.

73. Liaw MY, Lin MC, Cheng PT, et al. Resistive inspiratory muscle training: its effectiveness in patients with acute complete cervical cord injury. *Arch Phys Med Rehabil.* 2000;81:752–756.

74. Kigin CM. Breathing exercises for the medical patient: the art and the science. *Phys Ther* 1990;70:700–706.

75. Hornstein S, Ledsome JR. Ventilatory muscle training in acute tetraplegia. *Physiother Can* 1986;38:145–149.

76. Rutchik A, Weissman AR, Almenoff PL, et al. Resistive inspiratory muscle training in subjects with chronic cervical spinal cord injury. *Arch Phys Med Rehabil* 1998;79:293–297.

77. Lin KW, Chuang CC, Wu HD, et al. Abdominal weight and inspiratory resistance: their immediate effects on inspiratory muscle functions during maximal voluntary breathing in chronic tetraplegic patients. *Arch Phys Med Rehabil* 1999;80:741–745.

78. Bach JR, Alba AS. Non-invasive options for ventilatory support of the traumatic high level quadriplegic. *Chest* 1990;98:613–619.

79. Montero JC, Feldman DJ, Montero D. Effects of glossopharyngeal breathing on respiratory function after cervical cord transection. *Arch Phys Med Rehabil* 1967;48(12):650–653.

80. DiPasquale PA. Exhaler class: a multidiscplinary program for high quadriplegic patients. *Am J Occup Ther* 1986;40:482–485.

81. Hardman JG, Limbird LE, Molinoff PB, et al. *Goodman and Gilman's the pharmacological basis of therapeutics*, 9th ed. New York: McGraw-Hill, 1996:673–675.

82. Nicholas TE, Barr HA. Control of release of surfactant phospholipids in the isolated perfused rat lung. *J Appl Physiol* 1981;51:90–98.

83. Nicholas TE, Barr HA. The release of surfactant in rat lung by brief periods of hyperventilation. *Respir Phys* 1983;52:69–83.

84. Massaro GD, Fischman, CM, Chiang MJ, et al. Regulation of secretion in Clara cells: studies using the isolated perfused rat. *J Clin Invest* 1981;67:345–351.

85. Hardman JG, Limbird LE, Molinoff PB, et al., eds. *Goodman and Gilman's the pharmacological basis of therapeutics*, 9th ed. New York: McGraw-Hill, 1996:212, 214.

86. Claxton AR, Wong DT, Chung F, et al. Predictors of hospital mortality and mechanical ventilation in patients with cervical spinal cord injury. *Can J Anaesth* 1998;45(2):144–149.

87. Myllynen P, Kivioja A, Rokkanen P, et al. Cervical spinal cord injury: the correlations of initial clinical features and blood gas analyses with early prognosis. *Paraplegia* 1989;27(1):19–26.

88. Bach JR, Rajarman R, Ballanger F, et al. Neuromuscular ventilatory insufficiency: effect of home mechanical ventilator use v oxygen therapy on pneumonia and hospitalization rates. *Am J Phys Med Rehabil* 1998;77(1):8–19.

89. Bach JR, Alba AS. Tracheostomy ventilation: a study of efficacy with deflated cuffs and cuffless tubes. *Chest* 1990;97(3):679–683.

90. Bach JR. Non-invasive alternatives to tracheostomy for managing respiratory muscle dysfunction in spinal cord injury. *Top Spinal Cord Injury Rehabil* 1997;2:49–58.

91. Creamer KM, McCloud LL, Fisher LE, et al. Closing pressure rather than opening pressure determines optimal positive end-expiratory pressure and avoids overdistention. *Chest* 1999;116(Suppl):26S–27S.

92. Acute Respiratory Distress Syndrome Network. Ventilation with lower tidal volumes as compared with traditional tidal volumes for acute lung injury and the acute respiratory distress syndrome. *N Engl J Med* 2000;342:1301–1308.

93. Hirvela ER. Advances in the management of acute respiratory distress syndrome: protective ventilation. *Arch Surg* 2000;135:126–135.

94. Massaro GD, Massaro D. Morphologic evidence that large inflations of the lung stimulate secretion of surfactant. *Am Rev Respir Dis* 1983;127:235–236.

95. Thet LA, Alvarez H. Effect of hyperventilation and starvation on rat lung mechanics and surfactant. *Am Rev Respir Dis* 1982;126:286–290.

96. Guyton AC, Hall JE. *Textbook of medical physiology*, 9th ed. Philadelphia: WB Saunders, 1996:487.

97. Gardner BP, Watt JW, Krishnan KR. The artificial ventilation of acute spinal cord damaged patients: a retrospective study of forty-four patients. *Paraplegia* 1986;24(4):208–220.

98. Lamid S, Ragalie GF, Welter K. Respirator-dependent quadriplegics: problems during the weaning period. *J Am Paraplegia Soc* 1985;8(2):33–37.

99. Peterson P, Brooks CA, Mellick D, et al. Protocol for ventilator management in high tetraplegia. *Top Spinal Cord Injury Rehabil* 1997;2(3):101–106.

100. Bach JR, Saporito LR. Criteria for extubation and tracheostomy tube removal for patients with ventilatory failure: a different approach to weaning. *Chest* 1996;110:1566–1571.

101. Weese-Mayer DE, Silvestri JM, Kenny AS, et al. Diaphragm pacing with a quadripolar phrenic nerve electrode: an international study. *Pacing Clin Electrophysiol* 1996;19(9):1311–1319.

102. Miller HJ, Thomas E, Wilmot CB. Pneumobelt use among high quadriplegic population. *Arch Phys Med Rehabil* 1988;69(5):369–372.

103. Short DJ, Stradling JR, Williams SJ. Prevalence of sleep apnoea in patients over 40 years of age with spinal cord lesions. *J Neurol Neurosurg Psychiatry* 1992;55:1032–1036.

104. Burns SP, Little JW, Hussey JD, et al. Sleep apnea syndrome in chronic spinal cord injury: associated factors and treatment. *Arch Phys Med Rehabil* 2000;81:1334–1339.

105. Klefbeck B, Sternhag M, Weinberg, et al. Obstructive sleep apneas in relation to severity of spinal cord injury. *Spinal Cord* 1998;36:621–628.

106. Stradling JR, Crosby JH. Predictors and prevalence of obstructive sleep apnoea and snoring in 1001 middle aged men. *Thorax* 1991;46:85–90.

107. Bach JR, Tilton MR. Life satisfaction and well-being measures in ventilator assisted individuals wih traumatic tetraplegia. *Arch Phys Med Rehabil* 1994;75:626–632.

108. Wilcox NE, Stauffer ES. Follow-up of 423 consecutive patients admitted to the spinal cord center, Rancho Los Amigos Hospital, 1 January to 31 December 1967. *Paraplegia* 1972;10:115–122.

109. Geisler WO, Jousse AT, Wynne-Jones M, et al. Survival in traumatic spinal cord injury. *Paraplegia* 1983;21:364–373.

110. Bach JR. Inappropriate weaning and late onset ventilatory failure of individuals with traumatic spinal cord injury. *Paraplegia* 1993;31:430–438.

111. DeVivo MJ, Krause S, Lammertse DP. Recent trends in mortality and causes of death among persons with spinal cord injury. *Arch Phys Med Rehabil* 1999;80:1411–1419.

112. McKinley WO, Jackson AB, Cardenas DD, et al. Long term medical complications after traumatic spinal cord injury: a regional model systems analysis. *Arch Phys Med Rehabil* 1999;80:1402–1410.

113. Meyers AB, Bisbee A, Winter M. The "Boston Model" of managed care spinal cord injury: a cross sectional study of the outcomes of risk based, pre paid, managed care. *Arch Phys Med Rehabil* 1999;80:1450–1456.

114. Deming WE. *Out of the crisis.* Cambridge, MA: Massachusetts Institute of Technology, 1986.

115. Walton, M. *The Deming management method.* New York: Putnam, 1986:98.

116. Nolan TW, Schall MW, Berwick DM, et al. *Reducing delays and waiting times throughout the healthcare system.* Boston: Institute for Healthcare Improvement, 1996:78, 88, 89.

117. Matz R. Principles of medicine. *N Y State J Med* 1977;77:99–101.

10

GASTROINTESTINAL DISORDERS

DAVID CHEN
STEVEN B. NUSSBAUM

Alterations in function of the gastrointestinal (GI) system are generally less obvious than those changes often seen in other body systems after spinal cord injury (SCI). Certain aspects of GI function (e.g., gastric digestion, absorption) change very little after a SCI, whereas other aspects are significantly altered (e.g., bowel evacuation). However, these changes may have significant psychosocial implications and have the potential to influence the social, emotional, and physical well being of patients with SCI.

This chapter reviews the normal neuroanatomy, anatomy, and physiology of the GI system. In addition, the physiologic and functional changes that occur after SCI, management of the neurogenic bowel, and common GI complications that occur in patients with SCI are discussed.

NEUROLOGIC CONTROL OF THE GASTROINTESTINAL SYSTEM

Enteric Nervous System

In general, throughout the GI tract, there are five layers present within the GI wall. The serosa is the external layer of the wall. The next two layers contain the externally placed longitudinal and internally placed circular muscle layers that are responsible for the propulsive and mixing actions of the gut. The externally placed submucosal and internally placed mucosal layers are responsible for most of the secretory activity of the gut (1).

Electrical activity within the gut transmits through gap junctions and consists of slow-wave and spike potentials. Slow waves are slow changes in the resting membrane potential. Spike potentials, which are responsible for the rhythmic contractions in the GI tract, are action potentials that are 10 to 40 times as long as normal nerve fiber action potentials. Calcium-sodium channels, which take longer to open and close, are used in the GI tract to propagate action potentials instead of the more commonly used sodium channels (1).

The enteric (intrinsic) nervous system consists of the myenteric plexus and submucosal plexus. The myenteric plexus (Auerbach plexus), which is located between the longitudinal and circular muscle layers, controls motor activities such as tonic and rhythmic contractions. The submucosal plexus (Meissner plexus), which is located in the submucosa, controls local intestinal secretion and absorption. The enteric nervous system can

function independently but is partially controlled by the autonomic nervous system (1,2).

Neurotransmitters such as acetylcholine, norepinephrine, dopamine, cholecystokinin, and somatostatin can also influence the enteric nervous system. In general, acetylcholine is excitatory, and norepinephrine is inhibitory (1).

Autonomic Nervous System

In general, the parasympathetic (PS) nervous system increases peristalsis, stimulates secretions, relaxes sphincters, and increases gut motility (3). The short postganglionic fibers of the PS nervous system secrete the neurotransmitter acetylcholine and terminate near the neurons of the myenteric plexus and submucosal plexus. The vagus nerve (cranial nerve innervated) supplies the PS innervation from the esophagus to the mid-transverse colon. There is minimal parasympathetic innervation to the small intestine (1). The pelvic nerve, which originates in the lateral anterior gray columns of spinal cord segments S2 to S4, supplies the parasympathetic innervation from the mid-transverse colon to the rectum.

In general, the sympathetic nervous system decreases peristalsis, inhibits secretions, contracts sphincters, and decreases gut motility (3). These neurons of the sympathetic nervous system generally secrete the neurotransmitter norepinephrine. The preganglionic fibers originate in the intermediolateral column of the spinal cord between T5 and L2. The superior and inferior mesenteric (T9 to T12) and hypogastric (T12 to L3) nerves contain postganglionic sympathetic neurons. Unlike the PS nervous system, which has unequal distribution of innervation along the gut, the sympathetic nervous system neurons are equally distributed (1).

NORMAL PHYSIOLOGY AND ANATOMY OF THE GASTROINTESTINAL TRACT

Mastication

Mastication (chewing) aids digestion by breaking down large particles, thus increasing the surface area of food particles that is exposed to digestive enzymes. The motor branch of cranial nerve V supplies the motor control of mastication. Saliva excreted by the parotid, submandibular, and sublingual salivary glands aids mastication. The parotid gland secretes ptyalin, an enzyme that digests starch. The submandibular and sublingual glands secrete mucin for lubrication (4).

Deglutition (Swallowing)

Normal swallowing consists of the voluntary, pharyngeal, and esophageal stages. During the voluntary stage, food is sent posteriorly into the pharynx by the upward and backward pressure of the tongue against the palate. Food moves from the pharynx to the esophagus during the involuntary pharyngeal phase. During this phase, the soft palate is pulled upward to close off the nasal passages, and the palatopharyngeal folds pull together to allow only small particles that have been broken down to pass. Also, the vocal cords close, and the larynx is pulled anteriorly and upward, thus causing the epiglottis to close off the larynx. This helps to prevent aspiration. In addition, pharyngeal muscular peristaltic waves propel food into the esophagus. During the involuntary esophageal phase, vagally controlled peristaltic waves move food down the esophagus. When food particles reach the lower esophagus, the normally tonically constricted lower esophageal sphincter relaxes, allowing passage of esophageal contents into the stomach (4).

Stomach

The stomach's main functions are to serve as a reservoir for ingested food products, to mix food products with gastric secretions, to reduce solids to small particles, and to regulate the delivery of food products into the duodenum. When food enters the stomach, the gastric body and fundus relax, permitting increased storage capacity. The vagally controlled pacemaker potentials stimulate gastric contractions. Sympathetic input further modulates the contractions (5). Food particles are prevented from entering the duodenum by the tonically contracted pyloric sphincter. Neural signals from the distended stomach and the influences of gastrin, cholecystokinin, and secretin further influence the opening or closing of the pyloric sphincter (4).

Two types of secretory glands are located within the gastric mucosa. The oxyntic glands located in the body and fundus of the stomach secrete hydrochloric acid, pepsinogen, and intrinsic factor. Pepsinogen, when combined with hydrochloric acid, converts to pepsin, a proteolytic enzyme. Intrinsic factor is necessary for vitamin B_{12} absorption. The pyloric glands located in the antrum of the stomach secrete protective mucus (6).

Small Intestine, Pancreas, and Liver

The main purpose of the small intestine is to digest and absorb nutrients with help from products made by the liver and pancreas. In the small intestine, pancreatic amylase digests carbohydrates, numerous pancreatic enzymes digest proteins, and lipase digest fats. Segmental concentric contractions controlled by the myenteric plexus mix and propel food particles through the small intestine (6).

The products secreted by the pancreas have numerous functions in normal digestion. Insulin is secreted by the islets of Langerhans. Sodium bicarbonate is secreted to neutralize the acidic stomach contents. Trypsin and chymotrypsin digest proteins, amylase digests starches, lipase digests fats, secretin stimulates bicarbonate formation, and gastrin stimulates digestive enzymes (6).

The liver produces bile acids that emulsify large fat particles, thus aiding digestion. Bile acids are subsequently stored in the gallbladder and released under the influence of cholecystokinin and autonomic nervous input (6).

Colon (Large Intestine)

The colon starts in the right lower quadrant as the cecum. This then connects to the ascending, transverse, descending, and sigmoid colon. The rectum and anus mark the termination of the colon.

The primary function of the ascending colon is to absorb electrolytes and water, and the primary function of the descending colon is to store fecal material until evacuation (2). Absorbing water and electrolytes, secreting mucus for lubrication, forming the stool, and supporting the growth of symbiotic bacteria are other functions of the colon. Normal colonic transit takes between 12 and 30 hours from the ileocecal valve to the rectum (7).

Haustrations and mass movements are two types of colonic motility. Circular muscular contractions of the colon that cause mixing of the colonic contents are called haustrations. Haustrations generally do not cause forward movement of the stool (4). Mass movements are large areas of muscular contractions that propel stool forward within the colon. These mass movements last 10 to 30 minutes and occur only a few times a day (4,8).

Reflexes of the Gastrointestinal Tract

The gastrocolic, colocolonic, and rectocolic reflexes generally stimulate colonic motility. The gastrocolic reflex describes the increase in colonic activity after ingestion of a meal. The mechanism for this cholinergically mediated reflex, which is blunted by atropine, has not been well defined. The colocolonic intramural reflex is controlled by the myenteric plexus. This reflex, which occurs even when the colon is removed from the body, causes the muscle above the dilatation to constrict and those below the dilatation to relax, causing the stool to be propelled caudally. The rectocolic reflex, mediated by the pelvic nerve, is responsible for the colonic peristalsis that occurs in response to chemical or mechanical stimulation of the rectum or anal canal (9). This is taken advantage of clinically by use of digital stimulation and suppositories in performing the bowel program. The anorectal reflex describes the involuntary relaxation of the internal anal sphincter as stool passes into the rectum, thus allowing stool to pass into the anal canal.

Normal Defecation

The internal and external anal sphincter controls the anal canal. The internal anal sphincter is composed of involuntary smooth muscle and provides continence in the resting state by remaining tonically contracted. The external anal sphincter, innervated by the pudendal nerve (S2 to S4), is composed of striated muscle, provides voluntary control of defecation, and prevents incontinence along with the puborectalis during cough or Valsalva maneuver.

The sequence of events in normal defecation includes colonic contractions causing the stool to move from the colon to the rectum. Stool then distends the rectum, stretching the puborectalis muscle, which causes a reflex relaxation of the internal anal sphincter (anorectal inhibitory reflex). This then causes the conscious urge to defecate, but the external anal sphincter and puborectalis muscle prevent defecation (i.e., the holding reflex). Under voluntary control, the external anal sphincter and puborectalis muscles relax, allowing defecation. Abdominal musculature aids defecation by increasing intraabdominal pressure (9).

GASTROINTESTINAL CHANGES AFTER SPINAL CORD INJURY

The enteric nervous system remains functionally intact after a SCI. However, some ganglion cell loss has been seen within the wall of the colon (9). The autonomic nervous system control of the enteric nervous system is affected, depending on the level of injury the individual has suffered.

Dysphagia is a common problem following a cervical SCI. This dysphagia is almost always transient and usually related to surgical trauma, especially after an anterior spinal fusion. Tracheostomies and cervical immobilizing braces, such as halo braces, also contribute to dysphagia (10,11). Although some individuals with tetraplegia suffer from gastroesophageal reflux, esophageal function generally remains intact after a SCI (12).

Changes in gastric motility occur in tetraplegia but do not occur in paraplegia (9,13). In tetraplegia, dissociation of antral and duodenal motility occurs. In addition, gastric pacemaker potentials no longer originate in the antrum in most tetraplegic patients (14). This contributes to decreased gastric emptying often suffered by patients with tetraplegia. It is unclear whether the gastrocolic reflex is functional after a SCI. A study by Connell and colleagues (15) showed the presence of the gastrocolic reflex, but Glick and associates (16) reported the absence of the gastrocolic reflex after SCI.

It has been suggested that increased gallbladder disease may occur in injuries above T10. Because the sympathetic supply to the gallbladder originates between T7 and T10, abnormal gallbladder motility and enterohepatic circulation may be caused by decreased sympathetic input (17).

Anal sphincter tone is directly related to the SCI level. When a SCI occurs above the conus medullaris (T12), the anal sphincter becomes spastic. Voluntary control is lost but reflex activity is intact. This situation is commonly referred to as an *upper motor neuron bowel*. In lesions above T1, there is prolonged mouth-to-cecum transit time. In addition, SCI patients have delayed left colon and rectal transit times as compared with controls (7). When a SCI occurs below T12, the anal sphincter is denervated and therefore flaccid. Voluntary and reflex activity is lost, and a rounder stool shape is produced. This situation is commonly referred to as a *lower motor neuron bowel* (2).

Decreased colonic motility, especially of the descending colon, leading to constipation or an ileus commonly occurs after a SCI. Loss of normal autonomic control, use of narcotics, immobility, and loss of abdominal musculature all may contribute. In an individual with an upper motor neuron bowel, the spastic anal sphincter may contribute to constipation by preventing stool evacuation. In an individual with a lower motor neuron bowel, the descending colon, sigmoid colon, and rectal denervation with the resultant absence of peristalsis contribute to constipation.

BOWEL MANAGEMENT AFTER SPINAL CORD INJURY

The effective management of the neurogenic bowel is important to prevent potential GI complications and can have a significant influence on successful reintegration of the SCI patient to their home, school, or work, and for quality of life. Bowel dysfunction is considered by many patients with SCI to be a major life-limiting problem (18). More than one third of patients with SCI rated bowel and bladder issues as having the most significant effect on their lives (19). Fear of bowel accidents is a frequent cause of people with SCI not to participate in social and other outside activities.

An effective and successful bowel program implies the predictable, regular, and thorough evacuation of the bowels without the occurrence of incontinence and prevention of complications. An effective bowel management regimen takes into consideration diet and nutritional factors, use of pharmacologic agents when necessary, and a well-developed, appropriate program that is consistent with the neurologic condition and needs of the patient. Other factors, such as availability of caregiver assistance, the need and use of adaptive equipment, home accessibility, activity level and lifestyle, and return to work or school, must also be considered. It is important to emphasize that each SCI patient is unique and that differences in bowel programs between patients should be anticipated to meet individual needs.

Pharmacologic Agents

Although used routinely in the initial establishment of a bowel program in acute SCI, the routine long-term use of oral medications, suppositories, or other bowel preparations is not always required or necessary in patients with SCI to manage their bowels effectively. Through proper diet and fluid management, many patients are able to maintain adequate stool bulk, consistency, and colonic transit without oral medications or supplements. In many instances, evacuation of the formed stool from the rectum does not require the use of specialized bowel preparations or medications. The use of pharmacologic agents should be looked on as an adjunctive tool to facilitate an effective overall bowel program. Commonly used medications fall into four general categories: stool softeners, bulk formers, peristaltic stimulants and prokinetic agents, and contact irritants.

Stool Softeners

When fluid management and dietary alterations are not effective in maintaining sufficiently soft, yet formed stool to facilitate regular bowel movements, the use of oral medications to soften stool is often helpful. Docusate sodium (Colace) and docusate calcium (Surfak) are surface-active agents that act to emulsify fat in the GI tract and decrease the reabsorption of water in the colon, thereby increasing the water content of the stool. Keeping the stool soft, yet formed may decrease hemorrhoids in patients who strain to have a bowel movement. It is important to recognize that appropriate fluid intake is necessary for these agents to be effective. These agents are not stimulants or laxatives and, therefore, are not specifically intended to enhance bowel or colonic transit or peristalsis. The laxative and stool softener Peri-Colace combines casanthranol and docusate sodium.

Bulk Formers

Bulk-forming agents act to increase the bulk of stool in the bowels by the absorption of water and expansion of volume. The increased volume or bulk of the stool in the bowel lumen distends the bowel and stimulates peristalsis. Bulk-forming agents include psyllium (Fiberall, Metamucil, Naturacil), calcium polycarbophil (FiberCon), and methylcellulose (Citrucel). Excessive use of these agents can cause diarrhea, and if adequate amounts of fluid are not taken with the agents, gastric and bowel obstruction may occur.

Peristaltic Stimulants and Prokinetic Agents

Unlike bulk formers, peristaltic stimulants and prokinetic agents enhance bowel peristalsis and colonic transit by direct stimulation of the colonic intramural plexus.

Senna (Senokot) is a commonly used oral peristaltic stimulant in the management of neurogenic bowels in patients with SCI. Its mechanism of action is believed to be through the stimulation of the Auerbach plexus to induce peristalsis in the colon. Senna facilitates bowel movements about 6 to 12 hours after ingestion and frequently is used in establishing a bowel program in patients with upper motor neuron lesions. For an evening bowel program, senna should be taken at midday, and for a morning program, it should be taken at bedtime. Long-term complications of senna can include melanosis coli, a staining of the colonic mucosa seen on colonoscopy, and cathartic colon, which is a progressive decrease in responsiveness over time, which may lead to a dilated, atonic bowel (20).

Cisapride (Propulsid) is an oral agent commonly used in the treatment of gastroesophageal reflux disease, diabetic gastroparesis, and irritable bowel disease that has been reported in a number of small studies to have potential benefits in reducing constipation and colonic transit time in patients with chronic SCI (13,21,22). Cisapride acts by stimulating serotonin-4 receptors, enhancing the release of acetylcholine at the myenteric plexus, and increasing GI motility. Its routine use in the bowel management of individuals with SCI has not been established. Recently, there have been reports of severe adverse reactions, including cardiac arrhythmias and deaths, which prompted the U.S. Food and Drug Administration to expand the warnings for cisapride (ultimately, the manufacturer withdrew the product from the market in July 2000) (23).

Metoclopramide (Reglan), a cholinergic agonist and dopa-mine antagonist, is frequently used in patients with slow gastric emptying because of its ability to increase gastric motility and emptying without affecting colonic activity (24,25). However, one should be aware of its extrapyramidal side effects and avoid its use in patients also taking monoamine oxidase inhibitors or antidepressants.

Contact Irritants

Contact irritants increase peristalsis of the colon by direct irritation or stimulation of the colonic mucosa. Several agents in this category are commonly used in the bowel management of patients with SCI and may be available in a variety of forms, such as oral tablets, suppositories, and liquid enemas.

Bisacodyl (Dulcolax) is one of the most commonly used contact irritants. It is available as an oral tablet, suppository, and enema. The bisacodyl suppository may have a vegetable oil base (Dulcolax) or a polyethylene glycol base (Magic Bullet), and there are reports of decreased bowel care time with the polyethylene glycol-based preparations (26,27). It has also been reported that faster results are obtained with the enema-based preparations (Therevac, Fleet Bisacodyl) (26). Theravac-Plus combines the liquid form of bisacodyl with benzocaine that, through its local anesthetic effect, may decrease the amount of afferent stimulation that accompanies a bowel program, which is important in patients susceptible to autonomic dysreflexia. It is important to remember that for any of the contact irritant preparations to be effective, the rectal vault within the reach of the inserted finger should be clear of as much stool as possible before insertion of the suppository or enema so that the active agent may readily reach the bowel wall. The oral tablet form of bisacodyl is generally reserved for situations such as constipation and poor bowel program results, and is not recommended for regular scheduled use.

Glycerin suppositories are also commonly used in bowel programs in SCI patients to evacuate stool from the rectum. In addition to being contact irritants, they also act as lubricating agents. They do not produce an effect like that of bisacodyl or Therevac, but are often used during the transition off suppositories to digital stimulation alone to perform the bowel program. Carbon dioxide suppositories are still used in some patients with SCI to perform a bowel program. After insertion of the suppository, a chemical reaction of the active ingredients of the suppository results in the production of carbon dioxide, which expands the intraluminal volume of the lower colon, stimulating the colonic mucosa and producing peristalsis.

Laxatives

Many oral laxatives are available. Saline laxatives are salts, usually of magnesium, sodium, or potassium. These include milk of magnesia, magnesium citrate, and Fleets phosphosoda. The saline laxatives act by drawing fluid into the small intestine, stimulating colonic motility. Hyperosmolar laxatives, which include lactulose, sorbitol, and polyethylene glycol (Golytely, MiraLax, Colyte), are metabolized in the colon into short-chain amino acids and act osmotically to draw fluid into the colonic lumen. Polyethylene glycol preparations are used to assist in cleansing out the bowel and do not cause electrolyte disturbances. Lactulose (Chronulac) is an agent more commonly used to prevent and treat hepatic encephalopathy that has bowel effects similar to bulk-forming agents. Lactulose produces an osmotic effect in the colon, similar to that of many oral laxatives, without affecting stool bulk, resulting in bowel distention and peristalsis. Although it can assist in helping to clean the bowel, it causes cramping and increased flatulence.

Enemas should be used only when there is a great deal of bowel impaction despite the use of oral medications and suppositories. Persistent enema use may cause a dependency on higher volumes for stimulation. In addition, trauma and electrolyte disturbances may occur.

Diet and Nutrition

A patient's diet may significantly alter the effectiveness of their bowel management. When making bowel management recommendations, one should take into consideration the patient's premorbid dietary history, habits, and food intolerances.

No prospective studies have specifically addressed the issue of specific diets or the influence of special diets on the effective management of the neurogenic bowel in patients with SCI. Of the studies that have dealt with the subject of diet and its effect on bowel function, most have focused primarily on specific dietary components, the most common being fiber.

In able-bodied people, increased dietary fiber is frequently recommended to promote regular bowel movements and decrease constipation. Dietary fiber is a plant component commonly found in vegetables, fruits, grains, and cereals. The role of fiber in promoting these effects is believed to occur by increasing stool water content, which increases stool bulk (weight and volume) and subsequently results in decreased intestinal transit time.

There is a common belief that high-fiber intake should be uniformly recommended in patients with SCI in order to enhance regular bowel movements. However, no studies have shown convincing evidence that increased dietary fiber results in improved bowel function or better results with bowel programs in SCI patients. In fact, several studies have shown that increased fiber may have the opposite effect in SCI patients than that seen in able-bodied people. Menardo and colleagues reported that patients with chronic SCI who were receiving a standard amount of daily fiber showed significantly delayed left colonic transit (7). More recently, Cameron and associates reported that a nominal increase in dietary fiber in patients with recent SCI resulted in a significant increase in rectosigmoid and colonic transit time (28). They concluded that dietary fiber did not have the same effect on bowel function in SCI patients that it is believed to have in people with normal bowel function.

Although unproved, there is likely some benefit to the inclusion of a reasonable amount of fiber in the daily diet of patients with SCI. It has been recommended that a diet should include at a minimum 15 g of fiber daily (29). The effects on stool consistency, frequency of bowel movements, and response to the bowel program should be monitored, and gradual adjustments to the amount of fiber intake should be made depending on these observations. Given the lack of evidence for its benefit and the potential for negative effects, high-fiber diets (20 to 30 g daily) should probably be avoided.

Fluid intake has a significant effect on the water content of stool and, therefore, influences stool consistency. By maintaining a soft, formed consistency, the complications often seen with hard stools, such as constipation, obstruction, hemorrhoids, and anal fissures, can be prevented or minimized. There are no clearly established guidelines regarding the appropriate amount of fluids that should be included in the diet of an individual with SCI to optimize bowel function and management. It has been suggested that individuals with SCI should consume 2 to 3 liters of fluids daily to optimize stool consistency and facilitate effective bowel management (30). In determining the appropriate amount of fluids, however, one must take into account the method of bladder management being used and how this may affect urine volume and the frequency with which intermittent catheterization may need to be performed or altered or a urinary drainage bag emptied, so that the potential for bladder complications is not increased.

Other dietary and nutritional factors that should be considered in promoting effective bowel management include avoiding foods that are known to have a propensity to produce flatulence or significantly affect stool consistency. Caffeine and foods containing large amounts of spices and fat are known to cause diarrhea in some patients with SCI.

Overall Bowel Management

Taking into consideration the influence of diet and nutrition and the availability and need for appropriate medications, the primary consideration in the development and alteration of a bowel management regimen is the individual with a SCI. One also needs to consider the patient's personal goals and objectives (e.g., return to school or work), daily schedule, role of family caregivers, need for and availability of attendant care, and home bathroom accessibility when designing a program.

Bowel Program

A bowel program is a regularly performed routine intended on effectively evacuating the bowel in a timely and predictable manner, so that unplanned evacuations and the development of other GI complications are avoided or minimized. An effective bowel program should result in complete evacuation of stool within 1 hour of the routine (3).

The time of day that the program is performed should be consistent to facilitate predictable and complete evacuation. Factors to consider when establishing a schedule include preinjury patterns or habits of elimination, lifestyle and anticipated activities (e.g., work or school schedules), and availability of attendant care or caregiver assistance, if needed.

A bowel program should be initiated early during the acute care period or hospitalization after a new SCI. In doing so, common complications, such as abdominal distention (which may also cause respiratory compromise in higher-level injuries), obstruction, impaction, or diarrhea, may be avoided.

The procedures used for a bowel program and the need for medications depend on the level of neurologic injury, the extent of neurologic impairment, and the subsequent effect of the injury on bowel function. Bowel programs should optimally be performed in the sitting position, allowing gravity to assist. If performing this in bed, the patient should be in the right side-lying position to take advantage of gravity and the normal rectal curvature.

Patients with incomplete neurologic impairments may retain the ability to sense rectal fullness and the need to evacuate the bowels as well as the ability to contract the external anal sphincter. In these individuals, no special measures or maneuvers may be necessary to move the bowels and evacuate appropriately.

Those with lower lumbar and sacral level injuries usually manifest areflexic bowel function (i.e., lower motor neuron bowel). This is characterized by a flaccid rectum with absence of spinal-mediated reflex activity. In these individuals, manual removal of stool from the rectum is usually required to manage the bowels. Stool softeners and bulking agents may be necessary to maintain adequate stool consistency to facilitate easy removal. Contact irritant suppositories would not be useful in these patients and, theoretically, would not be effective, owing to the absence of spinal reflex activity in the rectum. In individuals with this type of bowel function, the program should initially be performed daily and may be required twice daily. Adjustment in frequency or schedule depends on results achieved.

Patients with higher-level SCI (cervical and thoracic) usually have reflexic bowel function (upper motor neuron bowel). This type of bowel function is characterized by the presence of reflex bowel activity in the rectum as a result of the preservation of spinal-mediated sacral reflex activity. This type of bowel activity may not be present for the first 4 to 6 weeks after injury but generally appears following the period of spinal shock.

In patients with this type of bowel function, stool evacuation occurs by means of reflex activity of the rectum in response to a stimulus administered in the rectum. Initially, the use of a contact irritant suppository with digital stimulation of the rectum is generally an effective stimulus. Digital stimulation is the insertion of a well-lubricated gloved finger by the individual or caregiver, or an adapted plastic device for those without adequate hand function, into the rectum, with rotation of the finger or device to provide physical stimulation to the rectal wall. Digital stimulation should be performed for about 15 to 20 seconds and repeated every 10 minutes during a bowel program until results are produced. As with patients with areflexic bowel function, this type of bowel program should initially be performed daily, with adjustments in frequency made depending on results. In many instances, patients are able to eliminate the use of contact irritants and rely only on digital stimulation to empty their bowels effectively. The use of stool softeners and bulking agents is at times necessary in individuals with reflexic bowel function to maintain adequate stool consistency to facilitate effective results with the bowel program and prevent complications such as diarrhea.

Despite similarities in neurologic injuries and bowel function, it is important to recognize that each individual is unique in his or her response to these GI management measures, and that there will be differences in bowel program details and frequency, medications required, and adaptive equipment needed from person to person. Periodically, the effectiveness of an individual's

bowel program needs to be reevaluated, with modifications made to the regimen. It is generally recommended that if changes are made to the bowel program, the routine should be maintained for three to five bowel care cycles before deciding whether the changes are effective or whether further changes are necessary (29).

For patients with an ineffective bowel program, there are options available, including an enema continence catheter (antegrade and retrograde) or a colostomy. The enema continence catheter is a specially designed catheter that is inserted into the rectum. A balloon is inflated to hold the catheter in place, and an enema is given. Once completed, the balloon is deflated and the catheter is removed; bowel contents then empty (31). The Malone procedure, an antegrade continence enema procedure, uses a segment of bowel, usually the appendix, to create a tunnel into the ascending colon to administer an enema (32). This provides a continent, independent catheterizable stoma. Both of these procedures have been described for children, with few reports in adults (33,34). These techniques, however, may preclude the need for a colostomy in patients with a persistent unsuccessful bowel program.

A colostomy is reserved for individuals as an adjunct treatment for a pressure ulcer or if there is severe constipation with a failure of establishing an adequate and timely bowel program (9). When performed to assist with wound healing, reversing the colostomy can be performed after healing occurs. When performed otherwise in candidates who understand the limitations of the procedure (i.e., body image), colostomies enhance the quality of life and reduce the time needed for bowel care (35–37). High placement of the stoma has been reported to allow the best visualization and self-management.

GASTROINTESTINAL COMPLICATIONS AFTER SPINAL CORD INJURY

GI-related medical complications are common both in the acute period after a new SCI and in the long term, and are a significant cause of morbidity and mortality in patients with SCI. GI disorders were the cause of death in the first postinjury year in 4.8% of all deaths reported by the Model Systems SCI program, which made it the sixth leading cause of death. Beyond the first year after injury, GI complications were the cause of death in 5.4% of deaths reported (38).

Numerous authors have reported on the high prevalence of chronic GI problems with constipation being one of the most frequently cited issues (39–43). GI-related complications are a frequent reason for rehospitalization after injury (18). Some other GI complications in patients with SCI include an acute abdomen, ileus, gastritis and ulcers, hemorrhoids, cholelithiasis, pancreatitis, and cancer.

Acute Abdomen

Acute abdominal emergencies are often a challenge to detect and diagnose in patients with SCI. During the early period after injury, acute abdomen has been reported in as high as 5% of new patients (44). One cause of an acute abdomen, GI hemorrhage, was reported in one large series to have occurred in more than 3% of patients in the acute period after SCI (45).

The diagnosis and therefore management of acute abdominal conditions are made difficult by the absence of the usual signs and symptoms of abdominal pathology, owing to impaired sensory, motor, and reflex functions. This often results in significant delay in diagnosing the problem and initiating treatment (46).

Clinical findings that may raise the suspicion for and can be helpful in identifying the occurrence of an acute abdomen in patients with SCI include constipation, abdominal spasticity, shoulder-tip pain, and abdominal pain with bloating. Bowel sounds that become hyperactive and then disappear may be suggestive of an obstruction (47,48). It is important to have an extremely high level of suspicion in evaluating these patients. Performing laboratory tests, ultrasonography, or a computed tomography scan of the abdomen early is often helpful to confirm the diagnosis.

Ileus

An adynamic ileus is one of the most common GI complications after SCI, especially in the acute period following injury, during which the incidence has been reported to be as high as 8% (43,49). In one series reported by Gore and colleagues, it was suggested that this condition was more common in complete neurologic injuries and in patients with cervical and upper thoracic level injuries (49). However, others have reported that the level of neurologic injury is not a factor when examining who is at risk for development of this condition (43).

In the acute period after SCI, an ileus frequently occurs within the first 24 to 48 hours of injury and generally resolves within 2 to 3 days of onset. This is most likely due to the loss of both sympathetic and parasympathetic activity during spinal shock. Management generally includes maintaining the patient NPO and using nasogastric decompression (without suction) until bowel sounds return. In situations in which an ileus persists or is accompanied by gastric dilatation or slow emptying, metoclopramide can be effective in enhancing return of GI peristalsis (50). If an ileus is prolonged, nutrition by other means is strongly recommended, so that the nutritional status of the individual is maintained. If ileus continues or develops in the chronic period after SCI, erythromycin may be tried (51). In severe cases, the use of neostigmine has been reported and, if severe, the patient may require surgical consultation (52).

Gastritis and Ulcers

Gastritis and the development of ulcers in patients with SCI are frequently reported complications, both in the chronic and acute periods after injury. Stinneford and coworkers reported that in their series of chronic patients, 61% reported symptoms of heartburn, and in those who underwent endoscopy and motility studies, common findings included evidence of inflammation and slowly propagating, abnormal peristalsis contractions (53). The clinical development of peptic ulcer disease in the acute or chronic period has been reported to occur in 4% to 20% of patients with SCI (18,43,53).

The risk for gastritis and ulcer disease appears to increase with higher neurologic levels and completeness of injuries (44). It has also been suggested that increased respiratory complications are a significant risk factor for peptic ulcer disease. The use of steroids in the acute period after SCI does not appear to be associated with an increased incidence of peptic ulcer disease (44).

The prophylactic use of antacids and histamine-2 antagonists in patients with acute SCI is routinely seen today in most trauma centers to prevent development of gastritis and ulcer disease. It has also been suggested that providing nutritional support to meet a new SCI patient's total energy requirement as early as possible decreases the risk for significant peptic ulcer disease (54).

Hemorrhoids

The chronic physical stimulation to the anus and rectum, which comes with the need to perform a bowel program in patients with impaired bowel function, unfortunately results in the frequent development of hemorrhoids in patients with SCI. It has been reported that 57% of patients more than 5 years after injury complained of symptomatic hemorrhoids (18). Bleeding is generally the presenting symptom, but prolapse of the rectal mucosa may also occur, resulting in the chronic secretion of fluid, which may result in skin breakdown in the perianal region. Smaller hemorrhoids generally respond to hydrocortisone suppositories or creams, which should be used after completion of the bowel program. For larger hemorrhoids or prolapsed internal hemorrhoids, sclerotherapy and elastic band ligation may be indicated. Rectal bleeding should not be attributed to hemorrhoids until anoscopy or a rectal examination is performed.

Cholelithiasis

It has been suggested that there is an increased risk for cholelithiasis in patients with SCI. Unfortunately, the true incidence and prevalence of this GI complication in the SCI population is unclear because many patients with gallstone disease are asymptomatic, and neurologic impairment of sensation often alters the clinical presentation, making the diagnosis challenging.

In one autopsy series, Apstein and Dalecki-Chipperfield reported a 29% prevalence of gallstone disease, compared with 11% in a noninjured control group (17). They found no difference in age, level, or duration of neurologic injury in patients with SCI with gallstone disease, compared with those without gallstones (17). In a larger prospective study using abdominal ultrasound, Apstein and associates reported a higher prevalence of gallstones in patients with SCI (34%) versus age-matched, non-SCI controls (17%) and found the difference significantly higher in patients younger than 40 years of age and in those with neurologic levels above T10 (55).

Although the reason for the apparent increased prevalence of cholelithiasis in SCI patients is not clearly known, theories include abnormal gallbladder motility due to impaired sympathetic innervation resulting in bile stasis, decreased intestinal transit leading to impaired enterohepatic circulation, and metabolic changes leading to abnormal biliary lipid secretion (17, 55).

Pancreatitis

In the differential diagnosis of an acute abdomen that develops in a patient with SCI, pancreatitis should be considered. Although the incidence of pancreatitis after SCI is not known, it has been suggested that the use of high-dose steroids may predispose patients with acute SCI to development of this condition and should be considered in individuals with unresolving ileus or recurrence of an adynamic ileus (44). Treatment of pancreatitis in the SCI patient is similar to that in the general population and includes resting the gut by maintaining the patient NPO, using of nasogastric suctioning to reduce gastric acids, and correcting of fluid and electrolyte imbalances. When the ileus has resolved, abdominal pain, if present, ceases, and the serum amylase or lipase has returned to near normal, gradual reintroduction of oral nutrition may begin initially with clear liquids, advancing to solid foods as tolerated.

Superior Mesenteric Artery Syndrome

Superior mesenteric artery syndrome is seen mostly in patients with tetraplegia who present with abdominal distention, discomfort, and recurrent emesis after eating (56,57). It is caused by obstruction in the distal part of the duodenum as it passes behind the superior mesenteric artery and in front of the spine and aorta. It often occurs in patients who are immobilized and have lost a significant amount of weight and retroperitoneal fat. It is worse in the supine position and in patients who are in a body jacket. Upper GI series reveal an abrupt cessation of barium in the third part of the duodenum. Treatment includes sitting the patient upright or using the left side-lying position after meals, providing nourishment to restore weight, and applying a lumbosacral corset to push the abdominal contents upward. Surgery is rarely indicated.

Cancer

It is uncertain whether colorectal cancer is increased after a SCI. In one study, the incidence of colorectal cancer was found to be 2 to 6 times higher than in the normal population, and in another study, the incidence was the same as in the normal population (58,59). As with the non-SCI population, routine screening for colorectal cancer should be performed. Rectal examination should be performed annually in patients older than 40 years. However, in SCI, false-positive results occur commonly because the individual is routinely performing a bowel program that may produce minor bleeding. Sigmoidoscopy or colonoscopy should be performed every 3 to 5 years routinely in patients older than 50 years of age (9).

CONCLUSIONS

Alterations in function of the gastrointestinal system after SCI and their impact on bowel function can have profound effects on the individual with SCI not only in terms of the physical changes and risk for secondary GI complications but also in terms of their potential to affect quality of life. An increased understanding and knowledge of the physiologic and functional changes to the GI system and an awareness of potential secondary complications that may occur after these injuries have improved the ability of health care professionals to more effectively manage and better educate patients and their families and caregivers in this area.

REFERENCES

1. Guyton AC. General principles of gastrointestinal function: motility, nervous control, and blood circulation. In: Guyton AC, ed. *Textbook of medical physiology* 8th ed. Philadelphia: WB Saunders, 1991:688–697.
2. Chen D, Nussbaum S. The gastrointestinal system following spinal cord injury and bowel management. In: Hammond M, ed. *Physical medicine and rehabilitation clinics of North America: spinal cord injury.* Philadelphia: WB Saunders, 2000:45–56.
3. Zejdlik CP. Reestablishing bowel control. In: *Management of spinal cord injury.* Boston: Jones & Bartlett, 1992:398–400.
4. Guyton AC. Transport and mixing of food in the alimentary tract. In: Guyton AC, ed. *Textbook of medical physiology* 8th ed. Philadelphia: WB Saunders, 1991:698–708.
5. Malagelada JR, Azpiroz F, Mearin F. Gastroduodenal motor function in health and disease. In: Sleisenger MH, Fordtran JS, eds. *Gastrointestinal disease* 5th ed. Philadelphia: WB Saunders, 1993:486–508.
6. Guyton AC. Secretory functions of the alimentary tract. In: Guyton AC, ed. *Textbook of medical physiology* 8th ed. Philadelphia: WB Saunders, 1991:709–725.
7. Menardo G, Bausano G, Corazziari E, et al. Large-bowel transit in paraplegic patients. *Dis Colon Rectum* 1987;30:924–928.
8. Nino-Murcia M, Stone JM, Chang PJ, et al. Colonic transit in spinal cord injured patients. *Invest Radiol* 1990;25:109–112.
9. Steins SA, Bergman SB, Goetz LL. Neurogenic bowel dysfunction after spinal cord injury: clinical evaluation and rehabilitative management. *Arch Phys Med Rehabil* 1997;78:S86–S100.
10. Martin RE, Neary MA, Diamant NE. Dysphagia following anterior cervical spine surgery. *Dysphagia* 1997;12:2–8.
11. Kirshblum S, Johnston M, Brown J, et al. Predictors of dysphagia after spinal cord injury. *Arch Phys Med Rehabil* 1999;80:1101–1106.
12. Singh RVP, Suys S, Villanueva PA. Prevention and treatment of medical complications. In: Benzel EC, Tator CH, eds. *Contemporary management of spinal cord injury.* Park Ridge: American Association of Neurologic Surgeons, 1995:209.
13. Rajendran SK, Reiser JR, Bauman W, et al. Gastrointestinal transit after spinal cord injury: effect of cisapride. *Am J Gastroenterol* 1992; 87:1614–1617.
14. Fealey RD, Szurszewski JH, Merritt JL, et al. Effect of traumatic spinal cord transection on human upper gastrointestinal motility and gastric emptying. *Gastroenterology* 1984;87:69–75.
15. Connell AM, Frankel H, Guttmann L. The motility of the pelvic colon following complete lesions of the spinal cord. *Paraplegia* 1963;1: 98–115.
16. Glick ME, Meshkinpour H, Haldeman S, et al. Colonic dysfunction in patients with spinal cord injury. *Gastroenterology* 1984;86:287–294.
17. Apstein MD, Dalecki-Chipperfield K. Spinal cord injury is a risk factor for gallstone disease. *Gastroenterology* 1987;92:966–968.
18. Stone JM, Nino-Murcia M, Wolfe VA, et al. Chronic gastrointestinal problems in spinal cord injury patients: a prospective analysis. *Am J Gastroenterology* 1990;85:1114–1119.
19. Hanson RW, Franklin MR. Sexual loss in relation to other functional losses for spinal cord injured males. *Arch Phys Med Rehabil* 1976;57: 291–293.
20. Gattuso JM, Kamm MA. Adverse effects of drugs used in the management of constipation and diarrhoea. *Drug Saf* 1994;10:47–65.
21. Binnie NR, Creasey GH, Edmond P, et al. The action of cisapride on the chronic constipation of paraplegia. *Paraplegia* 1988;26:151–158.
22. Geders JM, Gaing A, Bauman WA, et al. The effect of cisapride on segmental colonic transit time in patients with spinal cord injury. *Am J Gastroenterol* 1995;90:285–289.

23. Wysowski DK, Bacsanyi J. Cisapride and fatal arrhythmia. *N Engl J Med* 1996;335:290–291.
24. Dowling PM. Prokinetic drugs: metoclopramide and cisapride. *Can Vet J* 1995;36:115–116.
25. Segal JL, Milne N, Brunnemann SR, et al. Metoclopramide-induced normalization of impaired gastric emptying in spinal cord injury. *Am J Gastroenterol* 1987;82:1143–1148.
26. House JG, Steins SA. Pharmacologically initiated defecation of persons with spinal cord injury: effectiveness of three agents. *Arch Phys Med Rehabil* 1997;78:1062–1065.
27. Steins SA. Reduction in bowel program duration with polyethylene glycol-based bisacodyl suppositories. *Arch Phys Med Rehabil* 1995;76:674–677.
28. Cameron KJ, Nyulasi IB, Collier GR, et al. Assessment of the effect of increased dietary fibre intake on bowel function in patients with spinal cord injury. *Spinal Cord* 1996;34:277–283.
29. Consortium for Spinal Cord Medicine. *Neurogenic bowel management in adults with spinal cord injury.* Washington, DC: Paralyzed Veterans of America, 1998.
30. Rehabilitation Institute of Chicago. *Spinal cord injury: educational guide for individuals and families.* Chicago: Rehabilitation Institute of Chicago, 1998.
31. Shandling B, Gilmore RF. The enema continence catheter in spinal bifida: successful bowel management. *J Pediatr Surg* 1987;22:271–273.
32. Malone PS, Ransley PG, Kiely EM. Preliminary report: the antegrade continence enema. *Lancet* 1990;336:1217–1218.
33. Christensen P, Kvitzau B, Krogh K, et al. Neurogenic colorectal dysfunction-use of new antegrade and retrograde colonic wash-out methods. *Spinal Cord* 2000;38:255–261.
34. Yang CC, Stiens SA. Antegrade continence enema for the treatment of neurogenic constipation and fecal incontinence after spinal cord injury. *Arch Phys Med Rehabil* 2000;81:683–685.
35. Stone JM, Wolfe VA, Nino-Murcia M, et al. Colostomy as treatment for complications of spinal cod injury. *Arch Phys Med Rehabil* 1990;71:514–518.
36. Deshmukh G, Bunkel D, Sevo D, et al. Use or misuse of colostomy to heal pressure ulcers. *Dis Colon Rectum* 1996;39:737–738.
37. Kelly SR, Shashidharan M, Borwell B, et al. *Spinal Cord* 1999;37:211–214.
38. DeVivo M, Krause JS, Lammertse DP. Recent trends in mortality and causes of death among persons with spinal cord injury. *Arch Phys Med Rehabil* 1999;80:1411–1419.
39. Han RR, Kim JH, Kwon BS. Chronic gastrointestinal problems and bowel dysfunction in patients with spinal cord injury. *Spinal Cord* 1998;36:485–490.
40. Kirk PM, King, RB, Temple R, et al. Long-term follow-up of bowel management after spinal cord injury. *SCI Nursing* 1997;14:56–63.
41. Menter R, Weitzenkamp D, Cooper D, et al. Bowel management outcomes in individuals with long-term spinal cord injuries. *Spinal Cord* 1997;35:608–612.
42. DeLooze, D, Van Laere M, DeMuyuck M, et al. Constipation and other chronic gastrointestinal problems in spinal cord injury patients. *Spinal Cord* 1998;36:63–66.
43. Albert TJ, Levine MJ, Balderston RA, et al. Gastrointestinal complications in spinal cord injury. *Spine* 1991;16:S522–S525.
44. Berlly MH, Wilmot CB. Acute abdominal emergencies during the first four weeks after spinal cord injury. *Arch Phys Med Rehabil* 1984;65:687–690.
45. Chen D, Apple DF, Hudson LM, et al. Medical complications during acute rehabilitation following spinal cord injury: current experience of the model systems. *Arch Phys Med Rehabil* 1999;80:1397–1401.
46. Longo WE, Ballantyne GH, Modlin IM. Colorectal disease in spinal cord patients: an occult diagnosis. *Dis Colon Rectum* 1990;33:131–134.
47. Miller LS, Staas WE, Herbison GS. Abdominal problems in patients with spinal cord lesions. *Arch Phys Med Rehabil* 1975;56:405–408.
48. Juler GL, Eltorai IM. The acute abdomen in spinal cord patients. *Paraplegia* 1985;23:118–123.
49. Gore RM, Mintzer RA, Calenoff L. Gastrointestinal complication of spinal cord injury. *Spine* 1981;6:538–544.
50. Miller F, Fenzl TC. Prolonged ileus with acute spinal cord injury responding to metoclopramide. *Paraplegia* 1981;19:43–45.
51. Clanton LJ, Bender J. Refractory spinal cord injury induced gastroparesis: resolution with erythromycin lactobionate. A case report. *J Spinal Cord Med* 1999;22:236–238.
52. Trevisani GT, Hyman NH, Church JM. Safe and effective treatment of acute colonic pseudo-obstruction. *Dis Colon Rectum* 2000;43:599–603.
53. Stinneford JG, Keshavarzian A, Nemchausky BA, et al. Esophagitis and esophageal motor abnormalities in patients with chronic spinal cord injuries. *Paraplegia* 1993;31:384–392.
54. Kuric J, Lucas CE, Ledgerwood AM, et al. Nutritional support: a prophylaxis against stress bleeding after spinal cord injury. *Paraplegia* 1989;27:140–145.
55. Apstein MD, George B, Tchakarova B. Spinal cord injury is a risk factor for cholesterol gallstone disease: a prospective study. *J Am Paraplegia Soc* 1991;14:197–198.
56. Gore RM, Mintzer RA, Calenoff L. Gastrointestinal complications of spinal cord injury. *Spine* 1981;6:538–544.
57. Roth EJ, Fenton LI, Gaebler-Spira DJ, et al. Superior mesenteric artery syndrome in acute traumatic quadriplegia: case reports and literature review. *Arch Phys Med Rehabil* 1991;72:417–420.
58. Frisbie J, Chopra S, Foo D, et al. Colorectal carcinoma an myelopathy. *J Am Paraplegia Soc* 1984;7:33–36.
59. Stratton M, McKirgan L, Wade T, et al. Colorectal cancer in patients with previous spinal cord injury. *Dis Colon Rectum* 1996;39:965–968.

ENDOCRINOLOGY AND METABOLISM AFTER SPINAL CORD INJURY

WILLIAM A. BAUMAN
ANN M. SPUNGEN

Persons with chronic spinal cord injury (SCI) have several metabolic disturbances. Topics covered in this chapter include carbohydrate, lipid, bone, and calcium metabolism; thyroid and adrenal function; salt and water metabolism; and anabolic hormones. Adiposity, a state of insulin resistance, and hyperinsulinemia, hyperlipidemia, and hypertension are a constellation of findings that represent an atherogenic pattern of risk factors for coronary heart disease (CHD). Recognition of metabolic abnormalities in patients with SCI is the first step in improving clinical care. The application of appropriate interventions to correct or ameliorate these abnormalities holds the promise to improve longevity and quality of life in persons with SCI.

CARBOHYDRATE METABOLISM

Disorders of oral carbohydrate tolerance are more prevalent in persons with SCI than in the able-bodied population (1–4). In most persons with SCI who have a disorder in glucose tolerance, peripheral resistance of insulin to mediate glucose uptake may be demonstrated. The normal homeostatic response to glucose challenge in the presence of insulin resistance is increased pancreatic β-cell release of insulin to maintain the blood glucose concentration within the normal range. Even in the absence of any deterioration in glucose tolerance, insulin resistance and hyperinsulinemia are recognized as an atherogenic condition. If the compensatory response of the pancreas is insufficient, as may occur with advancing age, worsening of carbohydrate tolerance will ensue.

Duckworth and colleagues reported that 23 of 45 subjects with chronic SCI had diabetes mellitus diagnosed by response to a 100-g oral glucose load by criteria established by the National Diabetes Data Group (4,5). Twelve of 23 patients with diabetes were found to be hyperinsulinemic and insulin resistant as determined by the kinetics of glucose disappearance to an oral glucose challenge. Duration of injury was significantly longer in subjects with diabetes and insulin resistance than in those who had normal glucose tolerance and were insulin sensitive (4).

Bauman and Spungen performed a 75-g oral glucose tolerance test in 100 subjects with all levels of SCI and in 50 able-bodied controls (3). In subjects with SCI, 22% had diabetes employing criteria established by the World Health Organization, whereas only 6% of the control group had diabetes (6). Eighty-two percent of the controls had normal oral glucose tolerance, compared with 38% of those with quadriplegia and 50% of those with paraplegia. Subjects with SCI had significantly higher mean plasma glucose and insulin values at several points during the oral glucose tolerance test when compared with controls, suggesting a relative state of insulin resistance in those with SCI. The sum plasma glucose concentration after an oral glucose load as a function of age was compared in those with SCI and controls; the group with SCI had significantly higher sum plasma glucose values at younger ages. In subgroups, determinants of insulin sensitivity were measured: percentage of lean body mass, percentage of fat body mass, and cardiopulmonary fitness. Values for insulin sensitivity were significantly related to those of fitness ($\dot{V}O_2$) determined from a progressive incremental upper-body exercise stress test. Although failing to reach significance, insulin sensitivity was directly correlated with lean body mass and indirectly correlated with adiposity. Thus, in a relatively small subgroup of untrained subjects with paraplegia, the strongest determinant of insulin sensitivity was cardiopulmonary fitness, a marker of activity.

Bauman and associates also studied the relationship of oral carbohydrate tolerance with several variables, including level and completeness of lesion, gender, ethnicity, age, duration of injury, and calculated percentage of body fat (2). Of the total group of 201 subjects, 27 (13%) had diabetes mellitus and 56 (29%) had impaired glucose tolerance as determined by criteria of the Expert Committee on the Diagnosis and Classification of Diabetes Mellitus (2,7). These subjects were on average a decade younger than those reported in the previously mentioned study, 39 ± 1 versus 49 ± 2 years of age, respectively (2,3). The subjects with complete tetraplegia had significantly worse carbohydrate tolerance (Fig. 11.1) and were more frequently classified with a disorder in carbohydrate tolerance than the other neurologic deficit subgroups (complete tetraplegia, 73%; incomplete tetraplegia, 44%; complete paraplegia, 24%; incomplete paraplegia, 31%). Those with complete tetraplegia had significantly greater peak and sum plasma insulin concentrations after an oral glucose

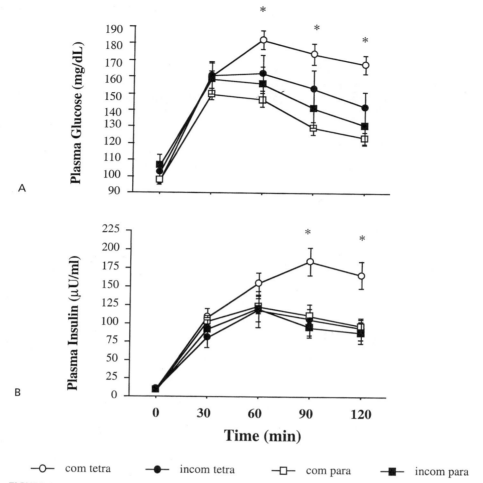

FIGURE 11.1. Comparison of oral glucose tolerance by neurologic deficit. **A**; Plasma glucose concentration versus time after a 2-hour oral glucose tolerance test. **B**; Plasma insulin levels versus time after a 2 hour oral glucose tolerance test. An asterisk (*) above the time point displays significant differences (*p* < 0.05) between the motor complete tetraplegia group and the three other neurologic deficit groups (incomplete tetraplegia, complete paraplegia, incomplete paraplegia). (From Bauman WA, Adkins RH, Spungen AM, et al. The effect of residual neurological deficit on oral glucose tolerance in persons with chronic spinal cord injury. *Spinal Cord* 1999;37:765–771, with permission.)

load compared with the other groups of lesser neurologic deficit. Oral carbohydrate tolerance was similar in men and women; however, the plasma insulin levels at the intermediate time points (30, 60, and 90 minutes) were significantly higher for men, suggesting a state of relative insulin resistance in men. Stepwise regression analyses demonstrated that peak serum glucose was significantly associated with increased percentage of total body fat, complete tetraplegia, older age, and male gender. The peak plasma insulin level was associated with increased percentage of total body fat and male gender. In this study, glucose tolerance appeared to be independent of the effects of ethnicity, and glucose abnormalities generally increased with advancing age.

About 6.6% of the U.S. population between the ages of 20 and 74 years have diabetes mellitus, with most cases classified as type II (8). At least three factors are involved in the pathogene-

sis of type II diabetes mellitus: a genetic predisposition, impaired insulin action, and a defect in pancreatic β-cell function (9). The genetic basis of type II diabetes is complex and multifactorial; however, the tendency to develop diabetes may be increased by environmental factors, such as those present in patients with SCI. Insulin resistance is generally present in individuals with a hereditary predisposition to develop impaired glucose tolerance or type II diabetes mellitus (10–12). If insulin resistance is present, the pancreas will compensate by increasing insulin release to maintain euglycemia, and hyperinsulinemia may ensue. To date, the natural course of impaired glucose tolerance, or "mild" diabetes, in patients with SCI has not been reported. The progression from impaired glucose tolerance to diabetes mellitus depends on a multiplicity of factors, including the genetic composition of the cohort, environmental factors, length of follow-up, and means of assessment.

Because the predominant peripheral action of insulin is on muscle, and paralysis results in an absolute decrease in the quantity and quality of muscle mass, it is important to address the known morphologic, physiologic, and biochemical effects of SCI on muscle. Denervation of skeletal muscle has been shown to cause insulin resistance (13). Electrical stimulation has been reported to improve structure and function of surviving muscle fibers (14–17). Using animal models, other investigators have reported the deleterious effect of denervation on postreceptor insulin action, exercise-induced glucose uptake, insulin receptor binding, receptor phosphorylation, the glucose transporter protein (GLUT-4), and protein kinase C activity (18–24).

After acute SCI, there is a rapid, severe atrophy of the denervated musculature. By 24 weeks of injury after traumatic complete SCI, the average cross-sectional area of the muscles of the leg was 45% to 80% of matched able-bodied controls (25). Of interest, there were differential changes in the atrophy of ankle plantar or dorsi flexor muscles but not of the thigh muscles (25). The relative cross-sectional area of type I fibers did not change, but there was a decrease of type IIa and an increase in type IIax + IIx (26). In subjects within 14 to 15 weeks of acute SCI who began a training program of functional electrical stimulation of the legs to perform cycle ergometry against increasing resistance, Baldi and coworkers demonstrated that muscle atrophy was prevented after 3 months and significant hypertrophy occurred by 6 months of training (27).

Subjects with tetraplegia were found to have a marked reduction in whole-body glucose transport that appeared to be due to a proportional reduction in muscle mass (28). In contrast to several previous studies in animal models of muscle denervation, the glucose transport system in skeletal muscle in those with tetraplegia remained remarkably intact despite severe morphologic changes, including a predominance of type IIb fibers (28). Lillioja and associates demonstrated a significant correlation between insulin resistance by the euglycemic clamp technique and percentage of type IIb muscle fibers (29). Type IIb muscle fibers are less sensitive to insulin action and have a reduced capillary density, which may also be responsible for a reduction in insulin-dependent, as well as insulin-independent, glucose uptake.

Prolonged inactivity has been shown to impair glucose tolerance and to be associated with hyperinsulinemia (30,31). Epidemiologic studies have demonstrated that the incidence rates for diabetes mellitus decline as energy expenditure and regular exercise increase (32,33). Placing healthy subjects on bed rest voluntarily for 7 days resulted in a moderate deterioration in oral glucose tolerance and increased plasma insulin levels both in the fasting state and in response to an oral glucose load (34). Obese, insulin-resistant subjects placed on bed rest have a further deterioration of carbohydrate tolerance (35). After bed rest, euglycemic clamp studies revealed a rightward shift of the insulin dose-response curve at which half-maximal stimulation occurred, requiring higher insulin concentrations to produce the same glucose uptake, with little change in the maximal response (34). Insulin-induced suppression of hepatic glucose output was not changed by bed rest. These investigators suggested that short-term immobilization and its effects on carbohydrate metabolism occur primarily in skeletal muscle (34). Bed rest does not appear to be associated with a decrease in insulin receptor

binding (35). Thus, postreceptor defects in insulin action may be operative. Single-leg casting for 1 week has been shown to reduce insulin-stimulated glucose uptake in the immobilized limb (36). In normal subjects, the carbohydrate intolerance of bed rest may be reversed within 1 week of ambulation (30,37). Goodyear and colleagues reported that the number and activity of the glucose transporter protein GLUT-4 were increased after exercise (38). Glycogen synthase activity was also increased after exercise, resulting in increased synthesis of glycogen and increased nonoxidative glucose disposal. In addition to the effects of insulin on glucose uptake by muscle, exercise appears to have an effect on peripheral glucose use. By hindlimb perfusion technique or the incubation of isolated skeletal muscle, muscle contraction, independent of insulin, increased glucose transport (39, 40). Thus, denervation appears to be responsible for a postreceptor defect in insulin action as well as for the loss of contraction-stimulated glucose disposal.

Because fasting plasma glucose has been shown to correlate highly with basal rates of hepatic glucose output, and the average fasting plasma glucose is only mildly elevated in subjects with SCI, peripheral insulin resistance is the major factor responsible for glucose intolerance in this disorder (41). Subjects with impaired glucose tolerance or diabetes mellitus may have fasting plasma glucose values within the normal range and be without symptoms of any carbohydrate disorder. In one study in which able-bodied individuals were screened for diabetes, 66% and 51% of those diagnosed with impaired glucose tolerance or diabetes mellitus, respectively, had fasting plasma values below 115 mg/dL (42).

There is a recognized association between adiposity and abnormalities in carbohydrate metabolism. Yalow and colleagues reported higher plasma insulin concentrations in obese individuals compared with lean controls (43). Studies have shown that the hyperinsulinism of obesity is due to decreased response of the peripheral tissues to insulin (44–46). It has been suggested that adipose tissue releases a cytokine, tumor necrosis factor-α (TNF-α), into the circulation, which may increase with obesity and depress the insulin receptor's tyrosine kinase activity, resulting in a reduced insulin action at the end organ (47). Caloric restriction may partially reverse these abnormalities. In adult-onset obesity, the size of the fat cell appears to correlate with insulin resistance (48,49). Adipocyte hypertrophy is associated with decreased insulin-mediated glucose uptake, presumably owing to a reduction in the number of insulin receptors as well as postreceptor defects (50,51). Studies of body fat topography in able-bodied individuals have suggested that distribution of body fat may be an important factor in the association of obesity with other metabolic disorders (52–59). In persons with SCI, the usual clinical measures of adiposity underestimate the degree of adiposity. Several methods of body composition have been employed in subjects with SCI and appear to offer reasonable estimates of total or regional body fat (60). Studies in able-bodied subjects have established associations between hypertension, hyperinsulinemia, obesity, and disorders of glucose tolerance (43,61–65). In persons with SCI, investigators have begun to establish associations between obesity (total and regional), level of activity, glucose intolerance, hyperinsulinemia, lipid abnormalities, and hypertension (1,3,66–68). Possibly reflecting a state of insulin resistance, an increased prevalence of hyperten-

TABLE 11.1. DIAGNOSTIC CRITERIA FOR DISORDERS OF CARBOHYDRATE METABOLISM[a]

	Fasting	At 120 min
Normal	<110	<140
Impaired	≥110, <126	≥140, <200
Diabetic	≥126	≥200

[a]All values are for venous plasma glucose concentration (mg/dL). From The Expert Committee on the Diagnosis and Classification of Diabetes Mellitus. Report of the Expert Committee on the Diagnosis and Classification of Diabetes Mellitus. *Diabetes Care* 1997;20:1183–1197, with permission.

sion has been reported in persons with chronic paraplegia (69). Hyperuricemia is also an inherent component of this metabolic syndrome (70). In a subset of subjects with SCI, hyperinsulinemia, hypertriglyceridemia, and hyperuricemia were also present (71).

Studies in subjects with SCI have relied on several diagnostic criteria (5–7). The presently accepted classifications for the diagnosis of the disorders of oral carbohydrate tolerance are those of the Expert Committee on the Diagnosis and Classification of Diabetes Mellitus (7) (Table 11.1). Any person with a potential genetic predisposition to diabetes or diagnosed as having impaired glucose tolerance should make an effort to reduce the risk for diabetes. Persons who are prediabetic have an atherogenic pattern of risk factors for CHD, possibly owing to obesity, hyperglycemia, and hyperinsulinemia, which may be present for several years before the emergence of diabetes and may contribute to CHD as much as diabetes itself (72). Intervention at any stage could prevent or delay progression of cardiovascular disease. Obesity, physical inactivity, and a high-fat diet are recognized risk factors for diabetes, all of which can be modified. Diet therapy should be instituted to achieve and maintain a desirable body weight. According to the recommendations of the Committee on Food and Nutrition of the American Diabetes Association, about 55% to 60% of total caloric intake should be in the form of carbohydrates and 0.8 g/kg body weight should be in the form of protein; total intake of fat should be restricted to less than 30% of total calories and cholesterol intake to less than 300 mg per day (73). Combining exercise with diet therapy has been shown to be of greater efficacy than either approach alone (74,75). The hypothesis that type II diabetes is preventable by drug therapy is an attractive concept but remains unproved. Two classes of medications, sulfonylureas and biguanides (76–78), have undergone limited clinical trials for prevention of diabetes with inconclusive results. Another class of agents, the thiazolidinediones, has been shown in human studies to decrease insulin resistance and improve carbohydrate handling in obese individuals with either normal or impaired glucose tolerance (79). This class of agents may hold particular promise in persons with SCI for the prevention of diabetes, as well as lipid abnormalities and hypertension, because all these disorders are associated with an insulin-resistant state (80). The general treatment of diabetes mellitus is beyond this discussion, but a description of the classes of pharmacologic agents and brief strategies for treatment has been provided in a prior review (1).

LIPID METABOLISM AND CARDIOVASCULAR DISEASE

Elevation in low-density lipoprotein (LDL) cholesterol and depression of high-density lipoprotein (HDL) cholesterol are the two important risk factors for CHD (81–84). Individuals with SCI are believed to have accelerated and premature CHD. Whiteneck and associates reported that cardiovascular diseases were the most frequent cause of death among patients with SCI more than 30 years after injury (46% of all deaths) and among those older than 60 years of age (35% of all deaths) (85). Using thallium scintillation stress testing, Bauman and coworkers found that asymptomatic CHD determined by upper-body exercise stress testing was present in 13 of 20 (65%) subjects with paraplegia (mean age, 52 years) and by dipyridamole infusion in 4 of 6 (67%) subjects with quadriplegia (mean age, 47 years) (86,87). Budoff and colleagues, using electron beam computed tomography, reported that the mean coronary artery calcium score of a group of 27 subjects with SCI was significantly greater than in a control group (88). Because these studies were of a relatively small sample size, a larger cohort in a future study is needed to determine more accurately the prevalence of CHD in the population with SCI (86–88). The lipid profile in patients with SCI should be determined, and if indicated, appropriate management to reduce risk for CHD should be instituted.

About 10% of the U.S. population has HDL cholesterol values less than 35 mg/dL, which is an independent risk factor for CHD, whereas about 24% to 40% of those with SCI have levels below this value (67,78,89–92). In subjects with SCI and in controls, a strong inverse correlation has been demonstrated between serum triglycerides and HDL cholesterol (67). This inverse relationship may reflect the effects of elevated plasma insulin (93,94). Indeed, a significant relationship was shown between serum HDL cholesterol and insulin sensitivity as determined by the minimal model method (67). Lower levels of serum HDL cholesterol have been found in subjects with chronic tetraplegia, relative to those with paraplegia, and subjects with motor complete injury have lower values of serum HDL cholesterol than those with incomplete injury for either category of level of lesion (66) (Fig. 11.2). Although men with SCI have been reported to have lower serum HDL cholesterol levels than controls, there was no significant difference found for women, who were predominantly premenopausal (92). Whites and Latinos with SCI had lower serum HDL cholesterol levels than ethnicity-matched able-bodied controls, whereas African Americans did not demonstrate any significant association of SCI with serum HDL cholesterol levels (92). African Americans have significantly higher serum HDL cholesterol values and a lower ratio of serum total to HDL cholesterol than whites or Latinos, as in the able-bodied population (95). Serum lipoprotein (a), a potentially atherogenic and thrombogenic serum lipoprotein fraction, does not appear to be significantly affected by age, duration of SCI, or level and completeness of lesion (96).

An increased level of cardiopulmonary fitness has been demonstrated to positively influence the serum HDL cholesterol level in subjects with or without SCI (67,80,90,97,98). Activity, independent of lipid values or other risk factors for CHD, may be an independent risk factor for CHD (99). Patients should be

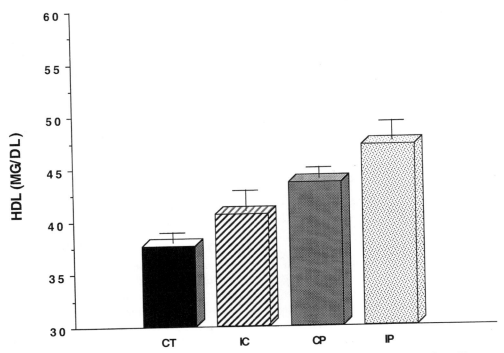

FIGURE 11.2. Serum high-density lipoprotein (HDL) cholesterol levels by neurologic deficit. CT, complete tetraplegia; IT, incomplete tetraplegia; CP, complete paraplegia; IP, incomplete paraplegia. All values are expressed in mean ± SEM. A significant inverse relationship was found for degree of neurologic deficit and serum HDL level (r = 0.19; *p* < 0.0001). (Drawn from data presented in Bauman WA, Adkins RH, Spungen AM, et al. The effect of residual neurological deficit on serum lipoproteins in individuals with chronic spinal cord injury. *Spinal Cord* 1998;36:13–17, with permission.)

strongly encouraged to reach and maintain the highest level of daily activity compatible with their injury.

In addition to immobilization, high-calorie or high-fat diets may increase plasma triglycerides and depress serum HDL cholesterol (100). Excessive alcohol intake may also depress serum HDL cholesterol levels (101). Mild to moderate alcohol consumption has been reported to increase serum HDL cholesterol levels (102). However, in obese subjects, this effect of alcohol to raise serum HDL cholesterol levels may not occur (103). Cigarette smoking has also been shown to be associated with insulin resistance and lower serum HDL cholesterol levels (104, 105). Current cigarette smoking is an independent risk factor for CHD and, when reduced or eliminated, decreases the risk for CHD (91). In a group of 250 male veterans with chronic SCI, Spungen and colleagues found that 76.8% had smoked cigarettes but only 31% were current smokers, which is comparable to the percentage of smokers reported in the general population (106,107). A low serum HDL cholesterol level is yet another medical indication to encourage a patient to avoid or discontinue cigarette smoking.

An inverse correlation generally exists between serum triglycerides and HDL cholesterol: the higher the triglycerides, the lower the HDL cholesterol (67,108). Persons with serum triglyceride concentrations above 200 to 250 mg/dL and HDL cholesterol values below 35 mg/dL should receive diet or pharmacologic therapy in an effort to raise the serum HDL cholesterol level. In individuals with hypertriglyceridemia, abstinence from alcohol should be achieved because drinking has been shown to raise serum triglyceride levels further (101,109). Several medications, including fibric acid derivatives, 3-hydroxy-3-methylglutaryl coenzyme A (HMG CoA) reductase inhibitors, and nicotinic acid, are available and effective by different mechanisms of action in raising the serum HDL cholesterol.

About 25% of the able-bodied population has an absolute elevation of the serum LDL cholesterol level. The level of serum LDL cholesterol in persons with SCI is similar to that reported in control groups. The recommendations of the National Cholesterol Education Program for therapy are based on the level of serum LDL cholesterol in association with the presence or absence of CHD or risk factors for CHD (91) (Table 11.2). Because persons with SCI may have at least two risk factors for CHD, or may have premature CHD, their target value for serum LDL cholesterol should reflect these considerations. A low-fat and low-cholesterol diet may be expected to reduce levels of serum LDL cholesterol between 10% and 20%. To maintain a therapeutic benefit, the patient must remain on diet therapy indefinitely. There are two classes of pharmacologic agents that are generally used to lower serum LDL cholesterol: HMG CoA reductase inhibitors and bile acid–binding resins. In the population with SCI, the bile acid–binding resins are less desirable because they may cause increased constipation and abdominal flatulence and interfere with the absorption of nutrients and medications as well as being less potent in their lipid-lowering potential.

TABLE 11.2. TREATMENT DECISIONS BASED ON LOW-DENSITY LIPOPROTEIN CHOLESTEROL LEVEL

	Patient Category	Initiation Level	LDL Goal
Dietary therapy	w/o CHD and <2 RFs	≥160 mg/dL	<160 mg/dL
	w/o CHD and ≥2 RFs	≥130 mg/dL	<130 mg/dL
	with CAD	>100 mg/dL	≤100 md/dL
Drug treatment	w/o CHD and <2 RFs	≥190 mg/dL	<160 mg/dL
	w/o CHD and ≥2 RFs	≥160 mg/dL	<130 mg/dL
	with CHD	≥130 mg/dL	≤100 md/dL

LDL, low-density lipoprotein cholesterol; w/o, without; RFs, risk factors.
From Expert Panel on Detection, Evaluation, and Treatment of High Blood Cholesterol in Adults (Adult Treatment Panel II). Summary of the Second Report of the National Cholesterol Education Program (NCEP). *JAMA* 1993;269:3015–3023, with permission.

The objective of the treatment of hyperlipidemia is to prevent or reduce the morbidity and mortality associated with CHD. To this end, several treatment programs in the general population have been reported to be successful (110–114). It is recommended that a complete lipid profile, including serum HDL cholesterol, be performed in all adults 20 years of age and older at least once every 5 years (91). If values exceed those recommended by the National Cholesterol Education Program, appropriate therapeutic intervention should be instituted (91).

BONE AND CALCIUM METABOLISM

Spinal cord injury produces immediate and permanent unloading of the gravity-bearing skeletal regions with structural and metabolic consequences. After acute immobilization, calciuria increases in 10 days, reaching a maximum between 1 and 6 months after injury (115–117). Hypercalcemia can occur in adults with acute SCI when bone resorption is increased in association with an impaired fractional excretion of calcium by the kidney. Multiple fractures place adults with SCI at increased risk for hypercalcemia. Children and adolescents with acute SCI may be particularly susceptible to hypercalcemia because of preexisting rapid bone turnover and elevated bone resorption (118). Other risk factors for hypercalcemia include recent paralysis, male gender, complete neurologic injury, high cervical injury, dehydration, and prolonged immobilization (116). The maximal urinary calcium level in those with SCI was between 2 to 4 times that of able-bodied subjects who were voluntarily placed on prolonged bed rest. Calciuria was not reduced by passive weight-bearing exercise or wheelchair activity (115). Mechanick and colleagues found that patients with complete SCI, compared with those with incomplete injury, had greater suppression of the parathyroid hormone (PTH)–vitamin D axis (119). After acute SCI, the PTH–vitamin D axis is suppressed with depressed PTH, 1,25-dihydroxyvitamin D, and nephrogenous cyclic adenosine monophosphate levels (120). Although urinary calcium was markedly elevated on a low-calcium diet (400 mg/d), increasing dietary calcium (to at least 1,160 mg/d) in a subset of subjects with acute SCI did not further increase either urinary or serum calcium concentrations (120). The finding of hypercalciuria and hypercalcemia after acute SCI has led to the misguided clinical practice of dietary restriction of calcium intake at time of acute injury, an ineffective and unnecessary intervention.

Symptoms of immobilization hypercalcemia usually develop relatively early after SCI, presenting between 4 and 8 weeks, but they may present earlier and up to 6 months after acute injury. The patients at increased risk for hypercalcemia have been previously mentioned, but it is worth reiterating that because of growth and the associated increased rate of bone turnover, children and young adults are at greatest risk. Hypercalcemia should be in the differential diagnosis of any patient with acute or subacute SCI who presents with nausea, vomiting, anorexia, fatigue, lethargy, polydipsia, polyuria, or dehydration (116). Serum calcium values should be followed with appropriate monitoring of the serum albumin concentration. In catabolic states, when reduction of the serum albumin concentration occurs, established formulas may be used for the correction of the total serum calcium values to estimate the biologically active free calcium level. However, a more direct and accurate approach would be to measure serially the ionized calcium concentration.

Treatment of hypercalcemia initially consists of fluids, intravenous normal saline at 100 to 150 ml/hr as tolerated, to enhance urinary excretion of calcium. While receiving intravenous fluid therapy, if bladder management is by intermittent catheterization, placement of an indwelling Foley catheter is recommended. To enhance calcium excretion, only if fluid balance can be meticulously determined, furosemide therapy may be considered once rehydration has been achieved. Additional medications and treatments have been used in attempts to lower the serum calcium concentration, including glucocorticoids, calcitonin, and etidronate (116,121). Recently, pamidronate administration (30 to 90 mg intravenously over 4 to 24 hours) has been used with efficacy (122,123). The advantages of pamidronate therapy include its rapid effectiveness in reducing the serum calcium level and that usually only a single dose is required, rather than the need for long-term intravenous fluids or oral medication administration.

Histomorphometry performed in rat models after immobilization suggests that bone loss occur in two phases, each by different mechanisms. In the first phase, which is the period immediately after immobilization (124,125), increased osteoclastic activity is evident, with peak activity between 3 and 5 days. There is a disruption of trabecular architecture, with loss of trabeculae and loss of connections between trabeculae. Bone resorption in the rat returns to normal levels by about 10 days of immobilization (126). During the second phase, which is characterized by a slower loss of bone, diminished osteoblastic activity appears to be responsible for the major fraction of bone loss. Chronic states of skeletal unloading result in a reduced pool of osteogenic cells within the bone marrow (127). The mechanisms by which the physical stress and strain placed on bone are transduced into bone cellular activity have not been elucidated.

A dramatic reduction in bone mineral content (BMC) and bone mineral density (BMD) has been amply documented in persons with chronic SCI (128–130). Osteoporosis generally involves the pelvis and lower extremities in persons with paraplegia, whereas bone is lost in the upper extremities as well in those with tetraplegia (131–135). In persons with incomplete SCI of the Brown-Séquard type, the mean bone density of the paretic knees was lower than that of the stronger knees, with leg strength and bone density moderately correlated (134). Bauman and colleagues studied eight pairs of male identical twins, one of whom had paraplegia (average duration of injury, 16 ± 9 years) (131). In the twins with paraplegia compared with their co-twins, there was a loss of bone density in the pelvis and lower extremities. The depletion of bone mineral appeared to be progressive over decades after injury. Garland and associates studied bone density in women with SCI stratified by age: less than or equal to 30 years, 31 to 50 years, and older than 50 years of age (132,133). Bone loss was greatest at the knee, with a loss of about 40% in the two premenopausal groups and about 50% in the postmenopausal group. Bone density of the hip was reduced by about 20% in the younger age group and by about 30% in the older age groups. Although the lumbar spine was slightly reduced in women in the younger group, density was increased about 10% in the women in the middle age group and further increased by 25% in the oldest women compared with controls. Perhaps the vertebral column in paralysis is generally spared bone loss because of its continued weight bearing function (135). However, a potentially confounding consideration is the possibility that the increase in vertebral BMD by dual-energy x-ray absorptiometry is an artifact due to neuropathic osteoarthropathy (loss of disk space, bone sclerosis, fragmentation, osteophytosis, and subluxation), masking actual vertebral osteoporosis (136). Deformities of the spine that reduce normal weightbearing on the vertebral bodies may place an individual with SCI at greater risk for osteoporosis of the spine (137–139). In the absence of spine deformity, a significant loss of spine density in a person with SCI would be unexpected, and thus secondary causes of osteoporosis should be considered.

Osteoporosis and increased risk for fractures are well-established complications of chronic SCI. Pathologic fractures of the long bones occur in individuals with SCI after negligible stress or trauma, such as during transfer maneuvers, range-of-motion exercises, bending, or minor falls. Several studies have addressed lower extremity fractures in patients with SCI (140–144). Attempts to improve bone mass and strength by modulating muscle tone, activity, or weightbearing have yielded negligible benefits (145–149).

Although disuse may be the primary cause of osteopenia in persons with SCI, there is reason to believe that nutritional deficiencies may be contributory, particularly involving calcium and vitamin D. Because of the tendency for calcium nephrolithiasis soon after acute SCI, individuals with chronic SCI are often instructed to restrict calcium intake, chiefly dairy products. This dietary restriction may also result in vitamin D deficiency because dairy products, especially milk, are fortified with vitamin D and generally serve as the main source of dietary intake of vitamin D (150). In addition, those with SCI may have reduced sunlight exposure or may receive anticonvulsants and other medications that induce hepatic microsomal enzymes, accelerating vitamin D metabolism (151–153). Regardless of the mechanism, reduced calcium and vitamin D intake would be expected to lower the serum calcium concentration and stimulate the release of PTH, resulting in increased bone resorption and accentuation of osteopenia. Bauman and colleagues reported that subjects with chronic SCI, relative to control subjects, had significantly lower 25-hydroxyvitamin D levels, the major storage form of vitamin D, which was negatively correlated with serum PTH (154). Serum 1,25-dihydroxyvitamin D levels were significantly elevated in patients with chronic SCI and positively correlated with PTH levels, suggesting a state of secondary hyperparathyroidism and associated increased bone turnover.

Bisphosphonates, which are analogues of pyrophosphate, markedly inhibit osteoclastic activity. This class of agents reduces osteoclast number by inhibition of osteoblast recruitment, adhesion, and lifespan as well as by reducing osteoclast activity. The utility of these agents, especially alendronate, has been demonstrated in the treatment of diseases with increased bone turnover. Animal studies have suggested that bisphosphonates reduce bone loss after skeletal unloading (155,156). Although removed from the market because of incidental reports of associated myeloproliferative disorders, disodium dichloromethylene diphosphate, when administered soon after acute SCI (therapy initiated on average within 17 to 18 days of injury), ablated resorptive hypercalciuria and prevented loss of BMC of the tibia and femur (157). Administration of tiludronate, a bisphosphonate, to subjects with paraplegia has been shown to reduce bone resorption by reducing the number of osteoclasts without impairing bone formation (158). The role of bisphosphonates in the treatment of bone loss in acute and chronic SCI remains to be defined. In the general able-bodied population, menopause is associated with osteoporosis of estrogen-sensitive bone, often initially presenting as fractures of vertebrae that consist predominantly of trabecular bone (159). In postmenopausal compared with premenopausal women with SCI, relatively more bone appears to be lost at the hip and knee, which is primarily cortical bone (132). Conceivably, estrogen and other antiresorptive agents, such as calcitonin and bisphosphonates, used to treat able-bodied women with postmenopausal osteoporosis, should be prescribed for postmenopausal women with SCI in an effort to reduce the osteopenia of the lower extremities (132,160,161).

THYROID FUNCTION

Any condition of traumatic stress in which caloric intake is reduced, especially a reduction of carbohydrate intake, will be associated with changes in serum thyroid hormone levels that have been referred to as several syndromes that are synonymous, including "low T_3," "euthyroid sick," or "systemic nonthyroidal illness" (162,163). Medications, specifically corticosteroid administration, frequently prescribed immediately after injury, may also alter serum thyroid hormone levels (164). Thus, acute SCI may be associated with thyroid function test changes.

Bugaresti and coworkers compared thyroid function tests in 18 patients with acute SCI and patients with spinal fractures without SCI (165). In the acute SCI group, but not in the acute spinal fracture group, transient reduction in serum triiodothyronine (T_3) was observed; reverse triiodothyronine (rT_3) was increased immediately after injury and persisted at day 7, suggesting a reduction in 5'-deiodinase activity. Claus-Walker and associates noted that T_3 and thyroxine (T_4) levels remained depressed for 2 to 6 months after traumatic tetraplegia (166). In a subsequent report, these investigators noted a depression in serum T_4 levels for only 2 months after injury that normalized thereafter (167). Low serum T_3 levels with relatively normal serum T_4 levels were reported by Prakash for 3 months after acute SCI, with greater depression in serum T_3 levels in those with higher cord lesions (168). In another report, patients with serum low T_3 levels were noted to have elevated serum rT_3 levels, confirming the syndrome (169).

After acute stress, there may also be associated changes in thyroid hormone binding that may lower serum thyroid hormone levels, although this has not been adequately studied in patients with SCI (170). Despite some controversy, current consensus holds that the low T_3 syndrome does not require treatment with replacement thyroid hormone, even though the observed changes may be dramatic and suggest hypothyroidism (171). There may be pituitary suppression of thyroid-stimulating hormone (TSH) release related to the stress of the illness, with a transient increase in serum TSH during the recovery phase (172). Indeed, in patients with diabetes mellitus and in fasting animals, there appears to be a decrease in the binding of T_3 to nuclear receptors and a reduction in postreceptor hormonal effects (173,174). Animal studies have suggested that functional recovery is improved if exogenous T_3 or thyrotropin-releasing hormone (TRH) is administered soon after acute SCI (175, 176). Administration of T_3 may have an effect on the neurons themselves, whereas the effect of TRH may be to attenuate a secondary mechanism of injury.

In subgroups of patients with chronic SCI, thyroid function tests have been associated with changes reminiscent of acute or chronic illness. In a study of 30 subjects with chronic SCI, mean serum T_3 and T_4 levels were lower, whereas T_3 resin uptake values were higher than those in able-bodied controls (177). The higher T_3 resin-binding capacity suggests increased binding of serum T_3 to thyroid-binding globulin (TBG). In nonthyroidal

systemic illness, TBG is usually within the normal range, but there appears to be a circulating inhibitor of serum binding of thyroid hormone, which is associated with a low thyroid hormone binding to TBG and the resin (178). In patients with active medical conditions, such as pressure ulcers, urinary tract infection, or pulmonary infection, a low T_3 syndrome was found. Of note, even when the group with SCI without coexistent medical conditions with normal serum T_3 levels were compared with the control group, those with SCI had lower serum T_3 levels (177). Serum TSH levels were generally in the normal range, which suggests a euthyroid state (177).

In a report of 63 men with SCI by Wang and colleagues, about 11% had low serum T_3 levels with normal serum T_4 and TSH levels (179). Patients with tetraplegia had lower serum T_3 levels than did those with paraplegia (179). Often, the prevalence of coexistent medical complications is increased in patients with higher cord lesions, which may result in a reduction in 5'-deiodinase activity and euthyroid sick syndrome. Huang and associates reported that the TSH response to TRH was normal in the SCI group as a whole (180). However, in a subgroup of eight, of the thirty subjects with SCI, the TSH and prolactin responses were elevated to TRH provocative stimulation, suggesting a reduction in central dopaminergic tone (180). Zeitzer and coworkers found that in two subjects with paraplegia and in two of three subjects with tetraplegia, circadian rhythm of TSH release was normally timed (181). Zhong and Bauman found no significant difference in T_3 or TSH levels between the SCI and non-SCI subjects in nine pairs of identical twins (unpublished observation). This study controlled for genetic variability in levels of thyroid hormone and suggests that thyroid function is normal in healthy, relatively young people with chronic SCI.

ADRENAL FUNCTION

Zeitzer and coworkers studied the circadian rhythm of serum cortisol levels with frequent blood sampling for 24 hours and found that both the 24-hour average and the circadian amplitude of the cortisol rhythm in patients with SCI were similar to those in able-bodied subjects (181). Other investigators have found a spectrum of results from low to high cortisol concentrations in subjects with SCI; however, these studies usually relied on one or two blood collections that may not accurately reflect secretion because of the inherent pulsatility of hormone release (182–186). Claus-Walker and colleagues found an altered circadian rhythm (185), but Nicholas and associates demonstrated a normal circadian rhythm (186).

The question arises as to whether appropriate release of cortisol occurs in response to stress in patients with SCI. An animal study suggests that afferent nerve feedback may also have an effect on cortisol secretion, a connection that would be absent in those with SCI (187). The purpose of dynamic studies of hypothalamic–pituitary–adrenal axis function is to define abnormalities in the functional relationships between the elements of the axis that may not be reflected in basal secretion. A problem with relying on observations of unstimulated plasma hormone levels as the basis for diagnosis of adrenal insufficiency is that hormone secretion is episodic, and a single value within the range of normal is inconclusive. Furthermore, a normal 8 a.m. serum cortisol value does not assess hypothalamic–pituitary–adrenal axis reserve.

Huang and associates performed provocative stimulation testing with corticotropin-releasing hormone or insulin-induced hypoglycemia in 25 men with SCI and 25 age-matched able-bodied men (188). The adrenocorticotropic hormone (ACTH) response to corticotropin-releasing hormone was less in patients with SCI than in the controls but did not reach significance. The cortisol response was significantly less in those with SCI, a difference that was obliterated if a correction for baseline values was made. Of the 25 subjects, 6 subjects failed to elicit a cortisol response to insulin-induced hypoglycemia associated with an absent or minimal ACTH response; another 11 subjects had a maximal cortisol response that was below the lower limit of normal. Wang and Huang tested adrenal reserve in men with SCI with an ACTH stimulation test of either high (200 μg) or low (1 μg) dose (189). These investigators found that there was a high prevalence of impaired adrenal reserve in patients with chronic SCI and concluded that the low-dose test is more sensitive for detecting subclinical adrenal insufficiency.

Although limited, these provocative studies of adrenal function suggest that a subset of patients with SCI may have an inadequate response to stress. However, it is appreciated that extrapolation from provocative testing of adrenal function to the physiologic ACTH–adrenal axis response to catastrophic stress is difficult (190). To address this concern adequately, it would be necessary to study patients with SCI who are under actual states of stress, such as during surgery, hypotension, or medical catastrophe, to more clearly elucidate whether adrenal replacement therapy is indicated. Given our present lack of knowledge of the adrenal response to life-threatening conditions in those with tetraplegia, if hypotension unresponsive to appropriate medical management occurs, the diagnosis of relative adrenal insufficiency may be considered with the administration of a glucocorticoid in high physiologic doses only during maximal stress, with subsequent rapid tapering of the dose.

SODIUM AND WATER METABOLISM

The orthostatic reflex that maintains blood pressure during upright posture by peripheral sympathetic system activation is absent in patients with complete tetraplegia. As such, because the normal increase in catecholamine release observed in able-bodied subjects is not present in patients with SCI, other homeostatic mechanisms must be operative to maintain blood pressure with upright position.

Mathias and coworkers noted a blunted plasma noradrenaline release and higher plasma renin activity to head-up tilt in subjects with tetraplegia than those in able-bodied subjects; there was a rise in plasma aldosterone, albeit delayed (191). In a subsequent report, Mathias and colleagues confirmed their earlier observations and, because values for plasma renin activity were unaffected by propranolol administration during upright posture, suggested that renin release is dependent on activation of renal vascular receptors and independent of the sympathetic nervous system (192). In subjects with tetraplegia, but not in able-bodied controls, sitting upright produced reductions in arterial blood pressure and a significant increase in plasma aldosterone and renin activity for identical changes in plasma osmolarity (193). Krooner and colleagues showed that blood pressure fell with upright posture in subjects with tetraplegia, unlike those with paraplegia and able-bodied controls (194). Plasma renin activity and aldosterone were higher with an associated fall in urinary sodium excretion in those with tetraplegia when sitting than in those with paraplegia or controls; in contrast to the other two groups, in those with tetraplegia, urine volume decreased with upright posture and increased with recumbency.

The effects of dietary sodium on plasma renin activity was studied in subjects with SCI. Plasma renin activity was higher at baseline and increased more rapidly to higher values in response to sodium restriction in subjects with tetraplegia than in those with paraplegia (195). Of interest, plasma atrial natriuretic peptide was higher in the group with tetraplegia during sodium loading or restriction (195). Caution is advised when treating patients with tetraplegia with an angiotensin-converting enzyme inhibitor because of the potential for catastrophic hypotension, as was reported in one case of an individual with volume depletion (196). Several studies have demonstrated that head-up tilt maneuver is associated with a several-fold rise in plasma vasopressin levels, in contrast to any noticeable rise in controls. This is likely due to the observed fall in blood pressure, a more potent stimulus to vasopressin release than is an elevated serum osmolality (197–199). Of note, patients with tetraplegia had vascular sensitivity to the pressor effects of intravenous infusion of vasopressin with a moderate elevation in mean arterial blood pressure, whereas controls did not (199).

Hypoosmolar hyponatremia has been reported to occur fairly frequently in patients with SCI (200). Often, patients with SCI are instructed to drink relatively large volumes of fluids (e.g., 3 to 6 L/d), but this should not result in dilutional hyponatremia because of the ability of the normal kidney to excrete much greater amounts of free water. Acute illness or stress in able-bodied subjects may stimulate the release of vasopressin, decreasing free water clearance, and this may have also been the case in those with SCI (201). In patients with tetraplegia with or without a history of hyponatremia, during maximal water diuresis when plasma vasopressin levels were suppressed, a reduction in osmolar clearance, free water clearance, and distal delivery of filtrate was demonstrated (200,202). In addition to an intrarenal defect in water handling, in subjects with hyponatremia, a resetting of the osmostat was noted, with plasma vasopressin rising before plasma osmolality reached the normal range to a hypertonic saline infusion (200,203). In a case report of a person with tetraplegia with hyponatremia who presented with a low threshold for vasopressin release, the threshold for release corrected to normal by a period of fluid restriction and restoration of the plasma osmolality to physiologic levels (204). Ample evidence exists to suggest that in patients with tetraplegia, there is a reduction in free water clearance in upright posture due to both vasopressin-dependent and vasopressin-independent mechanisms.

ANABOLIC HORMONES

Testosterone and growth hormone are anabolic hormones that have potent effects on protein preservation as well as specific hormonal functions necessary for optimal health and function. Testosterone has effects on muscle that differentiate male and female pubertal development. It is also important to realize that, during adulthood, testosterone has beneficial effects on a multiplicity of other tissues, including bone, fat, liver, kidney (erythropoietin production), and brain. Growth hormone has obvious developmental effects on bone and soft tissues. In the adult, growth hormone continues to exert a profound salutary influence on body composition, exercise tolerance and capacity, lipids, general metabolism, and the psyche. There is also an apparent synergistic interaction between testosterone and growth hormone that stimulates release and function. Thus, a deficiency state of one or both of these hormones has the potential for adverse consequences. Indeed, patients with SCI have body compositional changes that are similar to those reported in elderly people, including loss of lean tissue and increase of fat tissue mass. Strong correlations between altered body composition and the level of SCI have been observed. Although there were no differences in body weight between groups, successively higher complete spinal cord lesions were associated with decreasing lean body mass and body cell mass, as well as increasing body fat (205) (Fig. 11.3). The percentage of body fat in patients with SCI may be as much as 60 percent greater than in matched able-bodied controls (206). In an identical twin study, with one co-twin in each pair having SCI, Spungen and associates reported a loss of total body lean tissue that was continuous and directly

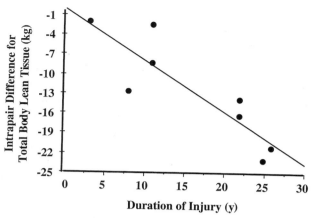

FIGURE 11.4. Associations between total body lean tissue and duration of injury. Total body lean tissue loss is represented by the intrapair difference (IPD) score: paralyzed twin − able-bodied twin (R = 0.87; slope = −0.782 ± 0.81; $p < 0.005$). (From Spungen AM, Wang J, Pierson RN Jr, et al. Soft tissue body composition differences in monozygotic twins discordant for spinal cord injury. *J Appl Physiol* 2000;88: 1310–1315, with permission.)

correlated with duration of injury (207) (Fig 11.4). Mollinger and colleagues demonstrated a correlation between level of SCI and degree of reduction in basal energy expenditure from predicted (208). Spungen and coworkers found that individuals with chronic paraplegia had a significant linear relationship between measures of lean body mass and energy expenditure (209). Related to these adverse body composition changes and inactiv-

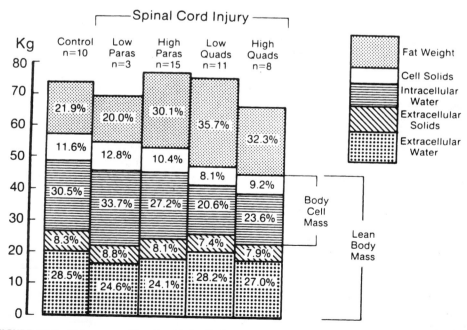

FIGURE 11.3. Body composition in able-bodied controls and four groups of subjects with complete spinal cord injury. Significant correlations were observed between higher levels of injury and diminishing lean body mass as well as increasing body fat. (From Rasmann Nulicek DN, Spurr GB, Barboriak JJ, et al. Body composition of patients with spinal cord injury. *Eur J Clin Nutr* 1988;42:765–773, with permission.)

ity, patients with SCI have a pattern of metabolic changes that is artherogenic, with adverse lipid changes, a reduction in metabolic rate, glucose intolerance, and insulin resistance (3,4,66–68, 92,109).

Although the literature provides conflicting data, there are subsets of men with SCI with relative or absolute androgen deficiency (210–215). The etiology of a relative deficiency of testosterone in those with SCI has not been elucidated. However, it is conceivable that prolonged sitting and euthermia of the scrotal sac and testis may itself have a deleterious local effect on testosterone production as well as on sperm development and ultimate function (216). In a group of 20 healthy subjects with SCI, Tsitouras and coworkers reported that a subset had reduced serum totals and free testosterone levels without a significant increase in serum gonadotropin concentrations (214). Of note, in those with SCI, serum testosterone levels did not decrease with age, as was observed in the able-bodied men, but did significantly decrease with duration of SCI (214). The lack of an age-associated finding in this study may have been because of the relatively small sample size and because the group with SCI already had low serum testosterone levels at younger ages. Bauman and associates reported that the mean serum testosterone level was significantly lower in those with SCI, relative to a control group, with a significantly greater percentage of subjects with SCI having low testosterone levels, and that serum testosterone levels declined with age (215). Wang and colleagues also reported on a subset of subjects with SCI who had low serum testosterone levels, but none had increased serum gonadotropin levels (179). In one report, direct stimulation of the testes for 2 days with pharmacologic levels of chorionic gonadotropin produced testosterone release similar to that in able-bodied controls (217). These studies suggest that in the subset of patients with SCI and hypogonadism, the defect may be pituitary in origin. It should be noted that acute or chronic illness has an adverse effect on serum testosterone levels. Furthermore, several medications are known to affect pituitary or testicular secretory function, such as psychotropic medications (218,219). Additional investigation should address paracrine factors within the testes as well as more subtle changes of the hypothalamus–pituitary–testicular axis in those with hypogonadism.

Growth hormone and its second messenger, insulin-like growth factor-I (IGF-I), have been reported to be depressed in patients with SCI. Bauman and colleagues reported a blunted growth hormone release, in subjects with SCI, to provocative stimulation with intravenous arginine (220). The average plasma IGF-I level was significantly lower in patients with SCI who were younger than 45 years of age than in able-bodied controls of the same age group (220). Similarly, Shetty and associates reported that the average plasma IGF-I level in patients with tetraplegia was depressed compared with ambulatory controls (221). In patients with postpoliomyelitis syndrome, lower plasma IGF-I levels were found to be a potent discriminator of those who had decreased capacity to perform activities of daily living, reduced functional independence, and increased pain (222). Thus, it would appear likely that a depression in plasma IGF-I in patients with SCI may have clinical associations in terms of reduced functional capacity. Furthermore, there appears to be a significant nonlinear relationship between plasma IGF-

I and serum total testosterone concentrations in healthy individuals with SCI (214). It is possible that growth hormone or IGF-I enhances testosterone secretion, as has been shown in animals, but the converse may also be operative, as has been demonstrated in adolescent males and adults (223–226). Baclofen, a frequently prescribed antispasmotic medication presumably acting centrally, has been reported to increase growth hormone release to provocative stimulation and normalizes plasma IGF-I levels in persons with SCI (227).

In the able-bodied population, replacement therapy for testosterone or growth hormone deficiency has been performed. Testosterone administration to elderly men has been associated with favorable body composition changes directly related to dose and duration of therapy, including an increase in lean mass and reduction of fat mass (228,229). In a study of older men with truncal obesity, testosterone therapy resulted in a 9.1% decline in visceral fat mass, with an associated fall in fasting serum glucose concentration (230). Testosterone replacement in older men was associated with a significant decrease in serum total and LDL cholesterol levels without a significant change in serum HDL cholesterol levels (231,232). In contrast, in young men with hypogonadism, physiologic testosterone tends to depress HDL cholesterol levels (233). Thus, it may be possible to reduce cardiovascular risk with physiologic replacement of testosterone in older men with relative deficiency states. As a separate concern, supraphysiologic levels of testosterone, while having a more favorable effect on body composition, are associated with an adverse lipid profile (234).

Exogenous administration of growth hormone has been demonstrated to have a beneficial effect in elderly people who have a relative growth hormone deficiency state (235–238), not dissimilar to those with SCI. This includes an increase in lean body tissue and a decrease in fat mass (235–238). Serum lipid values have been improved with growth hormone administration, with a reduction in LDL cholesterol and an elevation in HDL cholesterol levels, reducing cardiovascular risk (239,240). In addition, the metabolic rate increased after only 2 weeks of therapy with growth hormone, before any body composition changes, probably because of an increase in thyroid hormone levels (238,241, 242). The potential to reverse some of the adverse body composition, adverse lipid, and metabolic changes in those with SCI with growth hormone, growth hormone–releasing hormone analogues, or IGF-I administration remains to be investigated.

Another consideration is the exogenous administration of anabolic steroids for specific indications in patients with SCI. A recent report has demonstrated that oxandrolone administration increased diaphragm thickness by 11%, spirometry measures of pulmonary function by about 10%, maximal inspiratory and expiratory pressures by 12% to 24%, and fat-free mass by 5%; after therapy, the self-reported symptom of breathlessness decreased by more than 50% (243). Also, oxandrolone has been shown to be efficacious in accelerating healing of burns, and recently this agent has been suggested to be of use in healing of refractory pressure ulcers (244–246). Because lean body tissue is already depleted in patients with SCI, and the level of depletion is correlated with the level of neurologic deficit, serious illness may result in nitrogen wasting and muscle losses that may more rapidly lead to catastrophic respiratory events. Thus, the possibility exists that oral anabolic steroids may be efficacious for limited therapeutic interventions, especially when there is pulmonary compromise because of infection in patients with tetraplegia. Pressure ulcers that are refractory to healing (despite optimal nutrition and medical and surgical care) may also be an indication for a limited trial with these agents, although at present the therapeutic efficacy is unproved. Caution must be exercised whenever administering anabolic steroid agents. Oxandrolone, though, is generally associated with less hepatotoxicity than other drugs in this class because of its clinically relevant increased renal excretion (247). All oral anabolic steroid agents adversely affect the lipid profile (248,249). If prescribed for a relatively brief interval with a clear therapeutic endpoint, the benefits of therapy may outweigh the potential risks.

REFERENCES

1. Bauman, WA. Carbohydrate and lipid metabolism after spinal cord injury. *Top Spinal Cord Injury Rehabil* 1997;2:1–22.
2. Bauman WA, Adkins RH, Spungen AM, et al. The effect of residual neurological deficit on oral glucose tolerance in persons with chronic spinal cord injury. *Spinal Cord* 1999;37:765–771.
3. Bauman WA, Spungen AM. Disorders of carbohydrate and lipid metabolism in veterans with paraplegia or quadriplegia: a model of premature aging. *Metabolism* 1994;43:949–756.
4. Duckworth WC, Solomon SS, Jallepalli P, et al. Glucose intolerance due to insulin resistance in patients with spinal cord injuries. *Diabetes* 1980;29:906–910.
5. National Diabetes Data Group. Classification and diagnosis of diabetes mellitus and other categories of glucose intolerance. *Diabetes* 1979;28:1039–1057.
6. WHO Expert Committee on Diabetes Mellitus. Second report. *WHO Tech Rep Ser* No. 646, 1980.
7. The Expert Committee on the Diagnosis and Classification of Diabetes Mellitus. Report of the Expert Committee on the Diagnosis and Classification of Diabetes Mellitus. *Diabetes Care* 1997;20:1183–1197.
8. Harris MI, Hadden WC, Knowler WC, et al. Prevalence of diabetes and impaired glucose tolerance and plasma glucose levels in the US population aged 20 to 74 yrs. *Diabetes* 1987;36:523–534.
9. DeFronzo RA. The triumvirate: beta-cell muscle, liver-A collusion responsible for NIDDM. *Diabetes* 1988;37:667–687.
10. Eriksson J, Franssila-Kallunki A, Ekstrand A, et al. Early metabolic defects in persons at increased risk for non-insulin-dependent diabetes mellitus. *N Engl J Med* 1989;321:337–343.
11. Lillioja S, Mott DM, Spraul M, et al. Insulin resistance and insulin secretory dysfunction as precursors of NIDDM: prospective studies of Pima Indians. *N Engl J Med* 1993;329:1988–1992.
12. Warram JH, Martin BC, Krolewski AS, et al. Slow glucose removal rate and hyperinsulinemia precede the development of type II diabetes in the offspring of diabetic parents. *Ann Intern Med* 1990;113:909–915.
13. Campbell PJ, Mandarino LJ, Gerich JE, et al. Glucose uptake and response to insulin of the isolated rat diaphragm: the effect of denervation. *Diabetes* 1959;8:218–225.
14. Schmalbruch H, Al-Amood WS, Lewis DW. Morphology of long-term denervated rat soleus muscle and the effect of chronic electrical stimulation. *J Physiol* 1991;441:233–241.
15. Al-Amood WS, Lewis DM, Schmalbruch H. Effects of chronic electrical stimulation on contractile properties of long-term denervated rat skeletal muscle. *J Physiol* 1991;441:243–256.
16. Greve J, Muskat R, Schmidt B, et al. Functional electrical stimulation (FES): muscle histochemical analysis. *Paraplegia* 1994;31:764–770.
17. Grimby G, Broberg C, Krotkiewska I, et al. Muscle fiber composition in patients with traumatic cord lesion. *Scand J Rehab Med* 1976;8:37–42.
18. Sowell MO, Dutton SL, Buse MG. Selective in vitro reversal of the insulin resistance of glucose transport in denervated rat skeletal muscle. *Am J Physiol* 1989;257:E418–E425.
19. Turinsky J. Glucose and amino acid uptake by exercising muscles in vivo: effect of insulin, fiber population, and denervation. *Endocrinology* 1987;121:528–535.
20. Burant CF, Lemmon SK, Treutelaar MK, et al. Insulin resistance of denervated rat muscle: a model for impaired receptor-function coupling. *Am J Physiol* 1984;247:E657–E666.
21. Burant CF, Treutelaar MK, Buse MG. In vitro and in vivo activation of the insulin receptor kinase in control and denervated skeletal muscle. *J Biol Chem* 1986;261:8985–8993.
22. Didyk RB, Anton EE, Robinson KA, et al. Effect of immobilization on glucose transporter expression in rat hindlimb muscles. *Metabolism* 1994;42:1389–1394.
23. Henriksen EJ, Rodnick KJ, Mondon CE, et al. Effect of denervation or unweighting on GLUT-4 protein in rat soleus muscle. *J Appl Physiol* 1991;70:2322–2327.
24. Heydrick SJ, Ruderman NB, Kurowski TG, et al. Enhanced stimulation of diacyglycerol and lipid synthesis by insulin in denervated muscle: altered protein kinase C activity and possible link to insulin resistance. *Diabetes* 1991;40:1707–1711.
25. Castro MJ, Apple DF, Hillegass EA, et al. Influence of complete spinal cord injury on skeletal muscle cross-sectional area within the first 6 months of injury. *Eur J Appl Physiol Occup Physiol* 1999;80:373–378.
26. Castro MJ, Apple DF, Staron RS, et al. Influence of complete spinal cord injury on skeletal muscle within 6 mo of injury. *J Appl Physiol* 1999;86:350–358.
27. Baldi JC, Jackson RD, Moraille R, et al. Muscle atrophy is prevented in patients with acute spinal cord injury using functional electrical stimulation. *Spinal Cord* 1998;36:463–469.
28. Aksnes AK, Hjeltnes N, Wahlstrom EO, et al. Intact glucose transport in morphologically altered denervated skeletal muscle from quadriplegic patients. *Am J Physiol* 1996;271:E593–E600.
29. Lillioja S, Young AA, Cutler CL, et al. Skeletal muscle capillary density and fiber type are possible determinants of in vivo insulin resistance in man. *J Clin Invest* 1987;80:415–424.
30. Lipman RL, Raskin P, Love T, et al. Glucose intolerance during decreased physical activity in man. *Diabetes* 1972;21:101–107.
31. Lipman RL, Schnure JJ, Bradley EM, et al. Impairment of peripheral glucose utilization in normal subjects by prolonged bed rest. *J Lab Clin Med* 1970;76:221–230.
32. Helmrich SP, Ragland DR, Leung RW, et al. Physical activity and reduced occurrence of NIDDM. *N Engl J Med* 1991;325:147–152.
33. Manson JE, Nathan DM, Krolewski AS, et al. A prospective study of exercise and incidence of diabetes among US male physicians. *JAMA* 1992;268:63–67.
34. Stuart CA, Shangraw RE, Prince MJ, et al. Bedrest-induced insulin resistance occurs primarily in muscle. *Metabolism* 1988;37:802–806.
35. Misbin RI, Moffa AM, Kappy MS. Insulin binding to monocytes in obese patients treated with carbohydrate restriction and changes in physical activity. *J Clin Endocrinol Metab* 1983;56:273–278.
36. Richter EA, Kiens B, Mizuno M, et al. Insulin action in human thighs after one-legged immobilization. *J Appl Physiol* 1989;67:19–23.
37. Blotner H. Effect of prolonged physical inactivity on tolerance of sugar. *Arch Intern Med* 1945;75:39–44.
38. Goodyear, LJ, Hirshman MF, King PA, et al. Skeletal muscle plasma membrane glucose transport and glucose transporters after exercise. *J Appl Physiol* 1990;68:193–198.
39. Nesher R, Karl I, Kipnis DM. Dissociation of effects of insulin and contraction on glucose transport in rat epitrochlearis muscle. *Am J Physiol* 1985;249:C226–C232.
40. Ploug T, Galbo H, Richter EA. Increased muscle glucose uptake during contractions: no need for insulin. *Am J Physiol* 1984;247:E726–E731.
41. Campbell PJ, Mandarino LJ, Gerich JE. Quantification of the relative impairment in actions of insulin on hepatic glucose production and peripheral glucose uptake in NIDDM. *Metabolism* 1988;37:15–21.
42. Marigo S, Donadoni R. Diagnosis of diabetes mellitus and impaired

glucose tolerance. In: M Morsiani, ed. *Epidemiology and screening of diabetes.* Boca Raton, FL: CRC Press, 1989:27–28.

43. Yalow RS, Glick SM, Roth J, et al. Plasma insulin and growth hormone levels in obesity and diabetes. *Ann N Y Acad Sci* 1965;131:357–373.

44. Horton ES, Runge CF, Sims EA. Endocrine and metabolic effects of experimental obesity in man. *Recent Prog Horm Res* 1970;29:457–496.

45. Nagulesparan MPJ, Savage R, Unger R, et al. A simplified method using somatostatin to assess in vivo insulin resistance over a range of obesity. *Diabetes* 1980;28:1272–1284.

46. Rabinowitz D, Zierler KL. Forearm metabolism in obesity and its response to intra-arterial insulin: characterization of insulin resistance and evidence for adaptive hyperinsulinism. *J Clin Invest* 1962;41:2173–2181.

47. Hotamisligil GS, Murray DL, Choy LN, et al. TNF-α inhibits signaling from the insulin receptor. *Proc Natl Acad Sci U S A* 1994;91:4852–4858.

48. Krotkiewski M, Sjostrom L, Bjorntorp P, et al. Regional adipose tissue cellularity in relation to metabolism in young and middle-aged women. *Metabolism* 1975;24:703–710.

49. Stern J, Batchelor B, Hollander N, et al. Adipose cell size and immunoreactive insulin levels in obese and normal weight adults. *Lancet* 1972;2:948–951.

50. Olefsky JM. Decreased insulin binding to adipocytes and circulating monocytes from obese subjects. *J Clin Invest* 1976;57:1165–1172.

51. Olefsky JM. The insulin receptor: its role in insulin resistance of obesity and diabetes. *Diabetes* 1976;25:1154–1172.

52. Bjorntorp P. Metabolic implications of body fat distribution. *Diabetes Care* 1991;14:1132–1143.

53. DeFronzo RA, Ferrannini E. Insulin resistance: a multifaceted syndrome responsible for NIDDM, obesity, hypertension, dyslipidemia, and atherosclerotic cardiovascular disease. *Diabetes Care* 1991;14:173–194.

54. Kissebah AH, Vydelingum N, Murray R, et al. Relation of body fat distribution to metabolic complications of obesity. *J Clin Endocrinol Metab* 1982;54:254–260.

55. Randle P, Garland P, Hales C, et al. The glucose-fatty acid cycle: its role in insulin sensitivity and the metabolic disturbances of diabetes mellitus. *Lancet* 1963;1:785–789.

56. Reaven GM, Greenfield MS. Diabetic hypertriglyceridemia: evidence for three clinical syndromes. *Diabetes* 1981;30:66–75.

57. Salan L, Knittle J, Hirsch J. The role of adipose cell size and adipose tissue insulin sensitivity in the carbohydrate intolerance of human obesity. *J Clin Invest* 1968;47:153–165.

58. Vague J. The degree of masculine differentiation of obesities: a factor determining predisposition to diabetes, atherosclerosis, gout and uric calculus disease. *Am J Clin Nutr* 1956;4:20–34.

59. Vague J, Rubin P, Jubelin J, et al. Regulation of the adipose mass: Histometric and anthropometric aspects. In: Vague J, Boyer J, eds. *Regulation of the adipose tissue mass.* Amsterdam: Excerpta Medica, 1974:296.

60. Spungen AM, Bauman WA, Wang J, et al. Measurement of body fat in individuals with tetraplegia: a comparison of eight clinical methods. *Paraplegia* 1995;33:402–408.

61. Bauman WA, Maimen M, Langer O. An association between hyperinsulinemia and hypertension during the third trimester of pregnancy. *Am J Obstet Gynecol* 1988;159:446–450.

62. Bonora E, Zavaroni I, Alpi O, et al. Relationship between blood pressure and plasma insulin in non-obese and obese non-diabetic subjects. *Diabetologia* 1987;30:719–723.

63. Modan M, Halkin H, Almog S, et al. Hyperinsulinemia: a link between hypertension, obesity and glucose intolerance. *J Clin Invest* 1985;75:809–817.

64. Rose HG, Yalow RS, Schweitzer P, et al. Insulin as a potential factor influencing blood pressure in amputees. *Hypertension* 1986;8:793–800.

65. Welborn TA, Breckenridge A, Rubinstein AH, et al. Serum insulin in essential hypertension and in peripheral vascular disease. *Lancet* 1966;2:1136–1137.

66. Bauman WA, Adkins RH, Spungen AM, et al. The effect of residual neurological deficit on serum lipoproteins in individuals with chronic spinal cord injury. *Spinal Cord* 1998;36:13–17.

67. Bauman WA, Spungen AM, Zhong YG, et al. Depressed serum high density lipoprotein cholesterol levels in veterans with spinal cord injury. *Paraplegia* 1992;30:697–703.

68. Maki KC, Briones ER, Lanbein WE, et al. Associations between serum lipids and indicators of adiposity in men with spinal cord injury. *Paraplegia* 1995;33:102–109.

69. Yekutiel M, Brooks ME, Ohry A, et al. The prevalence of hypertension, ischemic heart disease and diabetes in traumatic spinal cord injured patients and amputees. *Paraplegia* 1989;27:58–62.

70. Vuorinen-Markkola H, Yki-Jarvinen H. Hyperuricemia and insulin resistance. *J Clin Endocrinol Metab* 1994;78:25–29.

71. Zhong YG, Levy E, Bauman WA. The relationships among serum uric acid, plasma insulin, and serum lipoproteins in subjects with spinal cord injury. *Horm Metab Res* 1995;27:292–285.

72. Haffner SM, Stern MP, Hazuda HP, et al. Cardiovascular risk factors in confirmed prediabetic individuals: does the clock for coronary heart disease start ticking before the onset of clinical diabetes? *JAMA* 1990;263:2893–2898.

73. Position statement: nutritional recommendations and principles for individuals with diabetes mellitus. *Diabetes Care* 1991;14:20–27.

74. Bourn DM, Mann JI, McSkimming BJ, et al. Impaired glucose tolerance and NIDDM: does a lifestyle intervention program have an effect? *Diabetes Care* 1994;17:1311–1319.

75. Pan X, Li G, Hu Y, et al. Effect of dietary and/or exercise interventions on incidence of diabetes in subjects with IGT: the Da-Qing IGT and diabetes study (abstract). *International Diabetes Federation Congress,* Kobe, Japan, November 1994.

76. Keen H, Jarrett RJ, McCartney P. The 10 year follow-up of the Bedford survey (1962-1972): glucose tolerance and diabetes. *Diabetologia* 1982;22:73–78.

77. Sartor G, Schersten B, Carlstrom S, et al. Ten-year follow-up of subjects with impaired glucose tolerance: prevention of diabetes by tolbutamide and diet regulation. *Diabetes* 1980;29:41–44.

78. Jarrett RJ, Keen H, Fuller JH, et al. Worsening to diabetes in men with impaired glucose tolerance ("borderline diabetes"). *Diabetologia* 1979;16:25–30.

79. Nolan JJ, Ludvik B, Beerdsen P, et al. Improvement in glucose tolerance and insulin resistance in obese subjects treated with troglitazone. *N Engl J Med* 1994;331:1188–1193.

80. Kersten S, Desvergne B, Wahli W. Roles of PPARs in health and disease. *Nature* 2000;405:421–424.

81. Castelli WP. Epidemiology of coronary heart disease: the Framingham study. *Am J Med* 1984;76(2A):4–12.

82. Castelli WP, Doyle JT, Gordon T, et al. HDL-cholesterol and other lipids in coronary heart disease: the cooperative lipoprotein phenotyping study. *Circulation* 1977;55:767–772.

83. Castelli WP, Leaf A. Identification and assessment of cardiac risk—an overview. *Cardiol Clin* 1985;3:171–178.

84. Goldbour U, Medalie JH. High density lipoprotein cholesterol and incidence of coronary heart disease: the Israeli ischemic heart disease study. *Am J Epidemiol* 1979;109:296–308.

85. Whiteneck GG, Charlifue SW, Frankel HL, et al. Mortality, morbidity, and psychosocial outcomes of persons spinal cord injured more than 20 years ago. *Paraplegia* 1992;30:617–630.

86. Bauman WA, Raza M, Machac J. Tomographic thallium[201] myocardial perfusion imaging after intravenous dipyridamole in asymptomatic subjects with quadriplegia. *Arch Phys Med Rehabil* 1993;74(7):740–744.

87. Bauman WA, Raza M, Spungen AM, et al. Cardiac stress testing with thallium-201 imaging reveals silent ischemia in individuals with paraplegia. *Arch Phys Med Rehabil* 1994;75:946–950.

88. Budoff MJ, Shariar A, Adkins RH, et al. Coronary atherosclerosis in persons with spinal cord injury. *J Spinal Cord Med* 2000;23:170(abst#22).

89. Brenes G, Dearwater S, Shapera R, et al. High density lipoprotein cholesterol concentrations in physically active and sedentary spinal cord injured patients. *Arch Phys Med Rehabil* 1986;67:445–450.

90. Hooker SP, Wells CL. Effects of low-and moderate-intensity training in spinal cord-injured persons. *Med Sci Sports Exerc* 1989;21:18–22.

91. Summary of the Second Report of the National Cholesterol Education Program (NCEP) Expert Panel on Detection, Evaluation, and Treatment of High Blood Cholesterol in Adults (Adult Treatment Panel II). *JAMA* 1993;269:3015–3023.

92. Bauman WA, Adkins RH, Spungen AM, et al. Is immobilization associated with an abnormal lipoprotein profile? Observations from a diverse cohort. *Spinal Cord* 1999;37:485–493.

93. Golay A, Zech L, Shi MZ, et al. High density lipoprotein (HDL) metabolism in noninsulin-dependent diabetes mellitus: measurement of HDL turnover using tritiated HDL. *J Clin Endocrinol Metab* 1987;65:512–518.

94. Reaven GM. NIDDM, abnormal lipoprotein metabolism, and atherosclerosis. *Metabolism* 1987;36[Suppl 1]:1–8.

95. Bauman WA, Adkins RH, Spungen AM, et al. Ethnicity effect on the serum lipid profile in persons with spinal cord injury. *Arch Phys Med* 1998;79:176–180.

96. Bauman WA, Adkins RH, Spungen AM, et al. Individuals with extreme inactivity do not have abnormal serum Lp(a) levels. *Horm Metab Res* 1998;30:601–603.

97. LaPorte RE, Brenes G, Dearwater S, et al. HDL cholesterol across a spectrum of physical activity from quadriplegia to marathon running [Letter]. *Lancet* 1983;1:1212–1213.

98. Hartung GH. Physical activity and high density lipoprotein cholesterol. *J Sports Med Phys Fitness* 1995;35:1–5.

99. Bauman A, Owen N. Habitual physical activity and cardiovascular risk factors. *Med J Aust* 1991;154:22–28.

100. Schlierf G, Reinhemer W, Stosberg V. Diurnal patterns of plasma triglycerides and free fatty acids in normal subjects and in patients with endogenous (type IV) hyperlipidemia. *Nutr Metabol* 1971;13:80–91.

101. Valimaki M, Taskinen MR, Ylikahri R, et al. Comparison of the effects of two different doses of alcohol on serum lipoproteins, HDL-subfractions and apolipoproteins A-I and A-II: a controlled study. *Eur J Clin Invest* 1988;18:472–480.

102. Hully S, Gordon S. Alcohol and high-density lipoprotein cholesterol: causal inference from diverse study designs. *Circulation* 1981;64(Suppl III):57–63.

103. Hagiage M, Marti C, Rigaud D, et al. Effect of a moderate alcohol intake on the lipoproteins of normotriglyceridemic obese subjects compared with normoponderal controls. *Metabolism* 1992;41:856–861.

104. Facchini FS, Hollenbeck CB, Jeppesen J, et al. Insulin resistance and cigarette smoking. *Lancet* 1992;339:1128–1130.

105. Criqui MH, Wallace RB, Heiss G, et al. Cigarette smoking and plasma high-density lipoprotein cholesterol. The Lipid Research Clinics Program Prevalence Study. *Circulation* 1980;62(Suppl 4):70–76.

106. Spungen AM, Almenoff PL, Alexander LR, et al. Prevalence of cigarette smoking in a group of male veterans with chronic spinal cord injury. *Mil Med* 1995;160:308–311.

107. Centers for Disease Control. Cigarette smoking among adults—United States. *MMWR Morb Mortal Wkly Rep* 1992;41:354–355.

108. Johansson J, Walldius G, Carlson LA. Close correlation between high-density lipoprotein and triglyceridemia in normotriglyceridemia. *J Int Med* 1992;232:43–51.

109. Steinberg D, Pearson TA, Kuller LH. Alcohol and atherosclerosis. *Ann Intern Med* 1991;114:967–976.

110. Frisk MH, Elo O, Haapa K, et al. Helsinki Heart Study. Primary-prevention trial with gemfibrozil in middle-aged men with dyslipidemia: safety of treatment, changes in risk factors, and incidence of coronary heart disease. *N Engl J Med* 1987;317:1237–1245.

111. Randomized trial of cholesterol lowering in 444 patients with coronary heart disease: the Scandinavian Simvastatin Survival Study (4S). *Lancet* 1994;344:1383–1389.

112. Shepherd J, Cobbe SM, Ford I, et al. Prevention of coronary heart disease with pravastatin in men with hypercholesterolemia. *N Engl J Med* 1995;333:1301–1307.

113. The Lipid Research Clinics Coronary Primary Prevention Trial results. I. Reduction in incidence of coronary heart disease. *JAMA* 1984;251:351–364.

114. The Lipid Research Clinics Coronary Primary Prevention Trial results. II. The relationship of reduction in incidence of coronary heart disease to cholesterol lowering. *JAMA* 1984;251:365–374.

115. Claus-Walker J, Campos RJ, Carter RE, et al. Calcium excretion in quadriplegia. *Arch Phy Med Rehabil* 1972;53:14–18.

116. Maynard FM. Immobilization hypercalcemia following spinal cord injury. *Arch Phys Med Rehabil* 1986;67:41–44.

117. Naftchi NE, Viau AT, Sell GH, et al. Mineral metabolism in spinal cord injury. *Arch Phy Med Rehabil* 1980;61:139–142.

118. Tori JA, Hill LL. Hypercalcemia in children with spinal cord injury. *Arch Phys Med Rehabil* 1978;59:443–447.

119. Mechanick JI, Pomerantz F, Flanagan S, et al. Parathyroid hormone suppression in spinal cord injury patients is associated with the degree of neurologic impairment and not the level of injury. *Arch Phys Med Rehabil* 1997;78:692–696.

120. Stewart AF, Adler M, Byers CM, et al. Calcium homeostasis in immobilization: an example of resorptive hypercalciuria. *N Engl J Med* 1982;306:1136–1140.

121. Meythaler JM, Tuel SM, Cross LL. Successful treatment of immobilization hypercalcemia using calcitonin and etidronate. *Arch Phys Med Rehabil* 1993;74:316–319.

122. Kedlaya D, Brandstatrer ME, Lee JK. Immobilization hypercalcemia in incomplete paraplegia: successful treatment with pamidronate. *Arch Phys Med Rehabil* 1998;79:222–225.

123. Massagli TL, Cardenas DD. Immobilization hypercalcemia treatment with pamidronate disodium after spinal cord injury. *Arch Phys Med Rehabil* 1999;80:998–1000.

124. Baron R, Vignery A, Lang R. Reversal phase and osteopenia: defective coupling of resorption to formation in the pathogenesis of osteoporosis. In: Frost HF, Jee WSS, Johnston CC, eds. *Osteoporosis: recent advances in pathogenesis and treatment.* Baltimore: University Park Press, 1981:311–320.

125. Tran Van P, Vignery A, Baron R. Cellular kinetics of the bone remodeling sequence in the rat. *Anat Rec* 1982;202:445–451.

126. Weinreb M, Rodan GA, Thompson DD. Osteopenia in the immobilized rat hind limb is associated with increased bone resorption and decreased bone formation. *Bone* 1984;10:123–128.

127. Manolagas SC, Jilka RL. Bone marrow, cytokines and bone remodeling. *N Engl J Med* 1995;332:305–311.

128. Biering-Sorensen F, Bohr H, Schaadt O. Bone mineral content of the lumbar spine and lower extremities years after spinal cord lesion. *Paraplegia* 1988;26:293–301.

129. Garland DE, Maric Z, Adkins R, et al. Bone mineral density about the knee in spinal cord injured patients with pathologic fractures. *Contemp Orthop* 1993;26:375–379.

130. Griffiths HJ, Zimmerman RE. The use of photon densitometry to evaluate bone mineral in a group of patients with spinal cord injury. *Paraplegia* 1973;10:279–284.

131. Bauman WA, Spungen AM, Wang J, et al. Continuous loss of bone during chronic immobilization: a monozygotic twin study. *Osteoporos Int* 1999;10:123–127.

132. Garland DE, Adkins RH, Ashford R, et al. Regional osteoporosis in females with complete spinal cord injury. *J Bone Joint Surg* (in press).

133. Garland DE, Adkins RH. Bone loss at the knee in spinal cord injury. *Topics in Spinal Cord Inj Rehabil* 2001;6:37–46.

134. Garland DE, Foulkes G, Adkins RH, et al. Regional osteoporosis following incomplete spinal cord injury. *Contemp Orthop* 1994;28:134–138.

135. Garland DE, Stewart CA, Adkins RH, et al. Osteoporosis after spinal cord injury. *J Orthop Res* 1992;10:371–378.

136. Jaovisidha S, Sartoris DJ, Martin EME, et al. Influence of sponylopathy on bone densitometry using dual energy x-ray absorptiometry. *Calcif Tissue Int* 1997;60:424–429.

137. Healey JH, Lane JM. Structural scoliosis in osteoporotic women. *Clin Orthop* 1985;195:216–223.

138. Velis KP, Healey JH, Schneider, R. Osteoporosis in unstable adult scoliosis. *Clin Orthop* 1988;237:132–141.
139. Velis KP, Healey JH, Schneider, R. Peak skeletal mass assessment in young adults with idiopathic scoliosis. *Spine* 1989;14:706–711.
140. Comarr AE, Hutchinson RH, Bors E. Extremity fractures of patients with spinal cord injuries. *Am J Surg* 1962;103:732–739.
141. Freehafer A, Coletta M, Becker CL. Lower extremity fractures in patients with spinal cord injury. *Paraplegia* 1981;19:367–372.
142. Ingram R, Suman R, Freeman P. Lower limb fractures in the chronic spinal cord injured patient. *Paraplegia* 1989;27:133–139.
143. Nottage WM. A review of long-bone fractures in patients with spinal cord injuries. *Clin Orthop* 1981;155:65–70.
144. Ragnarsson K, Sell G. Lower extremity fractures after spinal cord injury: a retrospective study. *Arch Phys Med Rehabil* 1981;62:418–423.
145. Hangartner TN, Rodgers MM, Glaser RM, et al. Tibial bone density loss in spinal cord injured patients: effects of FES exercise. *J Rehabil Res Dev* 1994;31:50–61.
146. Kaplan PE, Gandhavadi B, Richards L, et al. Calcium balance in paraplegic patients: influence of injury duration and ambulation. *Arch Phys Med Rehabil* 1978;59:447–450.
147. Kaplan PE, Roden W, Gilbert E, et al. Reduction of hypercalciuria in tetraplegia after weight-bearing and strengthening exercises. *Paraplegia* 1981;19:289–293.
148. Kunkel CF, Scremin E, Eisenberg B, et al. Effect of "standing" on spasticity, contracture, and osteoporosis in paralyzed males. *Arch Phys Med Rehabil* 1993;74:73–78.
149. Leeds EM, Klose J, Ganz W, et al. Bone mineral density after bicycle ergometry training. *Arch Phys Med Rehabil* 1990;71:207–209.
150. Miller BE, Norman AW. Vitamin D. In: Machlin LJ, ed. *Handbook of vitamins: nutritional, biochemical, and clinical aspects.* New York: Marcel Dekker, 1984:80.
151. Loomis WF. Skin-pigment regulation of vitamin D biosynthesis in man. *Science* 1967;157:501–506.
152. Conney AHL. Pharmacologic implications of microsomal enzyme induction. *Pharmacol Rev* 1967;19:317–366.
153. Hahn TJ, Hendin BA, Scharp CR, et al. Effect of chronic anti-convulsant therapy on serum 25-hydroxycalciferol levels in adults. *N Engl J Med* 1972;287:900–904.
154. Bauman WA, Zhong YG, Schwartz E. Vitamin D deficiency in veterans with chronic spinal cord injury. *Metabolism* 1995;44:1612–1616.
155. Kurokouchi K, Ito T, Ohmori S, et al. Changes in the markers of bone metabolism following skeletal unloading. *Environ Med* 1995;39:12–24.
156. Kurokouchi K, Ito T, Ohmori S, et al. Effects of bisphosphonate on bone metabolism in tail-suspended rats. *Environ Med* (in press).
157. Minaire P, Berard E, Meunier PJ, et al. Effect of disodium dichloro-methylene diphosphonate on bone loss in paraplegic patients. *J Clin Invest* 1981;68:1086–1092.
158. Chappard D, Minaire P, Privat C, et al. Effects of tiludronate on bone loss in paraplegic patients. *J Bone Miner Res* 1995;10:112–117.
159. Linsey R, Tohme J. Estrogen treatment of patients with established postmenopausal osteoporosis. *Obstet Gynecol* 1990;76:290–295.
160. Avioli LV. The role of calcitonin in the prevention of osteoporosis. *Endocrinol Metab Clin North Am* 1998;27:411–418.
161. Rossini M, Gatti D, Zamberlan N, et al. Long-term effects of a treatment course with oral alendronate of postmenopausal osteoporosis. *J Bone and Miner Res* 1994;9:1833–1837.
162. Chopra IJ. Euthyroid sick syndrome: is it a misnomer? *J Clin Endocrinol Metab* 1997;82:329–334.
163. McIver B, Gorman CA. Euthyroid sick syndrome: an overview. *Thyroid* 1997;7:125–132.
164. Gamstedt A, Jarnerot G, Kagedal B, et al. Corticosteroid and thyroid function: different effect on plasma volume, thyroid hormones and thyroid home-binding proteins after oral and intravenous administration. *Acta Med Scand* 1979;205:379–383.
165. Bugaresti JM, Tator CH, Silverberg JD, et al. Changes in thyroid hormones, thyroid stimulating hormone and cortisol in acute spinal cord injury. *Paraplegia* 1992;30:401–409.
166. Claus-Walker J, Vallbona C, Carter RE, et al. Resting and stimulated endocrine function in human subjects with cervical cord transection. *J Chron Dis* 1971;24:193–207.
167. Claus-Walker J, Halstead LS, Carter RE, et al. Biochemical responses to intense local cooling in healthy subjects and in subjects with cervical spinal cord injury. *Arch Phys Med Rehabil* 1976;57:50–54.
168. Prakash V. Low serum 3,3′,5-triiodothyronine (T3) and reciprocally high serum 3,3′,5′-triiodothyronine (reverse T3) concentration in spinal cord injury patients. *J Am Paraplegia* 1983;6:56–58.
169. Prakash V, Lin MS, Song CH, et al. Thyroid hypofunction in spinal cord injury patients. *Paraplegia* 1980;18:53–56.
170. Bermudez F, Surks MI, Oppenheimer JH. High incidence of decreased serum triiodothyronine concentration in patients with non-thyroidal disease. *J Clin Endocrinol Metab* 1975;41:27–40.
171. Gomberg-Maitland M, Frishman WH. Thyroid hormone and cardio-vascular disease. *Am Heart* 1998;135:187–196.
172. Bacci V, Schussler GC, Kaplan TC. The relationship between serum triiodothyroine and thyrotropin during systemic illness. *J Clin Endocinol Metab* 1982;54:1229–1235.
173. DeGroot LJ, Coeaoni AH, Rue PA, et al. Reduced nuclear triidothyro-nine receptors in starvation induced hypothroidism. *Biochem Biophys Res Commun* 1977;79:173–178.
174. Wiersinga WM, Frank HJL, Chopra IJ, et al. Alterations in hepatic nuclear binding of triiodothyronine in experimental diabetes mellitus in rats. *Acta Endocrinol* 1982;99:79–85.
175. Tator CH, van der Jagt RHC. The effect of exogenous thyroid hormones on functional recovery of the rat after acute spinal cord compression injury. *J Neurosurg* 1980;53:381–384.
176. Fadan AI, Jacobs TP, Smith TM. Thyrotropin-releasing hormone in experimental cord injury: dose response and late treatment. *Neurology* 1984;34:1280–1284.
177. Cheville AL, Kirshblum SC. Thyroid hormone changes in chronic spinal cord injury. *J Spinal Cord Med* 1995;18:227–232.
178. Chopra IJ, Huang TS, Beredo A, et al. Serum thyroid hormone binding inhibitor in nonthyroid illness. *Metabolism* 1986;35:152–159.
179. Wang YH, Huang TS, Lien IN. Hormone changes in men with spinal cord injuries. *Am J Phys Med Rehabil* 1992;71:328–332.
180. Huang TS, Wang YH, Chiang HS, et al. Pituitary-testicular and pitui-tary-thyroid axis in spinal cord-injured males. *Metabolism* 1993;42:516–521.
181. Zeitzer JM, Ayas NT, Shea SA, et al. Absence of detectable melatonin and preservation of cortisol and thyrotropin rhythms in tetraplegia. *J Clin Endocrinol Metab* 2000;85:2189–2196.
182. Cruse JM, Lewis Jr RE, Bishop GR, et al. Decreased immune reactiv-ity and neuroendocrine alterations related to chronic stress in spinal cord injury and stroke patients. *Pathobiology* 1993;61:183–192.
183. Naftchi NE. Alterations of neuroendocrine functions in spinal cord injury. *Peptides* 1985;6(Suppl 1):85–94.
184. Grant JMF, Yeo JD. Studies on the levels of 17 hydroxy-corticoids in 24-hour specimens of urine from five quadriplegic patients and two paraplegic patients admitted to the Royal North Shore Hospital, Sydney. *Paraplegia* 1968;6:29–31.
185. Claus-Walker JL, Carter RE, Lipscomb HS, et al. Analysis of daily rhythms of adrenal function in men with quadriplegia due to spinal cord section. *Paraplegia* 1969;6:195–201.
186. Nicholas JJ, Streeten DHP, Jivof L. A study of pituitary and adrenal function in patients with traumatic injuries of the spinal cord. *J Charon Dis* 1969;22:463–471.
187. Li C, McDonald TJ. Source of corticotropin-releasing hormone-like innervation of the adrenal glands of fetal and postnatal sheep. *Brain Res* 1997;76:87–91.
188. Huang TS, Wang YH, Lee SH, et al. Impaired hypothalamus-pitui-tary-adrenal axis in men with spinal cord injuries. *Am J Phys Med Rehabil* 1998;77:108–112.
189. Wang YH, Huang, TS. Impaired adrenal reserve in mjen with spinal cord injury: results of low- and high-dose adrenocorticotropin. *Am J Phys Med Rehabil* 1999;80:863–866.
190. Berrande G, Thomopoulos P, Luton JP. Failure of synthcen to diag-nose corticotropin insufficiency. *Ann Endocrinol (Paris)* 1998;59:27–30.
191. Mathias CJ, Christensen NJ, Corbett JL, et al. Plasma catecholamines,

plasma renin activity and plasma aldosterone in tetraplegic man, horizontal and tilted. *Clin Sci Molec Med* 1975;49:291–299.

192. Mathias CJ, Christensen NJ, Frankel HL, et al. Renin release during head-up tilt occurs independently of sympathetic nervous activity in tetraplegic man. *Clin Sci* 1980;59:251–256.

193. Wall BM, Williams HH, Presley DN, et al. Altered sensitivity of osmotically stimulated vasopressin release in quadriplegic subjects. *Am J Physiol* 1990;258:R827–R835.

194. Krooner JS, Frankel HL, Mirando N, et al. Haemodynamic, hormonal and urinary responses to postural change in tetraplegic and paraplegic man. *Paraplegia* 1988;26:233–237.

195. Sutters M, Wakefield C, O'Neil K, et al. The cardiovascular, endocrine and renal response of tetraplegic and paraplegic subjects to dietary sodium restriction. *J Physiol* 1992;457:515–523.

196. Schmitt JK, Koch KS, Midha M. Profound hyptotension in a tetraplegic patient following angiotension-converting enzyme inhibitor lisinopril: case report. *Paraplegia* 1994;32:871–874.

197. Sved AF, McDowell FH, Blessing WW. Release of antidiuretic hormone in quadriplegic subjects in response to head-up tilt. *Neurology* 1985;35:78–82.

198. Ozcan O, Ulus IH, Yurkuran M, et al. Release of vasopressin, cortisol, and beta-endorphin in tetraplegic subjects in response to head-up tilt. *Paraplegia* 1991;29:120–124.

199. Poole CJM, Williams TDM, Lightman SL, et al. Neuroendocrine control of vasopressin secretion and its effect on blood pressure in subjects with spinal cord transection. *Brain* 1987;110:727–735.

200. Leehey DJ, Picache AA, Robertson GL. Hyponatremia in quadriplegic patients. *Clin Sci* 1988;75:441–444.

201. Sica DA, Midha M, Zawada E, et al. Hyponatremia in spinal cord injury. *J Am Paraplegia Soc* 1990;13:78–83.

202. Wall BM, Williams HH, Presley DN, et al. Vasopressin-independent alterations in renal water exretion in quadriplegia. *Am J Physiol* 1993; 265:R460–R466.

203. Williams HH, Wall BM, Horan JM, et al. Nonosmotic stimuli after osmoregulation in patients with spinal cord injury. *J Clin Endocrinol Metab* 1990;71:1536–1543.

204. Wall BM, Williams HH, Presley DN, et al. Reversible changes in osmoregulation of vasopressin release due to impaired water excretion. *Am J Kidney Dis* 1991;18:269–275.

205. Rasmann Nulicek DN, Spurr GB, Barboriak JJ, et al. Body composition of patients with spinal cord injury. *Eur J Clin Nutr* 1988;42:765–773.

206. Bauman WA, Spungen AM, Wang J, et al. Quantification of adiposity by dual photon x-ray absorptiometry in individuals with paraplegia or quadriplegia. *J Am Parapleg Soc* 1993;16(1):55(abst).

207. Spungen AM, Wang J, Pierson Jr RN, et al. Soft tissue body composition differences in monozygotic twins discordant for spinal cord injury. *J Appl Physiol* 2000;88:1310–1315.

208. Mollinger LA, Spurr GB, El Ghatit AZ, et al. Daily energy expenditure and basal metabolic rates of patients with spinal cord injury. *Arch Phy Med Rehabil* 1985;66:420–426.

209. Spungen AM, Bauman WA, Wang J, et al. The relationship between total body potassium and resting energy expenditure in individuals with paraplegia. *Arch Phys Med Rehabil* 1993;73:965–968.

210. Bors E, Engle ET, Rosenquist RC, et al. Fertility in paraplegic males: A preliminary report of endocrine studies. *J Clin Endocrinol Metab* 1949;10:381–398.

211. Kikuchi TA, Skowsky WR, El-Toraei I, et al. The pituitary-gonadal axis in spinal cord injury. *Fertil Steril* 1976;27:1142–1145.

212. Naftchi NE, Via AT, Sell GH, et al. Pituitary-testicular axis dysfunction in spinal cord injury. *Arch Phy Med Rehabil* 1980;61:402–405.

213. Nance P, Shears AH, Mivner ML, et al. Gonadal regulation in men with flaccid paraplegia. *Arch Phys Med Rehabil* 1985;66:757–759.

214. Tsitouras PD, Zhong YG, Spungen AM, et al. Serum testosterone and growth hormone/insulin-like growth factor-I in adults with spinal cord injury. *Horm Metab Res* 1995;27:287–292.

215. Bauman WA, Zhang RL, Spungen AM. Depressed serum testosterone levels in subjects with SCI. Submitted to the 2001 Annual Meeting of the American Spinal Injury Association.

216. Brindley GS. Deep scrotal temperature and the effect on it of clothing,

air temperature, activity, posture and paraplegia. *Br J Urol* 1982;54: 49–55.

217. Bulat T, Tsitouras PD, Drexler, H, et al. Hypothalamic-pituitary axis in chronic spinal cord injured subjects. *J Spinal Cord Med* 1995;18: 293(abst).

218. Rinieris P, Hatzimanolis J, Markianos M, et al. Effects of 4 weeks treatment with chlorpromazine and/or trihexyphenidyl on the pituitary-gonadal axis in male paranoid schizophrenics. *Eur Arch Psychiatry Neurol Sci* 1988;237:189–193.

219. Rinieris P, Hatzimanolis J, Markianos M, et al. Effects of treatment with various doses of haloperidol on the pituitary-gonadal axis in male schizophrenic patients. *Neuropsychobiology* 1989;22:146–149.

220. Bauman WA, Spungen AM, Flanagan S, et al. Blunted growth hormone response to intravenous arginine in subjects with a spinal cord injury. *Horm Met Res* 1994;26:149–153.

221. Shetty K, Sutton CH, Mattson DE, et al. Hyposomatomedinemia in quadriplegic men. *Am J Med Sci* 1993;305:95–100.

222. Rao U, Shetty KR, Mattson DE, et al. Prevalence of low plasm IGF-I in poliomyelitis survivors. *J Am Geriatr Soc* 1993;41:697–702.

223. Chatelain PG, Sanchez P, Saez JM. Growth hormone and insulin-like growth factor I treatment increase testicular luteinizing hormone receptors and steroidogenic responsiveness of growth hormone deficient dwarf mice. *Endocrinology* 1991;128:1857–1862.

224. Illig R, Prader A. Effect of testosterone on growth hormone secretion in patients with anorchia and delayed puberty. *J Clin Endocrinol Metab* 1970;30:615–618.

225. Liu L, Merriam GR, Sherins RJ. Chronic sex steroid exposure increases mean plasma growth hormone concentration and pulse amplitude in men with isolated hypogonadotropic hypogonadism. *J Clin Endocrinol Metab* 1987;64:651–656.

226. Martin LG, Clark JW, Conner TB. Growth hormone secretion enhanced by androgens. *J Clin Endocrinol Metab* 1968;28:231–245.

227. Bauman WA, Spungen AM, Zhong YG, et al. Chronic baclofen therapy improves the blunted growth hormone response to intravenous arginine in subjects with spinal cord injury. *J Clin Endocrinol Metab* 1994;78:1135–1138.

228. Tenover JL. Effects of androgen supplementation in the aging male. In: Oddens BJ, Vermeulen A, eds. *Androgens and the aging male.* New York, Parthenon, 1996:191–204.

229. Tenover JL. Therapeutic perspective: issues in testosterone replacement in older men. Can replacement doses of testosterone produce clinically meaningful changes in body composition in older men? *J Clin Endocrin Metab* 1998;83:3439–3440.

230. Sih R, Morley JE, Kaiser FE, et al. Testosterone replacement in older hypogonadal men: a 12-month randomized controlled trial. *J Clin Endocrinol Metab* 1997;82:1661–1667.

231. Morley JE, Perry HM, Kaiser FE, et al. Effect of testosterone replacement therapy in older hypogonadal males: a preliminary study. *J Am Geriatr Soc* 1993;41:149–152.

232. Tenover JS. Effects of testosterone supplementation in the aging male. *J Clin Endocrinol Metab* 1992;75:1092–1098.

233. Zgliczynski S, Ossowski M, Slowinska-Srzednicka J, et al. Effect of testosterone replacement on lipids, and lipoproteins in hypogonadal and elderly men. *Atherosclerosis* 1996;121:35–43.

234. Meriggiola MC, Marcovina S, Paulsen CA, et al. Testosterone enanthate at a dose of 200 mg/week decreased HDL-cholesterol levels in healthy men. *Int J Androl* 1995;18:237–242.

235. Cuneo RC, Judd S, Wallace JD, et al. The Australian multicenter trial of growth hormone (GH) treatment in GH-deficient adults. *J Clin Endocrinol Metab* 1998;83:107–116.

236. Jorgensen JOL, Pedersen SA, Thuesen L, et al. Beneficial effects of GH treatment in GH-deficient adults. *Lancet* 1989;1:1221–1225.

237. Rudman D, Feller AG, Nagraj HS, et al. Effects of human growth hormone in men over age 60 years old. *N Engl J Med* 1990;323:1–6.

238. Salomon F, Cuneo RC, Hesp R, et al. The effects of treatment with recombinant human growth hormone on body composition and metabolism in adults with growth hormone deficiency. *N Engl J Med* 1989;321:1797–1803.

239. Binnerts A, Swart GR, Wilson JH, et al. The effect of growth hormone administration in growth hormone deficient adults on bone, protein,

carbohydrate and lipid homeostasis, as well as on body composition. *Clin Endocrinol* 1992;37:79–87.

240. Cuneo RC, Salomon F, Watts GF, et al. Growth hormone treatment improves serum lipids and lipoproteins in adults with growth hormone deficiency. *Metabolism* 1993;42:1519–1523.

241. Chong PKK, Jung RT, Scrimgeour CM, et al. Energy expenditure and body composition in growth hormone deficient adults on exogenous growth hormone. *Clin Endocrinol* 1994;40:103–110.

242. Moller J, Jorgensen JOL, Moller N, et al. Effects of growth hormone administration on fuel oxidation and thyroid function in normal man. *Metabolism* 1992;41:728–731.

243. Spungen AM, Grimm DR, Dumitrescu OL, et al. Improvements in diaphramatic width and pulmonary function following anabolic steroid therapy in subjects with tetraplegia. Accepted for presentation. *Am J Respir Crit Care Med* 1999;159:A586(abst).

244. Demling RH, DeSanti L. Oxandrolone, a anabolic steroid, signifi-cantly increases the rate of weight gain in the recovery phase after major burns. *J Trauma Inj Infect Crit Care* 1997;43:47–51.

245. Demling RH, DeSanti L. Closure of the "non-healing wound" corresponds with correction of weight loss using the anabolic agent oxandrolone. *Ostomy/Wound Management* 1998;44:58–68.

246. Spungen AM, Rasul M, Koehler KM, et al. Effect of anabolic steroid therapy on healing of long-standing pressure sores: nine case reports in patients with SCI. *J Spinal Cord Med* 1999;22:27.

247. Karim A, Ranney RE, Zagarella J, et al. Oxandrolone disposition and metabolism in man. *Clin Pharm Therap* 1973;14:862–869.

248. Haffner SM, Kushwaha RS, Forster DN, et al. Studies on the metabolic mechanism of reduced high density lipoproteins during anabolic steroid therapy. *Metabolism* 1983;32:413–420.

249. Thompson PD, Cullianane EM, Sady SP, et al. Contrasting effects of testosterone and stanzolol on serum lipoprotein levels. *JAMA* 1989;261:1165–1168.

NEUROGENIC BLADDER FOLLOWING SPINAL CORD INJURY

TODD A. LINSENMEYER

Voiding dysfunction is commonly encountered in persons with spinal cord disorders. These problems not only result in increased urinary tract infections (UTIs), bladder stones, and other lower urinary tract morbidity, but also can potentially lead to kidney complications including renal deterioration. Therefore, timely identification of the type of voiding dysfunction, proper decisions on the type of bladder management, and follow-up are important.

ANATOMY AND PHYSIOLOGY OF THE UPPER AND LOWER URINARY TRACTS

Discussions often focus on a person's "neurogenic bladder." However, it is important to remember that changes in the lower tracts, such as poor drainage or high bladder pressures, often have a direct impact on the kidneys. The urinary tract is divided into the upper and lower urinary tracts. The upper tracts are composed of the kidneys and ureters. The lower urinary tracts are composed of the bladder and urethra.

Upper Urinary Tracts

The kidney consists of two parts: the renal parenchyma and the collecting system. The renal parenchyma secretes, concentrates, and excretes urine into the collecting system. In this collecting system, urine drains from multiple renal calices into a renal pelvis. The place where the renal pelvis narrows and becomes the ureter is known as the ureteropelvic junction (1). This is of clinical significance because congenital narrowing or kidney stones can cause obstruction of the kidneys.

In the adult, the ureter is approximately 30 cm long. In addition to the ureteropelvic junction, there are two other areas of physiologic narrowing that take on clinical significance with respect to possible obstruction from stones: the lower part of the ureter where the iliac artery crosses over the ureter and the ureterovesical junction (2,3). The ureterovesical junction is where the ureters traverse obliquely between the muscular and submucosal layers of the bladder wall. It traverses for a distance of 1 to 2 cm before opening into the bladder. This submucosal tunnel is designed to allow urine flow into the bladder while preventing reflux into the ureter. Any increase in intravesical pressure simul-taneously compresses the submucosal ureter and effectively creates a one-way valve (4). Presence of ureteral muscle in the submucosal segment also has been shown to be important in preventing reflux (5). Unfortunately, this same configuration can inhibit drainage from the kidneys, if there are sustained high intravesical pressures.

Lower Urinary Tracts

Anatomically, the bladder is divided into the detrusor and the trigone. The detrusor is composed of smooth muscle bundles that freely crisscross and interlace with each other. Near the bladder neck, the muscle fibers assume three distinct layers. The circular arrangement of the smooth muscles at the bladder neck allows them to act as a functional sphincter. The trigone is located at the inferior base of the bladder and extends from the ureteral orifices to the bladder neck. The deep trigone is continuous with the detrusor smooth muscle; the superficial trigone is an extension of the ureteral musculature (4).

There is no clear demarcation of the musculature of the bladder neck and the beginning of the urethra in men or women. In women, the urethra contains an inner longitudinal and outer semicircular layer of smooth muscle. The circular muscle layer exerts a sphincteric effect along the entire length of the urethra, which is approximately 4 cm long (Fig. 12.1). In men, the penis is made up of two corpora cavernosa that contain the spongy erectile tissue and a corpus spongiosum that surrounds the urethra. The male urethra is divided into the posterior or prostatic urethra, extending from the bladder neck to the urogenital diaphragm, and the anterior urethra, which extends to the meatus. The junction between the anterior and posterior urethra is known as the membranous urethra.

Urinary Urethral Sphincters

Traditionally, the urethra has been thought to have two distinct sphincters, the internal and the external, or rhabdosphincter. The internal sphincter is not a true anatomic sphincter. Instead, in both men and women, the term refers to the junction of the bladder neck and proximal urethra, formed from the circular arrangement of connective tissue and smooth muscle fibers that extend from the bladder. This area is considered to be a func-

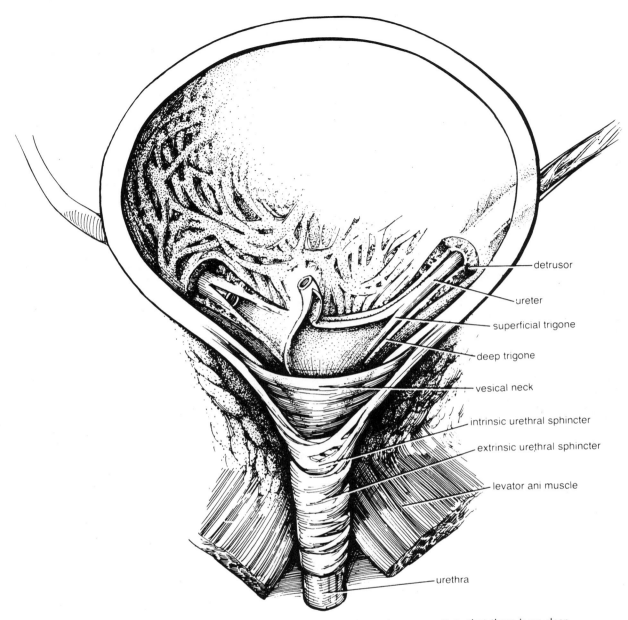

detrusor

ureter

superficial trigone

deep trigone

vesical neck

intrinsic urethral sphincter

extrinsic urethral sphincter

levator ani muscle

urethra

FIGURE 12.1. Anatomy of the bladder and related structures in women. Note that there is no clear demarcation between the bladder neck and sphincter mechanism. (From Hinman F Jr. Bladder repair. In: Hinman F Jr, ed. *Urological surgery.* Philadelphia: WB Saunders, 1989:433, with permission.)

tional sphincter because there is a progressive increase in tone with bladder filling so the urethral pressure is greater than the intravesical pressure. These smooth muscle fibers also extend submucosally down the urethra and lie above the external rhabdosphincter (6).

In men, the external sphincter, or urethral rhabdosphincter, often is diagrammatically illustrated as a thin circular band of striated muscle forming a diaphragm just distal to the prostatic urethra (i.e., membranous urethra). In an anatomic study, however, Myers et al. (7) reconfirmed earlier studies showing that the urethral external striated sphincter does not form a circular band but has fibers that run up to the base of the bladder. The

bulk of the fibers are found at the membranous urethra (8). This sphincter is under voluntary control. The striated muscular fibers in both men and women are thought to have a significant proportion of slow-twitch fibers with the capacity for steady tonic compression of the urethra. In women, striated skeletal muscle fibers circle the upper two thirds of the urethra (8).

Normal Urine Transport from the Kidneys to the Bladder

Urine transport is the result of passive and active forces. Passive forces are created by the filtration pressure of the kidneys. The normal proximal tubular pressure is 14 mm Hg and the renal pelvis pressure is 6.5 mm Hg, which slightly exceeds resting ureteral and bladder pressures. Active forces are due to peristalsis of the calices, renal pelvis, and ureter. Peristalsis begins with the electrical activity of pacemaker cells at the proximal portion of the urinary collecting tract (9).

For the ureter to efficiently propel the bolus of urine, the contraction wave must completely coapt the ureteral walls (6). Ureteral dilation for any reason results in inefficient propulsion of the urine bolus, which can delay drainage proximal to that point. This can result in further dilation and over time lead to hydronephrosis.

NEUROANATOMY OF THE LOWER URINARY TRACT

Bladder storage and emptying is a function of interactions between the peripheral parasympathetic, sympathetic, and somatic innervation of the lower urinary tract. Additionally, there is modulation from the central nervous system (CNS). Slight alterations in storage or emptying have significant clinical implications, not only because of potential morbidity but also because of the social embarrassment of urinary incontinence, no matter how infrequently it occurs.

Bladder Neuroanatomy

Efferent System

The parasympathetic efferent supply originates from a distinct detrusor nucleus located in the intermediolateral gray matter of the sacral cord at S2-4 (Fig. 12.2). Sacral efferents emerge as preganglionic fibers in the ventral roots and travel through the

pelvic nerves to ganglia immediately adjacent to or within the detrusor muscle to provide excitatory input to the bladder. After impulses arrive at the parasympathetic ganglia, they travel through short postganglionics to the smooth muscle cholinergic receptors. These receptors, called cholinergic, because the primary postganglionic neurotransmitter is acetylcholine, are distributed throughout the bladder. Stimulation causes a bladder contraction (10,11).

The sympathetic efferent nerve supply to the bladder and urethra begins in the intermediolateral gray column from T11-L2 and provides inhibitory input to the bladder. Sympathetic impulses travel a relatively short distance to the lumbar sympathetic paravertebral ganglia. From here, the sympathetic impulses travel along long postganglionic nerves in the hypogastric nerves to synapse at α- and β-adrenergic receptors within the bladder and urethra. The primary postganglionic neurotransmitter for the sympathetic system is norepinephrine. Variations in this anatomic arrangement do occur. Sympathetic ganglia sometimes also are located near the bladder, and sympathetic efferent fibers may travel along the pelvic and the hypogastric nerves (Fig. 12.2) (10,11).

Sympathetic stimulation facilitates bladder storage because of the strategic location of the adrenergic receptors (Fig. 12.3). β-Adrenergic receptors predominate in the superior portion (i.e., body) of the bladder. Stimulation of β-receptors causes smooth muscle relaxation. α-Receptors have a higher density near the base of the bladder and prostatic urethra; stimulation of these receptors causes smooth muscle contractions and therefore increases the outlet resistance of the bladder and prostatic urethra (10–12).

After SCI, several changes that alter bladder function occur to the bladder receptors. There is evidence that when smooth muscle is denervated, its sensitivity to a given amount of neuro-

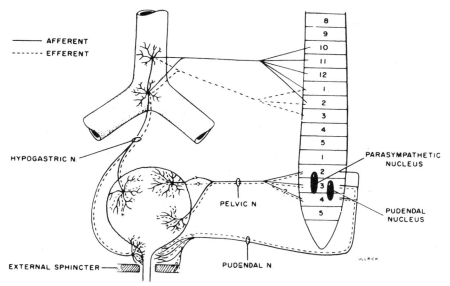

FIGURE 12.2. Peripheral innervation of the bladder and urethra. Sympathetic stimulation responsible for storage travels through the hypogastric plexus. Parasympathetic stimulation, causing bladder contractions, travels through the pelvic nerve. (From Blaivas JG. Management of bladder dysfunction in multiple sclerosis. *Neurology* 1980;30:73, with permission.)

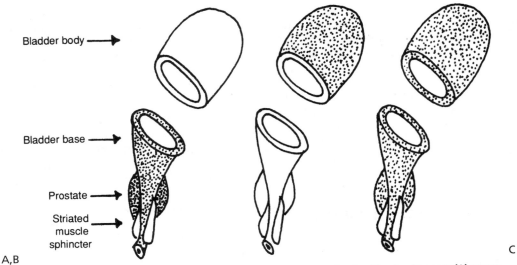

Bladder body ⟶

Bladder base ⟶

Prostate ⟶

Striated
muscle
sphincter ⟶

A,B

C

FIGURE 12.3. Location of bladder receptors. Bladder storage is maintained by simultaneous **(A)** sympathetic adrenergic receptors (contraction) and **(B)** β-adrenergic receptor (relaxation stimulation). Bladder emptying occurs with parasympathetic cholinergic receptor stimulation **(C)**.

transmitter increases (i.e., denervation supersensitivity). Therefore, smaller doses of various pharmacologic agents would be expected to have a much more pronounced effect in people with SCI, compared with those with nonneurogenic bladders (13). A change in receptor location and density may also occur. Norlen et al. (14) found that after complete denervation, there is a change from a β-receptor predominance to an α-receptor predominance. Because α-receptors cause contraction of smooth muscle, a change in receptors may be one reason some individuals have poor compliance of the bladder after SCI.

Animal studies have revealed that although the previously described long postganglionic neurons exist, there are ganglia close to the bladder and urethra in which there are both cholinergic and adrenergic fibers. This has been termed the urogenital short neuron system. These ganglia are composed of three cell types: adrenergic neurons, cholinergic neurons, and small intensely fluorescent cells. The small intensely fluorescent cells are believed to be responsible for this interganglionic modulation of the adrenergic and cholinergic neurons. Further work is needed to define this system in humans (15).

Afferent System

The most important afferents that stimulate voiding are those that pass to the sacral cord via the pelvic nerves. These afferents include two types: small myelinated A-delta fibers and unmyelinated (C) fibers. The small myelinated A-delta fibers respond in a graded fashion to bladder distention and are essential for normal voiding. The unmyelinated (C) fibers have been termed "silent C fibers" because they do not respond to bladder distention and therefore are not essential for normal voiding. However, these "silent C fibers" do exhibit spontaneous firing when they are activated by chemical or cold temperature irritation at the bladder wall. Additionally, the unmyelinated (C) fibers, rather than A-delta afferents, have been found to "wake up" and respond

to distention and stimulate bladder contractions in animals with suprasacral SCI.

Increased C-fiber afferent activity after SCI has been experimentally demonstrated by systemic administration of capsaicin, a neurotoxin that is known to disrupt the function of C-fiber afferents. In non-SCI animals (with A-delta afferents), there was no blockage of bladder contractions with bladder distention. However, in SCI animals, capsaicin completely blocked rhythmic bladder contractions induced with bladder distention. These findings have important potential therapeutic implications. There has been some success at blocking uninhibited contractions with the use of intravesical capsaicin, and preliminary results with another C-fiber neurotoxin, resiniferatoxin (RTX), are promising (16). RTX is 1,000 times as potent as capsaicin and has such a fast onset of action that its intravesical instillation does not cause bladder discomfort, which is often associated with intravesical capsaicin instillation (16).

Bladder Neurotransmitters

There are additional transmitters besides acetylcholine and norepinephrine, including nitric oxide (NO), vasoactive intestinal polypeptide (VIP), endogenous opioid peptides, and neuropeptide Y. These transmitters may work on their own or help modulate the classic neurotransmitters. NO and VIP have smooth muscle relaxant effects. The large number of receptors helps to explain the concept of "atropine resistance." It has been found that a single neurotransmitter-blocking agent such as atropine fails to suppress 100% of the bladder or urethral activity (13, 17). This explains why a combination of agents may be more effective than a higher dose of a single agent.

Urethral Sphincter Innervation

The external urethral sphincter (EUS) classically has been described as having somatic innervation, which allows the sphincter to be closed at will. Somatic efferents originate from a pudendal nucleus of sacral segments from S1-4. Somatic efferents then travel through the pudendal nerve to the neuromuscular junction of the striated muscle fibers in the EUS.

The internal urethral sphincter has been described as being under control of the autonomic system. This area has a large number of sympathetic α-receptors, which cause closure when stimulated. Animal studies have revealed that NO is an important neurotransmitter, mediating relaxation of the urethral smooth muscle (7,17).

The distinction between the internal and external sphincter is, however, becoming less clear. Elbadawi and Schenk (18) reported histochemical evidence of a triple innervation pattern of the external sphincter in five mammalian species, with dual sympathetic and parasympathetic autonomic components superimposed on the somatic component. Sundin and Dahlstrom (19) demonstrated sprouting and increasing adrenergic terminals after parasympathetic denervation in cats. Crowe et al. (20) reported a substantial invasion of adrenergic nerve fibers in smooth and striated muscle in the urethra in patients with SCI with lower motoneuron lesions.

Influences of the Central Nervous System on the Lower Urinary Tract

Facilitation and inhibition of the autonomic nervous system are under the control of the CNS. There are several theories of how this occurs. Denny-Brown and Robertson (21) suggested that micturition was primarily due to a sacral micturition reflex. According to their theory, descending nervous system pathways modulate this micturition reflex. De Groat (17), Barrington (22), and Bradley (23) thought that facilitative impulses to the bladder originated from a region of the anterior pons, termed the Barrington center.

De Groat (17) additionally stressed the importance of the sympathetic nervous system in facilitating urine storage. Carlsson (24) provided evidence that this pontine mesencephalic area also plays a role in coordinating detrusor and sphincter activity. Stimulation of the Barrington center significantly decreased electromyographic (EMG) activity in the periurethral striated sphincter while causing a bladder contraction (24). In humans, this center is felt to be responsible for causing sphincter relaxation, which in turn initiates a bladder contraction. Detrusor sphincter dyssynergia (DSD), intermittent contractions of the sphincter during a bladder contraction, occurs without coordination from this center.

Transection experiments in cats suggest that the net effect of the cerebral cortex on micturition is inhibitory. This also is true for the basal ganglia and corresponds to clinical findings of detrusor hyperreflexia in those with basal ganglia dysfunction (e.g., Parkinson disease). The cerebellum is thought to maintain tone in the pelvis floor musculature and influence coordination between periurethral striated muscle relaxation and bladder emptying (14,24).

NORMAL VOIDING PHYSIOLOGY

Micturition should be considered as having two phases: the filling (storage) phase and the emptying (voiding) phase. The filling phase occurs when a person is not trying to void. The emptying phase is defined as when a person is attempting to void or is told to void.

During filling, there should be very little rise in bladder pressure. As filling continues, low intravesical pressure is maintained by a progressive increase in sympathetic (a) stimulation of the β-receptors located in the body of the bladder that cause relaxation and (b) stimulation of the α-receptors located at the base of the bladder and urethra that cause contraction. Sympathetic stimulation also inhibits excitatory parasympathetic ganglionic transmission, which helps suppress bladder contractions. During the filling phase, there is a progressive increase in urethral sphincter EMG activity (25). Increased urethral sphincter activity also reflexly inhibits bladder contractions. When a bladder is full and has normal compliance, intravesical pressures are between 0 and 6 cm H_2O and should not rise to more than 15 cm H_2O. Filling continued past the limit of the viscoelastic properties of the bladder results in a steady progressive rise in intravesical pressure (26). This part of the filling curve usually is not seen in a person with normal bladder function, because this much filling would cause significant discomfort and not be tolerated.

When a patient is told to void (voiding or emptying phase), there should be cessation of urethral sphincter EMG activity and a drop in urethral sphincter pressure and funneling of the bladder neck. There is no longer reflex inhibition to the sacral micturition center from the sphincter mechanism. This is followed by a detrusor contraction. The urethral sphincter should remain open throughout voiding, and there should be no rises in intraabdominal pressure during voiding. In younger individuals, there should be no postvoid residua (PVR), although the amount of PVR may increase with aging (see later discussion).

CLASSIFICATION OF VOIDING DYSFUNCTION

Suprapontine Lesions

Any suprapontine lesion may affect voiding. Lesions may result from cerebrovascular disease, hydrocephalus, intracranial neoplasms, traumatic brain injury, Parkinson disease, and multiple sclerosis (MS). MS is unique among the suprapontine lesions because it also affects the white matter of the spinal cord and often has a relapsing and remitting nature. The expected urodynamic finding after a suprapontine lesion is detrusor hyperreflexia without DSD. Normally, the sphincter should remain relaxed during the bladder contraction. DSD occurs when the sphincter intermittently tightens during the contraction. Voiding dysfunctions may be very different from expectations because of various factors such as medications, prostate obstruction, and possible normal bladder function but poor cognition.

Suprasacral Spinal Cord Lesions

Traumatic SCI is the most common suprasacral lesion affecting voiding. Other suprasacral lesions include transverse myelitis, MS, and primary or metastatic spinal cord tumor. Patients with suprasacral spinal cord lesions would be expected to have detrusor hyperreflexia with DSD. However, because of partial lesions, occult lesions of the sacral cord, or persistent spinal shock, this is not always the case (27).

Traumatic suprasacral SCI results in an initial period of spinal shock, in which there is hyporeflexia of the somatic system below the level of injury and detrusor areflexia. During this phase, the bladder has no contractions even with various maneuvers such as the "ice-water filling" test, bethanechol supersensitivity testing, or suprapubic tapping. The neurophysiology for spinal shock and its recovery is not known. Recovery of bladder function usually follows recovery of skeletal muscle reflexes. Uninhibited bladder contractions gradually return after 6 to 8 weeks (28).

Clinically, a person with a traumatic suprasacral SCI may begin having episodes of urinary incontinence, as well as various visceral sensations, such as tingling, flushing, increased lower extremity spasms, or autonomic dysreflexia with the onset of uninhibited contractions. As uninhibited bladder contractions become stronger, the PVR decreases. Rudy et al. (29) reported that voiding function appears optimal at 12 weeks postinjury. However, detrusor hyperreflexia has been reported to have a delayed onset, up to 22 months postinjury (30). Eventually, all of these patients did develop uninhibited contractions. Comarr (31) considered the bladder "balanced" when the PVR test results were less than 20% of the total bladder capacity in patients with detrusor hyperreflexia. Graham (32) reports that 50% to 70% of patients will develop balanced bladders without therapy. Unfortunately, high intravesical voiding pressures usually are required for the development of a balanced bladder. These high pressures, however, may cause renal deterioration (see the "Hydronephrosis" and "Vesicoureteral Reflux" sections).

Traditionally, it has been thought that there is decreased activity of the EUS during acute spinal shock. However, Downie and Awad (33) noted in dogs that with surgical transection between T2 and T8, there was no change in the activity of the periurethral, striated musculature despite detrusor areflexia. In humans, Nanninga and Meyer (34) found that in 44 patients in spinal shock with suprasacral lesions, all had a positive bulbocavernosus reflex and 30 of 32 had sphincter activity despite detrusor areflexia within 72 hours of injury. Koyanagi et al. (35) noted that external sphincter electrical activity was not affected during acute spinal shock but was likely to increase after recovery from spinal shock. This increase was more marked in those with high suprasacral lesions, compared with those with low suprasacral lesions (35).

Detrusor external sphincter dyssynergia (DESD) also commonly occurs after suprasacral lesions. DESD is defined as intermittent or complete failure of relaxation of the urinary sphincter during a bladder contraction and voiding. This diagnosis should not be made during the filling phase if the sphincter fails to relax when there is no bladder contraction. Blaivas et al. (36) noted that DESD occurred in 96% of patients with suprasacral lesions and found several patterns of DESD. Rudy et al. (29) proposed that DESD is an exaggerated continence reflex. The continence reflex is the normal phenomenon of increasing urethral sphincter activity with bladder filling. They (29) believed that the patterns described by Blaivas et al. (36) represented variations of the single continence reflex.

In addition to DESD, internal sphincter dyssynergia also has been reported, often occurring at the same time as DESD.

Sacral Lesions

Various lesions may affect the sacral cord or roots. These include spinal trauma, herniated lumbar disk, primary or metastatic tumors, myelodysplasia, arteriovenous malformation, lumbar stenosis, and inflammatory process (e.g., arachnoiditis). In the series by Pavlakis et al. (37), trauma was responsible for conus and cauda equina lesions more than 50% of the time. The next most common cause was L4-5 or L5-S1 intervertebral disk protrusion. The incidence of lumbar disk prolapse causing cauda equina syndrome is between 1% and 15% (37). Damage to the sacral cord or roots generally results in a highly compliant acontractile bladder; however, particularly in patients with partial injuries, the areflexia may be accompanied by decreased bladder compliance, resulting in progressive increases in intravesical pressure with filling (38). The exact mechanism by which sacral parasympathetic decentralization of the bladder causes decreased compliance is unknown (38,39).

It has been noted that the external sphincter is not affected to the same extent as the detrusor. This is due to the fact that the pelvic nerve innervation to the bladder usually arises one segment higher than the pudendal nerve innervation to the sphincter (40). The nuclei also are located in different portions of the sacral cord, with the detrusor nuclei located in the intermediolateral cell column and the pudendal nuclei located in the ventral gray matter. This combination of detrusor areflexia and an intact sphincter helps contribute to bladder overdistention and decompensation.

Peripheral Lesions

There are multiple etiologies for peripheral lesions that could affect voiding. The most common lesion is a peripheral neuropathy secondary to diabetes mellitus. Other peripheral neuropathies that have been associated with voiding dysfunction include chronic alcoholism, herpes zoster, Guillain-Barré syndrome (GBS), and pelvic surgery (41,42). A sensory neuropathy is the most frequent finding in diabetes. Urodynamic findings including decreased bladder sensation, chronic bladder overdistention, increased PVR volumes, and possible bladder decompensation may result from bladder overdistention due to decreased sensation of fullness. Andersen and Bradley (43) reported that in their series, mean bladder capacity was 635 mL, with a range of 200 to 1,150 mL (43). An autonomic neuropathy also may be responsible for decreased bladder contractility. GBS and herpes zoster are predominantly motor neuropathies. Transient voiding symptoms, predominantly urinary retention, have been reported to occur in 0% to 40% of patients and are thought to be due to involvement of the autonomic sacral parasympathetic nerves. Detrusor hyperreflexia occasionally has been found in patients with GBS (44). Voiding dysfunctions resulting from pelvic surgery or pelvic trauma usually involve both motor and sensory innervation of the bladder (43).

COMPREHENSIVE EVALUATION OF VOIDING DYSFUNCTION

Neurourologic History

A thorough patient history is required to identify the neurologic diagnosis and associated medical problems. The urologic history should include the present bladder management (type, problems, and acceptance), fluid intake and output, and voiding complaints such as urgency, frequency, hesitancy, dysuria, incontinence, and autonomic dysreflexia. Although symptoms can help to determine what is bothering a person, whether or not a person is out of spinal shock, and problems with bladder management, it is important not to initiate treatment based on symptoms. Similar symptoms may occur from abnormal bladder function, abnormal sphincter function, or a combination of both. Therefore, symptoms alone are not able to differentiate abnormalities in voiding. Urodynamics is therefore needed to objectively evaluate voiding dysfunction after SCI.

Significant past medical history and social history include surgery or medications that may affect voiding, allergies, smoking and drinking history, other medical problems, lifestyle and sexuality, and living environment. The functional history is of particular significance for voiding dysfunction. One should ask about hand function, dressing skills, sitting balance, ability to perform transfers, and ability to ambulate. These factors are important considerations when developing bladder management strategies.

Neurourologic Physical Examination

The neurourologic physical examination should focus on the abdomen, external genitalia, and perineal skin. When performing the rectal examination, one must note that it is not the overall size of the prostate but the amount of prostate growing inward that causes obstruction. Therefore, urodynamic study, rather than rectal examination, is needed to diagnose outflow obstruction objectively. In women, one should examine for the location of the urethral meatus and whether there is a cystocele or rectocele.

The sensory examination should focus on determining the level of injury in patients with SCI. Particularly important is establishing whether the level of injury is above T6, which would make the patient prone to autonomic dysreflexia. Sacral sensation evaluates the afferent limb (i.e., the pudendal nerve) of the sacral micturition center.

The motor examination helps to establish the level of injury and degree of completeness in patients with SCI. Hand function should be assessed to determine the ability to undress or possibly perform intermittent catheterization (IC). Upper and lower extremity spasticity, sitting, standing, and ambulating need to be evaluated. Anal sphincter tone also should be evaluated. Decreased or absent tone suggests a sacral or peripheral nerve lesion, whereas increased tone suggests a suprasacral lesion. Voluntary contraction of the anal sphincter tests sacral innervation, suprasacral integrity, and the ability to understand commands.

Cutaneous reflexes that are helpful to the neurourologic examination are the cremasteric (L1-2), bulbocavernosus, and anal reflexes (S2-4). Absence of these cutaneous reflexes suggests pyramidal tract disease or a peripheral lesion. The bulbocavernosus reflex may be present only 70% to 85% of the time in neurologically intact people. A false-negative result often is due to a person being nervous and already having his or her anal sphincter clamped down at the time of the examination. Muscle stretch reflexes also should be evaluated. A sudden increase in spasticity may be an indication of a UTI.

Laboratory Evaluation

It is best to obtain a baseline urine sample for culture and sensitivity. A serum creatinine clearance is not as helpful as a 24-hour creatinine clearance because a significant amount of kidney damage must occur before there are changes in the serum creatinine clearance.

Urologic Assessment of the Upper and Lower Urinary Tract—Overview

Because patients with SCI usually have a neurogenic bladder, objective testing of the lower urinary tracts is important. As noted previously, changes in voiding from the lower tracts have a direct impact on the upper tracts. Therefore, there needs to be constant surveillance of the upper tracts and the lower tracts.

Upper Tract Tests

Various tests designed to evaluate the upper tracts are available. Some tests are better at evaluating renal function and others at evaluating renal anatomy. Those that evaluate anatomy include an abdominal x-ray (which is performed routinely as part of the cystogram), an intravenous pyelogram (IVP), and renal ultrasound. If more detailed imaging is needed, an abdominal computed tomography (CT) scan may be ordered. Tests that primarily evaluate renal function include a 24-hour urine creatinine clearance and quantitative renal scan (45,46).

There are no studies that show which test is best to use for monitoring the upper tracts. A renal scan is frequently used as the initial modality to monitor renal function.

Some institutions use renal ultrasound as their method of screening. We feel that renal scans are more sensitive at picking up changes in renal function than ultrasound. We use ultrasound only if a person is having symptoms such as recurrent UTIs and hematuria, if there is a question of a stone on x-ray, or if the patient has an abnormal renal scan. Other specific upper tract radiologic tests (e.g., IVP and CT scan) are generally recommended as further evaluation of abnormalities if found on renal scan or ultrasound.

The IVP traditionally has been used to visualize kidneys and ureters but has been replaced largely by ultrasound and renal scan. Reasons for not using IVP to screen patients include potential allergic reactions, radiation exposure, and patient inconvenience, specifically, getting an IVP laxative preparation the night before the test. Because an IVP with tomograms gives good anatomic detail, this test is often very helpful when there is a concern about possible kidney or ureteral tumors, possible ureteral stones, or equivocal ultrasound or renal scan findings.

The kidney ultrasound is helpful for detecting hydronephrosis and kidney stones (46). The major disadvantage of ultrasound is that it is user dependent and does not show renal function. Although some institutions use renal ultrasound for initial screening, many institutions use renal ultrasound as an adjunctive study if there is a possible anatomic abnormality or stone noted on KUB, IVP, or renal scan. If further anatomic definition is needed, CT should be considered.

The quantitative renal scan is an excellent way to monitor renal function and drainage. Many institutions use this as the primary modality to evaluate renal function. Attempts should be made to obtain the glomerular filtration rate (GFR) or effective renal plasma flow (ERPF) (46). If the nuclear medicine department does not have the capability to obtain a GFR or ERPF, a renal scan and a 24-hour urine creatinine clearance can be used to follow quantitatively year-to-year renal function. Serum creatinine clearance is not helpful for monitoring yearly kidney function because it may remain within the reference range despite moderate to severe renal deterioration (47).

Lower Urinary Tract Tests

Tests to evaluate the lower tracts include cystogram, cystoscopy, and urodynamics. Because each test involves instrumentation, it is best to obtain a urine culture and sensitivity and give antibiotics if the urine culture and sensitivity test result is positive before the testing. Some indications for cystoscopy in patients with voiding disorders include hematuria, recurrent symptomatic UTI, recurrent asymptomatic bacteriuria with a stone-forming organism (i.e., *Proteus mirabilis*), an episode of genitourinary sepsis, urinary retention or incontinence, pieces of eggshell calculi obtained when irrigating a catheter, and long-term indwelling catheter. Cystoscopy also is indicated when removing an indwelling Foley catheter that has been in place 4 to 6 weeks and changing to a different type of management, such as IC or a balanced bladder. Cystoscopy can reveal pubic hairs or eggshell calculi that may be missed on radiography and serve as a nidus for bladder stones. Urodynamics provides objective information on voiding function.

Urodynamics

Urodynamics is defined as the study of normal and abnormal factors in the storage, transport, and emptying of urine from the bladder and urethra by any appropriate method (48). When deciding on an appropriate urodynamic test, one must consider whether information is needed about the filling phase, emptying phase, or both phases of micturition. The physician's presence is important to help direct the urodynamic study. Typical decisions include how much water to put in the bladder, whether to repeat the study, and whether to have the patient sit or stand to void. Observing the patient during urodynamics also will help in getting an idea of factors that might influence the test, such as patient anxiety or inability to understand when told to void. Blood pressure monitoring is particularly important in patients with SCI prone to autonomic dysreflexia.

Evaluation of Bladder Filling (Storage Phase)

The bedside cystometrogram involves filling the bladder with water through a Foley catheter. The end of the catheter is connected to a 60-mL bulb syringe and water is poured through the open end of the syringe. It is sometimes attached by means of a Y connector to a manometer, which is used to measure the rise in water pressure. This test can be used to evaluate sensation, stability, and capacity, and as a screening test to determine whether a patient with SCI has come out of spinal shock. This test can also be used in combination with blood pressures to determine whether a person develops autonomic dysreflexia with bladder filling. A variant of this test is the "ice-water test" described by Bors and Comarr. A total of 50 mL of ice water is instilled through a catheter (balloon deflated). If a person is out of spinal shock, the bladder has a forceful contraction, expelling both the catheter and the water, constituting a positive test result. There are several limitations to the bedside cystometrogram, however. It is difficult to determine whether small rises in the water column are due to intraabdominal pressure (e.g., straining) or a bladder contraction. Most important, the voiding phase cannot be evaluated.

Evaluation of Bladder Emptying

One of the easiest screening tests to evaluate bladder emptying is a PVR; however, it should not be used to characterize the specific type of voiding dysfunction. PVR volume can be determined with catheterization or bladder ultrasound. PVR tests are often helpful to monitor the success of a medication once a urodynamic study has characterized the voiding dysfunction. Before injury, a younger person generally has no PVR, whereas an older adult person with no voiding complaints may have a PVR volume of 100 to 150 mL. Postinjury, a PVR volume of 100 to 200 mL is considered acceptable even in younger individuals if a person is clinically doing well. There are limitations to studying only the PVR volume, because a PVR volume within the reference range does not rule out a voiding problem. For example, a PVR test result may be normal despite significant outflow obstruction (e.g., DSD and benign prostate hypertrophy) due to a compensatory increase in the strength of detrusor contractions, or with no bladder contractions due to increasing intraabdominal pressure (e.g., Credé method and Valsalva maneuver). Caution also must be taken in interpreting a large PVR volume. It may be abnormal because it was not taken immediately after voiding, because of poor patient understanding or due to an abnormal voiding situation (e.g., the patient was given a bedpan at 3:00 a.m.).

A water-fill urodynamic study is necessary to measure both the filling and the emptying phase of micturition. A number of urodynamic parameters can be evaluated at the same time. Some of these include the EMG activity of the sphincter, the total pressure in the bladder (intravesical pressure), the urethral pressure, the intraabdominal pressure, and flow rate and volume of urine. Many urodynamic systems will also give a tracing of the detrusor pressure, which is actually generated from the machine by subtracting the total pressure in the bladder (i.e., the intravesical pressure) from the abdominal pressure. Thus, the intravesical pressure minus the intraabdominal pressure will give pressure due to the bladder contraction. These studies are often called multichannel urodynamics, because urodynamic machines are described by the number of parameters (called channels) they can measure. More sophisticated urodynamic studies also may incorporate videofluoroscopy and the use of various pharmacologic agents such as bethanechol.

Pharmacologic Testing

Pharmacologic testing sometimes is done in conjunction with this urodynamic test. Lapides et al. (49) popularized the bethanechol supersensitivity test. A 15-cm rise in pressure after subcutaneous bethanechol is given is considered positive. Wheeler et al. (50) pointed out that false-positive test results may be due to UTI, psychogenic stress, and azotemia. Therefore, when this test is used, it should be interpreted in light of the rest of the neurologic examination.

Normal Water-Fill Urodynamic Study

A water-fill urodynamic study evaluates two distinct phases of bladder function (Fig. 12.4). The first is the filling (storage) phase, during which water is being infused into the bladder. Urodynamic parameters that can be evaluated during this phase include bladder sensation, bladder capacity, bladder wall compliance, and bladder stability (i.e., whether there are uninhibited contractions). The second portion of the study is the voiding (emptying) phase. This phase begins when a person is told to void, or when an inpatient who has a neurogenic bladder begins to have an uninhibited contraction and voiding begins. Urodynamic parameters that can be evaluated during the voiding phase

include opening or leak point pressure (bladder pressure at which voiding begins), maximum voiding pressure, urethral sphincter activity (EMG or actual pressure), flow rate, voided volume, and PVR. In patients who have the potential for autonomic dysreflexia, changes in blood pressure before, during, and after voiding can also be evaluated.

With an empty bladder, there should be no sensation of fluid within the bladder. During the filling phase, the first sensation of fullness usually occurs with 100 to 200 mL in the bladder. The sensation of fullness occurs around 300 to 400 mL, and the onset of urgency usually occurs between 400 and 500 mL. There is, however, variability in bladder capacity, which ranges between 400 and 750 mL in adults. There should be little to no rise in the intravesical pressure, which indicates normal bladder wall compliance. Additionally, there should be no involuntary bladder contractions during this part of the study.

During the voiding phase, the detrusor pressures usually are less than 30 cm H_2O in women and between 30 and 50 cm H_2O in men. A normal maximum flow rate is between 15 and 20 mL per second and should not be less than 10 mL per second in any age group. The patient should have at least 150 mL in the bladder because the flow rate depends on the voided volume (51). The flow usually has a bell-shaped curve, progressively increasing to its maximum rate and then decreasing. The urethral sphincter should remain open throughout voiding, and there should be no rises in intraabdominal pressure during voiding. As previously discussed, there should be no PVR, although PVR levels increase with aging. A single elevated PVR level during urodynamic testing should be interpreted with caution, because the patient may be nervous and voluntarily may stop the urine stream. Several catheterized or ultrasound PVR tests should be done to confirm an increased urodynamic PVR level. Urody-

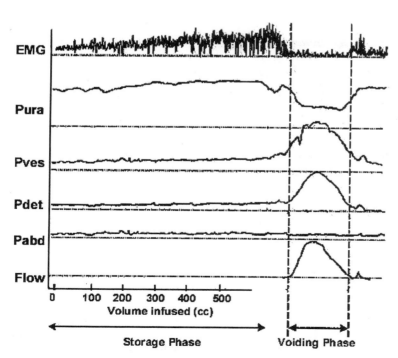

FIGURE 12.4. Normal urodynamic pattern.

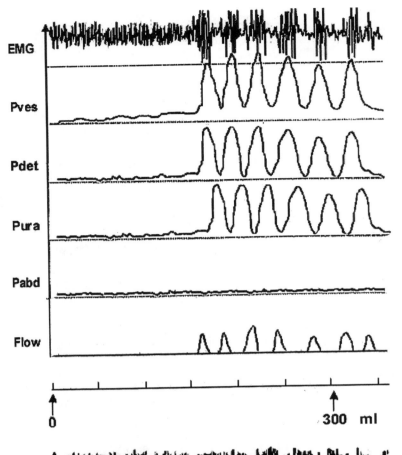

FIGURE 12.5. Urodynamics representing detrusor sphincter dyssynergia. Note: Sphincter, detrusor, and vesicle are contracting at similar times. Failure of relaxation of urethra when bladder (detrusor and vesicle) is contracting results in an intermittent urinary stream.

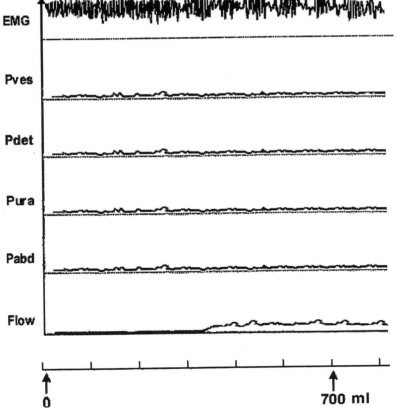

FIGURE 12.6. Urodynamics representing areflexic bladder. Note that there are no contractions. There may be a weak urinary stream as the bladder becomes distended.

namics is able to characterize specific types of voiding patterns. Examples of abnormal urodynamic study results are shown in Figs. 12.5 and 12.6.

There are no studies investigating the frequency with which monitoring should be done. Initial testing is often performed at 3 to 6 months postinjury or whenever the bladder comes out of spinal shock. The bladder is considered to come out of spinal shock when uninhibited bladder contractions begin to occur. This should be suspected if a person begins to have urinary incontinence or autonomic dysreflexia in the absence of a UTI. There may be so much spasticity of the sphincter that voiding does not occur, despite bladder contractions. This is why testing is needed even if it is not obvious that the bladder is out of spinal shock.

Institutions often have patients with SCI undergo a yearly evaluation for the first 5 to 10 years, and if their upper tracts are stable, then evaluations should occur every other year. However, some centers initially evaluate individuals every other year for the first 5 to 10 years and then begin to perform more intensive monitoring (yearly) after 10 years. There is general agreement that patients with an indwelling suprapubic or urethral catheter should undergo yearly cystoscopy even after 10 years, particularly because there is a much higher incidence of bladder stones (52).

Special Considerations in Children

Myelodysplasia is a common cause of pediatric spinal cord dysfunction resulting in a neurogenic bladder. Reflux and renal deterioration often occur during the first 3 years of life. McGuire et al. (53) reported a high incidence of renal deterioration in patients with urethral leak point pressures of more than 40 cm H_2O. Therefore, it is recommended that all myelodysplastic newborn children be evaluated as soon as possible (54). It is difficult to obtain high-quality water-fill urodynamic studies on children younger than 4 or 5 years. In younger children, it sometimes is necessary to use sedation or general anesthesia. It is important that children feel comfortable with the physician, nurse, and test. As a general principle, the amount of additional information gained from insertion of EMG needles usually is not enough to warrant the risk of obtaining poor urodynamic results from a crying, fearful child. This is particularly true if it is anticipated that the child will come back for follow-up studies.

MANAGEMENT OF VOIDING DYSFUNCTIONS

Management of voiding dysfunctions varies depending on the type of bladder and sphincter function that a person has after SCI. This section is divided into two broad categories: suprasacral injuries and sacral injuries. Within each of these categories, pharmacologic, surgical, and supportive treatment options are discussed. As previously discussed, the difference between the internal and external sphincter is becoming less distinct. Therefore, in the following discussion, *sphincter* refers to the sphincter mechanism, which in turn refers to both the internal and the external sphincter. One must remember that bladder and sphincter function frequently changes over time. A person may also have a combined suprasacral and sacral injury and varying de-

grees of "completeness" of injury. An initial evaluation and monitoring of the upper and lower tracts, as discussed previously, is therefore essential.

In addition to knowing the type of bladder and sphincter function that has resulted after an SCI, a number of goals should be kept in mind. These goals include the following:

- prevention of upper tract complications (e.g., deterioration of renal function, hydronephrosis, renal calculi, and pyelonephritis)
- prevention of lower tract complications (e.g., cystitis, bladder stones, and vesicoureteral reflux)
- development of a bladder management program that will allow a person to reintegrate most easily back into the community

Management of Suprasacral Injuries

Immediately after SCI, a person's bladder is in spinal shock and does not have any bladder contractions. Even in those with suprasacral injuries, in which one would expect the presence of uninhibited contractions, there is frequently a lack of contractions for several months, even up to 2 years postinjury.

When a person is first admitted to the hospital with an acute suprasacral SCI, there are usually a number of significant medical problems with large fluctuations in urine output in response to intravenous fluids and posttraumatic changes in fluid balances. During this time, it is best to manage the person's bladder with an indwelling catheter. Once a person is no longer receiving intravenous fluid, has a fluid output of less than 100 mL per hour, and does not have problems with orthostatic hypotension requiring increased fluids, IC can be started. IC is best started at a frequency of every 4 hours. The goal is to keep catheterization volumes from exceeding 400 mL. This can usually be accomplished by encouraging patients to have a daily 2-L fluid restriction. Sterile IC is frequently used in an inpatient setting to help decrease the spread of nosocomial infections. This can be accomplished using a sterile catheter and sterile catheter tray. Alternatively, a sterile catheter, which is self-contained in a sterile bag and can be pushed out through a closed bag, may be used. The urine then drains through the catheter into the bag. The advantage to using this system is that the urine is contained in a closed system.

When patients with suprasacral injuries come out of spinal shock, they begin having uninhibited bladder contractions. Several options are then available. Men can decide whether they would like to suppress the uninhibited contractions and perform IC or whether they would like to reflexly void. Women do not have the option of reflex voiding without needing to use diapers because there are no good external collecting devices for women.

Incontinence due to the Bladder

Intermittent Catheterization
Once patients are out of spinal shock, they will frequently begin having significant urinary incontinence because of the return of uninhibited bladder contractions. If a person is not sure what type of management to use and has good hand function, it is

best to encourage a trial of IC. Pharmacotherapy, such as an anticholinergic medication, is frequently needed to suppress the uninhibited bladder contractions, to prevent incontinence between catheterization. IC should be tried first because bladder capacity generally decreases with other types of management such as reflex voiding or an indwelling catheter. This is because the bladder is not intermittently distended, as it is with IC. If a person then develops a small bladder capacity, it is extremely difficult to increase bladder capacity if a person later decides to switch to IC.

IC has a long tract record and is considered to be one of the safest methods of management. Guttmann and Frankel (55) popularized sterile IC for patients with SCI in the 1960s with a low rate of complications. In the mid-1970s, Lapides et al. (56) reported on the effectiveness of clean IC (CIC). They attributed the success of CIC to the ease of performing CIC, compared with the sterile technique, so patients were more likely to catheterize themselves and prevent bladder overdistention than with the sterile technique (56). Maynard and Glass (57) reported that 80% of patients on CIC followed for 60 months continued on CIC, suggesting low morbidity and high patient acceptance. Recently, a retrospective study of 316 patients post-SCI followed for 18 years compared IC, spontaneous (reflex) voiding, urethral catheterization, and suprapubic catheterization. Although this was a retrospective study and patients did vary from one type of management to another during this time, the investigators reported that IC was found to be the safest method of management (58).

There are several major complications that can occur from IC. Urethral trauma can occur, particularly if there is a significant amount of sphincter spasticity. Although less frequent than with indwelling catheters, epididymitis and urethral stricture may occur. There have also been reports of the development of silent hydronephrosis and vesicoureteral reflux. One group of investigators noted that upper tract deterioration occurred in 28 of 85 individuals with chronic SCI who had initially had an areflexic bladder that changed to detrusor hyperreflexia with DSD (59). Another study that followed patients on IC for 8 years found that 7 of 40 had significant upper tract deterioration (60). These studies point out the importance of monitoring the upper and lower tracts.

The reason for these upper tract changes is felt to be high storage pressures due to uninhibited bladder contractions, combined with DSD and poor bladder wall compliance. Bladder wall compliance may also decrease (become poor) after SCI. This results in increased resting pressures, which can also cause stasis of the upper tracts. Although this can occur after IC, it has been found that decreases in bladder wall compliance are much less using IC than spontaneous reflex voiding or an indwelling catheter (61).

There has been controversy about using the sterile versus the clean technique. Although the clean technique works well in the outpatient setting, Anderson (62) reported that there was a high rate of significant bacteriuria despite antibiotic prophylaxis in the hospital setting and suggested that the sterile technique may be preferred in the acute spinal cord center (62). Outpatient sterile catheterization is difficult because a person requires a sterile catheterization kit and gloves for each catheterization. The outpatient sterile technique is now much more practical, with the development of sterile catheters in an enclosed urine bag, which in turn collect urine into the bag. However, many insurance companies do not pay for this type of catheter unless there are frequent complications from CIC.

The important principles of IC are to restrict fluids to 2 L a day and to catheterize frequently enough to keep the bladder from becoming overdistended (less than 400 mL). This usually requires a person to catheterize the bladder every 4 to 6 hours. They may have to add extra catheterizations if they increase their fluid intake. Because many patients with SCI do not have any sensation of bladder fullness, they catheterize at set intervals, as previously described. Ideally it would be best to catheterize by bladder volume. The Food and Drug Administration (FDA) recently approved a small handheld ultrasound device to measure bladder volumes. This is held over the bladder and indicates the amount of fluid in the bladder so a person can decide whether to catheterize (63). Use of prophylactic antibiotics in patients who perform IC is controversial (57,62). Relative contraindications to IC are women with significant adductor leg spasticity, patients with history of a urethral false passage, or those with poor hand-eye coordination, poor cognition, or poor motivation.

Pharmacologic Treatment Options for Incontinence due to the Bladder

There are a number of pharmacologic agents that can be used to suppress uninhibited bladder contractions. Their primary action is to block acetylcholine receptors competitively at the postganglionic autonomic receptor sites. Some agents such as oxybutynin also have a localized smooth muscle antispasmodic effect distal to the cholinergic receptor site and a local anesthetic effect on the bladder wall. It sometimes is helpful to combine an agent such as propantheline, with primarily anticholinergic effects, with one that also has local effects (64). Potential side effects of anticholinergic medications include dry mouth, pupillary dilation and blurred vision, tachycardia, drowsiness, and constipation from decreased gastrointestinal (GI) motility. Newer anticholinergic agents, which are more selective to the bladder such as terodiline and slow-release oxybutynin, have been developed to lessen anticholinergic side effects, particularly dry mouth.

Tricyclic antidepressants sometimes are used alone or in combination with anticholinergic agents. These medications, of which imipramine has been used most extensively, are thought to have a peripheral anticholinergic effect and a central effect. They have been found to suppress uninhibited bladder contractions, increase bladder capacity, and increase urethral resistance (65). There have been several reports of severe autonomic dysreflexia in patients with SCI secondary to overdistention of the bladder with urine (66).

Intravesical medications are gaining interest because oral anticholinergic medications have a number of side effects. Intravesical medications have the advantage of minimal to no systemic side effects. This is particularly helpful for patients with a neurogenic bowel, because anticholinergic medications frequently cause constipation, which could lead to fecal impaction. Anticholinergic medications may also cause a dry mouth, which can be particularly difficult to tolerate for patients trying to limit their fluid intake because of being on IC.

Oxybutynin is the anticholinergic medication of choice for intravesical instillation, because it has an anticholinergic effect and a topical anesthetic effect. Although this medication is effective at suppressing uninhibited bladder contractions, it has a disadvantage of only being effective for 4 to 6 hours. We have found 5 to 10 mg dissolved in 30 mL of normal saline instilled into the bladder four times a day to be effective. One study using this dose noted in the seven men studied an improvement in body image and enhanced sexuality because of the significant improvement in continence (67). Another investigator examined 32 patients, comparing standard dosages of intravesical Ditropan (0.3 mg/kg of body weight per day) with increasing dosages in steps of 0.2 mg/kg of body weight up to 0.9 mg/kg per day. Twenty-one (64%) of 32 patients became continent with the standard dose. Seven (22%) of the 11 incontinent patients became continent with a median dose of 0.7 mg/kg of body weight. Four (12.5%) of the 11 had no improvement and 2 of the 11 patients had side effects with a dose of 0.9 mg/kg of body weight per day (68). There is currently no commercial preparation for intravesical oxybutynin instillation. Therefore, a person has to dissolve the medication in sterile saline and instill it at 4- to 6-hour intervals. Many individuals abandon this because it is so labor intensive.

Intravesical instillations may, however, assume a more important role in helping to control uninhibited contractions with the development of longer acting agents. Of particular interest is afferent C-fiber neurotoxins. The prototype medication is capsaicin, which is effective at suppressing uninhibited contractions for several months at a time. In a double-blind placebo-controlled study of 20 patients with spinal cord lesions, bladder capacity increased from 169 ± 68 mL to 299 ± 96 mL and maximum detrusor pressure decreased from 77 ± 24 cmH$_2$O to 53 ± 27 cmH$_2$O when given capsaicin (69). Unfortunately, capsaicin frequently causes discomfort or suprapubic pain, urgency, hematuria, and autonomic dysreflexia, which can last up to 2 weeks after instillation.

A newer afferent C-fiber neurotoxin, RTX, is being investigated. It is a 1,000 times stronger than capsaicin and also is long acting. It has an extremely rapid onset of action at desensitizing the C-fiber afferent neurons, although it causes minimal discomfort when it is instilled. In one study, 14 patients with detrusor hyperreflexia were instilled with 100 mL (or the bladder capacity if lower than that volume) of 50 to 100 nmol/L RTX instillation in 10% alcohol in saline. Treatment improved or abolished incontinence in 9 (75%) of 12 patients. Mean cystometric capacity increased from 182 to 330 mL. Maximal detrusor pressure was not modified by treatment. The effects were long lasting, up to 12 months in seven patients (70). Other studies also appear very promising (16,71).

Other medications that have been reported, or are being investigated, to improve storage include intrathecal baclofen and prostaglandin inhibitors (72,73). Desmopressin acetate has been found to decrease the number of episodes of nocturia in patients with MS. However, further studies are needed to determine its usefulness because of potential risks of inducing hyponatremia and fluid retention (74). Potential side effects and contraindica-

tions must be weighed against potential benefits when using any pharmacologic agents for the treatment of incontinence due to the bladder (64,65).

Surgical Treatment Options for Incontinence due to the Bladder

Bladder Augmentation. Surgical treatment is sometimes needed to improve bladder capacity in adult patients who are incontinent and want to perform IC. The indications for surgical intervention include inability to tolerate or not wanting to take pharmacologic agents, severe detrusor hyperreflexia or poor bladder wall compliance, recurrent UTIs, autonomic dysreflexia, and continued upper tract deterioration despite aggressive pharmacotherapy and other types of management. Bladder augmentation is a surgical technique that is frequently used to create a large bladder capacity with low intravesical pressures. Because this is a surgical procedure, other alternatives such as pharmacologic treatment should first be tried.

An extensive preoperative evaluation is important. The history should include questions about any GI problems. Urodynamics should be performed to evaluate bladder and sphincter function. Various treatments may be needed to treat the sphincter if there is a low leak point pressure. Laboratory work should include liver and renal function tests. To help reduce the risk of significant acidosis and metabolic abnormalities, bladder augmentation is best reserved for those with serum creatinine clearance of less than 2.0 mg/dL. A cystogram should be done to evaluate for vesicoureteral reflux. Ureteral reimplantation may be considered if there is significant reflux. Upper tract evaluation is also important, both to rule out any problems and to serve as a baseline for follow-up postaugmentation (75).

There are a number of techniques of bladder augmentation in which different segments of bowel can be used. The most common type of bladder augmentation is the clam cystoplasty. This procedure involves isolating a piece of intestine, being careful to keep it attached to its mesentery, detubulizing it, and sewing it onto the bladder, which is first partially bivalved. Various bowel segments can be used and depend on the surgeon's preference.

There are predictable metabolic abnormalities depending on the segment being used. The stomach mucosa has secretory epithelium with little resorptive function. Gastric mucosa secretes hydrochloric acid in conjunction with systemic bicarbonate release. Therefore, hypochloremic metabolic alkalosis can result if the stomach is being used, particularly if there is poor renal function. However, the stomach has the least absorptive properties and best if one is concerned about metabolic acidosis from reabsorption of urinary solutes through the bowel wall. However, this is technically more difficult than an intestinal segment closer to the bladder.

The jejunal mucosa is different from the ileum and large intestine in that it secretes sodium and chloride and may result in hyponatremia, hypochloremia, and hyperkalemia. This segment is most likely to result in metabolic abnormalities and is rarely used in diversions. The ileum and colon have similar transport mechanisms. Ammonia and chloride are reabsorbed, which can lead to hyperchloremic metabolic acidosis (76).

The most frequent changes that occur after this are an increase in mucus noted in the urine, possible metabolic changes, abnormal drug absorption (particularly those that are absorbed by the GI tract and excreted unchanged by the kidneys such as Dilantin and certain antibiotics), osteomalacia from chronic acidosis and stones (particularly in those with urea-splitting organisms), and hyperchloremic metabolic acidosis. Long-term consequences of bowel attached to bladder are unknown. There have also been case reports of cancer including adenocarcinomas, undifferentiated carcinomas, sarcomas, and transitional cell carcinomas, and in those with bladder augmentations, ileal conduits and colon conduits (77,78).

Mast et al. (79) reported a 70% success rate at stopping incontinence (mean length of follow-up, 1½ years) and this was increased to 85% with the addition of an artificial sphincter in those with low sphincter resistance (79). Complications included recurrent UTI (59%) and stone formation (22%). Because of complications, however, further surgery was required for 44% of the patients. Another study evaluated clinical outcome and quality of life after enterocystoplasty in 18 patients with neurogenic bladders and 3 with contracted bladders due to radiation cystitis (80). Enterocystoplasty was performed using a 40-cm segment of terminal ileum. Their mean bladder capacities improved from 165 mL preoperatively to 760 mL postoperatively. At a mean of 36 months, 90% had acceptable continence rates and 95% reported improved quality of life (80).

Another method of surgically increasing bladder size without mucus formation and use of a bowel segment is a bladder autoaugmentation, also called a detrusor myomectomy. Through an abdominal approach, the bladder muscle is stripped away from the inner mucosal lining. Without this muscle lining, the bladder mucosa gradually stretches to become a large diverticulum, thereby increasing bladder capacity. Autoaugmentation has the advantage of not causing metabolic and absorption problems, as previously described for bladder augmentation using a bowel segment. However, this procedure is often technically difficult, particularly in patients with a neurogenic bladder who frequently have a small, heavily trabeculated bladder, and also offers only an approximate 25% increase in bladder capacity. The capacity does not immediately increase but gradually increases over time.

One investigator reported on bladder autoaugmentation in 50 men with neurogenic bladders. Bladder capacity increased over 1 to 6 months. One patient had a bladder rupture and two were reported to have "failed" due to psychological reasons (81).

Urinary Diversions. Although there are many types of surgical urinary diversions, they can be grouped into two general types: standard (noncontinent) and continent diversion. The most common standard noncontinent diversion is an ileal conduit. Ten to 15 cm of ileum, along with its mesentery, is isolated from the ileum. The isolated segment of ileum is closed off at one end and the other end is brought out through the abdominal wall and everted as a nipple stoma. The ureters are implanted onto the side of the ureters. Standard noncontinent diversions are primarily used in patients with SCI who need to have the urinary stream diverted from the perineum. Common indications include impaired healing of a pressure ulcer due to urinary incontinence or a urethral stricture or fistula.

Continent diversions may be used in patients who need to have their urinary stream diverted but are frequently used in patients who would like to perform IC but are not able to for various reasons, which may include a small bladder capacity or severe leg spasticity. Continent diversions are divided into two types: (a) orthotopic diversions, in which the bowel reservoir is anastomosed to the urethra, and (b) a continent catheterizable pouch.

Orthotopic diversions are much like bladder augmentations and are used to increase bladder capacity. Because they are attached to the urethra, people can catheterize themselves through their urethra in the same manner they would if they were catheterizing their bladder. Continent catheterizable pouches have the advantage that the stoma can be placed in a location that makes catheterization easier. For example, the stoma can be created within the umbilicus so people do not have to undress to catheterize themselves. The most difficult part of the continent diversion is the creation of a continent mechanism. The most commonly used bowel segment for this is the ileocecal valve. The right colon, with or without a segment of small bowel to increase volume, is used for the pouch and the terminal ileum is used to create the catheterizable limb (75,78).

Postoperatively, patients need to catheterize their pouch frequently to prevent rupture. Because there is an increase in mucus, patients need to be taught how to irrigate their pouch. Irrigations can be decreased over time, although a schedule of at least once a month is recommended. There may be malabsorption of bile salts due to the use of the ileocecal valve, which may cause diarrhea. This is best treated with oral administration of cholestyramine (76). Long-term follow-up of bladder augmentations and urinary diversions includes regular monitoring of the upper tracts and careful monitoring of blood chemistries and renal function. Cystoscopy is used to monitor for stones or tumors.

Other Surgical Options. Surgical methods also have been designed to interrupt innervation to the bladder. This can be performed centrally (e.g., subarachnoid block or cordectomy), peripherally (e.g., anterior or anteroposterior rhizotomy), or perivesically (e.g., extensive mobilization of the bladder) (82, 83). Although there usually is a successful short-term outcome, decreased compliance or detrusor hyperreflexia may return. This may be due to an increased sensitivity of receptors after decentralization (24). Impotence usually occurs after these procedures.

Neurostimulation is a relatively new area of research. Electrical stimulation has a number of uses in treating patients with voiding dysfunction. It has been used both to facilitate storage by decreasing uninhibited bladder contractions and to improve voiding by helping to trigger uninhibited contractions. Methods to inhibit bladder contractions had their widest use in able-bodied individuals with overactive bladders. Ohlsson and Frankenberg-Sommar (84) reported an average 49% increase in bladder capacity by stimulation of the pudendal nerve with anal and vaginal electrode plugs. Tanago (85) reported success at selective sacral root stimulation to increase sphincter tone, which in turn suppresses detrusor activity.

In patients with SCI with neurogenic bladders, investigators continue to try to improve voiding through the use of neurostimulation. Techniques include placing electrodes on the bladder itself, the pelvic nerves, conus medullaris, sacral nerves, and the sacral anterior roots. Of these, sacral anterior root stimulation has been most successful.

Brindley et al. (86) developed an anterior root stimulator that produces micturition by stimulating the sacral nerve roots. The largest experience is with the surgically implanted Finetech-Brindley sacral afferent stimulator, in which there have been an estimated 800 implants over 15 years (87). Prerequisites for successful neurostimulation include an intact sacral reflex arc and a detrusor capable of contracting. Stimulation of the sacral afferent nerves causes reflex activation of the efferent nerves to the sphincter. However, this reflex accommodates so that fatigue of the sphincter occurs and the pressure generated in the urethra is overcome by the bladder contraction. A posterior rhizotomy is often performed at the same time as the sacral implant to abolish uninhibited bladder contractions, abolish contractions of the sphincter, and improve bladder wall compliance. The disadvantage of the posterior rhizotomy is the loss of reflex erections and reflex ejaculations, loss of perineal sensation, and loss of reflex bladder contractions (87). Van Kerrebroeck (88) reviewed the worldwide experience with the Finetech-Brindley sacral stimulator. In 184 cases, of whom 170 were using the stimulator, 95% had PVR volumes of less than 60 mL. There was no deterioration of the upper tracts. Two thirds of men reported stimulated erections, although only one third used these for coitus (88). The FDA recently approved the extradural version of this device, which is known as the VOCARE Bladder System. Individuals must have a suprasacral injury with an intact sacral reflex arc so the stimulator can trigger uninhibited bladder contractions (see chapter 25 for details).

Supportive Treatment Options for Incontinence due to the Bladder

Indwelling Catheter. With shorter lengths of hospital stay, patients are often discharged from the hospital while their bladder is still in spinal shock. Both men and women with cervical injuries and poor hand function have much more independence as outpatients with an indwelling catheter than when they are dependent on others for IC. Indwelling catheters are particularly helpful at preventing bladder distention, which can provoke autonomic dysreflexia.

An indwelling catheter also may be an option for men who are unable to wear a condom catheter or who have contraindications to performing IC such as a urethral diverticulum. If an indwelling catheter is going to be used as a long-term bladder management option, some men prefer to switch to a suprapubic catheter so it is easier to have intercourse. An indwelling catheter is used more often in women than men with suprasacral injuries and poor hand function. This is because there is no satisfactory external collecting device for women.

Once the patient is out of spinal shock, an indwelling catheter can irritate the bladder and provoke uninhibited contractions in patients with suprasacral injuries. This in turn can cause high intravesical pressure, resulting in a functional obstruction at the ureteral orifices, which in turn may cause decreased drainage from the upper tracts. Therefore, use of an anticholinergic also should be strongly considered for patients who have an indwell-

ing bladder catheter in place, particularly if there is urodynamic evidence of detrusor hyperreflexia.

Principles of management include an oral fluid intake of at least 2 L a day, keeping the catheter taped to the abdomen of men when they are laying down to decrease the risk of a penile scrotal fistula, cleaning the urethral meatus of incrustations with soap and water twice a day, preventing reflux of urine into the bladder by never raising the drainage bag above the level of the bladder, and changing the Foley catheter every 2 to 4 weeks. Before removing an indwelling Foley catheter, to start IC or reflex voiding, we believe it is important to obtain urine culture and sensitivity tests and to treat the patient with an appropriate antibiotic for several days before and after catheter removal. This is to decrease the risk of bacteremia if the patient is unable to void and gets a distended bladder. If a Foley catheter has been in place for 4 to 6 weeks before switching a patient over to IC, cystoscopy is recommended to remove eggshell calculi and debris that may have collected in the bladder and may have the potential of becoming a nidus for large bladder stones. Prophylactic antibiotics are not recommended for a patient with an indwelling catheter because of the risk of developing resistant organisms.

Although there is a lack of prospective studies, risks are generally felt to be higher with an indwelling Foley catheter compared with IC (58). The most common complications of indwelling catheters include the development of bladder stones; hematuria; bacteremia, particularly if the catheter becomes obstructed; meatal erosions; penile scrotal fistulas; and epididymitis. Perhaps the highest risk with any type of indwelling catheter, compared with other types of management, is bladder stones (89). There is a reported significant increase in febrile UTIs, dysreflexia, and bladder stones, as well as a 54% incidence of urethral erosions in women with indwelling Foley catheters compared with IC (90). Care in using a small-caliber (16 French) catheter and keeping the leg bag from getting overfilled and pulling down on the catheter will decrease the frequency of urethral erosions.

A suprapubic catheter has been found to be safer than an indwelling Foley catheter because it decreases the risk of epididymitis, urethral stricture disease, and urethral irritation (58). In addition, it allows for a lower incidence of hypospadias and for easier access of the penis for sexual activity. The suprapubic tube is a good option if the patient requires an indwelling catheter, particularly for women, because it is easier to keep clean, minimizes inoculation of vaginal and fecal flora into the bladder, and is less cumbersome for participation in sexual activity.

Although many criticize the use of suprapubic catheters, one group of investigators evaluated complications in 44 individuals with SCI who had been treated with an indwelling suprapubic catheter. They found no renal deterioration and a low incidence of incontinence, UTI, and calculi (91). Another study retrospectively evaluated 32 patients with SCI with an indwelling catheter and 25 with SCI without a catheter. There was a statistically higher incidence of bladder stones, with no overall statistically significant difference in upper tract or lower tract complications between the two groups. The authors suggested that the decision to manage a person with quadriplegia should not be based on relative risks of complications of renal deterioration, but that the decision to avoid an indwelling catheter should reflect patient comfort, convenience, and quality of life (92). A controlled prospective study would be helpful to confirm their observations. As with any type of bladder management, one needs to carefully monitor for potential problems of the upper and lower urinary tracts.

Reflex Voiding. Another method of management that can be used in men with an intact sacral micturition reflex is reflex (spontaneous) voiding. This type of voiding involves having the person wear a condom catheter attached to a leg bag. The bladder has a spontaneous uninhibited contraction when it reaches a certain bladder volume. However, the volume that "triggers" the uninhibited bladder contraction is different for each person. One advantage to an external condom catheter and a leg bag is that is does not require good hand function. A caregiver can put on the condom catheter in the morning and not have to change it until the next day. Some assistance is needed, however, because the leg bag holds 1,000 mL and should be emptied when it is half full. Similar to an indwelling catheter, another advantage is that there is no limit on fluid intake, as there is with the use of IC as a method of bladder management. Major disadvantages are potential penile skin breakdown, having to wear an external condom catheter and leg bag, and possibly a slightly increased risk of bladder infections compared with IC.

Because men who reflexly void usually have DSD, their upper tracts and lower tracts have to be monitored. Although there is agreement that elevated voiding pressures cause upper tract problems, there is no consensus on what voiding pressure will cause this damage (93–96). A recent study revealed that the most important voiding parameter causing upper tract stasis, in those who reflexly void, was the duration of the bladder contraction (97). Since we have a better understanding of what is causing upper tract and lower tract problems and treatments are not without complications, it is best to treat a person if they are having or are beginning to have problems. Problems may include autonomic dysreflexia, recurrent bladder infections, vesicoureteral reflux, kidney or bladder stones, kidney infection, or deterioration in bladder function (progressively higher PVR levels) or renal function.

Various treatment options are available for patients who reflexly void and are having problems. Various methods to improve voiding secondary to outlet obstruction without the presence of DSD are discussed in the sections on pharmacologic treatment and surgical treatment for urinary retention due to the sphincter.

Incontinence due to the Sphincter

It would be extremely unusual for a person with a suprasacral injury to have urinary incontinence solely due to the sphincter. It is possible that this may occur if the person's bladder was still in spinal shock and urinary incontinence occurs due to overflow from an overdistended bladder. However, if urinary incontinence was found to be due to the sphincter in the absence of uninhibited bladder contractions, one should suspect a secondary sacral injury. Because DSD is common after suprasacral SCI, treatment of the sphincter should not be undertaken because of the risk of making the dyssynergia worse.

Retention due to the Bladder—Therapy Overview

As previously discussed, urinary retention occurs when patients are in spinal shock. As they have return of bladder contractions, they develop large PVRs. This may be due to weak bladder contractions or DSD. Treatment of DSD is discussed in detail in the section "Retention due to the Sphincter." IC or an indwelling urethral catheter is often used to help maintain bladder emptying.

Pharmacologic Treatment for Retention due to the Bladder

Bethanechol chloride, which provides relatively selective stimulation of the bladder and bowel and is resistant to rapid hydrolysis by acetylcholinesterase, may be used to increase bladder contractions (98). Even in patients with bladder contractions, bethanechol is not very helpful for treating retention in those with suprasacral injuries because it also worsens DSD. Sporer et al. (99) found that bethanechol increased external sphincter pressures by 10 to 20 cm H_2O in men with SCI. Therefore, it should not be used in those with DSD. Bethanechol also is contraindicated in patients with bladder outlet obstruction. Potential side effects and contraindications must be weighed against potential benefits when pharmacologic agents are used to improve emptying (100).

Two investigational agents to improve bladder emptying are prostaglandins and narcotic antagonists. Intravesical prostaglandin $F_{2\alpha}$ was noted to increase detrusor pressures in patients with SCI with suprasacral lesions (101). Narcotic antagonists are thought to block enkephalins, which are believed to inhibit the sacral micturition reflex (102).

Retention due to the Sphincter

Behavioral Treatment for Retention due to the Sphincter

Retention due to the sphincter is a common problem in patients with suprasacral SCI due to DSD. In addition to actual retention, DSD causing high PVRs can also cause outlet obstruction. This can result in high voiding pressures with uninhibited contractions being of long duration, which in turn can cause backpressure to the kidneys. Moreover, the forceful uninhibited contractions against the dyssynergic sphincter can cause autonomic dysreflexia in those with injuries at or above T6.

One method to help cause sphincter relaxation and trigger an uninhibited bladder contraction is suprapubic bladder tapping. Tapping is usually performed for 10 to 30 seconds; this briefly relaxes the sphincter. Because tightening of the sphincter reflexly inhibits the bladder from having a contraction, relaxation of the sphincter will frequently allow the bladder to have an uninhibited bladder contraction. Another method that has been described is using a scissoring action of the fingers in the rectum. This results in relaxing the anal and urethral sphincter. This technique is not very practical for voiding because it can also trigger a bowel movement, but it is sometimes used in situations in which there is difficulty passing a urethral catheter due to significant sphincter spasticity. Although both of these methods will frequently trigger voiding, they do not reduce voiding pressures. Additionally, both of these methods may cause autonomic dysreflexia in those with injuries at or above T6. For this reason, these methods are best reserved for triggering voiding after pharmacologic or surgical treatment for the sphincter has been undertaken.

Pharmacologic Treatment for Retention due to the Sphincter

α-Adrenergic blocking agents have been shown to be effective at improving bladder emptying in patients with DSD and prostate outlet obstruction (103,104). In those with prostate outlet obstruction, this is because the prostate smooth muscle is mediated by α-adrenergic stimulation (105). Placebo-controlled studies have shown a significant improvement in voiding in subjects taking phenoxybenzamine, prazosin, and more recently, terazosin (105).

α-Blocking agents may improve voiding in patients with sphincter dyssynergia secondary to an SCI due to several factors. After denervation, a supersensitivity of the urethra to α-adrenergic stimulation can occur. In addition, there may be a conversion of the usual β-receptors to α-receptors (25,106). Therefore, α-blockers also have the potential of improving bladder wall compliance. One study reported that bladder wall compliance improved by 73% with the use of α-blockers. There was also an improvement in maximum bladder pressure, and episodes of autonomic dysreflexia improved with terazosin treatment (107). An added benefit of α-blockers is their ability to blunt autonomic dysreflexia (108).

Scott and Morrow (108) found that phenoxybenzamine worked well at decreasing residual urine volume in patients with suprasacral SCI and autonomic dysreflexia but had variable effects on those without dysreflexia. When deciding which α-blocker to use, one must be aware that the manufacturer of phenoxybenzamine has indicated a dose-related incidence of GI tumors in rats. There have been no cases of GI tumors linked to phenoxybenzamine in humans in more than 30 years of use (109); however, the potential medicolegal issues of long-term use of phenoxybenzamine in young patients with SCI should be considered.

Three other drugs that have been used for striated external sphincter relaxation are baclofen, diazepam, and dantrolene. In our experience, these agents are not as effective as α-blocking agents and should not be used as the drugs of choice for external sphincter relaxation. Potential side effects and contraindications must be weighed against potential benefits when using pharmacologic agents to improve emptying (110).

Surgical Treatment Options for Retention due to the Sphincter

There are times when pharmacologic treatment cannot be used (the person has significant hypotension), a person does not want to be treated with medications, or an α-blocker is not effective. In these cases, surgical alternatives should be considered.

Transurethral sphincterotomy is a well established treatment for spinal cord injured men with DSD. Indications include vesicoureteral reflux, high urinary residual volumes with severe autonomic dysreflexia or recurrent UTIs, upper tract changes with

sustained high intravesical pressures, and poor compliance or side effects from medications being used to relax the outlet. Perkash (111) reported a more than 90% success rate at relief of dysreflexia symptoms, a decrease in residual urine, a decrease in infected urine, and a significant radiologic improvement. He stressed the importance of extending the incision to the bladder neck (111). Longitudinal studies have shown a 25% to 50% sphincterotomy failure rate. This has been attributed to various causes such as poor patient selection (i.e., those with detrusor areflexia or bladder contractions less than 30 cm H_2O, recurrent DSD, failure to recognize the need for a concomitant procedure (such as bladder neck incision or prostate resection), or new-onset detrusor hypocontractility (112).

The major concerns of many patients with SCI are that the procedure is irreversible, it is a surgical procedure, and they will have to wear a leg bag. The traditional electrocautery method of performing a sphincterotomy has been reported to at times be bloody, with hemorrhage requiring blood transfusion varying from 5% to 26%. This risk of bleeding has been largely eliminated with the use of Nd:YAG contact laser sphincterotomy. Perkash (113) reported that in 30 patients undergoing laser sphincterotomy, blood loss was 150 mL in one patient and less than 50 mL in the other 29 patients. The major advantages to a sphincterotomy and reflex voiding are that there are no fluid restrictions, the procedure is effective for the previously mentioned problems, and it will decrease attendant care in those who had previously performed IC (111).

Another method of treatment for DSD is the stainless steel woven mesh stent (e.g., UroLume Endourethral Wallstent, American Medical Systems), which holds the sphincter mechanism open. With an experienced team, this can be done under local anesthesia. Because the sphincter is not cut, the procedure is potentially reversible with removal of the stent. The stent becomes covered by epithelium in 3 to 6 months, preventing calcium incrustation. A multicenter study of 153 men with SCI revealed a significant decrease in voiding pressures and PVR urine volumes up to 2 years. Hydronephrosis resolved in 22 (78.6%) of 28 patients (114). There was no loss or erectile function. Complications included mild postoperative hematuria in 10 patients (7.1%), penile edema in 2 patients, incrustation of the stent in 3 patients, stent removal (usually due to stent migration) in 10 patients, and subsequent operation for bladder neck obstruction in 13 patients. Long-term follow-up studies are underway. This device is approved by the FDA for the treatment of urethral strictures and DSD.

Another method under investigation to decrease urethral sphincter pressure is botulinum toxin (BTX). BTX blocks acetylcholine release from the motor nerve terminals, thereby blocking neuromuscular transmission (115). It has an onset of action that may vary from 1 day to 1 week. Peak effect is usually present by 3 weeks. The medication may relax the sphincter for 3 or more months. Dykstra et al. (116) reported decreased DSD in 10 of 11 men with suprasacral SCI, with injection of BTX into the sphincter. Wheeler et al. (117) reported success at relaxing a person's sphincter to facilitate IC.

Pudendal block or neurectomy was used in the past in spine-injured men with DSD (118). This procedure largely has been replaced by sphincterotomy. Pudendal block or neurectomy is being used to relax the sphincter mechanism by some investigators working at perfecting electrical stimulation for voiding (85). A unilateral neurectomy is recommended over a bilateral procedure to help decrease the risk of impotence and fecal incontinence (82).

Supportive Treatment for Retention due to the Sphincter

Urinary retention in the absence of uninhibited contractions is usually due to DSD. Although unusual, some individuals with suprasacral injuries do have significant spasticity of the sphincter without uninhibited contractions. One possible mechanism for this occurring is that there is so much tone in the sphincter that it reflexly inhibits the bladder from contracting. IC is an excellent option for these individuals if they have good hand function. There are times when there is so much tone in the sphincter that it is very difficult to pass a catheter. If a person is properly trained, a catheter coudé (a catheter with a slight curve at the end) will sometimes pass easier than a regular catheter. A combination of pharmacologic agents is often helpful. Other options include an indwelling catheter or suprapubic catheter.

Sacral Lesions

Patients with sacral injuries are not expected to have bladder contractions. Incontinence due to a weak sphincter mechanism can occur, particularly with increased intraabdominal pressure such as performing a weight shift. Additionally, incontinence can occur if the pressure in the bladder is higher than that in the sphincter due to distention and poor bladder wall compliance (decreased compliance). The pressure at which this occurs is known as the abdominal leak point pressure. Myelodysplastic children have been found to have a much greater chance of upper tract deterioration with abdominal leak point pressures of more than 40 cm H_2O pressure (119). Some patients may have a combined suprasacral and sacral injury. These individuals have been found to have very unpredictable urodynamic findings (120).

Management options for those with complete sacral and peripheral injuries are similar both acutely and in the long term because bladder function usually does not have significant changes. However, there are changes in patients with incomplete injuries. Urodynamics is important in monitoring those with sacral injuries to ensure that there is not a return of uninhibited contractions that could impact the upper tracts.

Therapy for Incontinence of the Bladder

Because incontinence of the bladder is most likely due to bladder overdistention, IC is usually effective. α-Blockers have been shown to improve bladder wall compliance and may have some benefit. A surgical option that is usually effective in a person with a small bladder capacity and poor bladder wall compliance is bladder augmentation. Care should be taken not to try to "tighten the sphincter" in this situation. This may allow the incontinence to resolve, although there will then be increased intravesical pressure. This in time could lead to upper tract complications.

Behavioral Treatment Options for Incontinence due to the Outlet or Sphincter

Timed voiding sometimes is helpful in patients with mild incontinence who have normal bladder function, but an underactive urethral sphincter mechanism. The object is to have the patient void before the bladder reaches full capacity. At full capacity, intravesical pressure is more likely to overcome the urethral pressure, resulting in leakage.

Pelvic-floor (i.e., Kegel) exercises and biofeedback also may be tried in neurologically intact patients with mild to moderate stress incontinence due to the sphincter (121). There is a great variation in the number of sets and repetitions described by various authors, with the total number of exercise contractions varying from 8 to 160 per day (122). Exercises sometimes are combined with commercial biofeedback units (123). Patients have to be highly motivated, and effects may not be seen for 4 to 8 weeks.

Pharmacologic Treatment Options for Incontinence due to the Sphincter

α-Adrenergic agonists may be useful at improving minimal to moderate stress incontinence due to the sphincter. Wyndaele (66) reported success at decreasing urinary leakage around the Foley catheter in women with incomplete SCI with patulous urethras. Ephedrine and phenylpropanolamine are two commonly used agents. Ephedrine causes a release of norepinephrine and directly stimulates α-receptors and β-receptors. Phenylpropanolamine is pharmacologically similar to ephedrine but provides less CNS stimulation (124). Recently, phenylpropanolamine has been reported to increase the risk of hemorrhagic stroke (125). The FDA has issued a health warning and recommended that phenylpropanolamine be taken out of over-the-counter medications.

Before prescribing any type of α-adrenergic agonist, one must rule out detrusor hyperreflexia or poor bladder compliance with urodynamics; otherwise, increasing the urethral sphincter tone may increase intravesical pressures, which could result in poor drainage from the upper tracts. Additionally, it could provoke autonomic dysreflexia if there is an additional spinal cord lesion at or above T6.

A 4- to 6-week course of estrogen supplementation may be helpful in postmenopausal women with atrophy of the urethral epithelium or irritative symptoms from atrophic urethritis (126). Its beneficial effect may be due to improving the local mucosal seal effect or by increasing sensitivity or improving the number of α-adrenergic receptors (127). The risks of endometrial cancer, thrombosis, or withdrawal bleeding are negligible when estrogen supplementation is used topically for this short duration.

Periurethral collagen injection therapy has recently received FDA approval for those with intrinsic urethral sphincter deficiency. Although clinical trials have focused primarily on individuals without SCI, this therapy appears to be a promising method to increase urethral resistance to the flow of urine. Appell (128) reported that 80% of female patients treated by this method were continent after two treatments. The major contraindication in properly selected patients is an allergy to bovine collagen (128). This should also not be used in a person with forceful uninhibited bladder contractions, because obstructing the urethra could cause back pressure into the kidneys.

Surgical Treatment Options for Incontinence due to the Outlet or Sphincter

Artificial sphincters are used infrequently in the adult SCI population, because they potentially can cause upper tract damage in those with detrusor hyperreflexia and high intravesical pressure. In addition, there is an increased risk of prosthesis infection or erosion of the cuff in patients with SCI because of frequent episodes of bacteriuria. Light and Scott (129) reported that 24% of their patients with SCI developed infection requiring removal of the device. If an artificial sphincter is going to be used, surgery should be delayed at least 6 months to 1 year to make sure there is not going to be a return of sphincter function. Artificial sphincters are better tolerated in children with myelodysplasia (130).

For women with stress incontinence due to the sphincter or intrinsic sphincter damage, such as from a long-term indwelling catheter, various surgeries have been developed to anatomically improve the urethral support and position. These procedures can be performed transabdominally, transvaginally, and even without surgical incisions. One- to 3-year follow-up success rates have been reported to be 57% to 91% (131). A potential problem is that the operation works too well and causes retention. Patients therefore should be aware of the possibility of needing to perform postoperative IC. Other surgical options for those with intrinsic sphincter damage include surgical closure of the bladder neck, followed by urinary diversion with an abdominal stoma that can be catheterized or the insertion of a suprapubic tube.

Supportive Treatment Options for Incontinence due to the Outlet or Sphincter

Supportive options are similar to those for incontinence due to the bladder. Specifically, these include diapers, external condom catheters, and indwelling catheters.

Therapy for Retention due to the Bladder

The method of choice for patients with sacral injuries who have urinary retention due to the bladder is IC. Patients with sacral injuries are not expected to have uninhibited contractions, so there is less likelihood of the need for anticholinergic medications. Urodynamics is still needed to characterize bladder function, because there is sometimes a mixed lesion resulting in uninhibited contractions or poor bladder wall compliance.

Credé/Valsalva

Credé maneuvers involve pushing down over the lower abdomen onto the bladder to express urine from the bladder. Valsalva maneuvers involve using intraabdominal pressure to push out

the urine. These maneuvers, particularly the use of intraabdominal pressure, may cause exacerbation of hemorrhoids, rectal prolapse, or hernia. This type of management is therefore best reserved for those who are unable to perform IC and have decreased urethral sphincter activity. Care must be taken to ensure that the person does not have DSD because increasing intraabdominal pressure often worsens the dyssynergia (132). Vesicoureteral reflux is a contraindication to this type of voiding.

Pharmacologic Treatment for Retention due to the Bladder

Bethanechol chloride is sometimes prescribed for patients with sacral lesions with urinary retention. Light and Scott (98) reported that it failed to induce bladder contractions in patients with SCI with detrusor areflexia. Therefore, bethanechol is not helpful in those who have no bladder contractions.

Surgical Treatment Options for Retention due to the Bladder

There have been reports of surgically reducing the size of the bladder to decrease the PVR volume; however, there is no effective way surgically to augment bladder contractions by operating on the bladder itself (133). Sphincterotomy has been reported in spine-injured men with detrusor areflexia, although this is generally not recommended because of the high failure rate at decreasing PVR levels (134).

One investigator reported on wrapping a portion of the rectus muscle around the bladder. Neurostimulation was performed, causing the bladder to contract and squeeze out the urine (135). Traditional neurostimulation, as described with suprasacral lesions, is not effective in patients with sacral lesions because of the need for an intact sacral reflex arc and bladder contractions.

Supportive Treatment Options for Retention due to the Bladder

One of the many important and successful methods for the management of failure to empty due to the bladder is CIC. In patients unable to tolerate pharmacotherapy and unable to perform IC, an alternative is an indwelling catheter (see previous discussion).

Retention due to the Sphincter

Behavioral Treatment Options for Retention due to the Outlet or Sphincter

Timed voiding and biofeedback methods have not been reported as successful methods of treatment in patients with neurogenic DSD. Biofeedback has been reported to be successful in patients with voluntary pseudo-DSD. These patients, who often are children, voluntarily tighten their sphincters during voiding, resulting in large PVR volumes and UTI (136).

In patients with SCI with detrusor hyperreflexia and DSD, anal stretching or scissoring and suprapubic bladder tapping have been reported as ways to temporarily interrupt the dyssynergia and allow voiding (137).

Supportive Treatment Options for Retention due to the Outlet or Sphincter

Supportive treatment options for the outlet are the same as those for retention due to the bladder—specifically, IC or indwelling catheters. Occasionally, a person has so much sphincter spasticity that it is difficult to pass a catheter. Instillation of lidocaine jelly down the urethra 5 minutes before catheterization, administration of α-adrenergic blockers, or use of a catheter coudé often facilitates catheterization.

Pediatric Considerations

The same pharmacologic principles discussed in the general management section apply for children. The age of the child and decreased doses need to be considered. Similarly, the same surgical procedures discussed under management can be used in children. In the past, children with vesicoureteral reflux were treated with urinary diversion, but because of long-term complications of urinary diversion and the excellent success of IC and ureteral reimplantation, this is rarely used today. Surgical procedures for children with severe incontinence include an anterior fascial sling around the urethra and an artificial urinary sphincter (138). There have been reports of 90% long-term success rates with the use of the artificial sphincter in children (130). The Kropp procedure, in which a new urethra is formed from a portion of bladder and tunneled submucosally in the trigone, has been described and may be a good alternative to an artificial urinary sphincter (139).

CIC has been shown to be effective treatment for children with failure to empty. In those with incontinence due to the bladder, an anticholinergic medication often is also required (oxybutynin, 1.0 mg per year of age twice daily). It is thought that parents and children adjust to this program if it is started when the child is a newborn. There have been no reported cases of urethral injury, epididymitis, or UTIs requiring hospitalizations due to this procedure. Children usually can begin performing their own IC at age 5 years (138).

COMPLICATIONS OF VOIDING DYSFUNCTIONS

Urinary Tract Infections

Bacteriuria is a common problem in patients with voiding dysfunctions. Lloyd et al. (140) followed 181 new patients with SCI discharged from an acute SCI center initially with sterile urine and on various bladder management programs for 1 year. At 1 year, 66.7% to 100% had at least one episode of bacteriuria depending on their bladder management program (140). Maynard and Diokno (141) reported on 50 new SCI inpatients on IC and found 88% had one or more episodes of bacteriuria (i.e., any bacteria present). Asymptomatic bacteriuria has been found to be present in 10% to 25% of community-dwelling patients and 25% to 40% of nursing home patients older than 65 years (142). These numbers would be expected to be at least as high as, if not higher than, those for patients with a voiding disorder.

Traditionally, a UTI was defined as more than 100,000 organisms in a midstream urine sample (143). The probability increased from 80% to 90% if this was found in two separate specimens. There is increasing controversy, however, about the true definition of a UTI. This is based on studies showing that symptomatic patients often have less than 100,000 organisms, uncertainty about the significance of asymptomatic bacteriuria and the presence or absence of pyuria, and the potential impact of other factors such as high voiding pressures, frequency of voiding, and PVR. It has been found that 30% of able-bodied women with acute dysuria had less than 10,000 coliforms per milliliter and many had less than 200 coliforms per milliliter (144,145).

In patients with SCI, Rhame and Perkash (146) reported that any specimen with more than 1,000 coliforms per milliliter was significant. Donovan et al. (147) thought that the appearance of any count of the same organism for two consecutive days was significant. The National Institute on Disability and Rehabilitation Research (NIDRR) UTI consensus conference based the definition of significant bacteria on the method of urine collection and colony count. A significant bacteria count does not necessarily mean an infection, rather confidence that the bacteria cultured were from the bladder and not contamination: for those on IC, more than 10^2 CFU/mL; for those who did not use catheterization, more than 10^4 CFU/mL; and for those who used an indwelling catheter, any detectable pathogens (148). There is controversy over whether significant bacteriuria should be regarded as a UTI or colonization.

With regard to pyuria, Stamm et al. (145) found that 96% of patients with symptomatic infections had more than 10 leukocytes per cubic millimeter. Deresinski and Perkash (149) reported that 79% of 70 patients with SCI with symptoms and bacteriuria also had pyuria; however, 46% of asymptomatic patients also had significant pyuria. Anderson and Hsieh-ma (150) also found that gram-negative bacteria caused significant pyuria, but that this was not true of *Staphylococcus epidermidis* or *Streptococcus faecalis* even in high numbers.

Signs and symptoms of a UTI involving the lower tract may include dysuria, frequency, urinary incontinence, and hematuria. Unless a person has had acute retention or urologic instrumentation, fever is less likely when the lower urinary tract is involved. Whereas many patients with SCI have decreased or no bladder sensation, a lower UTI often will cause cloudy strong-smelling urine, increased abdominal or lower extremity spasticity, new onset of urinary incontinence, occasionally retention from increased DSD, or autonomic dysreflexia in those with a lesion above T6.

Patients with acute upper tract involvement may present with any of these signs and symptoms. They also usually will have fever and chills and an elevated serum white blood cell count. Those with sensation usually complain of costal vertebral angle tenderness. In the elderly, signs and symptoms may be subtler and patients may present simply with confusion or lethargy. UTIs should be considered in the differential diagnosis of new cognitive changes in a head-injured patient.

Treatment of Asymptomatic Urinary Tract Infection

Guidelines for treatment have been difficult to establish for asymptomatic bacteriuria because of controversy about whether this represents colonization, rather than infection. Ideally, the urine should be sterile; however, the side effects of antibiotics and development of resistant organisms need to be taken into account. Kass et al. (151) followed 225 children on CIC for 10 years and reported that in the absence of vesicoureteral reflux, bacilluria proved innocuous, with only 2.6% of subjects developing fresh renal damage. In high-grade reflux, however, 60% developed pyelonephritis (151). Lewis et al. (152) followed 52 patients with acute SCI during their initial hospitalization. Seventy-eight percent of patients had more than 100,000 organisms, but only 13% had symptoms and required antimicrobial therapy over 6 months. Of interest is that 35% of culture results changed weekly from positive to negative, negative to positive, or one organism to another, necessitating a short course of antibiotics (152).

An accurate characterization of voiding dysfunction such as voiding pressure, bladder compliance, and PVR, along with accurate characterization of level and completeness of injury, often is lacking in various studies discussing UTIs in patients with SCI. It is hoped that prospective evaluations considering these factors in relation to factors such as bacteriuria, pyuria, upper and lower tract anatomy, virulence of organisms, and types of bladder management will allow guidelines to be formulated for the treatment of asymptomatic bacteriuria. There is general agreement that asymptomatic bacteriuria in a patient with an indwelling Foley catheter should not be treated. Attempts should be made to eradicate asymptomatic bacteriuria in those with high-grade reflux, before urologic instrumentation, in hydronephrosis, or in the presence of urea-splitting organisms.

Treatment of Symptomatic Urinary Tract Infections

Once a urine culture has been obtained, empirical oral antibiotic treatment can be started for patients with minimal symptoms while waiting for the culture results. Patients usually do well with a 7-day course of antibiotics. In those with high fevers, dehydration, or autonomic dysreflexia, more aggressive therapy should be instituted. It is our opinion that these patients should be hospitalized, closely monitored, hydrated, and given broad-spectrum antibiotics (e.g., gentamicin and ampicillin) while waiting for the culture results and for the fever to defervesce. It is important to have an indwelling Foley catheter in place during intravenous or oral fluid hydration to keep the bladder decompressed. We believe that it also is beneficial to give an anticholinergic medication while the Foley catheter is in place; this will decrease the intrinsic pressure within the detrusor, allowing relaxation of the ureterovesical junction and improving drainage of the kidneys. On renal scans, Tempkin et al. (153) showed that there was improved drainage of the upper tracts in patients with SCI who were given anticholinergics. Patients with significant fever should be considered to have upper tract involvement (i.e., pyelonephritis) and therefore should continue receiving 2 to 3 weeks of oral antibiotics after the fever has resolved. In addition, these patients should undergo a urologic evaluation for the cause of urosepsis. Acutely, this should consist of a plain abdominal radiograph to rule out an obvious stone, followed by a renal ultrasound. If there is a question of a stone, hydronephrosis, or persistent fever, an IVP should be performed. Once the patient has been treated, it is often necessary to perform a cysto-gram to evaluate for reflux, a cystoscopy to evaluate the bladder outlet and bladder, and urodynamic testing to evaluate voiding function.

Complications of Urinary Tract Infections

In addition to acute lower tract infections (i.e., cystitis) and upper UTIs (i.e., pyelonephritis), the physician should be aware of other potential problems. Those from lower UTIs include epididymitis, prostatic or scrotal abscess, sepsis, or an ascending infection to the upper tracts. Complications that may occur include chronic pyelonephritis, renal scarring, progressive renal deterioration, renal calculi if there is a urea-splitting organism such as *Proteus*, papillary necrosis, renal or retroperitoneal abscess, or bacteremia and sepsis.

Role of Prophylactic Antibiotics

There is controversy over the role of prophylactic antibiotics (62,141,154). Anderson (62) reported a statistically significant difference in bacteriuria in SCI inpatients on a combination of oral nitrofurantoin and neomycin-polymyxin B solution compared with controls. Merritt et al. (155) reported a statistically significant decrease in bacteriuria with methenamine salt or co-trimoxazole compared with controls at 3 to 9 months, but not at more than 15 months. Maynard and Diokno (141) reported that antibiotic prophylaxis significantly reduces the probability of a laboratory infection, but not the probability of a clinical infection. Kuhlemeier et al. (154) evaluated vitamin C and a number of antimicrobial agents as prophylactic agents and found no beneficial effect in patients with SCI compared with controls. These studies seem to show that prophylactic agents do not have a long-term effect in decreasing bacteriuria compared with controls. The role of prophylactic antibiotics in patients with recurrent clinical infections, anatomic abnormalities such as vesicoureteral reflux, or hydronephrosis is not known. Prophylactic antibiotics should be considered before urologic testing requiring instrumentation, particularly in those with bacteriuria.

Hydronephrosis

Ureteral dilation for any reason results in inefficient propulsion of the urine bolus due to inability of the walls to coapt completely, as well as in decreased intraluminal pressure due to the increased ureteral diameter. Over time, this may result in further distention of the ureter with eventual hydronephrosis (6,156). There are several causes for ureteral dilation. It can occur transiently from a brisk diuresis effectively overloading the ureters, not allowing enough time for individual boluses to travel down the ureter. Another cause may be a mechanical obstruction such as a stone or stricture. Those with poor bladder wall compliance, DSD, or outlet obstruction may develop a functional obstruction due to high intravesical pressures. The elevated intravesical pressure increases the tension within the bladder wall, which in turn constricts the submucosal ureter and increases the hydrostatic force within the bladder. Ureteral dilation will occur if ureteral peristalsis is unable to overcome these increased pressures (157).

McGuire et al. (53) reported that 81% of myelodysplastic children with leak point pressures of more than 40 cm H_2O developed upper urinary tract changes, whereas only 11% with leak point pressures of less than 40 cm H_2O developed upper tract changes. Hydrostatic forces in the ureter and kidneys also may be increased by vesicoureteral reflux blocking the downward egress of urine (52). Teague and Boyarsky (158) identified another potential cause of ureteral dilation. They found that *Citrobacter* sp and *Escherichia coli* from human urine cultures injected into the lumen of dog ureters produced marked suppression of peristalsis and ureteral dilation, lasting up to 2 hours (158).

Vesicoureteral Reflux

Prince and Kottke (159) reported in an 8-year study that vesicoureteral reflux was one of the factors frequently associated with renal deterioration after SCI. Fellows and Silver (160) found that there was a definite association between the degree of reflux and renal damage. Vesicoureteral reflux in children has been associated with a congenital shortening or absence of the submucosal ureter, absence of ureteral muscle in the submucosal segment, or association with a paraureteral diverticulum of the bladder (161). In people with neurogenic voiding dysfunctions, high intravesical pressures are thought to be a major cause of reflux. Recurrent cystitis and anatomic changes in the oblique course of the intravesical ureter due to bladder thickening and trabeculation are believed to be other causes of reflux. Renal deterioration from reflux is thought to be secondary to recurrent pyelonephritis resulting in renal scars and back-pressure hydronephrosis.

The mainstay of treatment in those with reflux and voiding dysfunction is to lower intravesical pressures and eradicate infections. Ureteral reimplants are technically difficult to perform in a trabeculated bladder and have not been uniformly successful.

Renal Calculi

Approximately 8% of patients with SCI develop renal calculi (162). It has been reported that 98% of renal calculi in patients with SCI are composed either of calcium phosphate or magnesium ammonium phosphate. These stones are typically associated with UTIs (163). Bacteria develop a biofilm, made up of sheets of organisms that secrete an extracellular matrix of bacterial glycocalyces and host proteins. The growth of this biofilm develops in a well-defined sequence. Bacteria first attach to the urothelium. This is facilitated by urease-producing bacteria, particularly *P. mirabilis,* which is a urease inhibitor. This causes an increase in ammonia breakdown products, which alkalinizes the urine and irritates the urothelium facilitating further bacterial adherence to the urothelium. Eventually, urinary crystals such as struvite and apatite are incorporated into this biofilm, which leads to incrustation and stone development (164). This process is also accelerated by urease-producing bacteria, because urease alkalinizes the urine and promotes crystallization of struvite and apatite (164).

Kuhlemeier et al. (165) found that renal calculi were the single most important cause of renal deterioration. Without treatment, a patient with a staghorn calculus has a 50% chance of losing the involved kidney (166). DeVivo and Fine (162)

found that patients with SCI with calculi were more likely to have neurologically complete tetraplegia, infections with *Klebsiella* or *Serratia* organisms, a history of bladder calculi, and high serum calcium values. Another study reviewing 1,669 patients with SCI between 1982 and 1996 reported an incidence of struvite stones of 1.5%; 67% of these patients had complete SCI, 5% had lesions of the cervical cord, and 53% developed their first stone more than 10 years after injury. Only 22% had kidney stones within the first 2 years postinjury. It was noted that those with kidney stones had a higher incidence of indwelling catheters (49%), bladder stones (52%), and vesicoureteral reflux (28%) (165). Patients who present with persistent infections with *Proteus* organisms should be monitored for renal calculi. Urea-splitting organisms form alkaline urine, which in turn causes supersaturation and crystallization of magnesium ammonium phosphate.

Previously, a surgical pyelolithotomy or nephrolithotomy was performed to remove these stones. Newer techniques, including percutaneous nephrolithotomy and extracorporeal shock wave lithotripsy, have largely replaced open surgical procedures (168). Any of these procedures need to be combined with sterilization of the urinary tract for urea-splitting organisms. DeVivo and Fine (162) reported a 72% reoccurrence rate within 2 years of the first kidney stone. Investigations are underway on the use of acetohydroxamic acid as a prophylactic agent; limitations of this agent are reported side effects and high cost (169).

Renal Deterioration

Renal failure previously was the leading cause of death after SCI. The death rate from renal causes was reported in the 1960s to be between 37% and 76%. The use of IC and sphincterotomy has markedly reduced the rate of death from renal causes. Price and Kottke (159) followed 280 patients for 8 years and reported 78% had good function; 13%, mild deterioration; 4%, moderate deterioration; and 5%, severe deterioration. Factors most frequently associated with renal deterioration were vesicoureteral reflux, renal calculi, recurrent pyelonephritis, and recurrent pressure ulcers. Kuhlemeier et al. (165) evaluated 519 patients with SCI with renal scans for up to 10 years. They found that factors associated with statistically significant decreased ERPF were quadriplegia, renal stones, female patients older than 30 years, and a history of chills and fever presumably due to acute UTIs. Renal calculi were the most important cause. Factors not found to be statistically significant included years since injury, presence of severe pressure ulcers, bladder calculi, bacteriuria without reflux, and completeness of injury (165).

Bladder Cancer

Paraplegic patients have been found to have a 16 to 28 times higher risk for squamous cell bladder cancer than their able-bodied counterparts. These cancers seem to occur after a person has been injured for more than 10 years. Possible causes include chronic irritation from UTIs, stasis of urine, and bladder stones. Kaufman et al. (170) reported that five of six patients with squamous cell cancer had an indwelling Foley catheter in place for more than 15 to 30 years (average, 21 years). Although only two of the six had an obvious tumor on cystoscopy, three had gross hematuria, one had known invasive squamous cell cancer of the urethra, and only one had no signs or symptoms (170). These studies suggest that yearly cystoscopy should be performed in people who have had indwelling catheters for more than 10 years. Most centers do perform yearly cystoscopy on those with an indwelling catheter, primarily to rule out bladder stones.

REFERENCES

1. Grant JCB. *An atlas of anatomy,* 6th ed. Baltimore: Williams & Wilkins, 1972:181–189.
2. Olsson CA. Anatomy of the upper urinary tract. In: Walsh PC, Gittes RF, Perlmutter AD, et al, eds. *Campbell's urology,* 5th ed. Philadelphia: WB Saunders, 1986:12–29.
3. Kaye KW, Goldberg ME. Applied anatomy of the kidneys and ureters. *Urol Clin North Am* 1982;9:3–13.
4. Tanago EA. Anatomy of the lower urinary tract. In: Walsh PC, Gittes RF, Perlmutter AD, et al, eds. *Campbell's urology,* 5th ed. Philadelphia: WB Saunders, 1986:46–61.
5. Stephens FD, Lenaghan D. The anatomical basis and dynamics of vesicoureteral reflux. *J Urol* 1962;87:669–680.
6. Griffiths DJ, Notschaele C. Mechanics of urine transport in the upper urinary tract: 1. The dynamics of the isolated bolus. *Neurourol Urodyn* 1983;2:155–166.
7. Myers RP, Goellner JR, Cahill DR. Prostate shape, external striated urethral sphincter and radical prostatectomy: the apical dissection. *J Urol* 1987;138:543–547.
8. Delancey JO. Structure and function of the continence mechanism relative to stress incontinence. In: Leach GE, Paulson DF, eds. *Problems in urology,* vol 1. Philadelphia: JB Lippincott Co, 1991:1–9.
9. Gosling JA, Dixon JS. Species variation in the location of upper urinary tract pacemaker cells. *Invest Urol* 1974;11:418–423.
10. Fletcher TF, Bradley WE. Neuroanatomy of the bladder-urethra. *J Urol* 1978;119:153–160.
11. Benson GS, McConnell JA, Wood JG. Adrenergic innervation of the human bladder body. *J Urol* 1979;122:189–191.
12. Elbadawi A. Autonomic muscular innervation of the vesical outlet and its role in micturition. In: Hinman F Jr, ed. *Benign prostatic hypertrophy.* New York: Springer-Verlag New York, 1983:330–348.
13. Burnstock G. The changing face of autonomic neurotransmission. *Acta Physiol Scand* 1986;126:67–91.
14. Norlen L, Dahlstrom A, Sundin T, et al. The adrenergic innervation and adrenergic receptor activity of the feline urinary bladder and urethra in the normal state and after hypogastric and/or parasympathetic denervation. *Scand J Urol Nephrol* 1976;10:177–184.
15. Elbadawi A. Ultrastructure of vesicourethral innervation: III. Axoaxonal synapses between postganglionic cholinergic axons and probably SIF-cell derived processes in feline lissosphincter. *J Urol* 1985;133:524–528.
16. Chancellor MB, De Groat WC. Intravesical capsaicin and resiniferatoxin therapy. *J Urol* 1999;162:3–11.
17. de Groat WC. Mechanism underlying the recovery of lower urinary tract function following spinal cord injury. *Paraplegia* 1995;33:493–505.
18. Elbadawi A, Schenk EA. A new theory of the innervation of bladder musculature: part 4. Innervation of the vesicourethral junction and external urethral sphincter. *J Urol* 1974;111:613–615.
19. Sundin T, Dahlstrom A. The sympathetic innervation of the urinary bladder and urethra in the normal state and after parasympathetic denervation at the spinal root level. *Scand J Urol Nephrol* 1973;7:131–149.
20. Crowe R, Burnstock G, Light JK. Adrenergic innervation of the striated muscle of the intrinsic external urethral sphincter from patients with lower motor spinal cord lesion. *J Urol* 1989;141:47–49.
21. Denny-Brown D, Robertson EG. On the physiology of micturition. *Brain* 1933;56:149–190.
22. Barrington FJF. The relation of the hindbrain to micturition. *Brain* 1921;44:23–53.
23. Bradley WE. Physiology of the urinary bladder. In: Walsh PC, Gittes RF, Perlmutter AD, et al, eds. *Campbell's urology,* 5th ed. Philadelphia: WB Saunders, 1986:129–185.
24. Carlsson CA. The supraspinal control of the urinary bladder. *Acta Pharmacol Toxicol* 1978;43A[Suppl II]:8–12.
25. Bradley WE, Teague CT. Spinal cord organization of micturitional reflex afferents. *Exp Neurol* 1968;22:504–516.
26. Barrett DM, Wein AJ. Voiding dysfunction: diagnosis, classification and management. In: Gillenwater JY, Grayhack JT, Howards SS, et al, eds. *Adult and pediatric urology,* 2nd ed. St. Louis: Mosby–Year Book, 1991:1001–1099.
27. Kaplan SA, Chancellor MB, Blaivas JG. Bladder and sphincter behavior in patients with spinal cord lesions. *J Urol* 1991;146:113–117.
28. Yalla SV, Fam BA. Spinal cord injury. In: Krane RJ, Siroky MB, eds. *Clinical neuro-urology,* 2nd ed. Boston: Little, Brown and Company, 1991:319–331.
29. Rudy DC, Awad SA, Downie JW. External sphincter dyssynergia: an abnormal continence reflex. *J Urol* 1988;140:105–110.
30. Light JK, Faganel J, Beric A. Detrusor areflexia in suprasacral spinal cord injuries. *J Urol* 1985;134:295–297.
31. Comarr AE. Diagnosis of the traumatic cord bladder. In: Boyarski S, ed. *The neurogenic bladder.* Baltimore: Williams & Wilkins, 1967:147–152.
32. Graham SD. Present urological treatment of spinal cord injury patients. *J Urol* 1981;126:1–4.
33. Downie JW, Awad SA. The state of urethral musculature during the detrusor areflexia after spinal cord transection. *Investig Urol* 1979;17:55–59.
34. Nanninga JB, Meyer P. Urethral sphincter activity following acute spinal cord injury. *J Urol* 1980;123:528–530.
35. Koyanagi T, Arikado K, Takamatsu T, et al. Experience with electromyography of the external urethral sphincter in spinal cord injury patients. *J Urol* 1982;127:272–276.
36. Blaivas JG, Sinha HP, Zayed AAH, et al. Detrusor-external sphincter dyssynergia. *J Urol* 1981;125:542–544.
37. Pavlakis AJ, Siroky MB, Goldstein I, et al. Neurourologic findings in conus medullaris and cauda equina injury. *Arch Neurol* 1983;40:570–573.
38. Sharr MM, Carfield JC, Jenkins JD. Lumbar spondylosis and neuropathic bladder investigations of 73 patients with chronic urinary symptoms. *Br Med J* 1976;1:645.
39. Hackler RH, Hall MK, Zampieri TA. Bladder hypocompliance in the spinal cord injury population. *J Urol* 1989;141:1390–1393.
40. Sislow JG, Mayo ME. Reduction in human bladder wall compliance following decentralization. *J Urol* 1990;144:945–947.
41. Appell RA, Whiteside HV. Diabetes and other peripheral neuropathies affecting lower urinary tract function. In: Krane RJ, Siroky MG, eds. *Clinical neuro-urology,* 2nd ed. Boston: Little, Brown and Company, 1991:365–373.
42. Bradley WE. Autonomic neuropathy and the genitourinary system. *J Urol* 1978;119:299–302.
43. Andersen JT, Bradley WE. Abnormalities of bladder innervation in diabetes mellitus. *Urology* 1976;7:442–448.
44. Wheeler JS Jr, Siroky MB, Pavlakis A, et al. The urodynamic aspects of the Guillain-Barré syndrome. *J Urol* 1984;131:917–919.
45. Rao KG, Hackler RH, Woodlief RM, et al. Real time renal sonography in spinal cord injury patients: prospective comparison with excretory urography. *J Urol* 1986;135:72–77.
46. Lloyd LK, Dubovsky EV, Bueschen AJ, et al. Comprehensive renal scintillation procedures in spinal cord injury: comparison with excretory urography. *J Urol* 1981;126:10–13.
47. Kuhlemeier KV, McEachran AB, Lloyd LK, et al. Serum creatinine as an indicator of renal function after spinal cord injury. *Arch Phys Med Rehabil* 1984;65:694–697.
48. Abrams P, Blaivas JG, Stanton SL, et al. Standardization of terminology of lower urinary tract function. *Neurourol Urodyn* 1988;7:403–427.

49. Lapides J, Friend CR, Ajemian EP, et al. A new test for neurogenic bladder. *J Urol* 1962;88:245–247.

50. Wheeler JS Jr, Culkin DJ, Canning JR. Positive bethanechol supersensitivity test in neurologically normal patients. *Urology* 1988;31:86–89.

51. Linsenmeyer TA. Characterization of voiding dysfunction following recent cerebrovascular accident [Abstract]. *Arch Phys Med Rehabil* 1990;71:778.

52. Linsenmeyer TA, Culkin D. APS recommendations for the urological evaluation of patients with spinal cord injury. *J Spinal Cord Med* 1999;22(2):139–142.

53. McGuire EJ, Woodside JR, Borden TA, et al. Prognostic value of urodynamic testing in myelodysplastic patients. *J Urol* 1981;126:205–209.

54. Bauer SB. Urologic management of the myelodysplastic child. *Probl Urol* 1989;3:86–101.

55. Guttmann L, Frankel H. The value of intermittent catheterization in the early management of traumatic paraplegia and tetraplegia. *Paraplegia* 1966/1967;4:63–84.

56. Lapides J, Diokno AC, Silber SJ, et al. Clean, intermittent self catheterization in treatment of urinary tract disease. *J Urol* 1972;107:458–461.

57. Maynard FM, Glass J. Management of the neuropathic bladder by clean intermittent catheterisation: 5 year outcomes. *Paraplegia* 1987;25:106–110.

58. Weld KJ, Dmochowski RR. Effect of bladder management on urological complications in spinal cord injured patients. *J Urol* 2000;163:768–772.

59. Nanninga JB, Wu Y, Hamilton B. Long term intermittent catheterization in spinal cord injured patients. *J Urol* 1982;128:760.

60. Gerridzen RG, Thijssen AM, Dehoux E. Risk factors for upper tract deterioration in chronic spinal cord injury patients. *J Urol* 1992;147:416–418.

61. Weld KJ, Grandy MJ, Dmochowski RR. Differences in bladder compliance with time and associations of bladder management with compliance in spinal cord injured patients. *J Urol* 2000;163:1228–1233.

62. Anderson RU. Non sterile intermittent catheterization with antibiotic prophylaxis in the acute spinal cord injured male patient. *J Urol* 1980;124:392–394.

63. Binard JE, Persky L, Lockhart JL, et al. Intermittent catheterization the right way! (Volume vs. time directed). *J Spinal Cord Med* 1996;19(3):194–196.

64. Brown JH. Atropine, scopolamine and related antimuscarinic drugs. In: Gilman AG, Rall TW, Nies AS, et al, eds. *Goodman and Gilman's the pharmacologic basis of therapeutics,* 8th ed. New York: Pergamon Press, 1990:150–165.

65. Baldessarini RJ. Drugs and the treatment of psychiatric disorders. In: Gilman AG, Rall TW, Nies AS, et al, eds. *Goodman and Gilman's the pharmacologic basis of therapeutics,* 8th ed. New York: Pergamon Press, 1990:383–435.

66. Wyndaele JJ. Pharmacotherapy for urinary bladder dysfunction in spinal cord injury patients. *Paraplegia* 1990;28:146–150.

67. Vaidyanathan S, Soni BM, Brown E, et al. Effect of intermittent urethral catheterization and oxybutynin bladder instillation on urinary continence status and quality of life in a selected group of spinal cord injured patients with neuropathic bladder dysfunction. *Spinal Cord* 1998;36:409–414.

68. Haferkamp A, Saehhler G, Gerner HJ, et al. Dosage escalation of intravesical oxybutynin in the treatment of neurogenic bladder patients. *J Spinal Cord* 2000;38:250–254.

69. de Seze M, Wiart L, Joseph PA, et al. Capsaicin and neurogenic detrusor hyperreflexia: a double-blind placebo-controlled study in 20 patients with spinal cord lesions. *Neurourol Urodyn* 1998;17:513–523.

70. Silva C, Rio M Cruz F. Desensitization of bladder sensory fibers by intravesical resiniferatoxin, a capsaicin analog: long-term results for the treatment of detrusor hyperreflexia. *Eur Urol* 2000;38:444–452.

71. Lazzeri M, Beneforti P, Turini D. Urodynamic effects of intravesical resiniferatoxin in humans: preliminary results in stable and unstable detrusor. *J Urol* 1997;158(6):2093–2096.

72. Nanninga JB, Frost F, Penn R. Effect of intrathecal baclofen on bladder and sphincter function. *J Urol* 1989;142:101–105.

73. Cordozo LD, Stanton SL, Robinson H, et al. Evaluation of flurbiprofen in detrusor instability. *Br Med J* 1980;280:281–282.

74. Resnick NM. Geriatric incontinence. In: Diokno AC, ed. *The urology clinics of North America.* Philadelphia: WB Saunders, 1996;23:55–74.

75. Gray GJ, Yang C. Surgical procedures of the bladder after spinal cord injuries. *Top Spinal Cord Med* 2000;11(1):61–69.

76. Anderson B, Mitchell M. Management of electrolyte disturbances following urinary diversion and bladder augmentation. *AUA News* 2000;5:1–7.

77. Golomb J, Klutke CG, Lewin KJ, et al. Bladder neoplasms associated with augmentation cystoplasty: report of 2 cases and literature review. *J Urol* 1989;142:377–380.

78. McDougal WS. Use of intestinal segments and urinary diversion. In: Walsh PC, Retik AB, Vaughan ED, et al, eds. *Cambell's urology,* 7th ed. Philadelphia: WB Saunders, 1998:3121–3157.

79. Mast P, Hoebeke P, Wyndaele JJ, et al. Experience with augmentation cystoplasty. A review. *Paraplegia* 1995;33:560–564.

80. Kuo HC. Clinical outcome and quality of life after enterocystoplasty for contracted bladders. *Urol Int* 1997;58(3):160–165.

81. Stohrer M, Kramer G, Gopel M, et al. Bladder autoaugmentation in adult patients with neurogenic voiding dysfunction. *Spinal Cord* 1997;35(7):456–462.

82. Misak SJ, Bunts RC, Ulmer JL, et al. Nerve interruption procedures in the urologic management of paraplegic patients. *J Urol* 1962;88:392.

83. Hodgkinson CP, Drukker BH. Infravesical nerve resection for detrusor dyssynergia: the Ingelman-Sundberg operation. *Acta Obstet Gynecol Scand* 1977;56:408.

84. Ohlsson BL, Frankenberg-Sommar S. Effects of external and direct pudendal nerve maximal electrical stimulation in the treatment of the uninhibited overactive bladder. *Br J Urol* 1989;64:374–380.

85. Tanago EA. Concepts of neuromodulation. *Neurourol Urodyn* 1993;12:497–498.

86. Brindley Gs, Polkey CE, Rushton DN. Sacral anterior root stimulator for bladder control in paraplegia. *Paraplegia* 1982;20:365–381.

87. Creasey GH, Bodner DR. Review of sacral electrical stimulation in the management of the neurogenic bladder. *Neurol Rehabil* 1994;4:266–274.

88. Van Kerrebroeck PEV. World wide experience with the Finetech-Brindley sacral anterior root stimulator. *Neurourol Urodyn* 1993;12(5):497–503.

89. Donnelan SM, Boulton DM. The impact of contemporary bladder management techniques on struvite calculi associated with spinal cord injury. *Br J Urol Int* 1999;84:280–285.

90. McGuire EJ, Savastano JA. Comparative urological outcome in women with spinal cord injury. *J Urol* 1986;135:730–731.

91. MacDiarmid SA, Arnold EP, Palmer NB, et al. Management of spinal cord patients by indwelling suprapubic catheterization. *J Urol* 1995;154:492.

92. Dewire DM, Owens RS, Anderson GA, et al. A comparison of the urological complications associated with long term management of quadriplegics with and without chronic indwelling urinary catheters. *J Urol* 1992;147:1060–1072.

93. Kim YH, Katten MW, Boone TB. Bladder leak point pressure: the measure for sphincterotomy success in spinal cord injured patients with external detrusor-sphincter dyssynergia. *J Urol* 1998;159:493–497.

94. Wyndaele JJ. Urology in male spinal cord injured patients. *Paraplegia* 1987;25:267–269.

95. Killorin W, Gray M, Bennet JK, et al. The value of urodynamics and bladder management in predicting upper urinary tract complications in male spinal cord injury patients. *Paraplegia* 1992;30:437–441.

96. Gerridzen RG, Thijssen AM, Dehoux E. Risk factors for upper tract deterioration in chronic spinal cord injury patients. *J Urol* 1992;147:416–418.

97. Linsenmeyer TA, Bagaria SP, Gendron B. The impact of urodynamic parameters on the upper tracts of spinal cord injured men who void reflexly. *J Spinal Cord Med* 1998;21:15–20.

98. Light KJ, Scott FB. Bethanechol chloride and the traumatic cord bladder. *J Urol* 1982;128:85–87.

99. Sporer A, Leyson JFJ, Martin BF. Effects of bethanechol chloride on the external urethral sphincter in spinal cord injury patients. *J Urol* 1978;120:62–66.

100. Taylor P. Cholinergic agonists. In: Gilman AC, Rall TW, Nies AS, et al, eds. *Goodman and Gilman's the pharmacological basis of therapeutics,* 8th ed. New York: Pergamon Press, 1990.

101. Vaidyanathan S, Rao MS, Mapa MK, et al. Study of intravesical instillation of 1A(s)-15 methy prostaglandin F_2 in patients with neurogenic bladder dysfunction. *J Urol* 1981;126:81–85.

102. Booth AM, Hisamitsu T, Kawatani M, et al. Regulation of urinary bladder capacity by endogenous opioid peptides. *J Urol* 1985;133: 339–342.

103. Lepor H. Alpha blockers for the treatment of benign prostatic hypertrophy. *Probl Urol* 1991;5:419–429.

104. Scott MB, Morrow JW. Phenoxybenzamine in neurogenic bladder dysfunction after spinal cord injury: I. Voiding dysfunction. *J Urol* 1978;119:480–482.

105. Lepor H, Gup DI, Baumann M, et al. Laboratory assessment of terazosin and alpha 1 blockade in prostatic hyperplasia. *Urology* 1988; 32[Suppl 6]:21–26.

106. de Groat WC. Nervous control of the urinary bladder of the cat. *Brain Res* 1975;87:201–211.

107. Swierzewski SJ III, Gormley EA, Belville WD, et al. The effect of terazosin on bladder function in the spinal cord injured patient. *J Urol* 1994;151:951–954.

108. Scott MB, Morrow JW. Phenoxybenzamine in neurogenic bladder dysfunction after spinal cord injury: II. Autonomic dysreflexia. *J Urol* 1978;119:483–484.

109. Wein AJ. Prazosin in the treatment of prostatic obstruction: a placebo controlled study [Editorial Comment]. *J Urol* 1989;141:693.

110. Cedarbaum JM, Schleifer LS. Drugs for Parkinson's disease, spasticity and acute muscle spasms. In: Gilman AG, Rall TW, Nies AS, et al, eds. *Goodman and Gilman's the pharmacological basis of therapeutics,* 8th ed. New York: Pergamon Press, 1990:463–484.

111. Perkash I. Modified approach to sphincterotomy in spinal cord injury patients. *Paraplegia* 1976;13:247–260.

112. Yang CC, Mayo ME. External sphincterotomy; long term follow up. *Neurourol Urodyn* 1995;14:25–31.

113. Perkash I. Contact laser transurethral external sphincterotomy; a preliminary report. *Neurol Rehabil* 1994;4(4):249–254.

114. Chancellor MB, Rivas DA, Linsenmeyer T, et al. Multicenter trial in North America of UroLume urinary sphincter prosthesis. *J Urol* 1994;152:924–930.

115. Schurch B, Hauri D, Rodic B, et al. Botulinum-A toxin as a treatment of detrusor-sphincter dyssynergia in spinal cord injured patients. *J Urol* 1996;155:1023–1029.

116. Dykstra DD, Sidi AA, Scott AB, et al. Effects of botulinum A toxin on detrusor sphincter dyssynergia in spinal cord injury patients. *J Urol* 1988;139:919–922.

117. Wheeler JS Jr, Walter JS, Chintam RS, et al. Botulinum toxin injections for voiding dysfunction following SCI. *J Spinal Cord Med* 1998; 21(3):227–229.

118. Engel RME, Schirmer HKA. Pudendal neurectomy in neurogenic bladder. *J Urol* 1974;112:57–59.

119. McGuire EJ, Woodside JR, Borden TA, et al. Prognostic value of urodynamic testing in myelodysplastic patients. *J Urol* 1981;126: 205–209.

120. Weld KJ, Dmochowski RR. Association of level of injury and bladder behavior in patients with post-traumatic spinal cord injury. *Urology* 2000;55:490–494.

121. Kegel AH. Progressive resistance exercises in the functional restoration of the perineal muscles. *Am J Obstet Gynecol* 1948;56:238–248.

122. Wells TJ, Brink CA, Diokno AC, et al. Pelvic muscle exercise for stress urinary incontinence in elderly women. *J Am Geriatr Soc* 1991; 39:785–791.

123. Jeter KF. Pelvic muscle exercises with and without biofeedback for the treatment of urinary incontinence. *Probl Urol* 1991;5:72–84.

124. Hoffman BB, Lefkowitz RJ. Catecholamines and sympathomimetic drugs. In: Gillman AG, Rall TW, Nies AS, et al, eds. *Goodman and Gilman's the pharmacological basis of therapeutics,* 8th ed. New York: Pergamon Press, 1990:187–220.

125. Kernan WN, Viscoli CM, Brass LM, et al. Phenylpropanolamine and the risk of hemorrhagic stroke. *N Engl J Med* 2000;343(25):1826.

126. Walter S, Wolf H, Barlebo H, et al. Urinary incontinence in post menopausal women treated with estrogens. *Urol Int* 1978;33:135.

127. Hodgson BJ, Dumas S, Bolling DR, et al. Effect of estrogen on sensitivity of rabbit bladder and urethra to phenylephrine. *Investig Urol* 1978;16:67–69.

128. Appell RA. Periurethral collagen injection for female incontinence. *Probl Urol* 1991;5:134–140.

129. Light JK, Scott FB. Use of the artificial urinary sphincter in spinal cord injury patients. *J Urol* 1983;130:1127–1129.

130. Bosco PJ, Bauer SB, Colodny AH, et al. The long term results of artificial sphincters in children. *J Urol* 1991;146:396–399.

131. Kelly MJ, Leach GE. Long term results of bladder neck suspension procedures. *Probl Urol* 1991;5:94–105.

132. Barbalias GA, Klauber GT, Blaivas JG. Critical evaluation of the Credé maneuver: a urodynamic study 136. *Neurol Rehabil* 1992;2(2): 23–26.

133. Hanna MK. New concept in bladder remodeling. *Urology* 1982;19: 6.

134. Lockhart JL, Vorstman B, Weinstein D, et al. Sphincterotomy failure in neurogenic bladder disease. *J Urol* 1986;135:86–89.

135. Stenzl A, Ninkovic M, Kolle D. Restoration of voluntary emptying of the bladder by transplantation of innervated free skeletal muscle. *Lancet* 1998;351;1483.

136. Maizels M, King LR, Firlit CR. Urodynamic biofeedback: a new approach to treat vesical sphincter dyssynergia. *J Urol* 1979;122: 205–209.

137. Kiviat MD, Zimmermann TA, Donovan WH. Sphincter stretch: new technique resulting in continence and complete voiding in paraplegics. *J Urol* 1975;114:895–897.

138. Linsenmeyer TA, Zorowitz RD. Urodynamic findings in patients with urinary incontinence after cerebrovascular accident. *Neurol Rehabil* 1992;2(2):23–26.

139. Parres JA, Kropp KA. Urodynamic evaluation of the continence mechanism following urethral lengthening: reimplantation and enterocystoplasty. *J Urol* 1991;146:535–538.

140. Lloyd LK, Kuhlemeier KV, Fine PR, et al. Initial bladder management in spinal cord injury: does it make a difference? *J Urol* 1986;135: 523–527.

141. Maynard FM, Diokno AC. Urinary infection and complications during clean intermittent catheterization following spinal cord injury. *J Urol* 1984;132:943–946.

142. Romano JM, Kaye D. UTI in the elderly: common yet atypical. *Geriatrics* 1981;36(6):113–120.

143. Kass EH. The role of asymptomatic bacteriuria in the pathogenesis of pyelonephritis. In: Quinn EL, Kass EH, eds. *Biology of pyelonephritis.* Boston: Little, Brown and Company, 1960:399–418.

144. Stamey TA. Recurrent urinary tract infections in female patients: an overview of management and treatment. *Rev Infect Dis* 1987;9[Suppl 2]:S195–S210.

145. Stamm WE, Counts GW, Running KR, et al. Diagnosis of coliform infection in acutely dysuric women. *N Engl J Med* 1982;307: 463–468.

146. Rhame FS, Perkash I. Urinary tract infections occurring in recent spinal cord injury patients on intermittent catheterization. *J Urol* 1979;122:669–673.

147. Donovan WH, Stolov WC, Clowers DE, et al. Bacteriuria during intermittent catheterization following spinal cord injury. *Arch Phys Med Rehabil* 1978;59:351–357.

148. The prevention and management of urinary tract infections among people with spinal cord injuries; National Institute on Disabilities and Rehabilitation Research Consensus Conference Statement. January 27–29, 1992. *J Am Paraplegia Soc* 1992;15:194–204.

149. Deresinski SC, Perkash I. Urinary tract infections in male spinal cord injured patients: part 2. Diagnostic value of symptoms and of quantitative urinalysis. *J Am Paraplegia Soc* 1985;8:7–10.

150. Anderson RU, Hsieh-ma ST. Association of bacteriuria and pyuria during intermittent catheterization after spinal cord injury. *J Urol* 1983;130:299–301.

151. Kass EJ, Koff SA, Diokno AC, et al. The significance of bacilluria in children on long term intermittent catheterization. *J Urol* 1981;126: 223–225.

152. Lewis RI, Carrion HM, Lockhart JL, et al. Significance of asymptomatic bacteriuria in neurogenic bladder disease. *Urology* 1984;23: 343–347.

153. Tempkin A, Sullivan G, Paldi J, et al. Radioisotope renography in spinal cord injury. *J Urol* 1985;133:228–230.

154. Kuhlemeier KV, Stover SL, Lloyd LK. Prophylactic antibacterial therapy for preventing urinary tract infections in spinal cord injury patients. *J Urol* 1985;134:514–517.

155. Merritt JLM, Erickson RP, Opitz JL. Bacteriuria during follow up in patients with spinal cord injury: part II. Efficacy of antimicrobial suppressants. *Arch Phys Med Rehabil* 1982;63:413–415.

156. Gillenwater JY. Hydronephrosis. In: Gillenwater JY, Grayhack JT, Howards SS, et al, eds. *Adult and pediatric urology,* 2nd ed. St. Louis: Mosby–Year Book, 1991:789–813.

157. Staskin DR. Hydroureteronephrosis after spinal cord injury. *Urol Clin North Am* 1991;18:309–316.

158. Teague N, Boyarsky S. Further effects of coliform bacteria on ureteral peristalsis. *J Urol* 1968;99:720–724.

159. Price M, Kottke FJ. Renal function in patients with spinal cord injury: the eighth year of a ten year continuing study. *Arch Phys Med Rehabil* 1975;56:76–79.

160. Fellows GJ, Silver JR. Long term follow up of paraplegic patients with vesico-ureteric reflux. *Paraplegia* 1976;14:130–134.

161. Winberg J. Urinary tract infections in infants and children. In: Walsh PC, Gittes RF, Perlmutter AD, et al, eds. *Campbell's urology,* 5th ed. Philadelphia: WB Saunders, 1986:848–867.

162. DeVivo MJ, Fine PR. Predicting renal calculus occurrence in spinal cord injury patients. *Arch Phys Med Rehabil* 1986;67:722–725.

163. Burr RG. Urinary calculi composition in patients with spinal cord lesions. *Arch Phys Med Rehabil* 1978;59:84–87.

164. Griffith DP, Osborne CA. Infection (urease) stones. *Miner Electrolyte Metab* 1987;13:278–285.

165. Kuhlemeier KV, Lloyd LK, Stover SL. Long term followup of renal function after spinal cord injury. *J Urol* 1985;134:510–513.

166. Singh M, Chapman R, Tresidder GC, et al. Fate of unoperated staghorn calculus. *Br J Urol* 1973;45:581–585.

167. Donnellan SM, Bolton DM. The impact of contemporary bladder management techniques on struvite calculi associated with spinal cord injury. *Br J Urol Int* 1999;84(3):280–285.

168. Irwin PP, Evans C, Chawla JC, et al. Stone surgery in the spinal patient. *Paraplegia* 1991;29:161–166.

169. Rodman JS, Williams JJ, Peterson CM. Partial dissolution of struvite calculus with oral acetohydroxamic acid. *Urology* 1983;22:410–412.

170. Kaufman JM, Fam B, Jacobs SC, et al. Bladder cancer and squamous metaplasia in spinal cord injury patients. *J Urol* 1977;118:967–971.

PRESSURE ULCERS AND SPINAL CORD INJURY

KEVIN C. O'CONNOR
RICHARD SALCIDO

Despite advances in health care, pressure ulcers remain one of the most common and serious complications of spinal cord injury (SCI). Persons with SCI are vulnerable across their lifespan to tissue breakdown that can interfere with initial rehabilitation in the acute posttraumatic recovery phase and successful reintegration into the community, as well as lead to more serious medical complications and result in profound psychosocial consequences. Although most pressure ulcers are preventable, the prevention and management of pressure ulcers add significantly to the cost of care for patients with SCI. Because of this, health care providers who serve this population must understand all aspects of pressure ulcers.

STAGING/GRADING

The National Pressure Ulcer Advisory Panel (NPUAP) defines a pressure ulcer as an area of unrelieved pressure over a defined area, usually over a bony prominence, resulting in ischemia, cell death, and tissue necrosis (1). An adequate description of the pressure ulcer allows for communication among team members and following interventions in wound healing for both clinical outcomes and research purposes. Pressure ulcers are usually classified as stages, including macroscopic and morphologic criteria, specifically based on erythema of the skin and depth of the ulcer. The Shea scale included four grades (2). The Yarkony-Kirk scale included a distinct classification of a red area and a healed area to allow for recognition of sites of future breakdown (3). It also described the depth of a wound by the tissue observed at the base of the wound. The staging system of pressure ulcers most commonly used is based on the NPUAP Consensus Development Conference, which incorporates several of the most commonly used staging systems (Table 13.1) (1).

Pressure ulcers do not necessarily progress from stage I to stage IV, or heal from stage IV to stage I. Some of the limitations of pressure ulcer staging include the following: Stage I ulcer may be superficial or may be a sign of deeper tissue damage, and stage I ulcers are not always reliably assessed, particularly in patients with darkly pigmented skin. In addition, when an eschar is present, a pressure ulcer cannot be accurately staged until the eschar is removed, and it is difficult to assess pressure ulcers in patients with casts, support stockings, or other orthopedic devices (1).

Numerous techniques have been described to measure the size and depth of an ulcer. Generally, the ulcer is measured at its maximum dimensions and it is then diagrammed, traced, or photographed (4). Sinography may be used when clinical assessment of a tunneling ulcer is not adequate and is performed by instilling radiopaque dye into the wound and taking a plain x-ray, which allows determination of the depth and extent of the wound (5).

INCIDENCE AND PREVALENCE

It has been estimated that 50% to 80% of persons with SCI will, at some time after their injury, develop a pressure ulcer (6, 7). Reliable data on the incidence and prevalence of pressure ulcers after SCI, however, are difficult to obtain. There is a large body of literature associating the development of pressure ulcers with certain demographic characteristics, variables associated with SCI itself, and psychosocial variables. The associated demographic variables include age, gender, ethnicity, marital status, employment status, and educational achievement (8–14). Variables associated with the SCI itself include extent of the paralysis, completeness of the SCI, longer duration of SCI, and degree of functional independence (10–17). Psychosocial variables associated with the development of pressure ulcers include use of tobacco and alcohol, poor nutrition, and being less satisfied with life and one's activities (13,15,17–19). Many of the studies that have shown an association between the variables and the development of pressure ulcers have corresponding studies that show no association.

The most reliable data on pressure ulcer prevalence after SCI are available from model systems data. In the model systems, 32% to 40% of all patients admitted developed pressure ulcers during their initial rehabilitation (14,20,21). In addition, the prevalence of pressure ulcers increases with the duration of the SCI. In a study of complete injuries at the level of C4 and above, Whiteneck et al. (22) reported a 23% incidence of pressure ulcers for individuals 1 to 5 years after injury and 30% for individuals 6 or more years after injury (22). More recently, Yarkony and Heinemann reported a prevalence of 7.9% at 1 year after discharge and 31.9% at 20 years postdischarge (23). Finally, having a pressure ulcer itself is a risk factor for developing future ulcers (10,12).

TABLE 13.1. NPUAP STAGES OF PRESSURE ULCERS

Stage I: Nonblanchable erythema not resolved in 30 minutes; epidermis intact; reversible with intervention (not detectable in persons with darkly pigmented skin).
Stage II: Partial-thickness loss of skin involving epidermis, possibly into dermis; may appear as blisters with erythema, abrasion, or shallow crater.
Stage III: Full-thickness destruction through dermis into subcutaneous tissue that may extend down to, but not through, the underlying fascia. The ulcer presents clinically as a deep crater with or without undermining of adjacent tissue.
Stage IV: Full-thickness skin loss with deep tissue destruction through subcutaneous tissue to fascia, muscle, bone, joint, or supporting structures. Undermining and sinus tracts may also be associated with stage IV pressure ulcers.

NPUAP; National Pressure Ulcer Advisory Panel.

In summary, SCI-associated factors that are related to the development of pressure ulcers include the higher level and completeness of the SCI, a longer duration of the SCI, a decreased level of activity, and previous ulcers (12,13,23–25). Psychosocial factors that have not been found to be associated with pressure ulcers in SCI include age at onset, quality of life, depression, satisfaction with social support, and social integration (11, 26–29).

COSTS

Pressure ulcers are responsible for physical, social, vocational, and economic costs. Young and Burns (14) found a strong association with medical complications and the development of pressure ulcers in the SCI population. Functionally, when a pressure ulcer occurs, persons with SCI lose time from work, school, and social activities, establishing many concomitant problems. The loss of income, productivity, progress toward vocational goals, independence, self-esteem, and sense of self-worth are some of the financial ramifications of pressure ulcers (30). Actual costs to heal pressure ulcers are difficult to estimate; however, estimates for less serious pressure ulcers to heal range from $20,000 to $30,000, and the cost to heal a complex full-thickness pressure ulcer is estimated to be $70,000 (31).

LOCATION AND SEVERITY OF PRESSURE ULCERS

Pressure ulcers usually develop over bony prominences. Model systems data from patients with SCI undergoing hospitalization and rehabilitation show that the most common sites of ulcers were the sacrum (37.4%), the heels (15.9%), and the ischium (9.2%). Severe ulcers (stages III and IV) occurred most often at the same sites: sacrum (50.9%), heels (12.5%), and ischium (6.3%) (23). Data from patients who were discharged show a change in the sites of the development of pressure ulcers, with the most common sites after 1 year being the sacrum (20.5%), ischium (18.3%), heels (16.6%), and trochanters (12.4%), with

the most severe ulcers at the sacrum (25.0%), trochanters, (23.4%) and ischium (22.7%) (23). The increase in the percentage of ulcers at the ischium is associated with the patient's progression from lying down to spending more time in the sitting position (wheelchair mobility). At year two, however, the most common site was the ischium (24.3%), followed by the sacrum (20.3%) and trochanters (12.5%), with the highest number of severe ulcers found at the ischium (30.9%), followed by the trochanters (26.5%) and sacrum (17.6%). One ulcer was reported for 64.8%, two ulcers for 24.2%, and three ulcers for 4.7% of patients (23). More recently, the development of pressure ulcers was reported to be the most frequent secondary medical complication, at 15.2%, with neurologically complete patients being more likely to have pressure ulcers at multiple sites (26).

PATHOPHYSIOLOGY

The pathophysiology of pressure ulcers has been comprehensively described elsewhere (25). The primary factors leading to pressure ulcers include pressure, shear, moisture secondary to perspiration or incontinence, anemia and nutritional deficiencies, and aged skin (32). Moreover, there is a parabolic relationship between pressure and time, indicating that higher pressures require a shorter time to cause ulceration than lower pressures (33). Pressure is more concentrated in the area of the muscle and fat adjacent to the bone, and these tissues are more susceptible to pressure and may show signs of tissue damage before there is evidence of damage to the skin (33–35). For the patient with SCI, these factors may often result in pressure ulcer formation, compared with the able-bodied population, because of their impaired function, associated loss of mobility and sensation, and neurogenic bladder and bowel.

SCI itself is associated with unique changes that contribute to the pathophysiology of pressure ulcers. Patients with SCI have alterations in the skin collagen, which is responsible for the skin's tensile strength, which contributes to its increased susceptibility to pressure ulcer development. Specifically, the activity of lysyl hydroxylase, an enzyme involved in the biosynthesis of collagen, is lower in biopsies performed below the level of the injury than in those performed above the level of injury and in non-SCI controls (36). In addition, there is an increased urinary excretion of the metabolite glucosyl-galactosyl hydroxylysine immediately after traumatic SCI (37). This excess secretion stops during the second year after injury, but increases can again be detected 2 to 5 months before pressure ulcer development (36). In addition, the alterations in the autonomic nervous system after SCI may affect pressure ulcer development and healing. A decrease in the density of adrenergic receptors, in the skin below the level of injury, for patients with SCI may occur, which could cause an abnormal vascular response (38,39). Patients with SCI have been shown to have a slower reflow rate after pressure is removed, and this vascular response may predispose to ulcer formation through lower tissue oxygenation and lower nutrient availability (40).

As in the able-bodied population, changes that occur in the skin of the patient with SCI with age can make the individual more at risk for the development of pressure ulcers. With aging, there are changes in the skin that impair its ability to effectively distribute pressure and there are changes in collagen synthesis that result in lowered mechanical strength and increased stiffness (41). In addition, as a person ages, the elastin content of the skin decreases, which increases the mechanical load on the skin and aging skin becomes thinner (42). These factors may be exacerbated in the patient with SCI because of the impaired sensation and mobility (13,43,44).

RISK ASSESSMENT SCALES

Because all individuals with SCI are at risk for developing pressure ulcers, risk assessment scales have been studied as a means of helping to prevent the development of pressure ulcers in this population. Risk assessment scales assign numerical equivalents to risk factors for pressure ulcer development and stratify that person's risk based on an overall numerical score. In the general population (at risk for pressure ulcers), the two most commonly used scales are the Braden scale and the Norton scale (45). The Braden scale is composed of six subscales: activity, mobility, sensory perception, nutritional status, skin moisture, friction, and shear (43). Each subscale is rated from highest risk (denoted by the number one) to lowest risk (number four), with total scores ranging from 6 to 23; lower scores reflect greater risk for pressure sore development (Table 13.2). The Norton scale uses five variables to assess pressure ulcer risk: activity, mobility, incontinence, physical condition, and mental condition (Table 13.3) (46).

Both of these scales may have limited application in the SCI population because these particular scales have not been studied in persons with SCI and additional research is needed to generalize their use in SCI. Because of their limitations, several researchers have developed scales for use in the SCI population. Salzberg et al. (47) initially designed a scale using 15 risk factors for pressure ulcer development in SCI (e.g., restricted activity level, degree of immobility, complete SCI, urinary disease, impaired cognitive function, diabetes, cigarette smoking, residence in a nursing home or hospital, hypoalbuminemia, and anemia). They later modified the scale for use in the community setting, using nine risk factors [level of activity, level of mobility, complete SCI, urine incontinence or moisture, autonomic dysreflexia, pulmonary disease, renal disease, being prone to infections that cause breathing problems, and paralysis caused by trauma (as opposed to disease)] (24). Lehman (25) also evaluated common risk factors that can contribute to the development of pressure ulcers in the person with SCI, who is at home. These risk factors include: nutrition, past history of pressure ulcers, and social support issues. His evaluation of these factors was a prelude to the development of a risk assessment scale for use by the home care nurse. However, scales designed for use in the SCI population will require more extensive development and rigorous evaluation.

PRESSURE ULCER PREVENTION

Preventive techniques should begin from the onset of the SCI and continue through the early medical management period to the rehabilitation phase. When the patients are integrated into the home and community-based environment, a continuum of care that is geared toward the prevention of pressure ulcers is paramount. Continuous education of the staff and the patient is most important to the prevention of pressure ulcers. In addition, pressure ulcer prevention includes proper positioning, both in

TABLE 13.2. BRADEN RISK ASSESSMENT SCALE

Subscale				Score
Sensory perception	1. Completely limited	2. Very limited	3. Slightly limited	4. No impairment
Moisture	1. Constantly moist	2. Very moist	3. Occasionally moist	4. Rarely moist
Activity	1. Bedfast	2. Chairfast	3. Walks occasionally	4. Walks frequently
Mobility	1. Completely immobile	2. Very limited	3. Slightly limited	4. No limitation
Nutrition	1. Very poor	2. Probably inadequate	3. Adequate	4. Excellent
Friction and shear	1. Requires moderate to maximum assistance in moving	2. Moves freely or requires minimum assistance	3. Moves independently	
				Totals

TABLE 13.3. NORTON SCALE

Subscale				Score
Physical condition	1. Very bad	2. Poor	3. Fair	4. Good
Mental condition	1. Stupor	2. Confused	3. Apathetic	4. Alert
Activity	1. Bed	2. Chairbound	3. Walk with help	4. Ambulant
Mobility	1. Immobile	2. Very limited	3. Slightly limited	4 Full
Incontinent	1. Doubly	2. Usually urine	3. Occasional	4. Not
				Totals

bed and while sitting, maintaining a balanced diet and good overall nutrition, and avoiding medical complications.

Education

A comprehensive educational program for patients with SCI and their family or caregivers should begin during the initial rehabilitation phase and be updated throughout the course of care to include new self-care techniques and technology (45). Information should be presented at an appropriate level for the target audience, may include principles of adult learning, including explanation, demonstration, group discussion, and drills, and should be designed to meet the listener's needs, interests, and background (48,49). The educational program should include information on etiology and pathology, risk factors, comorbid conditions, proper positioning, equipment, complications, and the principles of wound prevention, skin care, and wound treatment (45). The educational program can be modified to include additional specific information regarding a particular treatment for those patients who have developed an ulcer (45). Studies have shown that compliance is greater and the treatment more successful when the patient actively participates in the learning process (50,51). In addition, it is important that family and caregiver education is comprehensive, because this may help decrease the incidence of new pressure ulcers (52).

Patients and their family or caregivers need to be instructed to inspect their skin at least twice daily, paying particular attention to the bony prominences, for the early signs of skin breakdown (53). Equipment such as a long-handled flexible mirror may assist in the skin inspection. In addition, education should be provided on proper inspection and maintenance of equipment that has been issued for pressure ulcer prevention so the equipment itself does not contribute to the development of the pressure ulcer.

Positioning and Equipment

Proper patient positioning and pressure relief should begin as soon as the emergency medical condition and spinal stabilization status allow (54,55). Pressure-decreasing procedures are aimed at reducing tissue ischemia to prevent pressure ulcers and to improve tissue healing once ulcers occur. As mentioned already, pressure ulcers occur over bony prominences. Depending on the patient's position, different bony prominences are at risk for the development of pressure ulcers. For example, when a person is sitting, the ischial tuberosities bear the weight of the upper body and are therefore at greatest risk. In persons lying on their side, the greater trochanters become at risk; in the supine position, the sacrum and the heels are at risk for pressure ulcer development. The prone position has a large surface area of low pressure and a smaller surface area of high pressure, although many patients cannot tolerate this position. All body assumable positions should be used for proper positioning, as tolerated by the patient (32). In measurements of transcutaneous partial pressure of oxygen and interface pressure, positioning patients at a 30-degree side-lying angle to the supine position reduces the interface pressure, and the transcutaneous partial pressure of oxygen returns to within the reference range (56,57).

Pillows can be used to assist in maintaining the desired position, to provide additional padding to bony prominences, or to suspend or provide pressure reduction over bony prominences with pillows proximally and distally placed, a technique known as bridging (58). Using this technique, one can achieve adequate pressure relief (59). Most persons can be treated with proper bed positioning and turns every 2 hours. Turning techniques should avoid shearing the soft tissues and patients should be alternated from side to side and placed prone if medically indicated and tolerated (41). Although it is common for a patient with SCI to extend the 2-hour turn schedule once home, with no increase in pressure ulcers probably secondary to improved tissue tolerance or perfusion, further research is needed to define which patients can and at what point can they increase their turning intervals.

With advances in technologies and difficulties that have risen in the acute care setting, including staffing, as well as medical conditions that prevent or limit turning, numerous beds and overlays have been developed to help prevent pressure ulcers. Although there is a large body of literature available on support surfaces, there is insufficient evidence to recommend one support surface over another for cost-effectiveness and appropriate patient characteristics of a specific mattress (45). Static support surfaces, which can be filled with foam, air, or gel, can be chosen for an individual without an ulcer without bottoming out on the support surface or for an individual with a pressure ulcer who can be positioned without weight bearing on the ulcer (45, 60,61). Examples of static support surfaces are listed in Table 13.4.

Dynamic support surfaces should be used if the individual cannot be positioned without pressure on the ulcer, if there is no evidence of ulcer healing, or if a new ulcer develops (60,62). Dynamic support surfaces include low-air-loss beds and overlays and air-fluidized beds. Examples of dynamic support surfaces are seen in Table 13.5. Performance characteristics of these surfaces are listed in Table 13.6.

Low-air-loss and air-fluidized beds should be used if there are multiple pressure ulcers, with large stage III or IV pressure ulcers, or after myocutaneous flap surgery (60). In comparison to air-fluidized beds, in general, low-air-loss beds and overlays are lighter and patient transfers are more easily managed (61). Air-fluidized beds are advantageous for excessive moisture, whether from the wound, perspiration, or incontinence, and the ceramic fluidized beads have a bactericidal effect due to the sequestration and desiccation of microorganisms (63,64).

The patient with SCI uses a wheelchair for mobility, and because the buttocks are at risk for the development of pressure

TABLE 13.4. EXAMPLES OF STATIC SUPPORT SURFACES

Foam	Air	Gel/Water
Eggcrate	Roho (Roho)	Rik Fluid Overlay (KCI)
Geo-Matt (Span America)	Sof-Care (Gaymar Industries)	
Comfortline (Hill-Rom)	First Step (Kinetic Concepts)	

TABLE 13.5. EXAMPLES OF DYNAMIC SUPPORT SURFACES

Low Air Loss Overlays	Low Air Loss Beds	Air Fluidized Beds
Micro Air (Invacare)	Flexicair (Support Systems International)	Clinitron (Support Systems International)
Clini-Care (Gaymar)	Kinair (Kinetic Concepts)	Skyton (Skytron)
First Step Select (KCI)	Mediscus (Mediscus Group)	FluidAir (Kinetic Concepts)

ulcers, care should be taken in prescribing the patient's wheelchair. While the patient is sitting, weight shifting will allow for reoxygenation of the tissues and is recommended every 15 to 30 minutes for 30 seconds (65,66). Weight shifts can be dependent, in which the patient's caregiver rotates the chair posteriorly so the patient's weight is no longer on the ischial tuberosities, but on the sacrum. Patients may use one or more of the following self-directed maneuvers aimed at shifting weight. The patient with or without assistance can perform weight shifts. To perform an anterior weight shift, the patient bends forward at the waist so his or her head is between the thighs and knees. To perform a lateral weight shift, the patient will remove the armrest on one side and lean to that side with his or her hand supporting the body weight on a stable surface and then the procedure is repeated on the other side. Finally, to perform a press-up weight shift, the most difficult weight shift, the patient will place his or her hands on the armrests and extend the elbows so the buttocks are suspended over the wheelchair cushion. All of these weight shift maneuvers will relieve the pressure from the buttocks and ischial tuberosities and redistribute it to other areas to allow reperfusion of the ischial areas.

Wheelchairs can also provide weight shifts through mechanical means and a power weight-shifting wheelchair system should be prescribed for individuals who are unable to independently perform an effective weight shift. The mechanical weight shift redistributes the pressure off of the buttocks and onto the back and a minimum of 45 degrees of backward tilt is required for adequate pressure distribution (67). Tilt-in-space mechanisms can be selected over reclining methods to avoid shear and if there is significant spasticity of spinal origin, which may be triggered with changes in body angles (68).

Proper positioning and alignment in the wheelchair can help prevent pressure ulcers on the buttocks. A significant reduction in the force on the buttocks while sitting can be obtained using armrests, which can support up to 10% of the body's weight (69). The sling-back wheelchair in the absence of patient trunk support promotes pelvic obliquity and kyphotic posture, with increased risks of pressure ulcers on the buttocks and sacrum, deformity, and pain (70). A wheelchair back support system can be prescribed to avoid these complications and keep the normal spinal curves intact. Wheelchair footplate adjustment must be tailored to the patient. Footplate adjustments for height and symmetry are important to ensure a more neutral sitting position of the pelvis, because any imbalance in the normal sitting position puts the patient at greater risk for pressure ulcer development (52,66,71).

Wheelchair cushions complement bed support surfaces in the prevention of pressure ulcers. Clinically useful computerized systems have been developed to evaluate the pressure exerted on various cushions, although they are limited in their ability to measure shear (72,73). The same materials available for support surfaces are now available in wheelchair cushions, including foam, air, and gel static cushions, as well as low-air-loss cushions. As with bed supports, the use of donut-shaped ring cushions should be avoided, because the ring will prevent perfusion of the central area (74). Examples of the different types of cushions are in Table 13.7.

Age-associated changes in the SCI patient's skin and mobility mean that the support surface, wheelchair, and wheelchair cushion initially prescribed may not be the most appropriate across the lifespan. It is therefore recommended that routine and regular assessment of each patient occurs before pressure ulcers develop, to determine whether a change in equipment or additional equipment is needed (72).

Nutrition

Normal tissue and skin integrity depend on adequate calorie, protein, and vitamin intake. Individuals who develop pressure ulcers often have significantly lower calorie and protein intake

TABLE 13.6. SUPPORT SURFACES CHARACTERISTICS

Performance Characteristics	Air Fluidized	Low Air Loss	Alternating Air	Static Flotation	Foam	Standard Mattress
Increased support area	Yes	Yes	Yes	Yes	Yes	No
Low moisture retention	Yes	Yes	No	No	No	No
Reduced heat accumulation	Yes	Yes	No	No	No	No
Shear reduction	Yes	?	Yes	Yes	No	No
Pressure reduction	Yes	Yes	Yes	Yes	Yes	No
Dynamic	Yes	Yes	Yes	No	No	No
Cost per day	High	High	Moderate	Low	Low	Low

From, AHCPR guidelines, 1994.

TABLE 13.7. EXAMPLES OF WHEELCHAIR CUSHIONS

Foam	Gel	Air	Alternating Air
Stimulite (Sepracor)	The Cloud (Otto Bock)	Roho (Roho)	Altern8 (Pegasus)
Combi (Jay Medical)	Jay (Jay Medical)	Nexus (Roho)	ErgoDynamic (ErgoAir)
Varilite (Cascade Designs)			

than those who do not develop pressure ulcers (53,75). For the purpose of assessing nutritional status, several blood chemistry tests are available and have been associated with the presence or development of pressure ulcers. For example, prealbumin is the most sensitive indicator for monitoring nutritional status because of its short half-life (2 to 3 days) and has been found to be significantly lower in patients with pressure ulcers, compared with those without pressure ulcers (76). In addition, decreases in total protein (less than 6.4 g/dL) and albumin levels (less than 3.5 g/dL) have similarly been found to be associated with pressure ulcer development (25,72,75,77). Factors associated with hypoalbuminemia include losses of protein and albumin in pressure ulcer exudate and the presence of a chronic inflammatory state (76,78,79).

Consequently, nutritional intake should be adequate to help prevent pressure ulcers and heal those that develop. Equations such as the Harris-Benedict equation have been used to estimate the spinal-injured patient's recommended caloric need, both with and without pressure ulcers (80). In addition, the Agency for Health Care Policy and Research (AHCPR) recommends that an individual without a pressure ulcer should consume 1.0-1.25 g of protein, per kilogram of body weight, per day. They also recommend that this amount should increase to 1.25-1.5 g/kg per day for a person with a pressure ulcer (45). However, indirect calorimetry is the best method of determining the energy expenditures in individuals with SCI who have pressure ulcers (81,82).

Other nutritional factors studied for wound healing include vitamins and minerals such as vitamins C and E and zinc. Vitamin C is an antioxidant that is necessary for the hydroxylation of proline and lysine during collagen formation and therefore may help with wound healing. However, supplementation of vitamin C has not been shown to accelerate healing of pressure ulcers and intake of vitamin C does not predict pressure ulcer development (66,83). Vitamin E is also an antioxidant; although it has been reported to improve the healing of pressure ulcers, there is limited scientific evidence of this (84). Zinc is involved in the structural integrity of collagen, and as with vitamin E, there are anecdotal reports of improved healing with supplementation; however, scientific evidence is limited (66,85).

Because catabolism, or loss of body protein, occurs with any open wound due to inflammation or infection, it is important to maintain adequate nutrition to prevent further loss of protein stores (86). With injury or chronic debilitation, there are decreased levels of the normal anabolic hormones, human growth hormone and testosterone (87,88). Because of this, several investigators have used the anabolic agent oxandrolone, combined with good nutrition, to restore weight and accomplish a significant increase in the healing rate of wounds (88–90). The use of these hormones for wound healing continues to be investigated.

Although inadequate nutritional intake has been found to correlate with the development of new pressure ulcers, in the patient who requires surgery, neither serum albumin nor total protein level has been found to correlate with postsurgical wound outcomes (13,29). Moreover, although wound closure is not advised in nutritionally depleted individuals, a particular serum albumin or total protein level has not been identified that would avert surgical intervention (86).

Finally, weight control is important for preventing pressure ulcers. Increases or decreases in weight may alter contributing factors to pressure ulcer development. For example, if an individual gains weight, he or she may become more susceptible to developing an ulcer from shear, particularly if his own strength or that of his caregiver is insufficient to transfer without sliding along the surface (43,52). Additionally, weight gain may cause a piece of equipment to no longer fit properly, such as a wheelchair, so the device itself can create a pressure risk. Given the limitations of most exercise facilities to adapt to the wheelchair user, weight control may become a challenge to patients with SCI with compromised energy expenditure.

Medical Complications

Cardiac disease, diabetes mellitus, vascular disease, immune deficiencies, collagen vascular diseases, malignancies, psychosis, and pulmonary disease are all factors that are associated with pressure ulcer development and may contribute to poor wound healing (91,92).

PRESSURE ULCER TREATMENT

General Principles

Treatment of the pressure ulcer in patients with SCI is not different from that in the non-SCI population. Pressure ulcers are most easily treated when the diagnosis is early and the interventions are promptly initiated. The general principles of pressure ulcer treatment are to relieve pressure, eliminate reversible underlying predisposing conditions, avoid friction, shear, and tissue maceration, and debride devitalized tissue. Treatment of the patient with SCI who has developed a pressure ulcer involves not only local wound care, but also an evaluation of causative factors and implementation of interventions, including additional equipment, to minimize the risk of both chronic wounds and repeated pressure ulcers.

Assessment

Before assessing the pressure ulcer itself, a comprehensive history and physical examination should be performed on any patient with a pressure ulcer (45). The pressure ulcer itself should be assessed in the context of the patient's overall physical and psychosocial health. Identification of comorbid factors may influence the plan of treatment, healing of the ulcer, and avoidance of additional and future pressure ulcers (45). In addition, every patient should be assessed for ulcer-related pain including during turning, dressing changes, and debridement (93–95). Up to 63% of patients report pain related to either the ulcer or its treatment and these studies also suggest that pressure ulcer pain changes over time (96,97).

To plan treatment of a pressure ulcer and to assess the effects of the treatment, the pressure ulcer should be monitored at every dressing change and the treatment should be reassessed at least weekly (45,98). Although frequently used alone as an assessment of pressure ulcers, concerns regarding pressure ulcer staging alone as the means of assessing the pressure ulcer include staff knowledge and ability to accurately apply the staging system, as well as its use to monitor changes in the status the pressure ulcer. Other assessment scales have been developed to assess pressure ulcers, including the Pressure Ulcer Scale for Healing Tool, the Pressure Sore Status Tool, and the Wound Healing Scale (99–101). Assessment of the pressure ulcer should include the location, depth, size, sinus tracts, undermining, tunneling, exudate, necrotic tissue, and the presence of granulation tissue and epithelialization. In addition to assessing depth, staging of the pressure ulcer may also be needed. At this time, all of these wound variables are considered important to determine the goal and plan of care. Specifically, these variables have been shown to be predictive of outcome in clinical studies and must be assessed for planning care and predicting outcome (102). The condition of the skin surrounding the pressure ulcer should also be assessed. A photographic record can be a useful aid in documenting progress of a pressure ulcer (103).

Physiology

Wound healing includes three overlapping phases: inflammation, tissue formation, and tissue remodeling. These events involve a complex array of cells including platelets, macrophages, neutrophils, fibroblasts, and epidermal cells, as well as a complex series of events including clotting, inflammation, granulation tissue formation, epithelialization, neovascularization, collagen synthesis, and wound contraction (104).

Managing Tissue Load

Primary tissue loads of sufficient intensity and duration are causative factors in the development of pressure ulcers. After the development of the primary pressure ulcer, extreme care must be taken to eliminate direct pressure on the wound, to avoid a delay in healing. Although the patient is restricted to bed mobility, a written repositioning schedule should be established to protect uninvolved areas, repositioning to avoid higher intensity or longer duration of pressure. Use of a specialized support sur-

face will provide an environment in which existing ulcers improve and may help prevent new ulcers from developing (77).

Debridement and Cleansing

Optimal wound healing can only occur in a clean wound (45). Cleaning the wound of inflammatory stimuli such as devitalized tissue and reactive chemicals involves debridement and cleansing. In addition, effective wound cleansing and debridement can reduce the bioburden and minimize colonization in pressure ulcers. Evidence is accumulating that effective debridement and cleansing improves wound healing. Chronic wounds may persist because of chronic inflammation secondary to devitalized tissue, wound exudate, and bacteria (105,106). Debridement can be accomplished in various ways; the most common methods include chemical, mechanical, autolytic, or surgically. Cleansing involves the use of specific types of fluid, usually saline based, to remove loosely adherent foreign material to facilitate wound healing (107).

Sharp debridement involves the use of a scalpel or scissors to remove the devitalized tissue and is the quickest way to remove devitalized tissue (108). In a multicenter study, Steed et al. (105) reported a lower rate of healing in those centers that performed less frequent debridement, independent of treatment. These findings suggest a correlation between aggressive wound debridement and improved wound healing. Mechanical debridement involves the use of woven cotton gauze in a wet-to-dry technique. Although various types of gauzes are available, the most effective gauze for mechanical debridement are those which are coarse and have large pores (109). Autolytic debridement is the process of keeping devitalized tissue hydrated and allowing reactive enzymes within the wound to digest the denatured tissues (110, 111). This can be accomplished using moisture-retentive dressings or hydrogels to moisturize the devitalized tissue. Mulder et al. (112,113) reported that when compared with a wet-to-dry gauze, a hypertonic gel was more effective in tissue removal and overall costs. When clinicians use autolytic debridement, the wound must frequently be cleansed to wash out partially degraded tissue fragments. Overall, autolytic debridement can be more selective and less traumatic to the surrounding tissue and healthy wound tissue than mechanical debridement (107). Enzymatic debridement uses commercially prepared enzymes such as Collagenase (Medical Services Group, Wayne, PA) and Accuzyme (Healthpoint, Fort Worth, TX), similar to autolytic debridement, to degrade devitalized tissue. However, although the commercial enzymes are expected to work faster, one study indicates that similar results can be achieved with hydrogel alone, which is much less expensive (114).

Wounds should be cleansed at each dressing change using a technique and solution that minimizes trauma to healthy wound tissue (45). Most wounds can be cleansed with normal saline, and for clean granulating wounds, a gentle flushing with isotonic saline will cleanse the wound (107). For dirty wounds, stronger cleansing solution may be required and clinicians can use commercial cleansing agents containing surfactants, such as Dermagran (Derma Sciences), Biolex (Bard Medical Division, CR Bard), and Ultra-Klenz Wound Cleanser (Carrington Laboratories). As the wound becomes cleaner, because surfactants are

TABLE 13.8. RELATIVE TOXICITY INDEXES OF NON–ANTIMICROBIAL AND ANTIMICROBIAL WOUND CLEANSERS

Product	Manufacturer	Toxicity Index
Non–antimicrobials		
Dermagran	Derma Sciences, Inc.	10
Shur-Clens Wound Cleanser	Convatec	10
Biolex	Bard Medical Division, CR Bard, Inc.	100
Cara-Klenz Wound and Skin Cleanser	Carrington Laboratories, Inc.	100
Saf-Clens Chronic Wound Cleanser	Convatec	100
Clinswound	Sage Laboratories, Inc.	1,000
Constant-Clens Dermal Wound Cleanser	Sherwood Medical-Davis and Geck	1,000
Curaklense Wound Cleanser	Kendall Healthcare Products Co.	1,000
Curasol	Healthpoint Medical	1,000
Gentell Wound Cleanser	Gentell	1,000
Sea-Clens Wound Cleanser	Coloplast Sween Corp.	1,000
Ultra-Klenz Wound Cleanser	Carrington Laboratories, Inc.	1,000
Antimicrobials		
Clinical Care Dermal Wound Cleanser	Care-Tech Laboratories, Inc.	1,000
Dermal Wound Cleanser	Smith and Nephew United, Inc.	10,000
MicroKlenz Antimicrobial Wound Cleanser	Carrington Laboratories, Inc.	10,000
Puri-Clens Wound Deodorizer and Cleanser	Coloplast Sween Corp.	10,000
Restore	Hollister, Inc.	10,000
Royl-Derm	Acme United Corp.	10,000
SeptiCare Antimicrobial Wound Cleanser	Sage Laboratories, Inc.	10,000

Adapted from Hellewell TB, Major DA, Foresman PA, et al. A cytotoxicity evaluation of antimicrobial and non–antimicrobial wound cleansers. *Wounds* 1997;9:15–20.

harmful to wound cells, the strength of the cleansing solution should be decreased (107). Although their benefit in addition to cleansing solutions has not been documented, antiseptic agents can be added to the cleanser, such as Dermal Wound Cleanser (Smith and Nephew United) and MicroKlenz Antimicrobial Wound Cleanser (Carrington Laboratories), which will dramatically increase the toxicity index of the solution (115). The relative toxicity of non-antimicrobial and antimicrobial wound cleansers are listed in Table 13.8.

Cleansers must be applied gently to minimize trauma to healthy tissue. Irrigation streams must keep the impact force below 15 psi. Wound irrigation pressures of 10 to 15 psi are superior to those of 1 or 5 psi. Direct application should only be with the smoothest and softest device available (107). As seen in Table 13.9, irrigation with a 35 mL syringe and a 19-gauge needle or angiocatheter meets these requirements.

TABLE 13.9. IRRIGATION PRESSURES BY VARIOUS DEVICES

Device	Irrigation Impact Pressure (PSI)
Bulb syringe	2.0
Piston irrigation syringe (60 mL) with catheter tip	4.2
Saline squeeze bottle (250 mL) with irrigation tip	4.5
Water-Pik at lowest setting (no. 1)	6.0
35-mL syringe with 19-gauge needle or angiocatheter	8.0
Water-Pik at middle setting (no. 3)	42
Water-Pik at highest setting (no. 5)	>50

Adapted from AHCPR, 1994.

Antibiotics

Topical antibiotics should be considered if no evidence of healing is seen after 2 to 4 weeks of optimal wound care and patient management. At this time, a 2-week trial of topical antibiotics such as silver sulfadiazine or triple antibiotic therapy is warranted and can often effectively reduce bacterial levels, thereby permitting healing (116).

Systemic antibiotics are generally only warranted when there is bacteremia, sepsis, advancing cellulitis, or osteomyelitis. Systemic antibiotics should be chosen based on blood culture and wound biopsy culture results. Care must be taken to not overlook other systemic causes of illness that may coexist with an otherwise noninfected wound (117).

Dressings and Adjunctive Therapies

Pressure ulcers require dressings to maintain physiologic integrity and to protect the wound. A dressing should be used that keeps the ulcer bed moist and the surrounding tissue dry (45, 118). Wet-to-dry dressings should be used for debridement and are not considered moist saline dressings (45). Interestingly, in a study that compared wet-to-dry dressings with hydrocolloid occlusive dressings, the wet-to-dry gauze dressings were found to have slower healing, take a longer time to change the dressing, and have a higher cost compared with the hydrocolloid occlusive dressing treatment (119). In comparisons of moist saline gauze treatment with hydrocolloid dressing treatments, however, there is no significant difference in healing rate (120–127). The hydrocolloid dressings, however, do show a significantly decreased cost of treatment, by consuming significantly less nursing time (119,128). Estimates note a tenfold increase in caregiver time for gauze versus hydrocolloid dressings, because of the differences in

TABLE 13.10. EXAMPLES OF DRESSINGS

Transparent Films	Hydrocolloids	Hydrogels	Foams	Alginates	Gauze Dressings
Tegaderm (3M Healthcare) Opsite (Smith and Nephew)	Restore (Hollister) Hollister Center PointLock Ultec (Kendall Healthcare)	Aquasorb (DeRoyal Woundcare) FlexiGel (Smith and Nephew) Carrasyn (Carrington)	Lyofoam (Ultra) Allevyn (Smith and Nephew) Kaltostat (Convatec)	Sorbsan (Bertek Pharmaceuticals) Algisite (Smith and Nephew)	Kendall Curity (Tyco Healthcare) Kendall Telfa (Kendall Healthcare) Xeroflo (Sherwood Medical)

the frequency of dressing changes (119). This factor is important for both inpatients and outpatients who may have limited assistance at home (129).

Although wounds heal better in a moist environment, excessive exudate can macerate surrounding tissue and prolong healing time (122). Foams, calcium alginates, and gauze dressings are absorbent and can be used on both deep and shallow wounds (45). The choice of which dressing to apply requires careful consideration of all factors, including cost, ease of use, size, location, and character of the wound, and evaluation of the goals and principles of the wound care. Examples of dressings are listed in Table 13.10.

Adjunctive therapies have long been described in the pressure ulcer literature. The AHCPR critically evaluated the strength of the literature on adjunctive therapies. Based on the clinical evidence available, only electrical stimulation merited recommendation and is to be considered for stage III and IV pressure ulcers that have proved unresponsive to conventional therapy, as well as for recalcitrant stage II ulcers (45). Hydrotherapy should be considered for pressure ulcers containing large amounts of exudate and necrotic tissue, where it can assist in debridement. However, once the wound is clean and has healthy granulation tissue, the agitating water may cause damage to the delicate new tissue and should be discontinued (45). The therapeutic efficacy of ultrasonography and hyperbaric oxygen, infrared, ultraviolet, and low-energy laser irradiation has not been sufficiently established for recommendation in the treatment of pressure ulcers (45). Currently, the Health Care Financing Administration uses a case-by-case evaluation of electrical stimulation for wound management for Medicare reimbursement (129).

Since the AHCPR recommendations were published, the strength of the scientific evidence for the use of electrical stimulation has advanced and there is also evidence that growth factors may be efficacious in the treatment of pressure ulcers (130–138). There are three new adjunctive therapies, since publication of the AHCPR guidelines, for the healing of pressure ulcers that have had initial evidence of efficacy: vacuum-assisted therapy (subatmospheric pressure therapy), normothermia, and constant tension approximation (129,139–142). Vacuum-assisted therapy, or subatmospheric pressure therapy, entails placing an open-cell foam into the wound, sealing the site with an adhesive drape, and applying subatmospheric pressure (125 mm Hg below ambi-

ent) that is transmitted to the wound in a controlled manner. This will increase blood flow in the wound and adjacent tissue and it will also increase clearance of bacteria from infected wounds, resulting in an environment that promotes healing (144). Normothermia employs the use of a radiant-heat dressing to hasten wound healing. In a small study involving patients with SCI with stage II and IV pressure ulcers, normothermia has been shown to decrease the mean wound surface area by 61% over a 4-week period (142). In one study on ulcers in patients with various comorbidities, constant tension approximation has been reported to increase the rate of healing through the use of a device for wound approximation. None of these new techniques have sufficient supporting evidence to recommend their use on pressure ulcers in SCI.

Surgical Management

In general, stage I and II pressure ulcers can be treated nonsurgically. Because of their high rate of recurrence and the long duration necessary for wound closure, stage III and IV pressure ulcers often require surgical intervention (45). In general, the goals of surgical wound closure can include: reduction in the time to heal, lower costs, improved patient hygiene and appearance, decreased amount of care needed, and prevention of secondary complications, including renal amyloidosis and Marjolin ulcer (145). Proper selection of the surgical candidate is important because of the cost, which can be expensive, and because of the postoperative recovery time, which can be extensive (117). In addition, if musculocutaneous flaps are performed, only a limited number can be performed, which may be detrimental if the individual has repeated pressure ulcers or additional risk factors are added with aging.

Operative procedures to repair pressure ulcers include direct closure, skin grafting, skin flaps, musculocutaneous flaps, fasciocutaneous flaps, and free flaps. The simplest type of repair that can adequately close the wound with a reasonable success rate should be chosen (117). Free flaps, skin flaps, and skin grafts are rarely used for pressure ulcers in patients with SCI, because they are poorly able to tolerate any future pressure or shear (117). Direct closure is rarely of benefit unless the source of the pressure has been eradicated and the wound is small (146). Musculocutaneous and fasciocutaneous flaps have become the coverage of choice for patients with SCI, who require surgical closure of the pressure ulcer. Because of their blood supply, these flaps are better able to withstand pressure and shear and can be particularly useful in osteomyelitis, by bringing highly vascularized muscle tissue into the area of infection (117,147,148).

Factors that impair postoperative healing include smoking, spasticity, nutritional concerns, and bacterial colonization. Smoking is one of the strongest inhibitors of wound healing as a result of carbon monoxide and nicotine, both of which are potent vasoconstrictors (117). In addition to compromises in arterial blood flow and oxygen delivery, smoking increases blood viscosity and increases oxidase release by neutrophils, all of which impair wound healing (149,150). Nicotine patches should not be used because they provide the same drug as cigarettes. Spasticity can also impair postoperative healing through repeated contraction of muscles, causing joint movement during the period of postoperative immobilization (151,152). In addition, significant contractures may impair pressure-relief efforts (153). Adequate nutrition must be maintained during the postoperative period to allow for wound healing, although serum albumin and total protein levels have not been found to correlate with postoperative wound outcome (154). Finally, exposure to bacterial contamination, particularly of urine and feces, increases colonization of wounds and is associated with slower rates of healing (61).

At the sacral area, the gluteus maximus muscle may be used in its entirety or in portions. At the ischium, a posterior thigh fasciocutaneous flap, inferior gluteus maximus myocutaneous flap, hamstring V-Y advancement flap, and tensor fascia lata fasciocutaneous flap can all be used to cover defects in this region (117). Prophylactic unilateral or bilateral ischiectomy is not recommended. Because weight is diverted to the contralateral ischium, unilateral ischiectomy is associated with the occurrence of a contralateral ischial ulcer (155). Bilateral ischiectomy will transfer weight bearing to the anterior pelvis and perineum, causing perineal ulcers and urethral fistulae (156,157). At the greater trochanter, the tensor fascia lata fasciocutaneous flap is considered the flap of choice in this area, although alternatives include the vastus lateralis, inferior gluteus maximus, and rectus femoris muscles (117). Girdlestone arthroplasty for ulcers that communicate with the hip joint may be necessary, although patients may experience a pistoning of the distal femur after this procedure, which may be detrimental to the flap (158).

Postoperatively, strict bed rest is prescribed with immobilization and pressure relief. Usually, a low-air-loss mattress or an air-fluidized bed is prescribed (117). The head of the bed should not be elevated more than 15 degrees to avoid risk of shear (93). Bed rest should be maintained postoperatively to allow sufficient time for the surgical site to heal (93). There is no consensus in the literature on the necessary length of immobilization, ranging from 2 to 6 weeks (117,159). A progressive sitting program is initiated after the period of immobilization, although there is no consensus regarding rate of progression in the sitting schedule. Overall, a 13% to 56% recurrence rate has been reported after surgical repair of pressure ulcers (158,160).

COMPLICATIONS

Pressure ulcers have been associated with many complications including, endocarditis, heterotopic bone formation, maggot infestation, perineal urethral fistulas, septic arthritis, sinus tract or abscess, squamous cell carcinoma in the ulcer, systemic complications of the treatment, and specifically in SCI, contractures (34,156,161–168).

Evidence of infection in a pressure ulcer includes the clinical signs of erythema, induration, purulence, and a foul odor. Swab cultures are not useful in determining the presence of infection of pressure ulcers and only reflect the bacteria on the surface of the pressure ulcer (169). Tissue biopsy can determine whether there are bacteria within the tissue, and if the bacterial count is more than 10^5, wound healing may be impaired (170). Advancing cellulitis is indicative of invasive tissue infection and must be treated with appropriate antibiotics. Approximately 25% of nonhealing pressure ulcers have underlying osteomyelitis (78, 171). Because the clinical diagnosis of osteomyelitis is unreliable, bone biopsy remains the definitive method to diagnose osteomyelitis and identify the organism (171,172). Bone scans have a high false-positive rate due to surrounding inflammation inherent in open wounds (171). Once the diagnosis is made, debridement and long-term antibiotic therapy are essential. Untreated, osteomyelitis can result in delayed healing, more extensive tissue damage, a longer length of hospitalization, and higher mortality rates (117).

In addition, once a pressure ulcer has occurred, there is the risk of recurrence. Niazi et al. (173) found a 35% recurrence rate of pressure ulcers regardless of whether the treatment was medical or surgical; however, Disa et al. (174) found that in 69% of patients and 61% of sores, a recurrent ulceration can occur. Smoking, diabetes mellitus, and cardiovascular disease were associated with the highest rates of recurrence in these studies. Patients with SCI often have misconceptions about pressure ulcers: One study found that 82% of people with SCI who had an ulcer did not believe they were at risk for the development of a future ulcer (6). Other factors, including age, employment status, and psychological well being are less well defined in their association with pressure ulcer recurrence (6,174,175).

Long-standing ulcers (20 years or more) can rarely (less than 0.5%) develop into Marjolin ulcers, a type of squamous cell carcinoma. Biopsy can identify the carcinoma that is suspected clinically with pain, increasing discharge, verrucous hyperplasia, and bleeding (176).

CONCLUSION

Pressure ulcers after SCI are an age-old problem. Even today, despite advances in education, equipment, and technology, as well as our understanding of their pathophysiology, pressure ulcers remain a significant psychological, financial, and functional barrier to many patients after an injury. However, with these advances, we have developed new ways of preventing and treating pressure ulcers. Further research is needed in all areas of pressure sore prevention and management to minimize its impact on the patient with SCI.

REFERENCES

1. National Pressure Ulcer Advisory Panel (NPUAP). Pressure ulcers prevalence, cost and risk assessment: consensus development conference statement. *Decubitus* 1989;2:24–28.
2. Shea JD. Pressure sores: classification and management. *Clin Orthop*1975;112:89–100.
3. Yarkony GM, Kirk PM, Carlson C. Classification of pressure ulcers. *Arch Dermatol* 1990;126:1218–1219.
4. Thomas AC, Wysocki AB. The healing wound: a comparison of three useful clinical methods of measurement. *Decubitus* 1990;3:18–25.
5. Hooker EZ, Sibley P, Nemchausky B, et al. A method for quantifying the area of closed pressure ulcers by sinography and digitometry. *J Neurol Nurs* 1988;20:118–127.
6. Rodriguez GP, Garber SL. Prospective study of pressure ulcer risk in spinal cord injury patients. *Paraplegia* 1981;19:235–247.
7. Richardson RR, Meyer PR. Prevalence and incidence of pressure sores in acute spinal cord injuries. *Paraplegia* 1981;19:235–247.
8. Krause JS. Skin sores after spinal cord injury: relationship to life adjustment. *Spinal Cord* 1998;36:51–56.
9. Young JS, Burns PE. Pressure sores and the spinal cord injured. *SCI Digest* 1981a;3:9–25.
10. Carlson CE, King BB, Kirk PM, et al. Incidence and correlates of pressure ulcer development after spinal cord injury. *J Rehabil Nurs Res* 1992;1:34–40.
11. Fuhrer MJ, Garber SL, Rintala DH, et al. Pressure ulcers in community-resident persons with spinal cord injury: prevalence and risk factors. *Arch Phys Med Rehabil* 1993;74:1172–1177.
12. Garber SL, Rintala DH, Hart KA, et al. Pressure ulcer risk in spinal cord injury: predictors of ulcer status over 3 years. *Arch Phys Med Rehabil* 2000;81:465–471.
13. Vidal J, Sarrias M. An analysis of the diverse factors concerned with the development of pressure ulcers in spinal cord injured patients. *Paraplegia* 1991;29:261–267.
14. Young JS, Burns PE. Pressure sores and the spinal cord injured: part II. *SCI Digest* 1981b;3:11–48.
15. Cull JG, Smith OH. A preliminary note on demographic and personality correlates of decubitus ulcer incidence. *J Psychol* 1973;85:225–227.
16. Lamid S, El Ghatit AZ. Smoking, spasticity and pressure sores in spinal cord injured patients. *Am J Phys Med* 1983;62:300–306.
17. Richards JS. Pressure ulcers in spinal cord injury: psychosocial correlates. *SCI Digest* 1981;3:11–18.
18. Young ME, Rintala DH, Rossi CD, et al. Alcohol and marijuana use in a community-based sample of persons with spinal cord injury. *Arch Phys Med Rehabil* 1995;76:525–532.
19. Anderson TP, Andberg MM. Psychosocial factors associated with pressure sores. *Arch Phys Med Rehabil* 1979;60:341–346.
20. Gunnewicht BR. Pressure sores in patients with acute spinal cord injury. *J Wound Care* 1995;4:452–454.
21. Mawson AR, Biundo JJ, Neville P, et al. Risk factors for early occurring pressure ulcers following spinal cord injury. *Am J Phys Med Rehabil* 1988;67:123–127.
22. Whiteneck GG, Carter RE, Charlifue SW, et al. *A collaborative study of high quadriplegia. Final report to the National Institute of Handicapped Research.* Englewood, CO: Rocky Mountain Regional Spinal Injury System, 1985.
23. Yarkony GM, Heinemann AW. Pressure ulcers. In: Stover SL, DeLisa JA, Whiteneck GG, eds. *Spinal cord injury: clinical outcomes from the model systems.* Gaithersburg, MD: Aspen Publishing, 1995.
24. Salzberg CA, Byrne DW, Cayten CG, et al. Predicting and preventing pressure ulcers in adults with paralysis. *Adv Wound Care* 1998;11:237–246.

25. Lehman CA. Risk factors for pressure ulcers in the spinal cord injured in the community. *Sci Nurs* 1995;12:110–114.
26. McKinley WO, Jackson AB, Cardenas DD, et al. Long-term medical complications after traumatic spinal cord injury: a regional model systems analysis. *Arch Phys Med Rehabil* 1999;80:1402–1410.
27. Carlson CE, Matthews-Kirk P, Stevens K, et al. Psychosocial factors associated with pressure sores after spinal cord injury [Abstract]. *Arch Phys Med Rehabil* 1990;71:788.
28. Fuhrer MJ, Rintala DH, Hart KA, et al. Depressive symptomatology in persons with spinal cord injury who reside in the community. *Arch Phys Med Rehabil* 1993;74:255–260.
29. Rintala DH, Young ME, Hart KA, et al. Social support and the well-being of persons with spinal cord injury living in the community. *Rehabil Psychol* 1992;37:155–163.
30. LaMantia JG, Hirschwald JF, Goodman CL, et al. Pressure sore readmission program: a method to reduce chronic readmissions for pressure sore problems. *Rehabil Nurs* 1987;12:22–25.
31. Braun J, Silvetti A, Zakellis G. What really works for pressure sores. *Patient Care* 1992;26:63–76.
32. Yarkony GM. Pressure ulcers: a review. *Arch Phys Med Rehabil* 1994;75:908–917.
33. Daniel RK, Wheatley D, Priest D, et al. Pressure sores and paraplegics: an experimental model. *Ann Plast Surg* 1985;15:41–49.
34. Rueler JB, Cooney TG. The pressure sore: pathophysiology and principles of management. *Ann Intern Med* 1981;94:661–666.
35. Nola GT, Vistnes LM. Differential response of skin and muscle in the experimental production of pressure sores. *Plast Reconstr Surg* 1980;66:728–733.
36. Rodriguez GP, Claus-Walker J. Biochemical changes in skin composition in spinal cord injury: a possible contribution to decubitus ulcers. *Paraplegia* 1988;26:302–309.
37. Rodriguez GP, Claus-Walker J, Kent MC, et al. Collagen metabolite excretion as a predictor of bone and skin related complications in spinal cord injury. *Arch Phys Med Rehabil* 1989;70:442–444.
38. Teasell RW, Arnold JM, Krassioukov A, et al. Cardiovascular consequences of loss of supraspinal control of the sympathetic nervous system after spinal cord injury. *Arch Phys Med Rehabil* 2000;81:506–516.
39. Rodriguez GP, Claus-Walker J, Kent MC, et al. Adrenergic receptors in insensitive skin of spinal cord injury patients. *Arch Phys Med Rehabil* 1986;67:177–180.
40. Hagisawa, Ferguson-Pell SM, Cardi M. Assessment of skin blood content and oxygenation in spinal cord injured subjects during reactive hyperemia. *J Rehabil Res* 1994;31:1–14.
41. Yarkony GM. Aging skin, pressure ulcerations, and spinal cord injury. In: Whitecock GC, ed. *Aging with spinal cord injury.* New York: Demos Publications, 1993:39–52.
42. Watelow J. Operating table: the root cause of many pressure sores? *Br J Theatre Nurs* 1996;6:19–21.
43. Bergstrom N, Braden B, Kemp M, et al. Multi-site study of incidence of pressure ulcers and the relationship between risk level, demographic characteristics, diagnoses, and prescription of preventative interventions. *J Am Geriatr Soc* 1996;44:22–30.
44. Rochon PA, Beaudet MP, McGlinchey-Berroth R, et al. Risk assessment for pressure ulcers: an adaptation of the National Pressure Ulcer Advisory Panel risk factors to spinal cord injured patients. *J Am Paraplegia Soc* 1993;16:169–177.
45. Bergstrom N, Bennett MA, Carlson CE. *Clinical practice guideline number 15: treatment of pressure ulcers.* Rockville, MD: US Dept of Health and Human Services, Public Health Service, Agency for Health Care Policy and Research; 1994. AHCPR publication 95-0652.
46. Norton D. Calculating the risk: reflections on the Norton scale. *Decubitus* 1989;2:24–31.
47. Salzberg CA, Byrne DW, Cayten CG, et al. A new pressure ulcer risk assessment scale for individuals with spinal cord injury. *Am J Phys Med Rehabil* 1996;75:96–104.
48. Maklebust J, Magnan MA. Approaches to patient and family education for pressure ulcer management. *Decubitus* 1992;5:18–26.

49. Warren VB, ed. *A treasury of techniques for teaching adults.* Washington: National Association for Public Continuing and Adult Education; 1977.

50. Engstrand JL. A nursing challenge: effective patient education. *AORN J* 1979;4:15–18.

51. Barnes SH. Patient/family education for the patient with a pressure necrosis. *Nurs Clin North Am* 1987;22:463–474.

52. Krouskop TA, Noble PC, Garber SL, et al. The effectiveness of preventative management in reducing the occurrence of pressure sores. *J Rehabil Res Dev* 1983;20:74–83.

53. Bergstrom N, Braden BA. A prospective study of pressure sore risk among the institutionalized elderly. *J Am Geriatr Soc* 1992;40: 747–758.

54. Parnham A. Interface pressure measurements during ambulance journeys. *J Wound Care* 1999;8:279–282.

55. Linares HA, Mawson AR, Suarez E, et al. Association between pressure sores and immobilization in the immediate post-injury period. *Orthopedics* 1987;10:571–573.

56. Defloor T. The effect of position and mattress on interface pressure. *Applied Nurs Res* 2000;13:2–11.

57. Seiler Wo, Allen S, Stahelin HB. Influence of the 30 degree laterally inclined position and the "Super-Soft" 3-piece mattress on skin oxygen tension on areas of maximum pressure-implications for pressure sore prevention. *Gerontology* 1986;32:158–166.

58. Land L. A review of pressure damage preventing strategies. *J Adv Nurs* 1995;22:329–337.

59. Bogie K, Nuseibeh I, Bader D. Transcutaneous gas tension in the sacrum during the acute phase of spinal cord injury. Proceedings of the Institute of Mechanical Engineers. Part H. *J Eng Med* 1992;206: 1–6.

60. Charles MA, Oldenbrook J, Catton C. Evaluation of a low-air-loss mattress system in the treatment of patients with pressure ulcers. *Ostomy Wound Manage* 1995;41:46–52.

61. Ferrell BA, Osterweil D, Christenson P. A randomized trial of low-air-loss beds for treatment of pressure ulcers. *JAMA* 1993;269:494–497.

62. Day A, Leonard F. Seeking quality care for patients with pressure ulcers. *Decubitus* 1993;6:32–43.

63. Sharbaugh RJ, Hargest TS, Wright FA. Further studies on the bactericidal effect of the air-fluidized bed. *Am Surg* 1973;39:253–256.

64. Sharbaugh RJ, Hargest TS. Bactericidal effect of the air-fluidized bed. *Am Surg* 1971;37:583–586.

65. Nixon V. Pressure relief. In: Nixon V, auth. *Spinal cord injury: a guide to functional outcomes in physical therapy management,* 1st ed. Rockville, MD: Aspen Publishers, 1985:67–75.

66. Bergstrom N, Bennett MA, Carlson CE. *Clinical practice guideline number 3. Pressure ulcers in adults: prediction and prevention.* Rockville, MD: US Dept of Health and Human Services, Agency for Health Care Policy and Research; 1992. AHCPR publication 92-0047.

67. Hobson DA. Comparative effects of posture on pressure and shear at the body-seat interface. *J Rehabil Res Dev* 1992;15:21–31.

68. Goossens RH, Snijders CJ, Holscher TG, et al. Shear stress measured on beds and wheelchairs. *Scand J Rehabil Med* 1997;29:131–136.

69. Gilsdorf P, Patterson R, Fisher S. Thirty-minute continuous sitting force measurement with different support surfaces in the spinal cord injured and able-bodied. *J Rehabil Res Dev* 1991;28:33–38.

70. Yarkony GM, Chen D. Rehabilitation of patients with spinal cord injuries. In: Bradden RL, ed. *Physical medicine rehabilitation,* 1st ed. Philadelphia: WB Saunders, 1996:1149–1179.

71. Koo TK, Mak AF, Lee YL. Posture effect on eating interface biomechanics: comparison between two seating systems. *Arch Phys Med Rehabil* 1996;77:40–47.

72. Salcido R, Hart D, Smith AM. The prevention and management of pressure ulcers. In: Braddon RL, ed. *Physical medicine rehabilitation,* 1st ed. Philadelphia: WB Saunders, 1996;630–648.

73. Barr CA. Evaluation of cushions using dynamic pressure measurement. *Prosthet Orthot Int* 1991;15:232–240.

74. Crewe RA. Problems of rubber ring nursing cushions and a clinical survey of alternative cushions for ill patients. *Care SCI Pract* 1987; 5:9–11.

75. Tourtual DM, Riesenberg LA, Korutz CJ, et al. Predictors of hospital acquired heel pressure ulcers. *Ostomy Wound Manage* 1997;43:24–30.

76. Bonnefoy M, Coulon L, Bienvenu J, et al. Implication of cytokines in the aggravation and malnutrition and hypercatabolism in elderly patients with severe pressure sores. *Age Aging* 1995;24:37–42.

77. Blaylock B. A study of risk factors in patients placed on specialty beds. *JWOCN* 1995;22:263–266.

78. Allman RM, Goode PS, Patrick MM, et al. Pressure ulcer risk factors among hospitalized patients with activity limitation. *JAMA* 1995;273: 865–870.

79. Segal JL, Gonzales E, Yousefi S, et al. Circulating levels of IL-2R, ICAM-1, and IL-6 in spinal cord injuries. *Arch Phys Med Rehabil* 1997;78:44–47.

80. Chin D, Kearns P. Nutrition in the spinal-injured patient. *Nutr Clin Pract* 1997;6:213–232.

81. Alexander LR, Spungen AM, Liu MH, et al. Resting metabolic rate in subjects with paraplegia: the effect of pressure sores. *Arch Phys Med Rehabil* 1995;76:819–822.

82. Liu MH, Spungen AM, Fink L, et al. Increased energy needs in patients with quadriplegia and pressure ulcers. *Adv Wound Care* 1996; 9:41–45.

83. terRiet G, Kessels A, Knipschild P. Randomized clinical trial of ascorbic acid in the treatment of pressure ulcers. *J Clin Epidemiol* 1995;48:1453–1460.

84. Houwing R, Overgoor M, Kon M, et al. Pressure-induced skin lesions in pigs: reperfusion injury and the effects of vitamin E. *J Wound Care* 2000;9:36–40.

85. Kohn S, Kohn D, Schiller D. Effect of zinc supplementation on epidermal Langerhans' cells of elderly patients with decubital ulcers. *J Dermatol* 2000;27:258–263.

86. Lawrence W. Clinical management of non-healing wounds. In: Cohen C, ed. *Wound healing.* Philadelphia: WB Saunders, 1992:541.

87. Jeevendra M, Ramos L, Shamos R, et al. Decreased growth hormone levels in the catabolic phase of severe injury. *Surgery* 1992;111: 495–502.

88. Demling R, DeSanti L. Oxandrolone, an anabolic steroid, significantly increases weight gain in the recovery phase after major burns. *J Trauma* 1997;43:47–51.

89. Demling R, DeSanti L. Closure of the "non-healing wound" corresponds with correction of weight loss using the anabolic agent oxandrolone. *Ostomy Wound Manage* 1998;44:58–68.

90. Fox M, Minor A. Oxandrolone: a potent anabolic steroid. *J Clin Endocr Metab* 1962;22:921–923.

91. Lazarus GS, Cooper DM, Knighton DR, et al. Definitions and guidelines for assessment of wounds and evaluation of healing. *Arch Dermatol* 1994;130:489–493.

92. Goodman CM, Cohen V, Armenta A, et al. Evaluation of results and treatment variables for pressure ulcers in 48 veteran spinal cord-injured patients. *Ann Plast Surg* 1999;42:665–672.

93. Black JM, Black SB. Surgical management of pressure ulcers. *Nurs Clin North Am* 1982;22:429–438.

94. Tudhope M. Management of pressure ulcers with a hydrocolloid occlusive dressing: results in twenty-three patients. *J Enterostomal Ther* 1984;11:102–105.

95. Dallam L, Smyth C, Jackson BS, et al. Pressure ulcer pain: assessment and quantification. *J Wound Ostomy Continence Nurs* 1995;22: 211–215.

96. van Rijswijk L. Full-thickness pressure ulcers: patient and wound healing characteristics. *Decubitus* 1993;6:16–21.

97. Day A, Dombranski S, Farkas C, et al. Managing sacral pressure ulcers with hydrocolloid dressings: results of a controlled, clinical study. *Ostomy Wound Manage* 1995;41:52–54.

98. van Rijswijk L, Braden BJ. Pressure ulcer patient and wound assessment: an AHCPR clinical practice guideline update. *Ostomy Wound Manage* 1999;45[Supple 1A]:56S–67S.

99. Thomas DR, Rodeheaver GT, Bartolucci AA, et al. Pressure ulcer scale for healing: derivation and validation of the PUSH tool. The PUSH Task Force. *Adv Wound Care* 1997;10:96–101.

100. Bates-Jensen B. New pressure ulcer status tool *Decubitus* 1990;3: 14–15.

101. Krasner D. Wound healing scale, version 1.0: a proposal. *Adv Wound Care* 1997;10:82–85.
102. Yarkony GM, Kirk PM, Carlson C, et al. Classification of pressure ulcers. *Arch Dermatol* 1990;126:1218–1219.
103. Cutler NR, George R, Seifert RD, et al. Comparison of quantitative methodologies to define chronic pressure ulcer management. *Decubitus* 1993;6:22–30.
104. Singer AJ, Clark RA. Cutaneous wound healing. *N Engl J Med* 1999; 341:738–746.
105. Steed DL, Donohoe D, Webster MW, et al. Diabetic ulcer study group. Effect of extensive debridement and treatment on the healing of diabetic foot ulcers. *J Am Coll Surg* 1996;183:61–64.
106. Burke DT, Ho CH, Saucier MA. Hydrotherapy effects on pressure ulcer healing. *Arch Phys Med Rehabil* 1997;183:61–64.
107. Rodeheaver GT. Pressure ulcer debridement and cleansing: a review of current literature. *Ostomy Wound Manage* 1999;78:1053.
108. Witkowski JA, Parish LC. Debridement of cutaneous ulcers: medical and surgical aspects. *Clin Dermatol* 1992;9:585–591.
109. Mulder GD. Evaluation of three nonwoven sponges in the debridement of chronic wounds. *Ostomy Wound Manage* 1995;41:62–67.
110. Flanagan M. The efficacy of a hydrogel in the treatment of wounds with non-viable tissue. *J Wound Care* 1995;4:264–267.
111. Bale S, Banks V, Haglestein S, et al. A comparison of two amorphous hydrogels in the debridement of pressure sores. *J Wound Care* 1998; 7:65–68.
112. Mulder GD, Romanko KP, Sealey J, et al. Controlled randomized study of a hypertonic gel for the debridement of dry eschar in chronic wounds. *Wounds* 1993;5:112–115.
113. Mulder GD. Cost-effectiveness managed care: gel versus wet-to-dry for debridement. *Ostomy Wound Manage* 1995;41:68–76.
114. Martin SJ, Corrado OJ, Kay EA. Enzymatic debridement for necrotic wounds. *J Wound Care* 1996;5:310–311.
115. Hellewell TB, Major DA, Foresman PA, et al. A cytotoxicity evaluation of antimicrobial and non-antimicrobial wound cleansers. *Wounds* 1997;9:15–20.
116. Kucan JO, Robson MC, Heggers JP, et al. Comparison of silver sulfadiazine, povidone-iodine and physiologic saline in the treatment of chronic pressure ulcer. *J Am Geriatr Soc* 1981;29:232–235.
117. Brown DL, Smith DJ. Bacterial colonization/infection and the surgical management of pressure ulcers. *Ostomy Wound Manage* 1999;45: 109S–118S.
118. Sebern MD. Pressure ulcer management in home health care: efficacy and cost-effectiveness of moisture vapor permeable dressing. *Arch Phys Med Rehabil* 1986;67:726–729.
119. Kim YC, Shin JC, Park CI, et al. Efficacy of hydrocolloid occlusive dressing technique in decubitus ulcer treatment: a comparative study. *Yonsei Med J* 1996;37:181–185.
120. Neill KM, Conforti C, Kedas A, et al. Pressure sore responses to a new hydrocolloid dressing. *Wounds* 1989;1:171–185.
121. Colwell JC, Foreman MD, Trotter JP. A comparison of the efficacy and cost-effectiveness of two methods of managing pressure ulcers. *Decubitus* 1993;6:28–36.
122. Xakellis GC, Chrischilles EA. Hydrocolloid versus saline-gauze dressings in treating pressure ulcers: a cost-effectiveness analysis. *Arch Phys Med Rehabil* 1992;73:463–469.
123. Banks V, Bale S, Harding K. The use of two dressings for moderately exuding pressure sores. *J Wound Care* 1994;3:132–134.
124. Banks V, Harding EF, Harding K, et al. Evaluation of a new polyurethane foam dressing. *J Wound Care* 1997;6:266–269.
125. Bale S, Squires D, Varnon T, et al. A comparison of two dressings in pressure sore management. *J Wound Care* 1997;6:463–466.
126. Honde C, Derks C, Tudor C. Local treatment of pressure sores in the elderly; amino acid copolymer membrane versus hydrocolloid dressings. *J Am Geriatr Soc* 1994;42:1180–1183.
127. Mulder G, Altman M, Seeley J, et al. Prospective randomized study of the efficacy of hydrogel, hydrocolloid and saline-moistened dressings on the management of pressure ulcers. *Wound Repair Regen* 1993; 1:213–218.
128. Bolton LL, van Rijswijk L, Shaffer FA. Quality wound care equals cost-effective wound care: a clinical model. *Adv Wound Care* 1997; 10:33–38.
129. Ovington LG. Dressings and adjunctive therapies: AHCPR guidelines revisited. *Ostomy Wound Care Manage* 1999;45:94S–106S.
130. Wood JM, Evans PE 3rd, Schallreuter KU, et al. A multicenter study on the use of pulsed low intensity direct current for healing chronic stage II and stage III decubitus. *Arch Dermatol* 1993;129:999–1009.
131. Gardner SE, Frantz RA, Schmidt FL. Effect of electrical stimulation on chronic wound healing. *Wound Repair Regen* 1999;7:495–503.
132. Robson MC, Phillips LG, Lawrence WT, et al. The safety and effect of topically applied recombinant basic fibroblast growth factor on the healing of chronic pressure sores. *Ann Surg* 1992;216:401–406.
133. Robson MC, Phillips LG, Thomason A, et al. Recombinant human platelet-derived growth factor-BB for the treatment of chronic pressure ulcers. *Ann Plast Surg* 1992;29:193–201.
134. Robson MC, Phillips LG, Thomason A, et al. Platelet-derived growth factor BB for the treatment of chronic pressure ulcers. *Lancet* 1992; 339:23–25.
135. Mustoe TA, Cutler NR, Allman RM, et al. A phase II study to evaluate recombinant platelet-derived growth factor-BB in the treatment of stage 3 and 4 pressure ulcers. *Arch Surg* 1994;129:213–219.
136. Rees RS, Robson MC, Smiell JN, et al. Becaplermin gel in the treatment of pressure ulcers: a phase II randomized, double-blind, placebo-controlled study. *Wound Repair Regen* 1999;7:141–147.
137. Kunimoto BT. Growth factors in wound healing: the next great innovation? *Ostomy Wound Manage* 1999;45:56–64.
138. Robson MC, Hill DP, Smith PD, et al. Sequential cytokine therapy for pressure ulcers: clinical and mechanistic response. *Ann Surg* 2000; 231:600–611.
139. Mullner T, Mrkonjic L, Kwasny O, et al. The use of negative pressure to promote healing of tissue defects: a clinical trial using the vacuum sealing technique. *Br J Plast Surg* 1997;50:194–199.
140. Argenta LC, Morykwas MJ. Vacuum-assisted closure: a new method for wound control and treatment: clinical experience. *Ann Plast Surg* 1997;38:563–576.
141. Deva AK, Siu C, Nettle WJ. Vacuum-assisted closure of a sacral pressure sore. *J Wound Care* 1997;6:311–312.
142. Kloth LC, Berman JE, Dumit-Minkel S, et al. Effects of a normothermic dressing on pressure ulcer healing. *Adv Skin Wound Care* 2000; 13(2):69–74.
143. Ger R. Wound management by constant tension approximation. *Ostomy Wound Manage* 1996;42:40–46.
144. Morykwas MJ, Argenta LC, Shelton-Brown EI, et al. Vacuum-assisted closure: a new method for wound control and treatment: animal studies and basic foundation. *Ann Plast Surg* 1997;38(6):553–562.
145. Daniel RK, Faibusoff B. Muscle coverage of pressure points: the role of myocutaneous flaps. *Ann Plast Surg* 1982;8:446–452.
146. Anthony JP, Hunstman WT, Mathes SJ. Changing trends in the management of pelvic pressure ulcers: a 12-year review. *Decubitus* 1992;5:44–51.
147. Daniel RK, Hall EJ, MacLeod MK. Pressure sores: a reappraisal. *Ann Plast Surg* 1979;2:53–63.
148. Mathes SJ, Feng LJ, Hunt TK. Coverage of the infected wound. *Ann Surg* 1983;198:420–429.
149. Read RC. Presidential address: systemic effects of smoking. *Am J Surg* 1984;148:706–711.
150. Fincham JE. Smoking cessation: treatment options and the pharmacist's role. *Ann Pharm* 1992;32:62–70.
151. Ger R, Levine SA. The management of decubitus ulcers by muscle transposition. An 8-year review. *Plast Reconstr Surg* 1976;58:419–428.
152. Herceg SJ, Harding RL. Surgical treatment of pressure sores. *Arch Phys Med Rehabil* 1978;59:193–200.
153. Haher JN, Haher TR, Devlin VJ, et al. The release of flexion contractures as a prerequisite for the treatment of pressure sores in multiple sclerosis: a report of ten cases. *Ann Plast Surg* 1983;11:246–249.
154. Goodman CM, Cohen V, Armenta A, et al. Evaluation of results and treatment variables for pressure ulcers in 48 veteran spinal cord injured patients. *Ann Plast Surg* 1999;43:572–574.
155. Arregui J, Canon B, Murray JE. Long-term evaluation of ischiectomy

in the treatment of pressure ulcers. *Plast Reconstr Surg* 1965;36: 583–590.

156. Hackler RH, Zampieri TA. Urethral complications following ischiectomy in spinal cord injury patients: a urethral pressure study. *J Urol* 1987;137:253–255.

157. Karaca AR, Binns JH, Blumenthal FS. Complications of total ischiectomy for the treatment of ischial pressure sores. *Plast Reconstr Surg* 1978;62:96–99.

158. Evans GR, Lewis VL Jr, Manson PN, et al. Hip joint communication with pressure sore: the refractory wound and the role of Girdlestone arthroplasty. *Plast Reconstr Surg* 1993;91:288–294.

159. Stal S, Serure A, Donovan W, et al. The perioperative management of the patient with pressure sores. *Ann Plast Surg* 1983;11:347–356.

160. Tavakoli K, Rutkowski S, Cope C, et al. Recurrence rates of ischial sores in para- and tetraplegics treated with hamstring flaps: an 8-year study. *Br J Plast Surg* 1999;52:476–479.

161. Schwartz IS, Pervez N. Bacterial endocarditis associated with permanent transvenous cardiac pacemaker. *JAMA* 1971;218:736–737.

162. Roche S, Cross S, Burgess I, et al. Cutaneous myiasis in an elderly debilitated patient. *Postgrad Med J* 1990;66:776–777.

163. Klein NE, Moore T, Capen D, et al. Sepsis of the hip in paraplegic patients. *J Bone Joint Surg* 1988;70:839–843.

164. Putnam T, Calenoff L, Betts HB, et al. Sinography in the management of decubitus ulcers. *Arch Phys Med Rehabil* 1978;59:243–245.

165. Berkwits L, Yarkony GM, Lewis V. Marjolin's ulcer complicating a pressure ulcer: case report and literature review. *Arch Phys Med Rehabil* 1986;67:831–833.

166. Johnson CA. Hearing loss following the application of topical neomycin. *J Burn Care Rehabil* 1988;9:162–164.

167. Shetty KR, Duthie EH Jr. Thyrotoxicosis induced by topical iodine application. *Arch Intern Med* 1990;150:2400–2401.

168. Dalyan M, Sherman A, Cardenas DD. Factors associated with contractures in acute spinal cord injury. *Spinal Cord* 1998;36:405–408.

169. Rousseau P. Pressure ulcers in an aging society. *Wounds* 1989;1: 135–141.

170. Sapico FL, Ginunas VJ, Thornhill-Joynes M, et al. Quantitative microbiology of pressure sores in different stages of healing. *Diagn Microbiol Infect Dis* 1986;5:31–38.

171. Lewis VL Jr, Bailey MH, Pulawski G, et al. The diagnosis of osteomyelitis in patients with pressure sores. *Plast Reconstr Surg* 1988;81: 229–232.

172. Sugarman B. Pressure sores and underlying bone infection. *Arch Intern Med* 1987;147:553–555.

173. Niazi ZB, Salzberg CA, Byrne DW, et al. Recurrence of initial pressure ulcer in persons with spinal cord injuries. *Adv Wound Care* 1997;10: 38–42.

174. Disa JJ, Carlton JM, Goldberg NH. Efficacy of operative cure in pressure sore patients. *Plast Reconstr Surg* 1992;89:272–278.

175. Heilporn A. Psychological factors in the causation of pressure sores: case reports. *Paraplegia* 1991;29:137–139.

176. Dumurgier C, Pujol G, Chevalley J, et al. Pressure sore carcinoma: a late but fulminant complication of pressure sores in spinal cord injury patients: case reports. *Paraplegia* 1991;29:390–395.

14

SPASTICITY FOLLOWING SPINAL CORD INJURY

MICHAEL M. PRIEBE
LANCE L. GOETZ
LISA-ANN WUERMSER

INCIDENCE AND PREVALENCE

Spasticity is a common sequela of upper motor neuron (UMN) spinal cord injury (SCI). In a study of 96 persons with acute SCI, Maynard et al. (1) found the incidence of spasticity to be 67%, with 37% requiring treatment by the time of discharge from rehabilitation. These figures increased to 78% and 49%, respectively, by the time of the first annual follow-up visit. Maynard et al. (1) also reported that the incidence of spasticity was higher in persons with cervical (82%) and upper thoracic (89%) SCI than in those with lower thoracic (45%) and lumbosacral (26%) SCI. In the same article, Maynard et al. (1) described a larger study of 466 persons with new traumatic SCI treated in model SCI systems and entered into the national SCI statistical center's database. Twenty-six percent were treated for spasticity by the time of discharge from rehabilitation. Again, persons with cervical and upper thoracic SCI had a higher incidence of anti-spasticity treatment (35%) than persons with lower thoracic (12%) and lumbosacral (5%) paraplegia (1). The overall incidence of antispasticity treatment in persons enrolled in the national database rose to 46% by the first annual follow-up.

Although in some cases spasticity may contribute to improve a person's function, when poorly controlled, spasticity may lead to various medical complications, impaired function, and decreased quality of life. In a cross-sectional study of 353 persons with SCI living in Sweden, Levi et al. (2) reported that 240 (68%) experienced spasticity. Of those with spasticity, 99 (41%) reported that spasticity constituted a significant problem by restricting activities of daily living or causing pain.

DEFINITION

Spasticity has been defined as "a motor disorder characterized by a velocity-dependent increase in tonic stretch reflexes (muscle tone) with exaggerated tendon jerks, resulting from hyperexcitability of the stretch reflex, as one component of the UMN syndrome" (3). Merritt (4) defined spasticity as "a condition of excessive reflex activity associated with involuntary movements and clonus, which may be accompanied by increased muscle tone." Young (5) expanded this definition by describing what he called *spastic paresis* as "a manifestation of excessive, involuntary motor activity including the Babinski response, velocity-dependent increase in tonic stretch reflexes, exaggerated phasic stretch reflexes, hyperactive cutaneous reflexes, increased autonomic reflexes, and abnormal postures."

Although spasticity has been described as being synonymous with hypertonicity, the previous descriptions define a more complex syndrome. An operational definition of spasticity for persons with SCI should include the following components: increased muscle tone, exaggerated tendon jerks, involuntary movements (spasms), clonus, and abnormal primitive reflexes (i.e., the Babinski response). In persons with incomplete SCI, the presence of inappropriate coactivation of muscles during voluntary movements should also be included as a manifestation of spasticity. Priebe et al. (6) reported that the different components of spasticity in persons with SCI, when assessed clinically, have only modest correlation to each other. This finding suggests that spasticity is a multidimensional problem and each component is unique. Therefore, the use of any single component as the measure of spasticity will underrepresent the magnitude and severity of spasticity in persons with SCI.

Spasticity is often characterized as either phasic or tonic. Phasic spasticity is typically seen as hyperactive tendon jerks, whereas tonic spasticity is seen as increased tone. Other components of spasticity are often a combination of phasic and tonic spasticity. For example, clonus, which is clearly phasic in nature, requires a degree of tone establishing a level of tension of the muscle before clonus can occur. When that tone is eliminated, for example, by flexing the knee when eliciting clonus from the ankle, clonus does not occur. Spasms may be either phasic or tonic, but again it is likely that phasic spasms require a level of underlying tone. The response to plantar stimulation can likewise appear either rapid and brief (phasic) or slow and sustained (tonic). Separating the phasic from the tonic components may be important because, as we describe later in this chapter, the mechanisms for each may very well be different. In addition, treatment for phasic spasticity may ultimately be different from that for tonic spasticity.

THE UPPER MOTOR NEURON SYNDROME

The UMN syndrome, which develops after lesions to cortical, subcortical, and spinal cord structures, has many components in common with our operational definition of spasticity. The UMN syndrome has been described as having both positive and negative symptoms. Positive symptoms, also called *abnormal behaviors,* include reflex release phenomena resulting in spasms and clonus, hyperactive proprioceptive reflexes (increased tendon jerks), increased resistance to passive stretch (increased tone), relaxed cutaneous reflexes (unmasked primitive reflexes, e.g., the Babinski response), and loss of precise autonomic control. Negative symptoms, also called *performance deficits,* include decreased dexterity and coordination, weakness or paralysis, and easy fatigability. Although the negative symptoms of the UMN syndrome are not usually considered part of what is called *spasticity,* it is often these symptoms that cause much of the functional impairment attributed to spasticity, particularly in persons with incomplete SCI.

MECHANISMS OF SPASTICITY

The mechanisms that lead to spasticity are only partially understood. To better understand the underlying mechanisms, we must differentiate phasic from tonic components. Although both of these components are likely due to a lowered threshold of phasic or tonic stretch reflexes, the mechanisms by which these changes occur are likely mediated by damage or relative preservation of different central nervous system (CNS) pathways. In most cases, there is interplay between phasic and tonic spasticity, resulting in what we see clinically as the constellation of signs and symptoms described as spasticity.

Phasic stretch reflexes, such as the deep tendon reflex, are monosynaptic reflexes. These reflexes are modulated by descending inhibitory signals and are thought to be transmitted through the medial vestibulospinal pathway. When inhibitory signals are lost due to spinal cord damage, the segmental reflexes are released and become hyperactive. Over time, denervation hypersensitivity occurs, leading to a decreased threshold for motor unit activation and a heightened response to stimuli.

Monoamines (serotonin and norepinephrine) are likely contributors to the denervation hypersensitivity seen after SCI. Both are produced supraspinally and transported through the spinal cord. After SCI, receptors for 5-hydroxytryptamine (5-HT) and norepinephrine increase, resulting in hypersensitivity. However, it appears that serotonergic receptors and noradrenergic receptors have opposite roles. The α_2-adrenergic agonists tizanidine and clonidine have been found to decrease spasticity, as can tricyclic antidepressants (noradrenergic agonists) (7). Selective serotonin reuptake inhibitors, however, have been reported to increase spasticity (8).

Tonic stretch reflexes, such as muscle tone, are generally described as polysynaptic reflexes. These reflexes are thought to be modulated by descending excitatory signals, which are transmitted through the lateral vestibulospinal and rubrospinal pathways. The vestibulospinal pathway facilitates extensor tone, and the rubrospinal pathway, which in humans only extends into the cervical spinal segments, facilitates flexor tone. These excitatory pathways are modulated by descending inhibitory signals from the brain. When the cortical input is disrupted to the nucleus, as in the case of brain injury or stroke, or when other descending inhibitory tracts are disrupted in the case of SCI, these pathways become hyperactive, leading to increased tone. Denervation hypersensitivity also occurs over time. When these pathways are completely disrupted, as in complete spinal cord transection, phasic segmental reflexes may become hyperactive, but increased tonic stretch reflexes are not seen, suggesting that some descending input is necessary for tonic spasticity to be present.

Multiple authors have described the presence of subclinical brain influence in persons with clinically complete SCI (9–12). They termed this "the discomplete syndrome." This syndrome is defined as neurophysiologic evidence of preserved suprasegmental control over reflex activity in persons with a clinically complete injury. Although they have no clinically apparent motor or sensory function below the level of their injury, these people are able to volitionally suppress their response to plantar stimulation, demonstrate volitional triggering of lower extremity (LE) spasms, or have preserved tonic vibratory reflexes (present only with preserved spinal cord function). This subclinical motor control manifests itself in the form of altered motor control, which may or may not be useful to the person with SCI. Altered motor control is defined as the reduced capacity to elicit and suppress muscle activity, including poor coordination, weakness, paralysis, and spasticity. The presence of the altered motor control and the discomplete syndrome argues that although the spinal cord is severely damaged, there are preserved axons traversing the injury site, which can be controlled by the brain.

The concept that spasticity is associated with abnormal descending motor input is supported by the data from the study by Maynard et al. (1), who found a significant difference in the need for spasticity treatment depending on the degree of incompleteness. Persons with Frankel grades B and C were more often treated for spasticity (50% and 52%, respectively) than persons with Frankel grades A or D (27% and 29%, respectively). This suggests that persons with a small degree of preserved spinal cord function have more spasticity than those with little or those with much preserved spinal cord function.

Kakulas (13) and others (14,15) have demonstrated that the spinal cord is usually not transected after traumatic SCI. The preserved tissue that traverses the injury site often includes intact functioning axons. These axons may represent altered pathways for descending motor control, which will be seen clinically as increased tone with spasms and may be an important target for manipulation for curative therapies. The presence of spasticity in persons with SCI may in fact be evidence of these preserved connections. Spasticity should be considered a form of altered motor control caused by a new spinal cord anatomy. If this anatomy and function is modulated and controlled, we may be able to restore a degree of volitional control below the site of injury in the future. This concept encourages therapeutic considerations for preserving cord function, rather than destroying the spinal cord to control spasticity. Likewise, attempts to modulate the abnormal motor control, harnessing spasticity for functional recovery, may play a key role in the eventual "cure" for SCI.

ASSESSMENT

Assessment of spasticity relies on instruments that can be classified as clinical, mechanical, or electrophysiologic. There is no one scale or instrument that is considered the gold standard for spasticity evaluation.

Clinical Assessment

The Ashworth Scale and the Penn Spasm Frequency Scale have become widely used both clinically and in research on spasticity and its treatment (16,17). These scales are relatively easy to use but rely on examiner interpretation of physical examination findings or patient self-report. These scales are ordinal in nature, which makes statistical manipulation more difficult. Because these are both five-point scales, they tend to group subjects within the middle grades. Both were originally designed to assess a different component of spasticity for specific intervention studies.

The Ashworth Scale was developed to assess hypertonicity in persons with multiple sclerosis (MS) (Table 14.1). This scale, which is graded from zero (no increase in muscle tone) to four (limb rigid in flexion or extension), has often been described as a one-to-five scale in the literature, which can lead to confusion if one isn't clear which scale is being used. The Ashworth Scale has been modified to improve its sensitivity in persons with hemiplegia by expanding the scale to include grades 0, 1, 1+, 2, 3, and 4 (18). The definitions for all categories, except 1+, are identical to those for the original scale. However, the interrater reliability of the modified Ashworth Scale has been shown to be no better than that of the original Ashworth Scale in the LEs of persons with SCI (19). The Ashworth Scale has been shown to have good interrater reliability in one study and only fair interrater reliability in another (19,20). Different techniques for assessing tone in the LEs, different methods of statistical handling of the data, and examiner experience may affect the reliability and reproducibility reported for the Ashworth Scale.

The Penn Spasm Frequency Scale is a five-point self-report scale, ranging from zero to four, originally developed as an outcome measure in trials of intrathecal baclofen (Table 14.2). Like the Ashworth Scale, this is an ordinal scale, making statistical manipulation of the data more difficult to interpret. Another critique of this scale is the intermingling of severity and ease of provocation (mild spasms induced by stimulation) and frequency of spontaneous spasms in a single scale.

In a study evaluating the association between clinical assessment tools for spasticity in SCI, Priebe et al. (6) found no correlation between the Ashworth Scale and the Penn Spasm Frequency Scale. In another study comparing self-report and the Ashworth Scale, Skold et al. (21) reported that spasticity could not be elicited in 40% of persons with SCI who reported spasticity. Both of these studies suggest that self-report and physical examination findings do not measure the same phenomena, and both should be assessed to obtain a complete understanding of the patient's spasticity.

Other components of spasticity are typically measured using a standard neurologic examination. Although five-point (zero to four) scales for muscle stretch reflex testing are widely used, Loubser et al. (22) have proposed a seven-point scale with an expanded upper range to better quantify the degree of clonus present (Table 14.3). Van Gijn (23) proposed an expanded scale

TABLE 14.1. ASHWORTH AND MODIFIED ASHWORTH SCALES

Ashworth scale
0	No increased tone
1	Slight increase in tone, giving a 'catch' when affected part is moved in flexion or extension
2	More marked increase in tone, but affected part easily flexed
3	Considerable increase in tone; passive movement difficult
4	Affected part rigid in flexion or extension

Modified Ashworth scale
0	No increased tone
1	*Slight increase in muscle tone, manifest by a catch and release or by minimal resistance at the end of the range of motion when the affected part is moved in flexion or extension*[a]
1+	*Slight increase in muscle tone, manifest by a catch, followed by minimal resistance throughout the remainder (less than half) of the range of motion*[a]
2	More marked increase in tone, but affected part easily flexed
3	Considerable increase in tone; passive movement difficult
4	Affected part rigid in flexion or extension

[a]Change compared with the Ashworth Scale.
From Ashworth B. Preliminary trial of carisoprodol in multiple sclerosis. *Practitioner* 1964;192:540–542; and Bohannon RW, Smith RB. Interrater reliability of a modified Ashworth scale of muscle spasticity. *Phys Ther* 1987;67:206–207, with permission.

TABLE 14.2. SPASM FREQUENCY SCORE

0	No spasms
1	Mild spasms induced by stimulation
2	Infrequent spasms occurring less than once per hour
3	Spasms occurring more than once per hour
4	Spasms occurring more than ten times per hour

From Penn RD. Intrathecal baclofen for severe spasticity. *Ann NY Acad Sci* 1988;531:157–166, with permission.

TABLE 14.3. MUSCLE STRETCH REFLEX SCALES

Standard scale
0	No reflex
1	Somewhat diminished, low normal
2	Average, normal reflex
3	Brisker than average, possibly indicative of disease
4	Very brisk, hyperactive, associated with clonus

An expanded scale
0	No response
1	Hypotonia
2	Normal response
3	Mildly hyperreflexia
4	Four beats of clonus
5	Unsustained clonus, more than four beats
6	Sustained clonus

From Loubser PG. Continuous infusion of intrathecal baclofen: long-term effects on spasticity in spinal cord injury. *Paraplegia* 1991;29:48–64, with permission.

TABLE 14.4. PLANTAR STIMULATION RESPONSE

0	No visible activity/flexor response (down-going toe)
1	Flicker of movement/extensor response (up-going toe)
2	Slight hip or knee movement
3	Knee lifted from support
4	Movement elicited by light touch

From van Gijn J. The Babinski sign and the pyramidal syndrome. *J Neurol Neurosurg Psychiatry* 1978;41:865–873, with permission.

to quantify the Babinski response to plantar stimulation (Table 14.4). Poor motor coordination with voluntary activity, although an important aspect of spasticity, does not have a useful clinical assessment scale. In general, clinical assessment tools are more useful for measuring involuntary and passive motor phenomena. Clinical scales to assess the fluidity and coordination of volitional movement are needed to better measure spasticity in persons with incomplete SCI.

Mechanical Assessment

Mechanical assessment is based on the theory that increased resistance to passive movement is due to a lowered threshold of tonic and phasic stretch reflexes. The various tools used to measure spasticity mechanically are designed to test the resistance to passive movement of a joint. Joint torque is a measure of the amount of resistance force opposing the movement of the limb over a specified angle. Differentiating the stiffness of a muscle due to its viscoelastic properties versus a change in the reflex activation is difficult without added surface electromyography (EMG). The pendulum test and isokinetic dynamometry have been used in persons with SCI to attempt to quantify spasticity (24–26). The pendulum test is performed by having the subject sit or lie on a table with his or her legs hanging freely over the edge at the knees. With the subject fully relaxed, the examiner extends one leg fully and drops it, allowing the leg to fall freely. The speed, quality of motion, number of oscillations, and the joint angular velocity can be measured. Lehmann et al. (27) and Hinderer et al. (28) described oscillation of the ankle joint, measuring joint compliance using surface EMG or torque, as a quantitative measure of spasticity in persons with SCI. Katz and Rymer (29) described the use of a servocontrolled motor that applies ramp and hold movements to the upper extremity in persons with hemiplegia. Through a series of studies, they demonstrated that spastic hypertonia in persons with hemiplegia is the result of a decrease in the stretch reflex threshold, rather than a change in reflex gain or changes in intrinsic viscoelastic properties of the muscle. Mechanical assessment appears to be most useful in evaluating the tonic components of spasticity.

Electrophysiologic Assessment

This assessment is based on the theory that spasticity is the result of a lowered threshold for activation of motor unit activity. The Hoffmann reflex (H reflex) and the H/M ratio (amplitude of H reflex to that of the compound motor action potential) can be employed to study spasticity in persons with SCI. These test the excitability of the motor neuron pool in the spinal cord and are best suited to studying the phasic components of spasticity.

Spasticity has been measured using surface EMG during clinical maneuvers. Sherwood et al. (30) described the Brain Motor Control Assessment (BMCA) as a clinical neurophysiologic assessment strategy for spasticity and altered motor control. The surface EMG data obtained during the BMCA have been shown to be reproducible and sensitive to change and correlated to the clinical examination, specifically the Ashworth Scale (31–33). Sherwood et al. (34) argue that surface EMG data, acquired under the controlled methods of the BMCA, are superior to the Ashworth Scale as an objective quantification of altered motor control and spasticity.

MANAGEMENT

Indications

Although up 80% of persons with SCI may have manifestations of spasticity, not all persons with spasticity require treatment. Decisions about whether to treat spasticity, either with medications, modalities, or procedures, should be based on several factors. These include the person's risk of developing debilitating contractures, interference of spasticity with function, and presence of pain related to spasms or tone. Hip extensor spasms may be powerful enough to catapult a person from a wheelchair or cause him or her to tip backward. Tonic quadriceps spasms may interfere with transfers to and from one's wheelchair. LE tone may be detrimental to gait in an ambulatory person with SCI. On the other hand, some persons report that they use LE tone to assist with functional activities such as transfers. Persons with incomplete SCI may use LE extensor tone to assist with standing and walking activities. Other reported benefits of spasticity, including maintenance of bone or muscle mass and prevention of deep venous thrombosis, remain unproved.

Identification and Amelioration of Nociception

When a person with SCI presents with spasticity, potential sources of nociception should be evaluated and, if present, treated before initiation of other treatments. Various underlying disease processes may exacerbate spasticity. Common causes of increased spasticity include urinary tract infections, bladder calculi, ingrown toenails, hemorrhoids, and bowel impaction. In addition, irritation from urethral catheters, fractures, menstruation, deep venous thrombosis, pressure ulcers, appendicitis, cholecystitis, or other acute abdominal processes, as well as any potentially painful process, should be considered possible causes. Changes in spasticity may also be an important presenting sign in syringomyelia (35,36). Careful neurologic examination should be undertaken to detect subtle changes in the person's baseline neurologic status.

PHYSICAL TREATMENT MODALITIES

Stretching

Stretching has long been the mainstay for the treatment of spasticity and the prevention of joint contractures. The relationship between spasticity and the development of contractures after acute or in chronic SCI has been assumed but only recently demonstrated (37,21). Stretching is believed to reduce motoneuron excitability and tone for up to several hours (38). The possible mechanisms underlying these phenomena are elucidated elsewhere (39). Stretching of spastic muscles should be completed at least daily but preferably twice a day or more often for persons with a high degree of tone. Particular emphasis should be given to muscles at risk for contractures. These include shoulder adductors, shoulder internal rotators, elbow flexors and finger extensors in the upper extremity, and hip flexors, knee flexors, and gastrocnemius soleus complex in the LE. Heating or warming muscle before doing stretching exercises, although not substantially impacting spasticity, is beneficial in reducing pain, promoting muscular and tendon lengthening, and temporarily reducing muscle spasm (40). Standing activities, including use of a tilt table or standing frame, provide prolonged stretch to joints, but further study is needed to provide clear evidence of a reduction in spasticity (41,42).

Posture and Positioning

Posture and positioning for persons who use wheelchairs and those at bed rest are extremely important for tone reduction and prevention of contractures. For wheelchair users, adequate low-back support to maintain lumbar lordosis and avoid sacral sitting should be provided. A positive seat plane angle, or "dump," and a reduction in the seat-to-back angle, or "squeeze," encourage proper upright posture and may reduce extensor tone. Sling-style sitting surfaces should be avoided because they encourage excessive internal femoral rotation. For those at bed rest, the "windswept" position and "frog leg" positions are felt to decrease tone but may contribute to contractures and increased risk for pressure ulcers if the person is not frequently repositioned.

Orthotic Management

Inhibitive casting, splinting, and orthotic management of muscles and joints at risk for contracture may be helpful in reducing tone as well. Inhibitive casting has long been used in persons with cerebral palsy (43). Prolonged stretch is believed to exert an inhibitory effect on motor neuron excitability, which is supported by a number of investigations (44–46). This may occur by reflex mechanisms involving secondary spindle endings and their group II afferents. Persons with SCI who are ambulatory and require bracing may have tone-reducing features incorporated into their orthoses. Examples include tone-reducing ankle-foot orthoses with neutral subtalar mediolateral and anteroposterior alignment, arch and metatarsal-supporting footplates, and slight toe dorsiflexion.

Cryotherapy

Cryotherapy may be an underused treatment for spasticity when applied focally to enhance function of specific muscle groups. Benefits have been shown for cold application provided sufficiently long to lower intramuscular temperature (usually about

20 minutes). These include elimination of clonus for up to several hours, reduction in tendon reflexes, and significantly enhanced strength of protagonist muscles (47–51). Ice packs or ice massages are effective methods of cold delivery often employed by therapists.

Electrical Stimulation

Electrical stimulation has been used to relieve spasticity via various mechanisms, usually with short-term effects. Electrical stimulation techniques have been applied transcutaneously to nerve, muscle, or sensory dermatome with reported benefits on F responses and the pendulum test (52–54). Improvements in gait patterns of persons with incomplete SCI have been reported, presumably due to stimulation of agonist and inhibition of antagonist muscles (55,56). Use of transcutaneous electrical nerve stimulation resulted in transient improvements in Ashworth Score and Achilles deep tendon reflex but not clonus or H-reflex amplitude (57). Increases in spasticity during and after functional electrical stimulation exercise have been noted (58, 59).

Using rectal probe electrostimulation for fertility studies, Halstead and Seager (60) and Halstead et al. (61) reported that men with SCI demonstrated marked reduction in tonic spasticity as measured by the Ashworth Scale, Penn scale, and pendulum test with preservation of phasic reflexes after electroejaculation. This was found to be independent of ejaculation, and women demonstrated similar improvements in spasticity after rectal electrostimulation. Effects lasted an average of 9 hours, with a range of up to 24 hours.

Spinal cord electrical stimulation has been proposed for the treatment of spasticity of spinal origin. Although the initial report showed substantial improvement in spasticity, lasting up to 2 years, subsequent reports have not reproduced this finding, with long-term benefits in less than 10% of patients (62,63).

PHARMACOLOGIC MANAGEMENT
Oral Medications

Because of the complex, multidimensional nature of spasticity, it is not surprising that no medication is universally beneficial to all patients. Persons with SCI presenting with signs of the UMN syndrome may complain of a far greater range of symptoms. Pain complaints and spasticity may at times be indistinguishable. Therefore, medical management of spasticity may require some amount of trial and error. Indeed, a recent comprehensive analysis of the available literature regarding medications for spasticity in SCI concluded that "there is insufficient evidence to assist clinicians in a rational approach to antispastic treatment for SCI" (64). Medications used for spasticity may exert anxiolytic and analgesic effects in addition to their antispasticity activity. Most share common side effects of sedation and asthenia of varying degrees. The person's age, comorbidities, and cognitive status should be carefully considered when choosing medication for spasticity. Commonly used medications are shown in Table 14.5.

Baclofen is currently considered by many to be an agent of

TABLE 14.5. ORAL MEDICATIONS FOR SPASTICITY

Medication	Dosage	Major Mechanism of Action
Baclofen	5 mg t.i.d.–40 mg q.i.d.	Presynaptic inhibition of GABA$_b$ receptors
Diazepam	5 mg q.d.–20 mg q.i.d.	Facilitates post-synaptic effects of GABA, increasing presynaptic inhibition
Dantrolene	25 mg q.d.–100 mg q.i.d.	Reduces calcium release, interfering with excitation contraction coupling in skeletal muscle
Tizanidine	2 mg q.d.–12 mg t.i.d.	α_2-Adrenergic agonist, increases presynaptic inhibition of motor neurons
Gabapentin	100 mg t.i.d.–1,200 mg q.i.d.	Unknown

Note: t.i.d., three times a day; q.i.d., four times a day; q.d., every day; GABA, γ-aminobutyric acid.

first choice for spasticity of spinal origin. Baclofen is an analog of γ-aminobutyric acid (GABA), a neurotransmitter that exerts inhibitory activity on monosynaptic and polysynaptic reflexes (39). Baclofen is believed to exert GABA agonist activity by binding presynaptically at the GABA$_b$ receptor. The clinically available compound is provided as a mixture of R($+$) and L($-$) isomers. Antispasticity and analgesic effects are believed to be related to the L($-$) isomer (65).

Multiple studies exist to support the efficacy of baclofen using both qualitative (Ashworth scores) and quantitative measures (vibratory inhibition index, pendulum test) in patients with SCI and MS (7,66). Baclofen reduces flexor spasms, increasing range of motion and decreasing spastic hypertonia. Herman and D'Luzansky (67) described a much greater effect on segmental reflexes (deep tendon reflexes, H reflex, manual muscle stretch) than intersegmental reflexes (spontaneous or provoked flexor spasms). One study showed no significant effect versus placebo on measures of ankle joint stiffness (28). A recent study in patients with MS demonstrated both central and peripherally mediated effects on ankle joint stiffness (68). They noted that the medication might unmask weakness, potentially interfering with ambulation.

Baclofen may be initiated at doses of 5 mg three times a day and titrated to doses of up to 120 mg per day or more. Relative effects of higher doses have not been compared. Baclofen has a short half-life (3½ hours) and four-times-a-day dosing may be needed to obtain steady plasma concentrations (67). The anxiolytic effect and analgesic properties of baclofen have been demonstrated (69–71). Reported side effects include sedation, fatigue, weakness, nausea, dizziness, paresthesias, and hallucinations. However, the emotional and psychological effects of baclofen have been studied and no major adverse effects were found (72).

If baclofen is to be discontinued, it must be tapered. Abrupt discontinuation has resulted in seizures, visual disturbances, and hallucinations (73). Baclofen is renally excreted and dosage should be adjusted accordingly in patients with impaired renal function, which may be present despite normal serum creatinine (74). Baclofen can occasionally affect liver function therefore, liver enzymes should be monitored.

Benzodiazepines are a class of medications known to have efficacy for spinal spasticity. They exert activity by binding at a site near the GABA$_a$ receptor on presynaptic neurons, enhancing GABA-mediated chloride conductance into nerve terminals and thereby increasing inhibitory activity of these neurons. Diazepam was once considered standard treatment for persons with SCI regardless of injury level, and many patients have been maintained on this drug for more than 10 years (75). It has been shown to be effective in clinical trials (76,77). Its use, although still common, has decreased because of its greater potential for side effects, which may include sedation, hypotension, depression, or tolerance, as well as weight gain (78,79). Tolerance may persist for long periods (months to years) after discontinuation (78). Diazepam affects cognitive performance measures, such as attention, concentration, and memory, and is therefore generally not used in persons with brain injury, stroke, or cerebral palsy. Diazepam is thought to be more effective in decreasing reflexes and treating painful spasms than pure tone (80). Doses in patients with SCI start at 2 to 5 mg twice a day and are slowly adjusted upward to 15 mg four times a day or more. A single nighttime dose may be helpful for treating nocturnal spasms that interfere with sleep.

Other benzodiazepines have been evaluated, including clonazepam, tetrazepam, and ketazolam. The latter has a long half-life, can be given once daily, and may be less sedating (81). However, accumulation of metabolites is markedly higher with ketazolam (78).

α_2-Adrenergic agonists, including clonidine and tizanidine, have been studied extensively for use in spasticity of spinal origin in recent years. These agents bind to presynaptic α_2-receptors on interneurons in the dorsal horn of the spinal cord. This results in depression of polysynaptic reflexes by either decreasing the release of excitatory amino acids such as glutamate and aspartate or facilitating the action of glycine, an inhibitory amino acid neurotransmitter.

Clonidine can be delivered either orally, via transdermal patch, or on occasion intrathecally. Oral doses are 0.05 to 0.1 mg twice a day. Oral clonidine has been shown to reduce the vibratory inhibition index of the H reflex (82) and provide a reduction in spasticity in several series (83–85). However, some patients in these series discontinued or adjusted their dosage due to side effects, including hypotension, sedation, and dry mouth. Transdermal patch therapy beginning at 0.1 mg/day per week and titrating upward to 0.3 mg/day per week was reported to give subjective benefit in 13 of 16 patients (86).

Tizanidine, which has a shorter half-life and lower incidence of hypotension than clonidine, has been shown to be effective for spasticity in a number of studies involving patients with SCI and MS. Nance et al. (7,87) demonstrated significant improvements in the Ashworth score and pendulum test results in patients with SCI and MS. Tizanidine appears to have no major effect on monosynaptic reflexes. Its action may be due to decreased firing rates of adrenergic neurons or inhibiting transmission in spinal nociceptive pathways.

Tizanidine should be started at 2 to 4 mg at bedtime and increased in 2-mg increments every 2 to 4 days. Typical effective doses for tizanidine range from 8 mg to 36 mg per day, usually given in three divided doses. However, smaller doses may be given more frequently if side effects are limiting effectiveness of the medication. Bradycardia has been observed with clonidine and to a lesser degree with tizanidine, which resolves with adjustment in dosage (88). Because of the somnolence seen, particularly in older adults, initial doses should be given at night and slowly titrated to effective levels. Tizanidine is metabolized by the liver, and 5% of patients experience elevated liver enzymes; therefore, LFTs should be monitored before and during treatment.

Gabapentin, an agent initially developed as an anticonvulsant, was also found to have antispasticity properties serendipitously in persons with SCI. Its use has recently increased for other interventions including neuropathic pain syndromes, although it lacks Food and Drug Administration (FDA) approval for indications other than partial seizures. Its mechanism of action is currently unknown. It is structurally related to the neurotransmitter GABA but does not interact with GABA receptors, has no metabolically active metabolites, and does not interfere with GABA uptake or degradation (89). Dosing in persons with SCI usually begins at 300 to 400 mg three times a day and may be titrated upward to a total dose of 3,600 mg per day. Because it is exclusively excreted renally, any alterations in renal function necessitate a decrease in dose. In animal studies, no lethal dose has been found. Blood levels and liver enzymes do not require monitoring.

In a multicenter, placebo-controlled study, gabapentin demonstrated improvements in spasticity scores as measured using surface EMG techniques (32). At doses of 400 mg three times a day, some improvements were noted, but all subjects had clinical improvements at higher doses of 1,200 mg three times a day. In another study, Ashworth scores and patient ratings of spasticity were significantly improved in 25 patients versus placebo at a dosage of 400 mg three times a day given for 2 days (90). More recently, Cutter et al. (91) demonstrated improvements in self-report scales and objective measures of spasticity in a randomized placebo-controlled study of persons with MS. Doses of gabapentin up to 900 mg three times a day were well tolerated in this study.

Dantrolene sodium is the only agent in common use that acts directly on muscle tissue. It exerts its effect by preventing neurally induced release of calcium ions from the sarcoplasmic reticulum along muscle fibers, thereby decreasing calcium-dependent excitation–contraction coupling. However, the drug acts on normal and spastic muscle, potentially resulting in weakness (92). Its antispasticity effects are felt to occur at doses less than those that would lead to clinical weakness. Some authors believe that

dantrolene exerts better activity at reducing tone than spontaneous spasms (92,93).

Dantrolene is initiated at 25 mg per day and titrated upward to a maximum of 100 mg four times a day. Dantrolene undergoes largely hepatic metabolism. The most worrisome side effect is hepatotoxicity, which can range from elevated LFT results (1.8% of patients) to fulminant hepatic failure in approximately 0.3% in patients treated for more than 60 days. Women older than 30 years on long-term treatment with doses exceeding 400 mg per day or taking medications with hepatic metabolism are at greatest risk (94). Dantrolene is considered to be less sedating than baclofen or diazepam and is therefore often used in persons with cerebral spasticity, including traumatic brain injury, cerebral palsy, or stroke. It may be of benefit in persons with concurrent SCI and traumatic brain injury.

Cyproheptadine is a nonselective serotonergic (5-HT) antagonist that has antihistamine activity and has long been safely used to treat itching from hives. Serotonin increases excitability of spinal motor neurons, and denervation hypersensitivity may exist on 5-HT receptors of spinal motor neurons, which can be antagonized by cyproheptadine (95,96). Barbeau et al. (97) demonstrated that cyproheptadine reduced clonus and spontaneous spasms in patients with SCI, although mild reductions in strength occurred as well. Nance (98) found that cyproheptadine was equal in efficacy to baclofen and superior to clonidine at reducing tone in terms of H reflex, and equivalent to both in other measures. Improvement in spastic gait patterns has been demonstrated in studies with cyproheptadine alone or in combination with clonidine (99–102). Cyproheptadine may be started at 4 mg at bedtime and increased by 4 mg every 3 to 4 days. The usual effective dose ranges from 16 mg to 24 mg per day in divided doses. The maximum recommended dose is 36 mg per day. Side effects are those typically associated with antihistamine use, including dry mouth and sedation. Significant fatigue may also occur, and excessive weight gain has been reported (99).

Opiates exhibit potent antispasticity activity in addition to their analgesic effects (67,103,104). Similar to benzodiazepines, opiates suppress polysynaptic reflexes to a greater extent than monosynaptic reflexes. Although sedation may limit their routine use, opiates may be used in certain settings. For example, in postoperative patients and those with fractures or other sources of severe pain, it is essential to assess and control the nociception as a major factor in controlling their spasticity. Opiates may be used to assist with spasticity control in this setting.

Use of amino acids, which act as inhibitory neurotransmitters in the spinal cord, such as *glycine*, and a precursor, *L-threonine,* has been investigated for spasticity in SCI. Glycine has been established as the chief inhibitory postsynaptic neurotransmitter in the spinal cord. When given intrathecally to rabbits, it has been shown to depress the H reflex (105). A small trial of oral glycine in human subjects provided subjective benefits (106). Oral L-threonine at 6 g per day was studied in 33 persons with spinal spasticity in a double-blind, placebo-controlled crossover study (107). Modest but significant reductions in the Ashworth score were noted.

The potassium channel-blocking agent *4-aminopyridine* has gained attention for its potential in improving neurologic function in persons with incomplete SCI. In a randomized, double-blind crossover trial of 26 persons with incomplete SCI, significant reductions in tone were noted compared with placebo (108). This effect was noted particularly at the higher of two doses. No improvement in spasm frequency was noted. Minimal side effects of light-headedness and nausea were noted. Other smaller studies have reported antispasticity effects of this agent as well (108,109).

Muscle relaxants such as carisoprodol and cyclobenzaprine do not have direct action on skeletal muscle but exert their effects through depression of brain-stem neuronal activity. Although they are sometimes prescribed to persons with SCI, no evidence exists to support their use or efficacy in spasticity of spinal origin (110). Orphenadrine citrate is an antimuscarinic antiparkinsonian agent with inhibitory action on motor neurons in the spinal cord and reticular formation. It is also used in acute musculoskeletal pain syndromes, although its exact mechanism of action is unknown. It was recently studied by intravenous administration in subjects with SCI. A significant reduction in Ashworth score and electrically elicited flexion-reflex threshold was observed compared with placebo (111).

Although not approved for clinical use, *marijuana,* or cannabis, is widely used by persons with SCI, who report diverse benefits including relief of spasticity (112,113). The active chemical, Δ9-tetrahydrocannabinol, was studied in double-blind placebo-controlled fashion in a group of patients with various CNS lesions including MS and SCI. Quadriceps EMG activity was reduced in patients with primarily extensor spasticity, and clinical measures of spasticity were significantly reduced (114).

The use of *herbal* or *homeopathic agents* has increased greatly. Although no studies currently exist, an increase in use among the SCI population has likely occurred simultaneously. Herbs such as kava (*Piper methysticum*) and valerian, for example, exert anxiolytic or sedative effects through GABA-ergic mechanisms and are believed to have spasmolytic or muscle relaxant effects (115). Their efficacy remains unstudied. However, because their potency may vary widely, practitioners should be alerted to their possible usage among their patients with SCI.

Intrathecal Medications

An alternative to oral antispasticity medication is intrathecal delivery. Recognizing that the delivery of medication across the blood–brain barrier is incomplete, delivery of drug directly into the CNS can improve spasticity control while decreasing side effects.

Morphine was the first medication studied for intrathecal delivery in the control of spasticity. Theoretically, by decreasing the afferent or sensory component, which drives spasticity, the efferent component would then decline. Small studies showed decreased spasticity, but tolerance often prevented long-term management (116). Today, morphine is not considered a first-line intrathecal medication for spasticity. However, patients may experience a decline in spasticity when intrathecal morphine is introduced for pain management, possibly allowing for a reduction in other antispasticity measures.

Intrathecal baclofen has been studied extensively in persons with SCI and is FDA approved for this indication. Baclofen, as

with other intrathecal medications, shows an incomplete ascent of drug in the spinal canal after injection. Differential concentrations of the drug when injected at L1 are as follows: lumbar, 4; cervical, 1; intracranial, less than 1. Therefore, control of spasticity is the best in the lower limbs, but less complete in the trunk and upper limbs (117). There is also minimal delivery of drug intracranially, resulting in fewer cognitive side effects than with oral dosing. Increasing doses may be necessary to improve spasticity control in the trunk and upper limbs.

Side effects of intrathecal baclofen are less severe than those of the same medication given orally. The package insert reports side effects of drowsiness, dizziness, nausea, hypotension, headache, seizures, and weakness. Long-term follow-up studies report adverse drug effects in about 12% of patients, but discontinuation of therapy in persons with SCI is uncommon (118–120). Pump complications are more common however and are discussed later in this chapter.

Although more commonly used for the primary or adjunctive treatment of pain, intrathecal clonidine may also be effective for the treatment of spasticity. It has been shown to decrease the amplitude of the polysynaptic spinal reflexes in a dose-dependent fashion, reducing spasticity and in most cases improving function (121). Dose requirements are generally low, in the range of 30 to 90 μg per day. A combination of clonidine and baclofen is another option, and the two medications can be safely combined in the pump reservoir. However, such use is not FDA approved (122). The most concerning side effect is hypotension. Systolic blood pressure has been reported to drop an average of 20 mm Hg, although these reports were with higher doses, often used in the treatment of pain.

There are three phases in the process of initiating treatment with intrathecal baclofen: (a) patient selection and trial; (b) pump implantation; and (c) follow-up rehabilitation and dose adjustment. Careful patient selection is critical to the success of an intrathecal baclofen program. The two major indications for intrathecal drug delivery are inability to control spasticity with oral medications and intolerable side effects to these medications. It is therefore imperative that factors that may worsen spasticity [e.g., kidney stones, heterotopic ossification (HO), and syringomyelia] be considered and ruled out before considering pump implantation. Patients should have failed oral medications before attempting intrathecal delivery. The mainstay of patient selection is the same as with any spasticity treatment programs—functional goals. It is useful to clearly define functional goals and endpoints of treatment before trial and implantation to guide the dosing of medication and make the expectations of results clear. During the trial, these functional goals should be considered and any improvement of functional activity during the trial should be noted. Patient reliability is also a key factor. Intrathecal baclofen carries with it a risk of severe withdrawal if the pump fails or a refill appointment is missed. Tachycardia, seizures, and even multiorgan system failure have been reported with intrathecal baclofen withdrawal. Each patient should be assessed for his or her ability to keep appointments before implantation.

Each candidate should undergo an intrathecal baclofen trial before pump implantation. During the trial, patients receive a 50-μg intrathecal injection of baclofen. Onset of action is at approximately 1 hour, with peak effect at 4 hours in most patients and loss of effect by 8 hours. Patients may experience reductions in spasticity, which are either more or less than desired. This is of no consequence, because the dosing can be carefully titrated after implantation. The results of the trial are essentially binary: either it is effective or it is ineffective. Efficacy is customarily defined as a decline in mean Ashworth score or Penn spasm scale score of two. If a patient fails the first day, subsequent trial days may be carried out with a 75-μg dose, then 100 μg. If there is no effect by the third day, implantation is not recommended. Failure may occur from inadequate delivery of drug throughout the intrathecal space secondary to poor cerebrospinal fluid flow, such as may be seen with myelographic block secondary to stenosis, syringomyelia, or spinal cord tethering. Because these conditions may also cause or increase spasticity, these should be considered and ruled out, preferably before the trial. The trial also gives an opportunity to assess for contracture versus rigidity and may give patients an opportunity to see the occasional usefulness of their spasticity.

If after the trial, the patient and physician have determined that intrathecal baclofen is the optimal treatment, the next step is implantation of the pump and catheter. Intrathecal pump systems are available in two major types. The first uses a controlled concentration of drug, with variable flow rate allowing dose adjustments. This highly programmable pump allows dose adjustments between refills and very precise dosing. Complex dosing of different doses at different times of the day is also possible. Dose changes are made via a telemetry programmer and are noninvasive. The major disadvantage of this type of pump is its high cost and the need for a programmer to make any adjustments. The second type of pump is a less expensive alternative using a continuous flow rate. Dose adjustments are made by altering the drug concentration. Adjustments cannot be made as precisely as with a variable flow rate pump and can only be made by refilling the pump. Both pumps are refilled during a simple office procedure using a percutaneous injection of drug into the pump's reservoir.

Pumps are implanted on the abdominal wall either subcutaneously or subfascially. The catheter is tunneled subcutaneously to the spine and customarily enters the spinal column at the L4-5 interspace. It is then threaded up to the level of L1. Recent studies have shown improved spasticity control of the upper limbs without sacrificing effect to the lower limbs by threading the catheter to T10. Hospital stays average 1 to 3 days. The starting dose for the pump is generally recommended to be twice the effective trial dose, unless a prolonged effect (more than 8 hours) is seen at the trial. Patients may initially see an increase in spasticity, driven by the postsurgical pain. Treatment with pain medications may be useful.

Once the patient is discharged from a surgical standpoint, rehabilitation and dose adjustment commence. Some patients may require no further physical therapy, whereas others may need extensive outpatient therapy or even qualify for inpatient rehabilitation if new functional goals are now obtainable. Oral spasticity medications should gradually be tapered as the intrathecal dose is increased, with recommended increases of 5% to 20% per adjustment and adjustments as frequent as every 24 hours. The average maintenance dose for the treatment of spasticity of spinal origin has been reported to be 400 to 600 μg per day, but with a range of 50 to more than 1,500 μg per day.

There is some controversy over whether tolerance to baclofen develops as it does with morphine. Akman et al. (123) showed that once patients have reached a stable dose, usually around 6 months, this usually remains for years, with increases usually needed only as battery life declines. However, other reports have shown that tolerance can develop, resulting in the need for high doses. Usually, this is observed in the first 6 to 12 months, with difficulty reaching a stable and efficacious dose.

Mechanical complications are not rare. On average 22% to 51% of all pump/catheter placements will fail unpredictably over the lifetime of the pump (118,119,124,125). Catheter dislodgment, kinking, or leakage may fail to deliver intrathecal baclofen but not register failure on the pump programmer. The pump itself can fail to deliver the programmed dose of baclofen from mechanical failure. This may also occur at the end of its battery life, averaging 3 to 7 years depending on the dose. In any of these cases, baclofen withdrawal can result. Presentation will be similar to that previously described for oral baclofen withdrawal, but with greater severity. When suspected, it can often be managed with oral baclofen until a complete pump evaluation is performed and any problem rectified. There is one case report of the successful use of dantrolene sodium for baclofen withdrawal unresponsive to oral baclofen (126).

Overdose is a relative term. Frank pump failure causing overdose is extremely rare with the newest generation of pumps. However, a dose increase may precipitate signs of excessive dosing such as respiratory depression, drowsiness, dizziness, nausea, hypotension, and weakness. Using the side-port to evaluate the catheter results in injection of all baclofen in the catheter into the intrathecal space, which can result in overdosage as well. Combining oral and intrathecal baclofen therapy may also produce signs of overdosage, particularly in the postimplantation period. Physostigmine was previously recommended for treatment, but fatal cardiac arrhythmias and seizures have been reported. Most overdoses can be managed by stopping the pump and supportive care.

Long-term follow-up studies have shown intrathecal baclofen to be highly effective and well tolerated, despite the pump complications mentioned. Studies have shown decreases in spasticity and functional improvements in the treatment of spasticity of spinal origin regardless of diagnosis, but most often treating traumatic SCI and MS (127). Penn (119), in a 7-year review, showed an average decline of more than two points on both the Ashworth Scale and Penn spasm scale, which was maintained an average of 75 months. It is important to make note of the method of evaluating spasticity when reviewing the literature on intrathecal baclofen. Gianino et al. (128) studied quality of life prospectively after intrathecal baclofen pump implantation. Although spasticity declined as expected, the quality of life index did not change, although the sickness impact profile improved significantly in both the physical and psychological subscales.

NERVE BLOCKS

Highly focused drug delivery in the form of peripheral nerve or motor-point block may be useful to manage focal areas of spasticity. Because spasticity is generally a multisite and multilimb problem in SCI, such focal treatments may be of less benefit than in other etiologies of spasticity. However, judicious use of such interventions, particularly in the upper limb or in persons with an incomplete injury, may achieve functional goals beyond those achieved by systemic treatment measures alone or may decrease the dosage needs of oral or intrathecal medication.

Nerve blocks using an anesthetic agent can be useful diagnostically but are of short duration. In contrast, injection of phenol or absolute alcohol causes destruction of the axon, without destruction of the endoneurial tubes, causing a much longer acting block (129). Nerve regrowth then occurs over weeks and months, with resulting return of motor function or spasticity. Length of effect varies by technique and study but can be up to several years, so this is considered a "permanent" block.

Aqueous solutions of phenol are commonly between 2% to 5%, with higher concentrations resulting in longer effect. Phenol blocks of the peripheral nerve can be performed several ways. Direct injection perineurally into the nerve trunk has shown highly variable results, with effects up to several years, but with a 10% risk of painful paresthesias. These can be avoided by injections into the motor branch, rather than into the mixed nerve. The closed technique uses a nerve stimulator to locate the motor branch, into which the phenol in then injected. Studies have been performed primarily in persons with brain injury and have shown effects for several months. An operative technique in which the nerve is exposed surgically and then is directly injected has been used with greater success and longer effect but is much more complicated. Perhaps the most commonly used technique is the motor-point block, whereby a nerve stimulator is used to locate the motor point and then the phenol is injected intramuscularly at the motor point. Effect has not been as great or as long-lasting as with an open injection, but this process is much easier to perform.

Botulinum toxin has gained immense popularity. It is technically easier to use than phenol secondary to excellent diffusion through muscle but is considerably more expensive. Botulinum toxin blocks neuromuscular transmission by inhibiting the release of acetylcholine into the synapse. Its onset of action is 4 to 10 days, and its length of effect is on average 3 to 6 months. Intramuscular injection is usually guided to the optimal location either by a nerve stimulator, as with phenol, or by seeking the motor endplate by EMG. Precise injection of botulinum toxin into the motor endplate has been shown to optimize the resulting paralysis. In an animal model, Shaari et al. (130) showed that injecting the toxin a mere 0.5 cm from the motor endplate reduces resulting paralysis by 50%. Therefore, precise injection technique leads to maximal muscle paralysis per unit of toxin injected. Side effects of botulinum toxin are few, although excessive dosing or intravenous injection can lead to widespread muscle weakness. The development of antibodies to botulinum toxin has been observed in other diagnostic groups, causing a decline in response to subsequent injections.

Advantages of phenol injections over the botulinum toxin are its low cost of drug and long-lasting effect. Disadvantages include the potential risk of paresthesias and risk of permanent weakness. In addition, intramuscular phenol does not diffuse through tissue well, so precise injection technique is even more

important. Follow-up stretching, which may include dynamic splinting or serial casting, is recommended to optimize the functional result from motor-point blocks.

ABLATIVE PROCEDURES

The history of surgical management has included a number of surgical interventions, many of them highly destructive (131). Both cordectomy and myelotomy have been performed to reduce spasticity, but with limited long-term success. If one considers the proposed theories on the origins of spasticity, it makes sense that further loss of descending inhibition would not ultimately be helpful. In an effort to improve the lives of persons with spasticity of other etiologies, or incomplete SCI, more selective procedures were developed.

Selective dorsal rhizotomy and the later developed dorsal root entry zone procedure have been proposed to control spasticity by decreasing the afferent component of spasticity. As with pharmacologic interventions with a similar mechanism of action, some degree of success may be obtained, but patient selection for optimal effect remains unclear. This treatment is most commonly used for the treatment of pain and may or may not result in decreased spasticity.

REFERENCES

1. Maynard FM, Karunas R, Waring WW. Epidemiology of spasticity following traumatic spinal cord injury. *Arch Phys Med Rehabil* 1990; 71:566–569.
2. Levi R, Hultling C, Seiger A. The Stockholm Spinal Cord Injury Study: 2. Associations between clinical patient characteristics and post-acute medical problems. *Paraplegia* 1995;33:585–594.
3. Lance JW. Symposium synopsis. In: Feldman RG, Young RR, Koella WP, eds. *Spasticity: disordered motor control.* Chicago: Mosby–Year Book, 1980:17–24.
4. Merritt JL. Management of spasticity in spinal cord injury. *Mayo Clin Proc* 1981;56:614–622.
5. Young RR. Treatment of spastic paresis. *N Engl J Med* 1989;320: 1553–1555.
6. Priebe MM, Sherwood AM, Thornby JI, et al. Clinical assessment of spasticity in spinal cord injury: a multidimensional problem. *Arch Phys Med Rehabil* 1996;77:713–716.
7. Nance P, Bugaresti J, Shellenberger K, et al. Efficacy and safety of tizanidine in the treatment of spasticity in patients with spinal cord injury. *Neurology* 1994;44[Suppl 9]:S44–S52.
8. Stolp-Smith KA, Wainberg MC. Antidepressant exacerbation of spasticity. *Arch Phys Med Rehabil* 1999;80:339–342.
9. Cioni B, Dimitrijevic MR, McKay WB, et al. Voluntary supraspinal suppression of spinal reflex activity in paralyzed muscles of spinal cord injury patients. *Exp Neurol* 1986;93:574–583.
10. Dimitrijevic MR, Fragenel J, Lehmkuhl D, et al. Motor control in man after partial or complete spinal cord injury. *Adv Neurol* 1983; 39:915–926.
11. Dimitrijevic MR, Dimitrijevic MM, Fragenel J, et al. Suprasegmentally induced motor unit activity in paralyzed muscles of patients with established spinal cord injury. *Ann Neurol* 1984;16:216–221.
12. Sherwood AM, Dimitrijevic MR, McKay WB. Evidence of subclinical brain influence in clinically complete spinal cord injury: discomplete SCI. *J Neurol Sci* 1992;110(July):90–98.
13. Kakulas BA. The applied neurobiology of human spinal cord injury: a review. *Paraplegia* 1988;26:371–379.
14. Kakulas BA. A review of the neuropathology of human spinal cord

injury with emphasis on special features. *J Spinal Cord Med* 1999; 22:119–124.

15. Bunge RP, Puckett WR, Becerra JL, et al. Observations on the pathology of human spinal cord injury. A review and classification of 22 new cases with details from a case of chronic cord compression with extensive focal demyelination. *Adv Neurol* 1993;59:75–89.

16. Ashworth B. Preliminary trial of carisoprodol in multiple sclerosis. *Practitioner* 1964;192:540–542.

17. Penn RD. Intrathecal baclofen for severe spasticity. *Ann NY Acad Sci* 1988;531:157–166.

18. Bohannon RW, Smith MB. Interrater reliability of a modified Ashworth Scale of muscle spasticity. *Phys Ther* 1987;67:206–207.

19. Haas BM, Bergstrom E, Jamous A, et al. The interrater reliability of the original and of the modified Ashworth Scale for the assessment of spasticity in patients with spinal cord injury. *Spinal Cord* 1996; 34:560–564.

20. Lee KC, Carson L, Kinnin E, et al. The Ashworth Scale: a reliability and reproducibility method of measuring spasticity. *J Neurol Rehabil* 1989;3:205–209.

21. Skold C, Levi R, Seiger A. Spasticity after traumatic spinal cord injury: nature, severity and location. *Arch Phys Med Rehabil* 1999;80: 1548–1557.

22. Loubser PG, Narayan RK, Sandin KJ, et al. Continuous infusion of intrathecal baclofen: long-term effects on spasticity in spinal cord injury. *Paraplegia* 1991;29:48–64.

23. van Gijn J. The Babinski sign and the pyramidal syndrome. *J Neurol Neurosurg Psychiatry* 1978;41:865–873.

24. Bajd T, Vodovnik L. Pendulum testing of spasticity. *J Biomed Eng* 1984;6:9–16.

25. Wartenburg R. Pendulousness of the legs as a diagnostic test. *Neurology* 1951;1:18–24.

26. Firoozbakhsh KK, Kunkel CF, Scremin AME, et al. Isokinetic dynamometric technique for spasticity assessment. *Am J Phys Med Rehabil* 1993;72:379–385.

27. Lehmann JF, Price R, deLateur BJ, et al. Spasticity: quantitative measurements as a basis for assessing effectiveness of therapeutic intervention. *Arch Phys Med Rehabil* 1989;70:6–15.

28. Hinderer SR, Lehmann JF, Price R, et al. Spasticity in spinal cord injured persons: quantitative effects of baclofen and placebo treatments. *Am J Phys Med Rehabil* 1990;69:311–317.

29. Katz RT, Rymer WZ. Spastic hypertonia: mechanisms and measurement. *Arch Phys Med Rehabil* 1989;70:144–155.

30. Sherwood AM, McKay WB, Dimitrijevic MR. Motor control after spinal cord injury: assessment using surface EMG. *Muscle Nerve* 1996; 19:966–979.

31. Sherwood AM, Priebe MM, Graves DE. consistency of multichannel surface EMG recordings: application in spinal cord injured subjects. *J Electrophysiol Kinesiol* 1997;7:97–111.

32. Priebe M, Sherwood A, Graves D, et al. Effectiveness of gabapentin in controlling spasticity: a quantitative study. *Spinal Cord* 1997;35: 171–175.

33. Zupan B, Stokic DS, Bohanec M, et al. Relating clinical and neurophysiological assessment of spasticity by machine learning. *Int J Med Inf* 1998;49:243–251.

34. Sherwood AM, Graves DE, Priebe MM. Altered motor control and spasticity after spinal cord injury: subjective and objective assessment. *J Rehabil Res Dev* 2000;37:41–52.

35. Schurch B, Wichmann W, Rossier AB. Post traumatic syringomyelia (cystic myelopathy): a prospective study of 449 patients with spinal cord injury. *J Neurol Neurosurg Psychiatry* 1996;60(1):61–67.

36. Kramer KM, Levine AM. Posttraumatic syringomyelia: a review of 21 cases. *Clin Orthop Rel Res* 1997;334:190–199.

37. Dalyan M, Sherman A, Cardenas DD. Factors associated with contractures in acute spinal cord injury. *Spinal Cord* 1998;36:405–408.

38. Burke D, Andrews C, Achby P. Autogenic effects of static muscle stretch in spastic man. *Arch Neurol* 1971;25:367–372.

39. Kirshblum S. Treatment alternatives for spinal cord injury related spasticity. *J Spinal Cord Med* 1999;22(3):199–217.

40. Lehmann J, Masock A, Warren C, et al. Effect of therapeutic tempera-

tures on tendon extensibility. *Arch Phys Med Rehabil* 1970;51: 481–487.

41. Bohannon RW. Tilt table standing for reducing spasticity after spinal cord injury. *Arch Phys Med Rehabil* 1993;74:1121–1122.

42. Kunkel CF, Scremin AME, Eisenberg B, et al. Effect of "standing" on spasticity, contracture and osteoporosis in paralyzed males. *Arch Phys Med Rehabil* 1993;74:73–78.

43. Carlson SJ. A neurophysiologic analysis of inhibitive casting. Physical and Occupational Therapy in Pediatrics, vol. 1. The Hayworth Press, Inc. 1985;4:31–42.

44. Devanandan MS, Eccles RM, Yokota T. Muscle stretch and the presynaptic inhibition of the group Ia pathway to motoneurons. *J Physiol* 1965;179(3):430–441.

45. Mark RF, Coquery JM, Paillard J. Autogenetic reflex effects of slow or steady stretch of the calf muscles in man. *Exp Brain Res* 1968;6: 130–145.

46. Robinson KL, McComas AJ, Belanger AY. Control of soleus motoneuron excitability during muscle stretch in man. *J Neurol Neurosurg Psychiatry* 1982;45(Aug):699–704.

47. Knuttson E. Topical cryotherapy in spasticity. *Scand J Rehabil Med* 1970;2:159–163.

48. Miglietta O. Action of cold on spasticity. *Am J Phys Med Rehabil* 1973;198–205.

49. Bell KR, Lehmann JF. Effect of cooling on H- and T-reflexes in normal subjects. *Arch Phys Med Rehabil* 1987;68:490–493.

50. Knuttson E, Mattsson E. Effects of local cooling on monosynaptic reflexes in man. *Scand J Rehabil Med* 1969;1:126–132.

51. Price R, Lehmann JF, Boswell-Bessette S, et al. Influence of cryotherapy on spasticity at the human ankle. *Arch Phys Med Rehabil* 1993; 73:300–304.

52. Rosche J, Paulus C, Maisch U, et al. The effects of therapy on spasticity utilizing a motorized exercise-cycle. *Spinal Cord* 1997;35: 176–178.

53. Robinson CJ, Kett NA, Bolam JM. Spasticity in spinal cord injured patients: 1. Short-term effects of surface electrical stimulation. *Arch Phys Med Rehabil* 1988;69:598–604.

54. Robinson CJ, Kett NA, Bolam JM. Spasticity in spinal cord injured patients: 2. Initial measures and long-term effects of surface electrical stimulation. *Arch Phys Med Rehabil* 1988;69:862–868.

55. Granat MH, Ferguson AC, Andrews BJ, et al. The role of functional electrical stimulation in the rehabilitation of patients with incomplete spinal cord injury—observed benefits during gait studies. *Paraplegia* 1993;31:207–215.

56. Pease WS. Therapeutic electrical stimulation for spasticity: quantitative gait analysis. *Am J Phys Med Rehabil* 1998;77:351–355.

57. Goulet C, Arsenault A, Bourbonnais D, et al. Effects of transcutaneous electrical nerve stimulation on H reflex and spinal spasticity. *Scand J Rehabil Med* 1996;28:169–176.

58. Glaser RM. Physiologic aspects of spinal cord injury and functional neuromuscular stimulation. *Cent Nerv Syst Trauma* 1986;3:49–61.

59. Douglas AJ, Walsh EG, Wright GW, et al. The effects of neuromuscular stimulation on muscle tone at the knee in paraplegia. *Exp Physiol* 1991;76:357–367.

60. Halstead LS, Seager S. The effects of rectal probe electrostimulation on spinal cord injury spasticity. *Paraplegia* 1990;29:43–47.

61. Halstead LS, Seager S, Houston J, et al. Relief of spasticity in SCI men and women using rectal probe electrostimulation. *Paraplegia* 1993;31: 715–721.

62. Barolat G, Myklebust JB, Wenninger W. Effects of spinal cord stimulation on spasticity and spasms secondary to myelopathy. *Appl Neurophysiol* 1988;51:29–44.

63. Midha M, Schmitt JK. Epidural spinal cord stimulation for the control of spasticity in spinal cord injury patients lacks long term efficacy and is not cost-effective. *Spinal Cord* 1998;36:190–192.

64. Taricco M, Adone R, Pagliacci C, et al. Pharmacological interventions for spasticity following spinal cord injury. *Cochrane Database Syst Rev* 2000;2:CD001131.

65. Sawynok J. GABA-ergic mechanisms of analgesia: an update. *Pharmacol Biochem Behav* 1987;26:463–474.

66. Bass B, Weinshenker B, Rice GP, et al. Tizanidine versus baclofen

in the treatment of spasticity in patients with multiple sclerosis. *Can J Neurol Sci* 1988;15:15–19.

67. Herman J, D'Luzansky S. Pharmacologic management of spinal spasticity. *J Neurol Rehabil* 1991;5:S15–S20.

68. Nielsen JF, Sinkjaer T. Peripheral and central effect of baclofen on ankle joint stiffness in multiple sclerosis. *Muscle Nerve* 2000;23:98–105.

69. Hinderer SR. The supraspinal anxiolytic effect of baclofen for spasticity reduction. *Am J Phys Med Rehabil* 1990;69:254–258.

70. Herman RM, D'Luzansky SC, Ippolito R. Intrathecal baclofen suppresses central pain in patients with spinal lesions. A pilot study. *Clin J Pain* 1992;8(4):338–345.

71. Terrence CF, Fromm GH, Tenicela R. Baclofen as an analgesic in chronic peripheral nerve disease. *Eur Neurol* 1985;24:380–385.

72. Jamous A, Kennedy P, Psychol C, et al. Psychological and emotional effects of the use of oral baclofen: a preliminary study. *Paraplegia* 1994;32(2):349–353.

73. Rivas DA, Chancellor MB, Hill K, et al. Neurological manifestations of baclofen withdrawal. *J Urol* 1993;150(6):1903–1905.

74. Aisen ML, Dietz M, McDowell F, et al. Baclofen toxicity in a patient with subclinical renal insufficiency. *Arch Phys Med Rehabil* 1994;75(1):109–111.

75. Broderick C, Radnitz C, Bauman W. Diazepam usage in veterans with spinal cord injury. *J Spinal Cord Med* 1997;20(4):406–409.

76. Corbett M, Frankel H, Michaelis L. A double-blind, cross-over trial of Valium in the treatment of spasticity. *Paraplegia* 1972;10:19–22.

77. Wilson L, McKechnie A. Oral diazepam in the treatment of spasticity in paraplegia: a double blind trial and subsequent impressions. *Scott Med J* 1966;11:46–51.

78. Higgitt A, Fonagy, Lader M. The natural history of tolerance to the benzodiazepines. *Psychol Med Monogr* 1988;13[Suppl]:1–55.

79. Frisbie JH, Aguilera EJ. Diazepam and body weight in myelopathy patients. *J Spinal Cord Med* 1995;18(3):200–202.

80. Davidoff RA. Antispasticity drugs: mechanisms of action. *Ann Neurol* 1985;17:107–116.

81. Basmajian JV, Shankardass K, Russell D. Ketazolam once daily for spasticity: double-blind cross-over study. *Arch Phys Med Rehabil* 1986;67:556–557.

82. Nance PW, Shears AH, Nance DM. Clonidine in spinal cord injury. *Can Med Assoc J* 1985;133:41–42.

83. Donovan WH, Carter RE, Rossi CD, et al. Clonidine effect on spasticity: a clinical trial. *Arch Phys Med Rehabil* 1988;69:193–194.

84. Maynard FM. Early clinical experience with clonidine in spinal spasticity. *Paraplegia* 1986;24:175–182.

85. Yablon SA, Sipski ML. Effect of transdermal clonidine on spinal spasticity. A case series. *Am J Phys Med Rehabil* 1993;72:154–157.

86. Weingarden SI, Belen JG. Clonidine transdermal system for treatment of spasticity in spinal cord injury. *Arch Phys Med Rehabil* 1992;73:876–877.

87. Nance PW, Sheremata WA, Lynch SG, et al. Relationship of the antispasticity effect of tizanidine to plasma concentration in patients with multiple sclerosis. *Arch Neurol* 1997;54(6):731–736.

88. Rosenblum D. Clonidine-induced bradycardia in patients with spinal cord injury. *Arch Phys Med Rehabil* 1993;74:1206–1207.

89. *Physicians' desk reference,* 53rd ed. Montvale, NJ: Medical Economics Company, 1999.

90. Gruenthal M, Mueller M, Olson W, et al. Gabapentin for the treatment of spasticity in patients with spinal cord injury. *Spinal Cord* 1997;35:686–689.

91. Cutter N, Scott D, Johnson J, et al. Gabapentin effect on spasticity in multiple sclerosis: a placebo-controlled, randomized trial. *Arch Phys Med Rehabil* 2000;81:164–169.

92. Herman R, Mayer N, Mecomber SA. The pharmacophysiology of dantrolene sodium. *Am J Phys Med* 1972;51:296–311.

93. Mayer N, Necomber SA, Herman R. Treatment of spasticity with dantrolene sodium. *Am J Phys Med* 1973;52:18–29.

94. Utili R, Boitnott JK, Zimmerman HJ. Dantrolene-associated hepatic injury. Incidence and character. *Gastroenterology* 1977;72:610–616.

95. White SR, Neuman RS. Facilitation of spinal motoneuron excitability by 5-hydroxytryptamine and noradrenaline. *Brain Res* 1980;188:119–127.

96. White SR, Fung SJ. Serotonin depolarizes cat spinal motoneurons in situ and decreases motoneuron after–hyperpolarizing potentials. *Brain Res* 1989;502:205–213.

97. Barbeau H, Richards CL, Bedard PJ. Action of cyproheptadine in spastic paraparetic patients. *J Neurol Neurosurg Psychiatry* 1982;45:923–926.

98. Nance P. A comparison of clonidine, cyproheptadine, and baclofen in spastic spinal cord injured patients. *J Am Paraplegia Soc* 1994;17:151–157.

99. Wainberg M, Barbeau H, Gauthier S. The effects of cyproheptadine on locomotion and on spasticity in patients with spinal cord injuries. *J Neurol Neurosurg Psychiatry* 1990;53:754–763.

100. Wainberg M, Barbeau H, Gauthier S. Quantitative assessment of the effect of cyproheptadine on spastic paretic gait: a preliminary study. *J Neurol* 1986;233:311–314.

101. Norman KE , Pepin A, Barbeau H, et al. Effect of drugs in walking after spinal cord injury. *Spinal Cord* 1998;36:699–715.

102. Fung J, Stewart JE, Barbeau H. The combined effects of clonidine and cyproheptadine with interactive training on the modulation of locomotion in spinal cord injured subjects. *J Neurol Sci* 1990;100:85–93.

103. Willer JC, Bussel B. Evidence for a direct spinal mechanism in morphine-induced inhibition of nociceptive reflexes in humans. *Brain Res* 1980;187:212–215.

104. Advokat C, Mosser H, Hutchinson K. Morphine and dextrorphan lose antinociceptive activity but exhibit an antispastic action in chronic spinal rats. *Physiol Behav* 1997;62(4):799–804.

105. Simpson R, Gondo M, Robertson C, et al. The influence of glycine and related compounds on spinal cord injury-induced spasticity. *Neurochem Res* 1995;20:1203–1210.

106. Stern P, Bokonjic R. Glycine therapy in 7 cases of spasticity. A pilot study. *Pharmacology* 1974;12:117–119.

107. Lee A, Patterson V. A double-blind study of L-threonine in patients with spinal spasticity. *Acta Neurol Scand* 1993;88:334–338.

108. Potter PJ, Hayes KC, Segal JL, et al. Randomized double-blind crossover trial of fampridine-SR (sustained release 4-aminopyridine) in patients with incomplete spinal cord injury. *J Neurotrauma* 1998;15(10):837–849.

109. Hansebout RR, Blight AR, Fawcett S, et al. 4-Aminopyridine in chronic spinal cord injury: a controlled, double-blind, crossover study in eight patients. *J Neurotrauma* 1993;10:1–18.

110. Ashby P, Burke D, Rao S, et al. Assessment of cyclobenzaprine in the treatment of spasticity. *J Neurol Neurosurg Psychiatry* 1972;35:599–605.

111. Casale R, Glynn CJ, Buonocore M. Reduction of spastic hypertonia in patients with spinal cord injury: a double-blind comparison of intravenous orphenadrine citrate and placebo. *Arch Phys Med Rehabil* 1995;76:660–665.

112. Dunn M, Davis R. The perceived effects of marijuana on spinal cord injured males. *Paraplegia* 1974;12:175.

113. Malec J, Harvey RF, Cayner JJ. Cannabis effect on spasticity in spinal cord injury. *Arch Phys Med Rehabil* 1982;63(3):116–118.

114. Petro DJ, Ellenberger C. Treatment of human spasticity with delta 9-tetrahydrocannabinol. *J Clin Pharmacol* 1981;21[Suppl]:8–9.

115. *Physicians' desk reference for herbal medicines,* 1st ed. Montvale, NJ: Medical Economics Company, 1998.

116. Erickson DL, Lo J, Michaelson M. Control of intractable spasticity with intrathecal morphine sulfate. *Neurosurgery* 1989;24:236–238.

117. Kroin JS, Ali A, York M, et al. The distribution of medication along the spinal canal after chronic intrathecal administration. *Neurosurgery* 1993;33:226–230.

118. Coffey RJ, Cahill D, Steers W, et al. Intrathecal baclofen for intractable spasticity of spinal origin: results of a long-term multicenter study. *J Neurosurg* 1993;78:226–232.

119. Penn RD. Intrathecal baclofen for spasticity of spinal origin: seven years of experience. *J Neurosurg* 1992;77:236–240.

120. Lewis KS, Mueller WM. Intrathecal baclofen for severe spasticity secondary to spinal cord injury. *Ann Pharmacother* 1993;27:767–774.

121. Remy-Neris O, Barbeau H, Daniel O, et al. Effects of intrathecal

clonidine injection on spinal reflexes and human locomotion in incomplete paraplegic subjects. *Exp Brain Res* 1999;129:433–440.

122. Middleton JW, Siddall PJ, Walker S, et al. Intrathecal clonidine and baclofen in the management of spasticity and neuropathic pain following spinal cord injury: a case study. *Arch Phys Med Rehabil* 1996;77: 824–826.

123. Akman MN, Loubser PG, Donovan WH, et al. Intrathecal baclofen: does tolerance occur? *Paraplegia* 1993;31(8):516–520.

124. Abel NA, Smith RA. Intrathecal baclofen for treatment of intractable spinal spasticity. *Arch Phys Med* 1994;75:54–58.

125. Teddy P, Jamous A, Gardner B, et al. Complications of intrathecal baclofen delivery. *Br J Neurosurg* 1992;6:115–118.

126. Khorasani A, Peruzzi W. Dantrolene sodium for the abrupt intrathecal baclofen withdrawal. *Anesth Analg* 1995;80:1054–1056.

127. Parke B, Penn RD, Savoy SM, et al. Functional outcome after delivery of intrathecal baclofen. *Arch Phys Med Rehabil* 1989;70:30–32.

128. Gianino JM, York MM, Paice JA, et al. Quality of life: effect of reduced spasticity from intrathecal baclofen. *J Neurol Nurs* 1998;30: 47–54.

129. Botte MJ, Abrams RA, Bodine-Fowler SC. Treatment of acquired muscle spasticity using phenol peripheral nerve blocks. *Orthopedics* 1995;18:151–159.

130. Shaari CM, Sanders I. Quantifying how location and dose of botulinum toxin injections affect muscle paralysis. *Muscle Nerve* 1993;16: 64–69.

131. Smyth M, Peacock W. The surgical treatment of spasticity. *Muscle Nerve* 2000;23:153–163.

IMMUNE FUNCTION FOLLOWING SPINAL CORD INJURY

DENISE I. CAMPAGNOLO
MARK S. NASH

Infections are a primary cause of death for persons with spinal cord injury (SCI) (1). Persons with SCI are 64 times more likely to die of septicemia and 36 times more likely to die of pneumonia than individuals from the general population having the same age, sex, and race (1). Once community integration after SCI is achieved, infection remains the most common reason for rehospitalization and emergency department visits (2,3). These data demonstrate the importance of understanding the various factors that impact on immunity and the acquisition of infections after SCI.

Several recent textbooks and reviews are devoted to the human immune response, and a complete review of this topic is beyond the scope of this chapter (4,5). Only the key elements needed to understand the deficiencies seen after SCI are briefly reviewed here. The immune system involves many widespread cells and soluble mediators that provide protection against foreign pathogens. The immune response has both nonspecific and specific functions. Nonspecific elements include mononuclear phagocytes, polymorphonuclear (PMN) leukocytes, and the complement system. These nonspecific components amplify and modify the immune response. The mononuclear phagocytes, as well as endothelial cells and some glial cells, act as antigen-presenting cells, whose function is to "present" antigens to T lymphocytes in the presence of major histocompatibility complex (MHC) proteins (Fig. 15.1). Thus, the nonspecific mononuclear phagocytes have an important role to play in the initiation of very specific T-lymphocyte responses. PMN leukocytes (basophils, eosinophils, and others) are important in all infection-mediated inflammatory reactions such as immediate hypersensitivity and immune complex reactions. The complement system is involved in the full development of immune reactions, serum sickness, and autoimmune disorders.

The elements of the immune system that provide specificity are the T and B-lymphocytes. Both recognize "self" from "nonself" and recognize the differences between non–cross-reacting antigens through receptors on their surface. Lymphocytes are unique in their ability to express specific receptors to unique antigens and then undergo clonal expansion. Soluble factors are small molecules, called *cytokines,* which interact with the immune system. Those produced by lymphocytes are called *lym-*

phokines, whereas those that act between neutrophils are designated *interleukins.* Virally infected cells produce interferons that prevent infection by another virus. Interferons are also produced by activated T cells, cause macrophage activation, and induce expression of MHC proteins on the surfaces of many cells. Tumor necrosis factor and colony-stimulating factors are examples of this (5).

Lymphocytes develop in the primary lymphoid organs: thymus and bone marrow. Secondary lymphoid tissues are areas of lymphoid filtering and have varying percentages of T and B cells. For example, the spleen has nearly equal percentages of T and B cells and is an important site of antibody production after intravascular infections such as bacterial sepsis. Lymph nodes provide regional response to antigens as mobile T cells clonally expand in area lymph nodes draining a site of infection (antigenic challenge). T-cell function is restricted, in that clones of a given T cell only interact with a specific antigen, although T cells are also long-lived and provide lasting immune memory. Their subclasses have several regulatory and effector actions. The cytotoxic T cells mainly combat virally infected cells and are involved in allograft rejection. They carry $CD8^+$ markers on their cell surface and are therefore said to be of the $CD8^+$ phenotype (Fig. 15.1). Another type of $CD8^+$ T cell is the so-called *suppressor T cell,* which many believe is involved in immune tolerance and disturbances of self-tolerance (4). Helper T cells are generally of the $CD4^+$ phenotype, are involved in delayed type hypersensitivity reactions, and trigger the B cell to develop into an antibody-secreting cell. The last type of lymphocyte that is discussed in this chapter is the natural killer (NK) cell. NK cells ($CD3^-CD56^+$) are large granulocytic lymphocytes. They demonstrate spontaneous cytolytic activity against a range of tumor-infected and virus-infected cells (4).

The terms "cell-mediated immunity" and "humoral immunity" need definition, because these terms commonly appear in immune-related literature. Cellular, or cell-mediated, immunity refers to immunity resulting from the transfer of T cells. The cellular arm of the immune system plays the most important role in protection against intracellular bacterial infections, viral infections, cancer, and in graft rejection (4,5). Humoral immunity refers to immunity that can be transferred by antibodies

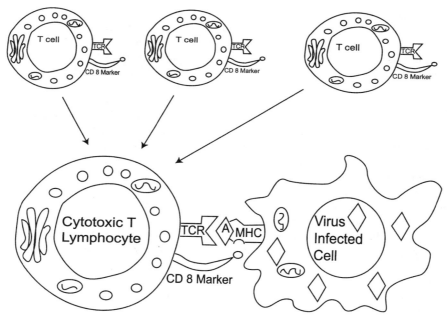

FIGURE 15.1. The depicted cytotoxic T lymphocyte (CTL) is one of many clones of an original T cell that has been sensitized to the viral antigen **(A)**. This CTL now has the capacity to interact with antigen–major histocompatibility complex proteins on the surface of this target cell (e.g., virus-infected cell). The result will be the conjugation of the CTL and target cell, followed by membrane damage and death of the target cell. The CTL is then recycled for continued immune surveillance and kill capability. (TCR, T-cell receptor; MHC, major histocompatibility complex.)

(immunoglobulins) present in plasma, lymph, and tissue fluids (4,5). Immunoglobulins B-cell protein products are constructed in various shapes and are categorized into five major classes or isotypes: IgG, IgM, IgD, IgE, and IgA. The function of these different isotypes varies but generally is involved with viral and bacterial opsonization and neutralization.

ASSESSMENT OF IMMUNE FUNCTION

The impairments of immune function found in persons with SCI have been identified using *in vitro* assays of immunity. The assays common to most studies discussed in this chapter are briefly summarized here.

1. Cytometry or cell enumeration determines the numbers and types of immunocytes in the compartment of the immune system being examined (e.g., peripheral blood and spleen). This process involves attaching antigen-specific monoclonal antibodies to the specific cell surface markers on immune cells. Once tagged by these antibodies, a fluorescence-activated cell sorter counts and separates the specific cell types. The quantity of immune cells, although important, does not provide information about their function. Functional competence is determined for individual cell populations with specific *in vitro* functional assays.

2. Lymphocyte proliferation assay (also called the mitogen assay). A mitogen is a compound that causes lymphocytes to divide or replicate (blastogenic response) (4,5). The mitogens typically used in clinical immunology laboratories are concanavalin A, phytohemagglutinin, and pokeweed. Mixed lymphocyte populations are incubated with one of these mitogens and ^{3}H-thymidine. The ^{3}H-thymidine is incorporated into the lymphocyte DNA as blastogenesis (replication) occurs. Thus, the lymphocyte's functional ability to undergo clonal expansion in response to a mitogen is measured by the release of the beta radiation measured by a scintillation counter.

3. NK cell cytotoxicity assay. NK cells are a subset of lymphocytes that do not require previous sensitization to kill target cells. Chromium-51–labeled cells of the human tumor cell line (K562) are used as targets and their death measured by release of the radioisotope. The death of the target cell provides a measure of the kill capability of the NK cells mixed with the target cells.

4. Phagocyte assay. Phagocytes are separated from whole blood by centrifugation. The composition of this cell population is predominantly neutrophils (PMN leukocytes). Previously opsonized *Staphylococcus aureus* bacteria are incubated with the PMN leukocytes at a bacteria to cell ratio of 100 : 1. Cell lysis is then performed and the supernatant placed on blood agar. The growth of *S. aureus* colonies after immediate cell lysis is a measure of the cell's ability to phagocytose bacteria. Intracellular killing ability of the PMN leukocyte is measured in the same way, except the cell lysis occurs after 1 to 2 hours of incubation.

IMMUNE RESPONSE FOLLOWING SPINAL CORD INJURY

A consistent and reproducible pattern of immune suppression has been found in persons with SCI. Abnormal immune findings have been reported by several independent investigators in 12 publications over the last 10 years (6–17). These findings include dampening of lymphocyte clonal expansion, reduction in the T helper : T suppressor ratio, impaired ability of NK cells to kill target cells, reduction in NK cell numbers, and impaired phagocytosis and altered patterns of cytokines and surface molecules. These immune parameters are summarized in Table 15.1 and are categorized by whether they affect the specific or nonspecific arms of the human immune response (Table 15.1). SCI also impairs T-cell blastogenesis in response to mitogen challenge. Clonal expansion of the T cell in response to mitogen is attempted after SCI, but the response is diminished, suggesting that clinically once exposed to a pathogen or antigen, the population of lymphocytes able to specifically combat that pathogen is unable to grow in number appropriately. Thus, the clinical response to infection is diminished. Similarly, NK cells provide the first line of defense against intracellular bacterial and viral infections, so a reduction in their number or function would potentially leave the host susceptible to infection. Controlled studies have established a clear association between immune parameter changes after SCI and clinical infection rates.

The Autonomic Nervous System and Its Effect on Immune Function

The regulation of immune responses to antigenic challenge is quite complicated and not entirely understood. It was once thought that the immune response was a self-regulated autonomous system. Indeed, some form of regulation is linked to the MHC molecules, whose genes are located on human chromosome 6 (5). We now know, however, that the age, nutritional status, and many other factors, including the integrity of the central nervous system (CNS), regulate the efficient response of the immune system to infection.

Convincing evidence documents regulation of the immune response by the CNS through central and peripheral neural connections, neurotransmitters, and neurohormones of the hypothalamic-pituitary axis and neuroendocrine systems. For example, primary and secondary lymphoid tissue is innervated ("hardwired") by postganglionic noradrenergic fibers of the sympathetic nervous system (SNS) (18,19). This, coupled with the finding of β_2-adrenergic receptors on the cell surface of many immunocytes, provides a direct avenue by which the CNS regulates the immune response, as well as a possible pathway by which disconnection of the CNS from this regulation can affect the immune response (20,21). Localized lesions of the CNS and chemical sympathectomy have been associated with alterations in *in vitro* immune response parameters in animal models (22). In experimental animals, adrenergic stress suppresses lymphocyte proliferation and NK cell activity in both adrenalectomized and hypophysectomized rats, showing the importance of direct lymphoid innervation from the autonomic nervous sytem (23, 24). The importance of this direct lymphoid "hardwiring" (as opposed to circulating hormonal influences) is supported by the finding that circulating hormone levels, although different from nondisabled subjects, did not differ from those of SCI subjects in a small study (25). Adrenergic stress also diminishes phagocytic activity and interferon-producing capacity (26,27). These same changes seen in experimental studies parallel immune abnormalities identified in persons with SCI (Table 15.1). The level of SCI (above or below the majority of sympathetic outflow levels) also influences immunity (8). This finding supports the role that decentralization of the SNS plays in orchestrating immunity after SCI (28).

Finally, psychological states and traits have been shown to alter immunity and affect susceptibility to illness. Schleifer et al. (29,30) demonstrated that stress in the form of conjugal bereavement reduced lymphocyte responsiveness to mitogens, as does major depressive disorders. Kiecolt-Glaser and Glaser (31) demonstrated reduced lymphocyte responsiveness after the stress of final examinations in a group of healthy medical students. It therefore follows that injury to the spinal cord could also effect the immune response both directly through disconnected "hardwiring" and through the many adverse physical and psychological complications of SCI.

Nonautonomic Effects of SCI on Immune Function

Efficient responses of the immune system to antigenic challenge are compromised by many drugs, chemicals, biologicals, diets, and activity levels. Therefore, unifying causes of immune dysfunctions are difficult, if not impossible, to identify. As previously stated, sympathetic dysfunction accompanying SCI is a suspected cause of depressed immune competence, although it is unlikely that it represents the sole cause. Because immune-altering states, conditions, and imprudent lifestyle choices are both common to those living with SCI and amenable to correction, the following sections address plausible causes for immune dysfunctions in persons with SCI beyond autonomic decentralization.

TABLE 15.1. IMMUNE PARAMETERS INFLUENCED BY SPINAL CORD INJURY

Specific arm of the immune response
Reduced $CD4^+$/$CD8^+$ (helper/suppressor) cell ratio (6,7)
In vitro lymphocyte transformation to mitogen challenge (6,8,9,10,11)
Nonspecific arm of the immune response
Reduced NK cell counts (6,9,10)
Depressed NK cytotoxicity (6,8,9,10,11)
Depressed T-cell function/activation (IL-2R) (9,12)
Depressed LFA-1 and VLA-4 (13)
Impaired neutrophil phagocytosis (14)
Elevated plasma IL-6, soluble IL-2R, and ICAM-1 (15,16,17)

Note: Immune alterations found in persons with spinal cord injury, categorized by whether they affect the specific or nonspecific arms of the human immune response.
[a]NK, natural killer; LFA-1, lymphocyte function–associated antigen-1; VLA-4, very late antigen-4; IL-6, interleukin-6; IL-2R, receptor for interleukin-2; ICAM-1, intercellular adhesion molecule-1.

Poor Diet

Imprudent dietary intake adversely influences various aspects of immune function. The dietary intake of persons with SCI is reportedly high in fat and low in protein content, with consumption of dietary fat exceeding 43% of total calories (32). This is higher than both the reference diet of persons without paraplegia and guidelines published by the American Heart Association, the Surgeon General's Report on Nutrition and Health, and other authoritative bodies (32). High dietary fat is associated with decreased killing capacity of NK cells, whose functions are strongly linked with autonomic dysfunction and whose killing capacity function is depressed after SCI (7,10,12,13,33). High-fat diets may also adversely influence graft versus host reactions (34,35). Protein malnutrition also adversely affects functions of both macrophages and mature lymphocytes (36–38). Many aspects of macrophage function appear to be impaired, including significantly decreased peritoneal numbers, a diminished ability to present antigens to lymphocytes, and reduced macrophage phagocytosis and killing. Low protein intake also impairs T-cell response to antigens and antibody production, findings that are corrected by nutritional repletion (36,37). Under similar protein restriction, others have shown depressed *in vitro* proliferative responses to mitogen stimulation, decreased complement levels, and impaired neutrophil chemotaxis (39).

Hyperglycemia

Glycemic state is known to influence both immune function and disease susceptibility. The first report of insulin resistance accompanying SCI appeared more than two decades ago and has since been verified by another study (40,41). Approximately 50% of persons with SCI exhibit traits of non–insulin-dependent diabetes. Therefore, it is worth noting that hyperglycemia in both diabetic and nondiabetic patients may depress granulocyte adherence, chemotaxis, phagocytosis, and microbicidal function (42–44). These abnormalities have profound clinical effects on postoperative nosocomial infection rates in those with blood glucose levels of more than 220 mg/dL, whose infection susceptibility is reversible with reestablishment of euglycemia (45).

Substance Abuse

Many prescription and over-the-counter medications used by persons with SCI are known to depress immune function. For example, pain formulations containing salicylates, nonsteroidal antiinflammatory drugs, and acetaminophen promote immune suppression. This is evidenced by delayed serum neutralizing antibody responses; increased nasal symptoms and signs after controlled rhinovirus infection; and delayed virus shedding, a response hypothesized to be mediated through drug affects on monocytes or mononuclear phagocytes (46). It has also been shown that diazepam (Valium) adversely influences immune function, including sustained depression of T-lymphocyte proliferation (47,48).

The administration of high-dose methylprednisolone immediately after acute SCI may also transiently suppress cellular immune function and elevate illness susceptibility in the acute care phases of injury. It is unlikely that immune changes identified chronically after SCI are due to this medication for the following reasons: (a) immune alterations were identified long before it was standard practice to use methylprednisolone (6) and (b) *in vitro* studies have shown that the effects of methylprednisolone on neutrophil function resolve after 5 days (50).

Inactivity and Its Immune Consequences

A sedentary lifestyle and low levels of fitness are common among many persons with SCI, which may influence their resting immune function and responses to stress imposed by physical activity (51). Many investigators find an association between resting immune dysfunction and low levels of fitness in persons without SCI, although some do not (52–57). Given that increased NK cell–specific number and killing capacity have been reported by several investigators after low-intensity but not high-intensity training, adverse immune responses to physical training are likely attributable to excessively intense exercise conditioning or competition stress, not exercise per se (52–54). This belief is supported by the well-defined relationship between high levels of fitness and immune suppression, in which exaggerated catecholamine and cortisol stress are observed during high-intensity activities, after which a period of immune downregulation ensues (59). These responses explain the convincing evidence that prolonged intense activity causes immune suppression and increased illness susceptibility, particularly upper respiratory tract infections (56,60). Because physical conditioning blunts the catecholamine responses to exercise stress in persons with and without SCI, one plausible benefit of exercise conditioning on immune function might be the blunting of exaggerated acute catecholamine and subservient immune responses to physical activity commonly experienced by deconditioned persons (61,62).

IMMUNE RESPONSES TO EXERCISE AFTER SCI

Four studies examined the effects of physical activity on acute and chronic adaptation of the immune system in persons with SCI. Two studies investigated the effects of exercise on persons with SCI during and immediately after electrically stimulated cycling (7,63). One of these investigations reported an acute leukocytosis, with augmentation of NK cell function in subjects with paraplegia but not tetraplegia (63). A study examining similar exercise responses in subjects with tetraplegia found no leukocytosis, but significant improvements in NK cell number and killing capacity in similar subjects (7). The latter findings were thought to be explained by β-endorphin response to either electrical current or exercise, as endogenous opioids have known inductive effects on numbers and cytotoxicity of NK cells (64). By contrast, an examination of the immune response to wheelchair marathon racing found a profound leukocytosis and augmentation of NK cell function, followed by a period of immune downregulation lasting up to 24 hours (65). In a single study examining the effects of rehabilitation therapy on subacute patients with SCI, rehabilitation was found to improve the depressed NK cell function and T-cell function observed immediately after hospitalization (12). The improvement in NK cell function positively correlated with changes in the Functional Independence Measure (FIM) scores obtained on these subjects. These studies suggest that acute and chronic physical activity either transitorily or chronically benefit immune functions, so long as the intensity and duration of activity are kept moderate.

AGING

Extensive clinical evidence documents decline of immune function (66), elevated incidence of infection, and increased susceptibility to neoplastic and autoimmune diseases accompanying aging (67–69). Declining structure and function of organ systems responsible for protection from infection accompany aging. This progressive breakdown of two mucocutaneous barriers—the skin and genitourinary tract—has been reported in older persons and is of particular consequence to infection susceptibility in persons aging with SCI. Age-related dysfunction of the genitourinary tract in persons without disability includes increased bacterial adherence to epithelial cells, elevated occurrence of nephrolithiasis, urinary stasis secondary to obstructive prostatitis in men and bladder prolapse in women; and increasing frequency of urinary tract infections (70).

Various cell-mediated and humoral responses to antigenic challenge are weakened by aging. One of the most consistently cited changes in functional immunity is diminishment of the *in vitro* proliferative response to mitogen stimulation (71). This mild to moderate decrease in cellular immunity is commonly attributed to age-related thymic involution and decreased thymic mass (72). Age-related thymic senescence also explains consistent reports that thymic-dependent immune reactions and T-cell function are more profoundly altered than thymic-independent immunity and B-cell function. T-cell–dependent changes characterized by altered number and diminished cell-mediated cytotoxicity also accompany aging, as the total number of circulating lymphocytes decreases by 15% to 20%, primarily due to decreased numbers of T cells, and not B cells and monocytes (73,74). No evidence suggests selective diminishment of the NK cell system with aging, and macrophage and B-cell function is at or near normal efficiency in the aged (75,76). These issues will most certainly impact on our aging population of persons with SCI.

In summary, injury to the spinal cord affects most organ systems in the body. Immune system changes have only come under scrutiny in the past decade and have been confirmed by independent clinical studies and parallel animal studies. Both specific and nonspecific arms of the immune system are altered after SCI, and both have integral parts to play in host defense. Therefore, it is not surprising that infection is a leading cause of death of persons with SCI. The causes of immune suppression are many and are intertwined with one another. The identification of the persons with SCI who are at risk immunologically is important, so interventions developed to augment immunity can be steered toward them. Possible interventions are already being explored (77,78). Future research on immune system changes and their impact on health after SCI may lead to decreased infectious morbidity and mortality in this population.

REFERENCES

1. DeVivo M, Stover S. Long term survival and causes of death. In: Stover SL, DeLisa JA, Whiteneck GG, eds. *Spinal cord injury clinical outcomes from the model systems.* Gaithersburg, MD: Aspen Publishers, 1995: 100–119.
2. Meyers AR, Branch LG, Cupples A, et al. Predictors of medical care utilization by independently living adults with spinal cord injuries. *Arch Phys Med Rehabil* 1989;70:471–476.
3. Davidoff G, Schultz S, Lieb T, et al. Rehospitalization after initial rehabilitation for acute spinal cord injury: incidence and risk factors. *Arch Phys Med Rehabil* 1990;71:121–124.
4. Kuby J. *Immunology.* New York: WH Freeman and Company, 1992.
5. Claman HN. The biology of the immune response. *JAMA* 1992;268: 2790–2796.
6. Nash MS, Fletcher MA. The physiologic perspective: immune system. In: Whiteneck GG, ed. *Aging with spinal cord injury.* New York: Demos Publications, 1992:159–181.
7. Nash MS. Immune responses to nervous system decentralization and exercise in quadriplegia. *Med Sci Sports Exerc* 1994;26(2):164–171.
8. Campagnolo DI, Keller SE , DeLisa JA, et al. Alteration of immune system function in tetraplegics. A pilot study. *Am J Phys Med Rehabil* 1994;73(6):387–393.
9. Cruse JM, Lewis RE, Bishop GR, et al. Neuroendocrine-immune interactions associated with loss and restoration of immune system function in spinal cord injury and stroke patients. *Immunol Res* 1992;11(2): 104–116.
10. Cruse JM, Lewis RE Jr, Bishop GR, et al. Decreased immune reactivity and neuroendocrine alteration related to chronic stress in spinal cord injury and stroke patients. *Pathobiology* 1993;61(3-4):183–192.
11. Kaplan AE. Spinal cord influences on immune responses demonstrated following interruption of the spinal cord as a result of injury [in Russian]. *Zh Vopr Neirokhir* 1977;6:40–43.
12. Kliesch WF, Cruse JM, Lewis RE, et al. Restoration of depressed immune function in spinal cord injury patients receiving rehabilitation therapy. *Paraplegia* 1996;34(2):82–90.
13. Cruse JM, Keith JC, Bryant ML Jr, et al. Immune system-neuroendocrine dysregulation in spinal cord injury. *Immunol Res* 1996;15(4): 306–314.
14. Campagnolo DI, Bartlett JA, Keller SE, et al. Impaired phagocytosis of staphylococcus aureus in complete tetraplegics. *Am J Phys Med Rehabil* 1997;76(4):276–280.
15. Segal JL, Brunnemann SR. Circulating levels of soluble interleukin 2 receptors are elevated in the sera of humans with spinal cord injury. *J Am Paraplegia Soc* 1993;16(1):30–33.
16. Segal JL. Spinal cord injury: are interleukins a molecular link between neuronal damage and ensuing pathobiology? *Perspect Biol Med* 1993; 36(2):222–240.
17. Segal JL, Gonzales E, Yousefi S, et al. Circulating levels of IL-2R, ICAM-1, and IL-6 in spinal cord injuries. *Arch Phys Med Rehabil* 1997; 78(1):44–47.
18. Livnat S, Felten SY, Carlson SL, et al. Involvement of peripheral and central catecholamine systems in neural-immune interactions. *J Neuroimmunol* 1985;10:5–30.
19. Felten SY, Felten DL, Bellinger DL, et al. Noradrenergic sympathetic innervation of lymphoid organs. *Prog Allergy* 1988;43:13–36.
20. Dulis BH, Wilson IB. The β-adrenegic receptor of live human polymorphonuclear leukocytes. *J Biol Chem* 1980;255:1043–1048.
21. Galant SP, Allred S. Binding and functional characteristics of beta adrenergic receptors in the intact neutrophil. *J Lab Clin Med* 1981; 98(2):227–237.
22. Madden KS, Livnat S. Catecholamine action and immunologic reactivity. In: Ader R, Felton DL, Cohen N, eds. *Psychoneuroimmunology,* 2nd ed. San Diego: Academic Press, 1991:283–305.
23. Keller SE, Weiss JM, Miller NE, et al. Stress-induced suppression of immunity in adrenalectomized rats. *Science* 1983;221:1301–1304.

24. Keller SE, Schleifer SJ, Liotta AS, et al. Stress-induced alterations of immunity in hypophysectomized rats. *Proc Natl Acad Sci* 1988;85:9297–9301.

25. Campagnolo DI, Bartlett JA, Chatterton R, et al. Adrenal and pituitary hormone patterns following spinal cord injury. *Am J Phys Med Rehabil* 1999;78(4):361–366.

26. Shavit Y, Lewis JW, Terman GW, et al. Opioid peptides mediate the suppressive effect of stress on natural killer cell cytotoxicity. *Science* 1984;188–190.

27. Palmblad J, Cantell K, Strander H, et al. Stressor exposure and immunological response in man: interferon-producing capacity and phagocytosis. *J Psychosom Res* 1976;20:193–199.

28. Campagnolo DI, Barlett JA, Keller SE. Influence of neurologic level on immune function following spinal cord injury: a review. *J Spinal Cord Med* 2000;23:121–128.

29. Schleifer SJ, Keller SE, Camerino M, et al. Suppression of lymphocyte stimulation following bereavement. *JAMA* 1983;250:374.

30. Schleifer SJ, Keller SE, Bond RN, et al. Major depressive disorder and immunity. *Arch Gen Psychiatry* 1989;46:81–87.

31. Kiecolt-Glaser JK, Glaser R. Stress and immune function in humans. In: Ader R, Felton DL, Cohen N, eds. *Psychoneuroimmunology,* 2nd ed. San Diego: Academic Press, 1991:847–868.

32. Levine AM, Nash MS, Green BA, et al. An examination of dietary intakes and nutritional status of chronic healthy spinal cord injured individuals. *Paraplegia* 1992;30:880–889.

33. Barone J, Hebert JR, Reddy MM. Dietary fat and natural-killer-cell activity. *Am J Clin Nutr* 1989;50:861–867.

34. Jeffery NM, Sanderson P, Sherrington EJ, et al. The ratio of n-6 to n-3 polyunsaturated fatty acids in the rat diet alters serum lipid levels and lymphocyte functions. *Lipids* 1996;31:737–745.

35. Sanderson P, Yaqoob P, Calder PC. Effects of dietary lipid manipulation upon graft vs host and host vs graft responses in the rat. *Cell Immunol* 1995;164:240–247.

36. Chandra RK. Interactions of nutrition, infection and immune response. Immunocompetence in nutritional deficiency, methodological considerations and intervention strategies. *Acta Paediatr Scand* 1979;68:137–144.

37. Hoffman-Goetz L, Kluger MJ. Protein deficiency: its effects on body temperature in health and disease states. *Am J Clin Nutr* 1979;32:1423–1427.

38. Rose AH, Holt PG, Turner KJ. The effect of a low protein diet on the immunogenic activity of murine peritoneal macrophages. *Int Arch Allergy Appl Immunol* 1982;67:356–361.

39. Conn CA, Kozak WE, Tooten PC, et al. Effect of exercise and food restriction on selected markers of the acute phase response in hamsters. *J Appl Physiol* 1995;78:458–465.

40. Duckworth WC, Solomon SS, Jallepalli P, et al. Glucose intolerance due to insulin resistance in patients with spinal cord injuries. *Diabetes* 1980;29:906–910.

41. Bauman WA, Spungen AM. Disorders of carbohydrate and lipid metabolism in veterans with paraplegia or quadriplegia: a model of premature aging. *Metabolism* 1994;43:749–756.

42. Bagdade JD, Stewart M, Walters E. Impaired granulocyte adherence. A reversible defect in host defense in patients with poorly controlled diabetes. *Diabetes* 1978;27:677–681.

43. Hostetter MK. Handicaps to host defense. Effects of hyperglycemia on C3 and Candida albicans. *Diabetes* 1990;39:271–275.

44. Venkatraman JT, Rowland JA, Denardin E, et al. Influence of the level of dietary lipid intake and maximal exercise on the immune status in runners. *Med Sci Sports Exerc* 1997;29:333–344.

45. Pomposelli JJ, Baxter JK 3rd, Babineau TJ, et al. Early postoperative glucose control predicts nosocomial infection rate in diabetic patients. *J Parenter Enteral Nutr* 1998;22:77–81.

46. Graham NM, Burrell CJ, Douglas RM, et al. Adverse effects of aspirin, acetaminophen, and ibuprofen on immune function, viral shedding, and clinical status in rhinovirus-infected volunteers. *J Infect Dis* 1990;162:1277–1282.

47. Descotes J, Tedone R, Evreux JC. Suppression of humoral and cellular immunity in normal mice by diazepam. *Immunol Lett* 1982;5:41–42.

48. Schlumpf M, Ramseier H, Lichtensteiger W. Prenatal diazepam induced persisting depression of cellular immune responses. *Life Sci* 1989;44:493–501.

49. Nash MS. The immune system. In: Whiteneck G, Charlifue SW, Gerhart KA, et al, eds. *Aging with spinal cord injury.* New York: Demos Publications, 1993:159–182.

50. Crockard AD, Boylan MT, Droogan AG, et al. Methylprednisolone-induced neutrophil leukocytosis—down-modulation of neutrophil l-selectin and Mac-1 expression and induction of granulocyte-colony stimulating factor. *Int J Clin Lab Res* 1998;28:110–115.

51. Washburn RA, Figoni SF. Physical activity and chronic cardiovascular disease prevention in spinal cord injury: a comprehensive literature review. *Top Spinal Cord Injury Rehabil* 1998;3:16–32.

52. Crist DM, Mackinnon LT, Thompson RF, et al. Physical exercise increases natural cellular-mediated tumor cytotoxicity in elderly women. *Gerontology* 1989;35:66–71.

53. Kusaka Y, Kondou H, Morimoto K. Healthy lifestyles are associated with higher natural killer cell activity. *Prev Med* 1992;21:602–615.

54. Nieman DC, Nehlsen-Cannarella SL, Markoff PA, et al. The effects of moderate exercise training on natural killer cells and acute upper respiratory tract infections. *Int J Sports Med* 1990;11:467–473.

55. Shephard RJ, Rhind S, Shek PN. Exercise and training: influences on cytotoxicity, interleukin-1, interleukin-2 and receptor structures. *Int J Sports Med* 1994;15[Suppl 3]:S154–S166.

56. Asgeirsson G, Bellanti JA. Exercise, immunology, and infection. *Semin Adolesc Med* 1987;3:199–204.

57. Tvede N, Kappel M, Halkjaer-Kristensen J, et al. The effect of light, moderate and severe bicycle exercise on lymphocyte subsets, natural and lymphokine activated killer cells, lymphocyte proliferative response and interleukin 2 production. *Int J Sports Med* 1993;14:275–282.

58. Nieman DC, Buckley KS, Henson DA, et al. Immune function in marathon runners versus sedentary controls. *Med Sci Sports Exerc* 1995;27:986–992.

59. McCarthy DA, Dale MM. The leucocytosis of exercise. A review and model. *Sports Med* 1988;6:333–363.

60. Pedersen BK, Tvede N, Christensen LD, et al. Natural killer cell activity in peripheral blood of highly trained and untrained persons. *Int J Sports Med* 1989;10:129–131.

61. Bloomfield SA, Jackson RD, Mysiw WJ. Catecholamine response to exercise and training in individuals with spinal cord injury. *Med Sci Sports Exerc* 1994;26:1213–1219.

62. Wolfel EE, Hiatt WR, Brammell HL, et al. Plasma catecholamine responses to exercise after training with beta-adrenergic blockade. *J Appl Physiol* 1990;68:586–593.

63. Klokker M, Mohr T, Kjaer M, et al. The natural killer cell response to exercise in spinal cord injured individuals. *Eur J Appl Physiol* 1998;79:106–109.

64. Kay N, Allen J, Morley JE. Endorphins stimulate normal human peripheral blood lymphocyte natural killer activity. *Life Sci* 1984;35:53–59.

65. Furusawa K, Tajima F, Tanaka Y, et al. Short-term attenuation of natural killer cell cytotoxic activity in wheelchair marathoners with paraplegia. *Arch Phys Med Rehabil* 1998;79:1116–1121.

66. Weksler ME. Senescence of the immune system. *Med Clin North Am* 1983;67:263–272.

67. Phair JP, Hsu CS, Hsu YL. Ageing and infection. *Ciba Found Symp* 1988;134:143–154.

68. Haddy RI. Aging, infections, and the immune system. *J Fam Pract* 1988;27:409–413.

69. Ries DT, Salerno E, Sank J, et al. Over-the-counter medications: quicksand for the elderly. *J Community Health Nurs* 1986;3:183–189.

70. Sobel JD, Kaye D. The role of bacterial adherence in urinary tract infections in elderly adults. *J Gerontol* 1987;42:29–32.

71. Murasko DM, Weiner P, Kaye D. Decline in mitogen induced proliferation of lymphocytes with increasing age. *Clin Exp Immunol* 1987;70:440–448.

72. Weksler ME. The thymus gland and aging. *Ann Intern Med* 1983;98:105–107.

73. Shigemoto S, Kishimoto S, Yamamura Y. Change of cell-mediated cytotoxicity with aging. *J Immunol* 1975;115:307–309.

74. Ligthart GJ, Schuit HR, Hijmans W. Subpopulations of mononuclear cells in ageing: expansion of the null cell compartment and decrease in the number of T and B cells in human blood. *Immunology* 1985; 55:15–21.

75. Krishnaraj R, Blandford G. Age-associated alterations in human natural killer cells. 1. Increased activity as per conventional and kinetic analysis. *Clin Immunol Immunopathol* 1987;45:268–285.

76. Ershler WB. Biomarkers of aging: immunological events. *Exp Gerontol* 1988;23:387–389.

77. Nash M. Immune dysfunction and illness susceptibility after spinal cord injury: an overview of probable causes, likely consequences and potential treatments. *J Spinal Cord Med* 2000;23:109–110.

78. Darouiche RO, Hull RA. Bacterial interference for prevention of urinary tract infection: an overview. *J Spinal Cord Med* 2000;23:136–141.

NEUROMUSCULOSKELETAL COMPLICATIONS OF SPINAL CORD INJURY

JAMES W. LITTLE
STEPHEN P. BURNS

After a spinal cord injury (SCI), secondary neuromusculoskeletal complications can develop over time. Complications can affect bones, joints, muscles, peripheral nerves, and the spinal cord (1). These complications can develop within weeks of or many years after SCI. They can be minor inconveniences, further disable the individual, or may be life threatening. SCI clinicians must understand these potential complications, because they can often prevent or treat them. This chapter reviews musculoskeletal SCI complications first and then neurologic complications.

MUSCULOSKELETAL COMPLICATIONS

Because musculoskeletal complications often present as pain, clinicians must distinguish musculoskeletal pain from visceral pain and neurologic pain (see chapter 26 for additional details on pain after SCI) (2,3). Musculoskeletal pain is usually mechanically aggravated by movement or use and relieved by rest. Most musculoskeletal pain is due to local pathology, but systemic arthritis or bone disease must be considered. Local swelling or tenderness, loss of joint motion, and joint instability suggest a musculoskeletal complication. Musculoskeletal complications are particularly common in patients using their upper limbs for weight bearing. The upper limbs are primarily designed for prehensile activities, but in persons with SCI, they are used for weight bearing, including transfers, wheelchair propulsion, and walking using crutches.

If pain is acute or subacute, referred nociceptive visceral pain must be promptly excluded, because it may indicate a need for urgent care—for example, urinary tract infection, peptic ulcer disease, and angina. In cervical and high thoracic SCI, visceral pain is often poorly localized, understates the underlying pathology, and manifests late. SCI clinicians must have a low threshold for pursuing additional diagnostic tests to rule out cardiopulmonary, gastrointestinal, and genitourinary causes of referred nociceptive visceral pain. Nonnociceptive neuropathic visceral pain is chronic. Clinicians must consider the possibility that nociceptive and neuropathic pain can coexist and potentiate each other.

Chronic neurologic pain can be of two types: (a) nociceptive neurologic pain due to either ongoing peripheral nerve irritation or nerve root or spinal cord irritation; and (b) chronic neuropathic pain due to abnormal pain generation within the central nervous system (CNS) without any ongoing nociceptive stimulus. Associated new weakness, sensory loss, or reflex changes are suggestive of acute or subacute nociceptive neurologic pain, rather than musculoskeletal pain, and may be due to peripheral nerve entrapment, radiculopathy, or a posttraumatic syrinx. Chronic neuropathic pain is often characterized by burning, tingling, or stabbing and has no clear association with movement or activity. Pain in anesthetic areas or associated with hyperesthesia or dysesthesia suggests chronic neuropathic pain.

Osteoporosis, Fracture

After SCI, there is rapid loss of trabecular bone in the lower limbs and pelvis, so homeostasis is reached by about 16 months with bone mass at 50% to 70% normal and near fracture threshold (4,5). Bone loss also occurs in the upper limbs of persons with tetraplegia, but spinal bone density is relatively preserved. The bone loss is due to enhanced osteoclastic activity with relative hypercalcemia, hypercalciuria, and suppression of the parathyroid hormone–vitamin D axis; bone loss continues over subsequent years due to aging. Overt symptomatic hypercalcemia is uncommon but is seen most often in adolescent boys with acute tetraplegia. Because of this hypercalcemia risk and a nephrolithiasis risk, low calcium intake has been advocated. In the long term, this dietary restriction, along with reduced sunlight exposure and medications that accelerate vitamin D metabolism, can lead to vitamin D deprivation and secondary hyperparathyroidism with further bone loss (6) (see chapter 11 for details).

The cumulative incidence of long-bone fractures is said to be about 2.5% more than 20 years after SCI; however, the true incidence is probably higher because not all fractures are recognized and these patients do not all present to SCI centers (7). Fractures are more common in complete versus incomplete SCI and in women versus men. These fractures are common because of the demineralized bone in SCI. Most fractures are due to falls during transfers, but in patients who are severely osteoporotic, fractures can result from minor stresses (e.g., prolong sitting or range-of-motion [ROM] exercises) or without any known

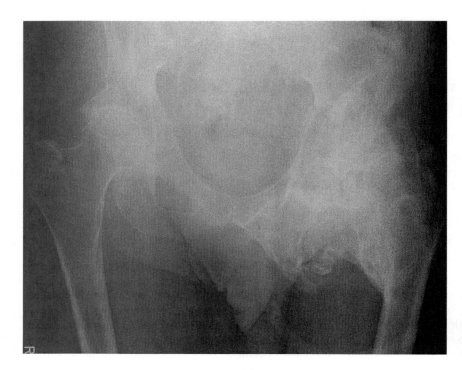

FIGURE 16.1. Lower limb fractures. This x-ray reveals a recent proximal tibiofibular fracture in a paraplegic man who fell during a transfer; he also has a healed supracondylar femur fracture.

etiology. Supracondylar and peritrochanteric femur fractures are most common, although femoral shaft, tibial, and humeral fractures are also common (Fig. 16.1) (8,9).

Fracture diagnosis in SCI individuals is subtler in the absence of pain. The patient may present with a swollen limb, malaise, and a low-grade fever. Other causes should be sought, but bony deformities, localized swelling, hematoma, and crepitus are evidence of a fracture. A plain x-ray will usually give a definitive diagnosis. Hospitalization is not always required and should be reserved for those who have severe swelling, who require surgery, or who require patient or family training to return home. Vascular studies should be performed if venous thrombosis or arterial injury is suspected.

The main goals of treatment are to minimize complications, to allow for bone healing with satisfactory alignment, and to preserve prefracture function (10–12). In patients with SCI not expected to ambulate, some degree of shortening and angulation is acceptable in full-time wheelchair users (10,12). Rotational deformity, however, is usually less acceptable. Most fractures are treated nonoperatively with soft-padded splints (11,12). A well-padded knee immobilizer is useful for femoral supracondylar, femoral shaft, and proximal tibial fractures; a well-padded ankle immobilizer can be used for distal tibial fractures. A soft splint can be made of a blanket wrapped around the fracture site and fixed with adhesive tape, but this is more difficult to keep clean and to remove and reapply (13). Circumferential casts should be avoided, but if they are used, they must be well padded and bivalved for skin inspection at least twice a day. Any skin breakdown that develops, even if superficial, must be treated aggressively; the source of the breakdown must be identified and eliminated.

Most fractures will heal using this approach. The patient does not need to remain in bed and should be mobile in the wheelchair within a few days. Having the legs flexed at the hip and knee in a wheelchair with feet flat on the footrests maintains functional positioning for healing. Callus formation is usually evident in 3 to 4 weeks; immobilization can usually be discontinued in 6 to 8 weeks and ROM exercises initiated, although weight bearing (tilt-table, standing, and stand-pivot transfers) should be delayed for a longer period (12–14). Nonunion of fractures occurs at a reported rate of 2% to 10%; however, this is not clinically significant in those who do not bear weight through their lower limbs (13–17). Increased spasms, venous thrombosis, and skin compromise can complicate fracture management in persons with SCI.

Methods commonly used for non-SCI fracture management (e.g., surgery, circumferential casting, and external fixation) are usually not indicated in the SCI population because of potential complications. Circumferential plaster casts or traction can cause skin breakdown because of sensory impairment (10,15,19). Surgical intervention for femoral shaft and distal femoral fractures is associated with a high complication rate because of bone quality, risk of osteomyelitis, and recurrent bacteremia (11,13–15, 18,20).

Surgical intervention may be indicated when conservative methods will not control rotational deformity. It may also be indicated for proximal femur fractures in patients who have severe muscle spasm; in patients for whom the splints are too bulky and interfere with function; if vascular supply is in danger, and if shortening and angulation will result in unacceptable function or cosmesis (10,12,13,17,18). Femoral neck and subtrochanteric fractures are probably the most difficult to manage and internal fixation may be considered if a minimal device such as an intramedullary rod can be used (12). Patients with femoral neck fractures can maintain prefracture mobility and may be mobilized without lower extremity (LE) immobilization, because splinting this area may be too difficult. Patients with intertrochanteric fractures can be seated in a wheelchair with their feet flat on the footrest and a pillow between the thighs. Femoral shaft and all other distal LE fractures, including tibial, ankle, and foot fractures, are usually treated with soft splints.

The cause of the fracture and the functional impact of the fracture must be considered. The patient may need acute or subacute rehabilitation for functional training; he or she may need additional assistance in the home and an alternate wheelchair, elevating leg rests, and wheelchair cushion. Deep venous thrombosis prophylaxis should be considered in all patients with SCI with lower limb fractures, for perhaps 7 to 14 days (21), although the optimal duration has not been established.

Spine

Spine fusion can lead to excessive stresses above or below the fusion. Those spine segments that are normally most mobile (i.e., C5-T1 and T12-L1) may be surgically fused, causing exaggerated forces on adjacent segments; spinal instability can develop. Such instability can lead to further bony and ligamentous destruction with resulting gross instability, referred to as Charcot spine or neuropathic spinal arthropathy (22–24). Charcot spine may present as worsening deformity with or without overlying skin breakdown, loss of sitting balance, increased spine pain, or neurologic change caudal to the SCI (e.g., loss of spasticity and loss of reflex bladder emptying). Diagnosis is usually evident on plain radiographs, with instability typically developing in the thoracic or lumbar spine, one to two segments caudal to a spinal fusion. Anterior and posterior surgical stabilization, with prolonged postoperative bracing, is often needed to prevent worsening deformity. Limited hip flexion ROM can amplify forces on the spine with sitting and may need to be corrected before spine surgery.

Other spine deformities are seen post-SCI, including cervical spine hyperlordosis or kyphosis, thoracic gibbous deformity, or scoliosis due to asymmetric strength or tone. Scoliosis is particularly common in pediatric SCI, when the cord injury occurs before puberty; as many as two thirds of such pediatric SCI cases will require surgery for scoliosis, in contrast to about 5% of adult-onset SCI (25).

New spine mechanical pain is often an indication of a spine complication or spine instrumentation failure (e.g., broken or displaced rod, plate, or screw). Other symptoms may include awareness of worsening deformity or a sensation of grinding or clanking with spine movements. X-rays plus or minus dynamic views, computed tomographic (CT) scan, and bone scan may be needed for evaluation. Spine biopsy may be needed to distinguish spine infection, spine tumor, and Charcot spine. Interventions for spine complications may include the use of a cervical or thoracolumbar brace, analgesics for pain, exercise and activity modification, and surgical stabilization for unstable spine or instrumentation failure. A seating system, which facilitates proper posture, can help prevent spinal deformities after SCI.

Shoulder

Shoulder pain is the most commonly reported painful joint after SCI. It is estimated that 30% to 50% of patient with SCI have shoulder pain of such severity that it interferes with self-care, and this prevalence increases with time since SCI (26–30). Pain during the first year after SCI is more common in tetraplegics, whereas pain in later years is more common in paraplegics. Shoulder pain can interfere with transfers, manual wheelchair propulsion, overhead reaching, and sleep; it can also limit vocational and recreational pursuits (31,32).

Shoulder pain in patients with SCI is believed to represent a form of overuse syndrome resulting from wheelchair propulsion, transfers, and other activities of daily living. Impingement syndrome after SCI results from upper limb weight bearing, which leads to upward humeral migration with glenohumeral laxity, articular wear and loss of cartilage, and subsequent arthritis or rotator cuff pathology. Use of an over-the-bed trapeze can also aggravate shoulder impingement.

Due to LE paralysis, people with SCI must rely extensively on their upper limbs to perform activities of daily living. Any further loss of upper limb function because of pain may have adverse effects on mobility and functional independence, as well as long-term health consequences (31,33).

It is estimated that two thirds of shoulder pain is due to chronic impingement syndrome, and half involves rotator cuff pathology (27). Complete or partial rotator cuff tears were found in 71% of symptomatic paraplegic patients (34). Bicipital tendonitis, subacromial bursitis, adhesive capsulitis, acromioclavicular degenerative joint disease, and cervical radiculopathy are other common causes of shoulder pain in chronic SCI (35–39). Other causes that are specific in the SCI population include muscle imbalance, spasticity, contractures, heterotopic ossification, and the presence of a syrinx. The specific cause of shoulder pain often results from a combination of factors unique to each patient.

The approach to shoulder pain in the patient with chronic SCI is similar to that for able-bodied persons, keeping in mind the special potential causes in SCI. A complete focused examination should include ROM, flexibility, strength, sensory testing, provocative tests for specific abnormalities, and a functional assessment. This includes an evaluation of the patient's posture, function (e.g., pressure releases, wheelchair mobility, and transfers), and home and work environments. Restrictions of scapulothoracic and glenohumeral motion should be identified. Sacral sitting in a wheelchair with thoracic kyphosis and cervical lordosis because of absent trunk muscles can lead to more flexed glenohumeral and more protracted scapulothoracic postures; this can lead to tendonitis or bursitis. Radiologic tests of the cervical spine or shoulder and electrodiagnosis should only be carried out if the diagnosis is unclear or to rule out a specific abnormality. X-rays may reveal superior migration of the humeral head with or without articulation to the acromion and narrowed glenohumeral joint space.

A recently developed questionnaire is useful for evaluating shoulder pain in patients with SCI. The Wheelchair User's Shoulder Pain Index (WUSPI) is a 15-item self-report instrument that measures shoulder pain intensity during various activi-

TABLE 16.1. WHEELCHAIR USER'S SHOULDER PAIN INDEX

1. Pushing wheelchair >10 min
2. Pushing wheelchair up ramps or on inclines
3. Sleeping
4. Loading wheelchair into car
5. Lifting object from overhead
6. Daily activities at work or school
7. Household chores
8. Wheelchair-car transfer
9. Wheelchair-tub transfer
10. Driving
11. Washing back
12. Bed-wheelchair transfer
13. Putting on T-shirt or pullover
14. Putting on pants
15. Putting on button-down shirt

Note: Listed in order of more to less pain for paraplegic individuals. From Curtis KA, Loach KE, Applegate EB, et al. Reliability and validity of the wheelchair user's shoulder pain index (WUSPI). *Paraplegia* 1995;33:595–601, with permission.

ties of daily living (Table 16.1) (31,39). Each item is scored using a 10-cm visual analog scale, which is anchored at the ends with "no pain" and "worst pain ever experienced." Individual item scores are summed to arrive at a total index score, which ranges from 0 to 150. The WUSPI is reported to be a valid and reliable measure of shoulder pain during functional activities in wheelchair users with no upper extremity weakness (39).

Early and aggressive management is needed; treatments can relieve pain, reduce inflammation, strengthen muscles, teach precautions, teach proper posture and proper biomechanics, minimize injurious activities, provide optimal equipment for mobility and self-care, and improve home and work environments. Relief of acute pain is achieved with pharmacologic intervention (e.g., nonsteroidal antiinflammatory drugs, acetaminophen, and muscle relaxants), rest, and modalities. Injection techniques into the subacromial bursa or appropriate space may be helpful. Unlike in an able-bodied individual, it is difficult for patients with SCI to completely rest a painful shoulder because of its role in functional activities. Decreasing stress imposed on the painful joint should be encouraged by using compensatory techniques, such as using a transfer board rather than performing lateral transfers, obtaining assistance when performing weight shifts, or using a power wheelchair. In some patients, complete rest may be required. Modalities such as ultrasound and transcutaneous electrical nerve stimulation, as well as acupuncture, may be helpful (40,41).

Once the pain has subsided, the emphasis of treatment is focused toward protecting the shoulder joint and preventing further problems. The main objective is to obtain a balance in strength and flexibility of the musculature surrounding the shoulder. Often overlooked for a well-balanced shoulder is maintenance of proper seated posture, as well as correcting or improving the patient's functional techniques and equipment. Exercise should then be prescribed to restore strength and balance of pectoral muscles; anterior muscles (e.g., pectoralis major) are tight and posterior muscles are overstretched and weakened.

Rowing and backward wheeling are exercises that can strengthen posterior scapular retractor and humeral depressor muscles (42). Recently, a study investigated the effectiveness of a 6-month exercise protocol on shoulder pain in wheelchair users. The study found that although the protocol resulted in decreased pain, these changes were not observed until 4 months into the study. The subjects in the treatment group actually experienced an initial increase in shoulder pain during the first 2 months (43).

Prescription of a wheelchair with a positive seat angle and a vertical, low backrest to allow lumbar lordosis while lessening thoracic kyphosis or cervical lordosis can lessen impingement, tendonitis, and bursitis (44). Diet instruction for weight loss is often indicated. Consider a power wheelchair prescription, if manual wheelchair propulsion is limited by pain. Surgery can be considered in those who fail conservative management; however, surgery involves months of postoperative healing and does not guarantee that pain will be eliminated or function restored (45).

Elbow, Wrist, Hand

Elbow pain is often due to overuse of elbows, as well as weight bearing and leaning on elbows (29,46,47). Olecranon bursitis and medial and lateral epicondylitis are common, and elbow degenerative joint disease can develop. Carpal instability, dorsal radiocarpal impingement, and scaphoid impaction syndrome are common with weight bearing through an extended wrist, as is carpal tunnel syndrome (CTS) (48). Overuse can also lead to ulnar nerve entrapment at the wrist (Guyon canal), de Quervain disease or other tenosynovitis, osteoarthritis, and stress fractures (see later discussion for a description of CTS and other nerve entrapments as complications of SCI).

In summary, many individuals with SCI develop upper extremity musculoskeletal pain from the cumulative trauma of functional activities they must perform. As patients age, they will either decrease their function or need to modify their equipment to accommodate their pain. An important aspect in treating any patient with SCI therefore is to analyze any repetitive motions the patient is required to perform and improve the patient's body mechanics and techniques used. Because many chronic upper limb musculoskeletal problems are due to overuse from functional activities, it is vital that proper exercise techniques and shoulder protection and conservation be learned early during acute rehabilitation and reinforced frequently. Often one hears the phrase "no pain, no gain," although the SCI team should teach their patients to "conserve it, to preserve it" (49).

Hip

Hip flexion contractures are particularly disabling in those for whom walking is a realistic goal. This is common in patients with fractures at the thoracolumbar junction (e.g., T10-L3); spine stabilization procedures at these levels will limit lumbar lordosis, so lumbar lordosis cannot be substituted for limitations of hip extension. In this setting, hip extension range is often critical for walking, because these patients often have hip extension weakness and must keep the upper body center of gravity behind the axis of rotation of the hip joint to maintain standing without upper limb weight bearing. Hip flexion contractures can result from myotendinous contracture of the iliopsoas, from hip joint capsule tightness, or from heterotopic ossification anterior to the hip joint. Clinicians can educate patients with SCI in the use of prone lying to prevent hip flexion contractures.

Hip subluxation and dislocation are most common in young pediatric patients with SCI and in those with hip adductor or flexor spasms (50). This hip instability can lead to pelvic obliquity, scoliosis, and pressures sores. Degenerative changes in the hip joint may be more common in those with cervical, rather than thoracic or lumbar, SCI and in those who are less active (29).

Knee, Ankle, Foot

Hamstring and ankle plantar-flexion contractures are common; preventing these contractures is important, particularly in those who will ambulate. Stretching, serial casting, nerve blocks, and surgical release may be needed. Overstretching of hamstring muscles must be avoided, because they aid pelvis stabilization in sitting.

Muscle

Muscle changes contribute to weakness after SCI. Muscles innervated caudal to an SCI, paralyzed from upper motoneuron–type weakness, undergo muscle fiber transformation from slow-twitch, fatigue-resistant oxidative type I fibers to fast-twitch, fatigable glycolytic type II fibers (51–53). Also, low levels of testosterone and growth hormone with reduced insulin-like growth factor (IGF-I) in some patients with SCI can contribute to reduced muscle mass (54). Treatment with anabolic steroids may be useful in some patients with SCI, although this is still considered experimental.

Aging leads to weakness in the able-bodied person; there is a 30% decline in strength between ages 60 and 90. Factors causing this strength decline include motoneuron loss, muscle atrophy, and impaired upper motoneuron recruitment (55–59). This aging-related weakness may be even more functionally significant in those with SCI because (a) there is less reserve for accomplishing functional tasks and (b) sprouting by motoneurons to compensate for loss at the time of SCI may lead to more weakness, if some spared motoneurons die with aging. Motoneuron loss with aging is largely a diagnosis by exclusion because electrodiagnostic studies are insensitive for identifying this cause. There are no well-established treatments, but ensuring adequate nutritional intake, avoiding muscle overuse, and providing compensatory rehabilitation may help.

NEUROLOGIC COMPLICATIONS

New weakness or new sensory loss is a reported secondary complication for about 20% to 30% of persons with SCI over time (60,61,62). Early and accurate diagnosis of a neurologic complication is aided by a baseline neurologic examination using standardized classification (e.g., American Spinal Injury Association classification), baseline magnetic resonance imaging (MRI) of

the spinal cord, and by serial quantitative strength testing (63–66). Electrodiagnostic tests, including peripheral motor and sensory nerve conduction studies, segmental H-reflex and F-wave studies, and long-tract somatosensory and motor evoked potential (MEP) studies, can help distinguish peripheral nerve from spinal cord complications (67). Timely diagnosis permits early treatment and can reverse neurologic decline (62).

Peripheral Nerve

Peripheral nerve entrapment is common in persons with SCI; this prevalence approaches 10% by clinical criteria but may be as much as 50% or more by electrodiagnostic criteria (62,68–70). Upper limb use such as with wheelchair propulsion, push-up transfers, and crutch walking increases the risk of peripheral nerve entrapment. Also, cervical cord injury may lead to a double-crush phenomenon, in which residual cord or root impingement proximally impairs axoplasmic transport and predisposes to distal nerve entrapment (71). CTS and ulnar nerve entrapment at the elbow are most common, although radial nerve entrapment at the spiral groove, peroneal nerve entrapment at the fibular head, and ulnar nerve entrapment at the wrist are also seen (62,70,72). Providing elbow pads or wrist splints, altering the biomechanics of transfers and wheelchair propulsion, as well as surgical decompression, may need to be considered.

CTS by electrodiagnostic criteria is noted in about half of patients with chronic SCI, with higher incidence rates seen at longer times after injury (30,68–70). Pressures within the carpal tunnel are within the reference range at rest in paraplegics; however, during functional activities, these pressures are greatly elevated (68,73–75). This is significant because individuals with SCI use their hands repetitively for functional activities in positions that will increase these pressures. This recurrent stress from transfers, wheelchair propulsion, and pressure reliefs increases the risk of median nerve compromise at the carpal tunnel, with cumulative events over years after injury. Electrophysiologic testing has revealed an incidence of CTS between 41% and 63% (68,69,73). Compressive neuropathy of the ulnar nerve at the wrist or elbow occurs less frequently than CTS but is also a function of repetitive trauma due to propelling a wheelchair and performing transfers.

Assessment includes inspection, palpation (e.g., for tenderness, crepitus, and joint instability), neurologic examination (e.g., for weakness, sensory loss, and reflex changes), and functional examination (e.g., to identify mobility, self-care, or vocational activities that load or stress joints). X-rays and electrodiagnostic studies may be needed to confirm the clinical diagnosis.

Treatments include analgesics, nonsteroidal antiinflammatory drugs, injections (anesthetic or corticosteroid), physical modalities (e.g., ultrasound and friction massage), exercises for stretching and strengthening, and functional training to correct poor technique, minimizing mechanical loads, optimizing equipment, and optimizing environment.

For CTS, rest is important, along with splinting (particularly at night), although rest from hand use is often difficult to achieve in persons with SCI. Steroid injection into the carpal tunnel may also be helpful. Techniques for transfers, pressure reliefs, and wheelchair propulsion should be modified to avoid end-range stresses at the wrist. The use of padded gloves while propelling the wheelchair can help protect the hands and wrists. If relief is not obtained, surgical release may be required; the postoperative recovery time must be weighed against the long-term benefits of the procedure.

Spinal Cord

Worsening myelopathy affects 5% to 20% of persons with SCI and can result from various causes (62). One of the most common is posttraumatic syringomyelia (PTS), a fluid-filled cyst elongating in the gray matter from the SCI level, causing additional cord damage. Another common cause is spinal canal or neuroforaminal stenosis due to residual bone fragments, spine instability, degenerative arthritis, or disk herniation (76,77). Other myelopathy may be due to arachnoiditis or meningeal scarring with myelomalacia or cord tethering with traction of spinal cord and root axons (78–82). Kyphotic deformity of the spine with traction on the cord and vitamin B_{12} deficiency can also cause worsening myelopathy in persons with SCI. Multiple sclerosis can develop in persons with SCI. The cause of worsening myelopathy is often identified with imaging (MRI, flexion-extension spine x-rays, myelogram CT scan) and blood studies such as vitamin B_{12}, methylmalonic acid, and thyroid-stimulation hormone blood levels (83–87). Slow-onset myelopathy may be mistaken for polyneuropathy and these myelopathies can predispose to peripheral nerve entrapment (62,71,88,89). Electrodiagnostic studies can often determine whether one or both are present and guide treatment (67). Patients with narrowed cervical canals are at high risk for new or worsening myelopathy with even minor trauma; they must be educated to avoid contact sports or other high-risk activities (90). Spine surgery may be needed for decompression or stabilization.

Posttraumatic Syringomyelia

A posttraumatic syrinx is evident in 3% to 8% of patients with SCI as neurologic decline, in 12% to 28% as an elongated cavity by MRI (Fig. 16.2), and in 17% to 20% as an elongated cavity at autopsy (61,64,89,91–98). In some, the cavity is multiloculated with glial septa. PTS has also been called ascending cystic degeneration or progressive posttraumatic cystic myelopathy. Posttraumatic cysts are small cystic structures that do not extend longitudinally and do not cause neurologic decline; as many as 39% to 59% of patients with SCI have such intramedullary cysts at the zone of cord injury (Table 16.2) (64,99,100).

A syrinx may develop at any time, from 2 months to decades after injury. It is one of the most common causes of worsening myelopathy after SCI, and it can be devastating because it may cause new disability after a person with SCI has successfully completed rehabilitation from their SCI (62).

The pathogenesis of posttraumatic syrinxes is unknown. The cavity begins at the level of the cord injury; it originates in the gray matter between the dorsal horns and posterior columns, which is a relatively avascular zone between the dorsal and ventral arterial supply (101). One initiating factor is likely cord hematoma with enzymatic lysis to an intramedullary cyst at the injury level (102,103). Other initiating factors may be arachnoiditis or

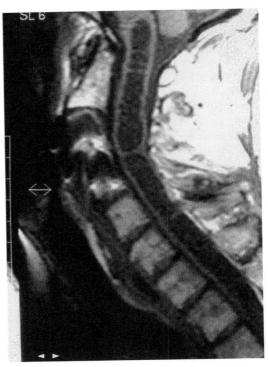

FIGURE 16.2. Posttraumatic syringomyelia. A large posttraumatic syrinx extends rostrally from the site of cord injury at T4 to the medulla on this T1-weighted magnetic resonance image. Despite extensive involvement of the cervical cord by this large dilating syrinx, the patient has full strength and function in his upper limbs.

meningeal scarring from subarachnoid bleeding or residual spinal canal stenosis and residual spinal kyphotic deformity; these deformities can lead to cord tethering, with resulting increased cord tension on spine flexion and to impaired cerebrospinal fluid (CSF) flow in the subarachnoid space (61,96,104,105). Patients with SCI with less than 15 degrees of residual kyphosis and less than 25% canal stenosis are half as likely to develop a posttraumatic syrinx (96). Cord tension may pull open cystic cavities and traction cord vessels, causing gray-matter ischemia; later, this myelomalacia due to gray-matter ischemia may coalesce into a syrinx (91,105). Cord tethering, cord tension, and impaired CSF flow can also result from spine fractures, spine angulation, disk protrusion, infectious meningitis, and spinal cord tumors; all can predispose to syringomyelia. Uncommon traumatic cyst-to-subarachnoid fistulas may allow more direct transmission of subarachnoid pressure surges to the cyst and lead to more rapid syrinx development (91,106,107).

Various factors lead to syrinx enlargement. The cyst may extend rostrally or caudally by dissecting through intermediate gray matter, often unilaterally (108). Posttraumatic syrinxes usually do not communicate with the fourth ventricle or the central canal (107,109–111). This longitudinal pressure dissection may result from pulsatile increases in subarachnoid fluid pressure due to coughing, sneezing, straining, Valsalva or Credé pressure over the abdomen, weight lifting, forward-lean pressure release, and quad coughing—i.e., intraabdominal or intrathoracic pressure increases, which are transmitted via valveless inferior vena cava and azygous veins to the epidural venous plexus (102,112–115). Subarachnoid pressure increases either pump fluid into the syrinx cavity via perivascular spaces (Virchow-Robin spaces) or cause a surge of fluid in the syrinx to "slosh rostrally" (110, 116–119). In an ovoid cavity, such as a spinal syrinx, pressure is greatest where the curvature is greatest; hence, syrinxes often extend at the poles and become long tubular structures (120). The perivascular spaces of Virchow-Robin may act as one-way valves, allowing fluid ingress from subarachnoid space into the syrinx but limiting egress; this may explain high pressures and high protein concentrations in some syrinxes (89,121). The dilated spinal cord may also be compressed against spondylitic encroachments, leading to additional neurologic decline (122).

Syrinxes due to spinal cord processes (e.g., cord injury, cord tumors, and arachnoiditis) usually originate in the gray matter and are lined with glial cells. Syrinxes that arise due to foramen magnum encroachment (e.g., Chiari I malformation) may originate in the central canal and are often referred to as hydromyelia; they likely represent impaired CSF flow at the fourth ventricle or foramen magnum (107). Because the two processes often cannot be distinguished by imaging studies, they may be referred to as syringohydromyelia or hydrosyringomyelia.

Early symptoms and signs of PTS are often nonspecific and variable; some patients with markedly elongated syrinxes that dilate the spinal cord may have minimal symptoms. The symptoms and signs are often unilateral early in the evolution of PTS, becoming bilateral later (89,92,123). A common presenting symptom of syringomyelia is pain, which is seen in 36% to 80% of patients with PTS (89,91,92,124). The pain is usually located at the site of the original injury or may radiate to the neck or upper limbs. The pain is described as an aching or burning, and is often worse when coughing, sneezing, straining, sitting rather than lying supine, or driving on a bumpy road. The next most common symptom is an ascending sensory loss level. This loss may be unilateral, bilateral, or intermittent in nature. Ascending sensory loss is found in 60% to 97%, typically as dissociated sensory loss with impaired pain and temperature sensation but intact touch, position, and vibration sense; loss of pain sensation can lead to a Charcot joint or neurogenic arthropathy (Fig. 16.3) (89,91,92,124). Worsening weakness is noted in 32% to 80% of patients with SCI who develop PTS (89,91,92,124,125) but rarely occurs in isolation (93,101). Muscle fasciculations and atrophy are noted later. An early sign of a syrinx is ascending loss of deep tendon reflexes and is often elicited before the onset of symptoms (126,127).

Less common clinical findings include increased or decreased spasticity, hyperhidrosis, autonomic dysreflexia, neck muscle fatigue with prolonged sitting, loss of reflex bladder emptying, worsening orthostatic hypotension, scoliosis, central or obstructive sleep apnea, new Horner syndrome, reduced respiratory drive, impaired vagal cardiovascular reflexes, and sudden death (89,128). With severe progression of a high cervical syrinx, one may see symptoms of diaphragmatic paralysis and cranial nerve involvement, including sensory loss in the trigeminal nerve distribution, dysphagia, dysphonia, and nystagmus. Symptoms may be postural and may be worse either in the sitting position or while lying supine, likely because of redistribution of fluid within the syrinx and distention of pain-sensitive structures (129). Loss

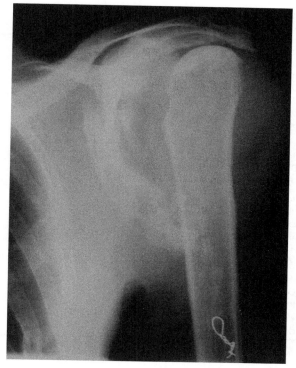

FIGURE 16.3. Charcot joint. The glenoid cavity and humeral head are massively eroded in this patient with Charcot joint due to posttraumatic syringomyelia for 45 years. He initially had a traumatic T2 paraplegia but later lost pain and temperature sensation in his upper limbs due to cervical cord involvement by the syrinx.

of protective pain and temperature sensation can lead to neurogenic arthropathy, pressure sores, and burns, often involving upper limbs.

PTS is variable in its manifestations and its rate of worsening. Long, dilating, rapidly developing syrinxes are most symptomatic, manifest as weakness and loss of function, but very long, very dilated syrinxes can manifest with minimal symptoms. There is no constant relationship between syrinx size on MRI and symptoms or degree of disability. Short dilating syrinxes can manifest as weakness and loss of function, particularly in regard to lower limb function mediated by long tracts in those with incomplete SCI. Short or long, dilating or nondilating syrinxes may be associated with neuropathic pain. With regard to natural history, syrinxes can spontaneously resolve; they can worsen then plateau; they can worsen intermittently; or they can worsen continuously. Syrinxes often worsen more rapidly if they show an early onset.

MRI is the gold standard for diagnosing PTS (Fig. 16.2). The characteristic finding is an intramedullary cyst with well-defined margins that is eccentric, extends beyond the limits of the original cord injury, does not communicate with the central canal or the fourth ventricle, and is isodense with CSF—that is, low-density T1-weighted image, high-density T2-weighted image. Syrinx MRI characteristics that are often associated with neurologic decline are syrinxes that are longer and wider, syrinxes with CSF flow from cardiac-gated images, syrinxes with poorly

TABLE 16.2. SPINAL CORD MAGNETIC RESONANCE IMAGING FINDINGS POST–SPINAL CORD INJURY

Posttraumatic syrinx:
- Eccentric, ovoid, or tubular intramedullary lesion
- Smooth, well-defined margins ± septa
- Often extends two or more spinal segments from SCI level
- Uniform signal intensity, isodense with CSF
- Often dilates the spinal cord

Posttraumatic cyst:
- Intramedullary fluid-filled cavity with well-defined margins
- Round, focal at SCI level—i.e., extends one segment or less
- Does not dilate the spinal cord
- Does not enlarge over time

Myelomalacia:
- Intramedullary lesion with ill-defined margins
- Extends one or more segments from SCI level
- Signal intensity between neural tissue and CSF on T1- and T2-weighted images
- May be due to ischemia with microcystic degeneration and gliosis

Arachnoiditis/meningeal scarring/cord tethering:
- Cord adhesion to canal wall
- Irregularly defined spinal cord
- Septations in or absence of subarachnoid space
- Abnormal flow-void signals in subarachnoid space

SCI, spinal cord injury; CSF, cerebrospinal fluid.

demarcated T2-weighted signal hyperintensity at the rostral extent, syrinxes with a flow-void sign on T2-weighted images, suggesting high pressure, and syrinxes associated with spinal stenosis (61,64,92,105,130–132). Limitations of MRI are that metal (e.g., rods, wires, plates, screws, and bullet fragments) may distort cord images, and there can be, although rarely, false-positive and false-negative MRI results for syrinxes. False-positive MRI results may include myelomalacia (e.g., ischemic cord damage or gliosis and microcystic degeneration), cord hemorrhage, and tumor (84,115,133). False-negative MRI results for PTS can occur when syrinx fluid is proteinaceous and the signal density is similar to neural tissue (133). Intravenous contrast agents with gadolinium can improve the distinction between syrinxes and intramedullary or extramedullary tumors, arteriovenous malformation, and multiple sclerosis plaques. CSF velocity imaging, obtaining images gated to the cardiac cycle, can also aid in distinguishing syrinxes from cystic myelomalacia and arachnoid cysts.

Other imaging studies can be useful for evaluating PTS and for distinguishing it from other progressive myelopathies. Conventional spine x-rays with flexion-extension views may help diagnose spinal instability, disk-space infection, and spinal stenosis. Metrizamide myelogram with immediate and delayed CT scans can aid in the diagnosis of PTS, arachnoiditis, and disk herniation.

Early electrodiagnostic findings in PTS include (a) prolonged segmental conduction on F-wave studies and (b) prolonged descending motor conduction on MEP testing (134,135). Later electrodiagnostic findings include (a) reduced compound muscle action potential amplitude, (b) enlarged motor-unit action potential (MUAP) amplitude consistent with motoneuron loss and

compensatory motor axon sprouting by spared motoneurons, and (c) reduced maximal firing rate of motor units during maximal voluntary effort consistent with reduced upper motoneuron input to lower motoneurons. Thus, there are often findings of mixed lower and upper motoneuron loss. Sensory nerve action potentials are preserved, except when there is an associated peripheral nerve entrapment, which occurs commonly (89,134). Muscle membrane instability is a late finding, presumably because the lower motoneuron loss is gradual and there is ongoing compensatory sprouting to minimize the number of denervated muscle fibers in a muscle.

Neurologic monitoring is essential to decide whether current treatment is adequate. Large syrinxes on MRI are often clinically asymptomatic. Some argue not to surgically decompress the syrinx until the patient becomes symptomatic. Others warn that early treatment is needed, or neuronal loss may advance silently and become irreversible. If nonoperative treatment is chosen, then close neurologic monitoring is needed to ensure that the patient is neurologically stable. The clinical neurologic examination may be inadequately sensitive to detect neurologic decline before irreversible damage has occurred. Neurologic monitoring can include pinprick self-exam by the patient, serial quantitative strength testing, serial electrodiagnostic studies (F waves, MEPs, MUAP amplitude), and serial MRI. Similar neurologic monitoring is needed postoperatively to ensure adequacy of the surgical decompression of the syrinx.

PTS can lead to neurologic decline of sufficient degree to cause functional loss. In severe cases, a fully independent person with paraplegia may become totally dependent for transfers and self-care with tetraplegia (109,136). Another common scenario for functional loss in PTS is the walking incomplete tetraplegic patient; such individuals regain walking and bowel and bladder control during initial rehabilitation and then lose walking and bowel and bladder control years later due a posttraumatic syrinx. In addition to disability from either ascending cord involvement or long-tract cord involvement in those with incomplete SCI, other factors can contribute to functional loss in PTS, including severe neuropathic pain, extensor spasms, and neuropathic joints. Noncystic myelopathy such as myelomalacia and cord tethering seemingly cause pain, sensory loss, and weakness, but the degree to which they cause functional decline is less clearly described.

Both conservative and surgical treatments have been advocated for PTS. Conservative treatments have not been carefully studied. Conservative treatment is often defined as clinical observation without any specific intervention. However, conservative management may also include activity restrictions; altering fluid dynamics in the spinal cord by reducing CSF production and by lowering venous pressures; percutaneous drainage of the syrinx, ensuring there are no secondary causes of myelopathy such as vitamin B_{12} deficiency; and providing rehabilitation interventions as needed (e.g., functional training and adaptive equipment). Activity restrictions include avoiding all maneuvers that might transmit venous pressures to the subarachnoid space: avoiding high-force exercise, avoiding Valsalva and Credé and quad coughing with direct compression over the inferior vena cava, and avoiding forward-lean pressure releases. Altering fluid dynamics in the spinal cord may include giving agents to reduce

CSF production; keeping the head of the bed elevated 20 degrees at night to lessen rostral slosh of fluid in the syrinx; using agents to promote venous dilation and lower venous pressures; and using agents to lessen fluid accumulation during the day because of orthostatic hypotension. Other treatable causes of myelopathy should be identified and addressed. Percutaneous drainage by tapping the syrinx with a needle under CT guidance and then withdrawing fluid from the syrinx has provided years of benefit in a few cases, but in most cases, there is reaccumulation of fluid within weeks (137,138). Whether a combination of these conservative measures can prevent neurologic decline without surgery has not been determined in clinical studies.

Surgical treatment is usually indicated if there is ongoing neurologic decline or severe intractable pain. Ideally, one should not wait until there is overt weakness to undertake surgery; if weakness develops due to a syrinx, prompt surgery should be considered because deficits can become irreversible if there is a prolonged delay before surgery (91,115,138). Surgical treatments have included (a) syringotomy or marsupialization to drain the syrinx, (b) shunting (syringosubarachnoid, syringopleural, or syringoperitoneal) (c) reconstructing the subarachnoid space with dissection of arachnoiditis or meningeal scarring and duraplasty, and (d) cordectomy (115,118,121,138–145).

Conservative nonoperative treatment is favored by some if there is no apparent or minimal neurologic decline, although in most studies, follow-up is for less than 10 years (91,92,146, 147). Rossier et al. (89) stated that "a patient, if followed long enough, will eventually show some signs of progression." Patients with a syrinx who are managed conservatively must be monitored closely; if they show significant decline, surgical treatment may need to be considered.

Surgery yields improved strength and improved pain control in some patients, whereas sensory recovery is not usually as favorable. Reduction of syrinx size on postoperative MRI usually predicts a good surgical result; however, complete resolution of the syrinx is not necessary for a good clinical outcome (148). With either shunting or arachnoid dissection or subarachnoid space reconstruction with duraplasty, there is recurrence of neurologic decline by 5 years in as many as 50% of patients (138, 145). In some, the failure is due to recurrence of the syrinx; shunts often occlude because of "collapse of syrinx cavity around the catheter tip with subsequent glial ingrowth into the shunt openings" (144). Shunts or duraplasty may fail even though the syrinx remains decompressed by MRI; cord tethering by the shunt or recurrent meningeal fibrosis may contribute. Patients with functional use in the lower limbs (i.e., American Spinal Injury Association [ASIA] class D or E) may be at particularly high risk for neurologic decline after shunting (147,149); the shunt tube may compromise descending motor axons coursing adjacent to the syrinx. Thus, ambulatory patients with SCI may benefit most from conservative treatment or arachnoid dissection or subarachnoid space reconstruction with duraplasty. Those with complete SCI (ASIA A) may benefit from cordectomy, which reportedly yields long-term neurologic stability in most patients (118,138).

Cervical or Lumbar Myeloradiculopathy

Late spinal cord or root compression is another common cause of neurologic decline in patients with SCI (62,67). Patients with SCI appear to have an increased risk for such decline; several factors likely contribute: (a) these patients often have congenital or degenerative spinal stenosis, (b) they may develop spinal instability in segments immediately rostral or caudal to a spine fusion, (c) they have altered spine biomechanics, which can lead to severe vertebral or disk degenerative changes, and (d) they may have residual bone fragments impinging cord or roots from the initial spine injury (26,76,77,150–152). Clinical findings are variable; they may have motor or sensory findings and they may have radicular or myelopathic findings. Quantitative myometry and electrodiagnosis can aid diagnosis of such late neurologic decline; serial studies help clinicians distinguish new abnormalities from those due to the original SCI. Such neurologic decline is often treated conservatively with a spinal orthosis, pain medications, and adaptive equipment. Persons with persisting cervical stenosis must be cautioned to avoid even minor cervical trauma, because this can cause irreversible neurologic decline. Surgery is considered if there is severe or rapid neurologic decline or uncontrolled pain (76,77).

Arachnoiditis/Meningeal Scarring with Spinal Cord Tethering

The normal cervical spinal cord ascends rostrally several centimeters with neck flexion (153). After SCI, arachnoiditis or meningeal scarring may tether the spinal cord, prevent this normal rostrocaudal sliding, and cause excessive cord tension or ischemia. MRI findings suggestive of tethering include a spinal cord displaced in the spinal canal or downward displacement of the medulla, with no syrinx present to explain the neurologic decline (Table 16.2) (79,80). Cord traction can be aggravated by a kyphotic spine deformity. Common symptoms of posttraumatic cord tethering include weakness (78%), sensory loss (58%), and worse pain (40%) (81). A trial of a rigid cervical brace that minimizes neck flexion may be beneficial, as has been useful for some with cervical spondylotic myelopathy. Untethering of the spinal cord from arachnoidal scarring with a dural graft to expand the subarachnoid space and prevent rescarring may relieve the symptoms of cord tethering and prevent further neurologic decline (79–81,84).

Vitamin B₁₂ and Other Nutritional Deficiencies

Nutritional deficiency is an uncommon cause of late neurologic decline in patients with SCI (87). Weakened muscles, innervated either at the zone of injury or below, may have a predilection for more weakness. SCI physicians must inquire about diet and medications in patients complaining of neurologic decline and obtain appropriate laboratory studies. Patients with SCI on vegetarian diets are at increased risk for vitamin B_{12} deficiency, as are older adults with SCI or those with prior gastric or intestinal resections (154,155). Some medications may interfere with vitamin absorption—for example, antibiotics, H_2-blockers, proton-pump inhibitors, and colestipol (156).

SUMMARY

SCI physicians must be aware of the musculoskeletal and neurologic complications that can develop in their spinal cord–injured patients. By monitoring for and diagnosing these complications, SCI physicians can initiate early treatment and often prevent further disability.

REFERENCES

1. Levi R, Hulting C, Nash M, et al. The Stockholm Spinal Cord Injury Study: 1. Medical problems in a regional SCI population. *Paraplegia* 1995;33:308–315.
2. Siddall PJ, Taylor DA, Cousins MJ. Classification of pain following spinal cord injury. *Spinal Cord* 1997;35:69–75.
3. Stormer S, Gerner HJ, Gruninger, et al. Chronic pain/dysesthesias in spinal cord injury patients: result of a multicentre study. *Spinal Cord* 1997;35:446–455.
4. Garland DE, Stewart C, Adkins R, et al. Osteoporosis following SCI. *J Orthop Res* 1992;10:371–378.
5. Szollar SM, Martin E, Parthemore J, et al. Densitometric patterns of spinal cord injury associated bone loss. *Spinal Cord* 1997;35:374–382.
6. Bauman WA, Garland DE, Schwartz E. Calcium metabolism and osteoporosis in individuals with spinal cord injury. *Top Spinal Cord Inj Rehabil* 1997;2:84–95.
7. McKinley WO, Jackson AB, Cardenas DD, et al. Long-term medical complications after traumatic spinal cord injury: a regional model systems analysis. *Arch Phys Med Rehabil* 1999;80:1402–1410.
8. Frisbie JH. Fractures after myelopathy. *J Spinal Cord Med* 1997;20:66–69.
9. Garland DE. Pathologic fractures and bone mineral density at the knee. *J Spinal Cord Med* 1999;22:335.
10. McMaster WC, Stauffer ES. Management of long bone fractures in the spinal cord injured patient. *Clin Orthop* 1975;112:44–52.
11. Ragnarsson KT, Sell GH. Lower extremity fractures after spinal cord injury: a retrospective study. *Arch Phys Med Rehabil* 1981;62:418–423.
12. Freehafer AA. Limb fractures in spinal cord injury. *Arch Phys Med Rehabil* 1995;76:823–827.
13. Freehafer AA, Mast WA. Lower extremity fractures in patients with spinal cord injury. *J Bone Joint Surg* 1965;46a:683–694.
14. Comarr AE, Hutchinson RH, Bors E. Extremity fracture in patients with spinal cord injuries. *Am J Surg* 1962;103:732–739.
15. Eichenholtz SN. Management of long bone fractures in paraplegic patients. *J Bone Joint Surg* 1963;47a:299–310.
16. Michaelis LS. *Orthopedic surgery of the limbs in paraplegia.* Berlin: Springer-Verlag, 1964.
17. Notthee WM. A review of long bone fractures in patients with spinal cord injuries. *Clin Orthop Related Res* 1981;155:65–70.
18. Freehafer AA, Hazel CM, Becker CL. Lower extremity fractures in patients with spinal cord injury. *Paraplegia* 1981;19:367–372.
19. Baird R, Kreitenberg A, Eltorai I. External fixation of femoral shaft fractures in spinal cord injury patients. *Paraplegia* 1986;24:183–190.
20. Azaria M, Anner A, Ohry A. Long bone fractures in spinal cord injured patients. *Orthop Rev* 1993;12:69–75.
21. Bick RL. International consensus recommendations. Summary statement and additional suggested guidelines. *Med Clin North Am* 1998;82:613–633.
22. Sobel JW, Bohlman HH, Freehafer A. Charcot's arthropathy of the spine following spinal cord injury: a report of 5 cases. *J Bone Joint Surg* 1985;67A:771–775.
23. Kalen V, Isono SS, Cho CS, et al. Charcot arthropathy of the spine in long-standing paraplegia. *Spine* 1987;12:42–47.
24. Standaert C, Cardenas DD, Anderson P. Charcot spine as a late complication of traumatic spinal cord injury. *Arch Phys Med Rehabil* 1997;78:221–225.
25. Dearolf WW, Betz RR, Vogel L, et al. Scoliosis in pediatric spinal cord-injured patients. *J Pediatr Orthop* 1990;10:214–218.
26. Nichols PJR, Norman PA, Ennis J. Wheelchair user's shoulder. *Scand J Rehabil Med* 1979;11:29–32.
27. Bayley JC, Cochran TP, Sledge CB. The weight-bearing shoulder. The impingement syndrome in paraplegics. *J Bone Joint Surg* 1987;69A:676–678.
28. Gellman H, Sie I, Waters RL, et al. Late complications of the weight-bearing upper extremity in the paraplegic patient. *Clin Orthop* 1988;223:132–135.
29. Wylie EJ, Chakera TM. Degenerative joint abnormalities in patients with paraplegia of duration greater than 20 years. *Paraplegia* 1988;26:101–106.
30. Sie IH, Waters RL, Adkins RH, et al. Upper extremity pain in post-rehabilitation spinal cord injured patients. *Arch Phys Med Rehabil* 1992;73:44–48.
31. Curtis KA, Roach KE, Applegate EB, et al. Development of the Wheelchair User's Shoulder Pain Index (WUSPI). *Paraplegia* 1995;33:290–293.
32. Curtis KA, Drysdale GA, Lanza RD, et al. Shoulder pain in wheelchair users with tetraplegia and paraplegia. *Arch Phys Med Rehabil* 1999;80:453–457.
33. Silfverskiold J, Waters RL. Shoulder pain and functional disability in spinal cord injury patients. *Clin Orthop* 1991;272:141–145.
34. Escobedo EM, Hunter J, Hollister M, et al. Prevalence of rotator cuff tears by MRI in individuals with paraplegia. *Am J Radiol* 1997;168:919–923.
35. Gellman H, Sie I, Waters R, et al. Late complications of the weight-bearing upper extremity in the paraplegic patient. *Clin Orthop* 1988;223:132–135.
36. Waring WP, Maynard FM. Shoulder pain in acute traumatic quadriplegia. *Paraplegia* 1991;29:37–42.
37. Campbell C, Koris M. Etiologies of shoulder pain in cervical spinal cord injury. *Clin Orthop* 1996;322:140–145.
38. Lal S. Premature degenerative shoulder changes in spinal cord injury patients. *Spinal Cord* 1998;36:186–189.
39. Curtis KA, Roach KE, Applegate EB, et al. Reliability and validity of the Wheelchair User's Shoulder Pain Index (WUSPI). *Paraplegia* 1995;33:595–601.
40. Dyson-Hudson TA, Shiflett SC, Kirshblum SC, et al. Acupuncture and Trager psychophysical integration in the treatment of shoulder pain in spinal cord injuries. *Arch Phys Med Rehabil* 2001;82:1038–1046.
41. Nayak S, Shiflett SC, Schoenberger NE, et al. Chronic pain following spinal cord injury: the efficacy of acupuncture in pain management. *Arch Phys Med Rehabil* 1999;80:1166.
42. Olenik LM, Laskin JJ, Burnham R, et al. Efficacy of rowing, backward wheeling and isolated scapular retractor exercise as remedial strength activities for wheelchair users: application of electromyography. *Paraplegia* 1995;33:148–152.
43. Curtis KA, Tyner TM, Zachary L, et al. Effect of a standard exercise protocol on shoulder pain in long-term wheelchair users. *Spinal Cord* 1999;37:421–429.
44. Hastings JD. Seating assessment and planning. In: Hammond MC, ed. *Topics in spinal cord injury medicine.* PM&R Clin NA 2000;11:183–207.
45. Robinson MD, Hussey RW, Ha CY. Surgical decompression of impingement in the weightbearing shoulder. *Arch Phys Med Rehabil* 1993;74:324–327.
46. Blankstein A, Shmueli R, Weingarten I, et al. Hand problems due to prolonged use of crutches and wheelchairs. *Orthop Rev* 1985;14:29–34.
47. Goldstein B. Musculoskeletal complications after spinal cord injury. In: Hammond MC, ed. *Topics in spinal cord injury medicine.* PM&R Clin NA 2000;11:91–108.
48. Schroer W, Lacey S, Frost FS, et al. Carpal instability in the weight bearing upper extremity. *J Bone Joint Surg Am* 1996;78:1838–1843.
49. Kirshblum S, Druin E, Planten K. Musculoskeletal conditions in chronic spinal cord injury. *Top Spinal Cord Inj Rehabil* 1997;2:23–35.
50. Rink P, Miler F. Hip instability in spinal cord injured patients. *J Pediatr Orthop* 1990;10:583–587.
51. Burnham R, Martin T, Stein R, et al. Skeletal muscle fibre type transformation following spinal cord injury. *Spinal Cord* 1997;35:86–91.
52. Thomas CK, Zaidner E, Calancie B, et al. Muscle weakness, paralysis,

and atrophy after human cervical spinal cord injury. *Exp Neurol* 1997; 48:414–423.

53. Gerrits HL, De Haan A, Hopman MTE, et al. Contractile properties of the quadriceps muscle in individuals with spinal cord injury. *Muscle Nerve* 1999;22:1249–1256.

54. Tsitouras PD, Zhong YG, Spungen AM, et al. Serum testosterone and growth hormone/insulin-like growth factor-I in adults with spinal cord injury. *Horm Metab Res* 1995;27:287–292.

55. Tomlinson BE, Irving D. The numbers of limb motor neurons in the human lumbosacral cord throughout life. *J Neurol Sci* 1977;34: 213–219.

56. Carlson BM. Factors influencing the repair and adaptation of muscles in aged individuals: satellite cells and innervation. *J Gerontol* 1995; 50A:96–100.

57. Larsson L. Motor units: remodeling in aged animals. *J Gerontol* 1995; 50A:91–95.

58. Bertoni-Freddari C, Fattoretti P, Paoloni R, et al. Synaptic structural dynamics and aging. *Gerontology* 1996;42:170–180.

59. Yue GH, Ranganathan VK, Siemionow V, et al. Older adults exhibit a reduced ability to fully activate their biceps brachii muscle. *J Gerontol* 1999;54A:M249–M253.

60. Bosch A, Stauffer E, Nickel V. Incomplete traumatic quadriplegia: a ten-year review. *JAMA* 1971;216:473–478.

61. Perrouin-Verbe B, Lenne-Aurier K, Robert R, et al. Post-traumatic syringomyelia and post-traumatic spinal canal stenosis: a direct relationship: review of 75 patients with a spinal cord injury. *Spinal Cord* 1998;36:137–143.

62. Bursell J, Little JW, Stiens SA. Electrodiagnosis in spinal cord injured patients with new weakness or sensory loss. *Arch Phys Med Rehabil* 1999;80:904–909.

63. Maynard FM Jr, Bracken MB, Creasey G, et al. International standards for neurological and functional classification of spinal cord injury. *Spinal Cord* 1997;35:266–274.

64. Sett P, Crockard H. The value of magnetic resonance imaging (MRI) in the follow-up management of spinal injury. *Paraplegia* 1991;29: 396–410.

65. Perkovitch M, Perl S, Wang H. Current advances in magnetic resonance imaging (MRI) in spinal cord trauma: review article. *Paraplegia* 1992;30:305–316.

66. Herbison GJ. Strength post-spinal cord injury: myometer vs manual muscle test. *Spinal Cord* 1996;34:543–548.

67. Little JW, Stiens SA. Electrodiagnosis in spinal cord injury. *Phys Med Clin North Am* 1994;5:571–593.

68. Gellman H, Chandler D, Petrasek J, et al. Carpal tunnel syndrome in paraplegic patients. *J Bone Joint Surg Am* 1988;70:517–519.

69. Davidoff G, Werner R, Waring W. Compressive mononeuropathies of the upper extremity in chronic paraplegia. *Paraplegia* 1991;29: 17–24.

70. Nemchausky BA, Ubilluz RM. Upper extremity neuropathies in patients with spinal cord injuries. *J Spinal Cord Med* 1995;18:95–97.

71. Baba H, Maezawa Y, Uchida K, et al. Cervical myeloradiculopathy with entrapment neuropathy: a study based on the double crush concept. *Spinal Cord* 1998;36:399–404.

72. Apple DF, Cody R, Allen A. Overuse syndromes of the upper limb in people with spinal cord injury. In: *Physical fitness: a guide for individuals with spinal cord injury*. Rehabilitation Research and Development Services, Department of Veterans Affairs, 1996:97–107.

73. Alijure J, Eltorai I, Bradley WE, et al. Carpal tunnel syndrome in paraplegic patients. *Paraplegia* 1985;23:182–186.

74. Tun CG, Upton J. The paraplegic hand: electrodiagnostic studies and clinical findings. *J Hand Surg* 1988;5:716–719.

75. Gelberman RH, Hergenroeder PT, Hargens AR, et al. The carpal syndrome. *J Bone Joint Surg* 1981;63a:680–683.

76. Anderson P, Bohlman H. Anterior decompression and arthrodesis of the cervical spine: long-term motor improvement. Part II. Improvement in complete traumatic quadriparesis. *J Bone Joint Surg Am* 1992; 74:683–692.

77. Bohlman H, Anderson P. Anterior decompression and arthrodesis of the cervical spine: long-term motor improvement. Part I. Improve-

ment in incomplete traumatic quadriparesis. *J Bone Joint Surg Am* 1992;74:671–682.

78. Gebarski SS, Maynard FW, Gabrielsen TO, et al. Posttraumatic progressive myelopathy. *Radiology* 1985;157:379–385.

79. Ragnarsson TS, Durward QJ, Nordgren RE. Spinal cord tethering after traumatic paraplegia with late neurological deterioration. *J Neurosurg* 1986;64:397–401.

80. Berrington NR. Posttraumatic spinal cord tethering: case report. *J Neurosurg* 1993;78:120–121.

81. Smith KA, Rekate HL. Delayed postoperative tethering of the cervical spinal cord. *J Neurosurg* 1994;81:196–201.

82. Falci SP, Lammertse DP, Best L, et al. Surgical treatment of posttraumatic cystic and tethered spinal cords. *J Spinal Cord Med* 1999;20: 173–181.

83. Silberstein M, Tress BM, Hennessy O. Delayed neurologic deterioration in the patient with spinal trauma: role of MR imaging. *Am J Neuroradiol* 1992;13:1373–1381.

84. Lee TT, Arias JM, Andrus HL, et al. Progressive posttraumatic myelomalacic myelopathy: treatment with untethering and expansive duraplasty. *J Neurosurg* 1997;86:624–628.

85. Karacostas D, Artemis N, Bairactaris C, et al. Cobalamin deficiency: MRI detection of posterior column involvement and posttreatment resolution. *J Neuroimaging* 1998;8:171–173.

86. Hemmer B, Glocker FX, Schumacher M, et al. Subacute combined degeneration: clinical, electrophysiological and magnetic resonance imaging findings. *J Neurol Neurosurg Psychiatry* 1998;65:822–827.

87. Vaidyanathan S, Soni BM, Oo T, et al. Syncope following intramuscular injection of hydroxocobalamin in a paraplegic patient. *Spinal Cord* 1999;37:147–149.

88. Yoshiyama Y, Tokumaru Y, Hattori T, et al. The "pseudo-polyneuropathy" type sensory disturbances in cervical spondylotic myelopathy. *Rinsho-Shinkeigaku* 1995;35:141–146.

89. Rossier AB, Foo D, Shillito J, et al. Post-traumatic syringomyelia: incidence, clinical presentation, electrophysiological studies, syrinx protein and results of conservative and operative treatment. *Brain* 1985;108:439–461.

90. Katoh S, Ikata T, Hirai N, et al. Influence of minor trauma to the neck on the neurological outcome in patients with ossification of the posterior longitudinal ligament (OPLL) of the cervical spine. *Paraplegia* 1995;33:330–333.

91. Edgar R, Quail P. Progressive post-traumatic cystic and non-cystic myelopathy. *Br J Neurosurg* 1994;8:7–22.

92. El Masry W, Biyani A. Incidence, management, and outcome of posttraumatic syringomyelia. *J Neurol Neurosurg Psychiatry* 1996;60: 141–146.

93. Schurch B, Wichmann W, Rossier AB. Post-traumatic syringomyelia (cystic myelopathy): a prospective study of 449 patients with spinal cord injury. *J Neurol Neurosurg Psychiatry* 1996;60:61–67.

94. Frisbie JH, Aquilera EJ. Chronic pain after spinal cord injury: an expedient diagnostic approach. *Paraplegia* 1990;28:460–465.

95. Isu T, Iwasaki Y, Nunomura M, et al. Magnetic resonance imaging of post-traumatic syringomyelia and its surgical treatment. *No Shinkei Geka* 1991;19:41–46.

96. Abel R, Gerner HJ, Smit C, et al. Residual deformity of the spinal canal in patients with traumatic paraplegia and secondary changes of the spinal cord. *Spinal Cord* 1999;37:14–19.

97. Wozniewicz B, Filipowicz K, Swiderska S, et al. Pathophysiological mechanism of traumatic cavitation of the spinal cord. *Paraplegia* 1983; 21:312–317.

98. Squier MV, Lehr RP. Post-traumatic syringomyelia. *J Neurol Neurosurg Psychiatry* 1994;57:1095–1098.

99. Backe HA, Betz RR, Mesgarzadeh M, et al. Post-traumatic spinal cord cysts evaluated by magnetic resonance imaging. *Paraplegia* 1991; 29:607–612.

100. Silberstein M, Hennessy O. Cystic cord lesions and neurological deterioration in spinal cord injury. *Paraplegia* 1992;30:661–668.

101. Biyani A, Masri WS. Post traumatic syringomyelia: a review of literature. *Paraplegia* 1994;32:723–731.

102. Williams B. Pathogenesis of post-traumatic syringomyelia [Editorial]. *Br J Neurosurg* 1992;6:517–520.

103. Silberstein M, Hennessy O. Implications of focal spinal cord lesions following trauma: evaluation with magnetic resonance imaging. *Paraplegia* 1993;31:160–167.
104. Caplan LR, Norohna AB, Amico LL. Syringomyelia and arachnoiditis. *J Neurol Neurosurg Psychiatry* 1990;53:106–113.
105. Asano M, Fujiwara K, Yonenobu K, et al. Posttraumatic syringomyelia. *Spine* 1996;21:1446–1453.
106. Van den Bergh R. Pathogenesis and treatment of delayed post-traumatic syringomyelia. *Acta Neurochir (Wien)* 1991;110:82–86.
107. Milhorat TH, Capocelli AL Jr, Anzil AP, et al. Pathological basis of spinal cord cavitation in syringomyelia: analysis of 105 autopsy cases. *J Neurosurg* 1995;82:802–812.
108. Hida K, Iwasaki Y, Imamura H, et al. Posttraumatic syringomyelia: its characteristic magnetic resonance imaging findings and surgical management. *Neurosurg* 1994;35:886–891.
109. Barnett HJM, Jouse AT. Post-traumatic syringomyelia (cystic myelopathy). In: Vinken, Bruyn, eds. *Handbook of clinical neurology*, vol 26. North Holland Publishing Company, 1976:113–157.
110. Jensen F, Reske-Nielsen E. Post-traumatic syringomyelia. *Scand J Rehabil Med* 1977;9:35–43.
111. Anton HA, Schweigel JF. Posttraumatic syringomyelia: the British Columbia experience. *Spine* 1986;11:865–868.
112. Williams B, Terry AF, Jones F, et al. Syringomyelia as a sequel to traumatic paraplegia. *Paraplegia* 1981;19:67–80.
113. Vernon JD, Silver JR, Symon L. Post-traumatic syringomyelia: the results of surgery. *Paraplegia* 1983;21:37–46.
114. Balmaseda MT, Wunder JA, Gordon C, et al. Posttraumatic syringomyelia associated with heavy weightlifting exercises: case report. *Arch Phys Med Rehabil* 1988;69:970–972.
115. Tator CH, Briceno C. Treatment of syringomyelia with syringosubarachnoid shunt. *Can J Neurol Sci* 1988;15:48–57.
116. Ball MJ, Dayan AD. Pathogenesis of syringomyelia. *Lancet* 1972;2:799–801.
117. Bertrand G. Dynamic factors of syringomyelia and syringobulbia. *Clin Neurosurg* 1972;20:322–333.
118. Durward QJ, Rice GP, Ball MJ, et al. Selective spinal cordectomy: clinicopathological correlation. *J Neurosurg* 1982;56:359–367.
119. Kruse A, Rasmussen G, Borgesen SE. CSF dynamics in syringomyelia: intracranial pressure and resistance to outflow. *Br J Neurosurg* 1987;1:477–484.
120. Martins G. Syringomyelia, an hypothesis and proposed method of treatment [Letter]. *J Neurol Neurosurg Psychiatry* 1983;46:365.
121. Shannon N, Symon L, Logue V, et al. Clinical features, investigation and treatment of post-traumatic syringomyelia. *J Neurol Neurosurg Psychiatry* 1981;44:35–42.
122. Shoukimas GM. Thoracic spine. In: Stark DD, Bradley WG Jr, eds. *Magnetic resonance imaging*, 2nd ed. Mosby–Year Book, 1992:1302–1338.
123. Kramer KM, Levine AM. Post-traumatic syringomyelia: a review of 21 cases. *Clin Ortho Related Res* 1997;334:190–199.
124. Lyons BM, Brown DJ, Calvert JM, et al. The diagnosis and management of post traumatic syringomyelia. *Paraplegia* 1987;25:345–350.
125. Tobimatsu H, Nihei R, Kimura T, et al. Magnetic resonance imaging of spinal cord injury in chronic stage. *Rinsho Seikei Geka* 1991;26:1173–1182.
126. Dworkin GE, Staas WE. Posttraumatic syringomyelia. *Arch Phys Med Rehabil* 1985;66:329–331.
127. Watson N. Ascending cystic degeneration of the cord after spinal cord injury. *Paraplegia* 1981;19:89–95.
128. Nogues MA, Gene R, Encabo H. Risk of sudden death during sleep in syringomyelia and syringobulbia. *J Neurol Neurosurg Psychiatry* 1992;55:585–589.
129. Quencer RM, Green BA, Eismont FJ. Post traumatic spinal cord cysts; clinical features and characterization with metrizamide computed tomography. *Radiology* 1983;146:415–423.
130. Wang D, Bodley R, Sett P, et al. A clinical magnetic resonance imaging study of the traumatized spinal cord more than 20 years following injury. *Paraplegia* 1996;34:65–81.
131. Quencer RM, Post MJD, Hinks RS. Cine MR in the evaluation of normal and abnormal CSF flow: intracranial and intraspinal studies. *Neuroradiology* 1990;32:371.
132. Jinkins JR, Reddy S, Leite CC, et al. MR of parenchymal spinal cord signal change as a sign of active advancement in clinically progressive posttraumatic syringomyelia. *Am J Neuroradiol* 1998;19:177–182.
133. Pojunas K, Williams AL, Daniels DL, et al. Syringomyelia and hydromyelia: magnetic resonance evaluation. *Radiology* 1984;153:679–683.
134. Little JW, Robinson LR, Goldstein B, et al. Electrophysiologic findings in post-traumatic syringomyelia: implications for clinical management. *J Am Paraplegia Soc* 1992;15:44–52.
135. Nogues MA, Stalberg E. Electrodiagnostic findings in syringomyelia. *Muscle Nerve* 1999;22:1653–1659.
136. Schlesinger EB, Antunes JL, Michelsen J, et al. Hydromyelia: clinical presentation and comparison of modalities of treatment. *Neurosurgery* 1981;9:356–365.
137. Peerless SJ, Durward QJ. Management of syringomyelia: a pathophysiological approach. *Clin Neurosurg* 1983;30:531–576.
138. Sgouros S, Williams B. Management and outcome of posttraumatic syringomyelia. *J Neurosurg* 1996;85:197–205.
139. Adelstein LJ. The surgical treatment of syringomyelia. *Am J Surg* 1938;40:384–395.
140. Suzuki M, Davis C, Symon L, et al. Syringoperitoneal shunt for treatment of cord cavitation. *J Neurol Neurosurg Psychiatry* 1985;48:620–627.
141. Barbaro NM, Wilson CB, Gutin PH, et al. Surgical treatment of syringomyelia: favorable results with syringoperitoneal shunting. *J Neurosurg* 1984;61:531–538.
142. Dautheribes LW, Pointillart V, Gaujard E, et al. Mean term follow-up of a series of post traumatic syringomyelia patients after syringo-peritoneal shunting. *Paraplegia* 1995;33:241–245.
143. Levi ADO, Sonntag VKH. Management of posttraumatic syringomyelia using expansile duraplasty. *Spine* 1998;23:128–132.
144. Batzdorf U, Klekamp J, Johnson JP. A critical appraisal of syrinx cavity shunting procedures. *J Neurosurg* 1998;89:382–388.
145. Klekamp J, Batzdorf U, Samil M, et al. Treatment of syringomyelia with subarachnoid scarring caused by arachnoiditis or trauma. *J Neurosurg* 1997;86:233.
146. Ronen J, Catz A, Spasser R, et al. The treatment dilemma in post-traumatic syringomyelia. *Disabil Rehabil* 1999;21:455–457.
147. Wiart L, Dautheribes M, Pointillart V, et al. Mean term follow-up of a series of post-traumatic syringomyelia patients after syringo-peritoneal shunting. *Paraplegia* 1995;33:241–245.
148. Grant R, Handley DM, Lang D, et al. MRI measurement of the syrinx size before and after operation. *J Neurol Neurosurg Psychiatry* 1987;50:1685–1687.
149. Wester K, Pedersen PH, Krakenes J. Spinal cord damage caused by rotation of a T-drain in a patient with syringoperitoneal shunt. *Surg Neurol* 1989;31:224–227.
150. Foo D. Spinal cord injury in forty-four patients with cervical spondylosis. *Paraplegia* 1986;24:301–306.
151. Fritz JM, Delitto A, Welch WC, et al. Lumbar spinal stenosis: a review of current concepts in evaluation, management, and outcome. *Arch Phys Med Rehabil* 1998;79:700–708.
152. Kojima A, Nakajima A, Koyama K. Cervical spondylosis in paraplegic patients and analysis of the wheelchair driving action: a preliminary communication. *Spinal Cord* 1997;35:768–772.
153. Breig A. *Biomechanics of the central nervous system: some basic normal and pathologic phenomena concerning spine, disks and cord.* Chicago: Year Book Publishers, 1960:76–95.
154. Lindenbaum J, Rosenberg IH, Wilson PWF, et al. Prevalence of cobalamin deficiency in the Framingham elderly population. *Am J Clin Nutr* 1994;60:2–11.
155. Davidsson T, Lindergard B, Mansson W. Long-term metabolic and nutritional effects of urinary diversion. *Urology* 1995;46:804–809.
156. Bradford GS, Taylor CT. Omeprazole and vitamin B12 deficiency. *Ann Pharmacother* 1999;33:641–643.

HETEROTOPIC OSSIFICATION

KRESIMIR BANOVAC
FILIP BANOVAC

DEFINITION

Heterotopic ossification (HO) is the formation of true bone at ectopic sites. HO was first described by Riedel (1) and has been described under many names including ectopic ossification, neurogenic ossifying fibromyopathy, myositis ossificans, and paraosteoarthropathy. After spinal cord injury (SCI), it is one of the most common orthopedic complications.

INCIDENCE

In adult patients with SCI, the incidence is approximately 50% (2–5), with up to 20% of patients suffering significant loss of range of motion (ROM) and 5% ankylosis. In children, HO is less frequent, approximately 18% (6). Both genders are affected, but men are more often affected than women (5). Most commonly, HO develops between 1 and 4 months after injury, with peak incidence at 2 months. Late onset of HO, however, may occur years after injury (7,8).

LOCATION AND PATHOLOGY

In approximately 90% of patients with SCI, HO develops around the hip. Less frequent locations include the knee, elbow, and shoulder (5,9). In the hip, HO is found most commonly on the anteromedial aspect of the joint (2). In the knee, it is usually around the medial epicondyle of the femur. HO is rare in the small joints of the hand and foot (10,11). Ossification is extraarticular and is always found below the level of the SCI (2). Histology of HO is similar to that of normotopic mature bone, with well-developed cortical and trabecular structures, as well as bone marrow (12–14). In the early stage of HO development, the central area contains undifferentiated mesenchymal cells surrounded with a denser cellular zone that gradually undergoes mineralization (15–17). The process of maturation of HO has a centripetal pattern, in which bone formation starts at the periphery and progresses to the central part of the lesion (16). In the process of HO formation, both membranous and endochondral ossifications are present, but usually membranous ossifications predominate (12).

ETIOLOGY

Several hypotheses have been proposed in the pathogenesis of HO, such as local trauma (18,19), spasticity (20,21), tissue hypoxia (15), necrosis (22,23), and humoral factors (24). Other variables were evaluated to define the factors responsible for the formation of HO. For example, advanced age, the completeness of the spinal cord lesion, the presence of a pressure ulcer, and increased spasticity are found to be positively related to the formation of HO (25,26). However, the etiology of HO after SCI remains uncertain. Based on experimental studies, it seems that at least two processes have an important role in the genesis of HO after SCI: the activation of pluripotential mesenchymal cells in the soft tissue and the local production of bone morphogenic proteins (BMPs) (27). Mesenchymal cells in muscle may switch their differentiation from a fibroprogenitor to an osteoprogenitor pathway under the influence of BMP, and then further proliferate and differentiate into bone-forming cells. The factors involved in triggering the activation of mesenchymal cells in muscle and local induction of BMP expression are presently unknown.

CLINICAL PRESENTATION

In the early stage of HO, fever is one of the first symptoms, although it is not always present. Fever tends to be higher at night, sometimes as high as 103°F. Several days later, joint swelling that limits ROM occurs. Patients with a preserved sensory function may have pain in the affected region. When the hip is involved, the entire thigh and knee may show edema. Some patients develop knee effusion, which is thought to be a transudate as a result of HO compression on lymphatic drainage and the hypertrophy of synovium in the knee (28,29). HO may coexist with deep venous thrombosis (DVT) (30–32) and pressure ulcers (25,26,33), but it does not necessarily precede these complications. In the late stage of HO, symptoms depend on the size and location of HO relative to joint structures. About 10% to 20% of patients with HO develop significant reduction of joint mobility that may affect transfers, routine bowel and bladder care, and other activities of daily living. In children, HO often has a benign course in which HO in soft tissue may resolve with time (34). This phenomenon is attributed to a higher turn-over rate of bone metabolism in children than in the adults.

Differential diagnosis for this clinical presentation includes a DVT, fracture of the lower extremity, impending pressure ulcer, septic arthritis, and cellulitis. Because DVT and a pressure ulcer may coexist with HO, one should always consider a combination of disorders occurring at the same time.

LABORATORY STUDIES

Blood test results may show an increased erythrocyte sedimentation rate (ESR) that may in the acute stage of HO develop in the range of 80 to 100 mm per hour. However, persons with SCI may have an elevated ESR secondary to other causes. C-reactive protein (CRP) may also be elevated in acute HO (35). One of the most commonly used tests in the diagnosis of HO is serum alkaline phosphatase (ALP) (9,15,36–41). It is thought that ALP plays an important role in the process of mineralization of biologic tissues. This enzyme is released from the membrane of osteoblasts into extracellular matrix, and in parallel, it increases in the serum. The increased serum level of ALP can be found in the early stage of HO and may further increase with the progression of bone growth (38). Although the level of ALP reflects the activity of osteoblasts during the formation of HO, in many patients, serum activity of ALP is not elevated (15,36, 37). Additionally, the diagnostic value of ALP in HO after SCI may be limited due to multiple skeletal injuries in these patients, which are also associated with an elevation of serum ALP. Similarly, surgical treatment of fractures and abdominal injuries with liver damage may result in a transient elevation of serum ALP. Although serum ALP level may rise with initial HO progression, the level does not correlate with the severity or number of lesions. Some patients with HO may also have an elevated serum creatine phosphokinase (CPK) level. In these patients, the origin of CPK is surrounding muscle tissue. The histology of muscles of these patients shows a destruction of myofibrils by invading immature HO (15).

Although the humoral control of bone metabolism is not entirely elucidated, it is likely that similar factors are involved in the formation of HO and normotopic ossification. Based on the assumption that some of the humoral factors may have a role in the pathogenesis of HO, several groups of investigators evaluated serum osteoinductive activity in patients with SCI (42–44). These studies tested *in vitro* osteoblastic activity and demonstrated contradictory findings. Similarly, a more specific evaluation of basic fibroblast growth factor in patients with SCI with and without HO revealed negative results (45).

In contrast to the blood tests, urinary tests for prostaglandin E_2 (PGE_2) levels have shown concomitant increases of PGE_2 with the progression of HO (46). This test offers a new diagnostic procedure in early diagnosis of HO but is presently not routinely available. Several studies were performed to determine the role of genetic predisposition on the development of HO (47–49). Human leukocyte antigens (HLA) A, B, and C were tested to identify the susceptibility of patients to HO. Results of these studies are contradictory, although it seems that appearance of HO after SCI is not associated in higher frequency with any specific HLA.

IMAGING

Different imaging studies have been used in the diagnosis of HO. It is clear that for effective management of HO, an early diagnosis is necessary before the development of calcified tissue. In this respect, imaging studies such as ultrasonography, computed tomography (CT), or bone scintigraphy have an important role in the diagnosis of early unmineralized HO. Although plain radiography is highly specific in the diagnosis of HO, this method lacks sensitivity in early diagnosis. Usually, HO is seen in the later stages of bone formation on plain radiographs; however, in early stages, an insufficient amount of calcium is present at the site of new bone formation to be detected by radiography. Therefore, other imaging methods are necessary for early diagnosis.

Ultrasonography in the early stage of HO formation reveals an echogenic peripheral zone and echolucent center (16). When HO develops in muscle, characteristic findings include a reduction of normal lamellar pattern of muscle fibers and an irregular echogenic tissue pattern, indicating muscle infiltration with liquid mass. Biopsy of this mass shows the presence of osteoid without evidence of mineralization (50). During the process of HO maturation, more calcified tissue can be identified on ultrasonography, first at the periphery of the lesion and later in the central part. The serial studies of patients with HO showed that within 2 weeks, the echolucent zone developed echogenic bands, indicating an increase of calcification of the tissue (16,51). At this stage, the first signs of bone formation can also be appreciated radiographically. The sonographic evaluation showed a maturation of HO similar to the "zone phenomenon" (16,51, 52) described by Ackerman (17) on the pathologic examination of myositis ossificans (17). Ackerman (17) demonstrated that osteoid and bone are first laid down in the peripheral zone, the second zone is formed of soft osteoid, and the central zone contains undifferentiated cells.

CT is not frequently used as a diagnostic test in patients with HO. The limited experience with CT in the diagnosis of HO has shown marked similarities in the development of soft tissue ossification to myositis ossificans (32,52,53). In both groups of patients, CT reveals a well-defined soft tissue mass with a dense shell of calcified density around a hypodense central area (Fig. 17.1). CT offers very precise delineation of the lesion and is frequently used in preoperative evaluation of the patients, along with MRI. Presently, experience with MRI in patients with HO after SCI is limited; it is mainly used in planning operative approaches.

Bone scintigraphy is one of the most commonly used diagnostic tests in the evaluation of early HO (5–7,31,38,54–56). It was introduced in 1974 for the diagnosis of myositis ossificans and since then has undergone several technical modifications (57). Presently, the test involves evaluation in three phases after the administration of radioactive material. Technetium-99m (^{99m}Tc) diphosphonate is used as radionuclide, which has a high affinity for newly developing bone. The first phase of the

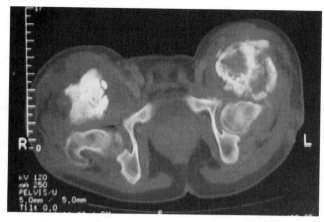

FIGURE 17.1. Computerized tomography (CT) of hip regions in a paraplegic patient with advanced stage heterotopic ossification. On the right leg, CT shows "zone phenomenon" with peripheral formation of bone; on the left leg, the entire soft tissue mass is ossified.

test represents the blood flow, when the images are obtained every 3 seconds. The second phase shows blood pooling in a hypervascular area, and the third phase is a whole-body scan obtained usually after 4 hours of administration of radioactive test substance (Fig. 17.2). The first two phases indicate hyperemia and blood pooling, which are precursors of the ossification process and are therefore most important to early diagnosis and monitoring the maturity of the HO.

It is well documented that immature HO after SCI can be detected by bone scintigraphy (4,5,38,55,58). Likewise, it was found that in the diagnosis of HO, bone scintigraphy is a more sensitive diagnostic test than plain radiography. Studies of the temporal relationship between bone scan and radiographic soft tissue calcification show that the radiographic HO follows positive bone scan results by an average of 3 weeks (36,38,55,58). Bone scintigraphy is used for the determination of maturity of HO before surgery (37), with a serial decrease or a steady state–uptake ratio being a reliable indicator of maturity. The value of this test in preoperative evaluation is limited, because of frequent finding of considerable activity of HO even after 2 years of medical therapy. The quantitative assessment of radioactive uptake at the site of HO, which is not routinely obtained,

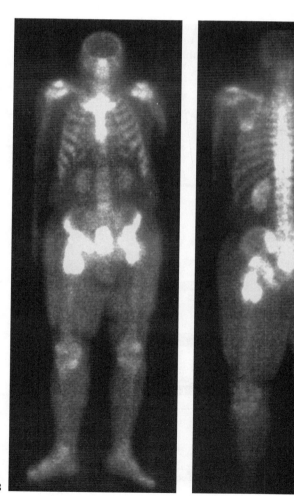

A,B

FIGURE 17.2. Bone scintigraphy with technetium-99m diphosphonate in a paraplegic patient with heterotopic ossification, showing the third phase of scintigraphy obtained 4 hours after administration of radioisotope. Anteroposterior view **(A)**; posteroanterior view **(B)**. Note an increased accumulation of radiotracer bilaterally around the proximal femur more on the right than on the left leg and predominantly anterior localization.

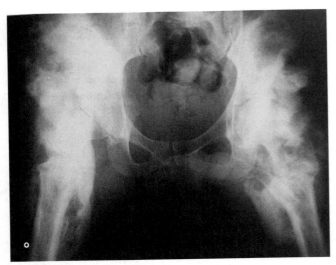

FIGURE 17.3. Heterotopic ossification around both hips in a paraplegic patient with bilateral hip joint ankylosis. Anteroposterior radiograph shows a massive formation of bone extending from the pelvis to the proximal femur bilaterally.

offers more precise preoperative measure of HO maturation (59, 60).

If not treated, HO becomes positive on radiography usually 2 to 3 weeks after the appearance of soft tissue swelling. The extent of tissue involvement by HO varies. In some patients,

only a small fragment develops around the joint, usually not causing joint dysfunction, whereas in others, a massive ossification can be found with bony bridges between proximal and distal regions of the joint, resulting in severe functional limitations or ankylosis of the joint (Fig. 17.3).

In most patients, the clinical course is characterized by a typical temporal presentation of clinical signs, symptoms, and laboratory findings. Initial abnormalities include the development of fever, soft tissue swelling, and an elevation of the ESR, then positive bone scintigraphy or ultrasound, and finally the elevation of serum ALP, which is followed by radiographic findings of immature HO (Fig. 17.4).

CLASSIFICATION

Several classifications for HO were recommended, which are predominantly based on radiographic findings. One classification often used to grade HO in patients with SCI is based on the degree of bone formation for other diagnostic groups, for example, in patients after undergoing total hip replacement (62). The Brooker classification uses four classes and can only be applied for HO around the hip and not the other locations. Another classification by Finerman and Stover (69) describes five different grades for HO around the hip and is based on radiographic evaluation. Garland and Orwin (54) proposed a radiographic classification for preoperative grading of the extent of bone formation in soft tissue. In this classification, there are five groups; grade 1, minimal; grade 2, mild; grade 3, moderate;

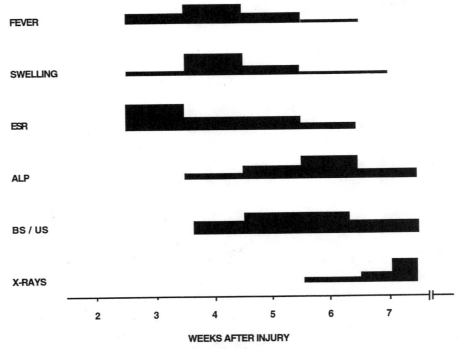

FIGURE 17.4. Development of clinical findings in patients with heterotopic ossification after spinal cord injury. (ESR, erythrocyte sedimentation rate; ALP, serum alkaline phosphatase; BS, bone scintigraphy; US, ultrasound examination.)

grade 4, severe; and grade 5, ankylosis. This classification can be used for any location of HO. Although it is simple to use, the differences between the categories are not sufficiently defined and the gradation of HO depends mainly on the subjective criteria of the examiner. There are no classifications that combine functional impairment and radiographic findings, which may be important in the decision-making process for further therapy.

On the basis of radiographic findings and clinical course, Garland proposed two classes of HO (54). Class I includes patients with radiographic progression of HO and elevated serum ALP level for 5 to 6 months; HO thereafter becomes inert. Class II is characterized by a radiographic progression of HO with persistent activity on the bone scan for an extended period. Some of the patients in class II ultimately require surgery. Few patients may develop HO several years after injury (58,61). The appearance of HO late after SCI is associated with a benign course and preservation of joint function (8).

APPROACH TO DIAGNOSIS

In patients with acute swelling of an extremity after SCI, first the complications such as bone fracture and DVT should be ruled out by radiographic examination and compression ultrasonography. After these tests, an ultrasonogram, CT scan, or bone scintigraphy will be the diagnostic test of choice for a diagnosis of HO. Serum ALP, the ESR, C-reactive protein, and CPK may be abnormal in acute HO; although other conditions such as recent skeletal trauma, surgery, concomitant infection, and inflammation should also be considered as sources for laboratory changes in the blood.

PROPHYLAXIS

There is no definitive protocol for prophylaxis against the formation of HO. Stover et al. (63) studied prospectively a dosage of etidronate of 20 mg/kg of body weight per day for 2 weeks, followed by 10 mg/kg per day for 10 weeks initiated 20 to 121 days after the injury. When treatment was completed, the HO in the treatment group was significantly less than that in the placebo group. Ossification did occur after the etidronate was discontinued, with both groups having equal incidence of HO, although with less functional deficits in the treated group. A limitation of this study is that only radiography was used to monitor the degree of HO.

TREATMENT
Medical

Because there is no definitive effective prevention of HO after SCI, the goal is to diagnose and treat HO in the initial stage of development before the formation of mineralized tissue (4,5, 38,55,64,65). Available medical therapy is directed toward the inhibition of mineralization of bone matrix. Etidronate is the only medication approved by the Food and Drug Administra-

tion for the treatment of HO after SCI. This drug blocks the late phase of bone formation, which is the stage of mineralization, preventing the conversion of amorphous calcium phosphate to hydroxyapatite (66). Etidronate has no effect on the early phase of ossification when nonossified bone matrix is produced by osteoblasts (66). In addition to its inhibitory effect on mineralization, it was found that etidronate has an antiinflammatory effect by reducing the production of cytokines (67,68). Clinically, this effect is seen as a rapid reduction in soft tissue swelling after initiation of therapy (65). A protocol initially designed for prophylaxis of HO by Stover et al. (63) in 1976 was subsequently adopted for the treatment of HO (69). The recommendation is to start with an oral dosage of etidronate of 20 mg/kg per day for 2 weeks, followed by a dosage of 10 mg/kg per day for 3 months. Newer therapeutic protocols have been recommended using higher doses of etidronate for an extended period (4,5,7, 14). Garland (14) recommended that high-dose etidronate (20 mg/kg per day) be used for up to 6 months or longer to prevent rebound formation of HO if treatment was for a shorter period of time. It has been shown that after cessation of 3 months of therapy with etidronate, a rapid increase in the growth of HO occurs ("rebound ossification") (63,64,69). The most common side effect of etidronate is gastrointestinal, including nausea and vomiting in 10% to 20% of patients (63). Administering the medication in divided doses 1 to 2 hours before meals improves this problem. Banovac et al. (65) introduced an improvement in treatment by using an intravenous loading dose of etidronate at the start of therapy to increase bioavailability of the drug, because only 2% to 5% of etidronate is absorbed in the gastrointestinal system after oral administration (70). Table 17.1 illustrates the dosages and time period of drug administration for this new protocol. Using this protocol, approximately 21% of patients develop a low degree of tissue ossification that is clinically not significant (4). In addition, the prolonged administration of etidronate for 6 months has a more sustained effect on preventing the formation of HO, with about a 5% incidence rate of "rebound HO" (8). In the later stages of HO when mature bone is formed, the treatment is mainly in the domain of surgery. In chronic stages of HO, etidronate may only limit the extent of formation of bone mass, having no effect on the size of already developed bone (63). In determining the effect of etidronate on bone fusion and fracture healing after SCI, a retrospective matched spine comparison of radiographs was made between 30 patients with SCI with HO treated with etidronate (within 8 weeks after injury) and 30 patients with SCI not treated with etidronate (71). Significant differences were found between the etidronate-treated group and the non–etidronate-treated group in the spine fracture line disappearing at 12

TABLE 17.1. ETIDRONATE THERAPY FOR ACUTE HETEROTOPIC OSSIFICATION

	Dose	Route	Time Period
Initial	300 mg	Intravenous	3 d
Maintenance	20 mg/kg/d	Oral	6 mo

weeks. Etidronate may delay the process of healing of a spinal fracture, although further study in this area is needed.

Nonsteroidal antiinflammatory drugs (NSAIDs) have been shown to be effective in the prevention of HO after pelvic fracture and hip arthroplasty surgery (72,73). Little is known about the effect of NSAIDs on the formation of HO after SCI. However, there are data to support a beneficial effect of these drugs in the prevention of HO recurrence after resection of HO (46, 74,75).

Radiation

Sautter-Bihl et al. (72) evaluated the effect of radiation therapy in patients with early HO formation. Different dosages of radiation were used to the hip, from single-dose 8 Gy irradiation up to 20 Gy in total from multiple doses, with most patients receiving 10 Gy in fractions of 2 to 2½ Gy. They reported that radiation therapy was an effective therapy as a primary treatment for early HO, because most patients showed no progression of their HO, with no adverse effects noted. There were also no differences in the fractionated regimen, compared with the single-dose treatment. The long-term risks, however, have not been studied.

Range of Motion and Exercise

Animal models have shown that new bone formation may occur after ROM, stretching, and forceful manipulation, which may cause soft tissue bleeding (19). However, there is limited documentation substantiating this relationship in the SCI population (51). Because most high-level persons with SCI undergo aggressive stretching as part of their rehabilitation, if this was a source of HO formation, one would expect a higher incidence of HO and more affected joints in the same individual than is currently documented. It is controversial whether an aggressive ROM exercise in the acute stage increases already present inflammation and induces additional tissue microtrauma, which may lead to increased formation of HO (77). Careful mobilization of affected joints is recommended and beneficial and does not appear to accelerate HO formation while maintaining or improving joint mobility (9,78). However, aggressive stretching should not recommence until the acute inflammatory signs have subsided. The goal is to maintain functional ROM for the individual.

Surgery

Surgery is a therapeutic option for a selected group of patients with HO (approximately 5% of patients). Surgical indications for resection are to improve mobility and activities of daily living (54,56,79) and to prevent or treat medical complications such as pressure ulcers or neurovascular compression (80). The main reasons for resection of HO around the hips and knees are limitations in sitting, positioning, and dressing. Surgical indications for the removal of HO around the elbow and shoulder are for improvements in feeding, hygiene, and dressing, as well as for clinical evidence of progressive ulnar nerve compression (32,81). Before surgery, it is recommended to wait for a period of 1½ to 2 years (14,54). This time interval is generally sufficient for

maximum maturation of HO. For clear indications, the surgery can be performed sooner (81). Serum ALP level may be a helpful test in determination of activity of HO, although many patients may have an increased serum level 2 years after injury (15,54). In addition, the ALP level may return to within the reference range before bone maturity is reached. Similarly, bone scintigraphy may not always reveal a significant reduction in bone uptake later in the disease. MRI or CT scan determines preoperative localization of HO.

Various surgical approaches have been used for the resection of HO (54). Wedge resection is the most common procedure, although bone resection is frequently associated with significant blood loss (52). Other complications include wound infection, neurologic or vascular injury, and recurrence. After resection, it is beneficial to start gentle ROM 72 hours postoperative and wait 1 to 2 weeks, until soft tissue swelling subsides, at which time active physical therapy can be commenced (54). Postoperatively, radiation, NSAIDs, and etidronate (20 mg/kg for 3 to 6 months) may be used as single or combination adjuvant therapy (13,54,76,78,81,82). Radiation therapy has been recommended as a secondary therapeutic modality after surgical removal of HO (54,81,82). Different radiation protocols have been used. One effective protocol is with a total dose of 1,000 centigray, divided in five consecutive fractions over a period of 1 week (81). This dosage of radiation substantially reduces the recurrence of HO after surgical resection. Kuijk et al. (83) described three patients that developed an osteonecrosis after surgery for HO, followed by radiation and use of an NSAID. The radiation was in the form of a single low dose. In short-term follow-up, no complication of the osteonecrosis was noted, although long-term problems have not been studied. This course of postoperative treatment (NSAID and radiation) may therefore not be appropriate. Further study in this area is needed.

Recurrence of HO after resection is common (13,54,79,84), but one should measure the success of the surgery by the functional improvement, such as wheelchair sitting, grooming, hygiene, feeding, and mobility capabilities. Recurrence may be lessened if HO is removed during a radionucleotide steady state. A proper wheelchair seating evaluation should take place after surgery of HO about the hip, to protect the skin and improve the sitting posture of the patients.

SUMMARY

HO is a soft tissue ossification often found after SCI. The incidence of HO after SCI is approximately 50%. The etiology of this condition is unknown. The pathology of HO is characterized by an extraarticular involvement of paralyzed extremities. The histology of HO is similar to that of normotopic mature bone with cortical bone and trabecular structure with bone marrow. Clinically, in the acute stage of HO, most common findings are fever, swelling of soft tissue, and reduction of ROM in affected joints. In the chronic stage, HO may limit the functional status of patients. In the early stage, the diagnosis of HO is based on bone scintigraphy, ultrasonography, or CT scan. In the chronic stages when HO contains mature bone, radiography is the diagnostic test. Serum ALP level, ESR, and C-reactive protein level may be used as complementary diagnostic tests. There is no definitive prophylaxis against the formation of HO. Treatment of HO in the acute phase is etidronate therapy and ROM exercises; at the stage of mature bone, the management of HO is in the domain of orthopedic surgery.

REFERENCES

1. Riedel B. Demonstrazion eines durch echttaegiges umhergehen total destruirten kniegelenkes von einen patienten mit stichverletzung des rueckens. *Verhandlungen der Deutschen Gesellschaft fur Chirurgie* 1983; 12:93–96.
2. Dejerine A, Cellier A. Paraosteoarthropathies of paraplegic patients by spinal cord lesion: clinical and roentgenologic study. *Clin Orthop Related Res* 1991;263:3–12.
3. Liberson M. Tissue calcification in cord lesions. *JAMA* 1953;152: 1010–1013.
4. Banovac K, Gonzalez F, Renfree KJ. Treatment of heterotopic ossification after spinal cord injury. *J Spinal Cord Med* 1997;20:60–65.
5. Banovac K, Gonzalez F. Evaluation and management of heterotopic ossification in patients with spinal cord injury. *Spinal Cord* 1997;35: 158–162.
6. Sobus KML, Alexander MA, Harcke HT. Undetected musculoskeletal trauma in children with traumatic brain injury or spinal cord injury. *Arch Phys Med Rehabil* 1993;74:902–904.
7. Garland DE. A clinical perspective on common forms of acquired heterotopic ossification. *Clin Orthop Related Res* 1991;263:13–29.
8. Banovac K. The effect of etidronate on late development of heterotopic ossification after spinal cord injury. *J Spinal Cord Med* 2000;23:40–44.
9. Stover SL, Hataway CJ, Zeiger HE. Heterotopic ossification in spinal cord-injured patients. *Arch Phys Med Rehabil* 1975;56:199–204.
10. Lynch C, Pont A, Weingarden SI. Heterotopic ossification in the hand of a patient with spinal cord injury. *Arch Phys Med Rehabil* 1981;62: 291–291.
11. Meythaler JM, Tuel SM, Cross LL, et al. Heterotopic ossification of the extensor tendons in the hand associated with traumatic spinal cord injury. *J Am Paraplegia Soc* 1992;15:229–231.
12. Hardy AG, Dickson JW. Pathological ossification in traumatic paraplegia. *J Bone Joint Surg* 1963;45B:76–87.
13. Stover SL, Niemann KMW, Tullos J. Experience with surgical resection of heterotopic bone in spinal cord injury patients. *Clin Orthop Related Res* 1991;263:71–77.
14. Garland DE. Surgical approaches for resection of heterotopic ossification in traumatic brain injured patients. *Clin Orthop Related Res* 1991; 263:59–70.
15. Rossier AB, Bussat P, Infabte F, et al. Current facts on para-osteoarthropathy (POA). *Paraplegia* 1973;11:36–78.
16. Cassar-Pulicino VN, McCleland M, Badwan DAH, et al. Sonographic diagnosis of heterotopic bone formation in spinal cord patients. *Paraplegia* 1993;31:40–50.
17. Ackerman LV. Extra-osseous localized non-neoplastic bone and cartilage formation (so-called myositis ossificans). *J Bone Joint Surg* 1958; 40A:279–298.
18. Naraghi FF, DeCoster TA, Moneim MA, et al. Heterotopic ossification. *Orthopedics* 1996;19:145–152.
19. Michelsson JE, Rauschning W. Pathogenesis of experimental heterotopic bone formation following temporary forceful exercising of immobilized limbs. *Clin Orthop Related Res* 1983;176:265–275.
20. Hernandez AM, Forner JV, de la Fuente T, et al. The para-articular ossification in our paraplegics and tetraplegics: a survey of 704 patients. *Paraplegia* 1978;16:272–275.
21. Garland DE. Heterotopic ossification. In: Nickel VL, Botte MT, eds. *Orthopedic rehabilitation.* New York: Churchill Livingstone, 1992: 453–469.
22. Elledge ES, Smith AA, McMahon WF, et al. Heterotopic ossification formation in burned patients. *J Trauma* 1988;28:684–687.
23. Evans EB. Heterotopic bone formation in thermal burns. *Clin Orthop Related Res* 1991;263:94–110.
24. Urist MR. Bone morphogenic protein: the molecularization of skeletal system development. *J Bone Miner Res* 1997;12:343–346.
25. Lal S, Hamilton BB, Heinemann A. Risk factors for heterotopic ossification in spinal cord injury. *Arch Phys Med Rehabil* 1989;70:387–390.
26. Bravo-Payno BB, Esclarin A, Arzoz T, et al. Incidence of risk factors in the appearance of heterotopic ossification in spinal cord injury. *Paraplegia* 1992;30:740–745.
27. Gonda K, Nakaoka T, Yoshimura K, et al. Heterotopic ossification of degenerating rat skeletal muscle induced by adenovirus-mediated transfer of bone morphogenic protein-2 gene. *J Bone Miner Res* 2000; 15:1056–1065.
28. Baron M, Stern J, Lander P. Heterotopic ossification heralded by a knee effusion. *J Rheumatol* 1983;10:961–964.
29. Good AK, Solsky MA, Gulati SM. Heterotopic ossification simulating acute arthritis: a patient with stable, chronic neurologic disease. *J Rheumatol* 1983;10:124–127.
30. Perkash A, Sullivan G, Toth L, et al. Persistent hypercoagulation associated with heterotopic ossification in patients with spinal cord injury long after injury has occurred. *Paraplegia* 1993;31:653–659.
31. Colachis SC, Clinchot DM. The association between deep venous thrombosis and heterotopic ossification in patients with acute traumatic spinal cord injury. *Paraplegia* 1993;31:507–512.
32. Banovac K, Renfree KJ, Hornicek FJ. Heterotopic ossification after brain and spinal cord injury. *Crit Rev Phys Rehabil Med* 1998;10: 223–256.
33. Hencey JY, Vermess M, Van Geertruyden HH, et al. Magnetic resonance imaging examinations of gluteal decubitus in spinal cord injury patients. *J Spinal Cord Med* 1996;19:5–8.
34. Sferopoulos NK, Anagnostopoulos D. Ectopic bone formation in a child with a head injury: complete regression after immobilization. *Int Orthop* 1997;21:412–414.
35. Sell S, Schieh T. C-reactive protein as an early indicator of the formation of heterotopic ossification after total hip replacement. *Arch Orthop Trauma Surg* 1999;119:205–207.
36. Hsu JD, Sakimura I, Stauffer ES. Heterotopic ossification around the hip joint in spinal cord injured patients. *Clin Orthop Related Res* 1975; 112:165–169.
37. Tibone J, Sakimura I, Nickel VL, et al. Heterotopic ossification around the hip in spinal cord–injured patients. *J Bone Joint Surg* 1978;60A: 769–775.
38. Orzel JA, Rudd TG. Heterotopic bone formation: clinical, laboratory and imaging correlation. *J Nucl Med* 1985;26:125–132.
39. Spielman G, Gennarelli TA, Rogers CR. Disodium etidronate: its role in preventing heterotopic ossification in severe head injury. *Arch Phys Med Rehabil* 1983;64:539–542.
40. Furman R, Nickolas JJ, Jivoff L. Evaluation of the serum alkaline phosphatase in the spinal cord and traumatic brain injured patients. *J Bone Joint Surg* 1970;52A:1131–1136.
41. Venier LH, Ditunno JF. Heterotopic ossification in the paraplegic patient. *Arch Phys Med Rehabil* 1971;52:475–479.
42. Binder SM, Rubins IM, Desjardins JV, et al. Evidence for a humoral mechanism for enhanced osteogenesis after head injury. *J Bone Joint Surg* 1990;72A:1144–1149.
43. Kurer MHJ, Khoker MA, Dandone P. Human osteoblast stimulation by sera from paraplegic patients with heterotopic ossification. *Paraplegia* 1992;30:163–168.
44. Renfree KJ, Banovac K, Hornicek FJ, et al. Evaluation of serum osteoblast mitogenic activity in spinal cord and head injury patients with acute heterotopic ossification. *Spine* 1994;19:740–746.
45. Wildburger R, Zarkovic N, Egger G, et al. Comparison of the values of basic fibroblast growth factor determined by immunoassay in the sera of patients with traumatic brain injury and enhanced osteogenesis and the effects of the same on the fibroblast growth in vitro. *Eur J Clin Chem Clin Biochem* 1995;33:693–698.
46. Schurch B, Capaul M, Rossier A. Prostaglandin E₂ measurements: their value in the early diagnosis of heterotopic ossification in spinal cord injury patients. *Arch Phys Med Rehabil* 1997;78:687–691.
47. Weiss S, Grosswasser Z, Ohri A, et al. Histocompatibility (HLA) antigens in heterotopic ossification associated with neurological injury. *J Rheumatol* 1979;6:88–91.

48. Minaire P, Betuel H, Girard R, et al. Neurologic injuries, paraosteoarthropathies, and human leukocyte antigens. *Arch Phys Med Rehabil* 1980;61:214–215.

49. Garland DE, Alday B, Venos KG. Heterotopic ossification and HLA antigens. *Arch Phys Med Rehabil* 1984;65:531–533.

50. Bodley R, Jamous A, Short D. Ultrasound in the diagnosis of heterotopic ossification in patients with spinal injuries. *Paraplegia* 1993;31:500–506.

51. Snoecx M, DeMuynck M, VanLaere M. Association between muscle trauma and heterotopic ossification in spinal cord injured patients: reflections on their causal relationship and the diagnostic value of ultrasonography. *Paraplegia* 1995;33:464–468.

52. Thomas EA, Cassar-Pullicino VN, McCall IW. The role of ultrasound in the early diagnosis and management of heterotopic bone formation. *Clin Radiol* 1991;43:190–196.

53. Zeanah WR. Myositis ossificans. *Clin Orthop Related Res* 1982;168:187–191.

54. Garland DE, Orwin JF. Resection of heterotopic ossification in patients with spinal cord injuries. *Clin Orthop Related Res* 1989;242:169–176.

55. Freed JH, Hahn H, Menter R, et al. The use of three-phase bone scan in the early diagnosis of heterotopic ossification (HO) and in the evaluation of Didronel therapy. *Paraplegia* 1982;20:208–216.

56. Garland DE. Clinical observations on fractures and heterotopic ossification in the spinal cord an traumatic brain injured population. *Clin Orthop Related Res* 1988;178:86–101.

57. Suzuki Y, Hisada K, Takeda M. Demonstration of myositis ossificans by ^{99m}Tc pyrophosphate bone scanning. *Nucl Med* 1974;111:663–664.

58. Prakash V, Lin MS, Perkash I. Detection of heterotopic calcification with ^{99m}Tc-pyrophosphate in spinal cord injury. *Clin Nucl Med* 1978;3:167–169.

59. Tanaka T, Rossier AB, Hussey RW, et al. Quantitative assessment of para-osteoarthropathy and its maturation on serial radionucleotide bone images. *Radiology* 1977;123:217–222.

60. Kim SW, Wu SY, Kim RC. Computerized quantitative radionucleotide assessment of heterotopic ossification in spinal cord injury patients. *Paraplegia* 1992;30:803–807.

61. Ditunno JF, Formal CS. Chronic spinal cord injury. *N Engl J Med* 1994;330:550–556.

62. Brooker AF, Bowerman JW, Robinson RA, et. al. Ectopic ossification following total hip replacement. *J Bone Joint Surg* 1973;55A:1629–1632.

63. Stover SL, Hahn HR, Miller JM. Disodium etidronate in the prevention of heterotopic ossification following spinal cord injury (preliminary report). *Paraplegia* 1976;14:146–156.

64. Garland DE, Alday B, Venos KG, et al. Diphosphonate treatment for heterotopic ossification in spinal cord injury patients. *Clin Orthop Related Res* 1983;176:197–200.

65. Banovac K, Gonzalez F, Wade N, et al. Intravenous disodium etidronate therapy in spinal cord injury patients with heterotopic ossification. *Paraplegia* 1993;31:660–666.

66. Francis MD, Russell RGG, Fleisch H. Diphosphonates inhibit formation of calcium phosphate crystals in vitro and pathological calcification in vivo. *Science* 1969;165:1964–1966.

67. Mahy PR, Urist MR. Experimental heterotopic bone formation induced by bone morphogenic protein and recombinant human interleukin-1b. *Clin Orthop Related Res* 1988;237:236–244.

68. Aida Y, Toda Y, Shimakosi Y, et al. Effect of disodium ethane-1-hydroxy-1,1-diposphonate on interleukin-1 production by macrophages. *Microbiol Immunol* 1986;30:1199–1206.

69. Finerman GA, Stover SL. Heterotopic ossification following hip replacement or spinal cord injury. Two clinical studies with EHDP. *Metab Bone Dis Related Res* 1981;4/5:337–342.

70. Recker RR, Saville PD. Intestinal absorption of disodium ethane-1-hydroxy-1-disphosphonate using a deconvolution technique. *Toxicol Appl Pharmacol* 1973;24:580–589.

71. Qian T, Kirshblum S, Campagnolo D, et al. Etidronate delays the healing of the spinal fracture in acute spinal cord injury patients. *Arch Phys Med Rehabil* 2000;81:197.

72. Sautter-Bihl ML, Liebermeister E, Nanassy A. Radiotherapy as a local treatment option for heterotopic ossifications in patients with spinal cord injury. *Spinal Cord* 2000;38:33–36.

73. Kjaersgaard AP, Schmidt SA. Total hip arthroplasty. The role of antiinflammatory medication in prevention of heterotopic ossification. *Clin Orthop Related Res* 1991;263:78–86.

74. McMahon JS, Waddell JP, Matron J. Effect of short course indomethacin on heterotopic bone formation after uncemented total hip arthroplasty. *J Arthroplasty* 1991;6:259–264.

75. Charnley G, Judet T, Garreay de Loubresse C, et al. Excision of heterotopic ossification around the knee following brain injury. *Injury* 1996;27:125–128.

76. Biering-Sorenson F, Tondevold F. Indomethacin and disodium etidronate for the prevention of recurrence of heterotopic ossification after surgical resection. Two case reports. *Paraplegia* 1993;31:513–515.

77. Crawford CM, Varghese G, Mani MM, et al. Heterotopic ossification: are range of motion exercises contraindicated? *J Burn Care Rehabil* 1986;7:323–327.

78. Wharton GW, Morgan TH. Ankylosis in the paralyzed patients. *J Bone Joint Surg* 1970;52A:105–109.

79. Subbarao YV, Nemchausky BA, Gratzer M, et al. Resection of heterotopic ossification and Didronel therapy—regaining wheelchair independence in the spinal cord injured patient. *J Am Paraplegia Soc* 1987;10:3–7.

80. Wainapel SF, Rao PU, Schepsis AA. Ulnar nerve compression by heterotopic ossification in a heard-injured patient. *Arch Phys Med Rehabil* 1985;66:512–514.

81. McAuliffe JA, Wolfson AH. Early excision of heterotopic ossification about the elbow followed by radiation therapy. *J Bone Joint Surg* 1997;79A:749–755.

82. Freebourn TM, Barber DB, Albe AC. The treatment of immature heterotopic ossification in spinal cord injury with combination surgery, radiation therapy and NSAID. *Spinal Cord* 1999;37:50–53.

83. Kuijk AA, Kuppevelt HJM, Schaal DB. Osteonecrosis after treatment for heterotopic ossification in spinal cord injury with the combination of surgery, irradiation and an NSAID. *Spinal Cord* 2000;38:319–324.

84. Meiners T, Abel R, Bohm V, et al. Resection of heterotopic ossification of the hip in spinal cord injured patients. *Spinal Cord* 1997;35:443–445.

DUAL DIAGNOSIS: TRAUMATIC BRAIN INJURY IN A PERSON WITH SPINAL CORD INJURY

ROSS D. ZAFONTE
ELIE ELOVIC

The spinal cord injury (SCI) medicine physician caring for the person with neurotrauma is often faced with the complex concerns of an individual with a dual diagnosis of SCI and traumatic brain injury (TBI). Neuromedical research in this area is minimal and data to guide clinicians are lacking. Institutional and community environments are often not equipped to handle one of these diagnoses, let alone both. Proper allocation of resources is challenging considering the wide spectrum that both disease processes can take.

Individuals with a dual diagnosis represent a tremendous challenge to the team of professionals treating them. Developing a treatment team comfortable in treating this complex group of persons is necessary. In today's environment, it becomes important, and perhaps critical, for the clinician to assist in the dedication of resources to further study the management of persons with a dual diagnosis. Epidemiological issues of TBI, clinical management of the person with a dual diagnosis, controversial neuromedical concerns, and outcomes are discussed.

EPIDEMIOLOGY OF TRAUMATIC BRAIN INJURY

It is never easy to discuss the issue of TBI epidemiology, because previous studies can be difficult to interpret. The landmark studies of the past had different inclusion criteria, making it difficult to compare and tabulate data. In addition, when reviewing the literature, one must not confuse a study's inclusion criteria with an actual definition of TBI. The reader is referred to a review of the epidemiology of TBI for detail [1].

The Centers for Disease Control and Prevention (CDC) estimated that 1.5 million Americans survive a TBI every year [2]. In the United States, 50,000 deaths per year result from TBI; this accounts for more than one third of all injury-related deaths [3]. There are approximately 230,000 hospital admissions each year as a result of TBI [4]. Most people who sustain a TBI survive, and there is an even larger pool of injured individuals with residual deficits. On a yearly basis, up to 90,000 persons develop a long-term disability secondary to TBI, and the CDC estimates that there are 5.3 million survivors of TBI in the

United States [5]. Financially, the costs of TBI can be staggering. An estimate from 1985 placed the direct and indirect cost in the United States at $37.8 billion [6]. Secondary to these potentially devastating costs, the government has recognized the need to study and increase prevention efforts and provide financial support to these processes. The Traumatic Brain Injury Act of 1996 provides $3 million per year funding for state surveillance systems. As a result, data collection is now occurring in an organized fashion in more than 15 states.

INCIDENCE

Numerous efforts have been made to determine the incidence of TBI in the United States [2,9–24]. A wide disparity exists between the studies relative to the actual incidence, based on location, population studied, time, and inclusion criteria. Cooper et al. [11] and Whitman et al. [13] reported the highest incidences of TBI, with rates of 249 per 100,000 population in the Bronx, New York, and 403 per 100,000 for inner city African Americans, respectively. Fife et al. [17], on the other hand, reported a rate of 152 per 100,000 in a more suburban community. Clearly, there has been a drop in hospital admissions secondary to TBI, and there has been some benefit from prevention programs. However, some of this drop is most likely secondary to hospital admission criteria. Changing the definition of brain injury to include emergency department and other outpatient visits without admission would give a much higher incidence. Schootman and Fuortes [25] estimated a rate of 540 out of every 100,000 in the United States from 1995 to 1997 using that criteria, whereas Guerrero et al. [26] reported a rate of 392 of 100,000 for emergency department visits alone.

INJURY SEVERITY

There is limited uniformity among authors describing TBI incidence and severity. To assist the SCI clinician in dealing with

TABLE 18.1. GLASGOW COMA SCALE

Score	Patient Response
Eye opening	
4	Eyes open on their own
3	Eyes open when asked in a loud voice
2	Opens eyes when pinched
1	Does not open eyes
Best motor response	
6	Follows simple commands
5	Pulls examiner's hands away when pinched
4	Pulls a part of the body away when pinched
3	Decorticate posturing when pinched
2	Decerebrate posturing when pinched
1	No motor response to pinch
Verbal response	
5	Carries on a conversation correctly and oriented
4	Seems confused or disoriented
3	Talks but makes no sense
2	Makes sounds that examiner cannot understand
1	Makes no noise

From Teasdale G, Jennett AB. Assessment of coma and impaired consciousness. *Lancet* 1974;2:81, with permission.

TABLE 18.2. RELATIONSHIP BETWEEN POSTTRAUMATIC AMNESIA AND INJURY SEVERITY

Length of Stay	Severity
Less than 5 min	Very mild
5–60 min	Mild
1–24 hr	Moderate
1–7 d	Severe
1–4 wk	Very severe
More than 4 wk	Extremely severe

TABLE 18.3. GLASGOW OUTCOME SCALE

Score	Category
1	Death
2	Persistent vegetative state
3	Severe disability
4	Moderate (disabled but independent)
5	Good recovery

From Jennett B, Bond MR. Assessment of outcome in severe brain damage: a practical scale. *Lancet* 1975;1:480–484, with permission.

the person who has a dual diagnosis, we discuss the most commonly encountered severity assessment scales.

The Glasgow Coma Scale (GCS) score, first described in 1974, is a widely used scale secondary to ease of use and potential prognostic value (Table 18.1) (27). Three parameters are tested: best motor score, eye opening, and verbal responsiveness. Scores on the GCS range from the lowest possible score of 3 to the highest possible score of 15. A score between 3 and 8 is considered a severe injury; between 9 and 12, a moderate injury; and between 13 and 15, a minor injury (27).

Najaryan (28) published a grading system based on the neurologic condition of the patient upon arrival to the emergency department. The patients are given a rating of I to IV based on their responsiveness and neurologic functioning. In 1974, Ommaya and Gennarelli (29) published a grading scale from I to VI based on severity of injury after a blow to the head. Grades I through III include injuries without loss of consciousness. Grades IV through VI involve loss of consciousness with increasing severity up to death with a grade VI lesion (29). Based on primate research, Gennarelli developed a grading system based on diffuse axonal injury (DAI). Grade 0 has no evidence of DAI. Grade 1 has DAI primarily in the parasagittal white matter, whereas a grade of 2 is given when the DAI also involves the corpus callosum. Finally, a grade of 3 is given if the DAI is also found in the superior cerebellar peduncle (30).

Russell and Nathan (31) was one of the first to recognize that posttraumatic amnesia (PTA) may be a good predictor of recovery and an assessment of injury severity (Table 18.2). A link between PTA and outcome related to the Glasgow Outcome Scale, as well as intelligence quotient performance, has been demonstrated (Table 18.3) (32,33). The length of PTA is con-

TABLE 18.4. THE GALVESTON ORIENTATION AND AMNESIA TEST

1. What is your name? (2) _____
   Where were you born? (4) _____
   Where do you live? (4) _____
2. Where are you now (city)? (5) _____
   Hospital? (5) _____
3. On what date were you admitted to the hospital? (5) _____
   How did you get here? (5)
4. What is the first event you can remember after the injury? (5) _____
   Can you describe in detail (e.g., date, time, companions) the first event you can recall after the injury? (5)
5. Can you describe the last event you recall before the injury? (5) _____
   Can you describe in detail (e.g., date, time, companions) the last event you can recall before the injury? (5)
6. What time is it now? (1 point for each half hour removed from the current time to a maximum of 5 points) _____
7. What day of the week is it? (1 point per day removed from correct one) _____
8. What day of the month is it? (1 point for each day removed from the correct one to a maximum of 15 points) _____
9. What is the month? (5 points for each month removed from the correct one to a maximum of 15 points) _____
10. What is the year? (10 points for each year removed from the correct one to a maximum of 30 points) _____

Total Error Points: _____
Total Score (100 minus total error points): _____

sidered the time that passes before the patient is able to form new continuous memory. Levin et al. (34,35) developed a scale called the Galveston Orientation and Amnesia Test (GOAT), which can be used to objectively assess the duration of amnesia (Table 18.4). When the patient scores more than 75 out of 100 consistently, he or she is out of PTA (34,35).

There has been a shift to a greater incidence of minor TBIs. It has been recently reported that up to 80% of all injuries are minor in origin (13–15,24). These data may be difficult to collect, because most mild injuries are not being captured in the state registries. Data that include emergency department visits give an extremely high incidence of mild brain injury, with an incidence of 1 to 1.5 million cases of emergency department treatments with discharge to home (2,26).

MORTALITY

According to Kraus (36), in 1990 TBI accounted for 75,000 deaths, accounting for 52% of the 148,480 injury-related deaths. In 1994, 51,350 people died in the United States secondary to TBI, with most of them dying from firearms or transportation issues (37). The mortality rate has dropped substantially (approximately 20%) from a rate of 24.7 per 100,000 in 1980 to 19.8 per 100,000 in 1994 (5). Choi et al. (38) noted that a low motor score on the GCS, together with the presence of a fixed or dilated pupil and older age, strongly predicted death or severe disability.

RISK FACTORS IN TRAUMATIC BRAIN INJURY

As with SCI, men are far more likely to have a TBI, all severity, when compared with women. Male to female incidence ratios vary from 2 to 3 : 1. Men are also more likely to die from their injury. When looking at mortality data, the ratio may become as high as 5 : 1. These differences may be explained in some part by gun-related violence, alcohol use, occupational hazards, and participation in contact sports (39,40).

According to the CDC, the leading cause of TBI-related mortality differs for the sexes. The leading cause of death of men between the ages of 15 and 84 is firearms, that for women aged 15 to 74 is transportation-related injuries. Among people older than 75 years, falls are the leading cause of TBI-related mortality for women, and it only becomes that for men when they reach age 85 (41).

Other important outcome differences have begun to be explored. Women who are hospitalized with a TBI have a significantly greater risk of poor outcome based on Disability Rating Scale scores (42). Recently, Farace and Alves (43) completed a metaanalysis involving eight studies and 20 variables, and women showed poorer outcomes on 85% of the variables studied.

A review of the literature regarding race has raised the issue of a potential relationship between race and TBI incidence and mortality. Although differences have been found, there has been no clear study that shows the difference is race specific and not related to some other confounding variable such as lower income

(10). There have been numerous publications that have documented a relationship between family income and an increase in incidence and mortality secondary to TBI (12,44,45).

Previous injury predisposes an individual to additional injury. Although this has been demonstrated in numerous studies, it is unclear whether this is a result of risk-taking behavior, premorbid conditions, or preselection by drugs or alcohol, or whether this is secondary to an actual deficit from the original injury. In all likelihood, it is probably a combination of all of the above (11,35,44).

The relationship between age and incidence of injury is high. Past work has often shown that the highest incidence of TBI occurs for people 15 to 24 years of age (1,13,14). More recently, reports from the state registries have demonstrated that the highest incidence actually occurs in people older than 75 years, and the next highest rate is for those 15 to 24 years old (46). Three recent papers that estimated the incidence of TBI based on emergency department and ambulatory visits have very different statistics by age. The two studies that only look at emergency department visits show that the younger a person is, the higher the incidence (26,47). The highest rate was reported for people 0 to 14 years old, with a rate of more than 1,200 per 100,000 for boys younger than 4 years. The study that included all ambulatory care visits had the highest rate for those 0 to 14 years of age, followed by 15 to 24, which was then followed by those older than 75 years (25). For the age-group consisting of people 75 years and older, falls were the number one cause for TBI, whereas transportation was first for the 15 to 24 year olds. For fatal injuries, the highest rate is reported for the older than 75 years group, whereas second to them are the 15 to 24 year olds. According to 1994 data from the CDC, firearms are the major cause of death for men aged 15 to 84. When men are older than 84, falls become the major source of fatal injury, whereas transportation is the leading cause of TBI-related death for those younger than 15 years. The picture is different for women. Up to age 74, transportation is the major source of TBI-related mortality, with falls being the greatest after age 75.

Age, as previously stated, is an important prognostic indicator. There is a progressive age-associated increase in mortality and morbidity (48). However, among survivors that require inpatient rehabilitation, although costs and length of stay are increased, similar outcomes can be achieved in an older population (49).

CAUSE OF INJURY

The etiology of TBI has been studied numerous times, because this is critical to assist in prevention efforts. Transportation remains the number one source of TBI, with falls being second (4,5,9,12,14,15,20). In special areas, such as the inner city, interpersonal violence may play a much larger part, may be far more important, and may even be the leading cause of TBI (10,13).

The etiology of TBI mortality has undergone drastic changes over the years. Air bags and seat belts have made a major impact in vehicle-related TBI mortality. As a result, there has been a 38% reduction in transportation-related TBI, from 11.1 per 100,000 in 1980 to 6.9 per 100,000 in 1994. Unfortunately, during that same time, firearm–related TBI deaths have increased 22%, from 6.9% to 8.4% and is now the leading cause of TBI-related mortality (5). The mortality rate of firearm-related TBI is more than 90% (9,50).

DUAL DIAGNOSIS

TBI can occur concurrently with SCI and vertebral injury; the remainder of this chapter discusses the issue of dual diagnosis. Data from the Spinal Cord Model Systems report that 28.2% of patients with SCI have at least a minor brain injury with loss of consciousness. They also report that 11.5% of patients with SCI have a TBI severe enough that cognitive or behavioral changes can be witnessed (51). Past studies have demonstrated that patients with an SCI are at high risk for having sustained a TBI as well. They demonstrated a rate of TBI between 24% and 59% when SCI is the primary injury (51,52–60). In addition, past research has demonstrated that the incidence of TBI increases with the level of the SCI (Table 18.5).

When the primary diagnosis is TBI, the incidence of SCI is relatively low, with studies reporting rates between 1.2% and 6% (Table 18.6) (58,61–64). Although it may be uncommon, the potential catastrophe of a missed SCI diagnosis makes it critical to be addressed, particularly with the obtunded or comatose patient with TBI. It is a vital part of acute management to avoid further injury to the patient while emergency treatment is being administered. Efforts at triage of patients for cervical spine evaluation have been somewhat helpful in clarifying matters; however, they sometimes give different answers. Gbaanador et al. (61) reported no relationship between severity of head injury and cervical spine injury (CSI), but Demetriades et al. (65) reported a higher incidence of CSI with lower GCS scores. With a GCS score between 13 and 15, 9 and 12, and less than 8, the incidence of CSI was 1.4%, 6.8%, and 10.2%, respectively (65).

How does one clear the spine in patients with multitraumas?

TABLE 18.5. PERCENTAGE OF TRAUMATIC BRAIN INJURY REPORTED WITH PRIMARY SPINAL CORD INJURY

Study	Year	Percentage
Meinecke (56)	1967	31% Calculated
Harris (57)	1967	44% Cervical
		23% Dorsal
		26% Lumbar
		33% Total
Silver (53)	1980	50%
Shrago (54)	1973	53% with C1–2
		9% with <C5
Steudel et al. (52)	1988	56%
Davidoff et al. (55)	1988	49%
Michael et al. (58)	1989	24%
Saboe et al. (59)	1991	26%
Model systems data (51)	1995	40%
Iida et al. (60)	1999	35% Moderate or severe

TABLE 18.6. PERCENTAGE OF SPINAL CORD INJURY REPORTED WITH PRIMARY TRAUMATIC BRAIN INJURY

Study	Year	Percentage
Gbaanador et al. (61)	1986	1.2%
Bayless and Ray (62)	1989	1.7%
Michael et al. (58)	1989	6%
Soicher and Demetriades (63)	1991	3.5% Cervical
Kach et al. (64)	1993	5.8% Stable cervical
		2.9% Unstable cervical
Model systems data	2000	4.1%

Bayless and Ray (62) suggest that cervical films may be avoided in the awake and asymptomatic patient. After reviewing the records of 333 consecutive trauma patients, Fischer (66) suggested that alert patients who had sustained blunt trauma require cervical spine radiographic evaluation only if they had signs or symptoms of cervical damage or neurologic injury. Bachulis et al. (67) reviewed the records of 5,000 trauma patients and recommended screening for patients with a decreased level of consciousness, patients whose injury suggests that they could have sustained a CSI, patients with neurologic deficits consistent with cervical injury, and patients with neck pain or tenderness. Grossman et al. (68) concluded from a national survey of trauma centers that CSI without fracture has a very low incidence of 0.7%. The rate of missed CSI was much lower, at 0.01%. There also was a general consensus about which patients required C-spine screening, but less so about which radiographic study was appropriate.

CLINICAL CONCERNS IN THE PERSON WITH A DUAL DIAGNOSIS

Advances in basic neurobiology research would add much to the knowledge of basic pathophysiology of TBI and SCI. It is well recognized that a primary concern of the rehabilitation team is the management of individuals with associated behavioral or cognitive disturbance. Because the primary and secondary injury phenomena associated with both injuries are so diverse, not one single entity can represent a pattern of care for such persons.

It remains important for the clinician to be aware of individuals with SCI who may have sustained mild or perhaps even less subtle TBI. The clinical variations and presentations of associated behavioral disturbance can be varied and pronounced. Deficits in arousal, attention, memory, and capacity for new learning, as well as initiation, can be observed. Of major concern to the rehabilitation team in dealing with a person with a dual diagnosis is the occurrence of agitation, aggression, disinhibition, and depression. The nature and severity of these disturbances can present in various ways. Their manifestation appears to be an interaction between preinjury cognitive, economic, and emotional statuses and the nature of the brain dysfunction and neuromedical variations during the time of care (69). Longer-term concerns can focus on depression, sleep disturbances, and difficulty integrating into the community.

Cognitive and Behavioral Disturbance in the Person with Dual Diagnoses

The Evaluation Process

No strong and traditional method for evaluating a patient with a dual diagnosis exists. A key factor is the incorporation of premorbid historical factors into any reasonable assessment of the patient's behavioral and cognitive status. Although typically thought of as a primary factor in determining TBI, posttraumatic alteration in consciousness is not necessarily present when individuals have TBI-related findings. Evaluation of preinjury parameters should include prior psychology-psychiatric disturbance, prior history of substance abuse, history of brain injury, and occult brain injury from assault or other etiology (70). Prior data support the conclusion that individuals with higher preinjury functional levels have better functional outcomes after TBI than individuals with less than optimal premorbid psychosocial integration into the community (71). Although no data are available, it would seem intuitive that this factor holds and perhaps is even magnified in individuals with dual diagnoses. Additional factors that should be considered should include a history of learning disability and family support.

The best known scale for TBI assessment was developed by Teasdale and Jennett (27), the GCS. This scale provides for a brief assessment tool that has been shown to be highly correlated with acute morbidity and mortality, and more grossly correlated with broad long-term functional outcome (72,73). It should be noted, however, that Williams et al. (74) demonstrated that among individuals with GCS scores between 13 and 14, persons with positive lesions on computerized axial tomography scan imaging appear to have outcomes that appear more like those of persons with moderate injuries. Some have classified these individuals as having "complicated" mild injuries.

Acute medical concerns that are associated with an impact on outcome include protracted elevated intracranial pressure, associated hypoxemia, or hypotension. Hypoxia and ischemia may be focal or rather diffuse and are noted to significantly affect mortality. This relative hypoperfusion remains a concern in persons with both severe brain injury and SCI, because it is well known that autodysregulation occurs after traumatic SCI as the relative mean arterial pressures are lowered. In an initial study of the question, Vale et al. (76) described the impact of maintaining perfusion on persons with SCI. No data exist that evaluate the role of hypoperfusion in persons with dual diagnoses (76).

Additional clinical findings that are important when evaluating the person with SCI and TBI include the best and worst GCS scores within 24 hours of injury, the duration of coma, and the length of PTA. Duration of PTA has been linked to functional outcome (77,78). This parameter may be challenging to measure retrospectively and the GOAT remains a valuable tool. Described by Levin et al. (34,35), the GOAT is an examination of orientation and recall that can be administered at the bedside (Table 18.4). As described previously, consecutive scores of more than 75 indicate emergence from PTA (34,35).

Imaging

Neuroimaging advances have made the demonstration of clinically suspected TBI cleaner; however, for most individuals with milder injury, static imaging test results including brain magnetic resonance imaging (MRI) and computed tomography (CT) scans are normal. CT imaging was noted to be superior to MRI in detecting hemorrhagic lesions in the first 72 hours after injury (79). The superiority of MRI is clearly present for detecting brain stem and deep lesions (79). Although prognostic of individuals who may remain in the vegetative state or who have more severe disabilities, the ability of MRI to predict a more specific functional outcome appears limited at present (80). Ventricular enlargement has been correlated with poor cognitive outcome (81,82). More promising are the functional imaging modalities such as functional MRI, single photon emission CT (SPECT), and positron emission tomography, which appears capable of demonstrating dynamic disorders. Although the lack of standardization in the interpretation of SPECT has led to some concerns, this diagnostic modality has been able to evaluate subtler lesions and address neurobehavioral outcome (83,84).

Clinical Data Interpretation

Specialists evaluating a patient with dual diagnosis should be well aware of the timing of any associated brain-stem abnormalities, evoked potential data and any obtained cerebrospinal fluid (CSF) markers. An important standardization of evaluation is the history of postinjury concerns or parameters, be they the rate of neurologic recovery, and neuromedical-associated morbid factors, such as return to surgery, hydrocephalus, posttraumatic hydrocephalus, or posttraumatic seizures. Behavioral disorders such as agitation or akathisia, pathologic tone, or persistent somatic complaints should be sought. No consistent formula for assessing cognitive parameters exists. Clearly, the GOAT, in conjunction with medical records, is used to support the evidence of suspected brain injury and the determination of PTA.

Formal neuropsychological testing may be battery based and may be of a great deal of assistance. The Halstead-Reitan neuropsychological test battery is widely used but is by no means given in its full form by all psychologists. This test's heavy reliance on sensory and motor functioning may not be appropriate for persons with SCI. Additional caveats include the concern of preinjury cognitive status, depression, and the effects of medications on cognition (85).

Diagnostic Concerns

Clinicians should be aware that persons with dual diagnoses certainly might become frustrating to staff and to the primary person caring for such individuals. Factors of symptom verification, emotional functioning, and grief awareness, as well as behavioral disturbance, are noted.

Careful scrutiny of all cases to evaluate for contributing factors in determining whether an individual has had an associated brain injury remains important. Response styles and veracity of the examinee cannot be overemphasized. In addition, a careful scrutiny of all data should be performed. Clinicians should monitor for elements of secondary gain, resistance to evaluation, violation of testing rules, and authenticity of effort (86). A number of tests can be given as screens for cognitive malingering or so-called simulation behaviors (87,88). These tests assist in evaluating the ability of responses but cannot be unilaterally employed to determine malingering.

Of concern, is the individual with a dual diagnosis who appears unaware of his or her situation and lacks common symptoms of grief and adjustment. Such individuals may report no or little emotional reaction and their interpretation may be accepted by the staff as an adequate or beneficial adjustment. As patients emerge from PTA, their awareness of deficits may well improve. A moral and ethical dilemma remains as to when to inform such individuals of personal losses that may have occurred as a result of their accident.

In contrast to the individuals just described are those individuals whose emotional liability, agitation, irritability, and impatience are clearly evident to the staff. Such persons may be labeled "uncooperative" or "noncompliant" when actually exhibiting evidence of posttraumatic agitation or posttraumatic behavioral disturbance. Concerns with disorders of memory and carryover also remain a substantial problem for individuals with dual diagnoses (89,90). Memory testing remains as a complex variety of tasks that involve arousal and initiation, acquisition, storage, and recall. The scope of these activities implicates areas from the nervous system that are diverse and involve frontal, temporal, and thalamic regions (91). Once a clear determination has been made that the person has a true memory, in addition to cognitive or behavioral dysfunction, a plan of action should be set forth by the team. Specifics related to this task are discussed.

Behavioral Disturbance and Agitation

Posttraumatic agitation receives potentially the greatest attention in the medical rehabilitation literature related to TBI. However, no clear agreement exists regarding the definition of the diagnosis of this state. The attention that this condition receives is likely secondary to the high intensity of staff utilization, frustration, and resource allocation that such patients require.

The incidence of posttraumatic agitation has ranged widely from 11% to 50%, largely because of an inconsistent definition of what posttraumatic agitation is (92). No data are available to describe the incidence of agitation among persons with a dual diagnosis. Sandel and Mysiw (93) proposed a definition that encompasses components of restlessness, aggression, and emotional dyscontrol, as well as cognitive changes. Their definition suggests that posttraumatic agitation is a subtype of delirium unique to survivors of TBI, in which the survivor is in a state of PTA and there was some combination of excessive behaviors that include aggression, akathisia, disinhibition, and emotional liability. These guidelines may be helpful in establishing further clarity of research into this area.

There is a need for a reliable measurement of acute behavioral dysfunction. The agitated behavior scale is the only instrument that is both reliable and validated as a measure of PTA in survivors of severe TBI. This instrument, which was developed by Corrigan and Bogner (94), is reasonably easy to administer and remains consistent with the previously described definition of posttraumatic agitation. Scores of 22 or more on this scale are considered indicative of posttraumatic agitation. Other scales can be employed to evaluate behavioral disturbance. One example is the overt aggression scale, which was developed for use in geriatric-psychiatric patients (95).

The evaluation of behavioral disturbance in the person with a dual diagnosis is complex. Not only must premorbid history be taken into account, but also the clinician caring for such persons must be aware of neuromedical causes of behavioral dysfunction. Issues such as seizures, posttraumatic hydrocephalus, new intracranial pathology, neuroendocrine disturbance, metabolic disturbance, hypoxemia, and infectious issues must be accounted for (96). Sleep disturbance also remains a profound cause of behavioral dysfunction (97). The individual with two neural disabilities may be at higher risk. Fichtenberg et al. (98) demonstrated that individuals with neural disability are at a high risk for post–acute sleep disturbance. Prigatano (99) discussed the instance of sleep disturbance in individuals with TBI and noted a significant impact of sleep on neurobehavioral function after TBI. Bilateral frontal lesions in animals have been demonstrated to result in permanent sleep dysfunction. Forebrain and brain stem interconnections act to form a rather complex network that participates in sleep generation (100,101). Sleep modulation occurs over a rather diffuse area, so it is easy to understand why individuals with TBI are likely to experience significant elements of sleep disturbance. This sleep disturbance can well lead to behavioral disturbance, depression, performance deficits, and irritability.

Medications That Impact Recovery

Medications can also play a role in the behavior that individuals with dual diagnoses exhibit. Such medications may exacerbate confusion or affect the learning of new behavioral strategies. It is important to closely monitor the medications because those frequently used for one disorder (SCI or TBI) can have a negative effect in a person with a dual diagnosis. In general, an approach that emphasizes reevaluation of all medications and a program of minimization should be accomplished.

Data suggest that anticonvulsant prophylaxis may be warranted for only the first week after TBI (102). Although this remains a point of discussion for some, no clear evidence supports long-term prophylaxis. Practice society guidelines of several organizations have advocated against long-term anticonvulsant prophylaxis (103). Long-term use of phenytoin has been associated with adverse cognitive effects, and the deleterious impact of phenobarbital on cognition and performance is well documented (104,105).

Antihypertensive agents such as methyldopa may have a significant sedative effect. Clonidine is an α_2-agonist with central activity that may impair cognition. Clonidine has been advocated for the treatment of spasticity in persons with SCI and brain injury (106,107). Barbeau et al. (108) employed clonidine to improve locomotor recovery in spinal-injured cats, whereas Goldstein (109) noted impaired motor performance in rats with cortical lesions.

Neuroleptic agents are relatively strong blockers of dopamine and also serve as cholinergic and adrenergic antagonists. By their very nature, neuroleptics block monoamine release and their use in persons with TBI raises some initial concerns. Feeney (110) first raised the issue that neuroleptics may impair some elements of recovery in the rodent model. Most neuroleptic agents act at the D2-receptor, which may in part explain their significant side-effect profile. Concerns remain with seizure thresholds, anticholinergic side effects, neuroleptic malignant syndrome, sleep disturbance, and detrimental effects on new learning and memory (111). Atypical antipsychotic agents are newer agents with both dopaminergic and serotonin blocking qualities (112). Although atypical antipsychotics appear to have a lower potential for extrapyramidal side effects, their effects on long-term cognitive outcome in the person with brain injury are not yet clear.

Gastrointestinal agents such as histamine-1–blocking agents may produce a sedative effect. Metoclopramide is often employed in the acute setting to enhance gastrointestinal mobility. Although this agent appears to raise esophageal pressure and promote pyloric relaxation, it also has significant dopaminergic antagonist effects. Such effects can produce deleterious cognitive responses and extrapyramidal side effects (113).

Benzodiazepines are commonly employed to assist persons with brain injury in managing their agitation, and in SCI, benzodiazepines are frequently used to treat spasticity. They act via the $GABA_a$ receptor. Benzodiazepines readily cross the blood brain barrier, producing anterograde amnesia and anxiolysis. These agents produce sedation but also decrease new learning and memory capacity.

Tricyclic antidepressant agents are often employed for persons with SCI to treat depression or pain. Care should be taken to monitor for anticholinergic side effects with these agents. Such effects can produce an element of drowsiness and affect new learning (114). Selective Serotonin Reuptake Inhibitor (SSRI) medications are frequently used for depression and arousal disorders, although concerns are raised regarding the potential of serotonin medications to exacerbate spasticity in person with SCI (115).

Lastly, anticholinergic agents, such as antihistamines, and other medications with anticholinergic activity can result in marked sedation and difficulty with new learning. Such agents should be avoided in routine employment, particularly as sleep-enhancing agents.

Impact on Rehabilitation

The cognitive and behavioral aspects of brain injury that may be present in the person who presents with an SCI have a dramatic impact on their ability to undergo comprehensive rehabilitation, as previously discussed. This includes from the perspective of the patient as well as from the rehabilitation staff. Comprehensive rehabilitation requires intensive new learning, mastering of new skills (e.g., mobility, self-care, and bowel and bladder issues), and adaptation to a new lifestyle. The proper setting for therapy will need to be determined. This includes whether the patient can tolerate therapy in an active gym or whether the patient requires a quiet setting to learn new tasks. In addition, individualized therapy may be more appropriate.

Treatment

The key to the treatment of posttraumatic agitation in a person with a dual diagnosis is a coordinated effort from a behavioral and pharmacotherapeutic intervention point of view (Fig. 18.1). Behavioral therapies should focus on those that are seen as relevant to the person and the situation manner. Patients often require a limitation of distracting environmental tasks and quiet

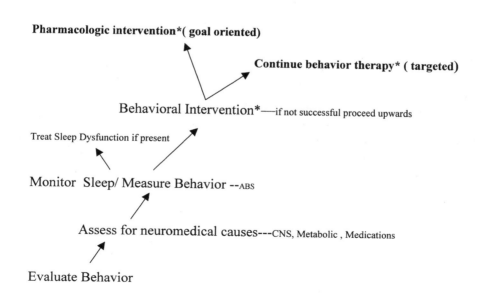

FIGURE 18.1. An approach to agitation.

environments (116,117). For patients who exhibit modifiable agitation, procedures such as time-out or slow-down periods have been employed to prevent aggression by preempting such episodes (118,119). Behavioral contracts can often be set up between parties, which clearly satisfy the rights and responsibilities for those individuals who are more aware.

There are virtually no prospective evaluations of pharmacologic intervention for the management of posttraumatic agitation. There is a serious limitation in the TBI literature and no studies looking at persons with a dual diagnosis exist. However, inferences can be made from retrospective case reports and inferential observations of several agents that have been employed successfully for the treatment of severe posttraumatic agitation. These are reviewed here.

Carbamazepine is described as the most commonly used pharmacologic agent in the management of posttraumatic agitation, but there is little evidence to support its efficacy (120). Several case studies have looked at the efficacy of carbamazepine in the management of agitation and aggressive disorders after brain injury (121). Carbamazepine used for neurobehavioral purposes should be titrated on the basis of clinical response, rather than rigidly adhering to "therapeutic drug levels." Valproic acid has been used as well in the treatment of posttraumatic agitation. Valproic acid may have a GABA-ergic or "antikindling-like" effect. Wroblewski et al. (122) reported a case series of posttraumatic patients with destructive and aggressive behaviors successfully treated with valproic acid.

Amantadine is a unique agent initially developed for treatment of influenza A. It has been used for the treatment of Parkinson disease and has now been advocated in brain injury for cognitive and neurobehavioral disorders. This agent appears to have presynaptic and postsynaptic dopamine-enhancing properties, as well as *N*-methyl-D-aspartate–receptor activity. Amantadine has been used by Chandler et al. (123) for the treatment of agitation, and it has also been described as improving arousal in a number of individuals (124). Adverse effects of amantadine include seizures, irritability, livedo reticularis, and hallucinations.

β-Blockers have been used in the treatment of organic brain syndrome, mental retardation, autism, dementia, and aggressive disorders after brain injury. Brooke et al. (125) evaluated the effects of β-blockers on 21 survivors of severe TBI in a double-blind placebo-controlled trial. They noted that the number of agitated episodes was unchanged by propranolol, but that the intensity of the agitation significantly decreased. There appears to be some differential between β-blockers: The more lipophilic β-blockers tend to produce a more sedative quality, and those that are more hydrophilic may treat some of the more peripheral manifestations of agitation.

Haloperidol remains the most classic of neuroleptic agents with strong antidopaminergic qualities. However, animal and human studies raise significant concerns about the negative effect of dopamine antagonists on motor recovery. It should be also pointed out that significant antiadrenergic effects exist with the use of neuroleptic agents (109,110). Given the potential side effects, which include seizures, extrapyramidal side effects, neuroleptic malignant syndrome, motor slowing, and impact on new learning and sleep, these agents do not appear to be first-line treatments for posttraumatic agitation (126). Clearly, the role of atypical antipsychotics needs to be further explored and their role in the management of agitation is not yet clear.

Benzodiazepines represent a commonly used treatment for agitation in TBI. However, major concerns are raised by their use. By their very design, benzodiazepines will produce an amnestic state that clearly is not beneficial to new learning. In addition, animal studies have suggested that persistent administration of benzodiazepines has resulted in reinduction of motor asymmetry weeks after the animal has recovered from a central nervous system (CNS) injury (127). The previously mentioned studies suggest that benzodiazepines contribute to the observed impaired recovery of motor and functional skills. When benzodiazepines are given on an intermittent basis, they may exacerbate the level of agitation, producing a so-called benzodiazepine psychosis.

Tricyclic antidepressants were first suggested as an intervention for posttraumatic agitation by Jackson (128). Cases described improvement in arousal and attention in survivors of severe TBI after initiating amitriptyline, protriptyline, and desipramine (129,130). In addition, Mysiw et al. (131) described the use of amitriptyline for posttraumatic agitation. Concerns have been raised regarding the potential anticholinergic properties of tricyclic antidepressants and their effect on cognitive recovery. However, these authors have not noted any significant impact of this in their work.

Trazodone and nefazodone have been used in the management of posttraumatic agitation. These agents have been used specifically to enhance sleep and produce a sedative quality at night. The efficacy of trazodone alone as a pure antiagitation agent is described in only one abstract, which looked at the effect of trazodone in improving agitation in a group of brain injury survivors who did not respond to amitriptyline (132). Trazodone has in general been used safely but can cause seizures, hypotension, hallucinations, cardiac dysrhythmias, and priapism. Boyeson et al. (133) also raised concerns about the impact of serotonin agents on motor recovery in the animal model. Although trazodone and nefazodone are very useful agents, thoughtful employment is necessary.

Additional agents have also been employed successfully for the treatment of agitated behavior disorders. Lithium, which is a membrane-stabilizing salt (134), has also effectively treated episodes of mania precipitated by brain injury (135). Care must be employed when using lithium because a compendium of side effects potentially exists. Buspirone has been described as effective in the treatment of anxiety and agitated-like disorders after brain injury in several case studies. The findings imply that most of the effects of buspirone are due to its anxiolytic properties, which are typically observed many weeks after initiation of therapy. The use of this agent in the acutely agitated patient is therefore in need of further investigation.

Memory Dysfunction

Memory deficits are extraordinarily common after TBI and may be exacerbated by the concomitant stress of individuals with dual diagnoses. It is in the realm of memory that many of the most frustrating defects exist after TBI. Poor performance on memory tasks can be related to retrieval, registration, or storage. Programs that focus on task-specific adaptations and the use of supportive devices are of greatest value.

The cholinergic system is one of the best known and most thoroughly studied components in memory. Evidence of the role acetylcholine plays in memory enhancement has come from studies in patients with Alzheimer disease, as well as nonhuman primates. There has been evidence that acetylcholine precursors and cholinergic agonists improve memory. Cardenas (136) completed her study of physostigmine in a double-blind clinical trial. More than 40% of patients demonstrated improved memory and long-term storage. An additional agent that has been employed in the treatment of memory disorders is tacrine, an anticholinesterase inhibitor. This agent has primarily been used in the Alzheimer disease population. Donepezil and rivastigmine are newer anticholinesterase inhibitors that have shown a positive impact in patients with Alzheimer disease. The use of donepezil in the treatment of posttraumatic memory disorders is underway.

Alertness and Arousal

Arousal is among the most basic of cognitive functions and the basis behind which all other higher level functioning is based. Whyte (137) defined *arousal* as "the general state of readiness of an individual to process sensory information and/or organize a response." Anatomically, the reticular activating system and limbic systems are involved in "general" and "goal-directed" arousal. Measures to evaluate a person's ability to respond have been reviewed, and the coma recovery scale has been found to be among the most favorable (138). After a careful examination of the potential neuromedical and pharmacologic confounding factors, one can consider augmentation via stimulants.

Neuromedical Complications

The role of the SCI medicine physician in dealing with the person with a dual diagnosis is complex. Several neuromedical complications clearly can occur and must be monitored. This discussion focuses on controversies that affect the person with a dual diagnosis including deep venous thrombosis (DVT), spasticity, and late CNS complications.

Deep Venous Thrombosis

Venous thromboembolism is a major complication associated with trauma. In a prospective study, Geerts et al. (139) found that 56.7% of the patients studied had DVT. The incidence of venous thromboembolism has been reported to be as high as 100% in individuals after traumatic SCI and has been reported to be as high as 54% in patients with major head injuries (140). A consequence of DVT can be the development of a serious and life-threatening pulmonary embolus (PE). The mortality rate of individuals developing a PE is high, because DVT is often clinically silent or presents with subtle nonspecific findings. Individuals suffering major head injuries and SCI have decreased awareness and limited sensation. Although statements

exist focusing on prevention for persons with SCI, this issue has not been well investigated in the TBI population. No studies focus on DVT in the dual-diagnosis population.

It is generally accepted that at least 90% of clinically important PEs result from DVT in the leg (141). The risk of developing DVT after TBI or SCI increases in direct proportion to the number of predisposing factors. Hammond and Meighen (142) described a number of risk factors for DVT, which include prolonged immobility and coma, protracted surgical procedures, paralysis, hypercoagulability, blood transfusion, pelvic and lower extremity fractures, femoral vein catheterization, disseminated intravascular coagulopathy, and sepsis.

Clinical examination to detect DVT is neither sensitive nor specific, yielding false-positive and false-negative results. The practitioner must maintain a high index of suspicion so the presence of the asymptomatic DVT is detected. The role of screening for DVT at the time of rehabilitation admission is not yet clear. Meythaler et al. (143) discussed the cost-effectiveness of duplex screening for DVT in the TBI population, whereas Lai et al. (144) described the incidence of symptomatic DVT to be low in the TBI population. Powell et al. (145) performed a retrospective study of 189 patients with SCI admitted to rehabilitation who underwent duplex scanning. These authors felt that screening examinations were important. However, others have felt that an unacceptable number of false-negative results occur with Impedance Plethysmography (IPG) or duplex screening. Rossi et al. (146) determined that D-dimer using an enzyme-linked immunosorbent assay method has a good negative predictive value for DVT, yet widespread use and standardization of this method is lacking.

Controversies in Prophylaxis and Treatment in the Dual-Diagnosed Patient

The Paralyzed Veterans of America (PVA) consortium group reviewed recommendations for prophylaxis among persons with SCI (147). Although reasonable evidenced-based recommendations have been made for persons with SCI, no such clarity exists for individuals with TBI. Although no studies appear to address the issue of the patient with a dual diagnosis, it is safe to assume that the risk of DVT is quite high. This risk is exacerbated by the amount of immobility required to treat both diagnoses in the acute care setting. Warbel et al. (148) noted that 10% of patients who had undergone a craniotomy experienced DVT risk factors of leg weakness, longer length of stay, and more postoperative days in the intensive care unit. Sonaglia et al. (149) noted that preoperative soluble fibrin polymers correlated with postoperative DVT in patients who underwent elective neurosurgery.

No clear data exist regarding safety for prophylaxis among individuals who have experienced traumatic intracranial lesions. Agnelli et al. (150) suggested that low-molecular-weight heparin (LMWH) and compression stockings are safe and effective prophylaxis for people who have required elective neurosurgery. Nurmohamed et al. (151) also noted that LMWH and compression stockings were safe in an elective neurosurgical population. The role of anticoagulants (either unfractionated or LMWH) in the treatment of DVT among persons with posttraumatic intracranial lesions is unclear. The risk of hemorrhagic complications with anticoagulation therapy in persons after intracranial surgery has prevented investigation of the use of anticoagulant agents during this period. Schaible et al. (152) evaluated the safety of anticoagulant therapy in Holtzman rats after craniotomy. They concluded that if therapy was initiated during the first 7 days, the risk of intracerebral hemorrhage was high. If, however, an additional 3 to 7 days elapsed before the initiation of anticoagulation, the incidence of hemorrhage declined significantly. This group suggested that anticoagulation could be safely initiated 10 to 14 days after craniotomy (152).

Spasticity

Spasticity is a common complication in the patient with SCI, TBI, or both. A comprehensive discussion regarding spasticity is covered in chapter 14. Proper positioning, casting, and splinting techniques are widely used to reduce tone and increase range. Among persons with dual diagnoses, special concerns, however, are raised. Persons with behavioral dysfunction may increase their restlessness or agitation when casting or splints are applied. Although devices that are not removable are often most beneficial for persons with TBI, sensory concerns may limit the use of such methods among persons with SCI.

As with other neuromedical problems, the use of pharmaceutical agents to treat spasticity in persons with dual diagnoses has not been adequately investigated. Several agents may have differential effects in the dual-diagnosis population. Diazepam, a GABA$_a$ analog has historically been employed in the treatment of spasticity. However, diazepam can produce sedation and has a noted effect on new learning. Lioresal, a GABA$_b$ agonist is noted to be effective in the treatment of spasticity of a spinal origin. No clear evidence exists demonstrating strong efficacy when the origin of the spasticity is central. At higher doses, Lioresal can produce sedation. Hallucination is a concern with abrupt withdrawal, and Lioresal can lower the seizure threshold. Tizanidine is an imidazoline derivative that has been employed to treat spasticity. Concerns exist about asthenia, hypotension, and sedation, which may limit its use in the dual-diagnosis population. Dantrium is a hydantoin derivative whose major function is to lower calcium flux across the sarcoplasmic reticulum. Additional medications such as clonidine, cyclobenzaprine, cyproheptadine, gabapentin, and vigabatrin are among other agents that have been used. Each carries a concern of sedation or exacerbation of motor dysfunction in the dual-diagnosis population. Of interest, a recent Cochrane database review revealed insufficient evidence to assist clinicians in a rational approach to antispasticity therapy for persons with SCI (153). Thus, the clinician must carefully evaluate the response of each patient, determine his or her tolerance to side effects, and make goal-oriented pharmacotherapeutic choices.

Local interventional therapy such as neuromuscular blockade, perineural blockade, and intramuscular administration of neurotoxin agents appears effective but requires a focus on the treatment goals. Spasticity of a more localized origin appears to respond favorably to these interventions, which do not carry the cognitive side-effect profile of the systemic medications. Intrathecal therapy with Lioresal has been found to be effective in the SCI and TBI population (154).

Late Central Nervous System Complications

Hydrocephalus

Hydrocephalus is the most common treatable CNS condition after TBI and can result in profound changes in some persons. The differentiation of hydrocephalus from *ex vacuo* ventricular dilation remains a challenge. Typically, hydrocephalus is described as communicating and noncommunicating. In communicating hydrocephalus, the ventricular system remains interconnected and CSF is free flowing from the ventricles to the cisterns. It is communicating hydrocephalus that occurs in most posttraumatic cases (155). The incidence of posttraumatic hydrocephalus varies according to the method employed to detect the ventricular enlargement. The incidence of posttraumatic ventricular enlargement in severe TBI averages 62%. However, most of this is believed to be posttraumatic *ex vacuo* phenomena and not true communicating hydrocephalus. The incidence of requiring a shunt is only 3% to 8% (156). The diagnosis of posttraumatic hydrocephalus is a challenging one and remains controversial. Persons may present with normal pressure, hydrocephalus-like symptoms of ataxia, incontinence, and dementia, although the degree of neurologic impairment and presentation varies widely. Persons may present with lethargy, motor incoordination, or even behavioral dysfunction. Static neuroimaging is moderately helpful, and serial CT scans can help evaluate progression of the process. The determination of which patients may benefit from shunting is also a point of controversy. Bontke et al. (156) advocated for lumbar puncture to evaluate for elevated CSF pressure, whereas other authors (157) discussed the use of CSF tap test, in which clinical response is monitored after 30 to 60 mL of fluid removal.

Neuroendocrine Disorders

Both anterior and posterior pituitary dysfunction can occur after CNS trauma. Panhypopituitarism is a rare situation that results in a significant decrease in arousal and awareness. Anterior pituitary dysfunction is associated with malaise, hyponatremia, hypothermia, and bradycardia. Hypothalamic dysfunction also leads to sleep regulatory, appetite, and satiety disorders.

Disorders of sodium metabolism are seen commonly after TBI. The syndrome of inappropriate secretion of antidiuretic hormone (SIADH) results in hyponatremia and is usually associated with posterior pituitary dysfunction. SIADH is most often treated with fluid restriction. Of note, although SIADH had been considered the most common cause of posttraumatic hyponatremia, an increasing appreciation for the identity of cerebral salt wasting (CSW) has begun. First described by Peters and Welt (158), CSW is a disorder of sodium metabolism that results in hyponatremia and evidence of dehydration exists as manifested by weight loss (159). Unlike with SIADH, hydration and oral sodium chloride are mainstays of therapy, so care must be taken to evaluate for the correct diagnosis. Central diabetes insipidus results in elevated serum sodium concentration and significant polyuria. Diabetes insipidus is traditionally treated with desmopressin.

Posttraumatic Epilepsy

Rates of posttraumatic epilepsy have varied depending on the criteria and definitions employed. Seizures have generally been divided into several categories. Early posttraumatic seizures occur within the first week, whereas late posttraumatic seizures occur after week one. Seizures that happen at the time of the injury are often referred to as impact seizures. The overall incidence of posttraumatic epilepsy has been reported to be 5%. Tempkin (102) demonstrated that routine use of prophylaxis for more than 1 week is not warranted. Risk factors for posttraumatic seizures include depressed skull fracture, early posttraumatic seizure, presence of a foreign body, dural tear, cerebral contusions, and PTA lasting more than 24 hours.

Central Dysautonomia

Autonomic dysfunction is a well-known sequela of SCI, yet central dysautonomia can be a vexing concern in persons with TBI. Caused by abnormal hypothalamic function, symptoms include rigidity, fevers, tachycardia, and sweating. The preoptic region and the anterior hypothalamus are the loci for hypothalamic control of temperature. Injuries impacting this area can produce findings of marked temperature dysregulation. Once other sources are evaluated for, β-blockers and bromocriptine have been reported to be of assistance (160,161).

DUAL DIAGNOSIS: OUTCOMES AND COMMUNITY INTEGRATION

Successful rehabilitation of persons with SCI requires that they have the ability to learn new skills and retain information pertaining to their care. Few studies have examined the actual effects of TBI on outcome among individuals with SCI.

Richards et al. (162) discussed the difficulty of making an unequivocal diagnosis of TBI among persons with SCI. In an earlier study, Richards et al. (163) collected outcome data on 150 persons with SCI. Evidence of TBI was sought by history and neuropsychological examination. Groups of persons with SCI alone and SCI and TBI where reevaluated 2 years later. Greater adjustment difficulties were noted among persons with dual diagnoses; however, the sample was not large enough to make conclusions (163). Brown and Vandergoot (164) evaluated quality-of-life parameters among persons with TBI and others living in the community. Unmet needs were stronger in the TBI group than in the SCI group. In Sweden, Kreuter et al. (165) noted that both SCI and TBI appear to negatively affect overall quality of life and mental well being.

A substantial concern for persons with neurodisability is substance abuse. Kolakowsky-Hayner et al. (166) reported that 81% of persons with TBI and 96% of persons with SCI reported preinjury alcohol use. Fifty-seven percent of persons with SCI and 42% of persons with SCI were heavy drinkers. It is likely that future data may reveal the importance of dealing with substance abuse among individuals with dual diagnoses.

Intuitively, it seems that the presence of a dual diagnosis would have a negative impact on all aspects of care. This would include an increase in the length of stay in acute rehabilitation, a decreased rate of discharge to home, and an increased rate of medical complications, thereby increasing rehospitalization rates. Medical issues may include pressure ulcers due to the ina-

bility to remember to perform a pressure relief, and bladder and bowel dysfunction due to the inability to perform these programs adequately. Unfortunately, there are few studies in this area, so the impact of a brain injury with an SCI has not been fully elucidated.

CONCLUSION

The care of the person with a dual diagnosis is complex and requires an interactive knowledge of two major disabilities. The approach to the individual with neurobehavioral dysfunction must be methodical and comprehensive. Further research is needed to delineate the appropriate treatment for neuromedical and neurobehavioral dysfunction associated with dual diagnoses.

REFERENCES

1. Elovic E, Antoinette T. Epidemiology and primary prevention of traumatic brain injury. In: Horn LJ, Zasler ND, eds. *Medical rehabilitation of traumatic brain injury.* Philadelphia: Hanley & Belfus, 1996.
2. Sosin DM, Sniezek JE, Thurman DJ. Incidence of mild and moderate brain injury in the United States, 1991. *Brain Inj* 1996;10(1):47–54.
3. Sosin DM, Sniezek JE, Waxweiler RJ. Trends in death associated with traumatic brain injury, 1979 through 1992. Success and failure. *JAMA* 1995;273(22):1778–1780.
4. Centers for Disease Control and Prevention. National Center for Injury Prevention and Control. Unpublished data analysis from the 1994 National Hospital Discharge Survey, 2000.
5. Division of Acute Care. Traumatic brain injury in the United States: a report to Congress. 1999.
6. Max W, Mackenzie EJ, Rice DP. Head injuries: costs and consequences. *J Head Trauma Rehabil* 1991;6:76–91.
7. Kalsbeek WD, McLaurin RL, Harris BS III, et al. The National Head and Spinal Cord Injury Survey: major findings. *J Neurosurg* 1980; Suppl:S19–S31.
8. Caveness WF. Incidence of craniocerebral trauma in the United States in 1976 with trends from 1970 to 1975. In: Thompson RA GJ, ed. *Advances in neurology.* New York: Raven Press, 1979:1–3.
9. Annegers JF, Grabow JD, Kurland LT, et al. The incidence, causes, and secular trends of head trauma in Olmsted County, Minnesota, 1935–1974. *Neurology* 1980;30(9):912–919.
10. Klauber MR, Barrett-Connor E, Marshall LF, et al. The epidemiology of head injury: a prospective study of an entire community—San Diego County, California, 1978. *Am J Epidemiol* 1981;113(5): 500–509.
11. Cooper K, Tabaddor K, Hauser WA, et al. The epidemiology of head injury in the Bronx. *Neuroepidemiology* 1983;2:70–88.
12. Jagger J, Levine JI, Jane JA, et al. Epidemiologic features of head injury in a predominantly rural population. *J Trauma* 1984;24(1): 40–44.
13. Whitman S, Coonley-Hoganson R, Desai BT. Comparative head trauma experiences in two socioeconomically different Chicago-area communities: a population study. *Am J Epidemiol* 1984;119(4): 570–580.
14. Kraus JF, Black MA, Hessol N, et al. The incidence of acute brain injury and serious impairment in a defined population. *Am J Epidemiol* 1984;119(2):186–201.
15. Tiret L, Hausherr E, Thicoipe M, et al. The epidemiology of head trauma in Aquitaine (France), 1986: a community-based study of hospital admissions and deaths. *Int J Epidemiol* 1990;19(1):133–140.
16. Gutierrez MI, Velasquez M, Levy A. Epidemiology of head injury in Cali, Columbia. In: Chiu WT, et al, eds. *Proceedings of the first international symposium of the epidemiology of head and spinal cord injury.* Taipei: 1994.

17. Fife D, Faich G, Hollinshead W, et al. Incidence and outcome of hospital-treated head injury in Rhode Island. *Am J Public Health* 1986;76(7):773–778.

18. MacKenzie EJ, Edelstein SL, Flynn JP. Hospitalized head-injured patients in Maryland: incidence and severity of injuries. *Md Med J* 1989;38(9):725–732.

19. Gabella B, Hoffman RE, Marine WW, et al. Urban and rural traumatic brain injuries in Colorado. *Ann Epidemiol* 1997;7(3):207–212.

20. Traumatic brain injury—Colorado, Missouri, Oklahoma, and Utah, 1990–1993. *MMWR Morb Mortal Wkly Rep* 1997;46(1):8–11.

21. Koskinen S, Leppanen L, Alaranta H, et al. Epidemiology of traumatic brain injury in Finland 1991–1995. In: Program and abstracts of the 3rd World Congress on Brain Injury; 1999; Quebec, Canada. Abstract.

22. Thurman DJ, Jeppson L, Burnett CL, et al. Surveillance of traumatic brain injuries in Utah. *West J Med* 1996;165(4):192–196.

23. Hillier SL, Hiller JE, Metzer J. Epidemiology of traumatic brain injury in South Australia. *Brain Inj* 1997;11(9):649–659.

24. Chiu WT, Yeh KH, Li YC, et al. Traumatic brain injury registry in Taiwan. *Neurol Res* 1997;19(3):261–264.

25. Schootman M, Fuortes LJ. Ambulatory care for traumatic brain injuries in the US, 1995–1997. *Brain Inj* 2000;14(4):373–381.

26. Guerrero JL, Thurman DJ, Sniezek JE. Emergency department visits associated with traumatic brain injury: United States, 1995–1996. *Brain Inj* 2000;14(2):181–186.

27. Teasdale G, Jennett B. Assessment of coma and impaired consciousness. A practical scale. *Lancet* 1974;2(7872):81–84.

28. Najaryan R. Emergency room management of the head injured patient. In: Becker DP, Gudeman SK, eds. *Textbook of head injury.* Philadelphia: WB Saunders, 1989:24–26.

29. Ommaya AK, Gennarelli TA. Cerebral concussion and traumatic unconsciousness. Correlation of experimental and clinical observations of blunt head injuries. *Brain* 1974;97(4):633–654.

30. Gennarelli TA, Thibault LE, Adams JH, et al. Diffuse axonal injury and traumatic coma in the primate. *Ann Neurol* 1982;12(6):564–574.

31. Russell WR, Nathan PW. Traumatic amnesia. *Brain* 1946;69:183–187.

32. Bishara SN. Post-traumatic amnesia and Glasgow Coma Scale related to outcome in survivors in a consecutive series of patients with severe closed-head injury. *Brain Inj* 1992;6:373.

33. Young B, Rapp RP, Norton JA, et al. Early prediction of outcome in head-injured patients. *J Neurosurg* 1981;54(3):300–303.

34. Levin HS, O'Donnell VM, Grossman RG. The Galveston Orientation and Amnesia Test. A practical scale to assess cognition after head injury. *J Nerv Ment Dis* 1979;167(11):675–684.

35. Levin HS, Mattis S, Ruff R. Neurobehavioral outcome following minor head injury. A three center study. *J Neurosurgery* 1987;66:234–243.

36. Kraus JF. Epidemiology of head injury. In: Cooper PR, ed. *Head injury.* Baltimore: Williams & Wilkins, 1993:1–24.

37. Centers for Disease Control and Prevention. National Center for Injury Prevention and Control. Unpublished analysis of data from multiple cause of death public use data. 2000.

38. Choi S, Narayan R, Anderson R, et al. Enhanced specificity of prognosis in severe head injury. *J Neurosurg* 1988;69:381–385.

39. Kraus JF, McArthur DL. Epidemiologic aspects of brain injury. *Neurol Clin* 1996;14(2):435–450.

40. Kraus JF, McArthur DL. Incidence and prevalence of, and costs associated with, traumatic brain injury. In: Rosenthal M, Griffith ER, Kreutzer JS, et al, eds. *Rehabilitation of the adult and child with traumatic brain injury.* Philadelphia: FA Davis Co, 1999:3–16.

41. Thurman D, Guerrero J. Trends in hospitalization associated with traumatic brain injury [see Comments]. *JAMA* 1999;282(10):954–957.

42. Wagner A, Hammond F, Sasser H, et al. The use injury severity variables to predict disability and community integration after traumatic brain injury. *J Trauma* 2000;49:411–441.

43. Farace E, Alves W. Do women fare worse? a metaanalysis of gender differences in traumatic brain injury outcome. *J Neurosurg* 2000;93:539–545.

44. Rimel RW, Jane JA, Bond MR. Characteristics of the head injured patient. In: Rosenthal M, Griffith ER, Bond MR, et al, eds. *Rehabilitation of the adult and child with traumatic brain injury.* Philadelphia: FA Davis Co, 1990:8–16.

45. Kraus JF, Fife D, Ramstein K, et al. The relationship of family income to the incidence, external causes, and outcomes of serious brain injury, San Diego County, California. *Am J Public Health* 1986;76(11):1345–1347.

46. Thurman D, Alverson C, Dunn K, et al. Traumatic brain injury in the United States; a public health perspective. *J Head Trauma Rehabil* 1999;14:602–615.

47. Jager TE, Weiss HB, Coben JH, et al. Traumatic brain injuries evaluated in U.S. emergency departments, 1992–1994. *Acad Emerg Med* 2000;7(2):134–140.

48. Teasdale G, Skene A, Parker L. Age and outcome of severe head injury. *Acta Neurochir* 1979;28:140–143.

49. Cifu D. Functional outcomes of older adults with TBI: a prospective multicenter analysis. *Arch Phys Med Rehabil* 1996;77:885–889.

50. Siccardi D, Cavaliere R, Pau A, et al. Penetrating craniocerebral missile injuries in civilians: a retrospective analysis of 314 cases. *Surg Neurol* 1991;35(6):455–460.

51. Go BK, DeVivo MJ, Richards JS. The epidemiology of spinal cord injury. In: Stover SL, Delisa JA, Whiteneck GG, eds. *Spinal cord injury: clinical outcomes from the model systems.* Gaithersburg: Aspen Publishers, 1995:21–51.

52. Steudel WI, Rosenthal D, Lorenz R, et al. Prognosis and treatment of cervical spine injuries with associated head trauma. *Acta Neurochir Suppl (Wien)* 1988;43:85–90.

53. Silver JR, Morris WR, Otfinowski JS. Associated injuries in patients with spinal injury. *Injury* 1980;12(3):291–224.

54. Shrago GG. Cervical spine injuries: association with head trauma. A review of 50 patients. *Am J Roentgenol Radium Ther Nucl Med* 1973;118(3):670–673.

55. Davidoff G, Thomas P, Johnson M, et al. Closed head injury in acute traumatic spinal cord injury: incidence and risk factors. *Arch Phys Med Rehabil* 1988;69(10):869–872.

56. Meinecke FW. Frequency and distribution of associated injuries in traumatic paraplegia and tetraplegia. *Paraplegia* 1968;5(4):196–209.

57. Harris P. Associated injuries in traumatic paraplegia and tetraplegia. *Paraplegia* 1968;5(4):215–220.

58. Michael DB, Guyot DR, Darmody WR. Coincidence of head and cervical spine injury. *J Neurotrauma* 1989;6(3):177–189.

59. Saboe LA, Reid DC, Davis LA, et al. Spine trauma and associated injuries. *J Trauma* 1991;31(1):43–48.

60. Iida H, Tachibana S, Kitahara T, et al. Association of head trauma with cervical spine injury, spinal cord injury, or both. *J Trauma* 1999;46(3):450–452.

61. Gbaanador GB, Fruin AH, Taylon C. Role of routine emergency cervical radiography in head trauma. *Am J Surg* 1986;152(6):643–648.

62. Bayless P, Ray VG. Incidence of cervical spine injuries in association with blunt head trauma. *Am J Emerg Med* 1989;7(2):139–142.

63. Soicher E, Demetriades D. Cervical spine injuries in patients with head injuries. *Br J Surg* 1991;78(8):1013–1014.

64. Kach K, Friedl HP, Imhof HG, et al. Unstable spinal injuries in craniocerebral trauma [in German]. *Helv Chir Acta* 1993;59(4):655–664.

65. Demetriades D, Charalambides K, Chahwan S, et al. Nonskeletal cervical spine injuries: epidemiology and diagnostic pitfalls. *J Trauma* 2000;48(4):724–727.

66. Fischer RP. Cervical radiographic evaluation of alert patients following blunt trauma. *Ann Emerg Med* 1984;13(10):905–907.

67. Bachulis BL, Long WB, Hynes GD, et al. Clinical indications for cervical spine radiographs in the traumatized patient. *Am J Surg* 1987;153(5):473–478.

68. Grossman MD, Reilly PM, Gillett T, et al. National survey of the incidence of cervical spine injury and approach to cervical spine clearance in U.S. trauma centers. *J Trauma* 1999;47(4):684–690.

69. Ricker J, Regan T. Neuropsychological and psychological factors in

acute rehabilitation of individuals with both spinal cord injury and traumatic brain injury. *Top Spinal Cord Rehabil* 1999;5:76–82.

70. Zasler N. Physiatric assessment in traumatic brain injury. In: Rosenthal M, Griffith ER, Kreutzer JS, et al, eds. *Rehabilitation of the adult and child with traumatic brain injury*. Philadelphia: FA Davis Co, 1999:117–130.

71. Putnam S, Adams K. Regression based prediction of long term outcome following multidisciplinary traumatic brain injury. *Clin Neuropsychol* 1992;6:383–392.

72. Teasdale G, Jennett B. Assessment and prognosis of coma after head injury. *Acta Neurochir* 1976;34:45–55.

73. Jennett B, Teasdale G, Braakman R. Prognosis of patients with severe head injury. *Neurosurgery* 1979;4:283–289.

74. Williams D, Levin H, Eisenberg H. Mild head injury classification. *Neurosurgery* 1990;27:422–428.

75. Miller J. Head injury. *J Neurol Neurosurg Psychiatry* 1993;56:440–447.

76. Vale FL, Burns J, Jackson AB, et al. Combined medical and surgical treatment after acute spinal cord injury: results of a prospective pilot study to assess the merits of aggressive medical resuscitation and blood pressure management. *J Neurosurg* 1997;87(2):239–246.

77. Katz DI, Alexander MP. Traumatic brain injury. Predicting course of recovery and outcome for patients admitted to rehabilitation. *Arch Neurol* 1994;51(7):661–670.

78. Zafonte RD, Mann NR, Millis SR, et al. Posttraumatic amnesia: its relation to functional outcome. *Arch Phys Med Rehabil* 1997;78(10):1103–1106.

79. Orrison WW, Gentry LR, Stimac GK, et al. Blinded comparison of cranial CT and MR in closed head injury evaluation. *AJNR Am J Neuroradiol* 1994;15(2):351–356.

80. Gentry LR, Godersky JC, Thompson B, et al. Prospective comparative study of intermediate-field MR and CT in the evaluation of closed head trauma. *AJR Am J Roentgenol* 1988;150(3):673–682.

81. Kurth SM, Bigler ED, Blatter DD. Neuropsychological outcome and quantitative image analysis of acute haemorrhage in traumatic brain injury: preliminary findings. *Brain Inj* 1994;8(6):489–500.

82. Anderson CV, Bigler ED. Ventricular dilation, cortical atrophy, and neuropsychological outcome following traumatic brain injury. *J Neuropsychiatry Clin Neurosci* 1995;7(1):42–48.

83. Jacobs A, Put E, Ingels M, et al. One-year follow-up of technetium-99m-HMPAO SPECT in mild head injury. *J Nucl Med* 1996;37(10):1605–1609.

84. Bavetta S, Nimmon CC, White J, et al. A prospective study comparing SPECT with MRI and CT as prognostic indicators following severe closed head injury. *Nucl Med Commun* 1994;15(12):961–968.

85. Prat R, Calatayud-Maldonado V. Prognostic factors in postraumatic severe diffuse brain injury. *Acta Neurochir (Wien)* 1998;140(12):1257–1260.

86. Sbordone RJ, Seyranian GD, Ruff RM. Are the subjective complaints of traumatically brain injured patients reliable? *Brain Inj* 1998;12(6):505–515.

87. Millis SR, Putnam SH. The Recognition Memory Test in the assessment of memory impairment after financially compensable mild head injury: a replication. *Percept Mot Skills* 1994;79(Suppl 1, Pt 2):384–386.

88. Coleman RD, Rapport LJ, Millis SR, et al. Effects of coaching on detection of malingering on the California Verbal Learning Test. *J Clin Exp Neuropsychol* 1998;20(2):201–210.

89. Santos ME, Castro-Caldas A, De Sousa L. Spontaneous complaints of long-term traumatic brain injured subjects and their close relatives. *Brain Inj* 1998;12(9):759–767.

90. Wilson BA. Recovery of cognitive functions following nonprogressive brain injury. *Curr Opin Neurobiol* 1998;8(2):281–287.

91. Giap B, Jong C, Ricker J, et al. The hippocampus anatomy, pathophysiology and regenerative capacity. *J Head Trauma Rehabil* 2000;15:875–894.

92. Wolf AP, Gleckman AD, Cifu DX, et al. The prevalence of agitation and brain injury in skilled nursing facilities: a survey. *Brain Inj* 1996;10(4):241–245.

93. Sandel ME, Mysiw WJ. The agitated brain injured patient. Part 1:

94. definitions, differential diagnosis, and assessment. *Arch Phys Med Rehabil* 1996;77(6):617–623.

94. Corrigan JD, Bogner JA. Factor structure of the agitated behavior scale. *J Clin Exp Neuropsychol* 1994;16(3):386–392.

95. Yudofsky SC, Kopecky HJ, Kunik M, et al. The overt agitation severity scale for the objective rating of agitation. *J Neuropsychiatry Clin Neurosci* 1997;9(4):541–548.

96. Mysiw WJ, Sandel ME. The agitated brain injured patient. Part 2: pathophysiology and treatment. *Arch Phys Med Rehabil* 1997;78(2):213–220.

97. Clinchot DM, Bogner J, Mysiw WJ, et al. Defining sleep disturbance after brain injury. *Am J Phys Med Rehabil* 1998;77(4):291–295.

98. Fichtenberg NL, Millis SR, Mann NR, et al. Factors associated with insomnia among post-acute traumatic brain injury survivors. *Brain Inj* 2000;14(7):659–667.

99. Prigatano GP. Sleep and dreaming disturbance in closed head injury patients. *J Neurol Neurosurg Psychiatry* 1982;45:78–80.

100. Viallablanca J, Marcus R, Omstead C. effects of frontal cortex ablation in cats. *Exp Neurol* 1976;53:31–39.

101. Nauta W. Hypothalamic regulation of sleep in rats. An experimental study. *J Neurophysiol* 1946;9:246–249.

102. Tempkin N. A randomized double blind trial of phenytoin following severe head injury. *N Engl J Med* 1990;323:497–502.

103. The Brain Trauma Foundation. The American Association of Neurological Surgeons. The Joint Section on Neurotrauma and Critical Care. Resuscitation of blood pressure and oxygenation. *J Neurotrauma* 2000;17(6-7):471–478.

104. Glenn M, Wrobleski B. Anticonvulsants for prophylaxis of posttraumatic seizures. *J Head Trauma Rehabil* 1986;1:73–74.

105. Masagli T. Neurobehavioral effects of phenytoin, carbamazepine and valproic acid: implications for use in traumatic brain injury. *Arch Phys Med Rehabil* 1991;71:219–226.

106. Maynard FM. Early clinical experience with clonidine in spinal spasticity. *Paraplegia* 1986;24(3):175–182.

107. Dall JT, Harmon RL, Quinn CM. Use of clonidine for treatment of spasticity arising from various forms of brain injury: a case series. *Brain Inj* 1996;10(6):453–458.

108. Barbeau H, Chua C, Rossingnol S. Noradrenergic agonists and locomotor training after cord transection in adult cats. *Brain Res Bull* 1993;30:387–393.

109. Goldstein L. Common drugs may influence motor recovery after stroke. *Neurology* 1995;45:865–871.

110. Feeney DM, Gonzalez A, Law W. Amphetamine, haloperidol and experience interact to affect rate of recovery after motor cortex injury. *Science* 1982;217:855–857.

111. Zafonte R, Elovic E, Mysiw WJ, et al. Pharmacology in traumatic brain injury: fundamentals and treatment strategies. In: Rosenthal M, Griffith ER, Kreutzer JS, et al, eds. *Rehabilitation of the adult and child with traumatic brain injury*. Philadelphia: FA Davis Co, 1999:530–555.

112. Elovic E. Atypical antipsychotics; risperidone and clozapine. *J Head Trauma Rehabil* 1996;11;89–92.

113. Meyers M. Gastrointestinal complications of traumatic brain injury In: Horn L, Zasler N, eds. *Medical rehabilitation of traumatic brain injury*. Philadelphia: Hanley & Belfus, 1996.

114. Cope DN. Psychopharmacologic aspects of traumatic brain injury. In: Horn L, Zasler N, eds. *Medical rehabilitation of traumatic brain injury*. Philadelphia: Hanley & Belfus, 1996:573–611.

115. Stolp-Smith KA, Wainberg MC. Antidepressant exacerbation of spasticity. *Arch Phys Med Rehabil* 1999;80(3):339–342.

116. Uomoto J, Brockway J. Anger management training for brain injury patients and their families. *Arch Phys Med Rehabil* 1992;73:674–679.

117. Crane A, Joyce B. Cool down: a procedure for decreasing aggression in adults with traumatic brain head injury. *Behav Res Treat* 1991;6:65–69.

118. Hanley W. behavioral management of brain damaged patients. *Rehabil Nursing* 1983;26:26.

119. Jacobs H. Behavioral management of aggressive sequelae in Reye syndrome. *Arch Phys Med Rehabil* 1986;67:558–562.

120. Fugate LP, Spacek LA, Kresty LA, et al. Measurement and treatment

of agitation following traumatic brain injury: II. A survey of the Brain Injury Special Interest Group of the American Academy of Physical Medicine and Rehabilitation. *Arch Phys Med Rehabil* 1997;78(9): 924–928.

121. Porcher E. Efficacy of the combination of buspirone and carbamazepine in early posttraumatic delirium. *Am J Psychiatry* 1994;151: 150–154.

122. Wroblewski BA, Joseph AB, Kupfer J, et al. Effectiveness of valproic acid on destructive and aggressive behaviours in patients with acquired brain injury. *Brain Inj* 1997;11(1):37–47.

123. Chandler MC, Barnhill JL, Gualtieri CT. Amantadine for the agitated head-injury patient. *Brain Inj* 1988;2(4):309–311.

124. Zafonte RD, Watanabe T, Mann NR. Amantadine: a potential treatment for the minimally conscious state. *Brain Inj* 1998;12(7): 617–621.

125. Brooke MM, Patterson DR, Questad KA, et al. The treatment of agitation during initial hospitalization after traumatic brain injury. *Arch Phys Med Rehabil* 1992;73(10):917–921.

126. Wilkinson R, Meythaler JM, Guin-Renfroe S. Neuroleptic malignant syndrome induced by haloperidol following traumatic brain injury. *Brain Inj* 1999;13(12):1025–1031.

127. Schallert T, Hernandez T, Bart T. Recovery of function after brain damage. Severe and chronic disruption by diazepam. *Brain Res* 1986; 379:104–111.

128. Jackson R, Corrigan J, Arnett J. Amitriptyline for agitation in head injury. *Arch Phys Med Rehabil* 1985;66:180–181.

129. Reinhard D, Whyte J, Sandel M. Improved arousal and initiation following tricyclic antidepressants use in traumatic brain injury. *Arch Phys Med Rehabil* 1996;77:80–83.

130. Wroblewski B. Protriptyline as an alternative stimulant medication in patients with brain injury. A series of case reports. *Brain Inj* 1993; 7:353–362.

131. Mysiw W, Jackson R, Corrigan J. Amitriptyline for posttraumatic agitation. *Arch Phys Med Rehabil* 1988;67:29–33.

132. Rowland T, Mysiw W, Bogner J. Trazodone for the treatment of postraumatic agitation. *Arch Phys Med Rehabil* 1992;73:963.

133. Boyeson MG, Harmon RL, Jones JL. Comparative effects of fluoxetine, amitriptyline and serotonin on functional motor recovery after sensorimotor cortex injury. *Am J Phys Med Rehabil* 1994;73(2): 76–83.

134. Glenn M. Lithium carbonate for aggressive behaviors or affective instability in 10 brain-injured patients. *Am J Phys Med Rehabil* 1989; 68:221–226.

135. Joshi P, Capozolli J, Coyle J. Effective management with lithium of a persistent, posttraumatic hypomania in a 10 year old child. *J Dev Behav Pediatr* 1986;6:352–354.

136. Cardenas D. Oral physostigmine and impaired memory in adults with brain injury. *Brain Inj* 1994;8:579–587.

137. Whyte J. Arousal and attention basic science aspects. *Arch Phys Med Rehabil* 1992;73:940–949.

138. O' Dell M. Standardized assessment instruments for minimally responsive brain injured patients. *Neurorehabilitation* 1996;6:45–55.

139. Geerts WH, Code KI, Jay RM, et al. A prospective study of venous thromboembolism after major trauma. *N Engl J Med* 1994;331(24): 1601–1606.

140. Mamen E. Pathogenesis of venous thrombosis. *Chest* 1992; 102[Suppl]:640–643.

141. Myllynene P, Kammonen M, Rokkanen P, et al. Deep venous thrombosis and pulmonary embolism in patients with acute spinal cord injury; a comparison with nonparalyzed patients due to spinal fractures. *J Trauma* 1984;25:541–543.

142. Hammond F, Meighen M. Venous thromboembolism in the patient with acute traumatic brain injury: screening , diagnosis and treatment issues. *J Head Trauma Rehabil* 1998;13:36–50.

143. Meythaler J, DeVivo M, Hayne J. Cost-effectiveness for routine screening for proximal deep venous thrombosis in acquired brain injury patients admitted to rehabilitation. *Arch Phys Med Rehabil* 1996; 77:1–5.

144. Lai J, Yablon S, Ivanhoe C. Incidence and sequelae of symptomatic

145. Powell M, Kirshblum S, O'Connor K. Duplex ultrasound screening for deep venous thrombosis in spinal cord injury patients at rehabilitation admit. *Arch Phys Med Rehabil* 1999;80:1044–1046.

146. Rossi R, Agnelli G, Taborelli P, et al. Local versus central assessment of venographies in a multicenter trial on the prevention of deep vein thrombosis in neurosurgery. *Thromb Haemost* 1998;82:1399–1402.

147. Clinical practice guidelines: prevention of thromboembolism in spinal cord injury. *J Spinal Cord Med* 1997;20:259–283.

148. Warbel A, Lewicki L, Lupica K. Venous thromboembolism; risk factors in the craniotomy patient population. *J Neurosci Nurs* 1999;31: 180–186.

149. Sonaglia F, Agnelli G, Baroni M, et al. Pre-operative plasma levels of soluble fibrin polymers correlate with the development of deep vein thrombosis after elective neurosurgery. *Blood Coagul Fibrinolysis* 1999;10(8):459–463.

150. Agnelli G, Piovella F, Buoncristiani P, et al. Enoxaparin plus compression stockings compared with compression stockings alone in the prevention of venous thromboembolism after elective neurosurgery. *N Engl J Med* 1998;339(2):80–85.

151. Nurmohamed M, van Riel A, Henkens C, et al. Low molecular weight heparin and compression stockings in the prevention of venous thrombosis after neurosurgery. *Thromb Haemost* 1996;75:233–238.

152. Schaible KL, Smith LJ, Fessler RG, et al. Evaluation of the risks of anticoagulation therapy following experimental craniotomy in the rat. *J Neurosurg* 1985;63(6):959–962.

153. Taricco M, Adone R, Pagliacci C, et al. Pharmacological interventions for spasticity following spinal cord injury. *Cochrane Database Syst Rev* 2000;(2):CD001131.

154. Meythaler J, Guin-Renfroe S, Hadley M. Continuously infused intrathecal baclofen for spastic hemiplegia: a preliminary report. *Am J Phys Med Rehabil* 1999;78:247–254.

155. Guyot LL, Michael DB. Post-traumatic hydrocephalus. *Neurol Res* 2000;22(1):25–28.

156. Bontke C, Zasler N, Baoke C. Rehabilitation of traumatic brain injury. In: Naryan R, ed. *Neurotrauma.* New York: McGraw-Hill, 1996: 841–858.

157. Damasceno BP, Carelli EF, Honorato DC, et al. The predictive value of cerebrospinal fluid tap-test in normal pressure hydrocephalus. *Arq Neuropsiquiatr* 1997;55(2):179–185.

158. Peters J, Welt L. A salt wasting syndrome associated with cerebral disease. *Trans Assoc Am Physicians* 1950;63:57–62.

159. Zafonte RD, Mann NR. Cerebral salt wasting syndrome in brain injury patients: a potential cause of hyponatremia. *Arch Phys Med Rehabil* 1997;78(5):540–542.

160. Meythaler J, Stinson A. fever of central origin in traumatic brain injury controlled with propranolol. *Arch Phys Med Rehabil* 1994;75: 816–818.

161. Russo RN, O'Flaherty S. Bromocriptine for the management of autonomic dysfunction after severe traumatic brain injury. *J Paediatr Child Health* 2000;36(3):283–285.

162. Richards J, Osuna F, Jaworski T, et al. The effectiveness of different methods of defining traumatic brain injury in predicting post discharge adjustment in a spinal cord injury population. *Arch Phys Med Rehabil* 1991;72:275–279.

163. Richards J, Brown L, Hagglund K, et al. Spinal cord injury and concomitant traumatic brain injury. *Am J Phys Med Rehabil* 1988;67: 211–216.

164. Brown M, Vandergoot D. Quality of life for individuals with traumatic brain injury : comparison with others living in the community *J Head Trauma Rehabil* 1998;13:1–23.

165. Kreuter M, Sullivan M, Dahlof A, et al. Partner relationships , functioning, mood and global quality of life in person with spinal cord injury and traumatic brain injury. *Spinal Cord* 1998;36:252–261.

166. Kolakowsky-Hayner SA, Gourley EV, Kreuter JS, et al. Pre-injury substance abuse among persons with brain injury and person with spinal cord injury. *Brain Inj* 1999;13:571–581.

venous thromboembolic disease among patients with traumatic brain injury. *Brain Inj* 1997;11:331–334.

19

REHABILITATION OF SPINAL CORD INJURY

STEVEN KIRSHBLUM
CHESTER H. HO
JAMIE G. HOUSE
ERICA DRUIN
CINDY NEAD
SUSAN DRASTAL

The neurologic impairment is not nearly as important as the quality of rehabilitation, the social support system, and possibly the personality and mind set of persons with SCI themselves that determine coping and ultimately satisfaction with life after injury.

—Sam Stover

Before the second half of the 20th century, persons who sustained a traumatic spinal cord injury (SCI) were given little hope for survival. However, since that time, there has been great progress in the medical care and rehabilitation of those who sustain an SCI, thus improving the life expectancy, functional capability, and community reintegration. Although the search for a cure has brought great success in terms of the basic understanding of injury to the spinal cord, rehabilitation is still what is available to enhance functioning after injury. Because of this, rehabilitation in the acute, subacute, and chronic phases after injury is of utmost importance.

Rehabilitation includes meeting the spine-injured patient's specific medical and rehabilitative needs and is extremely important to help the injured individual achieve his or her potential in terms of physical, social, emotional, recreational, vocational, and functional recovery. The history of spinal cord medical and rehabilitation care in SCI, including the emergency medical services, trauma care centers, the history of the subspecialty of SCI medicine (chapter 1), and the model systems of SCI, is covered elsewhere (1–3).

REHABILITATION IN ACUTE CARE

Rehabilitation should begin as soon as possible after injury. In the acute care hospital, once lifesaving measures have been taken, rehabilitation efforts are important to prevent medical and physical complications, such as atelectasis, thromboembolic disorders, pressure ulcers, and contractures. If early medical complications can be prevented, the rehabilitation course is facilitated and the total rehabilitation and cost of care is lessened, as well as the

degree of human suffering (4). The amount of complications appears to be inversely related to the quality of care available at the hospitals that provide early care (1).

Some of the medical aspects of the SCI specialist's acute recommendations are covered in chapters 6 and 8. The most important aspects in the acute period include bowel, bladder, and pulmonary management, deep venous thrombosis, and gastrointestinal prophylaxis, and proper positioning in bed with turning at least every 2 hours. Once the spine is stabilized, physical and occupational therapy will incorporate range of motion (ROM), including active, active-assistive, and passive ROM. This should be done at least daily, by staff or family, which will help prevent contractures. The shoulder, elbow, hip flexors, and heel cords are most important to range because they are the most frequently observed contractures on presentation to the acute rehabilitation unit and can potentially serve as a source of pain and functional limitation. In addition, light exercises of muscles that are innervated to maintain muscle strength can be performed to prevent disuse atrophy and weakness. Resting splints for paralyzed upper extremities (UEs) can help prevent contractures and increase comfort. Functional UE splints may also be useful for feeding and other self-care skills in the early period. Sitting tolerance can be initiated at the bedside in the acute care hospital. If the patient is sitting, a form of weight relief (shifts) must be performed every 20 to 30 minutes. If the patient is medically stable, mat training can begin in the therapy setting. Speech and language pathologists are frequently asked to perform bedside screening for dysphagia for those with cervical levels of injury. For persons with high-level tetraplegia, who have undergone tracheostomy, early introduction of communication aids (e.g., letter boards) can aid in communication and education in this critical acute care period.

Once the patient is medically stable and after spinal stabilization by surgery or the proper orthosis is in place, the patient should be transferred to a specialized spinal cord rehabilitation unit.

Rehabilitation Team

The interdisciplinary approach of the rehabilitation team is important for the optimal care of the individual with SCI. The team approach allows for an integrated effort of multiple professional disciplines working together with the patient and his or her family for the common goal of maximizing the potential of the patient. The physician specializing in the care of the persons with SCI, who is the team leader, is most commonly a physiatrist, preferably with subspecialty board certification in SCI medicine. Responsibilities of the physician include preventing and treating SCI-specific medical issues, formulating the therapeutic goals and prescriptions, solving team-member conflicts, and discussing prognosis with the patient and family. Members of the team include the rehabilitation nurse; physical, occupational, speech, recreational, and vocational therapists; psychologist; and the social worker or case manager. Additional team members include the orthotist, driving instructor, SCI educator, nutritionist, and rehabilitation engineer. Everyone should keep in mind that the patient and family are full members of the team.

The role of every member of the team is valuable. Although there is occasional overlap between the services, this serves as reinforcement for the patient, rather than as a duplication of services. This includes the training of transfers by the therapists and nurses, spinal cord education by all services, and everyone assisting in adjustment issues for the patient and family to help with reintegration into the community and preparation for discharge.

The rehabilitation nurse serves the usual nursing functions but has the added responsibility of serving as an educator, motivator, and listener and assists in the coordination of discharge planning. The rehabilitation nurse helps the patient and family to recognize medical issues and focus on prevention of complications. This includes training in bowel and bladder issues, monitoring of skin and nutritional needs, and reinforcing ROM and transfer techniques. Nurses are the front line in encouraging the patient to be an active participant in the rehabilitation process. For discharge, the rehabilitation nurse assists in listing the supplies and equipment for the patient. The more educated a patient and family are, the better the outcome in respect to health function and quality of life.

Physical and occupational therapists should work together to help the patient achieve an optimal level of self-care skills and mobility. A coordinated integrated program, encompassing ROM, strengthening, and functional training in all areas, providing patient and family education, and training with equipment, is just a part of the therapist's responsibilities. Other important aspects of care include an assistive technology evaluation and training (including environmental control units [ECUs]), a home evaluation and recommendations for modifications, and specialty equipment recommendations (e.g., wheelchair, cushion, orthoses, assistive devices, bed, and mattress). The therapist also serves as a motivator who is able to listen to the patient's frustrations and attempt to channel those emotions into the rehabilitation process. The most commonly used techniques in therapy are discussed later in this chapter, including ROM, mat activities, modalities, weight shifts, transfer training, wheelchair training, standing, and ambulation.

The speech pathologist will be needed if there is any suspicion of swallowing, communication, or cognitive deficits. A bedside evaluation for swallowing and a videofluoroscopic swallowing study may be performed, particularly for older patients who have sustained a high-level cervical injury, who have a tracheostomy tube, or may have undergone anterior approach spinal surgery (5). Training for swallowing and voice control can be undertaken.

Key areas detailed in other chapters include psychological, vocational, recreational, and driver training. The psychologist assesses the patients' cognitive status, particularly if there is a question of a brain injury, their adjustment to disability, and their current emotional status. The psychologist can help the team members and the patient and family identify problem issues and suggest appropriate interventions to assist in attaining the rehabilitation goals. Recreational therapy plays an important role in helping the patient focus on leisure activities that are possible as an inpatient, but also once discharged from the rehabilitation hospital. The team should encourage the patient to participate in previous recreational interests and search for new enjoyable activities. Spine-injured individuals often are unaware of the scope of activities that are available and may focus only on things that they can no longer participate in, rather than on the many activities that they can. Community outings frequently take place (e.g., to a shopping mall or movie theater) during the inpatient stay with therapists to start integrating the patient back into community settings.

The social worker or case manager (who in some institutions is a nurse) helps the patient and family with the insurance and financial issues, maximizing their benefits and resources, and identifying other resources to assist with the care that may be needed. The social worker or case manager should facilitate discharge planning and help ensure a smooth transition to the discharge destination. Home care equipment delivery and outpatient programs should be scheduled before the patient is discharged, and continuity of care should be ensured. Family counseling throughout this period is crucial.

Team conferences should be held as part of the team approach on a weekly basis to allow all members to address the clinical problems, report progress, update goals, and secure a proper and safe discharge. Frequently, a home evaluation performed early in the inpatient stay is particularly valuable to assess for home modifications and adaptive equipment that may be needed. In addition, a workplace evaluation may be recommended either as part of the inpatient stay or as part of the outpatient program.

As the length of stay shortens in acute rehabilitation, coordination of the entire team has become more important, to allow for a timely and safe discharge.

Inpatient Rehabilitation

There are many options to consider when choosing where to receive inpatient rehabilitation, so careful evaluation should be undertaken. Key areas to focus on include the experience of the staff, including the physicians, therapists, and nurses, and the number of spine-injured patients served by that facility per year. It is estimated that a minimum of 50 new annual patients with spinal cord disorders, traumatic and nontraumatic, should be admitted (1). This serves as a reference to the degree of expertise of services that may be available, including in the medical and therapeutic areas, the presence of full-time psychology, vocational, and SCI educational services, as well as an active peer support program. The ability for an individual to undergo rehabilitation with others that have similar impairments is extremely helpful. Additional opportunities available at larger centers include the use of trial equipment (e.g., multiple wheelchairs, cushions, and bathroom equipment), high-level assistive technology (ECUs), and a specialized seating clinic.

At admission, the SCI physician performs a comprehensive evaluation, establishing the motor, sensory, and neurologic level of injury (NLI), as well as the American Spinal Injury Association (ASIA) impairment classification (chapter 5). Based on this evaluation, there is a formulation of a problem list, and long-term and short-term goals should be set (Table 19.1). A specific

TABLE 19.1. SAMPLE PROBLEM LIST

Problem List	Interventions
Medical	
Respiratory	Monitor vital capacity. Perform incentive spirometry, assisted cough, deep breathing techniques, chest PT, and respiratory treatments.
Gastrointestinal	Stress ulcer prophylaxis.
Nutrition	Perform calorie count. Monitor weekly weights.
Neurogenic bowel	Initiate bowel program and adjust as needed. Patient and family training.
Neurogenic bladder	Proper intake and output. Discuss bladder options. Family training.
DVT prophylaxis	Check admission doppler study. Adequate pharmacological prophylaxis. Monitor LE circumference.
Skin	Proper mattress. Turn Q 2 degrees initially. Heel protectors. Frequent weight shifts in wheelchair. Proper cushion. Teach patient to use mirror to check skin.
Orthostasis	Change positions slowly. Ace wrap or LE stockings and abdominal binder. Use tilt table. Pharmacologic intervention if needed.
H.O.	Monitor hip and knee ROM. X-rays and bone scan if suspect.
Spasticity	Stretching/ROM. Modalities. Medications. Injections. Intrathecal baclofen.
Autonomic dysreflexia	Monitor closely.
Hypercalcemia	Monitor for symptoms. Fluids, medications.

Rehabilitation issues	
Mobility	ADL
Adjustment to disability	Cognitive
Communication	Swallowing
SCI education	Vocational
Sexuality	Driving
Recreation	Family training
Discharge planning	Equipment evaluation

LE, lower extremity; ROM, range of motion; SCI, spinal cord injury; PT, physical therapy; HO, heterotopic ossification; DVT, deep vein thrombosis; ADL, activities of daily living.

TABLE 19.2. SAMPLE PHYSICAL AND OCCUPATIONAL THERAPY PRESCRIPTION

Diagnosis: C7 ASIA A tetraplegia

Goals: (See outlined goals in Table 19.3)

Precautions: Skin, respiratory, sensory, orthostasis, safety, risk for autonomic dysreflexia and others as needed for the specific patient (e.g., bleeding if on Coumadin).

Physical therapy:
PROM to bilateral LE, with stretching of hamstrings and hip extensors.
Mat activities.
Tilt table as tolerated. Start at 15 degrees, progress 10 degrees every 15 min within precautions up to 80 degrees.
Sitting balancing (static and dynamic).
Transfer training from all surfaces including mat, bed, wheelchair, and floor.
Wheelchair propulsion training and management.
Teach and encourage weight shifting.
Standing table as tolerated.
Deep breathing exercises.
FES for appropriate candidates.
Family training.
Community skills.
Teach home exercise program.

Occupational therapy:
Passive, active assisted, active ROM/exercises to bilateral UEs.
Allow for some finger tightness to enhance grasp.
Bilateral UE strengthening.
Motor coordination skills.
ADL program with adaptive equipment as needed (dressing, grooming, feeding).
Functional transfer training (bathroom, tub, car, etc.).
Splinting and adaptive equipment evaluation.
Desktop skills.
Shower program.
Kitchen and homemaking skills.
Wheelchair training (parts and management).
Home evaluation.
Family training.
Teach home exercise program.

LE, lower extremities; ROM, range of motion; UE, upper extremity; FES, functional electrical stimulation.

therapy prescription for all of the team members who will be involved in the case based on the goals should be established (Table 19.2).

Therapy usually begins at a minimum of 3 hours per day. At first, some of the therapy may take place at the bedside, progressing as tolerated into the therapy gym. Mobilization begins slowly, with placement of the patient on a reclining wheelchair to help them get used to the upright position. The use of an abdominal binder and elastic wraps or stocking on the lower extremities (LEs) is recommended to prevent orthostasis. In therapy, a tilt table may be used. Over the course of days to weeks, the patient is usually able to tolerate increasing degrees of sitting upright, mobilizing in a standard wheelchair, and participating in an increasing amount of therapy.

Functional Goals

The most important factors in determining functional outcome are the motor level and the degree of impairment—that is, ASIA

TABLE 19.3. PROJECTED FUNCTIONAL OUTCOMES AT 1 YEAR POST–INJURY BY LEVEL

	C1–4	C5	C6	C7	C8–T1
Feeding	Dependent	Independent with adaptive equipment after setup	Independent with or without adaptive equipment	Independent	Independent
Grooming	Dependent	Minimum assistance with equipment after setup	Some assistance to independence with adaptive equipment	Independent with adaptive equipment	Independent
UE dressing	Dependent	Requires assistance	Independent	Independent	Independent
LE dressing	Dependent	Dependent	Requires assistance	Some assistance to independence with adaptive equipment	Usually independent
Bathing	Dependent	Dependent	Some assistance to independence with equipment	Some assistance to independence with equipment	Independent with equipment
Bed mobility	Dependent	Assists	Assists	Independent to some	Independent
Weight shifts	Independent in power, Dependent in manual wheelchair	Assists unless in power wheelchair	Independent	Independent	Independent
Transfers	Dependent	Maximum assistance	Some assistance to independent on level surfaces	Independent with or without board for level surfaces	Independent
Wheelchair propulsion	Independent with power, Dependent in manual	Independent in power; independent to some assistance in manual	Independent—manual with coated rims on level surfaces	Independent, except curbs and uneven terrain	Independent
Driving	Unable	Independent with adaptations	Independent with adaptations	Car with hand controls or adapted van	Car with hand controls or adapted van

POTENTIAL OUTCOMES FOR COMPLETE PARAPLEGIA

	T2–9	T10–L2	L3–S5
ADL (grooming, feeding, dressing, bathing)	Independent	Independent	Independent
BIB	Independent	Independent	Independent
Transfers	Independent	Independent	Independent
Ambulation	Standing in frame, tilt table or standing wheelchair / Exercise only	Household ambulation with orthoses / Can try ambulation outdoors	Community ambulation is possible
Braces	Bilateral KAFO forearm crutches or walker	KAFOs, with forearm crutches	Possibly KAFO or AFOs, with canes/crutches

UE, upper extremity; LE, lower extremity; AFOs, ankle-foot orthoses; KAFOs, knee-ankle-foot orthoses; BIB, bowel/bladder.

impairment classification (complete vs. incomplete status). Table 19.3 lists the functional goals expected for each key level of injury for a person with a motor complete injury to be achieved at 1 year. Table 19.4 lists equipment usually prescribed for persons with that level of injury. The ideal outcome may not always be achieved for each patient, because there is a significant amount of variability in individual outcomes despite similar levels of injury. The extent to which an individual can achieve, from a functional standpoint, is dependent on the age of the individual and coexistent conditions such as obesity, cognitive impairment, brachial plexus injury, or preexistent conditions. In addition, complications that may develop such as pain, spasticity, contractures, and depression may also interfere with achieving the expected long-term goals. Persons who are highly

motivated and those who have good social support may exceed the expected functional outcome for their respective level of injury.

Persons with motor complete injuries are usually expected to gain one motor level of function from their initial examination at 72 hours to 1 week (see chapter 7). Depending on the time of admission of the individual to the rehabilitation unit, this should be kept in mind when determining goals. For those with complete injuries, the most rapid recovery takes place in the first 2 months after injury, slows after 3 to 6 months, but still may show motor and functional recovery up to 2 years postinjury.

The projected long-term goals are the end point for the rehabilitation prescription to eventually achieve. The treatment team should be guided by long-term functional goals, but the rehabili-

TABLE 19.4. SUGGESTED EQUIPMENT FOR COMPLETE TETRAPLEGIC (EACH PATIENT VARIES)

	C1–4	C5	C6	C7	C8-T1
Orthotics					
Balanced forearm orthosis (mobile arm support)	X	?	—	—	—
Resting hand splint	X	X	X	—	—
Long opponens splint	X	X	—	—	—
Spiral splint	—	X	X	—	—
Powered tenodesis splint	—	X	—	—	—
Wrist-driven tenodesis splint	—	—	X	—	—
Rachet tenodesis splint	—	X	—	—	—
Short opponens splint	—	—	X	X	—
Universal cuff	—	X	X	X	—
Lumbrical bar	—	—	—	—	X
Mouth stick	X	?	—	—	—
Transfers/mobility					
Power/mechanical lift	X	X	X	—	—
Transfer board	X	X	X	X	X
Power wheelchair with tilt/recline	X	X	?	—	—
Power wheelchair	—	—	X	?	—
Manual wheelchair	X	X	X	X	X
Feeding					
Adapted equipment (plate, etc.)	X	X	—	—	—
Utensils with built-up handles	—	X	X	—	—
Grooming and dressing					
ADL splints (wash mitt, razor holders)	—	X	X	—	—
Dressing equipment (pant loops, sock aide, dressing stick, long shoehorn, etc.)	—	—	X	X	—
Gooseneck mirror	X	X	X	X	X
Communication					
Environmental control unit	X	X	?	—	—
Computer	X	X	X	X	—
Book holder	X	X	X	X	—
Bathing					
Grab bars	—	—	X	X	X
Reclining shower/commode chair	X	—	X	X	X
Tub seat/shower chair (padded)	—	X	X	X	X
Handheld spray attachment	X	X	X	X	X
Beds					
Full electric hospital bed	X	X	X	—	—
Full specialized mattress	X	X	?	?	—
Overlay mattress	—	—	X	X	?

tation program should be individualized to meet each person's strengths, weaknesses, and circumstances. Short-term goals are progressive steps that should be attained to achieve the long-term goals. Monitoring of the progress toward the functional goals at the team conference helps identify limiting factors, along with the patient's additional needs. The rehabilitation program can then be modified to help the patient meet individual expectations. Projected functional goals may not be attainable despite a good rehabilitation program. The patient should understand the goals projected to become an active participant in the program.

Length of stay has been decreasing, both for acute care and for rehabilitation. It is no longer possible to achieve all of the rehabilitation goals in the fewer rehabilitation days that are being

certified by third-party payers. Discharge planning should be discussed at the first team conference, ensuring a timely and most importantly a safe discharge.

C1-4 Level

The muscles available with lesions at or above C3 include the cervical paraspinal, sternocleidomastoid, neck accessory muscles, and partial innervation of the diaphragm. Functionally, this allows for neck flexion, extension, and rotation. At the C4 level, there is further innervation of the diaphragm and paraspinal muscles, with additional functional movement of scapular elevation and inspiratory strength.

Persons with motor levels at or above C3 will usually require long-term ventilator assistance, whereas most patients with lesions at C4 will be able to wean off the ventilator (chapter 9). For persons requiring a ventilator, two ventilators are recommended (6). Additional respiratory equipment will be needed, including a method for secretion management (suction, mechanical insufflator/exsufflator), backup batteries, and a generator in case of power failure. One should be in touch with the local power company and emergency services to alert them before being discharged.

Individuals with these high levels of injury, whether requiring a ventilator or not, are dependent in self-care activities and mobility. They should, however, be independent in instructing others in providing their care including performing weight shifts, ROM, positioning in bed, donning orthoses, transfers, and in setting up their ECU. In addition, they should be able to instruct in the use of a mechanical lift, which is frequently used to assist with transfers. These individuals should be independent in power wheelchair mobility, using breath control, mouth stick, and tongue or chin control mechanisms (chapter 38). For persons on a ventilator, a ventilator tray needs to be added to the wheelchair. If the patient can control a power chair, then both a power chair (power recline or tilt wheelchair) and a manual wheelchair should be prescribed. The manual wheelchair is to be used when accessibility for a power wheelchair is not available, in case the power wheelchair fails, or if the patient is unable for some reason to use the power wheelchair. Once properly set up, persons with these levels of injury should be independent in their ECU control (see later discussion).

Persons with a C4 NLI that have some elbow flexion and deltoid strength may be able to use a mobile arm support (MAS) or balanced forearm orthosis (BFO) to assist with feeding, grooming, and hygiene (Fig. 19.1). These devices may also enable patients who have limited shoulder flexion, by repetition, to increase the strength and endurance of this motion. Once the deltoid and biceps muscles have strength of 3 + /5 with adequate endurance, the MAS is no longer needed. A long straw or a bottle that the person can easily access to drink fluids is important to obtain.

Persons at this level require total assistance with their bowel and bladder management. It is often difficult to ensure that there is always a trained person to perform intermittent catheterization (IC), so other bladder options should be discussed. These persons are not able to drive but should have an adapted van for accessibility.

The benefit of specialized acute rehabilitation for persons with such high levels of injury is justifiable despite that they may not be able to tolerate 3 hours a day of therapy and having what may seem as limited goals. The SCI medical and nursing care during the first few months after injury are crucial for monitoring, treating, and preventing medical complications that can lead to future morbidity and mortality. The patient and family education, emotional and social support, and exposure to advanced technology that may allow independence in the proper environment (e.g., power mobility, ECU) may for the injured mean the difference between returning to their family and community versus spending their life in a nursing home.

C5 Level

The C5 level adds the key muscle group of the biceps (elbow flexors), as well as the deltoids, rhomboids, and partial innervation of the brachialis, brachioradialis, supraspinatus, infraspinatus, and serratus anterior. These muscles allow for shoulder flexion, extension and abduction, elbow flexion and supination, and weak scapular adduction and abduction. These movements allow the individual to be partially independent with skills such as feeding and grooming with splints. It is extremely important to prevent elbow flexion and forearm supination contractures caused by unopposed biceps activity. Continued stretching should be performed acutely and in the chronic phase after rehabilitation. A MAS may initially be needed, although the person should regain adequate strength to perform these activities without it.

The addition of the elbow flexors should allow for use of a joystick on a power wheelchair and can allow manual wheelchair propulsion on level surfaces with either rim projections (lugs)

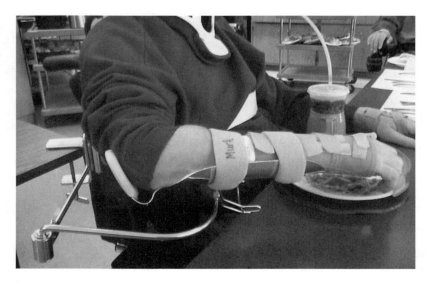

FIGURE 19.1. Balanced forearm orthosis. Also note the long-handled straw, plate guard, and Dycem.

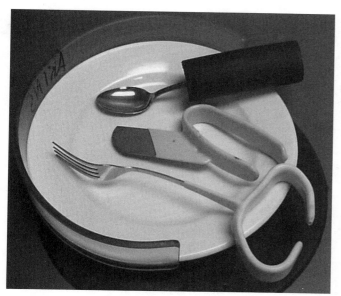

FIGURE 19.2. Adaptive feeding equipment. Dycem, plate guard, adapted utensils.

or plastic-coated hand rims with a protective glove. Power wheelchairs, with a power recline or tilt mechanism, are usually still required, in addition to the manual wheelchair. The lighter the manual wheelchair, the easier it is to propel.

A long-opponens splint, with a pocket for inserting different utensils, is extremely important to assist with many tasks including feeding, hygiene, grooming, and writing. Various adaptive devices are represented in Figs. 19.2, 19.3, and 19.4. Most functional activities will require the use of assistive devices; therefore, tendon transfers or the use of the implanted electrical stimulation devices may be considered after neurologic recovery is complete (chapters 25 and 28).

Persons at this level of injury will require almost total assistance for their bowel program. Performing this on a padded commode or shower chair is recommended. Bladder manage-

ment, as with all levels of injury, is a decision based on discussion with the SCI specialist and urologist, urodynamic results, amount of assistance available, and lifestyle circumstances. IC usually cannot be performed independently. If the patient is using a leg bag, electronic devices can help empty the bag. Driving a specially modified van is possible at this level (chapter 24).

C6 Level

The C6 level adds the key muscle group of the extensor carpi radialis longus, which performs wrist extension. Additional muscles partially innervated include the extensor carpi radialis brevis, supinator, pronator teres, and latissimus dorsi. Movements gained also include scapular abduction and radial wrist extension. Active wrist extension can allow for tenodesis, the opposition of the thumb and index finger with flexion as the tendons are stretched with wrist extension. One should avoid overly stretching the finger flexors initially after injury in C5 and C6 motor level patients to avoid potentially losing the tenodesis action. Tenodesis splints can be fabricated but are frequently discarded by patients.

Feeding, grooming, and UE hygiene are usually performed independently after assistance with setting up utensils; however, clothing modifications such as Velcro closures on shoes, instead of buttons, loops on zippers, and pullover garments are usually advised. Meal preparation is still required as well as other homemaking tasks.

Transfers may be possible using a transfer board and with loops for LE management, but usually requires assistance. Although persons with a C6 motor-level injury can propel a manual wheelchair with plastic-coated rims, a power wheelchair is often required for long-distance trips, particularly if the individual will be returning to the workplace. Driving a modified van is a goal, with a lift for access, allowing the patient be fully independent.

The person at this level of injury can assist with the bowel program but will require assistance. IC is possible for men after assistance with setup of assistive devices. Although the use of

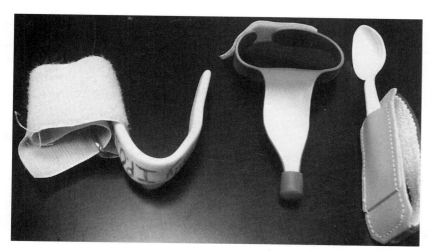

FIGURE 19.3. Adaptive utensils including **(from left to right)** a quad phone holder, typing peg, and universal cuff with a plastic spoon attached.

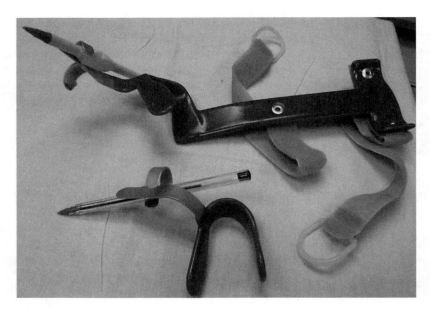

FIGURE 19.4. Adaptive writing utensils.

adaptive equipment may enhance independence for men, this technique is more difficult for women.

C7 and C8 Levels

The C7 level adds the triceps (elbow extensors) as the key muscle group; and C8, the flexor digitorum profundus (long finger flexors). At C7, elbow extension, ulnar wrist extension, and wrist flexion, as well as some finger extension, are added. At the C8 level, long finger flexors become functional, allowing for improved hand and finger function. Additional new muscles with some innervation at these levels include the flexor carpi radialis, extensor carpi ulnaris, pronator quadratus, flexor digitorum superficialis, abductor pollicis, and lumbricals.

The C7 level is considered the key level for becoming independent in most activities at the wheelchair level. Persons with a C7 motor level injury are usually independent for weight shifts, transfers between level surfaces, feeding, grooming, and upper body dressing. Uneven surface transfers may require some assistance, as well as lower body dressing. They should be independent in light meal preparation, although require some to total assistance for complex meal preparation and housecleaning. The person with this level of injury should be independent in manual wheelchair propulsion for indoor and outdoor terrain but may require some assistance for uneven surfaces. Most require plastic-coated rims to substitute for lack of grip. Driving should be independent in a modified van or the use of a car if they can transfer and load and unload their wheelchair independently.

Bladder care (i.e., IC) in men can be performed, although it is more difficult for women, particularly if LE spasticity is present. Bowel care, particularly suppository insertion, may still require assistance, although independence can be achieved with adaptive devices that aid in suppository insertion and digital stimulation. Padded elevated toilet seats allow the individual to perform bowel care duties independently with various adaptive equipment and protect against skin breakdown.

Thoracic Levels

It is best to separate persons with a thoracic injury into upper (T1-6) and lower level thoracic injuries (T7-12). All levels of paraplegia should be independent with activities of daily living including LE dressing and mobility skills at the wheelchair level on even and uneven surfaces. They should be able to drive a car with adaptations, although loading and unloading the wheelchair may still be difficult for the individual. Persons should be able to prepare meals in an adapted environment and perform light housekeeping but may still require assistance with heavy housekeeping.

Advanced wheelchair training (described later in this chapter) should be undertaken. For most thoracic-level injuries, ambulation is not a functional long-term goal. The lower the level of the injury, the greater the trunk control due to abdominal and paraspinal muscle innervation. Although individuals with high and mid-thoracic–level injuries may be interested in gait training and should undergo this if there are no medical contraindications (e.g., hip flexion contractures and LE fractures), ambulation is usually not an inpatient goal. Persons with lower thoracic levels of paraplegia can participate in ambulation training with bilateral LE orthoses as an exercise and short-distance ambulation (see the section on ambulation).

Persons with these levels of injury should be independent in their bowel and bladder programs, with any technique they choose.

Lumbar Paraplegia

The lower the level of injury, the greater the opportunity for the patient to become independent in ambulation. The greater the muscle strength and the less bracing necessary, the more functional the person will be for greater distances (see the section on ambulation).

L1-2 Levels

Muscles gained at these levels include the hip flexors and part of the quadriceps. Although the person can walk for short distances, a wheelchair will still be required. Persons with these levels of injury should be independent in their bowel and bladder programs, with any technique they choose. Bladder care is usually by IC. Individuals with these levels of injury can drive a car with hand controls.

L3-4 Levels

The knee extensors are fully innervated, with some ankle dorsiflexion regaining strength. Ambulation usually requires ankle-foot orthoses (AFOs) with canes and crutches. Bowel and bladder management depends on whether there is upper motor neuron (UMN) or lower motor neuron (LMN) damage. In either case, the person should be independent in his or her management. If there is a LMN injury, bowel management is by contraction of abdominal muscles and manual disimpaction. Suppositories will not be effective because of the loss of reflexes. Bladder management is usually performed via IC or Valsalva maneuver if postvoid residual urine test results are within the reference range and urologic workup reveals no contraindication to this method (chapter 12). Absorbent pads can be used. If there is a UMN injury, digital stimulation will usually suffice for bowel management, and bladder management is similar to that described for thoracic-level paraplegia.

L5 and Below

These individuals should be independent in all activities unless there are associated problems such as severe pain and cardiac conditions.

SPINAL ORTHOSES IN REHABILITATION

Spinal orthoses are commonly used after SCI to limit spinal movement, protect the spine during healing, and provide mechanical unloading (6,7). The goal of this section is to review the most frequently used spinal orthoses seen in the rehabilitation setting.

Numerous designs are available, providing different degrees of support for the different segments of the spine. Few spinal orthoses provide complete immobilization of the spine, but in general, the longer and better fitting the orthosis, the greater its effectiveness. When an orthosis is used to protect the spine during healing of a fracture or postoperatively after a surgical fusion, it generally is worn for 10 to 12 weeks (see chapter 6). To ensure that a patient's spinal stability is not compromised, one may place limitations on the patient's ability to participate in certain functional activities (e.g., certain types of transfers or weight shifts, prone or high-level position changes, and advanced wheelchair skills) while in the orthosis. These precautions must be clearly communicated between the physician and treating therapists.

Different nondescriptive eponyms are frequently used for orthotic devices. To reduce confusion, a descriptive nomenclature for orthotic devices was developed in which orthoses are named according to the body segments involved and the planes of movement restricted. Consequently, spinal orthoses are classified as cervical orthoses (COs), head cervical orthoses (HCOs), cervicothoracic orthoses (CTOs), thoracolumbosacral orthoses (TLSOs), lumbosacral orthoses (LSOs), and cervicothoracolumbosacral orthoses (CTLSOs) (7).

The COs are soft cervical collars made of cloth or foam rubber or a more rigid collar (Thomas collar). These are usually comfortable to wear and restrict neck motion primarily through sensory feedback, rather than by mechanical restriction (8). They have little indication for use in traumatic SCI, because they do not offer enough immobilization. Prefabricated HCOs, made of various plastic materials in different designs to provide greater support and restriction, include the Philadelphia, Aspen, and Miami collars, as well as other collars with a similar design (Fig. 19.5) (9). These collars are useful for spinal immobilization but do not stabilize the spine. HCOs are usually indicated for stable mid-cervical bony or ligamentous injuries, or postoperatively when rigid control is no longer required. If stabilization is required, a head cervicothoracic orthosis (HCTO) (i.e., a halo) is required for the cervical levels of injury.

Posterior cervical appliances are examples of CTOs that usually consist of chin and occipital pieces, which are connected by two to four adjustable metal uprights to sternal and back plates. Such devices may provide greater restriction of neck motion than previously mentioned collars (8). The sternal occipital mandibular immobilizer (SOMI) is lightweight and usually more comfortable than collars with metal uprights, because there are no posterior rods, making it easier to use in a patient who is bedridden. In addition, a headband that encircles the forehead can be used if the chin piece needs to be removed (e.g., during eating). The SOMI can be applied and easily fitted and provides substantial restriction of motion in the mid- to low-cervical region (8). The Yale orthosis is another type of CTO that is similar to an extended Philadelphia collar, thus increasing the restriction of motion. Sandler et al. (10) studied the mechanical restrictive properties of the different types of COs, including the soft collar, Philadelphia collar, Philadelphia collar with an extension, and a SOMI brace. They found that although the previous order of orthoses showed a progressive improvement in restriction of movement, the differences were not large.

Complications of bracing include pressure sores, muscle atrophy, allergic reactions to bracing materials, heat retention causing skin maceration, and skin discoloration. Monitoring the condition of the underlying skin is an extremely important aspect of brace management. Neck exercises within the brace may be appropriate for certain patients toward the end of their orthotic treatment. The length of bracing treatment must be closely followed, with regular physical examinations and radiographs (see chapter 6).

Maximum immobilization of the cervical spine is obtained by application of an HCTO, including the rigid halo and the semirigid Minerva orthosis. The Minerva orthosis is a custom-molded total-contact appliance made of plastic materials shaped over a positive body cast. It encloses the upper part of the trunk, the neck, and the back of the head and may have a band around

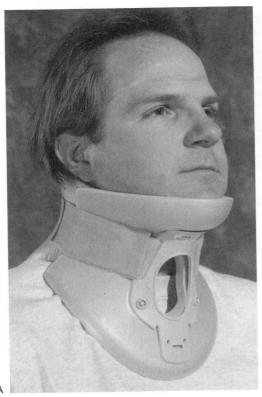 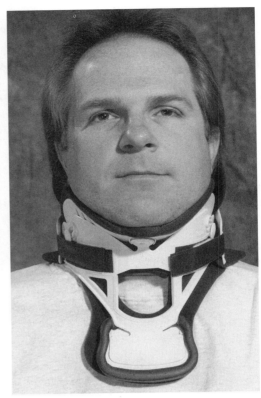

FIGURE 19.5. A; Philadelphia collar. **B;** Miami collar.

the forehead. It provides excellent restriction of lateral and rotational neck motions and limits flexion and extension. This brace may be the only true noninvasive orthosis that offers the support of the halo for injuries below C2. The halo, however, is still better at controlling the occiput to C2 levels (11).

A halo orthosis is frequently applied for external support after a period of cervical traction or after surgical spinal fusion (Fig. 19.6). Although the halo orthosis provides the maximum restriction of flexion and extension of the potentially unstable cervical spine, it does not guarantee maintenance of alignment and ultimate fusion. The halo consists of a halo ring, a vest, and upright posters. The ring is made of lightweight magnetic resonance imaging–compatible metal and should be large enough to provide a 1-cm clearance around the head. Four pins attach the ring to the head, two anterolaterally on the forehead and two posteriorly. The pins can be tightened if loosening occurs as long as resistance is felt; otherwise, they will require replacement to another site. To prevent infection, the pin sites should be cleaned two to three times daily with normal saline solution. The routine use of povidone iodine, hydrogen peroxide, hypochlorite solution, and chlorhexidine has been associated with increased infection, disruption of the healing process, or disruption of the normal flora of the skin (12). The use of ointments blocks the drainage of fluid at the pin site and increases the risk of infection (13). Superficial pin infections are treated with local care, oral antibiotics, and movement of the pin to another site.

The halo vest is made of prefabricated plastic material and is lined with sheepskin or a soft fabric. It must fit the body well to prevent pressure sores and loss of spinal reduction. Once the halo orthosis has been securely applied, the patient can usually get out of bed and participate in physical activities, either ambulatory or in a wheelchair. Most rehabilitation exercises do not cause any greater motion to the spine than does daily motion and activity. However, shoulder shrugging and overhead activities (shoulder abduction at more than 90 degrees) should be avoided because this can push on the straps of the vest and increase the load on the cervical spine (14,15).

Complications of the halo (in decreasing order of occurrence) include pin loosening, infection and discomfort; ring migration; and pressure sores (particularly under or over the scapula). Less frequent complications include nerve injury, dysphagia, perforation of the skull, brain abscess, degenerative changes of facets from immobilization, avascular necrosis of the dens, limitation of self-care activities and social activities, vascular compression of the duodenum, and a reduction of vital capacity.

Flexible LSO or TLSO corsets made of different fabrics with adjustable sets of straps are relatively ineffective in mechanically restricting motion but are usually comfortable and effective in reducing pain for various painful back disorders when spinal stability is not in question. When greater restriction of spinal motion is needed, various prefabricated, adjustable, and more rigid orthoses are used. These include the Knight-spinal LSO, Knight-Taylor TLSO, and hyperextension orthoses such as the attached to provide restriction of motion of the upper thoracic and cervical spine. A rigid, total-contact TLSO is particularly indicated for unstable fractures of the spine when surgical stabilization is not indicated or when the adequacy of the surgical stabilization is in question. Because of the total contact, this orthosis tends to be warm and somewhat uncomfortable. Often,

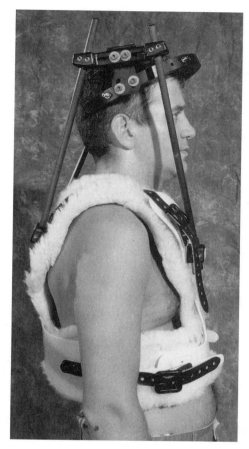

FIGURE 19.6. Halo device.

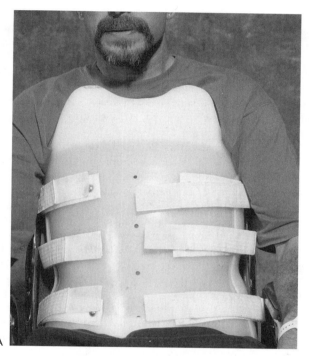

A

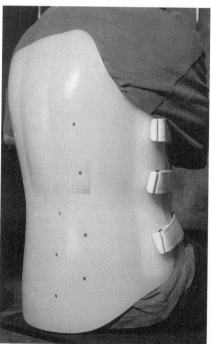

B

FIGURE 19.7. Custom molded (plastic) body jacket. **A;** Frontal view. **B;** Lateral view.

Jewett and CASH (cruciform anterior spinal hyperextension) braces. These orthoses effectively reduce gross motion and provide trunk support but are inadequate for treatment of unstable spinal fractures. The Jewett brace is occasionally used after surgical stabilization of fractures at the thoracolumbar junction. This prefabricated, adjustable orthosis uses a three-point pressure system in which pressure is applied anteriorly on the sternum above and on the pelvis or pubic bone below, by means of pads attached to a firm metal frame. Posteriorly, pressure is applied over the lower thoracic and upper lumbar spine by a pad that is attached to the anterior metal frame by adjustable straps. The Jewett and CASH braces provide no abdominal muscle support and limit only flexion. They are lightweight but may be uncomfortable because the corrective forces are spread over a relatively small area.

The most commonly seen TLSO posttrauma is the rigid design, custom-molded, total-contact TLSO; sometimes referred to as a body jacket (Fig. 19.7). It is prescribed for maximum restriction of flexion, extension, and rotation. This orthosis is usually made of plastic materials and is usually bivalved, with Velcro straps that attach the anterior and posterior halves. The jacket is molded to firmly fit the pelvis below and may extend anteriorly to the manubrium of the sternum and posteriorly to the mid-portion of the scapula. A cervical extension may be when the TLSO is initially fitted in the supine position, once the patient is able to sit, trimming may be required to protect against skin breakdown. In addition, if the patient loses a great deal of weight, a new brace may need to be fabricated.

It is unfortunate that as spinal orthoses provide a degree of immobilization of a fractured spine, they also restrict the general mobility of the patient with paralysis and thus may interfere with the rehabilitation program and achievement of functional goals in a timely manner. In general, COs and LSOs do not restrict a person's mobility significantly and therefore do not interfere with the achievement of rehabilitation goals. In contrast, more restrictive spinal orthoses, such as the halo orthosis or a custom-molded TLSO, will limit the person's ability to fully participate in the rehabilitation program and will delay the achievement of rehabilitation goals. Some consider that the patient should not initially go to an acute SCI rehabilitation unit until the orthosis is removed, at which time full advantage of rehabilitation can begin. However, the postacute period after an SCI is crucial to prevent medical complications and deal with social and psychological reactions to injury. Acute rehabilitation is indicated, even while wearing these restrictive orthoses, because persons with SCI can participate in these areas and make significant gains. They can exercise to strengthen innervated muscles, participate in training of bladder and bowel programs, engage in SCI educational programs and psychological counseling, train with adaptive equipment, and make preparations for discharge to home. Once the restrictive spinal orthosis is removed, achievement of goals in activities of daily living and mobility usually occurs swiftly. One should not however undergo wheelchair prescription while the restrictive orthosis, particularly a halo or TLSO, is in place and should wait until these braces are removed so the patient can adequately try the wheelchairs before final prescription. Rehabilitation may be facilitated by modern surgical stabilization techniques that eliminate or reduce the need for a spinal orthosis.

SPECIFIC ACTIVITIES IN THERAPY

A number of key aspects of the therapy program and the most important assistive devices are detailed.

Range of Motion

ROM prevents contractures and maintains functional capabilities. Decreased ROM of a joint can result from structural bony changes, as seen in heterotopic ossification or from soft tissue tightness in muscles and supportive tissue around the joint. Active assisted ROM and exercise should be performed at least daily in muscles with partial functional strength above and below the level of injury, and passive ROM in areas with minimal or no strength.

The level of injury will determine the areas requiring intervention with passive ROM. In both paraplegia and tetraplegia, the hips, knees, and ankles are of primary importance. The hips often develop flexion tightness or contractures secondary to frequent side lying and sitting in a wheelchair, as well as spasticity. Hip ROM should involve flexion and extension, abduction and

adduction, and internal and external rotation. The goal of ROM of the knee should be to maintain passive ROM through a 120-degree arc. Ankle ROM occurs in all planes, but prevention of heel cord tightness and contracture is of utmost importance for proper positioning of the feet on the wheelchair footplate (16). Stretching of the lumbar spine is initiated when tightness or spasticity interferes with function but is often avoided to provide the patient with increased postural stability and balance in the short and long sitting positions (1).

Tetraplegia introduces unique challenges not seen in paraplegia. Individuals with high-level tetraplegia (C1-4) lack active shoulder movement and can develop limited ROM with or without spasticity. Natural shoulder movements should be replicated with ROM exercises in flexion and extension, abduction and adduction, and internal and external rotation. Elbow flexion and supination contractures can develop in individuals without active triceps function (C5 and C6 motor-level patients). In addition to flexion and extension ROM, supination and pronation should be addressed. Existing wrist and hand motor function will determine whether a stretching or tightening program will be implemented. Individuals with high-level injuries and no motor function at the wrist or hand can have their wrist and fingers stretched to lie open and flat to accommodate the wheelchair arm tray. For those with active wrist extension and weak or no finger function, the finger flexors should not be fully stretched, but allowed to tighten somewhat and naturally curl to improve grip strength and function using a "tenodesis" action (1,16). Maintaining relative tightness of the long finger flexors can occur while performing finger ROM if done properly. The fingers are passively flexed when the wrist is extended and extended when the wrist is in flexion (17).

Mat Activities

Mat activity focuses on training for balance, strength, and endurance for reaching, sitting, and transferring. As one of the first steps in therapy, mat activities are crucial to bridge the gap between immobility and functional activities. The functional goals of mat activities include training for bed mobility; preparing the individual to sit up in a bed or wheelchair; preparing the individual for further complex functional activities, such as dressing and transfers; and preventing complications of a prolonged stay in bed, including deconditioning, pressure sores, atelectasis, pneumonia, orthostasis, and social isolation.

Mat activities are started with simple passive tasks, progressing to more active and complex tasks. Initially, the focus is on the achievement of bed mobility. ROM and strengthening exercises of the muscles used for functional activities, such as the shoulder stabilizers, are undertaken. As the individual progresses, rolling activities may begin. Individuals with or without strong biceps (C5) can achieve rolling. For those without strong biceps, supine to prone rolling can be achieved with the momentum of the outstretched UEs that rock from side to side. The individual then swings the arm over to the side to roll toward that side, with the rest of the body to follow this motion. Those with strong biceps will pull on a stabilizing object, to help roll the body over. Once rolling has been achieved, various prone and supine positions with the upper body propped up can be used, such as the prone-on-elbows, prone-on-hands, and supine-on-elbows positions. These positions will help strengthen important muscles in the UEs and the shoulders.

As the individual tolerates sitting up, static and dynamic balance training and pushing up on the mat should be started, in preparation for transferring into the wheelchair. In individuals with paraplegia, kneeling and the quadruped position can be part of the activities. All these can be achieved with strengthening of the trunk muscles, strengthening of the UEs, using the head and neck muscles for balance and positioning, hand-eye coordination, and safety training to teach the individual how to catch him- or herself from falling. These activities are also part of more complex functions that require a great deal of trunk balance in a sitting position, such as feeding or grooming.

Modalities

Modalities such as heat and cold and ultrasound can all be used above the level of the sensory loss. However, in areas that have diminished or no sensation, one must be extremely cautious before using such modalities. The risk of causing a burn is high, so alternatives should be sought. The use of fluidotherapy or whirlpool in neutral temperature is a good alternative for the extremities.

Weight Shifts

Weight shifts are essential to the prevention of pressure ulcers. Patients need to be instructed in proper pressure-relief techniques before sitting. After an SCI, sensory feedback is usually diminished or absent, leading to infrequent pressure relief over the ischial tuberosities and sacrum, thereby preventing adequate capillary perfusion. There is an inverse relationship between time and pressure, with tissue injury occurring with both high pressures over a short duration and low pressures over a prolonged duration (18). Shear forces and friction also play a role in the etiology of pressure ulcers and should be minimized whenever possible (19) (chapter 13).

The method of pressure relief will vary depending on the level of injury and functional capability of the patient. Individuals with injuries at C5 and above will usually require a power wheelchair with a tilt or recline mechanism. A full-body tilt seating mechanism is preferred to the reclining type to prevent the shear forces that occur at the body–seat interface (20). Some individuals with a C5 injury can perform an anterior weight shift, with loops attached to the back of their wheelchair (power or manual), allowing them to pull themselves back to the upright position by using their elbow flexors with the loops. Individuals with C6 tetraplegia lack innervation of triceps muscles and cannot support their body weight while straightening the elbows to provide pressure relief. Instead, they can use an alternative method, such as a lateral or an anterior (forward) weight shift. When performing a lateral weight shift, the person hooks an arm over the back of the chair or through an attached loop to stabilize the trunk and assist in returning to the initial sitting position. The forward-leaning position is accomplished by leaning forward with the chest toward the thighs, with an angle of more than 45 degrees from the wheelchair backrest. This position has been shown to be significantly more effective in pressure relief than tipping the wheelchair backwards to 35 or 65 degrees (21). Individuals with an injury at C7 and below have triceps function and are usually capable of performing independent push-up pressure relief.

Force-sensing array (FSA) pressure mapping is a method used to approximate capillary closing pressure (32 mm Hg) by measuring the interface pressure, defined as the perpendicular force per unit area between the body and support surface (22,23). FSA can be used to locate areas of high pressure in the patient's current wheelchair cushion and serve as a teaching tool to demonstrate which pressure-relief technique provides the best results. Studies have used FSA pressure mapping to compare various wheelchair cushions with tilting and upright positions (24).

Some authors recommend that patients perform a pressure relief for 1 minute every 30 minutes while in the wheelchair (25). Others suggest a 15-second pressure relief every 15 minutes. Regardless of the chosen time frame, it is critical to instill in all patients the importance of regularly scheduled weight shifts and daily skin integrity examinations. The use of a mirror will greatly enhance the ability to monitor the sacral area and ischial tuberosities.

Transfers

Transfers are complex activities that require motor planning, strength, and coordination. Proper technique allows for full realization of the patient's potential level of independence. With incorrect techniques, one may sustain overuse injuries and may cause more serious injuries if he or she falls.

There are many types of transfers, including transferring between different functional surfaces (e.g., bed to wheelchair, wheelchair to car, and commode or tub) and transfers between level (e.g., bed to chair) and uneven surfaces (e.g., floor to chair) (26). Different techniques require different muscle groups. Initially, transfer training can be started on the mat, with subsequent progression to functional surfaces. Transfer training involves multiple components, including training the patient, training the caregivers in case assistance is required, and educating the patient to be able to give clear instructions to caregivers about how to perform the transfer.

The presence of spasticity and contractures can influence the transfer technique used. For instance, in the presence of some spasticity, the individual may be able to bear weight even without antigravity motor strength. Therefore, transfer methods that require weightbearing through the LEs can be considered, for example, a stand-pivot transfer. Flaccid LEs will not allow standing without extensive bracing, thereby making transfers that require LE weightbearing impractical. However, excessive spasms may interfere with the safety of the transfers. Similarly, the presence of contractures in the weightbearing joints may present with restrictions on the method of transfers.

The wheelchair should be in proper position before the transfer begins. The footrest and the armrest need to be properly positioned so they are out of the way. The wheelchair should be positioned correctly next to the surface to be transferred to, at about 30 to 45 degrees to it. The brakes should be locked after the correct positioning of the wheelchair. Safety precautions

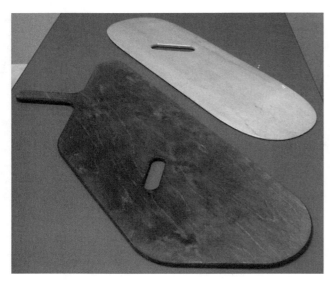

FIGURE 19.8. Different types of transfer boards.

and the avoidance of impulsive behavior are important to prevent injuries. The transfer technique and method chosen should consider the presence of pressure ulcers at surfaces such as the sacrum and the ischial tuberosity. For instance, transfers with a transfer (sliding) board may result in significant shearing force on the ischial tuberosity and therefore should be avoided in these situations.

Generally speaking, individuals with paraplegia should achieve independence with transfers, whereas those with tetraplegia may have varying levels of transfer independence. In most instances, those with an NLI at or below C7 can perform independent transfers, with or without the use of a transfer board, although some individuals with a C6 level of injury may also do so independently with its use (Fig. 19.8). Individuals with a C5 level of injury are expected to require the assistance of one person with or without a transfer board, whereas individuals with an injury at or above the level of C4 will be dependent.

The most commonly used transfer techniques include the following:

1. *Lift transfer* is for individuals who are completely dependent with transfers. If the individual is light, a one-person carry transfer can be performed. Otherwise, the transfer should be performed with more than one caregiver, for safety reasons.
2. *Lift transfer with a mechanical device* allows the transfer to be performed safely usually with one caregiver. A sling or a similar device is attached to a mechanical lift. The lift may be manual or electric; free standing, rolling, or attached to a structure (e.g., the ceiling).
3. *Stand-pivot transfer* allows the individual to be transferred from one seating surface to another. Individuals who require assistance can use this technique if they can bear weight through the LEs with sufficient extension ROM in the hips and knees. This weightbearing can be made possible with LE extensor spasticity. After the individual is stood up from the sitting position, he or she is pivoted on his feet by the care-

giver to the adjacent surface, where he will be lowered to a sitting position. This transfer requires good body mechanics and strong leverage by the caregiver.

4. *Transfer (sliding) board transfer* is a method that allows a transfer from one seating surface to another, with the use of a board that bridges the gap between them. This can be performed independently by individuals with good upper body strength and control and good sitting balance. This technique can also be used to assist a caregiver in transferring an individual who requires assistance. There is no weightbearing in the LEs. The board is a sturdy, smooth, flat board that is made of wood or plastic and comes in different sizes, styles and handgrips for different transfer situations. Body habitus affects the degree of ease with which this transfer can be performed. The use of the board may increase the level of independence in transfers while decreasing the pressure on the shoulder joints.
5. *Sit-pivot transfer* can be performed in patients with a strong upper body, good short sitting balance, and good control of head and shoulder movements. It allows transfer from one seating surface to another. The individual needs to push himself off of the surface with his UEs, with one arm for support on the original surface or wheelchair and the other on the surface to which he is transferring. The individual then pushes across the transfer surfaces with the UEs. The LEs may bear some weight and act as a pivotal point, but they do not provide any pushing force. The buttocks are not in contact with any surface throughout the transfer. Additional momentum can be gained by a quick twisting and turning movement of the head and shoulders opposite to the direction of the planned hip movement.
6. *Swivel-trapeze/overhead loops transfer* allows independent transfer from a bed to another surface and requires a very strong upper body. The individual will need an overhead swivel trapeze bar or loops to be attached to the bed, lifting his body up while pulling on the trapeze or loops, then swinging it across to another surface. This can be a source of shoulder pain as time goes on and is not recommended to be used on a constant basis.
7. *Lateral transfer* enables the individual with a very strong upper body to transfer from the wheelchair to another surface that allows the long sitting position, such as the mat, and vice versa. The individual needs to be able to tolerate the long sitting position, with hamstring flexibility and good sitting balance. With a lateral transfer, the individual positions the wheelchair laterally to the surface to be transferred to, placing his LEs on the mat. The patient then will carry out a long sitting push-up to transfer himself out of the wheelchair to the mat in the long sitting position.
8. *Floor-to-chair/chair-to-floor transfer* allows the individual to move between the floor and the chair safely. It is particularly useful in accidental situations such as a fall, when the individual can then return to the wheelchair independently. It may also be useful for social or recreational activities, allowing the individual to lower to the floor. It is a physically demanding technique, requiring a very strong upper body in both the arms and the shoulders. There are several approaches to this transfer. They include the side approach, which requires fi-

nesse and loose hamstrings (appropriate for those with an injury level of C7 or below), and the front approach and the back approach, which require very strong and neurologically intact UEs (appropriate for individuals with paraplegia).

The exact transfer technique used by individuals with SCI varies tremendously, with many possible variations and modifications of the different techniques described. For instance, an individual with a strong upper body who can stand with the help of devices such as a walker or crutches may be able to transfer from a wheelchair to another surface independently using a stand-pivot transfer. Furthermore, devices such as cushions to raise the seat height, frames, and mechanical devices that can help individuals with SCI to stand may be very helpful in transfers. Whatever technique and device that will provide the best functional solution to the individual is the best transfer technique, as long as it is safe and effective for the individual (and caregiver). This develops over time with training.

Wheelchair Training

Wheelchair training includes basic and advanced activities. Basic skills include wheelchair propulsion on level and uneven surfaces (e.g., inclines and carpets) and transfers in and out of the wheelchair while in the bathroom or getting into a car. The patient and family should be taught how to handle the chair on curbs and inclines, how to fold the wheelchair for placement into a car, and how to perform maintenance and simple repairs that may be needed. Advanced activities include negotiating uneven surfaces such as riding on rough terrain, independently negotiating ramps and curbs, performing "wheelies," negotiating elevators and escalators, being able to fall safely, and transfer from the floor to the wheelchair.

Standing

Standing can be achieved after SCI with the use of tilt tables or standing frames. After an acute SCI, standing has been shown to decrease hypercalciuria and may retard or lessen bone loss (27,28). In contrast, standing has not been shown to reverse osteoporosis after it has occurred in chronic SCI (29–32). Standing should proceed with caution in patients with chronic SCI because bone mineral density is often at or below fracture threshold (33). An increase in physical self-concept scores and a decrease in depression scores have been reported with standing after SCI (34). Standing may also decrease spasticity and enhance bowel and bladder programs secondary to the effect of gravity, as does ambulation (35) (see the next section). Tilt tables can be used early in the rehabilitation process to gradually obtain a vertical position, aiding in the treatment of orthostatic hypotension.

The decision to purchase a standing frame after rehabilitation depends on the motivation of the user to use it on a consistent basis. It is not recommended that one stand in the frame for more than 1 hour at a time if there is a great amount of edema that develops.

Ambulation and Lower Extremity Orthoses

The ability to walk is one of the first goals that many persons with SCI set for themselves. It is important that patients with SCI understand their prognosis in terms of achieving this goal, when it should be worked on, and the various levels of ambulation.

There are four general levels of ambulation: community ambulation, household ambulation, ambulation for exercise, and nonambulatory (36). Community ambulation is when the individual is independent in performing transfers, is capable of coming from the sit to stand position, and can ambulate unassisted in and outside the home at reasonable distances (more than 150 ft) with or without braces and assistive devices. Household ambulation is when the person can ambulate within the home with relative independence but may require assistance for transfers and is unable to ambulate outdoors for any significant distances. Ambulation for exercise is for a person that requires significant assistance for ambulation. For those who cannot achieve ambulation, standing can still take place.

Physiologic benefits of walking include potentially decreasing the progression of osteoporosis, reducing urinary calcinosis, reducing spasticity, aiding in digestion and improving bowel program because of the effect of gravity, and preventing pressure ulcers by allowing pressure relief on normally weightbearing areas (28,35,37–41). In addition, it enables reaching for objects not obtainable from the wheelchair level and affords access to areas that are not wheelchair accessible, such as through narrow doorways. There are also psychological benefits, which include allowing the individual to be at eye level with others.

Although ambulation after SCI has physiologic and psychological benefits, it also has significant drawbacks, including increased energy consumption; weightbearing through the UEs, which may predispose an individual to shoulder, elbow, and wrist problems; and poor long-term follow-through, resulting in wasted time, energy, and money. Studies have demonstrated that increased energy consumption, along with a decreased speed of ambulation, can make ambulation after SCI very inefficient when compared with the relatively normal energy expenditure and velocity of wheelchair use (42–44). The average speed of ambulation for a subject with paraplegia using a swing-through gait with crutches and bilateral knee-ankle-foot orthoses (KAFOs) was 64% slower than normal and the rate of oxygen uptake was 38% higher. Subjects with intact hip flexion and knee extension who used AFOs and crutches to ambulate in a reciprocal gait pattern demonstrated a rate of oxygen uptake that was 20% higher and a speed of ambulation that was 67% lower. In comparison, it was found that use of a wheelchair on a level surface proved a very efficient means of locomotion, with the average speed, rate of oxygen uptake, and oxygen cost approximating the values for normal walking (42).

There has been great disagreement regarding which patients, specifically at which level of injury, will be able to ambulate after training (45–47). Although there is no one definite level at which patients should not perform training with braces, there are factors that will contribute to difficulty in ambulation, including older age, higher weight, lack of motivation, inherent poor agility and coordination, and greater spasticity (48). Clinical experience and clinical studies have shown that most persons with an SCI at the T12 level and above who undergo gait training with orthoses and assistive devices will not become a community or household ambulator in the long term (43,49,50). Most individuals, even with levels to L2-3, will usually not continue braces exclusively for mobility. Some may therefore consider the training a waste of time and resources. However, we believe that all patients with the potential for ambulation be given a trial if they want to pursue this. The individual should not feel denied of the opportunity to walk and should be able to discover on his or her own whether this goal is feasible. However, for persons with thoracic-level injuries, training should not be initiated until transfer training and wheelchair activities are mastered.

Factors in addition to the neurologic examination (muscle strength) are important to consider when determining whether a patient is appropriate for ambulation; these include the ROM of the hips and knees, the degree of spasticity present, proprioception, orthostasis, cardiac stability due to the energy requirement involved, and motivation. To maintain standing in bilateral long leg braces, a patient must attain the "para-stance" position, a posture in which the weight line falls posterior to the hips and anterior to knees and ankles. Patients therefore need hip extension beyond neutral, full knee extension, and ankle dorsiflexion beyond neutral. This will allow the patient to be biomechanically stable in stance with orthoses without LE muscle strength. Skeletal factors such as the presence of scoliosis, leg length discrepancy, hip joint instability, and advanced osteoporosis should also be determined. Before gait training, proficiency with wheelchair-level activities should be attained because most individuals will use a wheelchair as their primary means of mobility, even after successful gait training.

There are various types of gait patterns that an individual with bilateral KAFOs may use with assistive devices. They include the reciprocal, swing-through, swing-to, and drag-to gait patterns. Individuals with active hip flexion best use a reciprocal gait pattern. Those without active hip flexion may also use this pattern if they are able to compensate by hiking the hip and performing a posterior pelvic tilt to advance one leg at a time. Another option is a swing-through gait pattern, which involves lifting the body and allowing the LEs to swing forward and land in front of the hands. As soon as the patient's feet land, the patient must immediately regain the para-stance position. Once stable, the hands are advanced and the patient is ready to again swing his LEs in front of his hands. A swing-to gait is similar to the swing-through gait, but rather than having the feet land in front of the hands, the feet now land slightly behind the hands. This allows the patient to more easily maintain his balance. For the patient who does not have the upper body strength to clear her feet for a swing-through or swing-to gait, a drag-to gait may be used. This is essentially the same as the swing-to gait pattern without the clearance, thereby making this a slower and less functional gait pattern.

The clinical examination has been used with good accuracy to determine a prognosis for ambulation (51–56). Those with higher level and neurologic complete injuries have a lower chance of ambulation. For individuals initially with sensory incomplete injuries, pinprick appreciation is a better prognosis

than is light touch alone. Motor incomplete lesions have the best prognosis for ambulation recovery (see chapter 7 for details).

Community ambulation requires bilateral hip flexors >3/5 and one knee extensor to be 3/5, with a maximum amount of bracing of one long leg brace and one short leg brace (50). Other methods have been described to determine the ability to ambulate. These include the description of the ambulatory motor index (AMI) by Waters et al. (67), which graded five muscles (hip flexors, hip abductors, hip extensors, knee flexors, and knee extensors) on a four-point scale (zero to three) (57). The sum of the scores is expressed as a percentage of the total score (30 points) and used as an indicator of paralysis, percent increase in O_2 consumption, velocity, heart rate, and cadence with ambulation. Waters et al. (57) reported that the AMI could be used as a reliable clinical indicator of functional mobility after SCI; with an AMI score of more than 60%, one would be a community ambulator and an AMI score of less than 40%, too much energy would be required for ambulation. In a subsequent study, Waters et al. (58) compared the AMI with ASIA muscles and found that although only two muscles were common to both AMI and ASIA key muscle groups (hip flexion and knee extension), there was good correlation.

Overall, as reported by Waters et al. (53–56) in multiple articles, community ambulation at 1 year is as follows: complete paraplegia, 5%; incomplete tetraplegia, 46%; and incomplete paraplegia, 76%. Prediction regarding ambulation at 1 year has been predicted based on the LE motor score (LEMS) at 30 days. For persons with incomplete tetraplegia, the chances of walking at 1 year with a 30-day LEMS of zero is zero; with a score of 1 to 9, 21%; a score of 10 to 19, 63%; and a score of more than 20, 100%. For persons with complete paraplegia, the chances of walking at 1 year with a 30-day LEMS of zero is less than 1%; and with a score of 1 to 9, 45%. For persons with incomplete paraplegia, the chances of walking at 1 year with a 30-day LEMS of zero is 33%; with a score of 1 to 9, 70%; and a score of more than 10, 100%.

A number of orthotic options exist to assist in ambulation, including mechanical orthoses, functional electrical stimulation (FES), and hybrid orthoses, a combination of a mechanical orthosis and FES (59). Clinical experience reveals that KAFOs are most frequently prescribed for ambulation. Hip-knee-ankle-foot orthoses (HKAFOs), including the hip guidance orthoses (HGOs) and the reciprocal gait orthosis (RGO), may enable persons with thoracic-level paraplegia to ambulate. The Parastep system is the simplest example of an FES system for walking. FES and hybrid systems for ambulation are discussed in chapter 25.

Craig-Scott Orthosis

The Craig-Scott orthosis (CSO), also called the Scott-Craig orthosis, is a double metal upright KAFO, but without the lower thigh and calf bands, so they are easier to don and doff (Fig. 19.9) (60). They are the most commonly prescribed KAFO for individuals with SCI. The CSO is a modified version of a conventional KAFO, designed to be as lightweight as possible and to capitalize on alignment stability to enhance upright activities in patients with low thoracic and lumbar SCI. The CSO has a

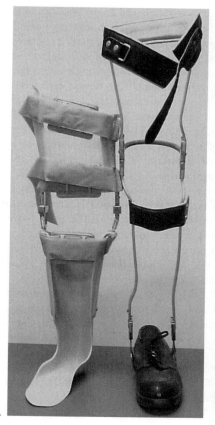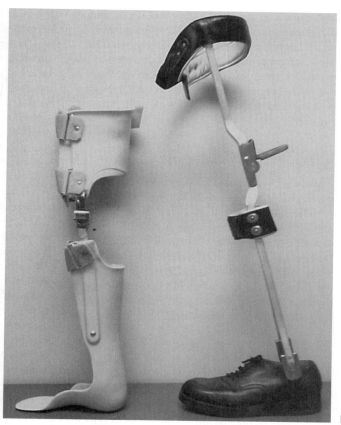

FIGURE 19.9. Knee-ankle-foot orthosis, **(left)** plastic molded, and **(right)** Craig-Scott orthosis. **A:** Frontal view. **B:** Lateral view.

rigid posterior thigh band, a rigid anterior tibial band, and an offset knee joint with a bail knee lock. A bail lock allows the medial and lateral locks to be disengaged at the same time by a posterior pressure, such as against the edge of a seating surface. This mechanism helps patients with paraplegia maintain bilateral UE support via crutches for stability. The ankle is set at 5 to 10 degrees of dorsiflexion and has a cushioned heel. These braces are designed for use with swing-through or swing-to gait.

Advantages of the CSO relative to the conventional or plastic KAFO are that they provide more stability, and the patient may be able to balance without using crutches. The cushioned heel may provide a softer landing and improve rollover techniques. The CSO allows for a more energy efficient gait relative to conventional KAFOs. The offset knee joint gives an extension force to the patient's knee, alleviating stress on the locking mechanism and making it easier to unlock. In addition, this type of joint has no sharp protruding edges when the knees are flexed during sitting. Lastly, the decreased medial upright height may lessen stimulation to the adductor longus tendon.

Disadvantages of the CSOs are that they are heavier and more expensive than conventional or plastic KAFOs. Standing from the floor may also be more difficult than with conventional KAFOs secondary to the fixed ankle and shoe. Lastly, a four-point gait is more difficult than with conventional KAFOs.

Conventional KAFOs

The KAFO uses drop locks as opposed to bail locks at the knee joint, which provides more stability around the knee joint, and has the extra calf and thigh bands. The KAFO is lighter than the CSO and therefore may provide more mobility. A four-point gait may be easier than with a CSO or plastic KAFO depending on the ankle adjustment. Standing from the floor is also easier than with the CSO. They are less expensive than the CSO and plastic brace. Progression from KAFO to AFO is also easier than with CSO, because the patient can train with the knees unlocked and the brace can be cut into an AFO if appropriate.

Disadvantages of the conventional KAFO are that they may provide less balance than CSO. The patient usually must keep one crutch in contact with the floor to maintain her balance. The conventional KAFOs are more difficult to don and doff, are more difficult to lock and unlock the knee joint, and allow for a less energy efficient gait than CSO.

Plastic KAFOs

The plastic molded KAFO is similar to the conventional KAFO as it compares to the CSO. Advantages of the plastic KAFO are that it is lighter and more cosmetic than the conventional KAFO and it allows for interchanging shoes. Disadvantages are that it is more definitive because adjustments available at the ankle joint are minimal. In addition, plastic does not absorb perspiration. There is increased potential for pressure sores, so this requires monitoring. This prescription may not be appropriate when the patient has increased LE tone, fluctuating edema, or decreased sensation. Because of the precise fit, weight changes are difficult to accommodate. Lastly, the plastic KAFO cannot easily be cut into an AFO if needed.

Vannini-Rizzoli Stabilizing Limb Orthosis

This is a leather boot that fits over a polypropylene AFO which encloses the lower leg, from 2 cm below the lower pole of patella to the toes (61). The ankle is placed in 10 to 15 degrees of plantar flexion to shift the ground reaction in front of the ankle and knee during standing, allowing for the stability of the knee upon standing. There are a number of varieties of boots, for winter and summer wear. The inside is padded to protect the skin. Ambulation is performed in a pendulum manner, using the stability of the assistive device and the patient shifts his torso toward one side, with the LEs to follow, and then the other side.

Swivel Walker

The swivel walker is for patients with neurologic levels below C6 to ambulate without the use of other assistive devices. It is a rigid body structure with fixation of the hips, knees, and ankles, provided by a leather chest pad, polypropylene sacral band, hinged knee bar, and foot clamp assembly. There are swiveling footplates beneath the body frame. Ambulation is achieved by alternately rocking sideways, which swivels the frame by lifting up one side. Movement is slow and restricted to level surfaces only. This is most commonly used in the pediatric population (see chapter 29).

Parawalker (Hip Guidance Orthosis)

The HGO is a rigid body brace with two KAFOs with a hip joint (62). There is minimal amount of abduction at the hips, low friction hip joints with flexion-extension stops. The shoe plate incorporates a rocker sole, placed in dorsiflexion. It allows for reciprocal walking, usually with crutches, for thoracic-level paraplegic individuals. The patient leans forward, placing the hips in full extension, and shifts their weight toward the stance side, allowing the opposite leg to swing forward under the influence of gravity. The knee joints are locked during ambulation with release mechanisms to allow the user to sit down.

Reciprocal Gait Orthosis

The current RGOs are a refinement of the original design and are referred to as the Louisiana State University (LSU) RGOs (63). These braces are joined bilateral KAFOs with offset knee joints, knee drop locks, posterior plastic AFOs, thigh pieces, a custom-molded pelvic girdle, hip joints, and a thoracic extension up to the xiphoid process of the sternum. The newer type of

hip joint has two locking positions: full hip extension and 20 degrees of flexion, which allows for normal upright posture, as well as forward to the center of gravity to better accommodate ambulation up an incline. The cable coupling mechanism provides hip stability, by preventing simultaneous bilateral hip flexion, yet allows free unilateral hip flexion-extension in a reciprocal fashion when a step is attempted.

RGOs are lighter and more cosmetic than CSOs and conventional KAFOs. They allow for more stability and a more acceptable gait pattern and are more energy efficient than CSOs or conventional or plastic KAFOs. There is also the opportunity to interchange shoes.

Disadvantages of the RGOs include that they are more difficult to don and doff than the CSOs and conventional and plastic KAFOs. One cannot adjust the ankle joint setting to increase the patient's balance. Problems from the plastic occur, including that it does not absorb perspiration, with increased potential for pressure areas. The braces may not be appropriate for persons with increased tone in their LEs and trunk. Fluctuating edema and weight changes are difficult to accommodate. RGOs require more cognitive and body awareness than other braces to use them effectively. Speed of gait is slower than when performing a swing-to or swing-through gait pattern with other braces. Falling can be dangerous because the hips are locked in extension. Scivoletto et al. (64) recently reported that 46% of subjects trained with RGOs no longer used them at 1-year follow-up (see chapter 29 for figure).

Advanced Reciprocating Gait Orthosis

A modification of the RGO has been described using a single encased cable, relative to a dual system, to reduce friction and allow the user to rise from the sitting position and sit from the standing position much easier than with RGOs. The person can stand with knees flexed without manually extending them, due to a compressed gas strut providing a knee extension moment to augment standing and control hip flexion during sitting. The hip and knee joints are connected via a knee lock actuating cable so the hip mechanism releases the knee lock (59).

Parastep

The Parastep is a portable FES system that allows reciprocal gait with a front-wheeled walker, which is connected by a cable to a microprocessor that is worn by the patient (65). Surface electrodes are placed on the quadriceps, the peroneal nerve, and the gluteal muscles. The stance phase is achieved through stimulation of the quadriceps, along with the gluteals and paraspinals as needed. The swing phase is achieved through stimulation of the peroneal nerve, resulting in a flexor withdrawal response.

Indications for the Parastep include a person with a UMN injury between T4-12 with good UE strength. ROM should be within functional limits, particularly hip extension and ankle dorsiflexion. The patient should be independent in transfers and have intact skin and lack of pain sensation in areas of electrode placement and stimulation. Contraindications include individuals with a LMN injury, significant osteoporosis, severe hypertension, fracture or rod implants, a pacemaker or cardiac disease, or a phrenic nerve pacemaker in place.

The potential benefits of the Parastep include an increased muscle strength/bulk in the LEs; independence in standing and ambulation; improved self-esteem and image; and an enhanced sense of well-being (32,33,66–68) (see chapter 25 for details).

Assistive Technology Devices

Assistive technology devices (ATDs) include any product or piece of equipment, whether acquired commercially or customized, that is used to increase, maintain, or improve functional capabilities of an individual with a disability. ATDs may be the key to independence for persons with SCI, becoming valuable tools for basic life skills and for improving social, recreational, and vocational activities. The person's level of injury will determine which ATD is appropriate. A comprehensive evaluation, by an assistive technology specialist, and trial period are important for the correct ATD to be prescribed.

Before prescribing assistive devices, one must identify the patient's capabilities and needed tasks. The assessment should incorporate a thorough current medical history and the individual's current functional status, level of cognition, and mood. This includes testing the patient's strength and ROM, as well as his positioning and sitting balance in bed and a wheelchair, degree of spasticity, auditory and visual capability, and cognitive status. The evaluator should also assess the patient's goals and try to match the goals to any environmental barriers that are determined. A trial process should follow, with a prescription and letter of justification to access the funding needed. The proper vendor, particularly for high-level ATDs, is crucial for proper service and delivery.

ATDs can be separated into low versus high level. Low-level technology includes everyday tools such as desktop and feeding items and telephone systems, and high-level technology includes complex electronic or battery-operated devices that require more detailed programming, trial, and means for funding. Low-level technology items are more affordable and may be commercially available or custom made for the client.

Low-Level ATDs

Desktop items are important for vocational and recreational activities and socialization. In individuals with an NLI of C1-4, these may include a computer with voice-recognition software or a mouth stick with a docking station. For word processing, voice-activated systems are available commercially, such as Dragon Dictate (IBM Systems). For those with a lower NLI (C5-7), items such as a wanchik's writer, typing pegs, or a universal cuff with a pen or pencil can be prescribed for writing (Figs. 19.3 and 19.4). Adaptive devices for reading in high-level–injured clients may include a battery-operated page turner, whereas for those individuals with lower levels of injury, a typing peg with or without a bookstand is appropriate.

Assistive devices for feeding are extremely important to allow an individual to feed himself. Items include an MAS or a BFO, with a table or wheelchair mount, for individuals with C4-5 levels of injury (Fig. 19.1). For persons with a C5-6 motor level,

items such as a plate guard or scoop dish, Dycem, long straw, horizontal or a vertical fork/spoon, universal cuff, or dorsal splint can be prescribed (Fig. 19.2).

Telephone access is an important basic skill to allow for socialization and to use in case of medical emergencies. In high-level injuries (C1-5), a stand-alone phone (e.g., Lifeline Corporation Telephone, Cambridge, MA) with an appropriate switch or mouth stick can be used, or setting up a phone system through an ECU (see later discussion). For lower levels of injury, a quad phone "C" clip with a typing peg or a gooseneck holder with a pen clip can be used (Fig. 19.3). A speakerphone or a headset phone can be used with these devices.

High-Level ATDs

Environmental Control Units

An ECU acts as a remote to control battery and electrical appliances in the person's environment with the use of a switch. The ECU is the control center that can control almost any aspect of the patient's environment, including radios, televisions, videocassette recorders, bed, computer, lights, fan, thermostat controls, and more. An ECU can allow the individual to remain home alone for a short period of time without assistance, because he is in full control of the environment. The correct ECU can enhance a person's life by giving her a sense of control, security, and independence.

The ECU has multiple components, including the control unit, display unit (auditory or visual), switch, and needed cables. The control method may be ultrasound, radio waves, or infrared light (69).

When addressing high-level ATDs, one must determine the type of adaptive switch for activation. A person can essentially use any body part to activate a switch as long as she can perform the activity consistently with accuracy. A reliable site can include the head, chin, mouth, shoulder, arm, or hand. Voice activation is also an option. The Bains Assistive Technology System (BATS) is an evaluation tool that can determine the proper switch for the individual, which includes four components: the patient, the task, the device, and the environment. The patient's overall capability (i.e., cognitive status and functional movements) and the environment should be evaluated to choose the appropriate switch. The switch can function as either a single (on/off activation), dual (e.g., allows scanning and selection options for an ECU or computer), or a multiple switch (e.g., joystick for greater capability). The switch operation can be either momentary (remains activated as long as pressure is maintained), latching (stays on or off until the switch is activated again), or proportional (degree of activity varies by amount of pressure applied).

One should address where the ATD will be used—home, school, work, and future environments anticipated. The switch can be mounted on the patient or on a wheelchair, bed, or desk and should be placed so the individual will be comfortable and easily able to activate it. Options for available switches are listed in Table 19.5.

Before prescribing an ECU, one should consider whether low-level technology or a commercially available device could meet the goal. An ECU can interface with other devices such

TABLE 19.5. TYPES OF SWITCHES AVAILABLE

Type of Switch	Mechanism of Action	Level of Injury
Eye blink	Infrared. Activated when light beam is interrupted by a timed sustained blink.	C1–3
Pneumatic	Dual mechanism. Activated by sip and puff into a straw, altering the air pressure.	C1–4
Rocker	Single or dual mechanism. Activated by gross movement of arm, hand, or wrist.	C4–6
Tongue touch keypad	Electrodes are embedded in a retainer worn in the patient's mouth and touched by the tongue activating the switch.	C1–5
Wobble	Single mechanism switch activated by tongue or chin, by movement up or down.	C1–3
Pillow, plate, cup	Single mechanism switch activated by touch of any part of the body.	C4–6
Sound activated	Converts a sound level to a switch activator.	C1–4
Mercury	Positional.	C1–4

as a power wheelchair. The client can use the switch already set up for driving the wheelchair as the means to access the ECU, by connecting a remote ECU package to the serial port in the wheelchair.

Computers

Persons with a SCI can access and use a computer in many ways (70). The computer can allow correspondence via letters, e-mail, and faxes, as well as to perform aspects of daily life including paying bills online and printing checks.

Individuals with a NLI below C5 can access the computer with their UEs, with or without typing pegs. If the patient is unable to use a traditional mouse, a trackball can be tried. For clients with a SCI from C1–4, it is imperative to perform a thorough evaluation, to recommend an access method that makes it easy to use. This may be a voice-activated or eye-gaze system or some type of operation with their mouth as the next best option.

An option for a keyboard, if the patient is unable to access a standard one, is a key guard, which fits over a standard keyboard with holes over the keys. Other nonstandard keyboards include on-screen, mini, enlarged, and alternate key arrangement. The on-screen keyboard graphically depicts a keyboard on the computer screen, which can be set up for scanning with a single switch or for people with only one functional hand. A mouse can point to the keys, and with a click of the mouse, the typed symbol appears in a word processing program. An added benefit is that there is word prediction, in which as soon as a letter is typed, a list of words that are most frequently used appears and the user chooses from the list, saving keystrokes. The user can also access the on-screen keyboard with a touch screen, mouth stick, or head pointer. Another option is a mini-keyboard, used for those with limited ROM who are unable to reach all of the keys on a standard keyboard. An enlarged keyboard is useful for people who have trouble with accuracy. This keyboard also requires very little pressure to activate the keys.

Additional options include a handheld pointing device, which may be used with an on-screen keyboard and a joystick. A touch pad can also be used, particularly if the user has functional use of one hand and can be accurate in pointing with one finger. One of the more sophisticated systems is the head pointer system. A camera is mounted on top of the monitor, pointed at the user, who has a reflective dot that reflects a small beam of light onto the computer screen. The beam of light is translated into a small arrow—a cursor. The user then moves his head very slightly to move the cursor. This system is used with an on-screen keyboard, and when the cursor is on a key, the user must "dwell" there for a predetermined period of time to activate the key in order for it to be typed. This method requires extremely good head and neck control. Lastly, one may use a foot mouse, perhaps useful for individuals with central cord syndrome, if they have no functional use of their hands but have use of their feet.

Software packages are available with additional accessibility options. Some examples include StickyKeys, which may save the user from having to use multiple keystrokes; adjustment of the acceptance rate of pressure on the keys, so the same letter will not be repeated if the user cannot remove his finger fast enough; and FilterKeys, which ignores brief or repeated keystrokes or slows down the repeat rate. Rate enhancement software—such as that in which a person programs in his own abbreviations and the entire word is then typed or that which uses word prediction in which the user is able to choose from a list of most frequently typed words—will speed the rate of typing.

Voice-recognition software has recently become less expensive and better technology is making this method of input a popular choice. Ventilator-dependent patients are able to use this method.

SPINAL CORD EDUCATION

All members of the team perform spinal cord education. A specific designated member can hold formal classes, commonly a nurse who coordinates the program for the patients and families. Topics should include anatomy and classification of the SCI; medical issues regarding bowel, bladder, skin, and autonomic dysreflexia; adjustment to disability issues; sexuality and fertility; and research topics in SCI. Because length of hospital stay is shorter, the importance of starting these classes as soon as possible is of great importance. However, formal classes alone are not sufficient. Bedside teaching by the nurses, reinforcing proper bowel and bladder techniques and the importance of skin checks with a mirror, cannot be overemphasized. Knowledge of recognizing the symptoms of autonomic dysreflexia and going through the steps of management may prove lifesaving once the patient is discharged. Reviewing proper techniques for ROM, proper placement of splints, and transfer techniques to all surfaces should be incorporated into therapy.

HOME MODIFICATIONS FOR PEOPLE WITH SCI

The home evaluation is an important aspect of the rehabilitation process, to allow the injured individual to return home. Before performing the home evaluation, it is helpful to have those individuals involved in the person's discharge submit a written floor plan of the residence. One should also discuss the key features of the home that the client feels most strongly about, because it is important to keep the home environment as similar as possible to the way it was before the accident.

The main areas of concern in the home evaluation include the entrances, bedroom, bathroom, kitchen, and general safety issues (71). The rehabilitation team should be familiar with contractors and architects in the local area and have information from previous clients who have used them available for the newly injured family members. In addition, family members may want to see other modified homes before going forth with their modifications.

The key pieces of information to know when performing the home evaluation is the patient's prognosis for functional recovery, social situation for return to home (i.e., how much assistance will there be), and financial considerations. The level of injury and prognosis will help determine whether the patient will require a wheelchair (power vs. manual) or whether the patient will be able to ambulate with assistance. This is important for measuring entranceways and doorways and deciding on ramps versus lifts. Understanding the social situation (family dynamics and home care availability) is important in making decisions for home modification, because the more a person with an SCI is alone, the more modifications will be needed. For instance, if there is someone home to help with meal preparation, then modifications to the kitchen may be kept to a minimum.

Entrances

The entire area, from the car to the front door, must be evaluated, ensuring that the surface is smooth and level. Outdoor walkways must accommodate a slope of 20 in. of length to every 1 in. in height, as the maximum grade. Ramps must recognize a 12-in. length for every 1 in. in rise. The ramp must be a minimum of 3 ft 6 in. wide, measured inside the railing. A low 4-in. curb should be provided on both sides of the ramp to serve as a guardrail. Handrails (between 2 ft 6 in. and 2 ft 8 in. in height) can be provided on both sides of the ramp to serve as a guard. Ramps should be of a nonslip material, fire-retardant construction and divided into 10- to 12-ft sections, with a 5-by-5-ft platform at any point where the ramp changes direction. The base of the ramp should terminate with a level section of the walkway or driveway.

The ramp entrance should be devoid of a storm door; if present, it should swing inward, away from the confined space of the porch landing or steps. A 5-by-5-ft exterior doorway landing at the top of the ramp for wheelchair maneuvering during door management should be constructed. The landing should be level with the living space floor.

The entranceway width should be at least 32 in. (measured from the door to the molding) if no turn is involved, with a 5-by-5-ft landing to allow space during door management. Door handles should be the lever type, which are easier to handle for people with limited hand function. Doors should be hung on offset hinges, which allow the door to swing clear of the doorway.

An individual with restricted mobility is particularly vulnerable to fire and other hazards. It is therefore recommended to provide two remotely located means of exit from any residence. An accessible secondary exit should provide the occupant with the ability to vacate the house in the event of an emergency.

Bedroom

The bedroom should be devoid of unnecessary furniture and should only contain the bed, dresser, and possibly a counter space for vocational or computer activities. The bedroom should accommodate an area of at least 10 by 14 ft and should allow at least one 5-by-5-ft area clear of furniture for maneuvering the wheelchair. A passageway with a minimum width of 3 ft should be provided on at least one side of the bed, with a passageway of a minimum of 4 ft provided at the end of the bed. A clear floor area, 4 ft in length, should precede dressers and closet space.

For closet access, if the person with an SCI has adequate arm and hand function, rods should be hung at a height of 3 ft 6 in. to 4 ft. Accessible shelves should be no higher than 4 ft 6 in. and no deeper than 1 ft 4 in. For a standard closet, bifolding or sliding doors are preferred, with recessed floor-mounted door tracks. A 4-ft clear floor space in front of the closet doors should allow for wheelchair maneuvering space. For a roll-in closet, the door should have a clearance width of 32 in. A minimum of a 5-by-5-ft area is needed, clear of shelving and hanging clothing, for wheelchair turning.

Work space may be provided in the bedroom. Equipment, such as stereo systems and computers, is easily accessible from a countertop. Counters should be constructed between 2 ft 6 in. and 2 ft 10 in. in height and a minimum depth of 2 ft. Knee space clearance should have a minimum height of 2 ft 3 in. and a minimum width of 3 ft. Countertop-level outlets should be provided.

Bathroom

Depending on the person's level of injury, the bathroom is most often the room that needs the greatest modifications. The accessible bathroom should be adjacent to the bedroom if possible and be a minimum of 8 by 10 ft. The swing of the bathroom door should be outward, into the bedroom, and away from the more confined space of the bathroom. A 5-by-5-ft area clear of fixtures, for wheelchair turning radius and maneuvering should be provided.

The sink should be mounted on a wall (no higher than 34 in. from the floor and projected approximately 2 ft 3 in. from the wall) without a cabinet beneath. The sink depth should not exceed 6½ in. Knee clearance should be provided below the sink that is at least 27 in. high, 30 in. wide, and 19 in. deep. A clear floor space, 30 in. wide 4 ft long, must be provided in front of the sink. Sink pipes or drains must be insulated to prevent scrapes and burns. To maximize knee space clearance, it is recommended that pipes be recessed, offset horizontally, or located behind the wall. Countertops provided should not have a height that exceeds 34 in.

A mirror should be hung for viewing from both a seated and a standing position, with the lower edge mounted no more than 3 ft 4 in. from the floor, and the top edge mounted no less than 6 ft 2 in.

A standard height (14-in. rim height) toilet is recommended for use with a standard rolling shower/commode chair or over-the-toilet commode. Space must be provided on both sides of the toilet to accommodate these commodes.

For a roll-in shower, it is recommended to construct a tiled, two- or three-sided shower, with no curb or threshold. The floor of the shower should be of nonslip material, a minimum of 5 by 5 ft, and slightly sloped for water drainage. A shower spray unit that can be used both as a fixed showerhead and as a hand-held spray is recommended. A thermostat control is an important feature. An adjustable-height extended (6 ft) shower hose with an on/off lever on the handle is preferred. A ceiling-hung track shower curtain is recommended for water containment. Lastly, a heat light and ventilating unit in the bathroom for temperature control due to the length of time for bowel, bladder, and personal hygiene routine should be added.

Kitchen

If the person with an SCI will be preparing meals, the counters should be 30 to 35 in. above the floor with 24 in. beneath for knee clearance. Providing a pullout surface for workspace can easily accommodate these specifications. All appliances need to be evaluated and recommendations made for access. The stove should contain front or side controls to avoid burns while reaching over the burners. Gas is preferred to electric, due to the visibility of knowing when the gas burner is on. The oven should be low enough for the person with an SCI to be able to reach inside, being careful not to roll the wheelchair too close. The microwave should be on a surface where the person with an SCI can reach inside. If the person with an SCI has difficulty pressing the recessed buttons, a microwave with a dial is preferred. The refrigerator or freezer should be a side-by-side model, keeping the most frequently used items on the lower shelves. A lazy Susan can be placed in the refrigerator and cabinets to allow easy access to items.

The sink should contain one-lever controls, preferably mounted on the side for easy access. The sink height should be 29 to 31 in. and with a shallow sink depth. The cabinets beneath the sink should be removed and the pipes well insulated to prevent burns. It is recommended that all lower kitchen cabinets have rollout shelves to facilitate access.

Floor-to-Floor Access

If the person with an SCI has adequate balance and is able to transfer to a seat, floor-to-floor access can be accomplished using a stair glide, which is a seat that glides along a track, mounted to the wall alongside an existing staircase. The stair glide does narrow the existing stairway and there needs to be adequate room for a caregiver to walk alongside the person with an SCI as he ascends or descends the staircase. Some models of stair glides have a seat that folds up that serves to not narrow the walk space of the staircase. Using a stair glide makes it necessary to have two wheelchairs, one at the bottom of the stair glide and one at the top. Some stair glides are made to incorporate turns and multiple levels with landings. A lift manufacturer should be contacted who is best able to meet the patient's needs. A backup power source is also needed, in the case of an electrical power outage and the stair glide is the only means of access to the outside. For people with poor balance who need to access another floor within the home, transferring to a stair glide is not possible, so a lift or elevator is the only option.

General Considerations

When discussing home modifications, many times the best place spatially for the person with an SCI would be in a garage or basement area. However, these areas should have stringent temperature control and must be well insulated. The area should be air-conditioned in warm weather and heated in cold weather, with controls for regulation that can be operated independently. Often, a zoned system is best, because it allows different areas of the house to be set for different temperatures. Many times, the patient will need to make one area of the house warmer or cooler than the rest of the house, due to the inability to regulate one's own body temperature.

There are a number of general recommendations that can be made for home modifications (Table 19.6). These are only general guidelines and recommendations for making the home accessible. The extensiveness of these modifications depends highly on the person's function, family wishes, and resources.

LONG-TERM FOLLOW-UP

Outpatient programs have recently taken on an even more important role than in previous decades because of the shortened inpatient length of stay. These include close monitoring of the medical status (i.e., bowel, bladder, skin, and respiratory management) and a comprehensive therapy program that includes not only physical and occupational therapies but also psychological and vocational counseling. With the shorter length of stay, there is less time to help the patient and family adjust to the disability and address all of the obstacles present that may interfere with social, vocational, and recreational reintegration.

Long-term follow-up with the SCI specialist is extremely important. Initially, visits should occur on a monthly basis, particularly while the person is on outpatient therapy. This allows for monitoring of medical issues, reevaluating the therapy program and setting updated goals, and prescribing equipment. Because patients go home from inpatient hospitalization earlier, frequently, medical issues that previously were experienced in the hospital now develop while at home. These include bowel, bladder, and spasticity changes, as well as the development of hetero-

TABLE 19.6. GENERAL RECOMMENDATIONS FOR ACCESSIBILITY IN THE HOME

- The minimum space for turning around is 5 ft by 5 ft for a manual wheelchair, and 6 ft by 6 ft for a power wheelchair.
- Doorway widths that require a "straight shot" (no turning involved) is 32 inches for a manual chair and 34 inches for a power wheelchair. This space increases to 36 inches if there is a turn involved.
- All thresholds should be no more than 1 inch to allow the person in the wheelchair to maneuver.
- Install carbon monoxide detectors and smoke alarms throughout the home.
- Low-pile carpeting or hard surface flooring is recommended for wheelchair maneuvering.
- Eliminate throw rugs, because they pose a hazard for people who are walking and are difficult for people in wheelchairs to roll over.
- Remove or rearrange furniture that will impede wheelchair access.
- Notify police and fire departments that an individual with a disability resides in the home and provide the bedroom location.
- An intercom system can be useful to allow for communication.
- Backup power should be provided if the person with a spinal cord injury is dependent on equipment for life support, such as a ventilator.
- Light switches should be at a height of no more than 36 inches.
- Fireplace/heater cautions: Wheelchairs are generally constructed of some type of metal, which may or may not conduct heat, so when a person in a wheelchair is seated near a fireplace or heater, care should be taken to cover the metal parts of the wheelchair that may contact the person's skin, to ensure that the person in the wheelchair does not get burned.
- Power door openers can be installed for people in wheelchairs, where a remote can be used, or install a push plate on the wall.

topic ossification and autonomic dysreflexia. After these issues are stabilized and outpatient therapy has switched to a maintenance-type program, visits should be every 3 to 6 months through the second year. For those patients who are medically stable, yearly visits are then recommended. The importance of these visits is to review any medical changes, monitor the neurologic examination to ensure that there is no deterioration, ensure that the equipment is being maintained, and prescribe any additional equipment that may be needed. Deterioration of the neurologic status may be secondary to a tethered cord, syringomyelia, or peripheral problems such as median or ulnar nerve entrapment or musculoskeletal complications. As more persons with SCI are surviving longer after their injury, the importance of their follow-up visits to maintain their quality of life cannot be overemphasized.

At times, readmission to the rehabilitation hospital for medical (e.g., pressure ulcer or autonomic dysreflexia) or rehabilitation issues may be needed. For medical issues, the SCI physician is able to care for the patient with consultation as required and the entire rehabilitation staff is most keenly aware of other issues that can occur in the patient with SCI. This includes the importance of maintaining the proper bowel and bladder programs, skin issues, and awareness of the signs and symptoms as well as the proper treatment of autonomic dysreflexia. In addition, many times, the person with SCI may require a "refresher course" in rehabilitation techniques that can best be taught in an intensive inpatient setting. Chapter 27 further outlines the changes over the life for those with SCI.

Unfortunately, some third-party payers will not cover SCI specialists to follow the person with an SCI after the acute rehabilitation stay. This may lead to an increase in secondary SCI-specific medical complications because issues such as heterotopic ossification, autonomic dysreflexia, spasticity, and bowel and bladder care are not commonly seen by the general practitioner. In addition, without experience regarding functional outcomes, the expenditures for equipment will often be higher.

REFERENCES

1. Ragnarsson KT, Stein AB, Kirshblum S. Rehabilitation and comprehensive care of the person with spinal cord injury. In: Capen DA, Haye W, eds. *Comprehensive management of spine trauma.* St. Louis: Mosby, 1998.
2. Stover SL, DeLisa JA, Whiteneck GG, eds. *Spinal cord injury: clinical outcomes from the model systems.* Gaithersburg, MD: Aspen Publications 1995.
3. Yarkony GM. Overview of spinal cord injury rehabilitation in the acute phase, the rehabilitation team, and classification of spinal cord lesion. In: Yarkony GM, ed. *Spinal cord injury: medical management and rehabilitation.* Gaithersburg, MD: Aspen Publications, 1994.
4. Ragnarsson KT, Gordon WA. Rehabilitation after spinal cord injury: the team approach. *Phys Med Rehabil Clin North Am* 1992;3:853–878.
5. Kirshblum S, Johnston M, Brown J, et al. Predictors of dysphagia after spinal cord injury. *Arch Phys Med Rehabil* 1999;80:1101–1106.
6. Kirshblum S, O'Connor K, Benevento B, et al. Spinal orthotics. In: Delisa JA, Gans B, eds. *Rehabilitation medicine: principles and practice.* Philadelphia, Lippincott, 1998:635–650.
7. Goldberg B, Hsu JD, eds. *Atlas of orthoses and assistive devices,* 3rd ed. St. Louis: Mosby, 1998.
8. Johnson RM, Owen JR, Hart DL, et al. Cervical orthoses in a guide to their selection and use. *Clin Orthop Related Res* 1981;154:34–45.
9. Askins V, Eismont FJ. Efficacy of five cervical orthoses in restricting cervical motion: a comparison study. *Spine* 1997;22:1193–1198.
10. Sandler AJ, Dvorak J, Humke T, et al. The effectiveness of various cervical orthoses. *Spine* 1996;21:1624–1629.
11. Sharpe KP, Rao S, Ziogas A, et al. Evaluation of the effectiveness of the Minerva cervicothoracic orthosis. *Spine* 1995;20:1475–1479.
12. Olson RS. Halo skeletal traction pin site care: towards developing a standard of care. *Rehabil Nurs* 1996;21:243–246.
13. Celeste S, Folcik MA, Dumas KM, et al. Identifying a standard for pin site care utilizing the quality assurance approach. *Orthop Nurs* 1984; 3:17–24.
14. Lind B, Sihlbom H, Nordwall A, et al. Forces & motions across the neck in patients treated with halo-vest. *Spine* 1988;13:162–167.
15. Koch RA, Nickel VL. The halo vest: an evaluation of motion and forces across the neck. *Spine* 1978;3:103–107.
16. Hanak M, Scott A. *Spinal cord injury: an illustrated guide for health care professionals.* New York: Springer-Verlag New York, 1983.
17. Pedretti LW. *Occupational therapy: practice skills for physical dysfunction,* 4th ed. St. Louis: Mosby, 1996.
18. Kosiak M. Etiology of decubitus ulcers. *Arch Phys Med Rehabil* 1961; 42:19–21.
19. Reichel S. Shearing force as a factor in decubitus ulcers in paraplegics. *JAMA* 1958;166:762–763.
20. Hobson DA. Comparative effects of posture on pressure and shear at the body–seat interface. *J Rehabil Res Dev* 1992;29(4):21–31.
21. Henderson JL, Price SH, Brandstater ME, et al. Efficacy of three measures to relieve pressure in seated persons with spinal cord injury. *Arch Phys Med Rehabil* 1994;75(5):535–539.
22. Landis E. Micro-injection studies of capillary blood pressure in human skin. *Heart* 1930;15:209–228.
23. Braddom R. *Physical medicine and rehabilitation.* Philadelphia: WB Saunders, 1996.
24. Burns P, Betz K. Seating pressures with conventional and dynamic

wheelchair cushions in tetraplegia. *Arch Phys Med Rehabil* 1999; 80(May):566–571.

25. Trombly A. *Occupational therapy: for physical dysfunction,* 4th ed. Baltimore, MD: Williams & Wilkins, 1995.

26. Hallin RP. Transfers and mobility for paraplegic and quadriplegic patients. *Lancet* 1967;87:130–132.

27. de Bruin ED, Frey-Rindova P, Herzog RE, et al. Changes of tibia bone properties after spinal cord injury: effects of early intervention. *Arch Phys Med Rehabil* 1999;80(2):214–220.

28. Kaplan PE, Roden W, Gilbert E, et al. Reduction of hypercalciuria in tetraplegia after weight-bearing and strengthening exercises. *Paraplegia* 1981;19:289–293.

29. Hangartner T, Rodgers MM, Glaser RM, et al. Tibial bone density loss in spinal cord injury patients: effects of FES exercise. *J Rehabil Res Dev* 1994;31:50–61.

30. BeDell KK, Scremin AME, Perell KL, et al. Effects of functional electrical stimulation-induced lower extremity cycling on bone density of spinal cord–injured patient. *Am J Phys Med Rehabil* 1996;75:29–34.

31. Leeds EM, Klose KJ, Ganz W, et al. Bone mineral density after bicycle ergometry training. *Arch Phys Med Rehabil* 1990;71:207–279.

32. Needham-Shropshire BM, Broton JG, Klose KJ, et al. Evaluation of a training program for persons with SCI paraplegia using the Parastep 1 ambulation system: part 3. Lack of effect on bone mineral density. *Arch Phys Med Rehabil* 1997;78:799–803.

33. Szollar S, Martin EM, Sartoris DJ, et al. Bone mineral density and indexes of bone metabolism in spinal cord injury. *Am J Phys Med Rehabil* 1998;77(1):28–35.

34. Guest RS, Klose KJ, Needham-Shropshire BM, et al. Evaluation of a training program for persons with SCI paraplegia using the Parastep 1 ambulation system: part 4. Effect on physical self-concept and depression. *Arch Phys Med Rehabil* 1997;78:804–807.

35. Kunkel CF, Scremin AM, Eisenberg B, et al. Effect of "standing" on spasticity, contracture, and osteoporosis in paralyzed males. *Arch Phys Med Rehabil* 1993;74:73–78.

36. Hussey RW, Stauffer ES. Spinal cord injury: requirements for ambulation. *Arch Phys Med Rehabil* 1973;54:544–547.

37. Rosenstein BD, Greene WB, Herrington RT, et al. Bone density in myelomeningocele: the effects of ambulatory status and other factors. *Dev Med Child Neurol* 1987;29:486–494.

38. Kaplan PE, Gandhavadi B, Richards L, et al. Calcium balance in paraplegic patients: influence of injury duration and ambulation. *Arch Phys Med Rehabil* 1978;59:447–450.

39. Bohannon RW. Tilt table standing for reducing spasticity after spinal cord injury. *Arch Phys Med Rehabil* 1993;74:1121–1122.

40. Ogilvie C, Bowker P, Rowley DI. The physiological benefits of paraplegic orthotically aided walking. *Paraplegia* 1993;31:111–115.

41. Merritt JL. Knee-ankle-foot orthotics: long leg braces and their practical application. *Phys Med Rehabil (State of the Art Reviews)* 1987;1:67–82.

42. Waters RL, Lunsford BR. Energy cost of paraplegic locomotion. *J Bone Joint Surg* 1985;67A:1245–1250.

43. Waters RL, Mulroy S. The energy expenditure of normal and pathologic gait. *Gait Posture* 1999;9:207–231.

44. Huang CT, Kuhlemeier KV, Moore NB, et al. Energy cost of ambulation in paraplegic patients using Craig-Scott braces. *Arch Phys Med Rehabil* 1979;60:595–600.

45. Zankel HT, Sutton BB, Burney TT. A paraplegic program under physical medicine and rehabilitation: one year's experience. *Arch Phys Med Rehabil* 1955;36:249–255.

46. Munro D. Two year end results in total rehabilitation of veterans with spinal cord and cauda equina injuries. *N Engl J Med* 1950;242:1–16.

47. Long C, Lawton EB. Functional significance of spinal cord lesion level. *Arch Phys Med* 1955;36:249–255.

48. Gordon EE, Vanderwalde H. Energy requirements in paraplegic ambulation. *Arch Phys Med* 1956;36:276–285.

49. Rossman N, Spira E. Paraplegic use of walking braces: a survey. *Arch Phys Med Rehabil* 1974;55:310–314.

50. Stauffer ES, Hoffer MM, Nickel VL. Ambulation in thoracic paraplegia. *J Bone Joint Surg* 1978;60A:823–824.

51. Crozier KS, Graziani V, Ditunno JF, et al. Spinal cord injury: prognosis for ambulation based on sensory examination in patients who are initially motor complete. *Arch Phys Med Rehabil* 1991;72:119–121.

52. Katoh S, El-Masry WS. Motor recovery of patients presenting with motor paralysis and sensory sparing following cervical spinal cord injuries. *Paraplegia* 1995;33:506–509.

53. Waters RL, Yakura JS, Adkins RH, et al. Recovery following complete paraplegia. *Arch Phys Med Rehabil* 1992;73:784–789.

54. Waters RL, Adkins RH, Yakura IS, et al. Neurologic recovery following incomplete paraplegia. *Arch Phys Med Rehabil* 1994;75:57–72.

55. Waters RL, Adkins RH, Yakura JS, et al. Motor and sensory recovery following incomplete tetraplegia. *Arch Phys Med Rehabil* 1994;75: 306–311.

56. Waters RL, Adkins R, Yakura J, et al. Functional and neurological recovery following acute SCI. *J Spinal Cord Med* 1998;21:195–199.

57. Waters RL, Yakura JS, Adkins R, et al. Determinants of gait performance following SCI. *Arch Phys Med Rehabil* 1989;70:811–818.

58. Waters RL, Adkins R, Yakura J, et al. Prediction of ambulatory performance based on motor scores derived from standards of the American Spinal Injury Association. *Arch Phys Med Rehabil* 1994;75:756–760.

59. Nene AV, Hermens HJ, Zilvold G. Paraplegic locomotion: a review. *Spinal Cord* 1996;34:507–524.

60. Lehmann JF, Warren CG, Hertling D, et al. Craig-Scott orthosis: a biomechanical and functional evaluation. *Arch Phys Med Rehabil* 1976; 57:438–442.

61. Lyles M, Munday J. Report on the evaluation of the Vannini-Rizzoli stabilizing limb orthosis. *J Rehabil Res Dev* 1992;29:77–104.

62. Butler PB, Major RE, Patrick H. The technique of reciprocal walking using the hip guidance orthosis (HGO) with crutches. *Prosthet Orthot Int* 1984;8:33–38.

63. Douglas R, Larson PF, D'Ambrosia R, et al. The LSU reciprocating gait orthosis. *Orthopedics* 1983;6:834–839.

64. Scivoletto G, Petrelli A, Di Lucente L, et al. One year follow up of spinal cord injury patients using a reciprocating gait orthosis: preliminary results. *Spinal Cord* 2000;38:555–558.

65. Chaplin E. Functional neuromuscular stimulation for mobility in people with spinal cord injuries. The Parastep I system. *J Spinal Cord Med* 1996;19:99–105.

66. Klose KJ, Jacobs PL, Broton JG, et al. Evaluation of a training program for persons with SCI paraplegia using the Parastep 1 ambulation system: part I. Ambulation performance and anthropometric measures. *Arch Phys Med Rehabil* 1997;78:789–793.

67. Jacobs PL, Nash MS, Klose KJ, et al. Evaluation of a training program for persons with SCI paraplegia using the Parastep 1 ambulation system: part 2. Effects on physiological responses to peak arm ergometry. *Arch Phys Med Rehabil* 1997;78:794–798.

68. Nash MS, Jacobs PL, Montalvo BM, et al. Evaluation of a training program for persons with SCI paraplegia using the Parastep 1 ambulation system: part 5. Lower extremity blood flow and hyperemic responses to occlusion augmented by ambulation training. *Arch Phys Med Rehabil* 1997;78:808–814.

69. Graf M, Holle A. Environmental control unit considerations for the person with high level tetraplegia. *Top Spinal Cord Inj Rehabil* 1997; 2:30–40.

70. Anson DK. *Alternative computer access: a guide to selection.* FA Davis Co, 1997.

71. Eberhardt K. Home modifications for persons with spinal cord injury. *OT Practice* 1998;November:24–27.

PSYCHOLOGIC ADAPTATION TO SPINAL CORD INJURY

JOYCE FICHTENBAUM
STEVEN KIRSHBLUM

Spinal cord injury (SCI) is one of the most devastating events that can occur to individuals and their families (1). Losses may be overwhelming (2). The many physical changes are immediate, unanticipated, and often permanent (3). Contending with altered mobility, adaptive equipment, accessibility concerns, bowel and bladder programs, disrupted sexual functioning, added dependency on others for assistance, limitations, and loss of spontaneity in many areas of functioning can tax a person's coping skills and psychological adjustment. SCI affects a person's physical, emotional, and vocational identity (4). A person who sustains an SCI is at risk for the "four D syndrome": dependency, depression, drug addiction, and if married, divorce (5).

There is a wide range of reactions to disability (6). An individual psychologically adjusts to a chronic illness or SCI through maximizing independence, achieving optimal health, developing responsibility for his or her care, rebuilding a sense of control, and finding ways to fulfill one's roles in life (3,4,7). This chapter reviews many of the psychological reactions and concerns that may occur after SCI.

EMOTIONAL REACTIONS FOLLOWING SCI

Stage Theories

Initially, theorists focused their efforts on responses of individuals with SCI soon after sustaining their injuries, rather than in the months or years that followed (1). Early efforts to characterize psychological adjustment to SCI included models of sequential processes or stage theories (3). Kübler-Ross suggested five stages, sequenced as denial, anger, bargaining, depression, and acceptance (8). Although this schema was originally developed to understand the reactions of the dying, it was readily applied to other populations including individuals with disabilities. Weller and Miller (9) presented four stages: shock, denial, anger, and depression. The intent of stage theories was to simplify and bring order to complex reactions. Often, however, they encouraged professionals to perceive more distress in patients than actually existed (10). Recently, stage theories have been criticized on two grounds: (a) the lack of empirical evidence and (b) their failure to take individual differences into account (3,4,11). Although not universal, some of the reactions proposed by these theories of loss may be seen in patients and their families after SCI.

Denial is a normal coping mechanism that individuals use when faced with overwhelming circumstances such as a serious illness or injury. It is painless relative to the other emotional reactions to disability, and it can be a temporary phase or part of one's coping style (12). The disability itself or its long-term implications may be denied. The denial of the permanence of disability can be unrelenting or it can wax and wane (13). Patients and family members may think, "This can't be happening," "it will get better in a matter of time," or "I know I will walk out of here" (14). The presence of denial often alarms rehabilitation personnel. However, initially, denial may not negatively impact rehabilitation because it is a verbal disavowal of a situation, rather than a behavioral one (15). Long-term denial, however, may lead to self-neglect and the development of secondary conditions (15,16).

Denial can be reconceptualized as hope and every patient has the right to use it (9,12). Resistance to using adaptive equipment may be an attempt to deny reality or it may be a way to maintain determination to do without certain devices (17). Patients who, despite the team's recommendation, insist on slowly propelling a manual wheelchair instead of using a power wheelchair may be denying their injuries or maintaining hope for sufficient recovery to forgo the use of power mobility. Hope can combat depression and anxiety or at least make them more manageable. The walls of denial are difficult to break though (12). For example, telling patients who believe they will walk out of the hospital that they won't, will engender conflict and anger. Focusing their therapies on skills they believe will be needed if they resume walking will result in increased motivation to participate.

Anger may come about when the patient realizes that something very serious is wrong (14). Statements beginning with the phrase "you should have" often suggest anger. Anger can be indicative of a motivated individual who is trying to exert some control over his or her destiny (9). Hostility may be directed toward health care providers, family members, or active people who serve as constant reminders of what was lost. Anger requires resolution (9).

Bargaining during the rehabilitation process is used to differentiate bearable outcomes. It takes many forms, changes over time, and is amenable to intervention. For example, in the inpatient rehabilitation setting, the desire to ambulate is often exchanged for the wish of the return of bowel and bladder function.

Depression

The views regarding depression secondary to SCI have changed over the years. Before 1987, stage theories were in vogue and depression was seen as a necessary component of SCI that stipulated whether a person would adjust to disability (18). The absence of depression was considered unhealthy and was suggestive of denial (18). Depression is the most frequent outcome variable studied post-SCI (18–21). Currently, depression is viewed as a complication that is amenable to treatment (18). It is related to poor adjustment and heightened mortality through suicide, substance abuse, or self-neglect (19).

Adaptation to SCI presents patients with experiences that could produce a grief reaction with a normal reactive dysphoric mood (3,18). Dysphoria is an affective state that can range from petulant to sad to melancholy to wretched (22). In general, it implies sadness, hopelessness, and helplessness (23). A transient depressed mood does not justify a diagnosis of major depression. It may occur in response to loss of relationships, questions about sexuality and ability to have children, loss of income, loss of dreams, and changes in plans for the future (5). Grief or bereavement may include feelings of depression and even vegetative signs but usually does not involve prolonged functional impairment, sense of worthlessness, and psychomotor retardation. Furthermore, feelings of guilt and thoughts of death are usually limited (24).

Methodological issues result in equivocal findings regarding the prevalence of depression. These research problems include inconsistent definition and use of diagnostic criteria, inaccurate measurement of depression, overlap of somatic symptoms of depression and medical illness, psychiatric illness before injury, sample differences, and timing of assessment across studies (18, 19,25).

Depressive symptomology is common in the medically ill and can pose diagnostic difficulties with a new spine-injured patient (26). Clinical depression is often assessed by a semistructured interview or a self-report measure such as the Beck Depression Inventory (27). Any self-report measure merely reflects a cluster of behaviors that may not reflect a diagnosable depressive or anxiety disorder. They should not be used to diagnose these disorders without a clinical interview, because self-report methods cannot necessarily differentiate between psychopathologic disturbances or normal responses to the physical effects of an injury (28).

Not all researchers have used self-report measures to quantify depression. Some have used various disciplines that observed and treated patients with SCI and assessed their level of depression and anxiety. Results indicated that staff tend to overestimate psychological morbidity, nurses the most and physicians and mental health professionals the least (29).

In postinjury depression studies, it is important to determine if psychiatric morbidity, such as schizophrenia, depression, or another mental disorder was present before the SCI because it may affect the reaction to the injury (30). Finally, when determining prevalence, intensity, or increase or decrease of depression over time, one must compare groups within the SCI population to account for individual differences based on specific characteristics in subpopulations (e.g., ventilator-independent vs. ventilator-dependent individuals).

Depressive disorders are the most common form of psychological distress in SCI (25). Given all the methodological precautions, depression is estimated to occur in 20% to 45% of the SCI population, with greater prevalence in women than in men (25,31–33). It is the most frequent postinjury diagnosis usually appearing within the first month (31). Depression is not a single entity, but a spectrum of disorders that vary by length of time symptoms are experienced and degree of severity. The unipolar disorders include major depression (approximately 15% of patients with SCI), depression not otherwise specified, adjustment disorder with depressed mood, depression secondary to a medical condition, and dysthymia. Of the various depressive disorders mentioned, adjustment disorders are generally encountered after SCI (34). An adjustment disorder with depressed mood is diagnosed when the constellation of symptoms does not meet the criteria for a depressive disorder or bereavement (31).

In comparison to dysphoria, depression is a disabling condition. Diagnosis requires persistent and pervasive loss of interest in other people, objects, or activities, in addition to a depressed mood. It is important, therefore, to determine whether the depression after injury is normal in terms of content and intensity or is pathologic in nature (26). Mourning or adjustment problems may turn into a major depressive episode when various psychosocial variables lead to despair. These include stressful events and their cognitive appraisal; the individual's coping resources, perceived social support availability, and degree of family conflict that develops over time (19).

Thirty percent of persons with SCI have been found to have higher levels of anxiety and depression up to 2 years post-injury (35). Two years after SCI, although depression somewhat decreases, suggesting a positive outcome over time, it is more frequently associated with perception of handicap, particularly social integration in terms of being less physically active, spending more time in bed at home, and being more isolated, rather than actual disability (3,36–39). Those who recover from depression have more social supports than those who remain depressed (36). Other studies, however, have not found that depression decreases with the passage of time (20,40,41). The presence of severe complications, a low level of autonomy, architectural barriers, poor education, unemployment, and insufficient family support can result in deprivation of a relatively normal lifestyle and may maintain or increase psychological distress postinjury.

Overall, risk factors for depression can be genetic, psychological, social, and environmental. They include a prior history of depression, family history of depression, family history of suicide attempts, suicidal ideation, chronic pain, female gender, lack of social support, multiplicity of life stressors, concurrent medical illness, and concurrent alcohol or substance abuse. Risk factors specific to SCI include complete neurologic injury and medical comorbidity with traumatic brain injury (31).

Social and environmental risk factors include a poor social network, few financial resources, vocational difficulties, inferior living arrangements, the need for personal and transportation assistance, and family disruption before injury.

Biologic factors that may contribute to depression include somatic effects of SCI such as fatigue and sleep disturbances, personal or family history of depressive illness, or presence of a general medical condition or medication that may cause or contribute to depression. Some medications that may cause or contribute to depression that are frequently used in SCI include metoclopramide, glucocorticoids, anabolic steroids, cimetidine, ranitidine, and clonidine (31). Medication-induced depression, however, is not very common. Sleep disturbance, a symptom of depression, can be affected in the hospital setting by interventions such as multiple awakenings for turning or intermittent catheterization. Again, because physiological symptoms of depression are often common somatic effects of SCI, it is important to ascertain the presence of other symptoms of depression, such as dysphoria and distractibility (31).

Psychological risk factors for depression and maladjustment for new spine-injured patients include psychological structure (e.g., narcissistic and antisocial personality features and behaviors), and a preinjury history of psychological or psychiatric impairment including: substance abuse, coping style, a poor social support system, poor problem-solving abilities, unresolved conflicts from previous losses or trauma, shame, hopelessness, bereavement, and having the opinion that death is better than living with SCI (5,31). Post-SCI predictors of depression are despondency, alcohol abuse, apathy, expressions of shame, stress, weight loss, anger, and destructive behavior (3).

Depression is accompanied by persistent and pervasive loss of emotional involvement with other people, objects, or activities (18). Accurate diagnosis of depressive disorders uses established diagnostic criteria for which clinicians are referred to the fourth edition of the *Diagnostic and Statistical Manual of Mental Disorders* (24). Any of the diagnosable depressive syndromes refer to a constellation of symptoms that can be grouped into behavioral, affective, and cognitive components. Distress or impairment in the areas of social, occupational, or other important areas of functioning is part of the criteria for diagnosis of a major depressive disorder.

Signs and symptoms of depression occur in the following spheres (18,24,31):

Affective/mood: sadness, emptiness, demoralization, irritability, loss of interest or pleasure in activities, apathy, hopelessness, helplessness, and inappropriate guilt or shame

Cognitive: poor attention and concentration, diminished ability to think, indecisiveness, recurrent thoughts of death, suicidal ideation, or self-criticality

Behavioral/somatic: appearance that is sad or weepy, decreased attention to self-care, changes in appetite, sleep, and energy levels, restlessness or agitation, being slowed down (psychomotor retardation), specific suicide plan or attempt

Assessment of "suicidality" should include questions about suicidal ideation, plan, and intent, access to lethal means, prior attempt(s), and comorbid alcohol or drug abuse (31). General suicide risk factors can be remembered by the mnemonic "sad persons" (31,42). They include *s*ex, being a white male; *a*ge, adolescent or elderly; *d*epression; *p*revious attempts; *e*thanol abuse; absence of *r*ational thinking and presence of disorganized or psychotic thinking; *s*ocial supports, which are poor; *o*rganized suicide plan; *n*ot being married; and *s*ickness, chronic illness or other disability (31). After SCI, variables related to suicide include postinjury despondency; expressions of shame, hopelessness, and apathy; a

history of preinjury family fragmentation; alcohol abuse; active involvement in causing the injury; and preinjury depression (43).

The suicide rate in individuals with SCI is two to six times greater than that for able-bodied persons (1). Suicide is the leading cause of death in individuals with SCI younger than 55 years, and 75% of the suicides occur within 4 to 5 years of injury (43–48). Depression, therefore, may be linked to mortality after SCI. In a study of suicide after SCI, the suicide rate was higher for those "marginally" injured (Frankel classification D or E) who showed a near-complete recovery (45). This may be because their right to grieve tends to be minimized; they receive less support, and have to contend with indefinite or uncertain degrees of loss, which may affect them upon return to their lives. Suicide rates may differ in studies because suicide, in general, is underreported. Death due to septicemia secondary to infection or a pressure sore that the patient left untreated may be suicide by self-neglect (45).

In a retrospective study by Kennedy et al. (49), when SCI was incurred as a result of a suicide attempt, comorbidity with psychiatric illness was found to exist. Schizophrenia and depression accounted for 59.8% of the psychiatric illness identified (49). Other categories included drug or alcohol abuse, personality disorders, bipolar disorder, and marital or work-related distress. In the group who received a psychiatric diagnosis, 94% attempted suicide by jumping. Although most individuals who sustain an SCI secondary to a suicide attempt do not reattempt suicide, 7.3% do. Because a significant proportion respond well to psychiatric and psychological treatment, it is imperative to provide interventions in the rehabilitation setting to those admitted as a result of self-harm (49).

Because mental health problems affect rehabilitation in general, psychological services need to be provided as part of SCI treatment (45,49). Although psychopharmacologic agents are helpful in treating neurovegetative and mood disturbance symptoms, they cannot address the cognitive aspects of depression or the social, environmental, and interpersonal concerns associated with depression. These are best addressed through psychotherapy. There are multiple psychotherapeutic modalities, including insight-oriented, psychodynamic, cognitive, marital, group, or family psychotherapy. The choice should be individually tailored. Spine-injured individuals who had high levels of anxiety or depression in the acute phase of hospitalization and who received group cognitive therapy had reduced symptoms with maintenance of up to 2 years (50–52). Depression and the contemplation of suicide can occur at any time and therefore should be assessed in outpatient, medical follow-up visits (31).

Pharmacologic Treatment of Depression

Pharmacologic intervention should be considered for patients whose mood disturbance is severe enough to interfere with their ability to perform in social, personal (activities of daily living), recreational, and vocational roles. Medications can and should be used as a complement to psychological counseling, particularly in the acute period after injury.

The treatment of a major depression after SCI with medication usually consists of three phases as proposed by Kupfer: the acute, continuous, and maintenance phases (53). In the acute phase, treatment lasts 4 to 12 weeks, during which time treatment is directed at reducing or eliminating the depressive symptoms. Treatment should continue, however, into the continuous phase (4 to 9 months), because discontinuation of the antidepressive medication during this time is associated with a high rate of relapse (53–57). During the maintenance phase, after 9 months, medication may need to be continued to prevent recurrence of symptoms (58). After 9 months, some medications may lose efficacy. In such situations, discontinuation with subsequent reinstitution of the same or another medication may be used (31). If the medication is to be discontinued, a slow tapering should be done, because the speed at which the medication is stopped may affect the likelihood of relapse (53,57). It is recommended to taper the medication over 3 to 4 weeks, with close monitoring of symptoms.

Treatment of depression is considered a long-term process because patients often experience high rates of relapse after discontinuation of medication (55,59,60). Recurrence rates for depression are estimated to be at least 50% for patients with one major depressive episode and 80% to 90% for those with two prior episodes (53,61). Medications may improve the patient's ability to function, but the depressive disorder may continue.

Many antidepressant medications are on the market. Most medications exert their effect by facilitating neurotransmission of serotonin or norepinephrine. The newer medications seem to be safer and better tolerated than the older tricyclic antidepressants and monoamine oxidase inhibitors, because of their side-effect profiles (31). The patient presenting with signs and symptoms, as well as the potential side-effect profile of each medication, should guide selection of a particular medication. Often the side effects of a medication will have therapeutic effects for some individuals. Table 20.1 lists some of the features of the

medications, which may help guide the clinician. Table 20.2 offers recommendations based on patient symptomatology.

The SCI clinician usually starts with pharmacologic treatment for the patient with depression. If the patient has suicidal ideation or presents with psychotic features, complex management is required, and the patient is best evaluated and treated by a psychiatrist. In addition, if the patient does not respond to one or two of the trials of antidepressant medications, a psychiatric evaluation is indicated.

In sum, although depressive disorders are seen frequently after SCI, all injured patients do not go through a period of depression. Each person reacts to his or her injury in an individualized manner (62). It is important to differentiate depressive behavior from a diagnosable depression because serious consequences such as weight loss, social problems, joblessness, need for more medical assistance, self-neglect, more time spent in bed, breakup of family, and suicidality can result from a major depression (18, 63). Therefore, although dysphoria or grief is understandable after injury, depression must be considered a maladaptive response to stress requiring diagnosis and treatment (1). Early detection of depressive symptomology is important because it is partly responsible for the individual response to rehabilitation, compliance, and ability to live in the community. Psychotherapy and counseling may improve mood as conflict resolution, hope, and problem solving are often amenable to intervention. Medications may be required for the short- and long-term management.

Anxiety

Anxiety (i.e., worry, dread, and tension) is often a psychological consequence of SCI. Some sources of anxiety include weaning from a ventilator, loss of an independent lifestyle, and concerns with loss of finances, being a burden, and the ability to be a

TABLE 20.1. ANTIDEPRESSANT DRUGS FOR PATIENTS WITH DEPRESSIVE DISORDER

Antidepressant	Usual starting dose (mg/d)	Usual maintenance dose (mg/d)	Sedation	Anticholinergic effects	Orthostatic hypotension	Activation
SSRIs						
Fluoxetine	20	20–40	+	0	0	+
Sertraline	20	100–200	+	0	0	+++
Paroxetine	20	20–60	+	0/+	0	+
Tertiary amines						
Amitriptyline	75	75–300	+++	+++	+++	+
Imipramine	75	75–300	++	++	++	+
Doxepin	75	75–300	+++	++	+++	+
Secondary amines						
Nortriptyline	10–50	50–200	++	+	+	+/0
Desipramine	75	75–300	+	+	+	0
Second-generation agents						
Trazodone	50	50–400	+++	0	++	0
Bupropion	200	300–450	0	0	0	++
Venlafaxine	75	150–375	+	0	0	+
Nefazodone	200	300–600	++	0	+	0
Mirtazapine	15	15–45	+++	0/+	0	0

SSRI, selective serotonin reuptake inhibitor. From the Paralyzed Veterans of America (PVA). *Consortium for spinal cord medicine. Depression following spinal cord injury: a clinical practice guideline for primary care physicians.* Washington: Paralyzed Veterans of America, 1998, with permission.

TABLE 20.2. GENERAL TREATMENT RECOMMENDATIONS

Symptom	Suggested Antidepressants
Decreased appetite/ weight loss	Mirtazapine, tertiary TCAs, some SSRIs (especially paroxetine)
Increased appetite/ weight gain	Fluoxetine, perhaps other SSRIs and new agents (except mirtazapine)
Insomnia	Sedating antidepressants: trazodone, nefazodone, mirtazapine, paroxetine, tertiary TCAs
Hypersomnia	Activating antidepressants: fluoxetine, venlafaxine, bupropion, sertraline, secondary TCAs
Psychomotor agitation	Sedating antidepressants: trazodone, nefazodone, mirtazapine, paroxetine, tertiary TCAs
Psychomotor retardation	Activating antidepressants: fluoxetine, venlafaxine, bupropion, sertraline, secondary TCAs
Fatigue/low energy	Activating antidepressants: fluoxetine, venlafaxine, bupropion, sertraline, secondary TCAs
Decreased concentration	Activating antidepressants: Fluoxetine, venlafaxine, bupropion, sertraline, secondary TCAs
Suicidal ideation	Avoid TCAs due to risk of overdose
Neuropathic pain and depression	Amitriptyline, nefazodone, any serotonergic antidepressant

TCA, tricyclic antidepressant; SSRI, selective serotonin reuptake inhibitor.
From the Paralyzed Veterans of America (PVA). *Consortium for spinal cord medicine. Depression following spinal cord injury: a clinical practice guideline for primary care physicians.* Washington: Paralyzed Veterans of America, 1998, with permission.

spouse or parent. Religious and existential fears concerning dying, death, and disability as punishment are also prominent. The transition from fear of death to fear of living with a disability is particularly salient in some patients.

Psychological distress, defined as the presence of both depression and anxiety, is often associated with age at SCI onset, education, completeness and level of injury, and gender (32). Older persons and those with low levels of education adjust poorly in comparison with younger and highly educated patients. Furthermore, men tend to be more anxious and women more depressed. People injured when young cope better with their disability than older adults who are often not provided with vocational, social, and leisure opportunities (64).

Acute stress disorder (ASD) and posttraumatic stress disorder (PTSD) are anxiety diagnoses that may limit adaptation to disability. They occur secondary to experiencing or witnessing a traumatic event that threatened the individual with death or serious bodily injury. Motor vehicle crashes, falls, and other etiologies of SCI can serve as stressors that lead to the development of ASD or PTSD. Gunshot wounds or other violent crimes

that result in threat to life or severe bodily injury, exposure to hideous sights, or the death of a loved one at the hands of violence may increase the likelihood of PTSD (65). When the onset of the disorder is within 4 weeks of the traumatic event and the symptoms last from 2 days to 4 weeks, the diagnosis is ASD. When onset occurs after the 4-week period, the diagnosis is PTSD (66).

The prevalence of PTSD after SCI has not been firmly established but is estimated to range from 12% to 17% (67). To meet the criteria for PTSD, the person has to experience sufficient symptoms in each of the following symptom clusters: (a) reexperiencing the trauma (e.g., intrusive and distressing recollections, flashbacks, and nightmares); (b) avoidance of the stimulus conditions that remind the person of the event or numbing of the individual's general responsiveness (e.g., avoiding thoughts and memories of the trauma, detachment, restricted range of affect, and a sense of foreshortened future); and (c) persistent symptoms of increased arousal (e.g., irritability, anger, difficulty sleeping, and hypervigilance). To meet the diagnosis, these symptoms must be present for 1 month and cause marked distress or impairment in functioning (24).

Symptoms of stress disorders such as nightmares and sleep disturbances not only leave the person fatigued but also secondarily affect cognitive processes such as attention, concentration, and the new learning and performance of daily routines (68). Heightened arousal symptoms such as an exaggerated startle response or angry outbursts may strain interpersonal relationships. Avoidance behaviors may affect an individual's ability to fully function within the family or return to the workforce. Overall, symptoms of PTSD often limit the achievements made after SCI (68). Furthermore, the development of comorbid psychopathology such as anxiety, depression, and cognitive problems may negatively affect rehabilitation as well (69).

Rehabilitation Goals as They Relate to Psychological Adaptation

The goals of rehabilitation are to preserve residual function, prevent serious complications, and develop compensatory structures so injured individuals can function in their environment (4). Assisting the injured person cope psychologically requires taking developmental, social, environmental, family, and preinjury personality factors into consideration (12).

According to Lewis and Lubkin (70), there are two illness roles: the sick role and the impaired role. The sick role is based on acute episodic illnesses that may require the individual to temporarily forgo major responsibilities while focusing on recovery. Although the sick role is often accepted during the acute phase of SCI, it applies neither to individuals with chronic illnesses nor those with long-term disabilities. The impaired role, on the other hand, encourages the individual to maintain normal behavior within the limits of the impairment through maximizing remaining potentialities and modifying life direction or methods used to achieve goals. Assisting individuals with SCI to move from the sick to the impaired role is a significant goal of rehabilitation.

Secondary Gains

During the acute rehabilitation phase, patients with SCI are exempted from roles they were expected to fulfill both at home and in the workplace. Role transitions are often difficult both during hospitalization and on return home (70). Individuals may choose to remain in the sick role to relieve themselves of stressful decision making and duties associated with their premorbid lifestyle and roles of spouse, parent, child, employer, or employee. Certain limitations may seem attractive to the patient. For example, patients may hold on to their beliefs that they are not capable of returning to their jobs, rather than return to an occupation that was disliked, mundane, or left them with little free time for family or avocations (70).

Spine-injured patients will often change their behaviors in an attempt to get their needs met under the conditions they now find themselves. In an attempt to tolerate dependency, once relatively independent individuals may resort to passive or regressive behavior. They may ask staff and family to take responsibility for them, rather than learn to direct their own care (70). Even when fully capable, they may refuse to do even the simplest tasks such as wiping their mouths after eating or raising the head of the bed by pushing a button. At times, they will test the patience of both staff and family. Patients may, for example, refuse to get up before a certain hour or they may strongly suggest that their spouse divorce them now rather than learn to live with a disabled mate. This may leave spouses bewildered and hurt, because they feel their love and ability to care for their injured partner is doubted. Limits may need to be set to promote independence. Communication within relationships should be encouraged.

Quality of Life

Quality of life (QOL) is a term often used in the SCI literature because it is considered "at risk" after the onset of disability. QOL can only be measured and evaluated by the person who is experiencing a particular life (e.g., is my life worth living) (71). Although it can be defined, it is often difficult to characterize. As noted by Glass et al. (6), QOL can be described as an estimation of happiness or satisfaction with subjective and objective aspects of life important to an individual.

Ratings of subjective measures of well being after SCI are lower than that of their peers, but the difference is relatively small. In a metaanalytic study by Dijkers (48), no relationship was found between disability in respect to level and completeness of injury and subjective QOL. Handicap, however, in terms of social stigma and lost opportunities did affect well being. According to Heinemann (1), when measures of QOL involve the extent to which an individual with SCI is able to direct his or her care, or perform activities independently, persons with paraplegia and incomplete injuries, initially, maintained a higher level of independence and QOL than those individuals with tetraplegia and complete injuries. Regardless of the level of injury, however, 3 years after discharge from rehabilitation, patients attained a relatively independent level of functioning and QOL improved or, at least, remained the same (1). Other factors found to positively affect QOL are emotional support, perceived control, perceived health status, physical and social activity, and self-esteem. A negative predictor is depression (64,72).

Objective measures of QOL after SCI include mortality, morbidity, and social variables such as residence, employment, economic stability, education, and marital status. Perceived health, level of functioning, and development of complications or secondary conditions are other objective variables that affect QOL (1).

The conclusions drawn by Pierce et al. (73) on predictors of life satisfaction after SCI suggest that the post-SCI level of participation (particularly mobility and social integration), the age at follow-up (which ranged from 1 to 20 years), and the perceived health status were predictive of QOL, in comparison with activity level and degree of disability. The model suggests that an individual's perceived health status is more important to his or her adaptation to SCI and perceived QOL than injury-related deficits.

Self-Neglect and Secondary Conditions

Self-neglect commonly occurs after SCI (74). It can encompass behaviors that range from overt and hostile to passive and inactive and can result in serious complications. Refusal of treatment; inattention to skin, bladder and bowel regimens; alcohol or drug abuse; refusal to participate in rehabilitation; and the contemplation of suicide are some behaviors frequently encountered. Macleod (75) found that self-neglect can be a symptom of an adjustment to a disability problem, a major depressive episode, or "existential suicide" (75). Existential self-neglect occurs years after the injury and is voiced by a clear and active decision to refuse further medical treatment. It is not prompted by feelings of depression or hostility.

Secondary conditions are "any additional physical or mental health condition that is causally related to a primary disabling condition" (76). They can occur as a result of self-neglect. Shackelford et al. (77) found a relationship between subjective measures of well being and the development of secondary disabilities, such as pressure ulcers. Patients however, may become depressed or anxious because they have a secondary condition. Frequently, referral to a mental health professional may promote better health care behaviors (78).

Violence-Induced SCI

Victims of violence, in general, and gunshot wounds in particular, tend to be different in terms of demographics, medical, and psychosocial status (79,80). They tend to be African Americans or Hispanics, are younger and usually single, or not living in a spousal type of relationship. They tend to have less education, no job to which they can return, and may also have a criminal or drug history (80,81). In terms of the psychosocial implications of violence-induced SCI, Gordon and Lewis (80) found that sociocultural differences between African American people with violence-induced SCI and rehabilitation caregivers often result in interpersonal difficulties, anger, hostility, and frustration (80). Some victims of violence report sadness and depression, in addition to the experiences of anger. Social and community reintegration problems occur due to family and friendship strains, limited financial funding, and fewer educational and vocational opportunities.

Patient interventions for inner-city men who sustain SCI through violence should include evaluation and psychotherapy that focuses on current psychosocial functioning and socioeconomic obstacles and use of psychotherapy groups, a substance-use relapse prevention program, and a return-to-work group when applicable (80). Staff interventions must include education about the impact of demographic, social, and cultural variables that affect adjustment to a violence-induced SCI. To reduce patients' perceived insincerity and staff's perception of noncompliant behavior, exploration about feelings of working with the inner-city population, which may include patients with a history of substance abuse or crime, may be additionally helpful (80).

Spinal Cord–Injured Ventilator-Assisted Persons

Mechanical ventilation is required by 41% of all patients with SCI during their acute hospitalization; however, most do not require ventilation on discharge from rehabilitation (82). Long after their injuries, ventilator-assisted and autonomously breathing persons with tetraplegia have reported that they are glad to be alive and are satisfied with their lives (82–84). The QOL of both groups was underestimated by health care professionals (83).

In a longitudinal follow-up study of high tetraplegia 14 to 24 years postinjury, Hall et al. (82) found 94% of the ventilator-assisted and 92% of the ventilator-independent (VI) subjects lived in private residences. The need for personal assistance was greater in the ventilator-assisted group than in the ventilator-independent group. Education was a priority, reports of substance abuse were few, and suicidal ideation was greater than in the general population and more common in the ventilator-assisted group than in the ventilator-independent group. Areas in which help was needed included socialization, financial status, personal attendant services, transportation, and employment.

Glass (84) studied the adaptation of six families to caring for a ventilator-dependent person at home with both interview and objective measures. Qualities found in these families were cohesiveness, good communication, and low levels of conflict.

Other Models of Adjustment

Researchers have been attempting to develop models of adjustment to disability (4,85). Adaptation can be conceived as a process that involves individual, family, cultural, temporal, and social variables (3,86). Predictors of positive adjustment include young age, female gender, internal locus of control, social skills, employment, access to transportation, financial security, assertiveness, good problem-solving skills, and resolution of compensation issues. Research has suggested that older age, low education, poor social support, male gender, and having an external locus of control are predictive of psychological morbidity after SCI (87). Ways of coping, locus of control, self-esteem, depression, social support, and attribution of "self" versus "other"

regarding the injury are some variables researched in an effort to predict adaptation to SCI (88).

VARIABLES AFFECTING SUCCESSFUL ADJUSTMENT

Age and Time Since Injury

Most traumatic SCIs occur in young adulthood, a time in life when people are completing their education, beginning a career, and developing a long-term relationship (2). Individuals injured at a younger age tend to experience successful adjustment and a better QOL than older individuals (15,48). This may be due to their flexible use of coping strategies, which may make life changes easier on them. Those injured as children may develop a self-concept that includes the knowledge of future limitations (89).

Krause and Crewe (90) suggested that age and time since injury operate in opposite directions, with younger persons having greater activity levels and greater opportunities to deal with the consequences of their injuries. Older persons at the time of injury, on the other hand, have more medical problems and more possibilities for satisfactory living and working arrangements. They were found to be less satisfied with activity level and sex life. Often with age, function declines and older adults are less able to manipulate the environment, which may result in an increase in frustration and irritability (17,91). Depression, which was greater in older injured persons, decreased with time since injury most likely as their experience with SCI increased (28,86).

Age and generation of the caregivers can be factors in the amount of interpersonal support the patient receives (17). The psychological burden of living with aging family members can even affect patients who are in their 20s and 30s. As caregivers age and begin to experience less energy and more biologic dysfunction of their own, people with SCI may experience increased concerns regarding their ability to continue to live in the community (17).

Social Support, Family, and Partner Relationships

Patients in rehabilitation have to ultimately decide whether to participate in treatment, how much energy to expend in each session, how to view their current life situation, and whether to persevere or give up (92). Their relationship to others, both in and out of the rehabilitation setting, may influence these decisions. Particularly for the newly injured, the quality of social support has a positive relationship with adjustment and an inverse relationship with psychological distress (1,2,15). Social support usually begins in the rehabilitation center, where they befriend other individuals with SCI with whom they can experience camaraderie and mutual support. Social supports that reinforce a person's self-worth enhance independent functioning, allowing individuals with SCI to engage in interactions in the community.

Many injured patients, particularly adolescents and young adults, have difficulty maintaining social relationships with friends they had before their injury. Some injured persons become apathetic or embarrassed (5). Others note their friends' discomfort and unnatural behaviors and allow them to drift away. As a result, social isolation develops. Because poor social integration and depression are associated, counseling services should be offered routinely to patients with SCI during medical follow-up visits (93). Promoting communication, developing social skills, and learning to counter friends' general misperceptions about disability can be useful (5).

SCI affects entire families. Losses include deprivation of personal space and time, financial concerns, isolation, changes in relationships, loss of spontaneity, and worry about the present and the future (94). Family members have to contend with role changes. Decker et al. (95) reported that these can be in the form of role confusion (e.g., becoming both spouse and attendant), role reversal (e.g., leaving a job to care for the injured party), and role overload (e.g., maintaining a job, childcare, and SCI responsibilities). Family members need to be reminded to maintain their own physical, social, and emotional health. Providing them with psychological support and finding support of other caregivers in similar situations may prove helpful.

Weller and Miller (96) applied stage theory to families. Denial may result in avoidance of meaningful conversation with staff members. Patient's anger and antagonistic behavior toward loved ones may confuse and hurt them and returning that anger may result in guilt. Preexisting difficult relationships may result in a defensive tendency to idealize the injured child. Depression may set in and result in attempts to escape newfound responsibilities. Some families, on the other hand, become overinvolved. Frequently, their attempts at doing too much stem from going through the *should*'s or *should not*'s as they relate to their guilt over their inability to prevent the injury (5). Limiting the ways they can participate will promote more positive outcomes than confrontation (12).

Holicky and Charlifue (97) corroborated the literature regarding the importance of spousal support as a contributing factor to life satisfaction, less depression, and good QOL for the injured individual. Spouses with an external locus of control, limited coping strategies (e.g., use of distancing and escape-avoidance), and minimal social support are at great risk for developing higher levels of depression in comparison to their injured partners. In addition, they show higher levels of caregiver burden and lower levels of life satisfaction and marital adjustment (98). When the spouse takes on the role of caregiver, discomfort with physical intimacy may lead to depression (5). Needs of spouses should be addressed, particularly when they fill the caregiver role, because they may experience more symptoms of stress and depression than their injured partners (99).

Premorbid Personality and Coping Styles

Although we cannot discount the roles of premorbid personality, resilience, and coping styles when discussing adjustment to disability, specific personality types are not associated with specific disabilities such as SCI (6). Extroversion and a cautious way of dealing with stressors and new situations are personality styles that commonly develop among wheelchair users after SCI. As a result, when compared with those with multiple sclerosis and

traumatic brain injury, individuals with SCI are found to more likely seek and accept assistance from others, to benefit from encouragement of health care providers, and to plan activities rather than act spontaneously (88). Interestingly, extroversion appears to be a good prognostic indicator even in the rehabilitation setting (28).

Use of active coping styles such as cognitive restructuring, emotional self-control, positive reevaluation, social support seeking, and use of problem-oriented strategies is more adaptive and appears to protect people against depression (28,100). In addition, active coping styles increase expectations of control. In contrast, emotion-focused coping such as escape-avoidance, wishful thinking, and unrealistic problem solving leave people vulnerable to psychological distress (28,100). Wishful statements such as "I'm going to walk out of here" only get results when coupled with the use of problem solving or solution-focused coping such as participation in therapies and with the ability to seek advice or assistance from others (100).

Locus of Control

Locus of control is significant when it comes to adapting to disability (10,14). People with an internal locus of control believe that their health and degree of recovery is based on their own behaviors; for example, these people have may say, "I developed a pressure sore because I did not do weight shifts." On the other hand, those with an external locus of control believe that what occurs in their lives is based on fate, chance, luck, or other people; these people might say, "I developed a pressure sore because the cushion was bad." Internal people believe they have personal control over events in their lives and by and large have fewer medical problems and lead more active and productive lives (2). After SCI those individuals who believe they are responsible for their own health are less depressed and behave more adaptively than those who are fatalistic (20,87). External people tend to do better in the structured rehabilitation environment, but on discharge when left to their devices, they may quickly develop problems or secondary conditions.

Search for Meaning, Self-Blame, and Attribution

The search for meaning often occurs in the face of SCI in an attempt to find some purpose for the injury or to place it in the context of one's life (101). The search is often accompanied by the question, "Why did this happen to me?" Bulman and Wortman (102) reported that individuals with SCI gave six reasons for their injury: God had a reason, chance, predetermination, a personal purpose (e.g., bringing the family together), probability, and it was deserved.

Attempts to understand the subjective experience of SCI have yielded several studies relating attribution of responsibility for the injury and the adjustment process. The effect of self-blame was found to be inconsistent. Individuals who accepted responsibility for the onset of their disability adjusted better than those who were true victims of a negative life event (102,103). Others, however, found that self-blame led to poorer adjustment, depression, hostility, and dysphoria (104,105). Brown et al. (106) reported that long-term mental health and vitality scores were not different for persons with SCI who held themselves accountable for their injury versus those who blamed others. Heinemann (1) concluded that although self-blame may be adaptive shortly after injury, it loses this function over time. Regardless of the actual circumstances, it is important for clinicians to keep in mind their own beliefs and biases regarding blame and responsibility if they are to help patients resolve their own conflict (105).

Integrity of the Self and Self-esteem

SCI results in lost integrity of the "self" (3). Individuals with SCI often rail against using adaptive equipment. For some, the wheelchair is the symbol of disability and serves as a mirror of negative societal values. After a long period of mandated bed rest, when it is seen as a means toward independence, a wheelchair is often viewed more positively. Learning whether the patient considers the wheelchair an enemy or a friend may be a useful way to gauge adaptation over time. Creating a new self-image is important after SCI (77). Lowered self-esteem leads to feelings of inferiority and insignificance. This will negatively affect goal setting, task mastery, and confidence in one's ability to live life in an effective manner (14). If an individual's self-esteem was low before the injury, the task of raising his or her self-worth is by far more difficult to do after the injury.

Motivation and Compliance

Motivation is directly related to the interaction between the personal characteristics of the patient, treatment team, and environment (107). A desire to understand their condition, to perform self-care, and to become positively dependent is associated with motivation. Positive dependency occurs when the patient recognizes and accepts help to achieve maximum independence (108). Success rather than failure, incentives, internal inducement based on the need to know, and mild anxiety promotes learning (109).

Compliance is the agreement between recommendations by the health care professionals and patient behavior (110). Compliance is related to the patient's motivation, locus of control, expectations, beliefs and values about achievable outcomes, environmental demands, and perceived ability to initiate and maintain behavioral changes in the face of multiple roles and commitments (3,110). For example, compliance with weight shifts may in part be environmentally determined. A patient may frequently do an anterior weight shift in a movie theatre but be less than willing to do so in the middle of a business meeting. Furthermore, compliance may be affected by comorbid conditions such as depression, substance abuse, and stress disorders (111).

Hope

During the rehabilitation process, communication, development of realistic expectations, and goal setting must be nurtured. One should not tell a patient who has expressed a death wish, "You owe it to your family to stay alive," "Don't be ridiculous," or "I would want to die too if I were in your situation." The injured individual needs reassurance that specific parts of the present situation will get better over time. Reassurance and hope, however, should not be false.

Hope is what enables us to move from the present, which may be filled with losses, to an imagined future that is better (112). Hope is defined as a cognitive set involving a sense of agency (will) and pathways for attaining one's goals. People with high hopes can clearly delineate goals and define alternative ways to reach them. In contrast, individuals with low hope come up with only vague goals and are uncertain about the routes to take to achieve them. Hopeful thinking generally develops from goal attainment. Hope after SCI may be sustained by working toward small incremental gains. Morse and Doberneck (113) delineated the multidimensional concept of hope based on four participant groups, one of which was persons with SCI. The components of hope are (a) a realistic assessment of the threat; (b) the envisioning of alternatives and the setting of goals; (c) bracing for negative outcomes; (d) an assessment of internal and external resources; (e) the solicitation of mutually supportive relationships; (f) seeking signs that reinforce selected goals; and (g) a determination to endure. Hopeful individuals use their determination to succeed in spite of their disability. "You just have to accept it; you can accept something without liking it" (113).

Substance Abuse

During hospitalization and after discharge, most persons with SCI use adaptive coping styles such as looking for comfort from others, information seeking, and reinterpretation of negative events, rather than maladaptive coping mechanisms such as alcohol and drug use (15). Substance use and abuse, however, are still frequently encountered in SCI rehabilitation settings. Prevalence data are contradictory, but for a substantial number of patients, SCI is, in part, a result of substance misuse (114). Mourer et al. (33) suggest that 40% of patients in their SCI center were drinking at the time of their accidents. Tate (115) reports that about 76% of her sample were self-reported drinkers before their injury and that the CAGE was found to be a reliable instrument with the SCI population (115). The CAGE is a four-question screening device for alcoholism. It is an acronym that stands for *c*ut down (have you ever felt you should cut down on your drinking?); *a*nnoyed (have you been annoyed by others criticizing your drinking?); *g*uilty (have you ever felt bad or guilty about drinking?); and *e*ye opener (have you ever taken a drink first thing in the morning to steady your nerves or to get rid of a hangover?). Two or more positive responses suggest a higher likelihood of alcoholism. Furthermore, Tate (115) reports that persons with SCI with higher CAGE scores had a higher incidence of medical complications.

Patients with SCI share substance abuse risk factors with the general population, such as family history, concomitant psychiatric problems, and personality features. The physical, psychological, and vocational difficulties they face after SCI may further enhance that risk (114,115). Misuse of prescription medication may occur independent of nonprescription substance abuse but does not appear greater in the SCI population when compared with the general adult population. Use of prescription medication irrespective of following dose guidelines was associated with depression and poor sense of psychological well being. As a result, clinical follow-up should be continued (116).

Alcohol and drug misuse contribute to SCI by increasing risk taking while intoxicated. Furthermore, they hamper learning and rehabilitation gains, interfere with self-care, place persons at risk for complications, contribute to mortality and morbidity, and limit long-term outcomes and capacity for independent living (1,117). Alcohol abusers and marijuana users perceive their health as worse than those who do not abuse substances. They are more depressed and experience more stress in their lives (118). Heavy drinkers before injury spend less time in educational and vocational activities while in a rehabilitation hospital, and alcohol users are less motivated to participate in their rehabilitation than nondrinkers (119). Postinjury abstinence by preinjury problem drinkers may result in depression and self-neglect, leading to, for example, urinary tract infections and pressure ulcers (117). Furthermore, the social support and coping skills of problem drinkers may limit their ability to deal with SCI and the lifestyle changes it necessitates. As a result of the significant problems associated with substance misuse, prevention and treatment programs need to be included in inpatient and outpatient SCI rehabilitation centers.

Developing and Maintaining a Positive Rehabilitation Outcome

One of the goals of rehabilitation is to help the injured person learn to be as independent as possible; that requires energy, motivation, and the will to do so. Rehabilitation team members often notice changes in a patient's mood, behavior, cognition, presentation of self, and coping abilities. In addition to referring them to rehabilitation psychologists for treatment, they can also serve to open the door to meaningful communication. Normalizing and empathizing benefit patients, families, and treatment team members. It lets people know that they are not losing their sanity and that expression, rather than suppression, of feelings is supported.

Caring and active listening without advising or trying to change a patient's perception are wonderful tools (5). You can neither cajole a person out of a dysphoric mood nor truly understand exactly how he or she feels. Although comparing one patient with another is usually well intentioned, it easily backfires. Although things could be worse, they could be better, too. Patients serve as mirrors for each other. They may ask themselves, for example, "Do I look like *that* sitting in my wheelchair?" All it takes for patients and their relatives to realize that things could be worse is to look around the therapy room at the seriousness of the injuries treated. Knowing that it could have been worse does not, however, necessarily improve one's ability to cope with one's own disability. One can derive a perspective from knowing others are in similar situations, although an individual's personal sense of loss is not diminished by this knowledge (13).

There is no single or right way to adjust to SCI, and programs should be tailored to meet the specific individual needs of patients (1). Patients with SCI need unconditional acceptance of them as people regardless of how they perform in therapy (92). Occupational and physical therapy are objective in nature. They assist in helping those with SCI become more functional. To help a patient adapt to a disability requires taking the patient's subjective world into consideration. Emotional health should be promoted by the rehabilitation team through customized teaching to meet the coping and learning styles of patients and through setting goals with, not for, the patients (2).

Negotiation, which is akin to bargaining, is another great tool. Patients will often fight for control or QOL concerns. Regressed patients may be acting childish in an attempt to cope with being dependent. Patients may refuse to go to the dining room and eat using adaptive equipment or to come to therapy unless you come and pick them up. The treating psychologist can help find out the specific need that the patient is attempting to have you fill. Negotiation will serve both the staff and the patient better than the stance of "I know best, I've treated hundreds of patients with this type of disability." Sometimes giving limited choices can be helpful. "I can't pick you up every day, but how about picking you up on Monday to start off the week." "I'll assist you in eating some of the meal, but only if you come to the dining room."

Rehabilitation professionals need to be aware of their own feelings concerning grief, powerlessness, control, disability, and loss if they are to maximize patients' adaptation (2). In addition, they need to watch for strong and unusual reactions when they share strong commonalities with their patients in terms of age, occupation, interest in sports, or other areas of emotional, social, environmental, or financial functioning. Often, a staff member can be heard to say, "That patient is exactly my child's age." This will ultimately bring out mothering behaviors or a desire to "fix" the patient's problems and may negatively affect the patient's rehabilitation.

Hope maintains all of us. We cannot give it to someone and we should not take it away. As indicated already, the treatment team can assist patients in regaining hope by helping them change their goals to more achievable ones or by helping them learn different ways of reaching their existing goals. When a difficult prognosis is given, the treatment team needs to support hope but not necessarily the time frame or the unrealistic goals the patient sets. People operate on multiple levels. Patients can hope they walk out of the rehabilitation hospital yet expect to go home independent at the wheelchair level.

CONCLUSION

Whether you use the term *adjust, adapt, accept,* or *tolerate,* there is a large discrepancy in terms of the length of time it takes a person to cope with SCI (6). Wright (120) suggests that years may pass before individuals are able to fully realize the implications of their disability on their lives. Adaptation continues to improve beyond the rehabilitation period (120). According to Dijkers (48), adjustment takes approximately 2 to 5 years. Trieschmann (4) views rehabilitation as a lifelong process of teaching people to live with their disability in their own environment. The process may go on indefinitely with no endpoint in sight. Adaptation is evident when disability is no longer the dominant concern in a person's life (1).

Although depression has been the factor most frequently studied in terms of adjustment to SCI, more attention must be given to other reactions such as anxiety and locus of control, as well as defense mechanisms such as denial and sublimation. Individual differences, although difficult to study, will affect how a person reacts to disability. The only thing individuals with SCI have in common is disability and the initial experiences that result. Extreme dependency, for example, is an immediate consequence after SCI regardless of patients' premorbid personality factors or how independent, dependent, depressed, or assertive they were before being injured (121).

Psychologists play an active role in promoting mental health after SCI. They work to reduce depression, anxiety, and self-neglect. The psychologist accomplishes this by maintaining the patient's motivation and hopefulness, promoting self-directed behavior, engaging patients in problem solving to find personally acceptable solutions, increasing a patient's sense of personal power, clarifying interpersonal and intrapersonal conflicts (e.g., loss of autonomy), promoting catharsis, and fostering a positive euthymic mood (3,75). Interventions to improve QOL need to concentrate on reducing barriers to participation and improving perception of health, rather than focusing on physical functioning (73).

Rehabilitation is a special field. Choosing to work with patients whose lives were changed in an instant often leaves staff open to the vulnerability that comes with the knowledge that at any moment, they too can be the victims of an injury. There is no current cure for SCI. Rehabilitation professionals assist patients in sustaining hope, becoming as independent as possible, and improving their QOL, mood, and sense of control. Treatment team members can negotiate, listen actively, empathize, support, and encourage. Individuals with SCI are just that—individuals. They will best be served by being treated in an unbiased, warm, honest, genuine, and nonjudgmental manner.

REFERENCES

1. Heinemann AW. Spinal cord injury. In: Goreczny AJ, ed. *Handbook of health and rehabilitation psychology.* New York: Plenum Press, 1995: 341–360.
2. Hulse L. Psychosocial health issues for individuals with spinal cord injury. *Spinal Cord Inj Psychosoc Process* 1997;10:3–7.
3. Steins SA, Bergman SB, Formal CS. Spinal cord injury rehabilitation. Individual experience, personal adaptation, and social perspectives. *Arch Phys Med Rehabil* 1997;78:65–72.
4. Trieschmann R. *Spinal cord injuries: psychological, social, and vocational rehabilitation,* 2nd ed. New York: Demos Publications, 1988.
5. Gill M. Psychosocial implications of spinal cord injury. *Crit Care Nurs Q* 1999;22:1–7.
6. Glass CA, Jackson HF, Dutton J, et al. Estimating social adjustment following spinal trauma. I: who is more realistic—patient or spouse? A statistical justification. *Spinal Cord* 1997;35:320–325.
7. Peters D. Individual and family growth and development. In: Lubkin IM, ed. *Chronic illness impact and interventions,* 4th ed. Massachusetts: Jones and Bartlett, 1998:26–52.
8. Kubler-Ross E. *On death and dying.* New York: Macmillan, 1969.
9. Weller DJ, Miller PM. Emotional reactions of patient, family, and staff in acute-care period of spinal cord injury. *Soc Work Health Care* 1977;2:369–377.
10. Trieschmann R. *Spinal cord injuries: the psychological, social, and vocational adjustment.* New York: Pergamon Press, 1980.
11. Keany KCM-H, Glueckauf RL. Disability and value change: an overview and reanalysis of acceptance and loss. *Rehabil Psychol* 1993;38: 199–210.
12. Moore AD, Patterson DR. Psychological intervention with spinal cord injured patients: promoting control out of dependence. *Spinal Cord Inj Psychosoc Process* 1993;6:2–8.
13. Langer KG. Depression and denial in psychotherapy of persons with disabilities. *Am J Psychother* 1994;48:181–194.
14. Bopp A, Lubkin I. Teaching. In: Lubkin IM, ed. *Chronic illness impact and interventions,* 4th ed. Massachusetts: Jones and Bartlett, 1998: 343–362.
15. Kennedy P, Lowe R, Grey N, et al. Traumatic spinal cord injury and psychological impact: a cross-sectional analysis of coping strategies. *Br J Clin Psychol* 1995;34:627–639.
16. Silverman J. Emotional care of the cord-injured and chronically ill patient. In: Constantian M, ed. *Pressure ulcers: principles and techniques of management.* Boston: Little, Brown and Company, 1981.
17. Trieschmann R. *Aging with a disability.* New York: Demos Publications, 1987.
18. Elliott TR, Frank R. Depression following spinal cord injury. *Arch Phys Med Rehabil* 1996;77:816–823.
19. Boekamp JR, Overholser JC, Schumber DSP. Depression following a spinal cord injury. *Int J Psychiatry Med* 1996;26:329–349.
20. Frank RG, Elliott TR. Life stress and psychological adjustment following spinal cord injury. *Arch Phys Med Rehabil* 1987;68:344–347.
21. Howell T, Fullerton DT, Harvey RF, et al. Depression in spinal cord injured patients. *Paraplegia* 1981;19:284–288.
22. Zuckerman EL. *The clinician's thesaurus,* 3rd ed. Pittsburgh, PA: The Clinician's Toolbox, 1993:109.
23. Tennen H, Hall JA, Affleck G. Depression research methodologies in the Journal of Personality and Social Psychology: a review and critique. *J Pers Soc Psychol* 1995;68:870–884.
24. American Psychiatric Association. *Diagnostic and statistical manual of mental disorders,* 4th ed. Washington: American Psychiatric Association, 1994.
25. Krause JS, Kemo B, Coker J. Depression after spinal cord injury: relation to gender, ethnicity, aging and socioeconomic indicators. *Arch Phys Med Rehabil* 2000;81:1099–1109.
26. Judd FK, Brown DJ, Burrows GD. Depression, disease and disability: application to patients with traumatic spinal cord injury. *Paraplegia* 1991;29:91–96.
27. Beck AT, Ward CH, Mendelson M, et al. An inventory for measuring depression. *Arch Gen Psychiatry* 1967;4:351–363.
28. Dias de Carvalho SA, Andrade MJ, Tavares MA, et al. Spinal cord injury and psychological response. *Gen Hosp Psychiatry* 1998;20: 353–359.
29. Cushman LA, Dijkers M. Depressed mood in spinal cord injured patients: staff perceptions and patient realities. *Arch Phys Med Rehabil* 1990;71:191–196.
30. Jacob KS, Zachariah K, Bhattacharji S. Depression in individuals with spinal cord injury: methodological issues. *Paraplegia* 1995;33: 377–380.
31. Consortium for Spinal Cord Medicine. *Depression following spinal cord injury: a clinical practice guideline for primary care physicians.* New York: Paralyzed Veterans of America, 1998.
32. Scivoletto G, Petrelli A, DiLucente L, et al. Psychological investigation of spinal cord injury patients. *Spinal Cord* 1997;35:516–520.
33. Frank RG, Chaney JM, Clay DL, et al. Dysphoria: a major syndrome factor in persons with disability or chronic illness. *Psychiatry Res* 1992; 43:231–241.
34. Mourer SA, Williams GN, Stimac DJ. Estimates of mental disorders in new spinal cord injuries: a brief report. *Spinal Cord Inj Psychosoc Process* 1996;9:69–72.
35. Craig AR, Hancock KM, Dickson HG. A longitudinal investigation into anxiety and depression in the first two years following a spinal cord injury. *Paraplegia* 1994;32:675–679.
36. Kishi Y, Robinson RG, Forrester AW. Prospective longitudinal study of depression following spinal cord injury. *J Neuropsychiatry Clin Neurosci* 1994;6:237–244.
37. Kennedy P, Rogers B. Anxiety and depression after spinal cord injury: a longitudinal analysis. *Arch Phys Med Rehabil* 2000;81:932–937.
38. Richards JS. Psychologic adjustment to spinal cord injury during first postdischarge year. *Arch Phys Med Rehabil* 1986;67:362–365.

39. Tate D, Forchheimer M, Maynard F. Predicting depression and psychological distress in persons with spinal cord injury based on indicators of handicap. *Am J Phys Med Rehabil* 1994;73:175–183.

40. Craig AR, Hancock KM, Dickson HG. Spinal cord injury: a search for determinants of depression two years after the event. *Br J Clin Psychol* 1994;33:221–230.

41. Hancock KM, Craig AR, Dickson HG, et al. Anxiety and depression over the first year of spinal cord injury: a longitudinal study. *Paraplegia* 1993;31:349–357.

42. Kaplan HI, Saddock BJ. *Comprehensive textbook of psychiatry,* 5th ed. Baltimore: Williams & Wilkins, 1989.

43. Charlifue SW, Gerhart K. Behavioral and demographic predictors of suicide following traumatic spinal cord injury. *Arch Phys Med Rehabil* 1991;72:448–492.

44. DeVivo MJ, Black BS, Richards JS, et al. Suicide following spinal cord injury. *Paraplegia* 1991;29:620–627.

45. Hartkopp A, Bronnum-Hansen H, Seidenschnur A, et al. Suicide in a spinal cord injured population: its relation to functional status. *Arch Phys Med Rehabil* 1998;79:1356–1361.

46. Judd FK, Brown DJ. Suicide following acute traumatic spinal cord injury. *Paraplegia* 1992;30:173–177.

47. Stover S, Fine PR. The epidemiology and economics of spinal cord injury. *Paraplegia* 1987;25:225–228.

48. Dijkers M. Quality of life after spinal cord injury. *Am Rehabil* 1996; Fall:18–24.

49. Kennedy P, Rogers B, Speer S, et al. Spinal cord injuries and attempted suicide: a retrospective review. *Spinal Cord* 1999;37:847–852.

50. Craig AR, Hancock KM, Dickson HJ, et al. Long-term psychological outcomes in spinal cord injured persons: results of a controlled trial using cognitive behavior therapy. *Arch Phys Med Rehabil* 1997;78:33–38.

51. Craig AR, Hancock KM, Chang E, et al. Immunizing against depression and anxiety after spinal cord injury. *Arch Phys Med Rehabil* 1998;79:375–377.

52. Craig AR, Hancock KM, Dickson HG. Improving the long-term adjustment of spinal cord injured persons. *Spinal Cord* 1999;37:345–350.

53. Kupfer DJ. Long-term treatment of depression. *J Clin Psychiatry* 1991;52:28–34.

54. Altamura AC, Percudani M. The use of antidepressants for long term treatment of recurrent depression: rationale, current methodologies, and future directions. *J Clin Psychiatry* 1993;54:29–37.

55. Kupfer DJ, Frank E, Perel JM. Five year outcome for maintenance therapies in recurrent depression. *Arch Gen Psychiatry* 1992;49:769–773.

56. World Health Organization, Mental Health Collaborating Centers. Pharmacotherapy of depressive disorders: a consensus statement. *J Affective Disord* 1989;17:197–198.

57. Prien RF, Kupfer DJ. Continuation therapy for major depressive episodes: how long should it be maintained? *Am J Psychiatry* 1986;143:18–23.

58. American Psychiatric Association. Practice guideline for major depressive disorder in adults. *Am J Psychiatry* 1993;150:1–26.

59. Montgomery SA, Montgomery DB. *Long term treatment of depression.* New York: Wiley-Liss, 1992:53–79.

60. Frank E, Kupfer DJ, Perel JM, et al. Three year outcomes for maintenance therapies in recurrent depression. *Arch Gen Psychiatry* 1990;47:1093–1099.

61. Angst J. Natural history and epidemiology of depression: results of community studies. In: Cobb J, Goeting N, Duphar Medical Relations 1-9, eds. *Prediction and treatment of recurrent depression.* Southampton, UK: Duphar Pharmaceuticals, 1990.

62. McColl MA, Skinner H. Measuring psychological outcomes following rehabilitation. *Revue Canadienne De Sante Publique* 1992;83[Suppl 2]:S12–S17.

63. Geisler WO, Jousee AT, Wynne-Jones M, et al. Survival in traumatic spinal cord injury. *Paraplegia* 1983;21:304–373.

64. Kreuter M, Sullivan M, Dahllof AG, et al. Partner relationships, functioning, mood and global quality of life in persons with spinal cord injury and traumatic brain injury. *Spinal Cord* 1998;36:252–261.

65. Nabors NA, Meadows EA. Posttraumatic stress disorder in violence-induced spinal cord injury. *Top Spinal Cord Inj Rehabil* 1999;4:62–69.

66. Kaplan HI. Posttraumatic stress disorder and acute stress disorder. *Trauma Response* 1998;4:9–12.

67. Radnitz CL, Tirch D. Substance misuse in individuals with spinal cord injury. *Int J Addict* 1995;30:1117–1140.

68. Williams GN. Post-traumatic stress disorder: implications for practice in spinal cord injury rehabilitation. *Spinal Cord Inj Psychosoc Process* 1977;10:40–42.

69. Meichenbaum D. *A clinical handbook/practical therapist manual for assessing and treating adults with PTSD.* Canada: Institute Press, 1994.

70. Lewis P, Lubkin I. Illness roles. In: Lubkin, IM, ed. *Chronic illness impact and interventions,* 4th ed. Massachusetts: Jones and Bartlett, 1998:77–102.

71. Sullivan J. Individual and family responses to acute spinal cord injury. *Crit Care Nurs North Am* 1990;2:407–414.

72. Kreuter M. Spinal cord injury and partner relationships. *Spinal Cord* 2000;38:2–6.

73. Pierce CA, Richards S, Gordon W, et al. Life satisfaction following spinal cord injury and the WHO model of functioning and disability. *Spinal Cord Inj Psychosoc Process* 1999;12.

74. Judd FK, Burrows GD. Liaison psychiatry in a spinal injuries unit. *Paraplegia* 1986;24:6–19.

75. Macleod MB. Self-neglect of spinal injured patients. *Paraplegia* 1988;26:340–348.

76. Pope AM. Preventing secondary conditions. *Ment Retard* 1992;30:347–354.

77. Shackelford M, Farley T, Vines CL. Identifying psychosocial characteristics of adults with SCI. *Spinal Cord Inj Psychosoc Process* 1997;10:49–52.

78. Krause JS. Intercorrelations between secondary conditions and life adjustment in people with spinal cord injury. *Spinal Cord Inj Psychosoc Process* 1998;1:3–7.

79. Waters RL, Sie IH, Adkins RH, et al. The neuropathology of violence-induced spinal cord injury. *Top Spinal Cord Inj Rehabil* 1999;4:23–28.

80. Gordon S, Lewis D. Psychological challenges of drugs, violence and spinal cord injury among African-American inner city males. *Spinal Cord Inj Psychosoc Process* 1993;6:49–52.

81. Waters RL, Adkins RH. Firearm versus motor vehicle related spinal cord injury: preinjury factors, injury characteristics, and initial outcome comparisons among ethnically diverse groups. *Arch Phys Med Rehabil* 1997;78:150–155.

82. Hall KM, Knudsen ST, Wright J, et al. Follow-up study of individuals with high tetraplegia (C1-C4) 14 to 24 years postinjury. *Arch Phys Med Rehabil* 1999;80:1507–1513.

83. Bach JR, Tilton MC. Life satisfaction and well-being measures in ventilator assisted individuals with traumatic tetraplegia. *Arch Phys Med Rehabil* 1994;75:626–632.

84. Glass CA. The impact of home based ventilator dependence on family life. *Paraplegia* 1993;31:93–101.

85. Wright BA. *Physical disability: a psychosocial approach.* New York: Harper & Row, 1983.

86. Glass CA, Jackson HF, Dutton J, et al. Estimating social adjustment following spinal trauma. II: population trends and effects of compensation on adjustment. *Spinal Cord* 1997;35:349–357.

87. Frank RG, Umlauf RL, Wonderlich SA, et al. Differences in coping styles among persons with spinal cord injury. A cluster analytic approach. *J Consult Clin Psychol* 1987;55:727–731.

88. Wheeler G, Krausher R, Cumming C, et al. Personal styles and ways of coping in individuals who use wheelchairs. *Spinal Cord* 1996;34:351–357.

89. Kennedy P, Gorsuch N, Marsh N. Childhood onset of spinal cord injury: self-esteem and self-perception. *Br J Clin Psychol* 1995;34:581–588.

90. Krause JS, Crewe NM. Chronological age, time since injury, and time

of measurement: effect on adjustment after spinal cord injury. *Arch Phys Med Rehabil* 1991;72:91–100.

91. Kemp BJ, Krause JS. Depression and life satisfaction among people ageing with post-polio and spinal cord injury. *Disabil Rehabil* 1991; 21:241–249.

92. Gans JS. Facilitating staff/patient interaction in rehabilitation. In: Caplan B, ed. *Rehabilitation psychology desk reference.* Rockville, MD: Aspen Publications, 1987:185–218.

93. Hammell KR. Psychosocial outcome following spinal cord injury. *Paraplegia* 1994;32:771–779.

94. Rehabilitation Research Training Center. Aging and spinal cord injury: caring for the caregivers. *Paraplegia News* 1994:46–49.

95. Decker SD, Schulz R, Wood D. Determinants of well-being in primary caregivers of spinal cord injured persons. *Rehabil Nurs* 1989; 14:6–8.

96. Weller DJ, Miller PM. Emotional reactions of patient, family, and staff in acute-care period of spinal cord injury. *Soc Work Health Care* 1977;3:7–17.

97. Holicky R, Charlifue S. Ageing with spinal cord injury: the impact of spousal support. *Disabil Rehabil* 1999;21:250–257.

98. Chan RCK. Stress and coping in spouses of persons with spinal cord injuries. *Clin Rehabil* 2000;14:137–144.

99. Weitzenkamp DA, Gerhart KA, Charlifue SW, et al. Spouses of spinal cord injury survivors: the added impact of caregiving. *Arch Phys Med Rehabil* 1997;78:822–827.

100. Moore AD, Bombardier CH, Brown PB, et al. Coping and emotional attributions following spinal cord injury. *Int J Rehabil Res* 1994;17: 39–48.

101. Thompson SC, Janigian AD. Life schemes: a framework for understanding the search for meaning. *J Soc Clin Psychol* 1988;7:260–280.

102. Bulman RJ, Wortman CB. Attributions of blame and coping in the "real world": severe accident victims react to their lot. *J Pers Soc Psychol* 1977;35:351–363.

103. Schulz R, Decker S. Long-term adjustment to physical disability: the role of social support, perceived control, and self-blame. *J Pers Soc Psychol* 1985;48:1162–1172.

104. Nielson WR, MacDonald MR. Attributions of blame and coping following spinal cord injury: is self-blame adaptive? *J Soc Clin Psychol* 1988;4:163–175.

105. Reidy K, Caplan B. Causal factors in spinal cord injury: patient's

evolving perceptions and association with depression. *Arch Phys Med Rehabil* 1994;75:837–842.

106. Brown K, Bell MH, Maynard C, et al. Attribution of responsibility for injury and long-term outcome of patients with paralytic spinal cord trauma. *Spinal Cord* 1999;37:653–657.

107. Jordon SA, Wellborn WR, Kovnick J, et al. Understanding and treating motivation difficulties in ventilator-dependent SCI patients. *Paraplegia* 1991;29:431–442.

108. Lubkin I. *Chronic illness: impact and interventions,* 3rd ed. Boston: Jones and Bartlett, 1995.

109. Redman BK. *The process of patient teaching in nursing,* 7th ed. St. Louis: Mosby, 1993.

110. Blevins D, Berg J, Dunbar-Jacob J. Compliance. In: Lubkin IM, ed. *Chronic illness impact and interventions,* 4th ed. Massachusetts: Jones and Bartlett, 1998:227–257.

111. Trosper RM. Psychological factors affecting noncompliant behavior: a case study. *Spinal Cord Inj Psychosoc Proc* 1998;11:70–74.

112. Snyder CR. To hope, to lose, to hope again. *J Pers Interpers Loss* 1996; 1:1–16.

113. Morse JM, Doberneck B. Delineating the concept of hope. *Image J Nurs Sch* 1995;27:277–285.

114. Radnitz CL, Schlein IS, Walezak S, et al. The prevalence of posttraumatic stress disorder in veterans with spinal cord injury. *Spinal Cord Inj Psychosoc Process* 1995;8:145–149.

115. Tate DG. Alcohol use among spinal cord-injured patients. *Am J Phys Med Rehabil* 1993;72:192–195.

116. Heinemann AW, McGraw TE, Brandt MJ, et al. Prescription medication misuse among persons with spinal cord injuries. *Int J Addict* 1992;27:301–316.

117. Heinemann AW, Hawkins D. Substance abuse and medical complications following spinal cord injury. *Rehabil Psychol* 1995;40:125–140.

118. Young ME, Rintala DH, Rossi D, et al. Alcohol and marijuana use in a community-based sample of persons with spinal cord injury. *Arch Phys Med Rehabil* 1995;76:525–532.

119. Heinemann AW, Goranson N, Ginsburg K, et al. Alcohol use and activity patterns following spinal cord injury. *Rehabil Psychol* 1989; 34:191–205.

120. Krause JS. Longitudinal changes in adjustment after spinal cord injury: a 15-year study. *Arch Phys Med Rehabil* 1992;73:564–568.

121. Bartol G. Psychological needs of the spinal cord injured person. *J Neurosurg Nurs* 1978;10:171–175.

VOCATIONAL ASPECTS OF SPINAL CORD INJURY

DENISE G. TATE
ANDREW J. HAIG
JAMES S. KRAUSE

The consequences of spinal cord injury (SCI) are often profound and dramatic, affecting a person's quality of life in several domains, including the vocational one. Employment opportunities are dramatically curtailed for the person with severe physical limitations. From a social policy vantage point, the employment of persons with SCI is desirable for several reasons. First, the individual will benefit both financially and psychosocially from an increased standard of living and greater social integration. Second, society will benefit from an increased productive capacity, a larger tax base, and a reduction in welfare program costs (2).

For decades, return to work has been a hallmark of successful rehabilitation. Despite the emphasis on returning to work in rehabilitation programs, less than 50% of persons with SCI obtain paid employment (3). This chapter is designed to provide an understanding of basic issues associated with vocational rehabilitation (VR) and employment for persons with SCI, as well as to describe the nature and scope of vocational services available, medical interventions in preparation for achieving vocational goals, and ergonomic solutions to return to work. This chapter concludes by providing recommendations for research and interventions in this area.

PREDICTION FACTORS AND EMPLOYMENT OUTCOMES IN SPINAL CORD INJURY

Most rehabilitation studies focus on predictive models of employment, vocational goals and outcomes, and the relationship of personality traits to these outcomes. A summary of these issues is provided.

Predictive Models of Employment

Numerous studies have identified several predictors of employment status after SCI (4–9). The main objective of this line of research has been to help rehabilitation professionals and policy makers recognize personal and environmental conditions that facilitate or constrain gainful employment after SCI (10–12). Multiple regression and discriminant analyses have been used to identify factors that identify and distinguish gainfully employed persons with SCI from others who are not employed. Table 21.1 summarizes key factors considered by various authors when determining prediction of employment for persons with SCI.

Broadly defining employment to include homemakers and students, one study conducted a discriminant analysis that correctly classified 90% of subjects with SCI as either employed or unemployed 3 years postinjury (5). Persons with SCI who returned to work were more likely to be young, white, women, and working at the time of injury and were more likely to have greater functional independence than those who did not return to work. Several years later, the same group of researchers revised this predictive model of employment with a sample of 154 persons with SCI 7 years postinjury (3). A discriminant function analysis was able to correctly classify 79% of the sample into one of four groups: homemaker, student, employed at some point during the follow-up period, and continuously unemployed. The model correctly classified 100% of the homemakers and 72% of the "employed" persons. Most classification errors occurred in attempting to discriminate the employed from the unemployed persons. The key predictors were gender, motivation, whether the patient's last job required ambulation, race, educational level, functional capacity, and whether the person had children.

A more recent study used covariance structure modeling to test hypothesized models of postinjury employment in a sample of 120 former patients with SCI of a large Canadian rehabilitation center (13). In this study, age, education, motivation, driving one's own vehicle, and social support were hypothesized to directly influence employment status, although internal locus of control (defined as one's perception that he or she is indeed in control of his or her life outcomes) and level of injury were hypothesized to have indirect paths to employment.

Several studies have reported that motivation to work is a strong predictor of postinjury employment status, among both individuals with SCI and other rehabilitation groups (3,7,14). Similarly, internal locus of control is frequently discussed as an important predictor of job search, and employment success has been significant in at least two studies of persons with SCI (10, 15). Trieschmann (16) suggests that persons with an internal

TABLE 21.1. PREDICTORS OF RETURN TO WORK AND EMPLOYMENT AFTER SPINAL CORD INJURY

Demographic Predictors	Studies Cited
Age	(4)
Gender	
Preinjury work status	(2,7)
Race	
Education	(22,23)
Marital status	
Injury level	(12,20)
TSI	
Psychosocial predictors	
Motivation	(2,6,13)
Social support	(12,16,17)
Loss of control	(9,14,15)
Violence as injury etiology	(7)
Functional predictors	
Functional independence	(4,21)
Driving	(12)
Ergonomic predictors	
Physical intensity of the preinjury occupation	(21)

Note: Numbers in parentheses refer to specific studies, as listed in the reference list.

locus of control are more likely to be employed after SCI because they can accept responsibility for their rehabilitation, whereas those with an external locus of control remain more overwhelmed by the disability and fail to either initiate or complete vocational training.

Social support has been a significant predictor of employment status and other forms of productivity after SCI (17,18). Social support aims to provide emotional reassurance, needed information about how to live independently in the community, and instrumental aid in various life activities (19). These benefits minimize stress and increase the individual's ability to work. In a study by McShane and Karp (13), strong motivation, greater social support, and driving one's own car were directly predictive of having paid employment.

Another important factor cited in the literature has been the neurologic level of injury. Findings have been controversial, with several studies showing a nonsignificant association with postinjury employment status (3,8,9,12,18,20). However, Goldberg and Freed (21) suggest that level of injury may be associated with motivation to work, but does not hold a direct relationship with employment status. Level of injury was indirectly associated with employment status, with patients who had more severe injuries being less likely to be employed.

In a recent study in the Netherlands by Tomassen et al. (22), the most important predictive factor for returning to gainful employment was functional independence as measured by the Barthel index. The chance of being employed post-SCI was 2.5 times higher for persons with a Barthel index of more than 15 (mildly disabled). The second most important predictive factor was the physical intensity of the preinjury occupation. Persons with less physically demanding occupations preinjury were more likely to be employed postinjury.

Five studies investigated the relationship between employ-

ment, race, and gender. Three of the studies used a narrow definition of employment (3,23,24), including only patients working for pay or those self-employed. In three of these studies, whites were more likely to be working, although the pattern for gender was mixed, with at least one study suggesting an interaction between race/ethnicity and gender (i.e., white men were more likely than white women to obtain gainful employment, whereas the opposite was true for African Americans). The remaining studies used a broad definition of employment, including patients who were working, self-employed, a homemaker, or a student (5,8). These studies found that when homemakers were classified with the employed group, persons with SCI who were white women were more likely to return to work.

These findings were described by Krause et al. (8) in a recent study about employment after SCI. Using model systems SCI data, the authors found that being white, younger at injury, having lived more years with SCI, having a less severe injury, and having more years of education before SCI were all predictive of being employed. Violence at injury was associated with lower employment rates (only 12.9% employed). Being employed at injury was associated with a greater probability of postinjury employment, but only in the first few years after injury. Among employed persons with SCI, women and those who had been injured fewer years averaged fewer hours spent at work.

Employment, Quality of Life, and Well-Being

Several studies have been conducted to identify the extent to which employment is related to valued rehabilitation outcomes, including quality of life and well-being. A series of studies by Krause (8,9) examined data gathered longitudinally from a cohort of 256 persons with SCI beginning in 1974. In the first study (8), the employed respondents reported having higher life satisfaction and self-rated adjustment scores than either the "unpaid productive" or the unemployed respondents. An additional finding was that persons who were younger and married were more likely to be working. Krause (8) found that productivity was related to more positive outcomes when correlating productivity with scores from the Life Situation Questionnaire (a measure of adjustment and quality of life after SCI). Participants who were gainfully employed reported better overall adjustment than participants who were performing nonpaid productive activities (e.g., attending school, homemaking, or volunteering), who in turn reported superior adjustment to those who were unemployed. One limitation of Krause's study, however, is that it did not differentiate between participation in an educational program and other types of productive activities (8).

In another study using the same participant sample, Krause (9) attempted to determine whether the enhanced life adjustment associated with employment was maintained after employment was terminated. The adjustment of participants who were currently employed was compared with that of two groups of unemployed participants: those who had worked at some time since the injury and those who had not been employed at any time since the injury. As expected, participants who were currently employed showed superior adjustment to both unemployed groups. The currently employed group had more education and reported greater positive feelings in life domains of economics, emotional distress, and general health, compared with either the continuously unemployed or the intermittently employed group. The basic findings of the two studies are the presence of a positive relationship between employment status, self-reported adjustment to disability, and satisfaction with various life domains. Surprisingly, however, there were essentially no differences in life adjustment between the two groups of unemployed participants. In other words, there appeared to be no carryover benefit of employment beyond the actual period of employment.

A third study by Krause and Crewe (25) reviewed factors associated with survival status in a 15-year follow-up of the original 1974 cohort of 256 persons with SCI. The deceased showed chronic, poor adjustment in several areas of life functioning before their deaths. Notably, there was a strong relationship between survival and being employed (25).

Krause (26) used a longitudinal design to investigate the direction of the relationship between employment and adjustment. Two competing hypotheses were tested: (a) a selective process whereby people who are better adjusted are more likely to become employed or (b) a facilitative process whereby being employed facilitates better adjustment. Participants were classified into four groups based on a cross tabulation of employment status: employed at both time 1 and time 2; employed at time 1, but unemployed at time 2; unemployed at time 1, but employed at time 2; and unemployed at both time 1 and time 2. Adjustment scores were compared between the four groups at both time 1 and time 2. The results suggested that employment facilitates better adjustment and that satisfaction scores increased after the transition from unemployment to employment. Declines in activity and satisfaction appeared to be associated with the negative transition from employment to unemployment.

In the most recent study, Krause and Anson (27) compared the life satisfaction, problems, and adjustment of participants with SCI who were either (a) gainfully employed, (b) unemployed, but attending school, or (c) unemployed and not attending school. They found that employed participants reported superior adjustment scores to the unemployed nonstudents on four of seven scales, but superior scores to the students on only one scale: career satisfaction. In contrast to the unemployed nonstudents, the students reported higher overall adjustment scores and fewer problems with skills deficits. The results point to the strong association of both education and employment with enhanced quality of life among people with SCI.

Postdisability productivity was moderately correlated with a standard life satisfaction measure in a random sample of 140 persons with SCI, representing 13 southeast Texas counties (28). In addition, individuals with SCI were asked to rate their satisfaction with 12 different life domains. Employment was rated as least satisfactory. In contrast, life satisfaction was more closely associated with self-assessed health, perceived control, and social support.

Personality Characteristics and Employment

Researchers and theorists have focused their attention on looking for links between preinjury and postinjury personality, identify-

ing more commonly observed traits, and identifying the relationship between personality and rehabilitation outcomes. The primary work on personality and SCI has been performed by Rohe et al., who conducted a series of studies on vocational interests among men with SCI (29–31). These studies clarified the predominant interest type among men with SCI along Holland's hexagonal personality typology. These interest types are realistic, investigative, artistic, social, enterprising, and conventional.

In the first of these studies, Rohe and Athelstan (29) obtained Strong Campbell Interest Inventories (SCII) of 134 men and 22 women with SCI within 1 year after injury. The participants were identified from four regional centers who participated in a collaborative study of psychological, social, and vocational aspects of SCI. Results indicated that men with SCI were significantly more introverted than men in general and that they preferred working with things rather than with data or people. Among the conclusions of this study were (a) vocations typically suitable for the physical limitations of men with SCI tend not to coincide with the interests of this group and (b) there seems to be a relationship between risk of injury and the interest in working with things, such as powerful machinery. The most common interests among the men in this sample were on the realistic theme of the SCII, a scale that reflects a preference for concrete activities, working with objects rather than people or data, and a liking for the use of tools (such as mechanical activities, carpentry, and construction work). Occupations in which the SCI participants had higher interests than a normative sample included skilled crafts, farmer, forester, and veterinarian. Interests in social and investigative activities and occupations (such as lawyer, social scientist, and psychologist) were lower than the normative sample. In addition, the SCI sample was more introverted (higher introversion-extroversion scores) and less comfortable in academic settings (lower academic comfort scores). Although the small sample size limited any generalizations with women, the same basic pattern of findings regarding lower interests in investigative, social, and academic interests also held for women.

In a second study addressing the issue of interest stability, Rohe and Athelstan (30) asked 117 men with SCI (an average of 9 years postinjury) and a matched control group of 130 nondisabled men to complete the SCII twice. The first SCII was completed using standard directions, and the second time, the directions were modified as participants were asked to complete it as they thought they would have before their injury. Correlations of actual and recalled interests suggested that interests tended to remain stable over time among persons with SCI (0.81 correlation rate between recalled and actual interests). Actual preinjury interest inventories were available for 14 participants and were also correlated with postinjury interests and recalled interests. These comparisons suggested that the recall method might have inflated the stability estimates, because a higher median correlation was obtained between recalled and postinjury interests than that obtained between actual preinjury interests and postinjury interests (62,81). Nevertheless, the salient outcome of this study was that those with SCI showed stability of interests essentially equal to that of nondisabled individuals over a similar time span.

In a later study, Rohe and Krause (32) conducted an 11-

year follow-up on the remaining sample of 79 participants that directly assessed the stability of interests over that time. The results parallel and reinforce those reported in the original study; they indicated that (a) the interests of men with SCI were as stable as those of similar-aged nondisabled samples, (b) anticipated age-related increases in scales associated with artistic and social interests and normative age-related decreases in scales associated with physically demanding and adventuresome activities did not occur, and (c) interests that reflect forceful interaction with the general public decreased.

Athelstan and Crewe (33) divided a sample of 126 persons with SCI into three groups based on degree of active involvement in the onset of disability: (a) active involvement (the "impudent" group), (b) passive involvement, and (c) "innocent victims" (27). No significant differences were reported between the groups on variables of sex, age, or educational level, although the "innocent victim" group contained significantly fewer persons with tetraplegia than the other two groups. The authors found that the active involvement group had the highest adjustment, whereas the innocent victims had the poorest adjustment. A significantly higher proportion of the active involvement group was employed, and as a whole, this group had significantly fewer hospitalizations for postrehabilitation medical problems. These authors suggest that the same characteristics that may predispose people to injury may facilitate adjustment postinjury; that is, having an external, action orientation may lead to active, energetic coping efforts.

Taken together, these studies suggest that personality characteristics are associated with vocational interests, which in turn are correlated with abilities. Abilities are associated with vocational success. Thus, personality may also be associated with vocational success.

In an investigation of the personality characteristics of 111 patients with diverse disabilities in rehabilitation programs, Malec (34) found that persons with traumatic SCI were more extraverted and less distressed than other patients, as measured by the Eysenck Personality Inventory (EPI) and the Symptom Checklist-90 (34). Extraversion, it was postulated, is correlated with the consistently intense risk-taking behavior that often precedes SCI. The author also suggests that more extroverted individuals may adjust to a changed body image and lifestyle with less distress, because they are less reliant on internalized models for coping than more introverted persons.

One problem with the foregoing studies of the relationship between personality and SCI is that each uses a different measure of personality, making it difficult to integrate findings across studies. Rohe and Malec (35) attempted to integrate several of these studies. They pointed out that Eysenck's extraversion construct does not refer to sociability, but to an external orientation toward learning by repeated, concrete experience. Presumably, the SCII introversion construct refers to social orientation. Thus, men with SCI are oriented toward "things" and prefer to work alone: They are "doers," not "thinkers."

As suggested by Rohe (36), several factors may combine to explain the vocational adjustment problems of men with SCI: (a) the discordance between preinjury vocational interests and postinjury functional limitations, (b) the relative stability of vocational interests over time, (c) the requirement of extensive education for many alternative occupations, and (d) the lack of interest in lengthy formal education.

In summary, studies that have investigated predictors of postinjury employment among persons with SCI have not considered the personality factors that appear to be prevalent in this group, particularly among men. On the other hand, studies that have investigated personality characteristics of persons with SCI have not demonstrated their relevance to important rehabilitation outcomes, such as employment. This is an important consideration, because significant employment difficulties are related to poor life satisfaction among persons with disabilities (37).

MEDICAL INTERVENTIONS TOWARD VOCATIONAL GOALS

Several studies emphasize the preventive nature of VR in the recovery process (38). In fact, the path to successful return to work for persons with SCI begins in the most intense of medical settings. Perhaps in the ambulance, in the intensive care room, or on awakening from anesthetic, the person with an SCI has his or her first thoughts of a changed future.

The distorted environment in which these first thoughts occur is within the medical model. At this early and vulnerable stage, the person with an SCI may develop an impression of a "used to be" person, or as a temporarily ill, but valued and skilled person who has a disability. If the literature on physician-patient communication in other areas of health care can be extrapolated to spinal cord medicine, it is clear that realistic encouragement and exposure to future possibilities by the physician will have a significant effect on the vocational outcome of SCI.

Medical interventions for VR progress from this early formative interaction through the inpatient rehabilitation unit to the outpatient multidisciplinary team setting, to a point at which the person with an SCI is medically stable and seeking improved function specific to a certain job. During the early phases of SCI rehabilitation, the VR counselor should meet with the injured individual, to provide support and guidance. The patient looks to this specialist for hope, particularly soon after injury in the initial adjustment period.

A primary role of the VR counselor as time from the injury progresses is to assist the person with SCI to develop employment skills using such tools as coaching, role-playing, or videotaping. He or she must also know what to do in response to questions about disability, either on an application or in an interview. The person will also need to know where to obtain business-specific information needed to target the job search, prepare for the interview, and learn how to obtain job leads through formal and networking channels.

For persons with SCI, a good job site assessment is critical to the success of the job placement process. It is the basis on which job accommodation recommendations are made. It may be done by the counselor or by an occupational therapist specialized in work assessment. The job must be analyzed for factors involved in the work environment, in the job tasks themselves, and for production expectations; for example, how is it determined that the employee is performing adequately? An analysis of the work site's physical factors may consider parking at the work site, rest rooms, cafeteria, and building accessibility.

The VR services provided by public and private agencies include vocational evaluation, functional assessment, work hardening and reconditioning, work capacity evaluation, job site analysis, job accommodations, job-seeking skills, employer development, employment skill training, job placement, and follow-up services. State VR agencies under the State Department of Education have played a key role in promoting employment opportunities for persons with severe physical limitations such as those with SCI. This role includes subsidizing their education, vocational assessment, transportation and personal care assistance costs, career development and training, and job placement, as well as helping to purchase equipment and other resources needed to obtain employment after SCI.

The primary purpose of VR is to assist and enable persons with SCI to increase their productivity, usually through competitive employment. The goal is to identify a feasible employment goal and then outline the VR services needed to achieve this goal. The VR process generally involves (a) individual assessment and planning, which may include interviewing, paper-and-pencil tests, and performance evaluation in real or simulated work situations; (b) service provision, which may include counseling, education, skill training, medical restoration, and procurement of adaptive equipment; and (c) job placement, which may include trial work placements, job development, marketing, and placement in permanent employment.

Employment is not so much a goal as a motivator for patients with SCI on the inpatient unit. Often, persons with SCI still require substantial medical care and their insurance only covers inpatient rehabilitation, because it applies to learning minimal skills to be discharged home. Employment and education directed toward survival are more relevant to the person with an injury when their eventual impact on quality of life—including work—is emphasized. When physical and educational gains can be related to work and other functions in society, the context of the hard work makes sense to the patient.

After the patient is discharged, VR services can occur in various settings. The state agencies are key in providing assistance and support to persons with SCI wanting to return to work or seek employment. These agencies can subsidize the cost of transportation, personal care, and equipment and devices needed for obtaining and maintaining employment. State agencies work with multiple community partners, both to increase awareness of services to consumers and to implement services. These partners include school systems, Centers for Independent Living (CILs), community mental health agencies, hospitals and health care clinics, substance abuse centers, local support groups, other state and county employment programs, and a whole host of social service agencies. State or private rehabilitation providers may also contract with community private not-for-profit organizations, which may provide work evaluation, community work adjustment programs, sheltered or transitional employment, job coaching, or other specialized job placement services.

Private rehabilitation counselors often contract with insurance carriers to provide VR services to those who qualify for these services through workers' compensation, auto no-fault, or long-term disability policies. These services are provided within the context of what the insurers will pay for the specific legislation involved. Consequently, private rehabilitation firms are usually very responsive to the payers' goals and objectives.

VR begins with the assessment of the person's vocational interests, wishes, abilities, needs, and potentials. The purposes of assessment are to identify the person's relative strengths and weaknesses, set goals, and plan a course of action. Assessment is also used to determine eligibility for services and to make predictions about a person's potential to benefit from rehabilitation. Assessment initially involves gathering data from various sources.

Conceptually, some vocational issues are best addressed early while on the inpatient unit. If ready, the person with SCI can benefit from discussions regarding his or her future. Psychologists, social workers, occupational therapists, vocational counselors, and peer counselors may orient the patient with SCI to work possibilities. Applications for Social Security or other disability programs should be processed early so the patient has the financial security to train for the best possible career, rather than the first job that comes along. With backlogs and underfunding, early application increases the likelihood that approval of funds for counseling, adaptive equipment, transportation, and training will occur on a timely basis during the process of outpatient rehabilitation. Insurers typically pay for equipment and assistive devices only once during the rehabilitation period. Because wheelchairs and other devices are typically prescribed from the inpatient unit, it is important for the team to consider the person's vocational needs when making their choices.

However, it is in the outpatient setting that coordinated vocational-medical rehabilitation takes a more active role. Here, persons with SCI can learn life skills in ways that prepare the individual for work. Once the person is living in the community, it may be easier to identify or deal with medical issues that may interfere with work. These issues typically include hidden "minor" musculoskeletal injuries, chronic pain, incontinence of bowel or bladder, recurrent bladder infections, spasticity, skin sores, and other problems. All can be managed based on work demands. In addition to SCI, occult traumatic brain injuries that interfere with cognition, judgment, or behavior can be detected and appropriate outpatient rehabilitation can begin. It is after discharge when depression, anxiety, alcohol and drug abuse, and other psychiatric issues often crop up. These problems and their treatment directly affect vocational success. Choice of medications, imposed activity restrictions, timing of surgical, or other interventions may either expedite or interfere with the VR process.

A well-coordinated outpatient rehabilitation team has much to offer the patient in terms of work adaptation. Depending on the vocational plan, different emphases can be placed in the areas of physical mobility skills, activities of daily living, and cognitive and speech language skills; orthotic and adaptive devices may be appropriate.

The service provision plan is formalized with an individualized written rehabilitation plan, which is jointly developed by the person with SCI and his or her vocational counselor. Once job placement has been achieved, follow-up services are provided for a minimum of 60 days, to provide support and consultation to the new employee and his or her employer. This helps to ensure that the employment situation is working out satisfactorily for all parties. As a result of the passage of the Technology-Related Assistance for Individuals with Disabilities Act of 1988, special emphasis has been placed on identifying the person's accommodation needs throughout the rehabilitation process. This enables the person with an SCI to participate more fully in his or her vocational evaluation, training, and job placement processes, as well as to maintain employment over time.

Finally, depending on vocational plans, direct work activity training may take place in the outpatient rehabilitation setting. General reconditioning is important for any job that has a significant physical component to it. The physical activity of some jobs is specific enough to require a creative job-simulation training program—that is, work hardening. If work hardening is indicated, not only should it include imitation of the job, but it should also look at specific muscle deficits and train those muscles aggressively. Without fatiguing exercise, muscles will not increase their capacity and secondary musculoskeletal disorders may occur. Occupational therapists may assess the work site and provide recommendations about physical skill deficits and ergonomic adaptation (39). Therapy can then focus on these areas. If there is a mismatch between the person's communication, cognitive or emotional status, and the job demands, consultation with a speech language pathologist, rehabilitation counselor, or psychologist may be indicated.

It is not unusual for a person to finish up his or her outpatient therapies—either via successful learning or running out of insurance benefits—months or years before he or she begins to think seriously about work. Barriers or lost opportunities may occur when medical or functional issues are taken as unchangeable when in fact therapies, equipment, or medical interventions may make a substantial difference. At this point, the VR counselor needs to redevelop ties with the health care system.

The vocational counselor may attempt to contact a number of different sources within the health care system including the primary physician, a specialist such as an orthopedic surgeon, or the physiatrist. The choice may be one of convenience, rather than logic. For instance, if the person is no longer being followed by a physiatrist on a frequent basis but has an appointment with a primary care physician in the next month, the primary care physician may be asked to deal with an issue. Although this may be appropriate for simple problems, in a trial of persons in the community seeking functional assistance, it was demonstrated that consultation with a physiatrist resulted in substantial and long-lasting functional and quality-of-life improvements in comparison to previous care directed by a primary care physician (40). Teamwork is even more effective. When patients were randomized to a physiatrist alone versus a physiatrist with a single-visit multidisciplinary assessment, results showed that the team came up with twice as many recommendations as the physiatrist alone and that the people evaluated by the team had improved outcomes in almost all measures (41). VR professionals may do best to seek out programs in which coordinated multidisciplinary assessments are available.

VR counselors are challenged to get timely access to their future clients. Because health care systems have tightened their budgets, many rehabilitation units contract out for their vocational services. The motivation to identify the need, remember the counselor's name, and make early contact is not high, particularly when reimbursement for private counselors is often absent. State agencies have substantial backlogs, and persons may not qualify for assessment until they have been disabled for a certain amount of time. This "dissociation of medical rehabilitation and VR" results in direct and indirect impacts on the employment of persons with SCI. The VR counselor is often forgotten or is involved in a very superficial way with the inpatient team. If a VR counselor is available, the team should consult him or her as early as possible and include vocational issues at team meetings.

The indirect effect of this "dissociation" is perhaps most alarming. Attending physiatrists and team leaders of a decade or more ago typically trained at inpatient units in academic centers. There was substantial VR presence on the inpatient units, so the physicians interacted on a frequent basis with vocational counselors through team meetings and informal "curbside consults." The physicians were constantly educated and reminded about how they interacted with the VR system. In contrast, physicians and staff trained in the current environment have little exposure to VR. As a result, we believe they are much less likely to identify vocational issues or to prescribe vocationally oriented rehabilitation services. Often, physicians have minimal interaction with vocational counselors on the inpatient unit and only random interaction with them in the outpatient setting, and therefore they have very little understanding of when and how to refer and coordinate with the vocational team. Although VR is clearly cost-effective, initiation of vocational services and meaningful interaction with physicians will not likely occur without substantial policy change.

In addition to VR agencies, many CILs successfully serve persons with SCI. The specific features of individual independent-living programs are determined by the needs of the persons served, the availability of existing community resources, the physical and social makeup of the community, and the goals of the program itself. Independent-living support services can be provided by various community-based programs such as self-help and information referral centers, generic service providers, transitional programs, and residential programs.

At a minimum, CIL services consist of peer counseling, information and referral, independent-living skills training, and advocacy. These services are primarily provided by other individuals with SCI who may or may not have professional training in those areas but who have personal experience in living with a disability. Many CILs also offer such services as housing assistance, personal assistant training and referral, sign language interpreter referral, and community awareness programs. In addition, with the 1992 Amendments to the Rehabilitation Act, many CILs are currently placing greater emphasis on systems advocacy and consumer empowerment. Systems advocacy aims at inclusion of people with disabilities in the policy-making roles that regulate delivery of medical, social, rehabilitation, or other services. Systems advocacy may be focused at the local, state, regional, or national level depending on the nature of the underlying issue being addressed.

ERGONOMIC SOLUTIONS TO EMPLOYMENT

At some point, the person with an SCI chooses a job. He or she hopefully chooses it because of its financial and professional reward. But physical impairments play a role in determining work. The manner in which a person goes about work after an SCI may put him or her at risk for secondary injuries.

Information on work-specific ergonomics for persons with SCI is almost nonexistent in the searchable literature. The National Institute on Disability and Rehabilitation Research has responded to this gap in knowledge by funding Rehabilitation Engineering Research Centers to address ergonomic solutions for employment (42). The primary task of these centers involves modeling of expert opinion (43,44). After extensive medical and ergonomic evaluation, usually involving videotaping of the potential work site, cases are brought to a group of experts including ergonomists, physiatrists, occupational medicine specialists, and rehabilitation engineers. The experts ask questions about (a) a person's present capabilities; (b) the job requirements as currently designed; (c) the person's capabilities of doing the current job; (d) work-related risks for future injury or illness; (e) types of work; (f) modifications that will help the person do the work safely and efficiently; and (g) the type of medical or rehabilitation interventions needed.

For a person with an SCI, capabilities may vary considerably based on the level and completeness of the injury and other associated medical factors. Although it is not possible to meaningfully screen each person regarding all work tasks, often a simple functional assessment involving basic common tasks in the area of vocational interest and capabilities can help the person with an SCI and the rehabilitation team to understand the task ahead.

Functional assessment can be applied to various domains such as mobility, interpersonal communication, sensory awareness, emotional stability, learning ability, general stamina, and motivity—that is, the capacity to initiate and control physical movements as required by specific task demands and situations. An adequate functional assessment, combined with an adequate analysis of the demands of a specific occupation, provides a major component in making decisions about the appropriateness or advisability of pursuing particular vocational objectives. Work experience, intelligence, personality, and other factors looked on favorably increase opportunities for job placement.

Job placement activities can be viewed as a continuum ranging from self-placement to the counselor assuming all placement responsibility. The skills and personality traits of the job seeker, the nature of the disability, and local market conditions can influence the extent of counselor involvement. In cases of severe disability, such as SCIs, counselor involvement is likely to be greater. Job site assessments are quite valuable in understanding the physical requirements of the job. Factors such as climbing, lifting, bending, twisting, grasping, reaching, repetition, force, and bimanual task requirements provide a basic understanding of the job as it is done by typical able-bodied persons. Often a person with an SCI can perform the job as others do, given adaptive devices. The Americans with Disabilities Act was passed in 1990 with extensive bipartisan support after 2 years of intensive lobbying by disability rights groups. This bill was to people with disabilities what the Civil Rights Act of 1964 was to African Americans (45).

The Americans with Disabilities Act prohibits discrimination against people with disabilities in employment, public services, public transportation, places of public accommodations (e.g., hotels and restaurants), and telecommunications. Businesses with more than 15 employees were required to make reasonable accommodations for qualified candidates with disabilities unless such accommodations would impose undue hardship. Such accommodations might include improving work site accessibility, equipment modification, work schedule modification, or provision of interpreters. The Americans with Disabilities Act defines job requirements by output, and not so much by a certain method of doing the work. A real understanding of the work output required in the job allows rehabilitation engineers, occupational therapists, and others to work with the person with SCI to make creative modifications.

Occasionally, the job is complex enough that more formalized measurement of task requirements is needed. Advanced measurements including videotaping, force measurements, and electromyographic monitoring may result in a most appropriate understanding of the work to be done. Substantial expertise is needed to gather the information and to interpret it in a meaningful way to others. Processing work and worker information can be a difficult issue. Physicians have little intuitive feel for a five-page report including statements such as "the job requires a 20-lb lift at 35 cm from the chest on a 25-second off cycle, 5-second on cycle, repeated for 30 minutes, five times a day." On the other hand, plant engineers may struggle with "T3 ASIA-A paraplegia." Yet the physician usually has the final say on work restrictions, and the plant engineer must agree to job adaptations. The real challenge is to distill this information down to the level where the persons who have the expertise and authority to make changes can understand it and therefore make informed decisions.

A primary goal of VR is to make the job accessible to the person with SCI. Over time, it is important that the job changes also minimize the chance of new injury and the risk of repetitive strain disorders. The modifications should consider the safety and productivity of the worker and others at the work site. It is beyond the scope of this chapter to discuss the multitude of specific modifications to specific work tasks. Typical VR interventions for persons with SCI may involve modification of the job site, adaptive equipment, or job policy changes.

Job site modifications may be as simple as eliminating barriers to a wheelchair or adjusting a desk height. Although others may be more complex—such as redesigning an assembly line—the total cost is usually minimal. Often the modification results in increased efficiency or safety for the able-bodied workers as well. When job site modifications involve changes in significant or complex structures or major electrical or plumbing systems, the modifier should have sufficient engineering background to ensure that the modifications will not cause fatigue, interfere with other functions, or become a hazard.

Adaptive equipment is often a simple, low-cost solution to employment. Commercially available physical assist devices may include sit-stand workstations, braces, reaching devices, grabbing devices, or tools with special handles. Industrial material-handling devices, which may not have been necessary for able-bodied workers, may have a place in adapting the workplace for persons with SCIs. They are usually beneficial, but they also may slow productivity, and the forces required to propel the lifted object through space may preclude their use in some settings. Electronic adaptations are coming to the forefront. Computer voice-recognition programs minimize the keystrokes needed during typing. Computerized memory programs can compensate for cognitive deficits and infrared remote controls are easily adapted to industrial settings.

Work policy changes may include alterations in the number of hours worked per day or the duration of breaks. Reassignment of occasionally performed physical tasks, such as lifting and climbing, to persons who are able to perform these tasks can allow the person in a wheelchair to perform the essentials of the work. More controversial is the alteration of job rotations. Manufacturers often rotate jobs on an hourly or daily basis to avoid repetitive strain injuries in workers. If a person with an SCI is able to perform one of the job rotations, but not the others, assignment of this person to the "easy" job may put others at risk for a disabling injury. The right solution involves estimating this added risk to others and using that information along with other facts to define whether the rotation is an "essential" component of the job according to the Americans with Disabilities Act.

Work policy changes are easy to adapt when the employer is small, the shop is nonunionized, and the worker has a good track record. In larger corporations, upper level management and high-level union leaders may disagree on the need for workforce diversity, the cost of not employing skilled workers who require adaptations, and the inevitability of disability for most workers. Often the power to make these changes lies with mid-level management and mid-level union personnel, and yet they have no responsibility for "big picture" issues such as workers' compensation losses, corporate philosophy, Americans with Disabilities Act requirements, or societal responsibility. They are under pressure to prove their personal effectiveness or to stifle any dissent or criticism among their workers and constituency. In most systems, financial rewards for adapting a work site accrue to the corporation, but not to the work unit. Risks of low productivity or worker dissent are borne by the work unit. Unfortunately, the mid-level management has little motivation to provide adaptation in most corporate cultures.

Recent efforts to increase the number of persons with SCI who are working include (a) Americans with Disabilities Act provisions requiring reasonable accommodations by employers; (b) increases from $500 to $700 per month in Substantial Gainful Activity (SGA) provisions that allow persons with SCI to work up to a specified limit without losing Social Security Disability Insurance (SSDI) and Supplemental Security Income (SSI) benefits; and (c) the Ticket to Work and Work Incentives Improvement Act of 1999 (46).

Recent changes in employment legislation, such as the Ticket to Work and Work Incentives Improvement Act of 1999, may prove helpful in increasing employment rates of persons with SCI receiving SSI or SSDI if they learn about relevant provisions. The most notable provision of this recent legislation allows continuation of Medicare (part A) benefits $4\frac{1}{2}$ years beyond the current 4-year maximum after return to work. It also allows states to expand the availability of Medicaid to more people, between the ages of 16 and 64, with disabilities who work. The Ticket to Work provisions increase beneficiary choice in obtaining rehabilitation and vocational services. Benefits can be restarted within 60 months of returning to work without a new application, if the person with an SCI is unable to work any longer because of his or her previous medical condition.

CONCLUSIONS AND RECOMMENDATIONS

The importance of the VR process in the lives of persons with SCI is clearly defined by the literature findings reviewed in this chapter. The concept of work is associated to one's self-worth and contribution to others and society. It can be viewed as an essential ingredient of one's self-esteem and self-identity, having significant effects on psychological and physical adjustment postinjury. Furthermore, these effects can be translated into financial and social costs to the individual, his or her family, and society at large.

The literature is replete with studies demonstrating that persons with SCI can be employed, and most of the research has focused on the identification of the characteristics of the person who succeeds in obtaining gainful employment. This research also suggests that some factors play an important role in predicting employment after SCI. These factors include age, race, gender, previous work status, education, motivation, locus of control, social support, neurologic level of injury, functional independence, etiology, marital status, and personality characteristics. The literature focuses almost exclusively on the personal variables to employment and VR, but little attention has been given to environmental variables such as employer attitudes, financial disincentives, and public policy. The only issue discussed under this category is that of social support. More research on this area is certainly needed. Furthermore, emphasis needs to be placed on environmental factors (e.g., physical barriers, attitudinal, social, political, and cultural) that preclude or facilitate employment and return to work. Disappointingly, this is not a new observation. About 20 years ago, a similar statement was made by Trieschmann (47):

> It seems that much of the literature has focused on statements that persons with SCI can work and on the identification of those factors within the person that predict success or failure in employment. However, there are many environmental variables that influence the employment rate, yet little research effort has been directed at the identification of these environmental factors and methods of modifying their effects (p. 123).

This chapter also reviewed outcomes from employment and VR. These included increased psychological adjustment, life satisfaction, quality of life, and well being. These findings varied particularly with respect to productivity. Postdisability productivity was moderately correlated with life satisfaction but life satisfaction was least associated with employment and most associated with perceived control and social support. More research with respect to these variables' role in relation to employment is needed.

Several factors preclude the assimilation of VR services to the extent and level required into our current ways of practicing rehabilitation for persons with SCI. These were pointed out with respect to medical interventions. Starting the process early and with guided communication between physicians, team members, VR counselors, and employers is highly recommended. It is also critical to ensure that all partners are integrated into this process, striving for a similar goal. These partners include schools, insurance case managers, community mental health agencies, and CILs, just to name a few.

Within the VR services provided to persons with SCI, there have been some substantial changes during the past 20 years. Environmental factors are given serious consideration when a counselor conducts a job assessment, evaluation, or adaptation. With the advent of assistive technologies, we are beginning to appreciate factors other than those dependent on the individual. Greater encouragement needs to be given to studies and interventions addressing this critical area of knowledge in rehabilitation. Although these studies and services can be helpful, by themselves they will not influence the employment of persons with SCI unless financial disincentives and broader environmental factors such as negative policies, attitudes, and values are changed accordingly.

ACKNOWLEDGMENTS

We wish to acknowledge the indirect contributions of Robert K. Heinrich, who wrote his doctoral dissertation on this topic. We also acknowledge the efforts of Liina Paasuke and Donald Anderson, who coauthored with Tate and Heinrich a similar chapter published in 1998 on VR, independent living, and consumerism. Selected information from that chapter has been included in this new one (1). Additional contributions for this chapter came from the Spine Program of the University of Michigan Health System and its medical director, Dr. Andrew Haig. Further support came from the Georgia Regional SCI System in Atlanta, Georgia, and the University of Michigan Model SCI Care System, two of the Model SCI Care Systems funded from 1995 to 2000 by the National Institute on Disability and Rehabilitation Research, Office of Special Education and Rehabilitative Services, Department of Education, Washington, DC. Finally, we thank Barbara Roderick for her clerical assistance in the timely preparation of this chapter.

REFERENCES

1. Tate DG, Heinrich RK, Paasuke L, et al. Vocational rehabilitation, independent living and consumerism. In: DeLisa JA, Gans BM, eds. *Rehabilitation medicine: principles and practice,* 3rd ed. Philadelphia: Lippincott–Raven Publishers, 1998:1151–1162.
2. Heinrich RK. *Personality characteristics and vocational outcomes of men with spinal cord injuries* [Unpublished dissertation]. Michigan: University of Michigan; 1995.
3. DeVivo MJ, Rutt RD, Stover SL, et al. Employment after spinal cord injury. *Arch Phys Med Rehabil* 1987;68:494–498.
4. Alfred WG, Fuhrer MJ, Rossi CD. Vocational development following severe spinal cord injury: a longitudinal study. *Arch Phys Med Rehabil* 1987;68:854–857.
5. DeVivo MJ, Fine PR. Employment status of spinal cord injured patients 3 years after injury. *Arch Phys Med Rehabil* 1982;63:200–203.
6. ElGhatit AZ, Hanson RW. Variables associated with obtaining and sustaining employment among spinal cord injured males: a follow-up of 760 veterans. *J Chronic Illness* 1978;31:363–369.
7. Goldberg RT, Freed MM. Vocational development, interests, values, adjustment and rehabilitation outlook of spinal cord patients: four year follow-up. *Arch Phys Med Rehabil* 1976;57:532.
8. Krause JS. The relationship between productivity and adjustment following spinal cord injury. *Rehabil Counseling Bull* 1990;33:188–199.
9. Krause JS. Employment after spinal cord injury. *Arch Phys Med Rehabil* 1992;73:163–169.
10. Crisp R. Locus of control as a predictor of adjustment to spinal cord injury. *Aust Disabil Rev* 1984;1(2):53–57.
11. Crisp R. Return to work after spinal cord injury. *J Rehabil* 1990;56(1):28–35.
12. DeJong G, Branch LG, Corcoran PJ. Independent living outcomes in spinal cord injury: multivariate analyses. *Arch Phys Med Rehabil* 1984;65:66–73.
13. McShane SL, Karp J. Employment following spinal cord injury: a covariance structure analysis. *Rehabil Psychol* 1993;38(1):2–41.
14. Goldberg RT, Bigwood AW. Vocational adjustment after laryngectomy. *Arch Phys Med Rehabil* 1975;56:521–524.
15. Ferington F. Personal control and coping effectiveness in spinal cord injured persons. *Res Nurs Health*, 1986;9:257–265.
16. Trieschmann RB. *Spinal cord injuries: psychological, social, and vocational rehabilitation,* 2nd ed. New York: Demos Publications, 1980.
17. Decker SD, Schultz R. Correlates of life satisfaction and depression in middle-aged and elderly spinal cord–injured persons. *Am J Occup Ther* 1985;39:740–745.
18. Kemp B, Vash C. Productivity after injury in a sample of spinal cord injured persons: a pilot study. *J Chronic Illness* 1971;24:259–275.
19. House JS. *Work stress and social support.* Reading, MA: Addison Wesley.
20. Felton J, Litman M. Study of employment of 222 men with spinal cord injury. *Arch Phys Med Rehabil* 1965;46:809–814.
21. Goldberg RT, Freed MM. Vocational development of spinal cord injury patients: an 8 year follow-up. *Arch Phys Med Rehabil* 1982;63:207–210.
22. Tomassen PC, Post MW, van Asbeck FW. Return to work after spinal cord injury. *Spinal Cord* 2000;38:51–55.
23. Krause JS, Sternberg M, Maides J, et al. Employment after spinal cord injury: differences related to geographic region, gender, and race. *Arch Phys Med Rehabil* 1998;79:615–624.
24. James M, DeVivo MJ, Richards JS. Postinjury employment outcomes among African-American and white persons with spinal cord injury. *Rehabil Psychol* 1993;38:151–164.
25. Krause JS, Crewe NM. Chronologic age, time since injury, and time of measurement: effect on adjustment after spinal cord injury. *Arch Phys Med Rehabil* 1991;72:91–100.
26. Krause JS. Employment after spinal cord injury: transition and life adjustment. *Rehabil Counseling Bull* 1996;39:244–255.
27. Krause JS, Anson CA. Employment after spinal cord injury: relationship to selected participant characteristics. *Arch Phys Med Rehabil* 1996;77:737–743.
28. Fuhrer MJ, Rintala DH, Hart KA, et al. Relationship of life satisfaction to impairment, disability, and handicap among persons with spinal cord injury living in the community. *Arch Phys Med Rehabil* 1992;73:552–557.
29. Rohe DE, Athelstan GT. Vocational interests of persons with spinal cord injury. *J Counseling Psychol* 1982;29:283–291.
30. Rohe DE, Athelstan GT. Change in vocational interests after spinal cord injury. *Rehabil Psychol* 1985;30:131–143.

31. Rohe DE, Krause JS. The vocational interests of middle-aged males with spinal cord injury. *Rehabil Psychol* 1999a:160–175.

32. Rohe DE, Krause JS. The five-factor model of personality: findings in males with spinal cord injury. *Assessment* 1999b;6:203–213.

33. Athelstan GT, Crewe NM. Psychological, sexual, social, and vocational aspects of spinal cord injury: a selected bibliography. *Rehabil Counseling Bull* 1979;22:311–319.

34. Malec J. Personality factors associated with severe traumatic disability. *Rehabil Psychol* 1985;30:165–172.

35. Rohe DE, Malec J. *A traumatic spinal cord injury personality: the new data* [Unpublished manuscript]. Rochester, MN: Mayo Clinic, Department of Psychiatry and Psychology; 1987.

36. Rohe DE. Personality and traumatic spinal cord injury. *Rehabil Rep* 1988;4:3–4.

37. Harris L, et al. *N.O.D/Harris Survey of Americans with Disabilities.* New York: Louis Harris and Associates, 1994.

38. Tate DG. Workers disability and return to work. *Am J Phys Med Rehabil* 1992;71(12):92–96.

39. Kanellos MC. Enhancing vocational outcomes of spinal cord–injured persons: the occupational therapist's role. *Am J Occup Ther* 1985; 39(11):726–733.

40. Haig AJ, Nagy A, LeBreck DB, et al. Patient-oriented rehabilitation planning in a single visit: first-year review of the "Quick" Program. *Arch Phys Med Rehabil* 1993;75:172–177.

41. Haig AJ, Nagy A, LeBreck DB, et al. Outpatient planning for persons with physical disabilities: a randomized prospective trial of physiatrist alone versus a multi-disciplinary team. *Arch Phys Med Rehabil* 1995; 76:341–348.

42. Armstrong T, Haig A, Levine S, et al. The Michigan Rehabilitation Engineering Research Center for Ergonomic Solutions to Employment. Available at: http://umrerc.engin.umich.edu/rerc.htm.

43. Armstrong T, Ahuja V, Franxblau A, et al. *Use of conceptual models for applying ergonomic technologies to overcome barriers to work.* Orlando, FL: Rehabilitation Engineering Society of North America, 2000.

44. Armstrong T, Ahuja V, Franxblau A, et al. *A model system for overcoming physical work barriers.* San Diego, CA: Human Factors Society, 2000.

45. Treanor RB. *We overcame: the story of civil rights for disabled people.* Falls Church, VA: Regal Direct Publishing, 1993.

46. Social Security Administration, Office of the Actuary. *Social Security Disability Insurance Program worker experience* [Actuarial study no 114]. Washington: Social Security Administration, SSA publication no 11-11543, 2000.

47. Trieschmann RB. *Spinal cord injuries.* New York: Pergamon Press, 1980.

22

SEXUAL FUNCTION AND FERTILITY FOLLOWING SPINAL CORD INJURY

TODD A. LINSENMEYER

Although this chapter focuses on sexual function and fertility after spinal cord injury (SCI), it is important to realize that acute SCI can have a significant impact on a person's body image and self-esteem, due to feelings of loss of control over one's life and surroundings. These broader issues should be addressed, in addition to the physical issues of sexual function.

In the acute period after SCI and during rehabilitation, a person experiences a tremendous amount of emotional and physical adjustment, and sexuality issues may not be raised. People with SCI often report that when they were first injured, they received little information on this topic. Therefore, medical professionals dealing with people with SCI must ensure that these issues are presented. Caregivers should inform the person with SCI that it is possible to enjoy a sexual relationship and to have children, opening the door for further detailed discussions. Ideally, classes should be established during rehabilitation that include other people with SCI who have successfully dealt with these sexuality issues.

OVERVIEW OF THE HUMAN SEXUAL RESPONSE CYCLE

Before discussing changes in sexual function after SCI, a clear understanding of the human sexual response cycle in able-bodied people is necessary. A number of physiologic changes occur in men and women during sexual activity. Masters and Johnson (1) determined that these changes occurred in a predictable manner and called this the "human sexual response cycle." Their description of the sexual response cycle was based on laboratory observations of more than 10,000 episodes of sexual activity in 382 women and 312 men. Their study is still considered the most definitive study of physiologic changes that occur with sexual activity.

The human sexual response cycle consists of four phases: the excitement phase, plateau phase, orgasm phase, and resolution phase (1). These represent generalized patterns that occur in women and men. A major difference between men and women is that men have a "refractory period" after orgasm, in which it is not possible to have a full erection or another orgasm. Women do not have a refractory period and may have multiple orgasms (1).

NEUROANATOMY AND PHYSIOLOGY

The Human Sexual Response Cycle in Able-Bodied Men

During the excitement phase, vasocongestion and erection of the penis may occur from psychogenic stimulation (erotic thoughts) or tactile stimulation to the genitalia. Psychogenic erections are mediated through the sympathetic system via the hypogastric plexus (T11-L2). Reflex erections result from sacral stimulation, which is mediated by the parasympathetic nervous system (S2-4). An erection often occurs within 3 to 8 seconds. When there is no stimulation, the penis is flaccid with equilibrium between the arterial inflow and the venous outflow. With stimulation, there is a relaxation of the arteriolar walls within the penis, allowing a rapid influx of blood.

The penis is made up of three compartments, which run up and down the length of the penis (Figs. 22.1 and 22.2). They consist of two corpora cavernosa, which lay side to side, and the corpus spongiosum, which lies underneath and between the two corpora cavernosa. Each corpus cavernosum is composed of a spongy network of endothelial-lined lacunae, which are designed to become engorged with blood to cause an erection. The corpus spongiosum contains a small amount of spongy tissue, as well as the urethra, which runs up its length. It expands at the distal end of the penis, covering the ends of the two corpora cavernosa, forming the glans (head) of the penis.

The spongy tissue within the corpora cavernosa is surrounded by the fascia of the corpora cavernosa. Both corpora cavernosa and the corpus spongiosum are in turn surrounded by a thick nondistensible fascia, the tunica albuginea. This arrangement causes compression of the venous outflow as the lacunae become engorged with blood. The compression of the venous outflow is very important to maintain an erection (2,3). If the excitement phase is prolonged, there is, in addition to penile tumescence, a thickening and elevation of the scrotal sac and partial testicular elevation and vasoconstriction (1). During the plateau phase, there is a further increase in penile and testicular vasocongestion. The testicles become fully elevated and rotated and may become 50% to 100% enlarged. There are secretions of a clear mucoid fluid from the bulbourethral (Cowper) glands, which occur and appear at the urethral meatus. Twenty-five percent of men develop a sex flush of their skin. There is an increase in respiratory rate and pulse.

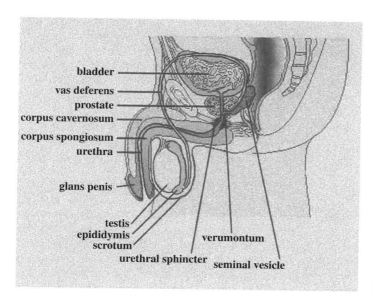

FIGURE 22.1. Male internal genitourinary organs.

During the orgasm phase, ejaculation occurs. Ejaculation is divided into two phases: the emission phase and the ejaculatory phase. The emission phase of ejaculation consists of peristalsis of smooth muscles of the vas deferens, seminal vesicles, and prostate, resulting in secretions traveling out through the ejaculatory ducts and being deposited into the posterior urethra. These events are dependent on sympathetic thoracolumbar outflow from the presacral and hypogastric nerves originating at T10 (thoracic) through L2 (lumbar). At the same time, this sympathetic stimulation via the hypogastric nerves closes the bladder neck. The bladder neck has a preponderance of α-adrenergic receptors, so sympathetic stimulation increases its tone. In this way, the bladder neck functions as a physiologic sphincter,

thereby preventing the ejaculate from going in a retrograde direction. The external sphincter, which is distal to the verumontanum, also remains closed during emission (4).

Also during the orgasm phase of the sexual response cycle, the second part of ejaculation (ejaculatory phase) occurs. This consists of a projectile ejaculate, which is produced by clonic contractions of the bulbospongiosus and ischiocavernous muscles of the pelvic floor (0.8-second intervals for three to four contractions and then slowing for two to four more contractions). This is due to sacral parasympathetic and somatic outflow from the pelvic nerves and pudendal nerves, respectively, originating at S1 through S4. During the ejaculatory phase, the bladder neck remains closed and the external sphincter opens. Because the ejaculatory ducts are between the bladder neck and external urethral sphincter, continued closure of the bladder neck and an opening of the external urethral sphincter produce an antegrade ejaculation. There continues to be an increase in respiratory rate and pulse rate (1,4,5).

The resolution phase is brought about by the sympathetic outflow during ejaculation. This outflow causes a direct contraction of the smooth muscle sinuses, forcing entrapped blood into emissary veins and resulting in decreased rigidity. This in turn promotes further venous outflow and detumescence of the penis (3). There is rapid loss of pelvic congestion. Approximately one third of men have a sweating reaction.

Changes in Human Sexual Response in Men after Spinal Cord Injury

During the excitement phase, men with complete upper motor neuron (UMN) injuries are unable to have psychogenic erections (less than 10%), because the SCI interrupts the pathways going from the brain down to the hypogastric plexus (T11-L2). These men should be able to obtain reflex erections, which are depen-

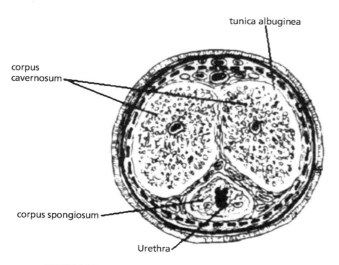

FIGURE 22.2. Transverse section through the penis.

dent on afferent and efferent impulses to and from the sacral spinal cord (S2-4). Studies have shown that more than 90% of men with complete and incomplete UMN lesions can achieve reflexogenic erections. Approximately 50% of men with incomplete UMN lesions can achieve a psychogenic erection (2,6,7). Although most men with UMN lesions are able to obtain reflex erections, these erections are often poorly sustained. Bors and Comarr (2) reported that only 44% of men with complete injuries and 56% of men with incomplete injuries were successful at having intercourse. Another investigator, although not specifying the level or completeness of injury, reported that only 40 (20%) of 186 men with reflex erections were able to have intercourse (6).

In men with complete lower motor neuron (LMN) lesions, reflex erections are believed lost, but up to 12% can achieve reflexogenic erections. Approximately 25% of individuals can develop psychogenic erections and a similar percent reported successful coitus (6). In men with SCI, the orgasm phase (ejaculation phase) of the sexual response cycle is also affected. Using a questionnaire, Talbot (6) found that in 408 men with SCI above T12, 75% reported erections, although only 10% reported having ejaculations. In a series of 529 men with SCI, Bors and Comarr (2) reported that only 5% of men with complete UMN lesions and 18% of those with LMN lesions had ejaculations. Thirty-two percent of men with incomplete UMN lesions, and 70% of men with incomplete LMN lesions had ejaculations. The degree of incompleteness was not specified (2). These authors suggested that patients with complete UMN lesions have less frequent ejaculations because increased parasympathetic sacral outflow inhibits emissions of spermatic fluid into the posterior urethra. This increased parasympathetic sacral outflow in men with UMN lesions may be secondary to the lack of inhibition of the sacral parasympathetic center from the cerebral cortex.

It is generally felt that most men with SCI have anejaculation; however, it is possible that a number of men have retrograde ejaculations. Because retrograde ejaculations would be expected to be undetected, they would therefore be unreported. Retrograde ejaculation may be due to lack of relaxation of the external sphincter (parasympathetic) or lack of closure of the internal bladder neck (sympathetic innervation). Although retrograde ejaculation does not pose a medical risk to the patient, urine contact with sperm has an adverse effect on sperm motility for those wishing to father a child (8).

Treatment Options for Erectile Dysfunction

A full review of erectile dysfunction in SCI has recently been published (9). The first type of treatment for erectile dysfunction was a penile implant. Unfortunately, there is a high complication rate with penile implants in men with SCI. The two most common complications are erosion of the implant out of the penis and infection, which have been reported to occur 8% to 33% of the time (10). Intracavernous injections of papervine (an opioid-related smooth muscle relaxant), phentolamine (an α-adregneric antagonist), and agents such as prostaglandin E₁ (PGE₁) (alprostadil) and prostaglandin E₂ (PGE₂) have been shown to be effective at producing an erection adequate for penetration in both able-bodied men and men with SCI. In one long-term study of 683 able-bodied men, sexual activity was reported to be possible after 94% of alprostadil injections (11). Men with SCI respond much more vigorously to these agents and therefore should received lower doses with careful titration to prevent priapism (prolonged erections requiring immediate treatment) (12,13).

Several agents have been applied topically to the penis with some success. These agents include nitroglycerin paste, minoxidil, and prostaglandins. These agents are not approved by the Food and Drug Administration (FDA) for this use. Intraurethral instillation of alprostadil (PGE₁) has been approved by the FDA (14). However, there are no large studies evaluating its effectiveness in men with SCI. One potential side effect in able-bodied men is hypotension. Therefore, it should be used with caution in men with injuries above T6 that already have low blood pressure. A number of oral agents are under investigation such as α-adrenergic agonists (yohimbine), serotoninergic receptor agonists (trazodone), L-arginine, and apomorphine (14). Sildenafil (Viagra) is an oral agent that has been approved by the FDA for treatment of erectile dysfunction and has been effective in studies for persons with SCI (15–17). However, it may cause symptomatic hypotension (T6 and above). Sildenafil is a selective inhibitor of type 5 (cyclic guanosine monophosphate [cGMP] specific) phosphodiesterase. Its mechanism of action is to decrease the catabolism of cGMP in the corpora cavernosa. The greater concentrations of cGMP within the corpora cavernosa cause smooth muscle relaxation within the sinuses, causing an erection. Sildenafil should be taken 60 minutes before intercourse. Headache is reported to occur in 14% (25-mg dose) to 30% (100-mg dose) of able-bodied men. Flushing has been reported in 13% (25-mg dose) to 20% (100-mg dose) of able-bodied men. These are identical to common signs and symptoms of autonomic dysreflexia, with the addition of severe uncontrolled hypertension during autonomic dysreflexia. Accurate diagnosis is needed because nitrates, which are often used to treat autonomic dysreflexia, can cause severe hypotension after the administration of sildenafil (15).

A vacuum pump and constriction rings can be used if a person has no erection. Negative pressure produced by the pump causes filling of the penis, with the erection maintained by the constriction ring at the base of the penis. Constriction rings alone to occlude venous outflow can be used if a person is having a poorly sustained erection. The erection however is sometimes not satisfactory; the penis may appear distended and may pivot due to the lack of filling below the ring. Premature loss of erection is the most common complaint. The rings should not be kept in place for more than 30 minutes, to prevent skin breakdown of prolonged venous congestion within the penis, and should not be used in men with sickle cell disease. Anticoagulants are a relative contraindication to their use (13).

Impact of Spinal Cord Injury on Male Fertility

As previously discussed, the human sexual response cycle is profoundly affected after SCI. Men wishing to father children are often unable to do so because of erectile and ejaculatory dysfunc-

TABLE 22.1. CAUSES OF POOR SEMEN QUALITY

Recurrent urinary tract infections
Scrotal hyperthermia
Long-term use of certain medications
Stasis of prostatic fluid
Sperm contact with urine (retrograde ejaculation)
Testicular denervation
Changes in the seminal fluid

tion. Even if a man is able to ejaculate, it has been found that semen quality, particularly sperm motility, is significantly impaired in most men after SCI. The exact cause is not known, although a review of the literature noted that various possible factors included recurrent urinary tract infections (UTIs), scrotal hyperthermia due to prolonged sitting in a wheelchair, long-term use of medications, stasis of prostatic fluid, and sperm contact with urine (retrograde ejaculation) (Table 22.1) (13). Other possibilities include the type of bladder management, testicular denervation, and changes in the seminal fluid (18–20). There is probably not one single cause for poor semen quality after SCI, but combinations of the various causes that result in poor semen quality. In an animal model, the Sprague Dawley rat, it has been found that sperm and testicular function undergo a profound decline during the first few weeks after SCI, with only partial recovery 4 to 6 months later (21). Research has shown that there is better sperm quality at least 6 months postinjury and that the semen quality does not decline with time after injury (22). Better sperm quality has been reported in cervical level injuries compared with sperm quality in thoracic level injuries, in men with incomplete injuries, and in men who use reflex voiding (23). Further research is needed to determine which of these factors, unidentified factors, or combination of factors has the most significant impact on semen quality. Until good semen quality can be maintained, assisted reproductive technologies will play an important role in allowing men with SCI to father children.

Parenting Issues for Men with Spinal Cord Injury

Being able to be a parent is an important issue for most people who have SCI. We asked 32 consecutive men who were coming in for routine urologic testing if they would like to have children; 13% of men responded that they would like to father a child "now" and another 67% said that they would like to have a child some time in the future. One study compared adult children reared from age two or younger by fathers with SCI with adult children reared by fathers without SCI. Subjects were matched on sex, father's age, education, and income. Seven objective tests assessed the major areas of psychosocial adjustment, personality, sex role identity, body image, values, interpersonal relationships, physical health patterns, athletic pursuits, recreational activities, and parent–child relations. Adult children of fathers with SCI were as psychologically well adjusted as children reared by fathers without SCI. No evidence was found that during childhood and adolescence, children experienced stigmatiza-

tion from peers by virtue of their father's disability, as has been previously cited in the literature. Children had significantly more positive attitudes toward fathers with SCI than fathers without SCI and responded more quickly and positively to both mothers' and fathers' requests (24,25).

Treatment for Ejaculatory Dysfunction

In men with SCI who want to father a child, there are a number of issues that should be addressed and it is important to do so using a team approach. Typical members of this team include a urologist, physiatrist, gynecologist, andrology lab technician, and in some cases a social worker. The couple should decide the length of time and methods they want to use before beginning to undergo the emotional roller coaster of attempts at having a child. The possibility of adoption should be discussed early, because there is a long waiting list. If adoption is a possibility, this process can be started early in case attempts at obtaining an ejaculate and having a child are unsuccessful.

Many strategies have been attempted to induce an ejaculate. These include the use of pharmacologic agents such as intrathecal neostigmine and subcutaneous physostigmine, vibratory stimulation, electroejaculation, and direct aspiration of fluid from the vas deferens or testicular biopsy (13,26,27). Gutmann and Walsh (26) reported a 59.7% success rate in obtaining ejaculates in 70 men with suprasacral SCI lesions using intrathecal neostigmine. Side effects included headaches, nausea, vomiting, and severe autonomic dysreflexia resulting in death from a cerebral hemorrhage. Intrathecal neostigmine is no longer used because of the invasive method of placement and significant side effects (28). Chapelle et al. (28) reported obtaining an ejaculate in 55.5% (75 of 135) of men with SCI using subcutaneous physostigmine. Fifteen of these men fathered children. All patients developed orthostatic hypotension if they did not remain in a strict decubitus position for 1 hour after the injection. Subcutaneous physostigmine is not being used in the United States to help increase ejaculations.

Vibratory stimulation is another modality that has been used to obtain an ejaculate. In 1965, Sobrero et al. (29) were the first to report the use of vibratory stimulation to obtain an ejaculate in humans, although Brindley (30) was largely responsible for popularizing the use of vibratory stimulation in men with SCI. Using a powerful Ling vibrator, Brindley (30) reported a 77% (48 of 62) success rate at obtaining an ejaculate if the person was more than 6 months postinjury (to ensure the person was out of spinal shock) and had hip flexion when scratching the soles of the feet. The use of a "department store" vibrator yielded a 30% success rate at obtaining an ejaculate. There have been recent advances in vibrator technology. Sonksen et al. (31) evaluated the effect of vibrator amplitude and frequency at obtaining ejaculates in men with SCI. They determined that changing the amplitude from 1 mm to 2.5 mm with a frequency of 100 Hz improved ejaculation rates from 32% to 96% in those with an ejaculation reflex (UMN lesion). Unfortunately, despite improvements, vibratory stimulation is not successful for men who do not have an intact sacral ejaculation reflex. Brackett et al. (32) reported that semen motility is somewhat better after vibratory stimulation (26%) versus electroejaculation (12%). Beckerman et al. (33) reported that side effects occurred in 5.9% of patients treated with vibratory stimulation. Side effects included autonomic dysreflexia (however, most investigators treated patients before vibratory stimulation), painful contractions of abdominal muscles, and superficial trauma to the glans penis resulting in bruising, bleeding, or superficial ulceration (33). Of most concern is significant autonomic dysreflexia. Therefore, men with SCI at or above T6 need to be premedicated and closely monitored during the procedure. A new handheld home unit (Ferticare) with an amplitude of 2.5 mm and frequency of 100 Hz has recently obtained FDA approval. This unit will allow couples to attempt to have children at home. However, those prone to autonomic dysreflexia (i.e., those with injury at T6 and above) should have medical supervision. If unsuccessful at producing a pregnancy due to poor semen quality, assisted reproductive technology can be used on semen obtained at home.

Electroejaculation has been one of the most common methods used to obtain an ejaculate, with excellent success rates (80% to 90%) at obtaining semen. Ohl et al. (18) reported that it was easiest to obtain ejaculates in men with SCI with thoracic level injuries (90% success), compared with men with cervical (60% success) or lumbar (50% success) level injuries (18). As with other techniques to obtain an ejaculate, autonomic dysreflexia is a potential problem in men with SCI above T6 (18). Rutkowski et al. (34) reported that ejaculation occurred in 97% of men with SCI using electroejaculation.

Other methods that have been described include the use of a radio-linked device to stimulate the hypogastric plexus and Teflon-coated needles for transperineal electroejaculation (35, 36). Aspiration of sperm from the vas deferens and testicular biopsies to obtain sperm are two other options that may become more useful. This is a result of new reproductive technologies that require only a few sperm and the ability to preserve sperm by freezing (37).

In general, in men with an intact sacral cord (UMN lesion), vibratory stimulation is usually first attempted. If this is not successful, electroejaculation may be attempted. If a person has an LMN injury, electroejaculation is sometimes successful. If neither of these techniques is successful, aspiration of sperm from the vas deferens or biopsy of the testicle itself may be attempted.

Assisted Reproductive Technologies

Despite poor semen quality, it is still possible for men with SCI to father children due to significant advances and increased availability of assisted reproductive technologies. The simplest method of assisted reproductive technology is intrauterine insemination (IUI) of sperm obtained from the injured man into the woman's uterus. Pregnancy rates per couple using IUI have varied between 10% and 14% (38). *In vitro* fertilization (IVF) has also been used to help achieve pregnancy. IVF has a 30% to 40% livebirth pregnancy success rate. For fertilization to occur, the sperm needs to have reasonable motility. Because a number of men have poor motility, IVF is not an option. One of the newest techniques involves injection of a single sperm directly into the ovum. This technique is called intracytoplasmic sperm injection (ICSI) and has pregnancy rates that are comparable to those of IVF. A significant advantage is that ICSI can be used even if there are very few sperm and if these sperm have poor motility. There is an increase in multiple births using assisted reproductive technology because several fertilized ova are placed in the uterus with the hope that at least one will implant. Birth defects have not been significantly increased with reproductive technologies (39). Overall, approximately 40% of men with SCI who have attempted to father children have done so. Rutkowski et al. (34) reported on the likelihood of pregnancy with the different combination of methods. There is significant optimism that continued advances in IVF, ICSI, and other new assisted reproductive technologies will continue to improve pregnancy rates.

Human Sexual Response Cycle in Women

The female reproductive organs are classified according to location: those that are external and those that are internal. The external organs include the mons pubis, major and minor labia, clitoris, and the vestibule of the vagina and vaginal orifice. The internal female genitalia include the ovaries, fallopian tubes, uterus, and vagina (Fig. 22.3) (5).

During the excitement phase, there is vasocongestion and tumescence of the external genitalia. The beginning of the excitement phase and first measurable sign of sexual arousal is an increase in vaginal epithelial blood flow. Blood flow increases 1.4 to 4 times the normal rate within 10 to 30 seconds of the onset of sexual stimulation, and vaginal lubrication begins to occur (40). This vaginal lubrication is considered to be the immediate counterpart to penile tumescence. This lubrication is felt to result from the increased vaginal blood flow, which creates an engorged condition. This in turn causes increased plasma transudation onto the vaginal epithelium. If this phase is prolonged, there is thickening of the vaginal walls, with expansion of the inner two thirds of the vagina and elevation of the cervix. The lower part of the vagina is supplied by the pudendal nerve (S2-3), whereas the afferent sensory fibers from the upper part of the vagina pass via the splanchnic (parasympathetic) nerves (S2-4) (5).

During the plateau phase, there is prominent vasodilation of the outer third of the vagina (called the orgasmic platform), as well as uterine and cervical elevation. Approximately 75% of women develop a "sex flush." There are also mucoid secretions from the Bartholin gland, analogous to the emission phase of ejaculation in men. During this phase, there is an increase in breast size and nipple erection. There is also an increase in respiratory rate and pulse rate.

During the orgasm phase, there are simultaneous rhythmic contractions of the uterus and of the outer one third of the vagina (orgasmic platform) and anal sphincter. These contractions are initially intense at short intervals (0.8 seconds) and may vary from 3 to 15 at a time. Unlike men, women are able to move back and forth from the plateau phase to the orgasm phase. Alternatively, they may move to the resolution phase.

During the resolution phase, there may be a return to the orgasm phase or gradual loss of pelvic vasocongestion and the vaginal orgasmic platform, as well as loss of clitoral tumescence. The vaginal transudation of fluid ceases and the fluid can be reabsorbed. There is rapid resolution of nipple erection and

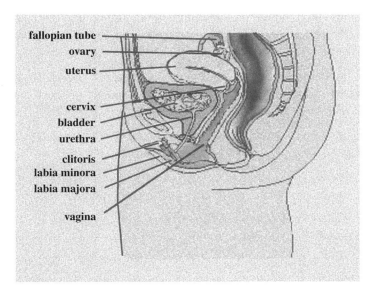

FIGURE 22.3. Anatomy of female internal genitourinary organs.

slower decline in breast size. About 30% to 40% of women have a sweating reaction during this phase.

Changes in Human Sexual Response in Women with Spinal Cord Injury

Until recently, little was known about the female sexual response cycle after SCI. During the excitement phase, it has been traditionally felt that women with complete injuries have predictable changes. Autonomic impulses coming down from the brain cannot pass the level of the lesion, so there should be no "psychogenic" vaginal lubrication (counterpart of erection). However, during the excitement phase, changes may occur above the level of injury, which may include an increase in blood pressure, pulse, and respiration. Because the upper chest receives some innervation from the cervical roots, even women with low complete cervical injuries may have some breast changes and the "sexual flush" above on the chest wall. Stimulation of the genitalia has the potential to cause autonomic dysreflexia in women with injuries at T6 and above (41). In a controlled laboratory setting comparing able-bodied women with women with complete and incomplete SCI, able-bodied women were found to have both psychogenic (audiovisual) and clitoral tactile stimulation that resulted in vaginal vasocongestion, increased vaginal vasoconstriction, and a significant increase in vaginal pulse amplitude (measure of vaginal lubrication) (42,43). Women with complete SCI were able to maintain reflexive (tactile), but not psychogenic, vaginal vasocongestion. They were able to have increased vaginal vasoconstriction and a significant increase in vaginal pulse amplitude (measure of vaginal lubrication) with tactile stimulation. Although women with both complete and incomplete UMN injuries had subjective arousal with audiovisual stimulation, only women with incomplete injuries (intact pinprick sensation, T11-L2) showed an increase in vaginal pulse (psychogenic lubrication) from audiovisual stimulation (43). These findings suggest that women with complete UMN injuries have reflex vaginal lubrication, whereas those with incomplete

SCI may have both psychogenic and reflex vaginal lubrication. The ability to have psychogenic lubrication is dependent on the ability to perceive pinprick sensation in the T11-L2 dermatomes (42,43). It has been proposed that the control of genital responses to psychogenic sexual stimulation is based on the sympathetic nervous system, the cell bodies of which lie at the levels of T11-L2 (44).

With regard to the orgasm phase, it has been noted that even women with complete lesions between C4 and T9 report that they have orgasms (45). Investigators in a controlled laboratory setting found that women with complete SCI experienced awareness of vaginal and cervical stimulation, orgasm, analgesia, and menstrual discomfort. They propose that there may be a functional genital afferent pathway that bypasses the spinal cord and projects directly to the brain via the vagus nerve (45). Approximately 50% of women who could stimulate themselves were able to achieve orgasm (47). The ability was not related to the type or degree of injury, but to the presence of greater sexual knowledge and higher sex drive. There was an increased time needed to achieve the orgasm relative to able-bodied women. Women with SCI at and below the T6 level were also studied in a laboratory setting. Fewer women with SCI at these levels of injury were able to achieve orgasm (44%), compared with able-bodied women (100%) (44). As with direct stimulation of the external genitalia, the onset of an orgasm has the potential to cause autonomic dysreflexia in women with injuries at or above T6 but it has not been documented in a controlled laboratory setting (46,47).

Women with complete LMN injuries, although not evaluated in a controlled laboratory setting, have reported that psychogenic lubrication occurs in up to 25% of women, but not reflex lubrication. Like women with incomplete UMN injuries, women with incomplete LMN injuries may also have both psychogenic and reflex vaginal lubrication (48). Women with complete LMN injuries affecting the S2-5 segments have a decreased ability to achieve orgasm (17%), compared with women with injuries at all other levels and with varying degrees of injury (59%) (44).

Impact of Spinal Cord Injury on Female Fertility and Childbearing

Unlike with men, SCI has not been found to impact adversely on female fertility. Immediately after SCI, amenorrhea occurs in 85% of women with cervical and high thoracic injuries and 50% to 60% of woman overall. Within 6 months postinjury, 50% of women have return of menstruation. The average duration of resumption of menstruation is 4.3 months, with a range of 1 week to 24 months (49). By 1-year postinjury, 90% of women have return of normal menstrual cycles. The same pattern of regularity or irregularity usually returns, although the menstrual cycle sometimes becomes regular. The level and completeness of injury do not appear to influence the menstrual cycle (6,50). Once menses returns, a woman does have the ability to have children. Women should be counseled regarding contraceptive use if they wish to avoid pregnancy. Menarche has been reported to occur normally in girls who have been injured as preadolescents. Women who are approaching menopause and have an SCI are likely to lose their menses (51).

Although fertility is not considered a problem after SCI, a number of potential prenatal, perinatal, and postnatal issues exist that one needs to be aware of in women with SCI (Table 22.2) (52). During the prenatal period, gastric motility normally decreases during pregnancy. This can be a particular problem in a person with a neurogenic bowel and already decreased intestinal motility. UTIs are an important potential complication and close consultation with an obstetrician needs to occur to decide on the best antibiotic if a woman does develop a UTI. Preventative measures include good fluid intake and extra care to prevent kinking of the catheter tubing, resulting in bladder distention in a person with an indwelling catheter, and frequent catheterizations to prevent bladder over-distention in those on intermittent catheterization. We prefer to switch women from "clean" to "sterile" intermittent catheterization using a self-contained "touchless" catheter and bag. There is also a higher risk of deep venous thrombosis during the prenatal and antenatal period, because of restricted venous return from the growing uterus in combination with the person's restricted mobility.

These problems may be a source of autonomic dysreflexia in women with injuries at T6 and above. There is also a risk of diminished respiratory function and possible accumulation of secretions that should be monitored, because the enlarging uterus may cause a decrease in the vital capacity. Premature onset

TABLE 22.2. POTENTIAL COMPLICATIONS OF PREGNANCY AFTER SPINAL CORD INJURY

Prenatal
Constipation, urinary tract infections, decreased vital capacity, deep venous thrombosis, pressure ulcers, increased spasticity, autonomic dysreflexia

Perinatal
Premature delivery, autonomic dysreflexia, deep venous thrombosis, pressure ulcers

Postnatal
Episiotomy skin break down, deep venous thrombosis

of labor is also a problem. Women with injuries at T10 and below do not sense labor pains. Labor may be signaled by an increase in spasticity. In those with injuries above T6, labor may be accompanied by autonomic dysreflexia. Autonomic dysreflexia may be confused with hypertension from preeclampsia and must be differentiated (52). A cesarean section is sometimes needed if there is a pelvic or spinal deformity or uncontrolled autonomic dysreflexia.

In the antenatal period, in addition to the previously stated problems, a high incidence of skin breakdown at the episiotomy site has been found; women are advised to use nonabsorbable sutures and leave them in place for several weeks (53).

Sexuality and Parenting Issues for Women with Spinal Cord Injury

One study reported a general decrease in sexual frequency and sexual desire. However, there was no relation between the extent of injury and whether a subject participated in sexual activities. Participation in activities was found to correlate with pre-SCI habits of subjects (54,55). In another study of 231 women with SCI, 69% were satisfied with their post-injury sexual experiences, although self-confidence, spasticity, and spontaneity were issues. Many women did not feel that they were provided with information about sexuality issues and felt a need for more literature, counseling, and peer support (56).

The literature is lacking regarding the impact of SCI on mothering. The first article that addressed this issue appeared in 1994 (57). Using a questionnaire, investigators evaluated six women with tetraplegia and 20 women with paraplegia, all of whom were in wheelchairs. The above-mentioned parents delivered a total of 47 children. The entire group of women felt that their family roles and relationships between family members did not differ from those of other families. No mothers felt that their children were unable to participate in regular activities because of their SCI. All the children who were able to independently fill out the questionnaire (n = 10) reported that they did not perceive their mothers to be any different from other mothers because of their mother's SCI. Fathers did not report that they felt they had any more responsibilities than fathers with able-bodied women. The above finding is similar to that of an informal study conducted by our department. We asked several women with SCI about the problems they encountered being a parent and having an SCI. None of them were able to think of any problems with childrearing due to their SCI. One noted that she did have problems going on field trips. Another responded that having a child actually provided a motivation to stay healthy. She reported that she couldn't afford not to catheterize her bladder and risk getting a bladder infection because she was so busy with her children.

CONCLUSION

Sexual function is significantly affected by SCI. Many people with SCI report a lack of discussions on this topic during their rehabilitation. It is hoped that further research, advances in treatment, and awareness in this area by caregivers will help people with SCI to have improved treatment options and be better educated in sexual function and infertility after their SCI.

REFERENCES

1. Masters WH, Johnson VE. *The human sexual response.* Boston: Little, Brown and Company, 1966.
2. Bors E, Comarr AE. Neurological disturbances of sexual function with special reference to 529 patients with spinal cord injury. *Urol Surv* 1960;10:191–222.
3. Saenz de Tejada I, Goldstein I, et al. Local control of penile erection: nerves, smooth muscle, and endothelium. *Urol Clin North Am* 1988; 15:9–15.
4. Linsenmeyer TA. Management of male infertility. In: Sipski ML, Alexander CJ, eds. *Sexual function in people with disability and chronic illness.* Gaithersburg, MD: Aspen Publishers, 1997:487–509.
5. Bracket NL, Bloch WE. Neurological anatomy and physiology of sexual function. In: Abae M, Singer C, Weiner WJ, eds. *Sexual dysfunction: a neuro-medical approach.* Armonk: Futura Publishing, 1994:1–8.
6. Talbot HS. The sexual function in paraplegia. *J Urol* 1955;73:91.
7. Comarr AE. Sexual function among the patients with spinal cord injury. *Urol Int* 1970;25:134–168.
8. Linsenmeyer TA, Wilmot C, Anderson RU. The effects of the electro-ejaculation procedure on sperm motility. *Paraplegia* 1989;27:465–469.
9. Monga M, Bernie J, Rajasekaran M. Male infertility and erectile dysfunction in spinal cord injury: a review. *Arch Phys Med Rehabil* 1999; 80:1331–1339.
10. Linsenmeyer TA. Evaluation and treatment of erectile dysfunction following SCI: a review. *J Am Paraplegia Soc* 1991;14:43–51.
11. Linet OL, Ogrine FG. Efficacy and safety of intracavernosal alprostadil in men with erectile dysfunction: the Alprostadil Study Group. *N Engl J Med* 1996;334:873–877.
12. Wyndaele JJ, de Meyer JM, de Sy WA, et al. Intracavernous injection of vasoactive drugs: one alternative for treating spinal cord injury patients. *Paraplegia* 1986;24:271–275.
13. Linsenmeyer TA, Pekash I. Infertility in men with spinal cord injury. *Arch Phys Med Rehabil* 1991;72:747–754.
14. Rivias DA, Chancellor MB. Management of erectile dysfunction. In: Sipski ML, Alexander CJ, eds. *Sexual function in people with disability and chronic illness.* Gaithersburg, MD: Aspen Publishers, 1997:429.
15. Goldstein I, Lue TF, Padma-Nathan H, et al. Oral sildenafil in the treatment of erectile dysfunction. *N Eng J Med* 1998;338:1397–1404.
16. Derry FA, Dinsmore WW, Fraser M, et al. Efficacy and safety all the oral sildenafil (Viagra) in men with erectile dysfunction caused by spinal cord injury. *Neurology* 1988;51:1629–1633.
17. Giuliano F, Hultling C, El-Masry WS, et al. Randomized trial of sildenafil for the treatment of erectile dysfunction in spinal cord injury. *Ann Neurol* 1999;46:15–21.
18. Ohl DA, Bennett CJ, McCabe M, et al. Predictors of success in electroejaculation of spinal cord injured men. *J Urol* 1989;142:1483–1486.
19. Frankel AJ, Ryan EL. Testicular innervation is necessary for the response of plasma testosterone levels to acute stress. *Biol Reprod* 1981; 24:491–495.
20. Brackett NL, Lynne CM, Weizman MS, et al. Endocrine profiles and semen quality of spinal cord injured men. *J Urol* 1994;151:114–119.
21. Linsenmeyer TA, Pogach LM, Ottenweller JE, et al. Spermatogenesis and the pituitary–testicular hormone axis in rats during the acute phase of spinal cord injury. *J Urol* 1994;152:1302–1307.
22. Brackett NL, Ferrell SM, Aballa TC, et al. Semen quality in spinal cord injured men: does it progressively decline postinjury? *Arch Phys Med Rehabil* 1998;79:625–628.
23. Brackett NL, Ferrell SM, Aballa TC, et al. An analysis of 653 trials of penile vibratory stimulation in men with spinal cord injury. *J Urol* 1998;159:1931–1934.
24. Buck FM, Hohmann GW. Personality, behavior, values, and family relations of children of fathers with spinal cord injury. *Arch Phys Med Rehabil* 1981;62:432–438.
25. Buck FM. Parenting by fathers with physical disabilities. In: Haseltine

FP, Cole SS, Gray DA, eds. *Reproductive issues for persons with physical disabilities.* Baltimore: Paul H. Brookes Publishing, 1993:163–185.
26. Gutmann L, Walsh JJ. Prostigmine assessment test of fertility in spinal man. *Paraplegia* 1971;9:39–51.
27. Chapelle PA, Blanquart F, Puech AJ, et al. Treatment of an ejaculation on total paraplegic by subcutaneous injection of neostigmine. *Paraplegia* 1983;21:30–36.
28. Chapelle PA, Roby BA, Yakovleff A, et al. Neurologic correlations of ejaculation and testicular size in men with a complete spinal cord section. *J Neurol Neurosurg Psychiatry* 1998;51:197–202.
29. Sobrero AJ, Harlan ES, Blair JB. Technique for the induction of ejaculation in humans. *Fertil Steril* 1965;16:765–767.
30. Brindley GS. Reflex ejaculation under vibratory stimulation in paraplegic men. *Paraplegia* 1981;19:299–302.
31. Sonksen J, Biering-Sorensen F, Kristensen JK. Ejaculation induced by penile vibratory stimulation in men with spinal cord injuries. The importance of the vibratory amplitude. *Paraplegia* 1994;32:651–660.
32. Brackett NL, Padron OF, Lynne CM. Semen quality of spinal cord injured men is better when obtained by vibratory stimulation versus electroejaculation. *J Urol* 1997;157:151–157.
33. Beckerman H, Becher MD, Lankhorst GJ. The effectiveness of vibratory stimulation in anejaculatory men with spinal cord injury. *Paraplegia* 1993;31:689–699.
34. Rutkowski SB, Geraghty TJ, Hagen DL, et al. A comprehensive approach to the management of male infertility following spinal cord injury. *Spinal Cord* 1999;37:508–514.
35. Brindley GS, Sauerwein D, Hendry WF. Hypogastric plexus stimulators for obtaining semen from paraplegic men. *Br J Urol* 1989;64: 72–77.
36. Ozkurkcugil C, Cardenas D, Hartsell C, et al. Electroejaculation using standard nerve stimulation equipment and Teflon coated needles. *Fertil Steril* 1993;60:1094–1095.
37. Bustillo M, Rajfer J. Pregnancy following insemination with sperm directly aspirated from vas deferens. *Fertil Steril* 1986;46:144–146.
38. Bennett CJ, Seager SW, Vasher EA. Sexual dysfunction and electroejaculation in men with spinal cord injury: review. *J Urol* 1988;139: 453–457.
39. Coulam CB, Opsahl MS, Sherins RJ, et al. Comparison of pregnancy loss patterns after intracytoplasmic sperm injection and other assisted reproductive technologies. *Fertil Steril* 1996;65:1157–1162.
40. Levin RJ. The physiology of sexual function in woman. *Clin Obstet Gynaecol* 1980;7:213–252.
41. Geiger RC. Neurophysiology of sexual response in spinal cord injury. *Sex Disabil* 1979;2:257–266.
42. Sipski ML, Alexander CJ, Rosen RC. Physiological parameters associated with psychogenic sexual arousal in woman with complete spinal cord injuries. *Arch Phys Med Rehabil* 1995;76:811–818.
43. Sipski ML, Alexander CJ, Rosen RC. Physiological parameters associated with psychogenic sexual arousal in woman with incomplete spinal cord injuries. *Arch Phys Med Rehabil* 1997;78:305–313.
44. Sipski ML. Sexual function in women with neurological disorders. *Phys Med Rehabil Clin North Am* 2001;12:78–90.
45. Whipple B, Gerdes CA, Komisaruk BR. Sexual response to self-stimulation in woman with complete spinal cord injury. *J Sex Res* 1996;33: 231–240.
46. Komisaruk BR, Gerdes CA, Whipple B. "Complete" spinal cord injury does not block perceptual responses to genital self-stimulation in woman. *Arch Neurol* 1997;54:1513–1520.
47. Sipski ML, Alexander CJ, Rosen RL. Orgasm in women with spinal cord injuries: a lab based experiment. *Arch Phys Med Rehabil* 1995;76: 1097–1102.
48. Sipski ML, Alexander CJ. Sexuality and disability. In: Delisa JA, Gans B, eds. *Rehabilitation medicine: principles and practice.* New York: Lippincott–Raven Publishers, 1998:1107–1113.
49. Jackson AB, Wadley V. A multi-center study of women's self-reported reproductive health after spinal cord injury. *Arch Phys Med Rehabil* 1999;80:1420–1428.
50. Reame NE. A prospective study of the menstrual cycle and spinal cord injury. *Am J Phys Med Rehabil* 1992;71:15–21.

51. Atterbury JL, Groome LJ. Pregnancy in woman with spinal cord injuries. *Nurs Clin North Am* 1998;33:603–613.
52. Burns AS, Jackson AB. Gynecologic and reproductive issues in women with spinal cord injury. *Phys Med Rehabil Clin N Am* 2001;12:183–187.
53. Verduyn WH. Spinal cord injured women, pregnancy and delivery. *Paraplegia* 1986;24:231–240.
54. Sipski ML, Alexander CJ. Sexual activities, response and satisfaction in women pre and post spinal cord injury. *Arch Phys Med Rehabil* 1994;74:1025–1029.
55. Zwerner J. Yes we have troubles but nobody's listening: sexual issues of women with spinal cord injury. *Sex Disabil* 1982;5:158–171.
56. Charlifue SW, Gehart KA, Menter RR, et al. Sexual issues of woman with spinal cord injuries. *Paraplegia* 1992;30:192–198.
57. Westgren N, Levi R. Motherhood after traumatic spinal cord injury. *Paraplegia* 1994;32:517–523.

23

RECREATIONAL AND THERAPEUTIC EXERCISE AFTER SPINAL CORD INJURY

MARK S. NASH
JOHN A. HORTON III.

Recreational and therapeutic exercises have long been cornerstones in the lives of many individuals living both with and without spinal cord injury (SCI). For those with SCI, these activities are intended to restore, remediate, or rehabilitate so as to enhance function, independence, and health. A justification for these therapies ought to be obvious. With respect to recreational exercise, most people who sustain SCI are young and active at the time of their injury, and their spared motor function may still permit involvement in sports and recreational leisure activities. With respect to therapeutic exercise, those with SCI were found to be at the lowest end of the human fitness spectrum nearly two decades ago and have not significantly increased their fitness in the ensuing years. Thus, although people without SCI have significantly improved their health and fitness, those with SCI have not.

Involvement in sports, recreation, and therapeutic exercise may be limited by motor function spared after injury as well as changes in autonomic function, fuel homeostasis, temperature regulation, and motor skill. In some cases, reintegration of sports and recreation into the lives of those with SCI requires special equipment, training, and opportunities. Similarly, participation in therapeutic exercise may require special adaptive equipment and, in instances of very high injuries, the use of electrical current to initiate purposeful movement of paralyzed muscles. Notwithstanding, there is considerable evidence that involvement in recreational and therapeutic exercise improves the activity, satisfaction, productivity, and health of its participants. Unfortunately, SCI may also increase the risk for injury and hasten the organ system deterioration as patients age with their injury and disability. Whether such imprudent involvement in sports or excessive exercise creates incipient disability, orthopedic deterioration, or neurologic dysfunction has been the topic of considerable discussion in recent years. Thus, this chapter investigates the advantages of exercise and then discusses the opportunities for participation in sports and recreational activities for those with SCI. Opportunities for therapeutic exercise using voluntary and electrically stimulated exercise are examined, and the adaptations to these therapies outlined. It is hoped that the information contained in this chapter will define a variety of interesting activities through which people with SCI can enhance their independence while not promoting injury or hastening of future disability.

THERAPEUTIC EXERCISE AND ITS BENEFITS AFTER SPINAL CORD INJURY

Sedentary lifestyles and low levels of fitness are common among patients with SCI, which may explain the significant risk for cardiovascular mortality now reported for people aging with spinal cord paralysis (1–3). Cross-sectional studies conducted 15 years ago placed survivors of SCI near the lowest end of the human fitness spectrum, with more recent evidence suggesting that people living with paraplegia have remained deconditioned and only marginally more fit than those with tetraplegia (4,5). To place the problem in proper perspective, nearly 25% of healthy young people with paraplegia fail to achieve a peak oxygen consumption of 15 mL·kg·min^{-1} on an arm ergometry stress test, a level of fitness only marginally sufficient to maintain independent living (6). No clinical or scientific evidence suggests that this level of fitness will improve without increasing their daily energy expenditure on a regular basis.

Several reviews published over the past decades have addressed the need for exercise in people living with SCI (7–10). Because many of these individuals now face the realities of their advancing age, the use and complications of exercise in both youth and advancing years after SCI requires examination. Of SCI survivors in the United States, 40% are now 45 years of age or older, and one in four has lived 20 or more years with disability (11). Although once thought of as a "static" medical condition unaffected by the passage of time, SCI is now viewed as a "dynamic" medical condition in patients whose needs, abilities, and limitations constantly change (12,13). These needs may be hastened or intensified by cumulative stresses imposed by decades of wheelchair propulsion, upper extremity weightbearing, and other essential repetitive activities (14,15). As fatigue, pain, weakness, joint deterioration, and even incipient neurologic deficits appear, the performance of essential activities mastered soon after injury (e.g., wheelchair locomotion, transferring, driving, and dressing) can again become challenging (13,16).

These life challenges and the secondary disabilities they foster further test the long-term survivor's adjustment, self-perception, and ability to participate in active, satisfying, productive, and rewarding pursuits (17). Prudent exercise intervention soon after SCI using well-designed exercise programs is clearly one way in which the apparently now-fated effects of longstanding paralysis might be minimized.

Many forms of exercise undertaken by people without SCI are effective for (a) increasing muscle mass, strength, and endurance; (b) reversing deconditioning and its cardiovascular disease risks; (c) lowering body fat; (d) reversing insulin resistance; and (e) attenuating the acute effects of physical stress. Unfortunately, the selection of exercise activities for people with SCI to accomplish the same goals is limited, and the consequences of imprudent exercise are more serious than those experienced by people without disability. It is important, therefore, to identify effective and available exercise activities that reduce the risks for physical dysfunction and cardiovascular diseases sustained by people with SCI while not increasing injury risks or hastening musculoskeletal deterioration. This chapter addresses how individuals with SCI can exercise and the common risks associated with their participation in exercise.

COMPLEX EXERCISE USING ELECTRICALLY STIMULATED CONTRACTIONS OF PARALYZED MUSCLES

Various forms of electrically stimulated exercise are available for use by people with SCI. These include site-specific stimulation of the lower extremities and upper extremities, leg cycling, leg cycling with upper extremity assist (hybrid cycling), lower body rowing, electrically assisted arm ergometry, electrically stimulated standing, and electrically stimulated bipedal ambulation either with or without an orthosis (18–38). Some of these applications can be used to strengthen muscles whose motor function is partially spared by SCI, whereas other applications use electrical current as a neuroprosthesis of the lower extremities and upper extremities (23,34,35,39–41).

Most electrical stimulation devices currently approved for use by the U.S. Food and Drug Administration (FDA) employ surface, not implanted, electrical stimulation. The three most common uses of surface electrical stimulation for exercise in those with SCI are (a) site-specific electrical stimulation of individual body segments, most often the knee extensors; (b) electrically stimulated cycling either with or without upper extremity assistive propulsion; and (c) electrically stimulated ambulation. Qualifications necessary to participate safely in exercise programs have been described, although those with lower motor neuron lesions are generally excluded from participation (26,42).

Cycling Exercise

Electrically stimulated cycling is a process of neuromuscular activation using sequentially activated contractions of the bilateral quadriceps, hamstrings, and gluteus muscles (43). Position sensors placed in the pedal gear provide feedback to a computer microprocessor that initiates muscle-firing sequences in a syner-

gistic pattern and also controls electrical current output necessary to sustain muscle contraction forces and programmed pedal rates (44). Improved fitness and gas-exchange kinetics and increased muscle mass have been reported after training using electrically stimulated cycling (24,28,45–47). For patients with incomplete injuries, mass gains were associated with increased voluntary and electrically stimulated isometric strength and endurance (47). Two specific improvements in circulatory function have also been reported after training. First, the adaptive left ventricular atrophy reported in people with tetraplegia is reversed after cycle training, with near normalization of cardiac mass (48). Second, lower extremity circulation after training is significantly improved, accompanied by a more robust hyperemic response to occlusion ischemia (49). Otherwise, reversal of osteopenia has been observed by some investigators, and an increased rate of bone turnover by another, although the site benefiting from training is usually the lumber spine and proximal tibia, and not the femur, which is most susceptible to fracture (50–52). Not all studies have found a posttraining increase in mineral density for bones located below the level of the lesion, although one of these studies enrolled subjects with longstanding paralysis and osteopenia that is likely irreversible by any known treatment (53). Otherwise, a study examining the appearance of lower extremity joints and joint surfaces using magnetic resonance imaging reported no degenerative changes induced by cycling and less joint surface necrosis than previously reported in sedentary people with SCI (54). Improved body composition favoring increased lean mass and decreased fat mass and an enhancement of whole-body insulin uptake and insulin-stimulated 3-*O*-methyl glucose transport in the quadriceps muscle have been observed (55,56). The latter finding, coupled with a report of increased expression of GLUT-4 transport protein, may be especially important for large numbers of people with SCI who show patterns of insulin resistance (56–58). When combined with simultaneous upper extremity arm ergometry, the acute cardiovascular metabolic responses are more intense and the gains in fitness greater than those observed with lower extremity cycling alone (28,29).

Bipedal Ambulation

The most complex form of electrical stimulation for reanimation of the paralyzed musculoskeleton involves activation of lower extremity muscle to achieve bipedal ambulation. Such stimulation can be used as a neuroprosthesis for those with motor complete injuries, or an assistive neuroprosthesis accompanying body weight support and pharmacologic intervention for those whose muscles can contract under voluntary control but lack strength necessary to support ambulation (34,35,59–62). The latter topic is sufficiently complex to be worthy of separate discussion and will thus not receive further attention herein.

Surface and implantable neuroprostheses for those with unspared motor function have been investigated for nearly 20 years, although the only method currently approved by the FDA uses surface electrical stimulation of the quadriceps and gluteus muscles to maintain an upright stance (35,63,64). The stepping motion for this ambulation neuroprosthesis is produced by a flexor withdrawal reflex initiated by introduction of a nociceptive electrical stimulus over the ipsilateral common peroneal nerve at the head of the fibula. This allows the hip, knee, and ankle to move into flexion, followed by extension of the knee joint initiated by electrical stimulation to the ipsilateral quadriceps muscle group. As muscle fatigue occurs, increasing levels of stimulation can be provided using bilateral switches mounted on the handles of the rolling walker.

Rates of electrically stimulated ambulation are relatively slow and distances of ambulation relatively limited (35,65). These responses are attributable to the inefficient way in which electrical current recruits muscle as well as the need for upper extremity stabilization to maintain upright posture. Despite the limitations of ambulation rate and distance, ambulation distances of up to 1 mile have been reported in some subjects after training (34, 35). Interestingly, upper extremity fitness is enhanced in people trained by electrically stimulated ambulation, despite the targeting of lower extremities for electrically stimulated contractions (34,66). Other adaptations to training include significantly increased lower extremity muscle mass, resting blood flow, and augmented hyperemic responses to an ischemic stimulus (67, 68). Despite these positive benefits, no change in bone mineralization of the lower extremity has been observed (69). In addition, use of these devices requires some trunk stabilization; they are thus seldom used in individuals with injuries above the midthoracic spine (34).

Voluntary Arm Exercise Training

There is clear evidence that upper extremity exercise conditioning results in increased peak oxygen uptake, although the magnitude of the increase varies based on level of spinal lesion (70–84). It is thus possible for people with low tetraplegia to train on an arm ergometer, although special measures must be taken to affix the hands to an ergometer. It is understood that gains in endurance and work capacity of subjects training with tetraplegia do not approach those of their paraplegic counterparts (85). Thus, level of injury is a key determinant of the extent to which gains in fitness are made after SCI (86,87).

Although the fitness benefits of arm training are widely reported for people with paraplegia, their performance is limited by circulatory dysregulation accompanying thoracic SCI (88–90). It is widely reported that individuals with injuries below the level of sympathetic outflow at the T1 spinal level have a significantly lower stroke volume (SV) at rest and during exercise than people without paraplegia, as well as a higher resting heart rate (HR) (91–93). The significant elevation of resting and exercise HR is reported by many investigators to compensate for a lower cardiac SV imposed by any or all of the following: pooling of blood in the lower extremity venous circuits, diminished venous return, or frank circulatory insufficiency (92,94). Additionally, higher resting catecholamine levels and exaggerated catecholamine responses to physical work have been reported in paraplegics with middle thoracic (T5) cord injuries. These resting and exercise catecholamine levels exceed those of both high-level injury paraplegics and healthy people without SCI (95,96). Hypersensitivity of the supralesional spinal cord is believed to regulate this unusual adrenergic state and dynamic, which contrasts the downregulation of adrenergic functions observed in people with high thoracic and cervical cord lesions (95, 96). To date, downregulation of adrenergic responses to exercise has been reported after training conducted by subjects with tetraplegia, but not paraplegia (97).

Hjeltnes first reported an excessive cardiovascular "strain" in people with paraplegia as an exaggerated percentage of HR reserve needed to satisfy physical responses to work challenge (88). Others have since reported similar findings and have included circulatory dysregulation imposed by mid-thoracic paraplegia as a limiting factor in the performance of activities of daily living (93,98,99). This finding is consistent with reports in which subjects with paraplegia require higher levels of oxygen consumption to perform at the same work intensity as subjects without SCI (79,89,93,95,100). As the sympathetic nervous system regulates hemodynamic and metabolic changes accompanying exercise, the elevated oxygen consumption and HR response to work in paraplegics with injuries below T5 may be a consequence of the reported adrenergic overactivity in people with paraplegia (95, 96,101). Thus, although the performance of physical activities by people with paraplegia is compromised by orthopedic and muscular decline of the shoulder complex, it is also limited by the unique and insufficient circulatory responses imposed by thoracic SCI, by impaired work capacities, and by the excessive oxygen cost of the subpeak work.

Among the most important benefits of arm exercise in people with paraplegia is a positive association between fitness and cardiovascular risk. One such study examined the relationship between peak oxygen consumption ($\dot{V}O_{2\,peak}$) attained on arm exercise and serum lipids, lipoproteins, and apolipoproteins in nine subjects with SCI (4). Significant inverse relationships were observed between $\dot{V}O_{2\,peak}$ and the following: total cholesterol ($Chol_{TOT}$)–to–high-density lipoprotein cholesterol (HDL-C) ratio; serum triglycerides (TG); and the low-density lipoprotein cholesterol (LDL-C)–to–HDL-C ratio. Direct significant association was found between $\dot{V}O_{2\,peak}$ and the HDL-C–to–apolipoprotein A-1 ratio. These findings suggest a direct association between cardiovascular risk indices and fitness similar to that observed for people without paraplegia. In a second study, blood samples were analyzed for $Chol_{TOT}$, TG, HDL-C, and LDL-C in subjects undergoing wheelchair ergometry training conducted at either 50% to 60% or 70% to 80% of the HR reserve. The high-intensity training group alone experienced increased HDL-C with decreased TG, LDL-C, and $Chol_{TOT}$–to–HDL-C ratio (78). High intensities, duration, and frequencies of exercise training may be required to invoke beneficial exercise-related lipid and lipoprotein changes in people without disability (102). These findings suggest that similar higher intensities may also be required to effect desirable reductions of elevated blood lipids commonly reported in people with paraplegia.

Despite the apparent logic for doing so, few studies have examined exercise strengthening of the upper extremities of people with paraplegia. In a study of Scandinavian men (most of whom had incomplete low thoracic lesions), a weight-training program with special emphasis on the triceps (for elbow extension during crutch walking) was undertaken for 7 weeks with modest but significant increases in $\dot{V}O_{2\,max}$ observed after training, accompanied by increased strength of the triceps brachii (103). Another study examined the effects of high-intensity arm ergometry conducted at 80 revolutions per minute in subjects assigned to high intensity (70% of their $\dot{V}O_{2\,peak}$) or low intensity (40% of their $\dot{V}O_{2\,peak}$) for 20 or 40 minutes per session, respectively (104). Strength gains were limited to subjects assigned high-intensity training and occurred only in the shoulder joint extensors and elbow flexors. Otherwise, no changes in shoulder joint abduction or adduction strengths were reported, and none of the muscles that move or stabilize the scapulothoracic articulation or chest were stronger after training. These results suggest that arm crank exercise is ineffective as a training mode for upper extremity strengthening because it fails to target muscles most involved in performance of activities of daily living.

Although one study has reported strengthening of five subjects with paraplegia and five with tetraplegia three times weekly for 9 weeks using a hydraulic fitness machine, exercises were limited to two maneuvers: (a) chest press, chest horizontal row; and (b) shoulder press, latissimus pull (105). Significant increases in $\dot{V}O_2$ and power output measured by arm ergometry testing were observed at the conclusion of the study, although no testing was conducted that directly measured strength gain in any muscle groups undergoing training. Also, the maneuvers used for training employed concentric but not eccentric actions, which neglected the need for eccentric strength in the performance of activities of daily living.

Another study focused the training on strengthening the scapular retractor muscles, comparing seated rowing and a standardized scapular retraction exercise, and did so only for concentric actions (106). The authors found that higher levels of retractor activation were obtained during retro than forward wheelchair locomotion and suggested that rowing was effective for improving scapular retractor activity and cardiorespiratory fitness. A recent study observed a decrease in subject-reported shoulder joint pain after resistance training when using elastic bands, although upper extremity strength was not examined as a study outcome (107).

We believe that greater emphasis needs to be placed on strengthening of people with SCI as well as testing of hypotheses that increased strength attenuates pain and either preserves or improves function as people age with SCI.

HAZARDS AND COMPLICATIONS ASSOCIATED WITH RECREATIONAL AND THERAPEUTIC EXERCISE

Complications arising from exercise are unfortunately omitted from most chapters and monographs examining the benefits of exercise in people with SCI. Special consideration is required when designing, instituting, or performing exercise programs for people with SCI. Some of the risks encountered will be similar to those experienced by people without paralysis, although complications such as general overuse may be exaggerated in people with SCI, and their occurrence will likely compromise daily activities to a far greater extent than similar injuries arising in people without SCI.

Trauma, Accidents, and Reinjury

Heightened awareness and prevention, better equipment, better training programs, and skilled individuals all decrease the likeli-

hood that injury will be sustained during sports competition and recreation. Nonetheless, it is plausible that such participation can result in secondary injury to the spine, spinal cord, or other body parts. Although no evidence has suggested that activity restrictions are warranted for those with SCI, several reports have documented the various and common injuries in sports for people with disabilities and their prevention. There has not been much documentation concerning these types of injuries among people with SCI who participate in sports activities; however, it is well documented that winter skiing, hockey, and other recreational activities are causes of SCI in people who had not been previously injured. Such injuries, for a person with an existing spinal cord injury, may alter the level of function or cause as yet unknown effects on body systems. For example, air embolism and the effects of extended decompression have been reported to alter neurologic function in people with and without SCI. Given that the influence of injury on the paralyzed body is more profound than that in those without physical disability and that the rates of healing are slower, prudence must be exercised in risking additional injury due to trauma.

Upper Extremity Injuries, Pain, and Deterioration

Individuals with paraplegia commonly depend on their upper extremities for daily activities including wheelchair locomotion, body transfers, and weight shifts for pressure ulcer prevention. Thus, the consequences and necessary treatments for shoulder pain and injury affect independence. The most commonly reported symptom of upper extremity physical dysfunction among people with SCI is upper extremity pain, and the most common site is the shoulder joint (108–114). This is also the location for commonly experienced rotator cuff dysfunction and tears as well as impingement (115,116). Although a single cause of shoulder pain has not been identified, many studies attribute pain to deterioration and injury resulting from insufficient shoulder strength, range, and endurance (113–115,117).

Pain that accompanies wheelchair locomotion and other wheelchair activities reportedly interferes with functional activities, including, but not limited to, upper extremity weightbearing for transfers, high-resistance muscular activity in extreme ranges of motion, wheelchair propulsion up inclines, and frequent overhead activities (108,112–114). All instigate or exacerbate shoulder pain (115). Several studies have examined activities that cause (or worsen) upper extremity pain and have reported that wheelchair propulsion and depression transfers cause the most pain and increase the intensity of existing pain more than other daily activities (83,108,112) (see chapters 16 and 26 for a full review). Given evidence that wheelchair locomotion is a major source of pain and dysfunction in people with SCI, one must question its use as the basis for the design of an exercise training program, unless this training is specific to an athletic event in which training specificity and skill acquisition are sought.

Special warnings for people undergoing upper extremity exercise are warranted. The most serious of these is overuse injury of the arms and shoulders (114,118,119). As noted, the shoulder joints are ill designed to perform locomotor activities but must do so in individuals unable to walk. As the upper extremities must also be used to perform the essential activities of wheelchair propulsion, weight relief, and depression transfers, injuries to the arms may profoundly influence normal daily activities in people with SCI (120,121).

Immune Suppression and Infections

A spinal level–dependent immune dysfunction has been reported after spinal cord injury by various investigators (122–130). Specific immune deficiencies affected by SCI are detailed in chapter 15. Notwithstanding, significant depression of T- and B-cell function has been reported in people without SCI undergoing intense and prolonged exercise (131). Further, an association has been defined between this immune deficiency and increased illness and infection susceptibility reported after athletic competitions (132). Given that people with SCI may start with increased susceptibility due to immune dysfunction and experience organ system dysfunction of the lungs and bladder that normally leads to infection, intense work may worsen their immune profiles and place them at greater risk for infection. To date, a single study has examined the effects of wheelchair racing on subjects with paraplegia and has found suppression of natural killer (NK) cell function and heightened levels of the stress hormone cortisol following racing, which resolved almost 24 hours after completion of exercise (133). Interestingly, the depressed NK cell function reported acutely after SCI is attenuated by moderate activity rather than complete inactivity, suggesting that the intensity of activity may determine whether improved or depressed immune function accompanies physical activity (126,132). Because infection susceptibility may also be related to competition stress and overtraining just before competition, training schedules that provide consistent intensities and duration may decrease the likelihood of an adverse outcome of sports participation (134).

Thermal Dysregulation

Individuals with SCI often lack vasomotor and sudomotor responses below the level of injury and are thus challenged to maintain thermal stability in both hot and cold environments (135–137). Altered sensation below the level of injury may also delay preventive measures normally taken when tissues become numb or frozen during winter sports. The same considerations should be taken when exercising in an environment controlled for temperature and humidity (138,139). Those who participate in outdoor exercise should be especially careful to prevent hyperthermia by paying attention to hydration and, if possible, limiting the duration and intensity of activities performed in intemperate environments. Proper clothing is of extreme importance.

Electrical Current

Several special concerns are engendered for individuals who are exercising under the control of electrical current. The foremost concern involves episodes of autonomic hyperreflexia, which can occur in individuals having injuries above the T6 spinal cord

level (140,141). Because the sympathetic system above this level is partially dissociated from the inhibitory influences of brain control, the nociceptive effects of electrical current may provoke a reflex adrenergic response, with accompanying crisis hypertension (141–143). The recognition of these episodes, withdrawal of the offending stimulus, and the possible administration of a fast-acting peripheral vasodilator may be critical in preventing serious medical complications. In such cases, prophylaxis with a slow calcium-channel antagonist or α_1-selective adrenergic antagonist may be needed (144–146). It should be cautioned that wheelchair racers sometimes induce dysreflexia as an ergogenic aid by restricting urine outflow through a Foley catheter, although such practices may be risky (147). Otherwise, fracture and joint dislocation may be caused by asynergistic movement of limbs against the force imposed by either electrical stimulation or the device used for exercise (148). These activities are therefore contraindicated for individuals with severe spasticity or spastic response to the introduction of electrical current (26). Postexercise hypotension may result from lost vasomotor responses to orthostatic repositioning, although these episodes can abate after upper limb training (149). Otherwise, skin burns may be caused by electrical stimulation, which are normally prevented through use of fresh electrodes with surfaces completely covered by gel conductor.

RECREATIONAL AND SPORTS ACTIVITIES

Most professionals trace the evolution of sports for this population to Sir Ludwig Guttmann at the Stoke Mandeville Hospital in England. By involving young people who sustained injury during World War II, Sir Guttmann and colleagues used sporting events as a rehabilitation tool to facilitate recovery and re-entry into society. In 1948, the first Stoke Mandeville Games, which originally involved only disabled British veterans, were held. The evolution of this competition had a broad impact on people with SCI. In 1952, the first international competition for wheelchair athletes occurred under the Stoke Mandeville sponsorship. This event also sparked the formation of the International Stoke Mandeville Games Federation (now named the International Stoke Mandeville Wheelchair Sports Federation), which has subsequently established links to the International Olympic Committee.

Beginning in 1960, 400 athletes from 23 countries participated in the first Paralympic Games held in conjunction with the Olympic Games in Rome, Italy. This event has continued, and since the 1988 games in Seoul, South Korea, the Paralympic Games have been held in the same venue about 2 weeks after the Olympic Games. The games in Sydney, Australia (2000) included about 5,000 athletes from 128 countries competing in 18 events. The Salt Lake Winter Games of 2002 are slated to stage competition in six winter sports. The International Paralympic Committee now touts representation of more than 10,000,000 disabled athletes worldwide (150). Two major national organizations representing most of the wheelchair athletes, Wheelchair Sports USA and Disabled Sports USA, boast 3,500 and 60,000 participants in their respective memberships (151, 152).

Recreational Activities

In the United States, with the 1990 passage of the Americans with Disabilities Act, any new public access facility is required to provide access to the disabled population (153). This has facilitated participation in numerous recreational activities by the disabled. Around the world, increasing awareness of the abilities and interests of this population has allowed for greater access as well. Currently, most recreational activities are virtually unlimited in their accessibility to the disabled. Common activities include fishing, bowling, golf, hand cycling, swimming, and sailing. Sports that enjoy lesser participation include horseback riding, mountain climbing, karate, scuba diving, water skiing, white water kayaking, sky diving, and flying (Figs. 23.1, 23.2, and 23.3). Many of these activities can be pursued on a competitive as well as recreational level. Table 23.1 contains a representative list, with the affiliated websites, of the associated United States organizations related to a wide variety of recreational sports activities.

Within each of these activities, there is a relative need for adaptive equipment. Some activities, such as billiards or bowling, require minimal adaptations for those with paraplegia; however, for individuals with high-level tetraplegia, adaptive devices are required and available. This is true of fishing as well as hunting. Many states have enacted special legislative initiatives to ensure that the most neurologically involved of people can participate in hunting activities. For snow skiing activities, adaptive skiing platforms must be used to facilitate participation. The designs of these platforms have improved substantially in recent years and are quite functional in performing their tasks and often compatible with conventional ski lift equipment. Many companies specialize in production of adaptive equipment to provide increased participation in recreational activities. Like sports in a broader sense, recreational activities now have become a common ground of participation that should continue to facilitate this same integration in the workplace and schoolroom as well.

Competitive Activities

Wheelchair sports have elevated from a curiosity involving a few disabled soldiers in the 1940s to well-established, high-performance competitive events involving thousands of athletes from all over the world. The scope of events included in the Paralympics has also expanded significantly. Just as it was once thought that women did not have the endurance to allow competition in full-court basketball or a marathon, wheelchair athletes were limited to short propulsion distances. As the technology of competition wheelchairs has progressed, the distances have expanded, and competition is now held for both sexes in the 5,000-meter, 10,000-meter, and marathon distances. Performance in all Paralympic events has also consistently improved over the years, similar to the able-bodied competition, with times for events dramatically decreased as training, technique, technology, and fitness improve in these highly trained athletes.

This chapter discusses three key areas of sports participation: sports organizational structure, rules and classification systems, and equipment changes for enhanced participation. Each of these areas has been key in promoting success achieved by wheelchair athletes.

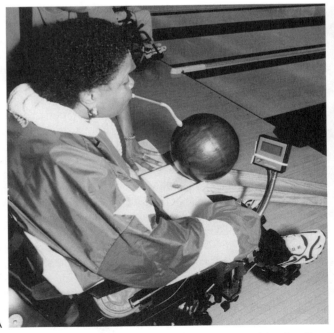
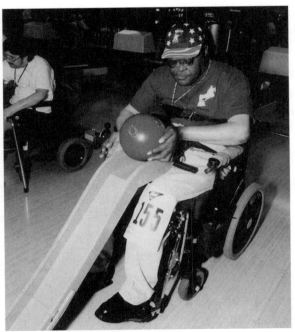

FIGURE 23.1. A,B; Leisure sports activity. Bowling: Two different levels of tetraplegia. (Courtesy of Sports 'N Spokes/Paralyzed Veterans of America.)

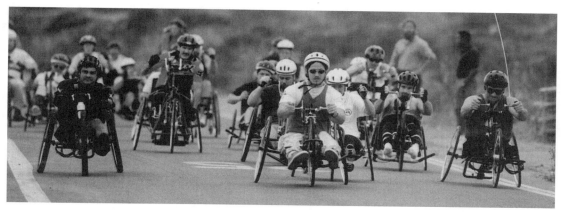

FIGURE 23.2. Hand cycling. (Courtesy of Sports 'N Spokes/Paralyzed Veterans of America.)

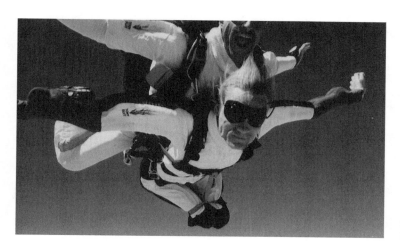

FIGURE 23.3. Skydiving. (Courtesy of Sports 'N Spokes/Paralyzed Veterans of America.)

TABLE 23.1. RECREATIONAL SPORTS—U.S. ORGANIZATIONS

Activities	Website
Aerobics—Disabled Sports USA	www.dsuas.org
American Canoe Association	www.acanet.org
Bowling—American Wheelchair Bowling Association	www.amwheelchairbowl.qpg.com
Billiards—National Wheelchair Billiards	www.nwpainc.com
Camping—National Park Services, Office of Special Programs	www.nps.gov
Disabled Sports—USA	www.dsusa.org
Flying—International Wheelchair Aviators	www.wheelchairaviators.org
Freedom's Wings International	www.freedomswings.org
Fishing—Paralyzed Veterans of America	www.pva.com
Handicapped Scuba Association	www.hsascuba.com
Horseback Riding—North American Riding for the Handicapped Association	www.narha.org
Hunting—NRA Disabled Shooting Services	www.nrahq.org
POINT—Paraplegics on Independent Nature Trips	www.turningpoint1.com
Sailing—National Ocean Access Project	www.dsusa.org
Special Olympics International	www.specialolympics.org
U.S. Rowing Association	www.usrowing.org
U.S. Wheelchair Swimming, Inc.	www.wsusa.org
Water Sports—American Water Ski Association	www.usawaterski.org
Wheelchair Sports—USA	www.wsusa.org

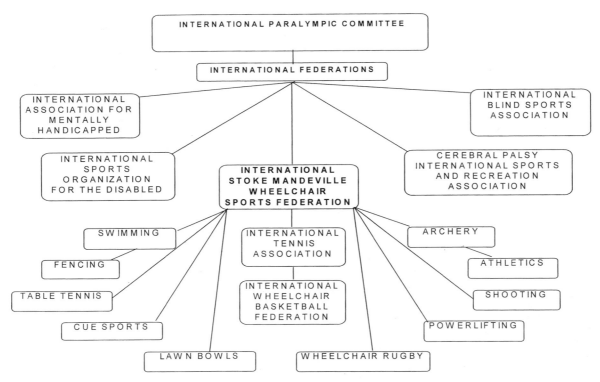

FIGURE 23.4. International Paralympic Sports Organization.

Organization

The International Olympic Committee has established the International Paralympic Committee (IPC) as the international representative organization for all athletes with disabilities (Fig. 23.4). The IPC coordinates international sporting events, including the world championships and Paralympic Games. It also functions as an international non-profit organization made up of 160 individual national paralympic committees and five disability-specific international sports federations. With respect to the individuals with tetraplegia and paraplegia, the International Stokes Mandeville Wheelchair Sports Federation is the specific International Sports Federation that governs the activities of competition. Beneath the umbrella of the Stokes Mandeville Wheelchair Sports Federation are the International Federations for tennis, wheelchair basketball, archery, athletics, shooting, powerlifting, wheelchair rugby, lawn bowling, cue sports, table tennis, fencing, and swimming (Fig. 23.1). All of these international organizations have associated national organizations with which they are loosely affiliated.

The United States Olympic Committee (USOC) was the first and only national committee designated to assume the responsibilities as the United States Paralympic Committee (USPC) (Fig. 23.5). This is accomplished through the Committee on Sports for the Disabled (COSD). Six national organizations for people with disabilities are associated with the COSD. These include organizations for blind athletes, the Special Olympics for the cognitively impaired, cerebral palsy athletes, dwarf competitors, and amputee athletics. It is through Wheelchair

Sports USA that most paraplegic and tetraplegic competitors are represented. These U.S. organizations are loosely affiliated with their respective international counterparts. The sport-specific national organizations controlled by Wheelchair Sports USA are listed in Table 23.2.

An additional organization with strong representation by athletes with spinal cord injury is Disabled Sports USA, which was established in 1967 by disabled Vietnam veterans. This organization offers nationwide sports rehabilitation programs to anyone with a permanent disability, including visual impairments, amputations, dwarfism, multiple scoliosis, head injury, cerebral palsy, other neuromuscular and orthopedic conditions, and SCI. Activities organized by Disabled Sports USA include snow skiing as well as fitness and special sports events. Disabled Sports USA is a member of the U.S. Paralympic Committee and is the national governing body of winter sports for all athletes with disabilities and of summer sports for amputee athletes.

Many other regional and sport-specific wheelchair and disabled sports organizations provide a national base for competitive activities. More specific information regarding the goals, activities, and participatory restrictions can be found at the websites for each of the parent U.S. Disabled Sports Organizations, which are listed in Table 23.1.

Collegiate Level Sports

Intercollegiate competition within the United States dates its beginnings to 1959 when the National Wheelchair Basketball

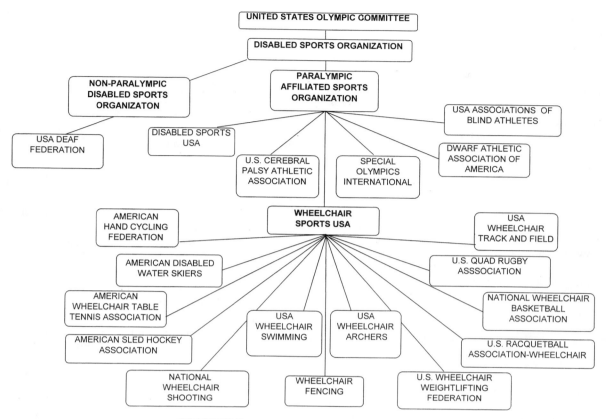

FIGURE 23.5. USA Paralympic Sports Organization.

Association (NWBA) was formed. The competitions held by the NWBA sparked the interest of a number of midwestern colleges, and in 1970, four universities (Southwest State University–Minnesota, Southern Illinois University, University of Wisconsin–Whitewater, and University of Illinois) organized the NWBA Intercollegiate Conference. The first intercollegiate basketball tournament was held in 1977. The NWBA has subsequently reorganized as the National Wheelchair Basketball Association Central Intercollegiate Division. The six-member institutions (the listed schools plus Edinboro University in Pennsylvania and University of Texas–Arlington) and three-affiliate institutions (Oklahoma State University, University of Arizona, and Wright State University), offer varying levels of competitive athletics. All offer wheelchair basketball competition, and some

TABLE 23.2. COMPETITIVE SPORTS—U.S. ORGANIZATIONS

Activities	Website
Wheelchair Archery, USA	www.wsusa.org
Wheelchair Athletics of the USA	www.wsusa.org
National Wheelchair Basketball Association	www.nwba.org
International Wheelchair Basketball Federation	www.iwbf.org
U.S. Fencing Association	www.usfa.org
Association of Disabled American Golfers	www.toski.com/golf/adag/
American Handcycle Association	www.ushf.org
American Sled Hockey Association	www.sledhockey.org
U.S. Quad Rugby Association	www.quadrugby.com
International Wheelchair Tennis Federation	www.itftennis.org
American Wheelchair Table Tennis Association	www.wsusa.org
National Wheelchair Softball	www.wsusa.org
U.S. Wheelchair Swimming	www.usa-swimming.org
United States Wheelchair Weightlifting	www.wsusa.org

provide for a much wider interaction. Athletes from the Central Intercollegiate Division have consistently represented their respective national teams in the Paralympic Games and in World Championship activities. The member organization websites show full listings of their athletic offerings.

In contrast to the NCAA, the Central Intercollegiate Division of the NWBA provides for no organized scholarship "skill-based" programs. Financial aid through grants, academic scholarship, tuition waiver programs, and so forth is member institution specific, and most financial assistance is provided through vocational rehabilitation programs and individual student loan programs. Most of these wheelchair and disabled sports activities are not sponsored by athletic departments of their respective institutions, and all member institutions currently provide these sporting activities through their student services and recreation departments. To achieve a more inclusive program, most of these member institutions also offer a variety of recreational opportunities for disabled students as well as the cited higher-level competitive activities. These programs are not unlike intramural programs sponsored by most athletic departments within the NCAA member institutions.

Classification and Disability Categories

Athletes with disability differ widely in their impairments. Conducting competition among these different athletes is challenging if one is to make these competitions fair. Classification is the method used to address the relative uniqueness of these widely differing athletes and to level the playing field of their competition.

Originally, competitors were segregated into a disability classification. An example of disability-type classification might be quadriplegic, C5 level versus paraplegic, T12 level. This method would not allow interimpairment competition despite relative functional similarities. This method of diagnosis-specific classification is evolving, and in most cases, athletes are now placed in a classification based on their functional ability. This method takes into consideration an athlete's ability to perform sport-related tasks. In doing so, people with different disability categories, such as cerebral palsy and paraplegia, can be placed in the same event, such as a 1,500-meter wheelchair race or 100-meter freestyle swim, because they have similar sport-related function.

The process of classification is rather complex. Specially trained observers and often a panel of evaluators are used to classify disabled athletes. A classification is also not "set in stone." The classification is performed a number of times throughout the athlete's career, and competitors may actually move into different classifications depending on their increase or decrease of function, acquisition of skill, or functional deterioration. During the Paralympic Games, classification documents are submitted by the athletes and verified by officials. Often, some of these athletes are reclassified during the course of the competition based on their observed function. Reclassification efforts may cause a challenge by the athlete, and therefore, a protest system is in place to reconsider the accuracy and fairness of the evaluation.

Of the 18 medal sports at the 2000 Paralympic games, Judo and goal ball were limited to participation by vision-impaired athletes only. Similarly, football (soccer) was played by cerebral palsy athletes only. The remaining sports-specific classification systems allow for interdisability group competitions. Examples of classification systems and criteria are described next.

Archery

Classification is divided into three standard classes: archery standing; archery wheelchair 1 (people with poor or nonexistent trunk control); and archery wheelchair 2 (people with lower-body paralysis or absence and have trunk control).

Track and Field Athletics

These classifiers are rather complex in name: T11 to T54 and F11 to F58, with "T" denoting track classifications and "F" denoting field classifications (Fig. 23.6). Examples include classes 11 to 13, which cover the visual impairment category; class 20 covers intellectually disabled athletes; classes 32 to 38 cover cerebral palsied athletes of differing levels; and classes 51 to 58 cover the different levels of spinal cord injury. Some of the examples in this section are T51, which describes mild weakness in the shoulders, able to bend elbows normally, limited ability to straighten elbows, can bend the wrist backward but not forward, no movement in the fingers, no trunk or leg function; T54, with describes normal arm and hand function, trunk function from some to normal, and some leg function possible; F51, which classifies athletes with mild weakness in the shoulders, able to bend the elbows normally, limited ability to straighten elbows, can bend the wrist backwards but not forward, no movements to the fingers, no truck or leg function; and finally, F58, which describes normal arm and hand function, normal trunk function, and can have more leg function than allowable for an F57 athlete.

Wheelchair Basketball

Individual players are assigned a point value from 1 to 4.5 depending on their physical function. The points for the collective

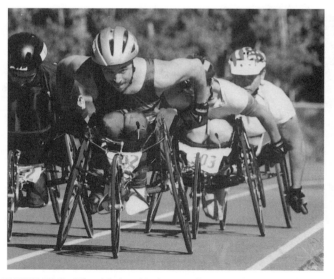

FIGURE 23.6. Wheelchair athletics—track racing. (Courtesy of Sports 'N Spokes/Paralyzed Veterans of America.)

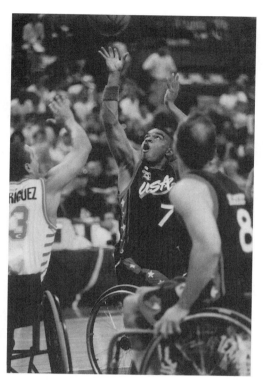

FIGURE 23.7. Wheelchair basketball. (Courtesy of Sports 'N Spokes/ Paralyzed Veterans of America.)

Wheelchair Tennis

Wheelchair tennis players must be diagnosed as having a mobility-related disability and must have a permanent or substantial total loss of function in one or two lower extremities. Sponsors of tennis competitions specify no other eligibility requirements.

Sitting Volleyball

A maximum of one minimum disability player is allowed on the court at any one time, with the remainder of the team requiring a higher level of disability. Different classes include the following:

Class A: minimal disability, including amputation of fingers, shortening of one arm or leg, fusion of an ankle or wrist, as well as high-level cerebral palsy.
Class B: middle-level disability, related to skills and functions required for volleyball, including below-the-elbow and transtibial amputations and other comparable disabilities.
Class C: severely impaired, including above-elbow or transfemoral amputations and other comparable impairments.

Wheelchair Rugby (Quad Rugby)

Players are grouped within a point system ranging from 0.5 to 3.5 points based on the highest level of functional ability (Fig. 23.8). The 0.5 range classifies the ability to scoop a ball on to the lap, and to use the back quarter of the wheel to stop, start, or turn. The person usually passes the ball forward and to the side with a two-hand toss and has poor balance. The person with 3.5 points has some trunk function, is stable in the wheelchair, and has very good ball control. The four players on the court must have a maximum of 8 points, in sum, to compete.

Winter Sports

Functional classifications are based on medical documentation and disability of the athlete. This is based on observation during practice or competition as well as functional tests, including (a)

team members are summed and must total less than 14 points for all five players on the court at any one time. Subclassifications are given when a player falls between classes, and a ½ point above or below a particular classification is allowed; however, the team total of 14 points on the court at any one time does not change (Fig. 23.7).

Powerlifting

Athletes are classified by weight classes, and all disabilities compete together. Wheelchair athletes must have a minimum 10% loss of function in their lower limbs, must be able to extend the arms fully with no more than a 20-degree loss of range with either elbow, and must be able to perform an approved lift according to the powerlifting rules.

Shooting

Two main classifications for shooting exist. Pistol and rifle competitors classified as SH1 do not require a shooting stand, whereas the designation SH2 is reserved for competitors lacking the ability to support the weight of the weapon with their arms and requiring a shooting stand.

Swimming

Swimming allows for competition within all disabilities categories. S1 to S10 performers have physical disability; S11 to S13 have visual impairment, and S14 swimmers have a cognitive impairment. The prefix S within a classification system denotes freestyle, backstroke, and butterfly. SB denotes the breaststroke, and SM is used for the individual medley.

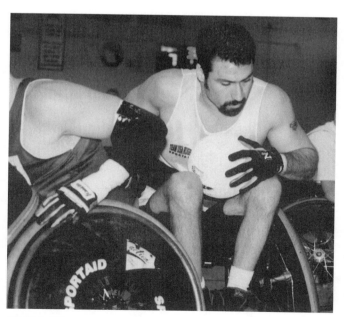

FIGURE 23.8. Quad rugby. (Courtesy of Sports 'N Spokes/Paralyzed Veterans of America.)

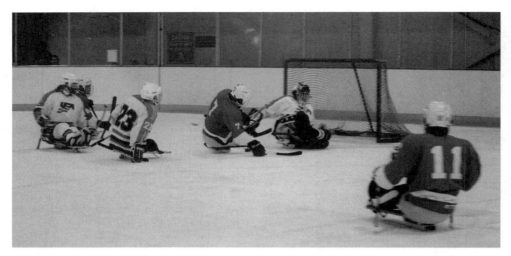

FIGURE 23.9. Sledge hockey. (Courtesy of Sports 'N Spokes/Paralyzed Veterans of America.)

test of hand, arm, and shoulder function, including strength, flexibility, coordination, and range of movement; (b) sitting balance in the sagittal plane; (c) sitting balance in the frontal plane; and (d) sitting balance in the frontal and sagittal planes with assessment and stability of the trunk and pelvic motions.

A standardized testing board performs all of these functional tests before the event. Examples of winter sports include ice sledge speed racing, Nordic sledge hockey (Fig. 23.9), and skiing (Fig. 23.10).

Complete classification guidelines for all sports involved in the Paralympic Sports movement are available at their website, *www.paralympic.org/ipc/handbook.*

Equipment Considerations

Technologic advancement has been directly linked to improved performance in the nondisabled population. From body suits

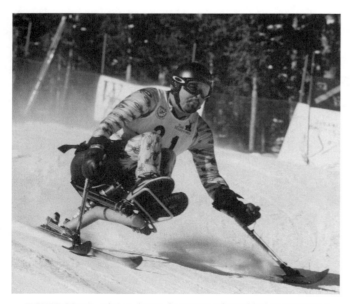

FIGURE 23.10. Alpine skiing. (Courtesy of Disabled Sports USA.)

used in swimming and speed skating to new materials employed for pole-vaulting poles and skis, these and other advances have meant dramatic changes in sport performance. This link may be even stronger when it comes to the performance of wheelchair competitors.

In the past, heavy wheelchairs with fixed armrests, sling seats, and hard rubber tires were used for all events. Beginning in 1967, the University of Illinois wheelchair basketball team began using pneumatic tires and lighter-weight stainless steel "sports chairs." This resulted in two successive national championships, in part because of superior technology (154). In the late 1970s and early 1980s, three companies were formed, which have transformed the concept of the wheelchair. These companies, Quickie Designs (Fresno, California), Shadow (Longmont, Colorado), and Sopur (Malsch/HD, Germany), all began rethinking the concept of the wheelchair. Lighter, stronger, and directed to sport specific usage, these wheelchairs continue to evolve (155).

Specific chair types are now recognized:

Racing wheelchairs. Racers now almost exclusively use a three-wheeled configuration with variable wheelbases depending on the racing event (sprint versus endurance). These custom chairs are tightly fitted to the athletes, who are positioned, generally in a kneeling position, to maximize the propulsive stroke with significantly less consideration for handling characteristics.

Basketball wheelchairs. Ultra-lightweight rigid frames with antitip devices in the front and sometimes in the rear as well. These chairs use high-pressure pneumatic tires that have spoke guards in place and are mounted with significant camber. The participant is limited in the maximum seat height (Fig. 23.11).

Tennis wheelchairs. Wheelchair tennis is a very fast sport requiring the ultimate in agility for the wheelchair user. These chairs have a single front caster with two rear wheels positioned with extreme degrees of camber to increase maneuverability and maximize lateral stability. The athlete is positioned with "pinch," causing the trunk to lean toward the thighs, which enhances balance and control. These chairs often have handles to assist the player in leaning and reaching tasks and to enhance racquet power.

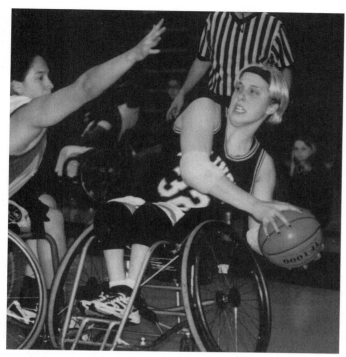

FIGURE 23.11. Example of a wheelchair basketball wheelchair (note camber, front rigging, and clear spoke guards). (Courtesy of Sports 'N Spokes/Paralyzed Veterans of America.)

Quad rugby chairs. This sport combines elements of team handball and rugby and is played by athletes with limited upper extremity function. Significant contact is permitted, and the chairs reflect this function. The rear wheels are radically cambered to increase stability and improve handling, but also help to shield the players' upper extremities from contact. A protective framework extends across the front of the chair to protect the lower extremities. The players are also positioned with extreme levels of "pinch" to facilitate stability and maneuverability.

Hand cycles. These devices are among the fastest-growing recreational activities for wheelchair users. The user is in a seated position with legs extended and propels the device with a crank apparatus and gearing similar to a conventional bicycle. More akin to a recumbent bicycle, these devices are unique in that they use the upper extremities for propulsion, steering, and gearing (156).

CONCLUSIONS

Individuals living with SCI experience severe physical deconditioning, significant musculoskeletal decline, and elevated risk for cardiopulmonary diseases. Many could benefit from sustained reconditioning exercise. Those with higher levels of cord injury may require electrical stimulation to perform exercise, which poses special restrictions on use and unique risks from participation. Nonetheless, qualified individuals benefit from chronic exercise through improved cardiovascular and musculoskeletal function. Positive benefits of training on bone density, regulation of orthostatic tolerance, and affect have been reported in

studies with limited numbers of subjects, and require well-controlled investigations for confirmation. Those with spared motor control of the upper extremity can perform arm or wheelchair exercises and participate in recreational sports. Greater emphasis needs to be placed on strengthening the upper extremity to preserve shoulder and arm functions for performance of daily living as these individuals age with their paralysis. Risk for injury or illnesses associated with imprudent exercise must be managed to ensure that the desirable benefits of physical activity can be sustained.

This chapter has presented activities of therapeutic and recreational exercise as separate entities, although such may not always be the case. Many individuals performing therapeutic exercise improve their fitness to the point of seeking participation in recreational exercise, or select activities that allow them to enjoy fraternity and fitness with others. Conversely, many individuals participating in recreational sports benefit through better fitness and health. The challenge remains, as in people without disability, to create a lifetime commitment to the maintenance of health and a healthy lifestyle, which includes adequate exercise. Whether this goal is accomplished by therapeutic exercise without competition or by competition that benefits the mind and body is unimportant. More important is that people with SCI understand the benefits of both, participate as their interest and abilities allow, and avail themselves of resources that will allow them safe and fulfilling participation in either.

Organizations that facilitate and foster participation with an extremely wide variety of activities have been discussed. Technology has advanced and has become much more readily available as the wheelchair industry matures and satisfies demand of the public for better equipment that satisfies more diverse sports and health needs. This allows participants to increase function, improve performance, and decrease risk for injury. Finally, with increased participation and improved access to facilities, options for participating in an active lifestyle exist in any type of setting—from the most leisurely activity to the most aggressive competition—and at any age—from junior sports teams to collegiate-level involvement to masters events. The opportunities are available and should be taken to maximize the enjoyment life affords as a healthy individual no matter what level of ability.

REFERENCES

1. Bauman WA, Adkins RH, Spungen AM, et al. Is immobilization associated with an abnormal lipoprotein profile? Observations from a diverse cohort. *Spinal Cord* 1999;37:485–493.
2. Washburn RA, Figoni SF. High density lipoprotein cholesterol in individuals with spinal cord injury: the potential role of physical activity. *Spinal Cord* 1999;37:685–695.
3. Berg A, Keul J, Ringwald G, et al. Physical performance and serum cholesterol fractions in healthy young men. *Clin Chim Acta* 1980;106:325–330.
4. Bostom AG, Toner MM, McArdle WD, et al. Lipid and lipoprotein profiles relate to peak aerobic power in spinal cord injured men. *Med Sci Sports Exerc* 1991;23:409–414.
5. Dearwater SR, LaPorte RE, Robertson RJ, et al. Activity in the spinal cord-injured patient: an epidemiologic analysis of metabolic parameters. *Med Sci Sports Exerc* 1986;18:541–544.
6. Noreau L, Shephard RJ, Simard C, et al. Relationship of impairment and functional ability to habitual activity and fitness following spinal cord injury. *Int J Rehabil Res* 1993;16:265–275.

7. Davis GM. Exercise capacity of individuals with paraplegia. *Med Sci Sports Exerc* 1993;25:423–432.

8. Figoni SF. Perspectives on cardiovascular fitness and SCI. *J Am Paraplegia Soc* 1990;13:63–71.

9. Glaser RM. Exercise and locomotion for the spinal cord injured. *Exerc Sport Sci Rev* 1985;13:263–303.

10. Phillips WT, Kiratli BJ, Sarkarati M, et al. Effect of spinal cord injury on the heart and cardiovascular fitness. *Curr Probl Cardiol* 1998;23:641–716.

11. Gerhart KA, Bergstrom E, Charlifue SW, et al. Long-term spinal cord injury: functional changes over time. *Arch Phys Med Rehabil* 1993;74:1030–1034.

12. Menter RR. Aging and spinal cord injury: implications for existing model systems and future federal, state, and local health care policy. In: *Spinal Cord Injury: the model.* Proceedings of the National Consensus Conference on Catastrophic Illness and Injury. Atlanta, GA, The Georgia Regional Spinal Cord Injury Care System, Sheperd Treatment of Spinal Injuries, Incorporated, 1990.

13. Zola IK. Toward the necessary universalizing of a disability policy. *Milbank Q* 1989;67[Suppl 2, Pt 2]:401–428.

14. Curtis KA, Drysdale GA, Lanza RD, et al. Shoulder pain in wheelchair users with tetraplegia and paraplegia. *Arch Phys Med Rehabil* 1999;80:453–457.

15. Ohry A, Shemesh Y, Rozin R. Are chronic spinal cord injured patients (SCIP) prone to premature aging? *Med Hypotheses* 1983;11:467–469.

16. Waters RL, Sie IH, Adkins RH. The musculoskeletal system. In: *Aging with spinal cord injury.* New York: Demos Publications, 1993:53–72.

17. Gerhart KA, Bergstrom E, Charlifue SW, et al. Long-term spinal cord injury: functional changes over time. *Arch Phys Med Rehabil* 1993;74:1030–1034.

18. Figoni SF, Glaser RM, Rodgers MM, et al. Acute hemodynamic responses of spinal cord injured individuals to functional neuromuscular stimulation-induced knee extension exercise. *J Rehabil Res Dev* 1991;28:9–18.

19. Rodgers MM, Glaser RM, Figoni SF, et al. Musculoskeletal responses of spinal cord injured individuals to functional neuromuscular stimulation-induced knee extension exercise training. *J Rehabil Res Dev* 1991;28:19–26.

20. Billian C, Gorman PH. Upper extremity applications of functional neuromuscular stimulation. *Assist Technol* 1992;4:31–39.

21. Bryden AM, Memberg WD, Crago PE. Electrically stimulated elbow extension in persons with C5/C6 tetraplegia: a functional and physiological evaluation. *Arch Phys Med Rehabil* 2000;81:80–88.

22. Mulcahey MJ, Betz RR, Smith BT, et al. Implanted functional electrical stimulation hand system in adolescents with spinal injuries: an evaluation. *Arch Phys Med Rehabil* 1997;78:597–607.

23. Scott TR, Peckham PH, Keith MW. Upper extremity neuroprostheses using functional electrical stimulation. *Baillieres Clin Neurol* 1995;4:57–75.

24. Hooker SP, Figoni SF, Rodgers MM, et al. Physiologic effects of electrical stimulation leg cycle exercise training in spinal cord injured persons. *Arch Phys Med Rehabil* 1992;73:470–476.

25. Nash MS, Bilsker MS, Kearney HM, et al. Effects of electrically-stimulated exercise and passive motion on echocardiographically-derived wall motion and cardiodynamic function in tetraplegic persons. *Paraplegia* 1995;33:80–89.

26. Ragnarsson KT, Pollack S, O'Daniel W Jr, et al. Clinical evaluation of computerized functional electrical stimulation after spinal cord injury: a multicenter pilot study. *Arch Phys Med Rehabil* 1988;69:672–677.

27. Krauss JC, Robergs RA, Depaepe JL, et al. Effects of electrical stimulation and upper body training after spinal cord injury. *Med Sci Sports Exerc* 1993;25:1054–1061.

28. Mutton DL, Scremin AM, Barstow TJ, et al. Physiologic responses during functional electrical stimulation leg cycling and hybrid exercise in spinal cord injured subjects. *Arch Phys Med Rehabil* 1997;78:712–718.

29. Raymond J, Davis GM, Climstein M, et al. Cardiorespiratory responses to arm cranking and electrical stimulation leg cycling in people with paraplegia. *Med Sci Sports Exerc* 1999;31:822–828.

30. Laskin JJ, Ashley EA, Olenik LM, et al. Electrical stimulation-assisted rowing exercise in spinal cord injured people: a pilot study. *Paraplegia* 1993;31:534–541.

31. Cameron T, Broton JG, Needham-Shropshire B, et al. An upper body exercise system incorporating resistive exercise and neuromuscular electrical stimulation (NMS). *J Spinal Cord Med* 1998;21:1–6.

32. Davis R, Houdayer T, Andrews B, et al. Paraplegia: prolonged closed-loop standing with implanted nucleus FES-22 stimulator and Andrews' foot-ankle orthosis. *Stereotact Funct Neurosurg* 1997;69:281–287.

33. Triolo RJ, Bieri C, Uhlir J, et al. Implanted functional neuromuscular stimulation systems for individuals with cervical spinal cord injuries: clinical case reports. *Arch Phys Med Rehabil* 1996;77:1119–1128.

34. Graupe D, Kohn KH. Functional neuromuscular stimulator for short-distance ambulation by certain thoracic-level spinal-cord-injured paraplegics. *Surg Neurol* 1998;50:202–207.

35. Klose KJ, Jacobs PL, Broton JG, et al. Evaluation of a training program for persons with SCI paraplegia using the Parastep 1 ambulation system: part 1. Ambulation performance and anthropometric measures. *Arch Phys Med Rehabil* 1997;78:789–793.

36. Kobetic R, Triolo RJ, Marsolais EB. Muscle selection and walking performance of multichannel FES systems for ambulation in paraplegia. *IEEE Trans Rehabil Eng* 1997;5:23–29.

37. Ferguson KA, Polando G, Kobetic R, et al. Walking with a hybrid orthosis system. *Spinal Cord* 1999;37:800–804.

38. Phillips CA, Gallimore JJ, Hendershot DM. Walking when utilizing a sensory feedback system and an electrical muscle stimulation gait orthosis. *Med Eng Phys* 1995;17:507–513.

39. Carroll SG, Bird SF, Brown DJ. Electrical stimulation of the lumbrical muscles in an incomplete quadriplegic patient: case report. *Paraplegia* 1992;30:223–226.

40. Dimitrijevic MM. Mesh-glove. 1. A method for whole-hand electrical stimulation in upper motor neuron dysfunction. *Scand J Rehabil Med* 1994;26:183–186.

41. Mulcahey MJ, Smith BT, Betz RR. Evaluation of the lower motor neuron integrity of upper extremity muscles in high level spinal cord injury. *Spinal Cord* 1999;37:585–591.

42. Phillips CA. Medical criteria for active physical therapy: physician guidelines for patient participation in a program of functional electrical rehabilitation. *Am J Phys Med* 1987;66:269–286.

43. Glaser RM. Functional neuromuscular stimulation: exercise conditioning of spinal cord injured patients. *Int J Sports Med* 1994;15:142–148.

44. Petrofsky JS, Phillips CA. The use of functional electrical stimulation for rehabilitation of spinal cord injured patients. *Cent Nerv Syst Trauma* 1984;1:57–74.

45. Hooker SP, Scremin AM, Mutton DL, et al. Peak and submaximal physiologic responses following electrical stimulation leg cycle ergometer training. *J Rehabil Res Dev* 1995;32:361–366.

46. Barstow TJ, Scremin AM, Mutton DL, et al. Changes in gas exchange kinetics with training in patients with spinal cord injury. *Med Sci Sports Exerc* 1996;28:1221–1228.

47. Scremin AM, Kurta L, Gentili A, et al. Increasing muscle mass in spinal cord injured persons with a functional electrical stimulation exercise program. *Arch Phys Med Rehabil* 1999;80:1531–1536.

48. Nash MS, Bilsker S, Marcillo AE, et al. Reversal of adaptive left ventricular atrophy following electrically-stimulated exercise training in human tetraplegics. *Paraplegia* 1991;29:590–599.

49. Nash MS, Montalvo BM, Applegate B. Lower extremity blood flow and responses to occlusion ischemia differ in exercise-trained and sedentary tetraplegic persons. *Arch Phys Med Rehabil* 1996;77:1260–1265.

50. BeDell KK, Scremin AME, Perell KL, et al. Effects of functional electrical stimulation-induced lower extremity cycling on bone density of spinal cord-injured patients. *Am J Phys Med Rehabil* 1996;75:29–34.

51. Mohr T, Podenphant J, Biering-Sorensen F, et al. Increased bone mineral density after prolonged electrically induced cycle training of paralyzed limbs in spinal cord injured men. *Calcif Tissue Int* 1997;61:22–25.

52. Bloomfield SA, Mysiw WJ, Jackson RD. Bone mass and endocrine adaptations to training in spinal cord injured individuals. *Bone* 1996; 19:61–68.

53. Leeds EM, Klose KJ, Ganz W, et al. Bone mineral density after bicycle ergometry training. *Arch Phys Med Rehabil* 1990;71:207–209.

54. Nash MS, Tehranzadeh J, Green BA, et al. Magnetic resonance imaging of osteonecrosis and osteoarthrosis in exercising quadriplegics and paraplegics. *Am J Phys Med Rehabil* 1994;73:184–192.

55. Hjeltnes N, Aksnes AK, Birkeland KI, et al. Improved body composition after 8 wk of electrically stimulated leg cycling in tetraplegic patients. *Am J Physiol* 1997;273:R1072–1079.

56. Hjeltnes N, Galuska D, Bjornholm M, et al. Exercise-induced overexpression of key regulatory proteins involved in glucose uptake and metabolism in tetraplegic persons: molecular mechanism for improved glucose homeostasis. *FASEB J* 1998;12:1701–1712.

57. Bauman WA, Spungen AM. Disorders of carbohydrate and lipid metabolism in veterans with paraplegia or quadriplegia: a model of premature aging. *Metabolism* 1994;43:749–756.

58. Duckworth WC, Solomon SS, Jallepalli P, et al. Glucose intolerance due to insulin resistance in patients with spinal cord injuries. *Diabetes* 1980;29:906–910.

59. Barbeau H, Ladouceur M, Norman KE, et al. Walking after spinal cord injury: evaluation, treatment, and functional recovery. *Arch Phys Med Rehabil* 1999;80:225–235.

60. Norman KE, Pepin A, Barbeau H. Effects of drugs on walking after spinal cord injury. *Spinal Cord* 1998;36:699–715.

61. Remy-Neris O, Barbeau H, Daniel O, et al. Effects of intrathecal clonidine injection on spinal reflexes and human locomotion in incomplete paraplegic subjects. *Exp Brain Res* 1999;129:433–440.

62. Stein RB, Belanger M, Wheeler G, et al. Electrical systems for improving locomotion after incomplete spinal cord injury: an assessment. *Arch Phys Med Rehabil* 1993;74:954–959.

63. Graupe D, Salahi J, Kohn KH. Multifunctional prosthesis and orthosis control via microcomputer identification of temporal pattern differences in single-site myoelectric signals. *J Biomed Eng* 1982;4: 17–22.

64. Kralj A, Bajd T, Turk R. Electrical stimulation providing functional use of paraplegic patient muscles. *Med Prog Technol* 1980;7:3–9.

65. Gallien P, Brissot R, Eyssette M, et al. Restoration of gait by functional electrical stimulation for spinal cord injured patients. *Paraplegia* 1995; 33:660–664.

66. Jacobs PL, Nash MS, Klose KJ, et al. Evaluation of a training program for persons with SCI paraplegia using the Parastep 1 ambulation system. 2. Effects on physiological responses to peak arm ergometry. *Arch Phys Med Rehabil* 1997;78:794–798.

67. Jaeger RJ. Lower extremity applications of functional neuromuscular stimulation. *Assist Technol* 1992;4:19–30.

68. Nash MS, Jacobs PL, Montalvo BM, et al. Evaluation of a training program for persons with SCI paraplegia using the Parastep 1 ambulation system. 5. Lower extremity blood flow and hyperemic responses to occlusion are augmented by ambulation training. *Arch Phys Med Rehabil* 1997;78:808–814.

69. Needham-Shropshire BM, Broton JG, Klose KJ, et al. Evaluation of a training program for persons with SCI paraplegia using the Parastep 1 ambulation system. 3. Lack of effect on bone mineral density. *Arch Phys Med Rehabil* 1997;78:799–803.

70. Cowell LL, Squires WG, Raven PB. Benefits of aerobic exercise for the paraplegic: a brief review. *Med Sci Sports Exerc* 1986;18:501–508.

71. Davis GM, Kofsky PR, Kelsey JC, et al. Cardiorespiratory fitness and muscular strength of wheelchair users. *Can Med Assoc J* 1981;125: 1317–1323.

72. Davis GM, Shephard RJ, Leenen FH. Cardiac effects of short term arm crank training in paraplegics: echocardiographic evidence. *Eur J Appl Physiol* 1987;56:90–96.

73. DiCarlo SE, Supp MD, Taylor HC. Effect of arm ergometry training on physical work capacity of individuals with spinal cord injuries. *Phys Ther* 1983;63:1104–1107.

74. Franklin BA. Exercise testing, training and arm ergometry. *Sports Med* 1985;2:100–119.

75. Franklin BA. Aerobic exercise training programs for the upper body. *Med Sci Sports Exerc* 1989;21:S141–148.

76. Gass GC, Watson J, Camp EM, et al. The effects of physical training on high level spinal lesion patients. *Scand J Rehabil Med* 1980;12: 61–65.

77. Hoffman MD. Cardiorespiratory fitness and training in quadriplegics and paraplegics. *Sports Med* 1986;3:312–330.

78. Hooker SP, Wells CL. Effects of low- and moderate-intensity training in spinal cord-injured persons. *Med Sci Sports Exerc* 1989;21:18–22.

79. Knutsson E, Lewenhaupt-Olsson E, Thorsen M. Physical work capacity and physical conditioning in paraplegic patients. *Paraplegia* 1973; 11:205–216.

80. Miles DS, Sawka MN, Wilde SW, et al. Pulmonary function changes in wheelchair athletes subsequent to exercise training. *Ergonomics* 1982;25:239–246.

81. Pachalski A, Mekarski T. Effect of swimming on increasing of cardio-respiratory capacity in paraplegics. *Paraplegia* 1980;18:190–196.

82. Pollock ML, Miller HS, Linnerud AC, et al. Arm pedaling as an endurance training regimen for the disabled. *Arch Phys Med Rehabil* 1974;55:418–424.

83. Taylor AW, McDonell E, Brassard L. The effects of an arm ergometer training programme on wheelchair subjects. *Paraplegia* 1986;24: 105–114.

84. Yim SY, Cho KJ, Park CI, et al. Effect of wheelchair ergometer training on spinal cord-injured paraplegics. *Yonsei Med J* 1993;34: 278–286.

85. DiCarlo SE. Effect of arm ergometry training on wheelchair propulsion endurance of individuals with quadriplegia. *Phys Ther* 1988;68: 40–44.

86. Drory Y, Ohry A, Brooks ME, et al. Arm crank ergometry in chronic spinal cord injured patients. *Arch Phys Med Rehabil* 1990;71: 389–392.

87. Hjeltnes N. Cardiorespiratory capacity in tetra- and paraplegia shortly after injury. *Scand J Rehabil Med* 1986;18:65–70.

88. Hjeltnes N. Oxygen uptake and cardiac output in graded arm exercise in paraplegics with low level spinal lesions. *Scand J Rehab Med* 1979; 9:107–113.

89. Hooker SP, Greenwood JD, Hatae DT, et al. Oxygen uptake and heart rate relationship in persons with spinal cord injury. *Med Sci Sports Exerc* 1993;25:1115–1119.

90. Hopman MT, Oeseburg B, Binkhorst RA. The effect of an anti-G suit on cardiovascular responses to exercise in persons with paraplegia. *Med Sci Sports Exerc* 1992;24:984–990.

91. DeBruin MI, Binkhorst RA. Cardiac output of paraplegics during exercise. *Int J Sports Med* 1984;5:175–176.

92. Hopman MT, Pistorius M, Kamerbeek IC, et al. Cardiac output in paraplegic subjects at high exercise intensities. *Eur J Appl Physiol* 1993; 66:531–535.

93. Van Loan MD, McCluer S, Loftin JM, et al. Comparison of physiological responses to maximal arm exercise among able-bodied, paraplegics and quadriplegics. *Paraplegia* 1987;25:397–405.

94. Hopman MT, Oeseburg B, Binkhorst RA. Cardiovascular responses in paraplegic subjects during arm exercise. *Eur J Appl Physiol* 1992; 65:73–78.

95. Schmid A, Huonker M, Barturen JM, et al. Catecholamines, heart rate, and oxygen uptake during exercise in persons with spinal cord injury. *J Appl Physiol* 1998;85:635–641.

96. Schmid A, Huonker M, Stahl F, et al. Free plasma catecholamines in spinal cord injured persons with different injury levels at rest and during exercise. *J Auton Nerv Syst* 1998;68:96–100.

97. Bloomfield SA, Jackson RD, Mysiw WJ. Catecholamine response to exercise and training in individuals with spinal cord injury. *Med Sci Sports Exerc* 1994;26:1213–1219.

98. Janssen TW, van Oers CA, van der Woude LH, et al. Physical strain in daily life of wheelchair users with spinal cord injuries. *Med Sci Sports Exerc* 1994;26:661–670.

99. Janssen TW, van Oers CA, Veeger HE, et al. Relationship between physical strain during standardised ADL tasks and physical capacity in men with spinal cord injuries. *Paraplegia* 1994;32:844–859.

100. Davis GM, Shephard RJ. Cardiorespiratory fitness in highly active versus inactive paraplegics. *Med Sci Sports Exerc* 1988;20:463–468.

101. Ehsani AA, Heath GW, Martin WH 3d, et al. Effects of intense exercise training on plasma catecholamines in coronary patients. *J Appl Physiol* 1984;57:155–159.

102. Blair SN, Kohl HW 3d, Paffenbarger RS Jr, et al. Physical fitness and all-cause mortality: a prospective study of healthy men and women. *JAMA* 1989;262:2395–2401.

103. Nilsson S, Staff PH, Pruett ED. Physical work capacity and the effect of training on subjects with long-standing paraplegia. *Scand J Rehabil Med* 1975;7:51–56.

104. Davis GM, Shephard RJ. Strength training for wheelchair users. *Br J Sports Med* 1990;24:25–30.

105. Cooney MM, Walker JB. Hydraulic resistance exercise benefits cardiovascular fitness of spinal cord injured. *Med Sci Sports Exerc* 1986;18:522–525.

106. Olenik LM, Laskin JJ, Burnham R, et al. Efficacy of rowing, backward wheeling and isolated scapular retractor exercise as remedial strength activities for wheelchair users: application of electromyography. *Paraplegia* 1995;33:148–152.

107. Curtis KA, Tyner TM, Zachary L, et al. Effect of a standard exercise protocol on shoulder pain in long-term wheelchair users. *Spinal Cord* 1999;37:421–429.

108. Gellman H, Sie I, Waters RL. Late complications of the weight-bearing upper extremity in the paraplegic patient. *Clin Orthop* 1988;132–135.

109. Sie IH, Waters RL, Adkins RH, et al. Upper extremity pain in the postrehabilitation spinal cord injured patient. *Arch Phys Med Rehabil* 1992;73:44–48.

110. Escobedo EM, Hunter JC, Hollister MC, et al. MR imaging of rotator cuff tears in individuals with paraplegia. *AJR Am J Roentgenol* 1997;168:919–923.

111. Goldstein B, Young J, Escobedo EM. Rotator cuff repairs in individuals with paraplegia. *Am J Phys Med Rehabil* 1997;76:316–322.

112. Nichols PJ, Norman PA, Ennis JR. Wheelchair user's shoulder? Shoulder pain in patients with spinal cord lesions. *Scand J Rehabil Med* 1979;11:29–32.

113. Pentland WE, Twomey LT. The weight-bearing upper extremity in women with long term paraplegia. *Paraplegia* 1991;29:521–530.

114. Pentland WE, Twomey LT. Upper limb function in persons with long term paraplegia and implications for independence: Part I. *Paraplegia* 1994;32:211–218.

115. Burnham RS, May L, Nelson E, et al. Shoulder pain in wheelchair athletes: the role of muscle imbalance. *Am J Sports Med* 1993;21:238–242.

116. Lal S. Premature degenerative shoulder changes in spinal cord injury patients. *Spinal Cord* 1998;36:186–189.

117. Curtis KA, Roach KE, Applegate EB, et al. Reliability and validity of the Wheelchair User's Shoulder Pain Index (WUSPI). *Paraplegia* 1995;33:595–601.

118. Burnham R, Chan M, Hazlett C, et al. Acute median nerve dysfunction from wheelchair propulsion: the development of a model and study of the effect of hand protection. *Arch Phys Med Rehabil* 1994;75:513–518.

119. Burnham RS, Steadward RD. Upper extremity peripheral nerve entrapments among wheelchair athletes: prevalence, location, and risk factors. *Arch Phys Med Rehabil* 1994;75:519–524.

120. Perry J, Gronley JK, Newsam CJ, et al. Electromyographic analysis of the shoulder muscles during depression transfers in subjects with low-level paraplegia. *Arch Phys Med Rehabil* 1996;77:350–355.

121. Reyes ML, Gronley JK, Newsam CJ, et al. Electromyographic analysis of shoulder muscles of men with low-level paraplegia during a weight relief raise. *Arch Phys Med Rehabil* 1995;76:433–439.

122. Campagnolo DI, Bartlett JA, Keller SE, et al. Impaired phagocytosis of *Staphylococcus aureus* in complete tetraplegics. *Am J Phys Med Rehabil* 1997;76:276–280.

123. Campagnolo DI, Keller SE, DeLisa JA, et al. Alteration of immune system function in tetraplegics: a pilot study. *Am J Phys Med Rehabil* 1994;73:387–393.

124. Cruse JM, Keith JC, Bryant ML Jr, et al. Immune system-neuroendo-crine dysregulation in spinal cord injury. *Immunol Res* 1996;15:306–314.

125. Cruse JM, Lewis RE Jr, Bishop GR, et al. Decreased immune reactivity and neuroendocrine alterations related to chronic stress in spinal cord injury and stroke patients. *Pathobiology* 1993;61:183–192.

126. Kliesch WF, Cruse JM, Lewis RE, et al. Restoration of depressed immune function in spinal cord injury patients receiving rehabilitation therapy. *Paraplegia* 1996;34:82–90.

127. Nash MS. Immune responses to nervous system decentralization and exercise in quadriplegia. *Med Sci Sports Exerc* 1994;26:164–171.

128. Segal JL. Spinal cord injury: are interleukins a molecular link between neuronal damage and ensuing pathobiology? *Perspect Biol Med* 1993;36:222–240.

129. Segal JL, Brunnemann SR. Circulating levels of soluble interleukin 2 receptors are elevated in the sera of humans with spinal cord injury. *J Am Paraplegia Soc* 1993;16:30–33.

130. Segal JL, Gonzales E, Yousefi S, et al. Circulating levels of IL-2R, ICAM-1, and IL-6 in spinal cord injuries. *Arch Phys Med Rehabil* 1997;78:44–47.

131. Nieman DC, Buckley KS, Henson DA, et al. Immune function in marathon runners versus sedentary controls. *Med Sci Sports Exerc* 1995;27:986–992.

132. Nieman DC, Nehlsen-Cannarella SL, Markoff PA, et al. The effects of moderate exercise training on natural killer cells and acute upper respiratory tract infections. *Int J Sports Med* 1990;11:467–473.

133. Furusawa K, Tajima F, Tanaka Y, et al. Short-term attenuation of natural killer cell cytotoxic activity in wheelchair marathoners with paraplegia. *Arch Phys Med Rehabil* 1998;79:1116–1121.

134. Nash MS. The immune system. In: Whiteneck G, Charlifue SW, Gerhart KA, eds. *Aging with spinal cord injury.* New York, Demos Publications, 1993:159–182.

135. Gass GC, Camp EM, Nadel ER, et al. Rectal and rectal vs. esophageal temperatures in paraplegic men during prolonged exercise. *J Appl Physiol* 1988;64:2265–2271.

136. Gerner HJ, Engel P, Gass GC, et al. The effects of sauna on tetraplegic and paraplegic subjects. *Paraplegia* 1992;30:410–419.

137. Sawka MN, Latzka WA, Pandolf KB. Temperature regulation during upper body exercise: able-bodied and spinal cord injured. *Med Sci Sports Exerc* 1989;21:S132–S140.

138. Ishii K, Yamasaki M, Muraki S, et al. Effects of upper limb exercise on thermoregulatory responses in patients with spinal cord injury. *Appl Human Sci* 1995;14:149–154.

139. Price MJ, Campbell IG. Thermoregulatory responses of spinal cord injured and able-bodied athletes to prolonged upper body exercise and recovery. *Spinal Cord* 1999;37:772–779.

140. Bergman SB, Yarkony GM, Stiens SA. Spinal cord injury rehabilitation. 2. Medical complications. *Arch Phys Med Rehabil* 1997;78:S53–58.

141. Comarr AE, Eltorai I. Autonomic dysreflexia/hyperreflexia. *J Spinal Cord Med* 1997;20:345–354.

142. Arnold JM, Feng QP, Delaney GA, et al. Autonomic dysreflexia in tetraplegic patients: evidence for alpha-adrenoceptor hyper-responsiveness. *Clin Auton Res* 1995;5:267–270.

143. Ashley EA, Laskin JJ, Olenik LM, et al. Evidence of autonomic dysreflexia during functional electrical stimulation in individuals with spinal cord injuries. *Paraplegia* 1993;31:593–605.

144. Chancellor MB, Erhard MJ, Hirsch IH, et al. Prospective evaluation of terazosin for the treatment of autonomic dysreflexia. *J Urol* 1994;151:111–113.

145. Steinberger RE, Ohl DA, Bennett CJ, et al. Nifedipine pretreatment for autonomic dysreflexia during electroejaculation. *Urology* 1990;36:228–231.

146. Vaidyanathan S, Soni BM, Sett P, et al. Pathophysiology of autonomic dysreflexia: long-term treatment with terazosin in adult and pediatric spinal cord injury patients manifesting recurrent dysreflexic episodes. *Spinal Cord* 1998;36:761–770.

147. Webborn AD. "Boosting" performance in disability sport. *Br J Sports Med* 1999;33:74–75.

148. Hartkopp A, Murphy RJ, Mohr T, et al. Bone fracture during electri-

cal stimulation of the quadriceps in a spinal cord injured subject. *Arch Phys Med Rehabil* 1998;79:1133–1136.

149. Lopes P, Figoni SF, Perkash I. Upper limb exercise effect on tilt tolerance during orthostatic training of patients with spinal cord injury. *Arch Phys Med Rehabil* 1984;65:251–253.

150. Extracted from information available at *www.paralympic.org.*

151. About Disabled Sports, USA. *www.dsusa.org,* 3 February, 2000.

152. About Wheelchair Sports, USA. *www.wsusa.org.*

153. Americans With Disabilities Act, 42 USC 2101 et seq, 1990.

154. LaMere TJ, Labanowich S. The History of Sports Wheelchairs—part I and part II. *Sports "N" Spokes* 1984;4:5.

155. Tiessen J. Lighter stronger faster: revolutionizing technology for athletes with a disability. In: *Commemorative Program from Xth Paralympic Games.* Oakville, ON, Canada: Disability Today Publishing Group, Inc. 1996:65–72.

156. Cooper R, Boninger M, Shimada S, et al. *Elite athletes with impairments in exercise and rehabilitation and medicine.* Champaign, IL: Human Kinetics, 1990.

DRIVING ASSESSMENT IN SPINAL CORD INJURY PATIENTS

BETH E. ANDERSON

"This is the first time I have felt normal since I have been hurt." To any driver rehabilitation specialist, such statements are common. Driving, more than other activities of daily living, signifies independence, freedom, and a first step into adult responsibilities. Losing the ability to drive can be devastating on many levels. In addition to the potential economic impact from the inability to drive to work or to handle everyday household chores, there is the psychological impact of depending on others for rides (1, 2). At most neurologic levels of injury, individuals with spinal cord injury have the potential to return to independent driving with the appropriate adaptive equipment.

A driver rehabilitation specialist is most often an occupational therapist by training but may be an individual with a nonmedical background in driver education with additional training in adaptive driving equipment. Some programs employ both specialists as a team for a comprehensive program. Occupational therapists are well suited to the position because of their experience with adaptive equipment and activity analysis. Certification and continuing education for these professionals are available through the Association of Driver Rehabilitation Specialists (*www.driver-ed.org*) (3).

The timing for a return to driving will vary by individual and to some extent by the level and type of injury. The person must be medically stable. The evaluation should not occur until the physician has discontinued the use of a cervical collar, which would impair the person's ability to turn the head to check traffic. The use of a thoracolumbosacral orthosis (TLSO) or similar thoracic brace may impede transfer ability and positioning behind the wheel. The person should also be psychologically ready to return to the road. This may require additional time if the person was injured in a motor vehicle accident.

A person with a complete paraplegic injury and no additional complications will probably require mechanical hand controls and a few additional minor pieces of equipment to operate a car with an automatic transmission. The cost of this equipment is about $1,000. If there is no evidence of lower extremity return, the evaluation could occur within 3 months of injury because there is little likelihood the equipment recommendations would change.

The issues differ for people with tetraplegic injuries or incomplete motor injuries at any level. Depending on the person's functional abilities, the cost of equipping a vehicle for a person with a cervical level injury can be as low as $1,000 or as high as $70,000. It is important for the person to plateau in function before being evaluated for driving because any gain in motor function or increase in strength can mean a difference in equipment costs of thousands of dollars. For a person with an incomplete injury, further recovery may mean the difference between requiring and not requiring equipment. It is not uncommon to wait at least 6 months to evaluate a person who is still experiencing functional return.

Funding and overall independence are two other reasons to wait. A person may need time to explore potential funding sources for adaptive equipment and vehicle purchase. In addition, if the goal is independent driving, the person must be potentially independent in the community.

PRE-DRIVING ASSESSMENT

Every person should undergo a pre-driving or clinical assessment. The main components of this assessment are history, vision screen, physical skills, wheelchair or mobility equipment, and reaction time (2,3). If the individual also has a history of brain trauma, cognitive and perceptual screens should be included; however, these are not addressed in this chapter.

History

The history section should include both the medical history and driving history. The level of the spinal cord injury and whether it is a complete or incomplete injury and the secondary medical problems that could impact driving should be considered. These could include additional injuries, such as extremity fractures or peripheral nerve damage, or unrelated conditions such as cataracts, diabetes, and heart disease. Seizure history should also be discussed because most states have regulations indicating the length of time the person must be seizure free before driving. In Georgia, for example, seizure patients cannot resume driving until they have been seizure free for 6 months. Some states require the physician to report the patient's condition to the licensing agency. The state agency that regulates driver's licenses can provide specific information.

If the person has problems with dizziness, the cause should

TABLE 24.1. COMMON MEDICATIONS THAT CAN IMPAIR DRIVING ABILITIES

Symptoms	Medication Trade Names
Pain	Percocet, Lortab, Vicodin, etc.
Antidepressant	Paxil, Prozac, Wellbutrin, etc.
Antiseizure	Neurontin, Tegretol, Klonopin, etc.
Antispasm	Baclofen, Valium, Zanaflex, etc.
Sinus	Claritin-D, Allegra-D, etc.

TABLE 24.2. VISION SCREEN CHECKLIST

Near acuity	Binocular or each eye (e.g., right eye 20/30, left 20/50)
Far acuity	Binocular or each eye (e.g., right eye 20/30, left 20/50)
Color perception	Pass/fail
Depth perception (stereopsis)	Pass/fail
Fusion	Pass/fail
Horizontal phoria	WFL or esophoria or exophoria
Vertical phoria	WFL or hyperphoria or hypophoria
Saccades	
Pursuits	
Near-point convergance	

WFL, within functional limits.

be determined. It is not uncommon for people with spinal cord injury to experience orthostatic hypertension when they first arise. However, because this usually passes within a few minutes, it would not be expected to affect driving. If the person experiences problems with dizziness once up in the wheelchair from conditions such as low blood pressure or vertigo, these must be resolved before resuming independent driving. All medications should be listed, with attention paid to those that might cause drowsiness, fatigue, dizziness, altered judgment, or altered vision (Table 24.1). Each individual is affected differently by medications, and the cumulative effect of multiple medications that cross the blood–brain barrier is difficult to predict.

If the driving history includes possession of a valid driver's license or permit, any license restriction should be recorded. The amount of driving experience the patient had before the injury, whether the environment was rural or urban, and any recent at-fault motor vehicle accidents and tickets should be noted. An initial discussion of the type of vehicle the patient owns and any plans to modify that vehicle are also important. If the patient does not own an appropriate vehicle, it is important to wait to purchase one until all recommendations have been made.

The vision screen includes tests designed to determine whether the person can meet the state requirements in addition to detecting other deficits that may impact driving. Most states have minimum requirements for distance acuity, and many states also have minimum requirements for visual fields. Other tests, which frequently make up a vision screen, include contrast sensitivity, depth perception, color recognition, night vision and glare recovery, phoria, and fusion. Vision-testing machines may include slides that test phoria and fusion. Two slides are used to test for phoria, or eye alignment in vertical and horizontal positions. Separate images are presented to each eye, and the subject is asked where the images are relative to each other. The fusion slide is similar but includes one unique image and one identical image presented to each eye. The subject is required to overlap the identical images and will appear to see three images rather than the four that are present. Both tests examine aspects of binocular vision.

Because deficits can be a result of a functional problem or a central nervous system deficit, such as cranial nerve palsy, it is beneficial to look at ocular motility function. The problem may be a preexisting one, to which the person may have already accommodated, but it is important for the evaluator to be aware of any deficits. The assessment should include fixation, saccadic eye movement, and pursuit eye movement. Patients should be able to fix their gaze on a target for at least 10 seconds. Saccadic

eye movements allow rapid redirection of line of sight and are tested by having subjects move their gaze between two targets over multiple trials. Pursuit eye movement, the final component, involves fixation of gaze on a moving target. These skills are needed to track vehicles in traffic and to look quickly between the road and the mirrors and other objects in the driving environment, such as signs and traffic signals (4). Many clinics use vision-testing machines, which include most of the tests mentioned. Common models include the Optec series by Stereo Optical Co., Inc. (Chicago, IL) and the Keystone View (Reno, NV). The American Automobile Association (AAA; Heathrow, FL) and Porto Clinic/Glare (Intext; Scranton, PA) make night-vision tests (Table 24.2).

Physical Examination

The physical skills section should include an assessment of upper and lower extremity strength, sensation, range of motion for extremities and neck, sitting balance, spasticity, transfer skills, and wheelchair-loading skills. Patients who can ambulate and require an assistive device such as a rolling walker or crutches should be asked if they can load that equipment into the car. Whether they can ambulate household distances versus community distances should be noted. Other factors, such as pain, sitting tolerance, and skin condition, should be discussed because they can play a part in determining the person's endurance. Driving equipment predictions are made based on the physical assessment; therefore, an accurate picture of the patients' abilities and deficits is crucial to their success as a driver (Table 24.3).

Upper extremity strength can be tested by a gross muscle test of key muscles to determine motor level. The key muscles by injury level according to the American Spinal Injury Association (ASIA) are C5 elbow flexors, C6 wrist extensors, C7 elbow extensors, C8 finger flexor to the middle finger, and T1 small finger abductors (5). Unlike formal ASIA testing, the person should be tested in a position seated as if driving. In addition, it is helpful to test shoulder flexion, extension and abduction, horizontal adduction and adduction, and shoulder internal and external rotation. These motions provide the force needed to turn the steering wheel and to operate hand controls. Grasp strength should be measured when present, and areas of the

TABLE 24.3. PHYSICAL EXAMINATION

Upper extremity function	Includes strength, ROM, sensation for each limb
Lower extremity function	Includes strength, ROM, sensation for each limb
Neck ROM	
Sitting balance	Static, dynamic
Spasticity	Can use Ashworth scale
Assistive devices	For ambulation, include distance walked
Pain	Where and to what degree it affects function
Sitting tolerance	Includes weight shift frequency
Car transfer skill	Can be done by FIM score; includes assistive device if needed
Wheelchair loading skill	

ROM, range of motion; FIM, functional independence measure.

body lacking sensation for pain or temperature should be noted because these areas may have to be protected from injury.

Lower extremity strength primarily affects the ability to operate the standard accelerator and brake pedals; however, it is often absent in patients with spinal cord injury. If strength is present, the person should again be tested in a seated position. The most important gross motions to be tested by level are L2 myotome, hip flexors; L3 myotome, knee extensors; L4 myotome, ankle dorsiflexors; and S1 myotome, ankle plantar flexors (5). Some amount of adduction and abduction of the hip or inversion and eversion at the ankle may be required to move the foot from the accelerator to the brake and back. Exact requirements depend on the layout of the pedals in the vehicle of choice.

If functional lower extremity strength is present, it is important to determine whether the person also has lower extremity sensation, particularly proprioception. A person with an incomplete injury may have enough lower extremity function to operate the original equipment manufacturer (OEM) pedals. Reaction time and foot placement may be tested in the clinic or in the car.

AAA makes an in-clinic reaction tester with two pedals that can be placed on the floor to simulate the vehicle. Brake reaction time can also be tested using an in-vehicle reaction timer such as the VC 1000 (also available through AAA). Because reactions are tested with the actual OEM pedals and with the dynamic forces acting on the body, this may be an advantage over the in-clinic test. The average brake reaction time is 0.50 to 0.75 seconds. The testing process involves an emergency stop from at least 25 mph. The driver must focus on a light mounted on the windshield and is prevented from looking at his or her feet. The device records the time to initiate braking and bring the vehicle to a complete stop, the speed of the vehicle, the braking distance, and the stopping distance. Traveling at 30 mph, the average braking distance on smooth, dry pavement is 38 feet (6). With inadequate proprioception, the patient may not be able to locate the pedals without looking at his or her feet. This would disqualify them from driving without adaptations. Multiple trials are recommended to determine whether fatigue affects performance. This same test could be performed on a

vehicle with adaptive equipment if, for example, the person's ability to perform an emergency stop using mechanical hand controls was questionable. Failure might result in a recommendation for electronic hand controls. If a modified van is being used, it should be noted that the stopping time and distance will be affected by the higher gross vehicle weight (3).

Active-range limitations should be noted during the strength tests. Passive-range limitations may affect positioning. If the person has impaired lower extremity range due to spasticity, edema, or heterotropic ossification, it may be difficult to position the legs under the steering wheel. If there are contractures in the hand, custom orthotics may be required to interface with the steering wheel or hand controls. Cervical fusion surgery or tight neck and shoulder muscles may result in limited neck rotation, which would affect the person's ability to check traffic. This, combined with decreased active trunk rotation, may necessitate the use of additional mirrors (7).

Sitting balance is often impaired as a result of the lack of trunk and abdominal muscle strength. Any person who cannot maintain an upright position against moderate side-to-side resistance or who cannot return to an upright position without using the arms should use a chest strap or other lateral support when driving (8). A small study (n = 13) was conducted of the seated postural stability of wheelchair users as measured through the use of a tilt platform. This study "revealed that SCI subjects lost balance at perturbation levels seen during normal braking maneuvers. In fact, the majority of SCI subjects became unstable at levels below which inertial belts are designed to lock" (9). The rate of change in the speed or direction of the vehicle also appears to influence stability. Most subjects lost their balance when the rate of change was rapid. The subjects with paraplegic injuries were more stable than those with tetraplegic injuries, and all were less stable than the able-bodied control group (9).

The presence of spasticity or abnormal tone should be determined, including which muscles are affected and what positions or conditions trigger the spasticity. Hypertonicity is a potentially dangerous complication for the operator of a motor vehicle. For example, adductor spasms can cause the person's knees to squeeze the steering wheel, possibly preventing it from turning. Extensor spasms might cause a foot to hit the floor pedals, activating the accelerator or brake. The physician should be consulted if abnormal tone interferes with safety and if there are no equipment solutions, such as pedal blocks, to prevent possible accidents (7).

Transfers

The person's ability to transfer to a car and load a wheelchair should be discussed during the clinical assessment and eventually observed in a vehicle. The level of injury, patient's weight and conditioning, and type of wheelchair affect these skills. In some cases, the wheelchair is chosen before the person has given much thought to transportation. Seating specialists should educate themselves about the different options in loading devices in order to assist the patient in wheelchair selection. A knowledgeable seating specialist can suggest options that make the manual chair smaller and lighter, making it easier to load. In some cases, this

TABLE 24.4. MANUAL WHEELCHAIR COMPONENTS

Reduce Frame Width	Reduce Frame Height	Reduce Overall Weight
Quick-release wheels	Quick-release push handles	Easily removable backs
Scissor wheel locks	Quick-release casters	Adjustable tension backs
	Folding front end	Short, fixed back
	Fold-down back	Sling back

means more removable parts, which may increase the time and complexity of the loading process. They should also question the person about his or her transportation plans so that the suggestion of a folding chair can be made if appropriate (10) (Table 24.4). If the person has been injured for several years, the wheelchair should be examined for appropriateness and condition. They should be questioned about its age and their plans for replacing it. If this is to occur soon, it is better to obtain the new wheelchair first rather than make vehicle equipment recommendations that may have to be changed.

BEHIND-THE-WHEEL ASSESSMENT

The behind-the-wheel assessment involves vehicle entry and exit, operation of primary controls, and operation of secondary controls. Primary driving controls operate the steering, accelerator, and brake. Secondary controls operate other vehicle functions and can be divided into two categories: those functions, such as the turn signals, that have to be activated while the vehicle is in motion; and those functions, such as the gear selector, that can be operated at rest (Table 24.5). If possible, the person should be evaluated in the type of vehicle they will eventually need, but the more important issue is for them to use the appropriate driving equipment (2).

A static assessment, either in a vehicle or in the clinic, may help the evaluator rule out certain equipment, but it should not be used to finalize primary equipment. The environment in a moving vehicle is dynamic. Forces act on the body and the wheelchair when the vehicle is accelerating, braking, and turning (8,11). Even the terrain can affect a person's ability to operate the equipment. A person who can push a hand-control lever

TABLE 24.5. SECONDARY CONTROLS

Used in Motion	Used at Rest
Turn signals	Gear selector
Horn	Ignition
Dimmer	Headlights
Wiper low/pulse	Windows
	Door locks
	Interior lights
	Climate controls
	Lift controls
	Lockdown release

forward to hold the brake at a flat intersection might not be able to maintain full braking when stopped on a steep uphill grade. In that circumstance, gravity is pulling the person, the arm, and the vehicle toward the rear. Some electronic or *servo* hand controls (controls that use a motor or force such as a vacuum or compressed air to move the pedals) allow the driving specialist to prescribe the direction of the braking motion. Some controls can be positioned such that the accelerator and brake operate in a side-to-side motion. These variations can only be confirmed by operating the equipment in a real-world environment (3). Specific equipment is discussed in the next section.

The behind-the-wheel evaluation often begins in a parking lot or driving range for safety. The experienced driver has to learn new motor patterns to operate the adaptive equipment but will be familiar with the overall driving task. The new driver will require extensive training to learn road rules and to pass the state driving test in addition to training with adaptive equipment. In this first phase, the primary driving equipment suggested by the results of the preassessment is introduced, and the person should be allowed to practice turns, lane control, braking, acceleration, and emergency-stopping maneuvers. A figure-of-eight steering maneuver can be included that involves a rapid full turn to the left followed by a full turn to the right once the car has made a complete circle. This maneuver stresses the person's lateral stability, coordination, and strength. Revisions to the wheelchair seating system or addition of a chest strap to the automotive seat may be required if stability cannot be maintained (8).

If the driving specialist is satisfied that the choice and setup of the vehicle equipment are appropriate, the evaluation can proceed to a variety of driving environments of increasing complexity. The route typically consists of residential streets, secondary roads with increasing levels of traffic, and finally limited access roads. Maneuvers such as parking, backing straight, three-point turns, and U-turns may be included. Hill stops and starts should be demonstrated for hand control users so that they will learn how to start on a hill without rolling back.

At the end of the evaluation, the driver rehabilitation specialist determines whether the equipment used was appropriate and, if not, what additional equipment may be needed. If additional training is indicated, there should be an indication of how much training time the person is expected to require. Training time can range from a few hours for mechanical hand controls and standard steering to more than 40 hours for joystick drivers. Even the behind-the-wheel evaluation may stretch over several sessions if the equipment issues are complex.

EQUIPMENT RECOMMENDATIONS BY LEVEL OF INJURY

Equipment recommendations include adaptive driving equipment, vehicle selection, and structural vehicle modifications. They may include recommendations for modifications or replacement of mobility equipment. The seating specialist and the driving specialist need to collaborate when possible on prescriptions to ensure that the patient has a mobility device that is compatible with the vehicle and driving equipment. It is important for each specialist to be aware of the equipment and options that can aid the patient. The most important instance of this is when a new wheelchair is being prescribed for a person who already drives a van from his wheelchair. In this case, changes in chair dimensions or style may require significant modifications to location of the existing driving equipment, resulting in added expense.

Vehicle Selection

The process begins with careful consideration of vehicles currently available to the patient. In general, an automatic-transmission vehicle with power steering and power brakes is required. The only exception is for a patient with a very incomplete injury who has enough function in all four limbs to operate a manual-transmission vehicle. Other factory options that facilitate modification include tilt steering wheel, power windows, and door locks and possibly a power driver's seat. Air conditioning, front and rear in the case of a van, is recommended to compensate for patients with spinal cord injury to regulate their body temperature. This can be life threatening, depending on the climate (2).

For most people with paraplegia, an automatic-transmission car is an option if there is no problem with transfers. If the person transfers well enough, other classes of vehicles, such as sport utility vehicles, are also possibilities. These are more difficult to transfer into because they usually sit higher from the ground. In all cases, the patients should try transferring to the specific vehicle they are considering before making a final decision. Transfer aids are available that can raise the person up to the level of a full-sized truck seat, but these are costly. If transfers or chair loading become more difficult because of shoulder pain, weight gain, medical complications, or age-related factors, a van may be considered.

For patients who cannot or who choose not to load the chair independently, a loading device may be considered. A person may not want to load the chair into a vehicle for space reasons (e.g., family members may occupy all the available seats, leaving no space to stow the wheelchair, or the patient may not want to pass the wheels and frame across his or her body and risk getting dirt on business attire). Most loading devices are designed to pick up a folding manual wheelchair. Car-top devices fold the wheelchair and stow it in a rooftop carrier (Fig. 24.1). There are also lifts that can stow the folding chair behind the driver's seat in an extended-cab three-door pickup truck. The person who can ambulate short distances also has the option of devices to load the chair into the trunk, in a sliding side door, or into the rear of a minivan or sport utility vehicle. Some of these devices even load certain power upright wheelchairs and scoot-

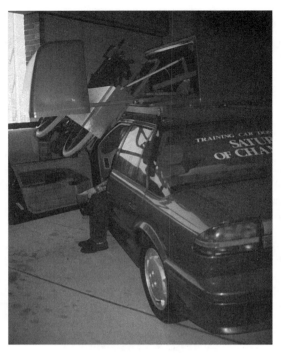

FIGURE 24.1. Braun chair-topper device.

ers. The height, width, length, and weight of the wheelchair will also affect its compatibility with loading devices and vehicles (10) (Table 24.6).

Most patients with tetraplegia choose a modified van. These patients may perform independent car transfers but may not be efficient enough to make them practical. The patient who uses a manual chair may lack the fine motor control and strength to disassemble and load it. Patients with tetraplegia frequently use power chairs for community mobility. Most power chairs cannot be disassembled into a car, and those that can are too heavy to be practical for routine use. For the person who uses both a manual and a power wheelchair, it is important to determine which chair is most practical for independent community use because not every vehicle solution can be used with both types. For example, patients who choose a lowered floor minivan may not be able to push the manual chair up the ramp but would be able to drive the power chair up the ramp. Even if they can enter the vehicle with both types of chair, it may not be possible to use a single-tiedown system that would accommodate both chairs because of differences in frames and seat heights.

There are some alternatives to modified vans for the wheelchair driver. One company, Braun (Winamac, Indiana), currently modifies a full-sized extended cab pickup truck. A Canadian company, Elaine Lift (KVB manufacturing: Smith Falls, Ontario, Canada), modifies some models of large sport utility vehicles. These vehicles make up a very small percentage of the total number of adapted vehicles. However, if there is a vocational need for a truck, they may be a more appropriate choice. Both have removable driver's seats to allow an able-bodied person to drive if necessary.

If a replacement vehicle is required, it is essential that an

TABLE 24.6. COMPATIBILITY OF VEHICLES WITH LIFTS FOR MOBILITY DEVICES

Vehicle	Type of Mobility Device	Location in Vehicle	Loading Device
Sedan	Folding manual W/C	In trunk	**Bruno Wheelchair-lifter** AWL-100
	Folding manual W/C	On rear bumper	**Bruno Back-saver** AWL-1600—will hold chair up to 70 lb
	Folding manual W/C	On roof	**Tip Top Mobility Wheelchair Lift** Attaches to frame and wheel
	Folding manual W/C	On roof	**Braun Chair Topper** Attaches to seat
Pickup truck	Folding manual W/C	Extended cab, driver-side door	**Bruno Cab-sider** PUL-1700
	Rigid manual W/C Folding manual W/C Power W/C	Bed	**Bruno Out-rider** PUL-1100 under 200 lb; can be paired with **Pow'r Topper** to have covered storage; recommended for power devices
Minivan and some sports utility vehicles	Folding manual W/C	Rear hatch	**Bruno Wheelchair-lifter** AWL-150
	Manual folding W/C Rigid manual W/C	Driver-side sliding door	**Bruno Scooter-lift II** VSL-900C-driver side sliding has a narrower opening limiting device width
	Power W/C < 200 lbs Power W/C Rigid manual W/C	Passenger side sliding door Rear hatch	**Bruno Curb-sider** VSL-600-power swing in to van, lose rear couch
	Power W/C	Rear hatch	**Bruno Curb-sider XL** VSL-650—will lift chairs up to 235 lb; lose rear couch
	Power W/C	Rear hatch	**Bruno Curb-sider Super XL** VSL-670—will lift chairs up to 300 lb; lose rear couch
Full-size van	Manual folding W/C Power W/C	Rear door	All devices listed above for rear hatch application
	Manual folding W/C Rigid manual W/C Power W/C < 200 lb	Passenger side door	**Bruno Scooter-lift II** VSL-900C—lose center couch; may have to modify step well

W/C, wheelchair.

evaluation be completed before purchase. Not every vehicle within a particular category is appropriate for structural modification. In some cases, a vehicle may be initially modified for dependent passenger use with the plan of eventual conversion for a wheelchair driver's use. Certain modifications may be performed more economically during the initial modification, whereas others can be added easily when the person is ready to drive. The driver rehabilitation specialist and the mobility equipment modifier can provide this information. It is crucial that patients obtain their personal wheelchair before starting modifications to the driver's area to ensure an appropriate fit.

Adaptive Driving Equipment

C1 to C4 Complete Tetraplegia

The C1 to C4 injury levels are not compatible with independent driving. There must be functional use of at least one extremity to operate a driving system. Patients with this injury level, however, do have transportation equipment needs that should be addressed. Usually, a person with a high-level tetraplegic injury operates a power wheelchair with a tilt or recline mechanism.

If that person is to use the chair for independent community mobility, there must be a way to transport the person and the wheelchair into the community.

Although it may be possible to perform a dependent transfer of the person to a passenger car or truck using a lift or sliding board, the bigger problem is providing adequate head, trunk, and upper extremity support for comfort and safety once in the vehicle seat. If the person is ventilator dependent, this becomes even more difficult. It is usually easier to transport the person seated in the wheelchair, which is already set up to provide the proper support. If the person can be transferred, the power wheelchair cannot be dismantled for easy transport. Even a manual tilt or recline wheelchair may be difficult to transport in a car. A structurally modified, full-sized van or lowered-floor minivan is usually required. The most common modifications to a full-sized van are a lowered floor in the cargo or center seat area and a raised roof and raised doors. The combination of structural vehicle modifications required is based on the seated height and overall dimensions of the person and the wheelchair. If possible, the doorway should be tall enough to allow the wheelchair user to enter in a fully upright position. An unmodified full-sized van has a door opening of 47½ to 48 inches, with an interior height of about 53 inches.

After the person is inside the van, it is important to have at least 2 inches of head clearance. Few adults have a seated height low enough to fit in an unmodified van. For the dependent passengers, the lowered floor drops their eye height to a point where they may be able to see out the side windows. A van with a raised roof alone tends to provide poor visibility because the person's head is usually above the original roofline. Depending on the seated height of the person, a combination of these modifications may be needed.

Floors are usually lowered 4 to 8 inches. This is done primarily on full-sized Ford vans. When a floor is lowered, the gas tank must be relocated, usually to the rear aft of axle position, and the spare tire is usually mounted on the back door. A raised roof may also be chosen to allow the caregivers to stand upright when providing assistance to the wheelchair user, particularly helpful if suctioning or catheterization must be performed. The primary disadvantage to a raised roof is increased overall vehicle height, which makes the vehicle difficult to fit in a garage or carport and more difficult to take into the community because it may not fit through drive-through windows or into parking decks. It also raises the vehicle's center of gravity, affecting the handling. A support cage should be added to restore the vehicle's structural integrity.

Entry to a full-sized van is accomplished by means of a platform lift. Lifts can be fully automatic or semiautomatic, the latter requiring the operator to unfold the lift platform manually. There are four main types of lifts: single-post, dual-post, swing, and under-vehicle lifts. The first two types are the most common; the swing lift is the least common (12). The single-post lift has one support arm mounted toward the rear of the vehicle (Fig. 24.2). In many models, the platform folds either manually or automatically, allowing able-bodied people to enter without having to deploy the lift. Because the left side of the doorway is clear and allows the footrests more clearance, the lack of a forward post makes it easier to turn and position the wheelchair forward facing. This feature also allows the front passenger seat

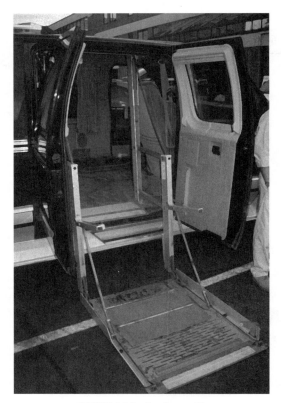

FIGURE 24.3. Dual-post lift.

to be adjusted for greater comfort or to be removed to allow the wheelchair occupant to ride up front if the floor has been modified to accommodate it. This can also be accomplished with an under-vehicle lift. The dual-post lift has greater platform stability, and some models can handle greater loads than the single-post style (Fig. 24.3). Under-vehicle lifts provide a completely clear door opening, an advantage with a long chair. Their primary disadvantage is a lower vehicle ground clearance because the lift is mounted under the vehicle frame. The primary advantage of the swing lift is the ability to load the platform parallel rather than perpendicular to the van, which decreases the space needed to park and load the van. This type of lift may not have a long enough platform for some wheelchairs and may require additional door height for head clearance.

Of vans smaller than full size with better gas mileage, the lowered-floor minivan has become increasingly popular since being introduced in the late 1980s. The floor can be lowered 8, 10, or 12 inches, with the 10-inch drop being the most common. Entry is gained by use of a folding ramp that deploys from the passenger-side sliding door. A few models use a rear-entry ramp or a slide-under floor ramp. Frequently, the vehicle is equipped with a kneeling feature, lowering the vehicle to decrease the angle of the ramp (Fig. 24.4).

The door openings on most minivans measure 53 inches, although a few models meet the Americans with Disabilities Act (ADA) requirement of 56 inches. The floor is lowered from the front firewall back to the rear seats, returning to original depth

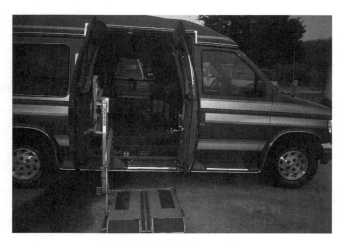

FIGURE 24.2. Single-post lift.

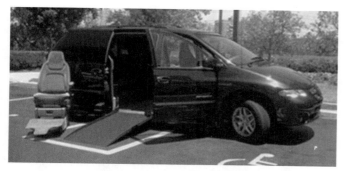

FIGURE 24.4. Lowered-floor minivan with removable driver's seat.

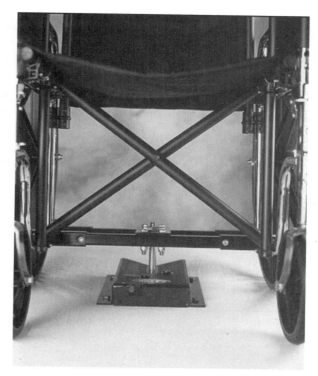

FIGURE 24.5. EZ Lock automatic lockdown.

in front of the rear wheel wells. A lowered-floor minivan can accommodate a passenger in the cargo or front passenger position if equipped with a removable front passenger seat. Because the minivan has less interior space and it may be difficult for a large power chair to turn into a forward-facing position, this should be attempted before purchase (12).

The final issue is ground clearance. A lowered-floor minivan sits lower to the ground than an unmodified vehicle. If the patient travels rough terrain, such as dirt roads, this should be factored into the final decision.

Once inside a van, the passenger and wheelchair must be secured. The two primary styles of lockdowns or tiedowns are manual and automatic. In either case, the brand chosen should be crash tested and compatible with the patient's wheelchair base. There are several types of manual lockdowns, but all consist of a strap system that hooks to the frame of the wheelchair. It is essential that the straps attach to parts of the wheelchair that are not removable. There are two front and two rear straps, which are attached to track bolted to the floor of the van. Some wheelchair bases, particularly midwheel drive styles, may not be compatible with every strap-type lockdown because the cowling on the base makes it difficult to find attachment points.

The primary advantage of a manual system is the ability to secure different chairs, which is useful if the passenger uses both a manual and power chair. Manual systems are also less costly than automatic systems.

The most common automatic lockdown has two parts: one that bolts to the frame of the chair, and a second that bolts to the floor of the van (Fig. 24.5). Where the two parts meet, they interlock and are released by a button. The primary advantage of the automatic system is ease of use. It is faster, has an alarm that sounds if the user is not properly secured, and does not require the person securing the wheelchair to bend over or crawl around the wheelchair attaching the straps. Less training is required to operate the automatic system, and less operator error is possible, an advantage if multiple caregivers or friends must be instructed in the lockdown procedure. Whichever system is chosen, it is not complete without an automotive lap and shoulder belt to secure the person in the wheelchair to the van. Belts attached to the wheelchair itself and belts secured by Velcro are not acceptable.

C5 Complete Tetraplegia

C5 tetraplegia is the highest level of injury leaving the patient with potential to drive. The driving evaluation should be postponed until the patient plateaus in strength, usually at least 8 months to 1 year from the time of injury. A power wheelchair is usually used for community mobility. The tilt or recline switch on the wheelchair should be disabled while operating a vehicle to prevent accidental activation. The same vehicle consideration mentioned previously will apply, with some additional modifications specific to driving. The van will need power door openers, and the lift or ramp must be fully automatic to allow the wheelchair user to open and close the vehicle independently. Remote controls, toggle switches, and magnetic switches mounted in the brake light are the most common switch access methods.

Most patients with a C5 injury will not transfer efficiently or independently and so will be driving from their wheelchair. The seating specialist should give extra consideration to lateral stability because the dynamic forces affecting the body in the moving vehicle are much greater than the ones seen when operating the chair in the clinic (8). Options such as tapered 90-degree leg rests, making the chair shorter or narrower, allow the chair to fit under the steering wheel more easily and may allow the person to sit closer to the wheel. A swing-away joystick may be needed to facilitate placement of primary driving controls. By keeping these issues in mind, the seating specialist can provide valuable assistance even before the person is ready to drive (see Table 24.7).

The driver's floor must be lowered in addition to lowering the floor in the cargo area, making it possible to drive the wheel-

TABLE 24.7. POWER WHEELCHAIR COMPONENTS

Feature	Advantage
Swing-away joystick mount	Allows proper placement of driving controls
Flip-back armrests	Allows proper placement of driving controls
Tapered legrests	Decreases need for engine cover modifications
Flexible antitip bars	Allows the chair to get into and out of a sloped driver's area
Adjustable rear wheel placement	Allows the overall length of the chair to be decreased and decreases the turning radius
Mid-wheel drive	Decreases the turning radius; these chairs can be very "tippy" and may need additional stabilizers
Adjustable seat-to-floor height	Allows chair to be raised to increase visual field or lowered to fit under steering wheel
"Transportable" wheelchairs	Can be disassembled for transport in a car. The frame weighs 65 lb, so this may not be practical.

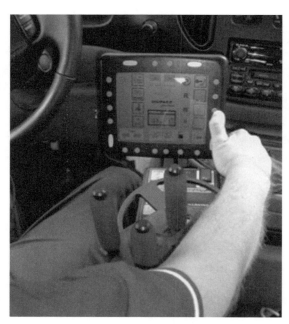

FIGURE 24.6. DS 2000 steering controller with tri-pin orthotic and Electronic Mobility Corporation (Baton Rouge, LA) Gold Series touchpad.

chair up under the steering wheel. In a full-sized van, the driver's floor may be sloped down from the cargo area and lowered up to 3 additional inches in order to drop the driver's eye level and knee height down to the appropriate height. Lowered-floor minivans have a consistent floor level from the front firewall back to the rear axle and are not usually appropriate for drivers sitting taller than 53 inches. Eyes should be even with the rear-view mirror and below the tint band of the windshield for proper visibility. The knees must fit under the steering wheel and not interfere with its motion.

In full-sized vans, the engine cover may have to be modified to provide enough room for the foot rests. The seat-belt retractor may also need to be recessed to provide additional clearance. An automatic lockdown is used in the driver's area along with a modified hands-free seat belt. Additional lateral supports or a chest strap may be required to provide additional stability when driving.

Some patients with a C5 motor level injury on one side and a C4 or higher level injury on the other side can drive. If only one extremity is to be used, a multiaccess driving system in which the steering, accelerator, and brake are operated by a single control lever would be used. These systems are complex and costly. If both upper extremities can be used, one will perform steering, and the other will operate an accelerator and brake—most often, an electronic or servo hand control. If there is a difference in strength, the stronger arm is generally used for steering.

In most cases, the person will have good deltoid function but will lack horizontal adduction past zero degrees. Shoulder rotation may also be weak. Most people at this level are unable to turn a standard steering wheel a full turn in each direction, even with the steering effort or force reduced. If the person cannot make consistent turns at all speeds using the reduced-effort steering, they will require a servo steering system. Low-

speed maneuvers, such as parking, require greater strength than turns at higher speed. One of the most common systems, the DS 2000 by Electronic Mobility Corporation (Baton Rouge, LA), uses a 6-inch wheel that can be mounted in any plane. It is frequently placed at the end of the wheelchair armrest in the location and orientation similar to the wheelchair joystick (Fig. 24.6). Two turns of the controller wheel are equal to one turn of the original steering wheel. A lever that requires less than 1 lb of force operates the electronic hand controls for accelerator and brake.

A tri-pin orthotic is frequently used to keep the person's hand in contact with both the steering and hand controls (Fig. 24.7).

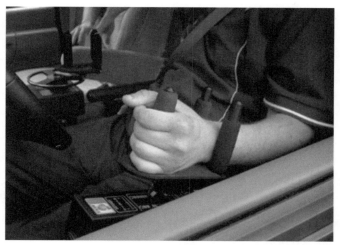

FIGURE 24.7. EGB with tri-pin orthotic.

The rear pins press on the dorsal and volar sides of the wrist with the forearm in a neutral position, and the front pin rests in the web space of the hand. Wrist supports may be worn to maintain a stable wrist position in the absence of active wrist extension. There can be a tendency to flex the biceps while driving, which can cause the hand to pull up out of the tri-pin. In such cases, the wrist support may be modified to interface with the driving orthotic to assist in keeping the hand in contact with the device, or a different style of orthotic may be tried. It should be noted that the person with this injury level lacks sensation in the hand and forearm, making it difficult to determine whether the hand is resting in the orthotic. These driving systems are complex and should never be prescribed without actual behind-the-wheel experience.

Most patients with C5 injuries require extensive modifications of secondary controls. They often do not have the fine motor control or reach required to operate the original controls. In some cases, the primary controls may block access to some of the vehicles systems, such as the thermostat and fan switches. Modifications for secondary controls can be as simple as an extension on a switch or as complex as a touch pad. Touch-pad systems can replace a single function or operate multiple systems through a single switch. The most complex systems control everything from gear selection to temperature controls. Simple touch-pad systems may control two to eight functions. A single switch that scans several functions with auditory cues may be used to activate secondary controls that have to be accessed while in motion. Less commonly used are voice-recognition systems that allow direct selection of secondary controls (2).

C6 Complete Tetraplegia

The C6 level of tetraplegia is often the most varied in physical performance. Most people are power chair users in the community and still require a van for transportation. If they do not transfer independently, they require the same driver's lowered-floor modifications mentioned previously. If they can transfer efficiently, a six-way power driver's seat may be considered (Fig. 24.8). This type of seat backs up from the steering wheel, turns 90 degrees, and can be raised or lowered to make a transfer easier. The patient backs into the van facing the passenger side door and maneuvers the wheelchair into an automatic lockdown positioned against the driver's sidewall of the van. The patient is thus seated parallel to the transfer seat. The lockdown is installed behind the seat to secure the unoccupied wheelchair; this position should never be used for passenger transport. A level or downhill transfer is usually possible in both directions, and the person can generally position the wheelchair closer to this seat than to the seat of a car. The transfer seat is operated by toggle switches that control forward and backward motions in addition to swivel and height adjustments. It is necessary for the user to reposition the legs several times as the seat moves back into position under the steering wheel. A person with long legs may not have enough room between the seats to do this, particularly in a lowered-floor minivan. A chest strap, such as the Grandmar (International Medical Equipment Corporation: Chico, California), can be added to provide lateral stability in the automotive seat.

A weak person with this level of injury may still lack the

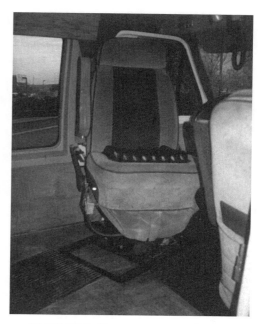

FIGURE 24.8. Six-way power-transfer seat.

active range to turn a full-sized steering wheel and thus require servo steering and an electronic accelerator and brake. The main advantage of a C6 injury over a C5 injury is in wrist strength; patients with C6 injury seldom require extra wrist support.

The stronger person at this level may be able to turn a full-sized steering wheel but will probably need the force or effort reduced. This is particularly true in a lowered-floor minivan because rack-and-pinion steering is often more difficult to turn (12). The same type of orthotic, the tri-pin, is likely to be used, although in this instance, it would be mounted on the rim of the OEM steering wheel. The location should be determined during the behind-the-wheel evaluation. In most cases, it will be placed in the lower right quadrant of the wheel, allowing the driver's arm to hang relaxed at his or her side when steering straight.

These individuals may be able to use mechanical hand controls with a modified handle to provide additional wrist support. It is important to determine whether they have adequate endurance and strength to apply and hold the brake in the most challenging situations, on a hill and during an emergency stop. Electronic hand controls are still needed in many cases. If reach and access are not a problem, simple extensions for the secondary controls may be the only modifications, although touch pads and sequencing switches are still common.

C7 to C8 Complete Tetraplegia

Most patients with C7 and C8 tetraplegic injuries have enough shoulder strength to turn the standard steering wheel and may not require reduced-effort steering. Minimal grasp strength may be present; hence, an orthotic, such as the tri-pin, the V-grip, or the U-grip, is still used for steering control in most cases. This prevents the person from losing control of the wheel should an emergency occur such as a tire blowout. Smaller than the tri-pin, both the V-grip and U-grip have two points of contact:

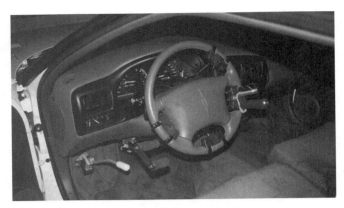

FIGURE 24.9. V-grip orthotic.

one in the palm, and one on the dorsum of the hand. The user keeps the wrist in extension to maintain contact (Fig. 24.9).

The presence of triceps makes the use of mechanical hand controls for braking and acceleration appropriate. Added wrist support may be needed if the person cannot grip the handle. A padded handle provides more friction and may be easier to maintain contact with.

There are four types of mechanical hand controls: the push right angle, push twist, push pull, and push rock. All require the user to push the control lever toward the dashboard to apply the brake. The primary difference is the method of applying the accelerator. With the most commonly used style, the push-right control, the lever is pushed toward the thigh. The push-twist control requires the user to twist the handle and hold it, which can be difficult with decreased grasp. With the push-pull style, the user pulls back toward his or her trunk to accelerate. Because it does not allow the user to depress the accelerator and brake simultaneously as all other styles do, this is useful for the driver who tends to ride the brake; however, it does make starting on a hill more difficult. The push-rock style has a vertical lever that is rotated back toward the driver's lap for acceleration.

In most cases, the hand controls are mounted on the left side of the steering wheel. This allows easier activation of the turn signals with the left hand. The left hand can depress the brake while the right operates the gear selector. Decreased strength or limited range of motion on the right can make steering difficult. In that instance, the hand controls can be mounted on the right side because they require less range and strength to operate. When that is done, some additional modifications to the secondary controls, such as the turn signals, may be needed.

Most secondary controls do not require modification. It is important to observe the person operating the controls in their chosen vehicle because minor modifications, such as switch extensions, may be needed. Activating turn signal–mounted windshield wipers can be difficult because they must be twisted, but adding a small tab to turn it into a lever can solve the problem. The most difficult control may be a floor-mounted gear selector because the driver may have trouble depressing the release button to move the handle. Similar problems exist for a hand-operated parking brake, which requires depression of a small button to release. An extension lever can be added to depress a foot-operated parking brake.

Some patients with C7 and C8 level injury can transfer independently. Wheelchair loading tends to be the primary difficulty because the person may lack the fine coordination and strength required for dismantling the chair and lifting it. A loading device may be used, but it will only be compatible with certain types of wheelchairs. If the patient uses a power chair or cannot manage the car transfer, a van could be modified to allow driving from the wheelchair or equipped with a power driver's seat. If the patient can transfer, the wheelchair is locked down behind the driver's seat for safety. In a full-sized van, the roof may need to be raised or the floor lowered to provide adequate head clearance for the transfer.

Complete Paraplegia

Assuming no additional orthopedic complications, patients with injuries at the paraplegic level have full function of their upper extremities. Standard steering is used, with the possible addition of a steering knob to make one-handed turns easier, and mechanical hand controls are to control speed. A parking brake extension may be needed if the lever is not hand operated. A chest strap is required for a person who does not have adequate motor return in his or her trunk and abdomen.

The choice of hand control style may be dictated by the available space in the driver's area rather than the hand function. A person with long legs or a small car may not have room for the lever to move far enough toward the thigh to get adequate acceleration with the push-right control style. The push-twist or push-rock control is often used in these cases.

Vans are sometimes recommended in cases in which the patient uses a power wheelchair or if there are complications such as shoulder pain that limit the patient's ability to transfer or load the chair. Power transfer seats are often used. Occasionally, an electronic hand control is required for a very large person who is driving from the wheelchair if there is not enough space in the driver's area to operate mechanical hand controls (5).

Incomplete Injuries

The person with an incomplete spinal cord injury can have an extremely varied functional picture. An accurate clinical assessment will give the evaluator a picture of the level at which the person is functioning regardless of the level of cord lesion. The evaluator must keep in mind that sensory and motor functions are not always preserved to the same extent.

It is important to note that some of the clinical syndromes present their own unique challenges. A person with a central cord lesion may be able to use the existing pedals but may be unable to steer because of proximal upper extremity weakness. A person with Brown-Séquard syndrome may have enough strength to use the OEM pedals but, because of the contralateral loss of sensation, may not be able to feel themselves touch the controls.

A person may present with intact left lower extremity function but impaired function on the right. In this case, a left-foot accelerator could be used, allowing the left foot to activate the pedals without having to reach across the body. The person could present as hemiplegic. Depending on which side has intact function, modifications to pedals or secondary controls may be needed. Any of the previously mentioned equipment may be appropriate for the person with an incomplete injury. It is also possible that no equipment will be needed. In this case, it is critical to test the reaction time and endurance of the lower extremities to support the lack of modifications (2,13).

Incomplete injuries can continue to improve over a varied period of time; thus, periodic reassessment is suggested because changes to the adaptive equipment may be needed. Formal reassessment is often required to remove legally a restriction on the patient's license for the equipment in question.

Driving evaluation is an essential component of a comprehensive spinal cord injury program. Information on transportation should be available to all patients. Evaluation services in the United States and Canada can be located through the membership directory on the Association for Driver Rehabilitation Specialist's website, *www.driver-ed.org*. Facilities are listed by state, and most include a description of the types of services offered. Vendors who belong to the National Mobility Equipment Dealers Association are a valuable resource to answer technical questions about equipment and the costs of vehicle modification (*www.nmeda.org*).

REFERENCES

1. DeJong, G, Branch, LG, Corcoran, PJ. Independent living outcomes in spinal cord injury: multivariate analysis. *Arch Phys Med Rehabil* 1984; 65:66–73.

2. Monga TN, Ostermann HJ, Kerrigan AJ. Driving: a clinical perspective on rehabilitation technology. In: *Physical medicine and rehabilitation: state of the art reviews*. Philadelphia: Hanley & Belfus, 1997:11(1): 69–92.

3. Pierce S. A roadmap for driver rehabilitation. *OT Practice* 1996;1(10): 30–38.

4. Scheiman M. Screening for visual acuity, visual efficiency and visiual information procession problems. In: Scheiman, M, ed. *Understanding and managing vision deficits: a guide for occupational therapists*. Thorofare, NJ: Slack, 1997:113–152.

5. Maynard FM. *International standards for neurological and functional classification of spinal cord injury*, 5th ed. Chicago: American Spinal Injury Association, 1996.

6. *How to drive: a text for beginning drivers*, 9th ed. AAA Association Communication, 1997.

7. Havard AB, Shipp MK. *Disabilities and their implications for driver assessment and training*. Ruston, LO: Louisiana Tech University, 1999.

8. Babirad J. Considerations in seating and positioning severely disabled drivers. *Assist Technol* 1989;1:31–37.

9. Kamper, D, Parnianpour, M, Barin, K, et al. Postural stability of wheelchair users exposed to sustained, external perturbations. *J Rehabil Res Dev*, 1999;36(2):121–132.

10. Strano CM. Physical disabilities and their implications driving. *Work: A Journal Of Prevention Assessment & Rehabilitation* 1997;8:261–266.

11. Linden M, Sprigle S. Development of instrumentation and protocol to measure the dynamic environment of a modified van. *J Rehabil Res Dev* 1996;33(1):23–29.

12. Holicky R. Big vans, minivans: pros and cons. *New Mobility* 1995; 6(22):50–53.

13. Tanner RW, Zura RD, Chen VT, et al. A system for adaptive transportation. *J Burn Care Rehabil* 1990;11:543–551.

NEUROMUSCULAR ELECTRICAL STIMULATION IN SPINAL CORD INJURY

JOHN CHAE
RONALD J. TRIOLO
KEVIN L. KILGORE
GRAHAM H. CREASEY
ANTHONY F. DIMARCO

The application of neuromuscular electrical stimulation (NMES) in patients with spinal cord injury (SCI) is broadly categorized as functional or therapeutic. *Functional neuromuscular stimulation* (FNS) is the use of NMES to activate paralyzed muscles in precise sequence and intensity to restore the function of the muscle. Devices or systems that provide FNS are essentially substituting for paralyzed muscles and, therefore, are also appropriately called *neuroprostheses. Therapeutic neuromuscular stimulation* is the use of repetitive NMES of paralyzed muscles to prevent complications of immobility. Although therapeutic neuromuscular stimulation may have functional implications, it does not directly fulfill the functional role of the paralyzed muscle.

This chapter focuses on the application of NMES in patients with tetraplegia and paraplegia secondary to traumatic SCI. The physiology of NMES is reviewed. The components of NMES systems and their evolution in design, with emphasis on development of neuroprosthesis systems, are presented. A review of the clinical implementation of NMES systems focuses on neuroprosthetic applications for the upper extremity, lower extremity, bladder, and pulmonary system. Therapeutic applications are reviewed and include cardiovascular deconditioning, muscle atrophy, osteoporosis, and deep venous thrombosis. Finally, perspectives on the future developments and directions are presented.

PHYSIOLOGY OF NEUROMUSCULAR ELECTRICAL STIMULATION

Excitation of Nervous Tissue by Neuromuscular Electrical Stimulation

The action potential produced by NMES is identical to the action potential produced by natural physiologic means, with the same "all-or-none" property. The lowest level of charge that will generate an action potential is termed the *stimulus threshold*. The stimulus threshold of any neuron is inversely proportional to the diameter of the neuron. Therefore, large-diameter neurons, such as alpha motor neurons, which have the lowest thresholds for stimulation are activated first, followed by activation of small-diameter neurons, such as C pain fibers (1,2). This property of NMES is referred to as the *reverse recruitment order*. Note that this is the reverse of the physiologic size principle, whereby normally smaller muscle fibers are recruited initially, and then larger fibers (3).

The stimulus current diminishes as a function of the distance from the stimulating source (2,4). Therefore, neurons furthest away from an electrode are least likely to receive stimulation at a level above threshold. The threshold for direct muscle fiber excitation is about 100 to 1,000 times higher than the threshold for nerve stimulation (2). Therefore, it is unlikely that direct muscle stimulation occurs as a result of any of the electrical stimulation paradigms described in this chapter. Although FNS systems are often described as involving stimulation of a "muscle," technically, they stimulate the nerves innervating the muscle, resulting in muscle contraction.

Muscle Response to Neuromuscular Electrical Stimulation

Muscle fibers are divided into three groups based on their contractile properties (Table 25.1). At one end of the spectrum are the fast-twitch glycolytic (type II) fibers, which generate high levels of force but fatigue rapidly (4,5). At the other end of the spectrum are the slow-twitch oxidative (type I) fibers, which generate lower forces but are fatigue resistant (4,5). Fatigue resistance is probably the most desirable quality for most NMES applications involving the skeletal muscle. However, because large fibers have lower threshold for stimulation, large type II fibers are recruited preferentially by NMES. Furthermore, disuse atrophy tends to convert type I to type II fibers (6). Fortunately, this muscle atrophy, with the concomitant change in fiber type, can be reversed with chronic NMES (7). Human studies have demonstrated that cyclic NMES of paralyzed muscles can in-

TABLE 25.1. CHARACTERISTICS OF SKELETAL MUSCLE FIBERS BASED ON THEIR METABOLIC AND MECHANICAL PROPERTIES

	Slow Oxidative (Type I)	Fast Oxidative Glycolytic (Type IIa)	Fast Glycolytic (Type IIb)
Muscle color	Red	Red	White
Motor unit strength	Low	High	High
Contractile speed	Slow	Fast	Fast
Rate of fatigue	Slow	Intermediate	Fast
Major source of adenosine triphosphate	Oxidative phosphorylation	Oxidative phosphorylation	Glycolysis
Oxidative capacity	High	Intermediate	Low
Glycolytic capacity	Low	Intermediate	High

crease muscle bulk and stimulated joint torques (8,9). All current neuroprosthetic applications use some form of muscle conditioning patterned after these studies. The effects of NMES on muscle physiology are presented in detail in the therapeutic neuromuscular electrical stimulation section.

Successful stimulation of muscle for functional purposes requires that the lower (alpha) motor neuron (LMN) be intact. In SCI, there is frequently some damage to the LMN pool at the level of the injury (10). If most or all of the LMNs to a particular muscle are damaged, then it will not be possible to obtain functional levels of force from the muscle with NMES. NMES mediated exercise does not reverse atrophy in fibers in which the LMN has been damaged. Extensive LMN damage is therefore a contraindication to NMES, and diseases or traumas that involve peripheral nerve damage (such as amyotrophic lateral sclerosis or brachial plexus injury) are not likely to benefit.

Force generated by NMES is modulated and influenced by various factors. To maintain smooth contraction and yet maximize fatigue resistance, the ideal stimulation frequency ranges between 12 and 16 Hz for upper extremity applications and 18 and 25 Hz for lower extremity applications. As the duration or amplitude of a stimulus pulse is increased, the stimulus threshold is reached for neurons further away from the stimulating electrode, leading to activation of more neurons and greater force generation. Factors external to stimulation parameters that influence force generation include movement of the electrode with respect to the target nerve, inherent length–tension characteristics of muscle, changes in the tendon moment arm as a function of joint angle, and volume conduction of current that may recruit muscles beyond the target muscle (11,12).

Safe Stimulation of Living Tissue

The parameters for safe stimulation and materials for safe electrodes for implanted systems have been experimentally established (2). Improper stimulation can result in electrochemical changes in the electrode material, leading to corrosion or dissolution of metal ions. Therefore, balanced biphasic stimulation should always be used with intramuscular stimulation to avoid this phenomenon. Tissue damage is also related to the charge per unit area of stimulation, not the voltage of the stimulus.

Therefore, it is safer to use constant current rather than constant voltage stimulation for electrodes within muscle or nerve tissue because it provides control of the charge density.

However, there are other factors to consider when transcutaneous electrodes are used. The electrode–tissue contact area is generally not constant because electrodes often pull away from the skin, which significantly decreases the electrode–tissue contact area. When constant current stimulation is used, this leads to high current densities, which can burn the underlying tissue. When using constant voltage stimulation, the increased resistance results in decreased current delivered to the tissue. Although this may be safer, it results in variations in the stimulation delivered to the muscle, changing the force output. Even with good skin contact, transcutaneous NMES may still result in warming and reddening of the skin, which is generally benign. However, if the current densities are too high, burning of the tissue can occur, even with good electrode–skin contact. Therefore, transcutaneous stimulation should be used with caution and with frequent examination of the skin when applied to patients with impaired sensation or cognition.

Intramuscular electrodes eliminate the risk for direct skin reaction to the applied stimulus but carry a risk for muscle tissue damage if the stimulus is improperly applied. Safe stimulation parameters with this type of electrode are biphasic pulses with amplitude of 20 mA and pulse duration of 200 μs. Frequency is typically in the range of 10 to 50 Hz, although frequency is not a factor in adverse tissue response to stimulation. Intramuscular NMES using these parameters has been applied for human use since the 1980s without any evidence of current related muscle damage (13).

Most direct nerve stimulation is accomplished using a nerve cuff electrode that encompasses the nerve trunk. Nerve tissue damage can occur through the same electrochemical mechanism as muscle tissue damage, but it can also occur through mechanical movement of the cuff relative to the nerve. In addition, tissue growth around nerve cuff electrodes can result in compression of the nerve and therefore secondary damage (14). Despite these potential problems, nerve cuffs have been used safely in many applications (15–17). Stimulation of nerves typically requires about one tenth of the current necessary for intramuscular stimulation.

SYSTEM COMPONENTS AND EVOLUTION IN DESIGN

The user of any neuroprosthesis must communicate his or her intent to the device through a variety of input devices to control the resulting limb movement (18,19). Once the user delivers a command to the system, the device must interpret the command and activate the appropriate stimulation channels. Optionally, the user can be made aware of what the system is doing through a feedback system. Most clinically applied FNS systems operate open loop; that is, they are unresponsive to the environment and do not automatically correct for errors that arise between the intended and actual motions of the limbs. Closed-loop systems require a sensor processor to monitor the actions of the limbs and allow the control processor to adjust stimulus levels automatically without conscious input from the user. Finally, the user can be informed of the orientation and state of his or her body (rather than the state of the device) through substitute sensory feedback. In this scheme, sensor signals are used to modulate tactile stimulation to sensate areas, or provide other indications of the status of the limbs and joints and their interaction with the environment (20,21).

FNS systems can be completely external or implanted. Despite the required surgery, implantable systems offer the advantages of placing the stimulating electrodes in close proximity to nerves, thus greatly increasing the selectivity and efficiency of activation while reducing the current required. For long-term clinical application, implanted systems such as these provide major advantages over other systems, including improved convenience, cosmesis, reliability, and repeatability (22).

Electrodes for FNS applications are classified according to the location of their stimulating surfaces. They are usually designed to activate nerves in the periphery, but increasing attention is being paid to developing new technologies to stimulate the spinal cord, motor cortex, or other regions of the brain. Most clinically available electrodes fall into three broad classes: transcutaneous electrodes applied to the skin, muscle-based electrodes, and nerve-based electrodes. Alternatively, lead wires connecting the electrodes to the stimulus generating circuitry are described by the course they take and the tissues through which they pass. Electrode leads can be classified as external, percutaneous, or implanted. All transcutaneous electrodes use external leads, whereas muscle- and nerve-based electrodes can be connected to either percutaneous or implanted lead wires.

Transcutaneous electrodes deliver electrical charge to the motor nerve through the skin. They are applied to the surface of the skin over the *motor point*, the location exhibiting the best contraction from the target muscle at the lowest levels of stimulation. NMES with transcutaneous electrodes offers several distinct advantages: (a) the electrodes are generally easy to apply and remove, (b) the stimulation technique is noninvasive and therefore reversible, (c) the use of transcutaneous electrodes can be easily learned and applied in the clinic, and (d) stimulators and transcutaneous electrodes are relatively inexpensive and commercially available. Stimulation with transcutaneous electrodes is the most widely used technique for therapeutic applications (23) and has been successfully employed to produce stand-

ing, stepping, and grasping motions and to assist with respiratory function (24–26).

Despite their apparent convenience when applied individually in small numbers, transcutaneous electrodes have several disadvantages: (a) they cannot produce isolated contractions of small muscles; (b) daily doffing and donning can complicate use, especially if electrode positions vary slightly from day to day; (c) an increasing number of electrodes are used; and (d) in many cases, cutaneous pain receptors are excited, and patients with preserved or heightened sensation may find it difficult to tolerate transcutaneous stimulation at the levels required to produce a motor response.

Muscle-based electrodes bypass both the high resistance of the skin and the cutaneous sensory fibers. They require significantly lower currents, exhibit greater muscle selectivity, and are better tolerated than transcutaneous stimulation. Intramuscular electrodes can be introduced either percutaneously or in an open surgical procedure and allow access to deep nerves and muscles (8,27,28). Early movement of the electrode tip away from the target nerve within the first 6 weeks after implantation is the most frequently observed failure mode of these devices (29). Epimysial electrodes are sutured directly to the epimysium or fascia to eliminate this early movement and provide immediate and permanent fixation. Because they are installed surgically, they are used almost exclusively with implanted stimulators but have also been connected to percutaneous leads (30).

Nerve-based electrodes have a more intimate contact with neural structures and therefore require even less current than muscle-based electrodes to produce a contraction. They take the form of epineural electrodes, which are sutured to the connective tissue surrounding a motor nerve; cuff electrodes that envelope the nerve; and penetrating intraneural probes, which are still laboratory-based investigational tools. Epineural and nerve cuff designs have both been employed as stimulating electrodes in FNS systems to restore motor function in SCI and stroke (17, 31). Cuff electrodes have also been configured to record from afferent nerves in attempts to use the natural sensors in the body to provide feedback signals to control and adjust the stimulation (32).

Electrodes are connected to stimulating or recording circuitry through lead wires. Percutaneous leads have been designed to connect chronically indwelling intramuscular and epimysial electrodes to circuitry external to the body while maintaining a barrier to infection. The leads are made of multiple strands of insulated stainless steel that are helically wound to form a thin, flexible cable of small-enough diameter for the tissue to heal around as it exits the skin.

Although they facilitate donning and doffing of neural prosthesis by eliminating the need to apply individual electrodes, percutaneous leads require continual attention from the user. They must be cleaned, dressed, and properly inspected and maintained in order to reduce the risk for complications. These leads are subject to breakage at areas of high shear stress. Although the electrode failure rate is low during the first few months after implantation, the cumulative 1-year failure rate can vary between 56% and 80%, which limits the use of percutaneous electrodes to short-term applications (<3 months) (33, 34). Other potential complications of using percutaneous intramuscular electrodes include formation of granulomas from retained electrode fragments and electrode-related infections, which are treated with oral antibiotics, minor outpatient surgical procedure, or both. Based on 20 years of experience in our laboratory with patients with SCI, stroke, and traumatic brain injury, cases of granuloma formation and electrode infection occurred at a rate of 1 per 5.5 years of research subject participation. Cases that required outpatient surgical treatment occurred at a rate of 1 per 18.5 years of subject participation. Although they can remain functional for years without infection or complication, percutaneous leads are usually reserved for acute and subacute applications and are generally considered to be ill suited for long-term clinical use.

Implanted leads can be of larger dimensions than percutaneous lead wires because they need to be more robust and resistant to failure and are not required to cross the skin. To allow repair or revision of implanted FNS systems, provisions have been made in several designs to isolate system subcomponents from each other using high-reliability implantable connectors (35). In-line connectors permit the surgical removal and repositioning of individual electrodes with minimal dissection and without extensive exposure of larger implanted circuit packages. Implantable electronic components can also be designed as passive devices, which derive their power from the radiofrequency signals providing the communication channels to external command or control processors. Systems using this configuration eliminate the need for additional surgery to replace internal batteries.

UPPER EXTREMITY NEUROPROSTHESES
Objectives of Upper Extremity Systems

FNS has been used to provide grasp and release for patients with a SCI at the cervical level (22,36–38). The objectives of these systems are to reduce the need of individuals to rely on assistance from others, to reduce the need for adaptive equipment, to reduce the need to wear braces or other orthotic devices, and to reduce the time it takes to perform tasks. FNS systems make use of the patient's own paralyzed musculature to provide the power for grasp and the patient's voluntary musculature to control the grasp. Typically, patients use the neuroprosthesis for such tasks as eating, personal hygiene, writing, and office tasks. These systems are now available clinically, and although they do not provide normal grasp function, they do enable patients to perform tasks more independently.

Candidate Selection

Most upper extremity neuroprostheses have been targeted for individuals with C5 and C6 motor levels. For these patients, the provision of grasp opening and closing using FNS provides a distinct functional benefit. At the C4 motor level, control of elbow flexion and shoulder stability must be provided by stimulation of the biceps or brachialis, or by mechanical or surgical means. FNS has been applied to a limited extent to these individuals, but there are no clinically deployed systems for this population to date. For individuals with C7 or C8 motor level function, there are other surgical options, such as tendon trans-

fers to provide function, and FNS is usually not indicated at the present time.

Electrical stimulation is delivered to intact lower motor neurons, as described earlier in this chapter, and is not used to activate denervated muscle directly. For C5 and C6 injuries, the muscles most likely to sustain LMN damage are the wrist extensors. Peckham and Keith found that between 80% and 100% of the muscles necessary for grasp had sufficient intact innervation to generate functional levels of force (39). In many cases, other paralyzed muscles can be used to substitute for the function that is not available (40).

FNS can be applied at any time after injury, but it is typically applied after neurologic stability has been achieved. Joint contractures must be corrected, or functional ability will be limited. Spasticity must be under control. Individuals who are motivated and desire greater independence are the best candidates for neuroprostheses. In addition, most current neuroprosthetic systems still require assistance in donning the device; therefore, it is necessary for the individual to have good attendant support.

Operating Principles

All existing upper extremity neuroprosthetic systems consist of a stimulator that activates the muscles of the forearm and hand and an input transducer and control unit. The control signal for grasp is derived from an action that the user has retained voluntary control over, which can include joint movement, muscle activity, respiration, or voice control (36,37,41–51). A coordinated stimulation pattern is developed so that the muscles are activated in a sequence that produces a functional grasp pattern. Two basic grasp patterns are generally provided for functional activities: lateral pinch and palmar prehension (52). Other grasp patterns have been described for use in neuroprostheses, including a pinch grip between the index and thumb and parallel extension grasp with finger extension and thumb abduction (53, 54). The user typically has control over grasp opening and closing but does not have direct control over the activation of each muscle. This design simplifies the control task required by the user.

Clinically Evaluated Applications

There are three commercially available neuroprosthetic systems designed to provide upper extremity function for patients with SCI: Handmaster (NESS Ltd., Ra'anana, Israel), FESMate (NEC Medical Systems, Tokyo, Japan), and Freehand (NeuroControl, Cleveland, Ohio) (55). The primary technical distinctions between these systems are their relative invasiveness. The Handmaster uses transcutaneous stimulation, FESMate uses percutaneous electrodes, and the Freehand system uses implanted electrodes and an implanted stimulator.

Transcutaneous Neuroprosthesis

Nathan from BeerSheva, Israel has developed a splint, which incorporates transcutaneous electrodes for grasp, as shown in

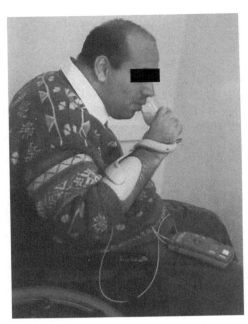

FIGURE 25.1. The Handmaster system, which consists of an arm splint with built-in transcutaneous electrodes and a control unit.

Fig. 25.1, called the Handmaster (37,38). The brace fixes the wrist in neutral, making it applicable primarily to C5 level tetraplegic patients who do not have a tenodesis grasp. A clinical study of the Handmaster was performed by Snoek and colleagues (38). Ten C5 to C6 quadriplegic individuals were evaluated for fitting of the neuroprosthesis, and four participated in the functional training. Each user underwent 2 weeks of muscle conditioning using the stimulator, and then 6 to 12 weeks of functional training. Functional performance was assessed in at least four tasks, which included pouring water from a can, opening a jar, opening a bottle, and inserting and removing a videotape. The results show that all four of the subjects could perform at least two tasks independently using the Handmaster that they could not perform without assistance using their hand with a splint. Three of the subjects demonstrated improvement in pouring from a can and opening a bottle. Other improved tasks included shaving, putting on socks, and handling a hammer. In this group, only one subject continued to use the Handmaster at home. Evaluation of a similar transcutaneous stimulation unit demonstrated a significant therapeutic benefit from the stimulation (56). The Handmaster has the European Community (CE) Mark in Europe and is approved by the U.S. Food and Drug Administration (FDA) as a therapeutic device.

Percutaneous Neuroprosthesis

The FESMate system uses up to 30 percutaneous electrodes to provide palmar, lateral, and parallel extension grasp patterns, and was developed by Handa and colleagues of Sendai, Japan (27,50,54). Percutaneous systems were developed to address the problems of specificity and repeatability encountered with transcutaneous stimulation systems (39,47,57,58). The implantation

is minimally invasive, requiring needle insertion only, with no surgical exposure. Grasp opening and closing is controlled by a switch operated by the opposite arm or by respiration using a sip-puff control. This system is primarily available in Japan. A formal assessment of outcomes with respect to disability and user satisfaction has not been reported.

Implanted Neuroprosthesis

An upper extremity neuroprosthesis was first implanted in 1986 by Peckham and colleagues in Cleveland and is now known as the FreeHand system (13,22) (Fig. 25.2). The FreeHand system consists of eight implanted electrodes and an implanted receiver-stimulator unit. It provides lateral and palmar grasp to patients with C5 and C6 tetraplegia (59). A radiofrequency inductive link provides the communication and power to the implant receiver-stimulator. The proportional control of grasp opening and closing is achieved using shoulder motion, which is measured using an externally worn joystick on the chest and shoulder (42). The FreeHand system has FDA approval in the United States and the CE Mark as a neuroprosthesis providing hand function for SCI.

A multicenter study was conducted to evaluate the safety, effectiveness, and clinical impact of the implanted neuroprosthesis on 50 individuals with SCI (22,60). The inclusion criteria for participants in the study were the following:

- The subject must have a traumatic SCI resulting in tetraplegia at the American Spinal Injury Association (ASIA) C5 or C6 functional motor level or ASIA impairment (formerly Frankel) grade A or B (International Classification grade 0, 1, or 2, Co or Cu) occurring at least 1 year before implantation.
- LMN innervation of key muscles of the forearm and hand or their substitutes must be demonstrated, as indicated by a grade 4 response to transcutaneous electrical stimulation. Key muscles are the thumb abductors, adductors, flexors, and extensors and the finger flexors and extensors.
- Participants must be at least 16 years old or skeletally mature (as indicated by fused growth plates); have shoulder and elbow strength adequate to position the hand for functional activities; have good tolerance and stability seated in a wheelchair; be in good physical and mental health; be motivated; and be willing and able to return to the clinic for periodic evaluations.

Exclusion criteria included cardiac pacemaker, history of chronic systemic infection or illness that increased surgical risk, uncontrolled spasticity, extensive and irreversible contractures in upper-extremity joints, diabetes, immune disease, heart disease or cardiac arrhythmia, and breast masses with a high probability of being cancerous.

Preoperatively, candidates were evaluated through a comprehensive physical examination, including a renal ultrasound and dental examination within 6 months of the implant surgery. Paralyzed muscle excitability was evaluated using transcutaneous stimulation applied to each muscle in the forearm and hand. Each candidate underwent a 1-month muscle-conditioning program using transcutaneous stimulation to build muscle strength. Postoperatively, the treated arm was immobilized in a cast for 3 weeks to allow electrode encapsulation and wound healing.

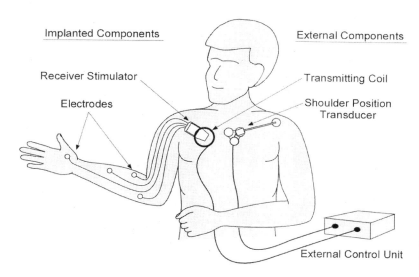

Implanted Components   External Components

Receiver Stimulator   Transmitting Coil

Electrodes   Shoulder Position Transducer

External Control Unit

FIGURE 25.2. The FreeHand system, which consists of an implanted stimulator and electrodes, an external power and control unit, and a shoulder position sensor.

After cast removal, muscle conditioning using the neuroprosthesis was initiated to build fatigue resistance in the muscles. After about 4 weeks of daily muscle conditioning at home, training and evaluation using the neuroprosthesis were performed during a 1- to 3-week inpatient stay. Follow-up studies were performed 6 months and 1 year after implantation.

The neuroprosthesis produced increased pinch force in every patient. In a test of grasp and release ability using six objects of different sizes and weights, 49 of the 50 participants (98%) moved at least one more object with the neuroprosthesis than they could without it (61,62). The direct impact of the neuroprosthesis in the performance of activities of daily living was tested in 28 patients. Each participant was tested in 6 to 15 tasks, which included eating with a fork, drinking from a glass, writing with a pen, dialing a phone, using a computer diskette, and brushing teeth. Every participant received training both with and without the neuroprosthesis to achieve their maximum independence using each method. If necessary, participants were provided with splints or adaptive equipment to perform the task. Therefore, the independence provided by the neuroprosthesis was directly compared with the maximum independence that could be provided by any other means. All 28 participants improved in independence in at least one task, and 78% were more independent using the neuroprosthesis in at least three tasks tested. All participants preferred to use the neuroprosthesis in at least one task tested, and 27 (96%) preferred to use the neuroprosthesis in at least three tasks tested. Satisfaction and daily use of the neuroprosthesis at home were measured through surveys and device data logging (63). More than 90% of the participants were satisfied with the neuroprosthesis, and most used it regularly. Follow-up surveys indicate that usage patterns are maintained at least 4 years after implantation.

Adverse events due to the implanted components and surgical installation were few. Four patients experienced a localized infection at the site of an electrode. In three cases, the electrode was removed, the infection resolved, and, where necessary, the electrode replaced. The fourth patient delayed seeking medical attention until the infection had progressed along some of the

electrode leads such that explantation of the entire system was considered prudent. There have been no cases of neuroprosthesis failure, and less than 1% experienced lead failures. In one patient, one channel on one implanted receiver-stimulator malfunctioned; however, the patient continued to use the neuroprosthesis with no functional deficit.

Summary of Upper Extremity Clinical Neuroprosthetic Applications

Neuroprostheses have been demonstrated to provide increased independence for patients with C5 and C6 level injuries. The different commercially available neuroprosthetic systems provide the patient and clinician with a variety of choices, depending on the individual's needs and goals. If the primary goal is muscle conditioning and contracture prevention, transcutaneous stimulation provides a noninvasive option that is relatively easy and inexpensive to implement. If the individual wants to maximize functional capability, implanted systems, in conjunction with surgical reconstruction, provide the greatest functional potential and have shown the greatest long-term use. For those individuals who are unwilling to undergo surgery or who have not yet achieved neurologic stability after injury, percutaneous or even transcutaneous stimulation systems may provide the individual with an opportunity to evaluate the function provided by neuroprostheses before making the more long-term commitment of an implanted system.

Current Research in Upper Extremity Neuroprostheses

Current research in the application of neuroprosthetics to the upper extremity in SCI includes the provision of additional function through the stimulation of more muscles, evaluation of new methods of control, new technologic advances, and the development of systems for C3 and C4 level injuries.

Additional Function

All three commercially available neuroprosthetic systems focus on the provision of grasp and release, but it has been shown that stimulation of additional muscles can provide even more function. Overhead reach can be provided by stimulation of the triceps muscle, and subjects can combine triceps activation with stimulated grasp function to gain improved functional abilities (37,64–66). Stimulation of the pronator quadratus muscle can develop adequate pronation that can be opposed by voluntarily generated supination (67). Stimulation of the finger intrinsic muscles can improve grasp function (68).

New Control Methods

A number of alternative methods for controlling a neuroprosthesis have been pursued. The use of wrist position to control grasp has been shown to be a better method of control for some patients when compared with control of grasp using shoulder position (45). Activation of voluntary antagonists has been used to control elbow angle and forearm supination and pronation (66,67). The use of the myoelectric signal from either forearm or neck muscles has been shown to be a viable method of control (45,46,48,49).

Technologic Advances

Technologic advances include implanted control transducers, new electrode technology, and use of devices that minimize surgical invasiveness (32,69–72). A second-generation implanted neuroprosthetic system has undergone clinical feasibility testing in four subjects and is shown in Fig. 25.3 (73). This system consists of an implanted stimulator-telemeter, 10 implanted electrodes, and an implanted wrist-position sensor. This neuroprosthesis provided increased independence for each subject, including grasp and release, elbow extension, and forearm pronation for C6 level injuries.

Application to C3 through C4 Injuries

Neuroprosthetic applications for high-level tetraplegia have been demonstrated clinically (37,50,51,54,74). Transcutaneous or percutaneous stimulation has been used to provide hand and elbow motion. Braces are used to support the shoulder. User control of both hand and arm function is provided through voice command, sip-puff control, or voluntary shoulder movements. Functional ability has been demonstrated in activities such as eating, drinking, and writing.

Treatment Strategy of Cervical Level Injury Using Surgical Reconstruction and Neuroprosthetics

Functional independence can be maximized for patients with cervical level injuries through a combination of surgical reconstruction and neuroprosthetics. These steps should be taken in conjunction with conventional therapeutic treatment that maximizes both passive and active movement.

C3 through C4 Injuries

Neuroprosthetic application for C3 through C4 injuries is still undergoing research. However, the preliminary results indicate that elbow flexion is a key component of the treatment. Surgical reconstruction is aimed at providing shoulder stability and elbow flexion. At present, although the results are encouraging, the application of FNS to this group of patients cannot yet be recommended with the expectation of functional outcome. There are no surgical reconstruction options because of the limited musculature under voluntary control.

C5 Injuries

Surgical reconstruction in this group of patients is focused on providing strong wrist extension through the transfer of the

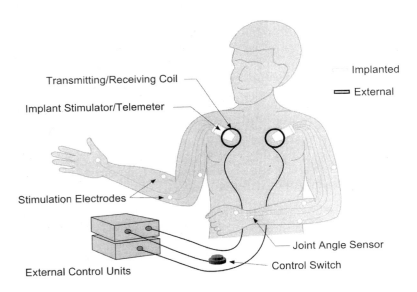

Transmitting/Receiving Coil

Implant Stimulator/Telemeter

Implanted

◻ External

Stimulation Electrodes

Joint Angle Sensor

External Control Units

Control Switch

FIGURE 25.3. The second-generation bilateral hand neuroprosthesis system provides elbow extension by stimulating the triceps and enhanced hand grasp control by using an implantable wrist angle transducer.

brachioradialis muscle. This eliminates the need for a wrist brace and provides a functional tenodesis grasp. Neuroprostheses provide grasp opening and closing as well as enhanced wrist extension. The transfer of the posterior deltoid tendon to the triceps tendon can provide elbow extension, which can be augmented through electrical activation of the triceps muscle. A strong C5 patient who does not have extensive lower motor neuron damage should, after these interventions, have voluntary wrist extension and elbow extension and stimulated grasp opening and closing.

C6 Injuries

Surgical reconstruction in this group is focused on providing strong elbow extension through the transfer of the posterior deltoid to the triceps, and augmenting weak wrist extension when necessary. Neuroprostheses provide strong pinch and grasp opening and may augment elbow extension and forearm pronation. Alternatively, thumb or finger flexion can be provided through tendon transfer procedures, and the neuroprosthesis can provide grasp opening and augmented pinch strength.

C7 Injuries

Surgical reconstruction in this group is focused on providing voluntary finger flexion through tendon transfers. Elbow extension can be augmented through tendon transfers if necessary. At present, neuroprosthetics are not typically applied to this group of patients because of the function that can be gained by tendon transfers alone.

LOWER EXTREMITY NEUROPROSTHESES

FNS can provide individuals paralyzed by thoracic or low cervical SCI with the ability to perform many activities that were previously impossible or difficult from the wheelchair, including standing, transfers, stepping short distances, and simple mobility functions such as side and back stepping (75–77). Preliminary clinical trials of lower extremity neuroprostheses suggest that continuous open-loop stimulation of the trunk, hip, and knee extensors can allow people with paraplegia to overcome physical obstacles, negotiate architectural barriers, and exert greater control over their environment by affording them the ability to reach and manipulate objects that are otherwise inaccessible from the wheelchair (78–80).

Neuroprostheses for Standing and Transfers

Standing with FNS has been achieved with relatively simple systems consisting of two to six channels of continuous transcutaneous stimulation (81,82). Transcutaneous electrodes can be easily applied and removed without invasive procedures, although daily variation in electrode placement can adversely affect the repeatability of the stimulated responses. Nevertheless, multichannel transcutaneous stimulation systems have been successful at producing standing and stepping movements in people with SCI in both laboratory and clinical settings (25,83,84).

Lower extremity FNS systems employing percutaneous intramuscular electrodes have also been successful in providing lower extremity functions to individuals with paraplegia (29,85). Patients with SCI using 16 or fewer channels of percutaneous intramuscular stimulation can perform simple mobility and one-handed reaching tasks while standing (86). Percutaneous approaches to most muscles of the lower extremities have been defined, allowing the generation of more complex movements than with transcutaneous stimulation alone (87). More recently, totally implanted pacemaker-like neuroprostheses for standing after SCI have undergone feasibility and initial clinical testing. Exercise and standing have been reported with a cochlear implant, and a 12-channel system for activation of the L2 through S2 motor roots has been applied to a handful of volunteers (88, 89). For long-term clinical application, implanted systems such as these provide major advantages over transcutaneous and percutaneous stimulation, including improved convenience, cosmesis, reliability, and repeatability (22).

Figure 25.4 shows an individual with complete motor and sensory mid-thoracic paraplegia using the implanted standing system. The implanted components of the standing and transfer system include an eight-channel receiver-stimulator with in-lead

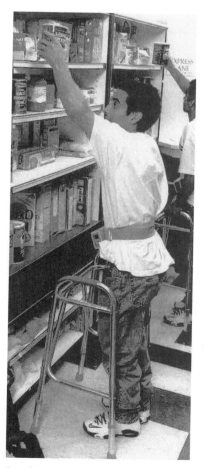

FIGURE 25.4. Standing with continuous stimulation to the trunk, hip, and knee extensors with an eight-channel implanted neuroprosthesis. Balance must be maintained by one extremity on an assistive device.

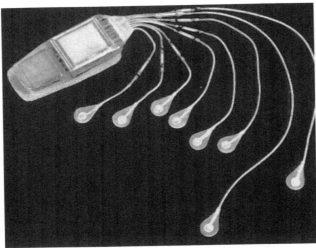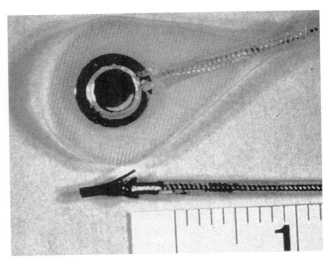

FIGURE 25.5. Implanted components of the standing/transfer neuroprosthesis. Depicted are the implanted eight-channel stimulator/receiver with in-lead connectors and epimysial electrodes (*left*) and a magnified view of epimysial and intramuscular electrodes used with the system (*right*).

connectors to epimysial or surgically implanted intramuscular electrodes (28,35,59,90) (Figs. 25.4 and 25.5). In a single surgical procedure, epimysial electrodes are installed bilaterally in the vastus lateralis, semimembranosus or posterior portion of the adductor magnus, and gluteus maximus. The intramuscular electrodes are inserted at L1 to L2 to activate the lumbar spinal roots for the erector spinae muscles. Surgical installation of the system is typically accomplished in less than 8 hours, and no appreciable blood loss or other postoperative complications, including infection, have been reported. A system-level diagram of the standing system and a composite x-ray of the internal components of the neuroprosthesis are shown in Fig. 25.6.

After a critical period of bed rest and restricted activity to promote healing immediately after implantation, an 8-week program of progressive resistance and endurance exercise with the implanted system is initiated. Upon completion of reconditioning exercise, patterns of stimulation are constructed for the sit-to-stand and stand-to-sit transitions, followed by a 2- to 3-month period of rehabilitation. System users progress from standing in parallel bars to a walker, to standing pivot transfers and swing-through gait. Balance training includes stand-to-retrieve tasks and releasing a hand to manipulate the controls of a wearable external control unit that provides power and command information to the implanted receiver-stimulator through an inductive link established by a transmitting coil placed on the surface of the skin above the implant.

The wearable external controller is programmed through a clinical interface suitable for use by nontechnical personnel (91, 92). The external controller is small and lightweight enough to be worn under the clothing and can operate for up to 4 hours on a single charge. Neuroprostheses recipients interact with the system through a series of buttons on the enclosure of the external controller or through remote switches worn on a ring or attached to the walker, crutch, or other support device. Users select a preprogrammed pattern of stimulation for exercise or

function from a series of menu options. To stand, a single activation of one switch initiates the stimulation sequence to raise the body from the seated position. After a short delay to allow the user to position the hands comfortably on an assistive device, stimulation to the trunk, hip, and knee extensors is increased to levels sufficient to raise the body from the seated position and maintained continuously to keep the body upright during standing. Another depression of the switch reverses the process and lowers the user to a seated position in a controlled fashion.

Continuous stimulation to the extensor musculature braces the body against collapse while the hands are used for balance (93). Stepping can be achieved with 16 channels of stimulation through the addition of a second implant to activate the hip flexors and ankle dorsiflexors (94,95). To date, a total of 12 such surgically implanted neuroprostheses for standing or stepping have been successfully installed at Case Western Reserve University and the Cleveland Veterans Association Medical Center. Multicenter clinical trials of the technology for FDA approval are underway (96). Long-term follow-up of at least 2 years has been completed on five subjects, indicating that stimulation thresholds are stable and internal components are reliable, with survival rates of epimysial electrodes in the extremities exceeding 91% and of intramuscular electrodes in the lumbar spine of 100% (97,98). No failures of the implanted stimulator, connectors, and lead wires have been observed.

Initial results from the clinical trials of the implanted standing systems show that the stimulated responses of the knee, hip, and trunk extensors are sufficiently strong and fatigue resistant for functional use. After completing the program of reconditioning exercise, ASIA total motor scores with stimulation are 16% to 21% (mean, 18.3%) greater than without FNS. Subjects who completed the exercise protocols were able to stand for sufficient lengths of time to complete various activities ranging from standing transfers to working at a counter. The amount of practice and training, body size, hip and trunk extensor strength, and

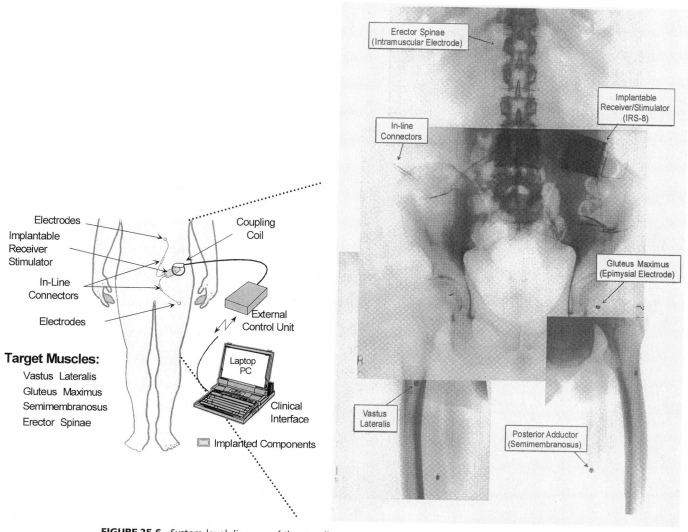

FIGURE 25.6. System-level diagram of the standing neuroprosthesis (*left*) and composite x-ray showing implanted components (*right*).

quadriceps endurance appear to be important influences on standing duration, which can vary from 3 minutes to longer than 20 minutes. Measures of stimulated strength and endurance are summarized in Fig. 25.7. Mean isokinetic knee extension moments (at 30 degrees per second), produced by epimysial electrodes in the vastus lateralis, exceed 35 Nm. Mean isometric hip extension moments, generated by the gluteus maximus and hamstrings, approach 20 Nm each and appear to be additive when stimulated simultaneously. The vastus lateralis exhibits good fatigue resistance after exercise with the neuroprosthesis, as evidenced by the ratio of final knee extension moment after 40 minutes of cyclic isokinetic contractions (1 second on, 3 seconds off). High endurance (fatigue ratios > 0.75) generally coincides with better performance in terms of standing duration.

All lower extremity FNS systems still require assistive devices, such as crutches, walkers, or additional bracing, to provide supplemental support or allow the upper extremities to inject the corrective forces necessary to maintain a stable upright posture. The magnitudes of these corrective forces can be quite small—on the order of 10% of body weight or less (99). They can be produced routinely by a single extremity without undue exertion, freeing the other hand to perform reaching tasks or other functions, as illustrated in Fig. 25.4 (100). FNS can readily generate the muscle forces and joint moments required for rising from a chair into a standing posture with minimal assistance from the upper extremities. Producing the postural corrections necessary to maintain balance in the presence of intrinsic (voluntary motions) or extrinsic (unanticipated environmental perturbations) destabilizing disturbances, however, remains a major challenge to the designers of FNS systems. Practical and robust control systems to provide standing balance (i.e., the maintenance of standing posture), even for the brief periods of time typically required for completing simple reaching activities, has been an elusive goal and is still an active area of research.

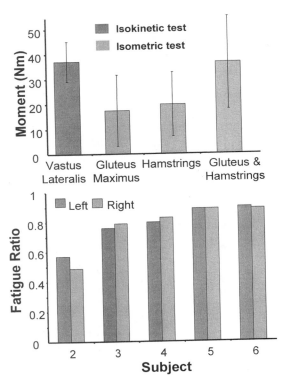

FIGURE 25.7. Summary of stimulated strength (*top*) and endurance (*bottom*) for early recipients of the implanted standing/transfer neuroprosthesis. Mean peak isokinetic (30 degrees per second) knee-extension moments and isometric hip-extension moments generated with electrical stimulation are significant and sufficient for function. Individual fatigue ratios (peak final to initial knee-extension moment during 40 minutes of cyclic contractions) show good endurance properties.

The distribution of support forces between upper and lower extremities while standing with continuous stimulation has been monitored in the course of initial clinical trials of the implanted standing system. The distribution of body weight in six early recipients of the standing neuroprosthesis is illustrated in Fig. 25.8. Most subjects were able to stand with little upper extremity

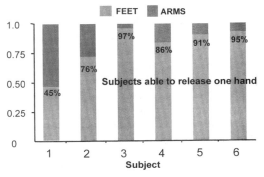

FIGURE 25.8. Distribution of mean vertical support forces during quiet standing with neuroprosthesis for the first six system recipients. The lower extremities typically support more than 85% of body weight, and these subjects are able to release one upper extremity from a support device to manipulate objects in the environment.

effort while stimulated contractions of the knee, hip, and trunk extensors prevented collapse. In the four later cases, balance was maintained through light touch on a support surface typically less than 10% of body weight. All but the earliest subjects were able to release one hand intermittently from a walker or other assistive device, and all were able to perform standing transfers with the neuroprosthesis. Users and their assistants reported a preference for FNS-assisted transfers over conventional methods when moving to and from high surfaces, whereas conventional pivot or sliding transfers were still the method of choice for level transfers (101). Transfers to heights impossible to perform by conventional lifting transfers required moderate effort or assistance with the neuroprosthesis.

Although the upper extremity corrective forces required for balance with open-loop stimulation can be quite small, on the order of the weight of the arms themselves, this is not true for all users of currently available standing neuroprostheses, who exhibit a great deal of variability in their standing performance. The support forces imposed on the arms while upright depend on many variables, including postural alignment and the stimulated moment produced at the joints. Increasing stimulated hip extension consistently decreases the vertical support forces placed on the upper extremities, and the same hip extension moment is more effective at decreasing the forces on the arms at more erect standing postures. At more erect postures (5 and 10 degrees of hip flexion), small amounts of active stimulated hip extension moment produce large decreases in arm-support forces. At more flexed postures (15 to 25 degrees), much more hip extension is required to reduce the arm-support forces by similar amounts (102,103). These results indicate that strong stimulated hip extension and the ability to assume an erect posture will be prerequisites for advanced systems providing postural corrections to destabilizing events.

The metabolic energy cost associated with quiet standing with continuous FNS is less than three times the basal metabolic rate during able-bodied standing and close to twice that of standing with knee-ankle-foot orthoses (104). This is a level comparable to tub bathing, piano playing, or fishing and results primarily from the stimulated activity of the lower extremity musculature, rather than from upper extremity exertion (105). Control strategies that minimize high levels of continuous stimulation to prepare for, or respond to, a change in postural demand need to be considered to keep energy expenditures at reasonable levels.

Neuroprostheses for Ambulation

Functional Neuromuscular Stimulation–Only Systems

Pioneering work in the application of FNS for restoration of standing and walking function to individuals with complete and incomplete SCI was conducted in the 1970s and 1980s in Ljubljana, Slovenia. The techniques developed by Kralj, Bajd, and others continue to be employed in many laboratories and clinics around the world (106). Using as few as two transcutaneous stimulation channels per leg, standing and reciprocal walking is produced by activation of the quadriceps muscles and the triggering of a flexion withdrawal reflex. A pair of transcutaneous electrodes is placed over the quadriceps on the anterior thigh.

A second pair of electrodes is located distally over the dermatomes of the peroneal, sural, or saphenous sensory nerves. Standing is achieved by simultaneously activating the quadriceps bilaterally in response to a command input, such as the simultaneous depression of switches on the handles of a rolling walker or crutches. A stride is produced by maintaining activation to the quadriceps of the stance leg while initiating a flexion withdrawal in the contralateral limb. Depression of the crutch- or walker-mounted switch on the swing leg stimulates the afferent sensory fibers and triggers a spinal reflex arc that causes hip, knee, and ankle flexion. To complete the stride, activation of the knee extensors on the swinging leg is initiated while the reflex is still active and flexing the hip. The stimulus producing the flexion reflex is then removed, leaving the user in double-limb support once again with bilateral quadriceps stimulation. Some paralyzed subjects have been reported to walk at speeds approaching one fourth of normal and to ascend a curb or step with transcutaneous stimulation.

Two additional stimulus channels to the gluteal muscles can be added to extend the hips (107). Complicating issues with this system include active flexion generated by the rectus femoris when the quadriceps muscle is stimulated with transcutaneous electrodes. This makes erect standing difficult and results in an anterior pelvic tilt with compensatory lordosis or excessive weight on the arms to maintain an upright posture. Not all patients exhibit a flexion withdrawal reflex that is strong or repeatable enough to be used for stepping. Because it is a mass flexion pattern resulting from synergistic activity of a group of muscles triggered by a single stimulus, the swing-limb motion is difficult to control. Reflex stepping can be effective in well-selected individuals, although it tends to be jerky, and the reflex can habituate with repeated activation, limiting the number of steps that can be taken at one time.

The Slovenian group has fit transcutaneous stimulation systems to more than 50 patients with several years of follow-up and has developed extensive prescriptive criteria for individuals with various neurologic deficits. Patients with incomplete injuries are first evaluated for conventional orthoses alone before adding FNS. Individuals with high-level injuries are considered for combinations of orthoses and stimulation, and those with mid- to low-level paraplegia are candidates for the transcutaneous FNS system without orthoses. These systems and implementation procedures have been successfully transferred to clinical practice, and a commercially available transcutaneous stimulation system (Parastep, Sigmedics, Inc., Northfield, IL) for standing and stepping has received FDA approval (25,26).

An increasing number of SCIs are resulting in neurologically incomplete lesions (108). With help of FNS, many of these individuals can become functional walkers because some of their motor, sensory, and proprioception function has been preserved. However, the high variability of the incomplete SCI population requires caution in the application of FNS (109). Voluntary strength can improve with exercise and therapy augmented with electrical stimulation. In these cases, increased stride length and reduced physiologic cost index during walking can be achieved. Alternatively, the quality of stimulated responses can improve while volitional function remains unchanged, necessitating a neuroprosthetic application of FNS. In some patients, an exaggerated extensor tone can provide safe standing, but the patients are unable to initiate a step. In such patients, peroneal stimulators may be useful to inhibit extensor tone and help initiate a step (110,111). When needed, hip abductors, hamstrings, and trunk extensors are included in stimulation patterns (112).

These approaches have been extended through the use of implanted electrodes for personal mobility functions, such as transfers; standing; one-handed reaching; forward, side, and back stepping; and stair ascent and descent. This approach involves individual activation of a number of muscles (typically eight or more) rather than the use of synergistic patterns such as the flexion withdrawal reflex, or extensive bracing. Marsolais and colleagues synthesized complex lower extremity motions by activating up to 48 separate muscles with chronically indwelling helically coiled fine-wire intramuscular electrodes with percutaneous leads under the control of a programmable microprocessor-based external stimulator (113). Some well-trained subjects are able to walk 300 meters repeatedly at 0.5 m/sec with this system (114). All components are worn by the user, freeing him or her from cabling to a walker or other assistive device. Freely articulating ankle-foot orthoses are used to protect the ligaments and structure of the foot and ankle. The quality of the motions produced by FNS with this system depended on the availability, strength, and endurance of paralyzed muscles; the ability of the therapist or engineer to specify patterns of stimulation for ambulation; and the subject's experience with the device.

Standing and stepping can be achieved in patients with complete paraplegia with 16 channels of stimulation (the four listed above for standing, plus the tibialis anterior, tensor fascia latae, sartorius and iliopsoas bilaterally). These systems rely on two eight-channel devices, as shown in Fig. 25.9. Users of the standing systems depicted in Figs. 25.4 and 25.6, with complete thoracic level injuries below the level of T4, can have the second implant installed to activate the additional muscles required for walking in a second surgical procedure. This neuroprosthesis is still being tested in the laboratory and is not yet clinically or commercially available. Other multichannel implanted systems for walking in paraplegia have also been reported to provide standing and swing-through gait (31,115).

Hybrid Systems Combining Functional Neuromuscular Stimulation and Orthoses

One method to achieve ambulation after SCI involves combining FNS with conventional bracing (77,116–119). The energy required to operate these hybrid systems is less than with braces alone, but increases rapidly with walking velocity. At slow to moderate speeds, energy consumption for both modes of walking is still less than with FNS alone. However, energy consumption for FNS walking decreases as walking speed increases, suggesting that as velocities approach normal, the differences between walking modalities will be minimized or reversed (with brace walking requiring more energy than FNS). The energy saving effect of hybrid systems is primarily a result of their ability to constrain the motions of the joints, reduce the degrees of freedom of movement, and provide mechanical stability. For static activities such as quiet standing, individuals with paraplegia can assume a stable posture with little or no muscular exertion

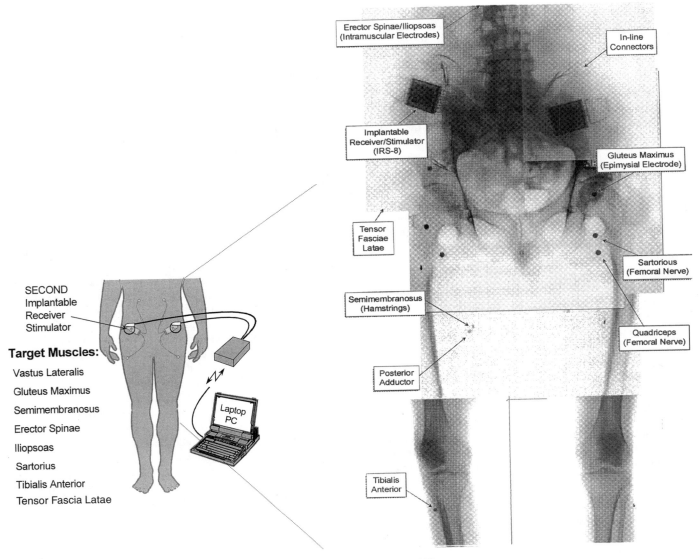

Erector Spinae/Iliopsoas
(Intramuscular Electrodes)

In-line
Connectors

Implantable
Receiver/Stimulator
(IRS-8)

Gluteus Maximus
(Epimysial Electrode)

Tensor
Fasciae
Latae

Sartorious
(Femoral Nerve)

Semimembranosus
(Hamstrings)

Quadriceps
(Femoral Nerve)

Posterior
Adductor

Tibialis
Anterior

SECOND
Implantable
Receiver
Stimulator

Target Muscles:

Vastus Lateralis

Gluteus Maximus

Semimembranosus

Erector Spinae

Iliopsoas

Sartorius

Tibialis Anterior

Tensor Fascia Latae

Laptop
PC

FIGURE 25.9. Dual-implant walking mobility system.

by locking the knees of a brace and hyperextending the hips, thus avoiding the fatigue associated with continuous stimulation. FNS is quite effective at introducing large impulsive forces into the biomechanical system through activation of large lower extremity muscles, which reduces the upper extremity exertion required for walking with conventional braces. Combining FNS and bracing in a hybrid orthosis takes advantage of the positive aspects of each technology and minimizes the potential shortcomings (120,121).

The Louisiana State University Reciprocating Gait Orthosis (LSU-RGO) hybrid system consists of a four-channel transcutaneous stimulator and a flexible copolymer electrode cuff that locates and maintains the transcutaneous electrodes over the rectus femoris and hamstrings. Because walking is accomplished with the knees locked, stimulating the hamstrings extends the hip and flexes the contralateral hip through the action of the reciprocating mechanism. Conversely, the rectus femoris is used to flex the hip actively, rather than extend the knee, and to assist with contralateral hip extension through the reciprocating mechanism. Rectus femoris and contralateral hamstrings are activated simultaneously to initiate a step on the depression of a walker-mounted switch. Hybrid systems of this type have been fitted to more than 50 patients to date with complete or incomplete thoracic or low-level cervical injuries at LSU and collaborating centers. Similar systems employing a hip-guidance orthosis or alternative reciprocating mechanism have been devised and tested in various centers in North America and Europe (122). Follow-up studies on RGO-based hybrid orthoses showed that up to 41% of system recipients used it for gait, whereas 66% used it for exercise (123,124).

Hybrid orthoses for walking in paraplegia is motivated primarily by the need to improve hip and trunk stability and forward progression. The simplest hybrid system uses a reciprocating gait orthosis for support against gravity through mechanical locks at the joints. Stimulation assists the patient in getting into stance and powering the reciprocal motion during walking (125). Other hybrid systems use the brace to provide mechanical support only at certain times in the gait cycle. With the joints passively locked by gravity, stimulation switches off and is only reactivated when the joint becomes unstable. In this way, stimulation duty cycle is reduced, and the onset of fatigue can be delayed (126). A third type of hybrid system regulates joint position with a controllable friction brake, hand-controlled mechanical joint locks, or externally powered joint actuators (127,128).

Hybrid systems are reliable and simple to implement in clinical environments with orthotic and prosthetic fabricating capacity. Standing with the knee joints of the brace locked allows all stimulation to be removed, postponing the onset of fatigue. The orthotic component of these may also protect the insensate joints and osteoporotic bones of users with long-standing SCI from possible damage resulting from the loads applied during weightbearing and ambulation. However, the bracing employed by hybrid systems can potentially encumber individuals in the execution of activities of daily living for which they were not designed. For example, locking the knees can hinder the completion of more complex movements useful for personal mobility, such as stair climbing. Similarly, the thoracic component can prohibit lateral bending and trunk rotation while sitting in the wheelchair. The devices are usually worn outside the clothing, and donning, doffing, and cosmetic aspects are similar to those of conventional braces.

Metabolic Costs of Functional Neuromuscular Stimulation Ambulation Systems

The study of energy consumption during locomotion with hybrid or FNS-only neuroprostheses is complicated by several factors that make generalization difficult. Most reports involve a small number of subjects with varying experience with the technology, and well-controlled or randomized trial are almost impossible to perform because raters and subjects alike can not be blinded to the status of their neuroprosthesis system. Furthermore, energy consumption during ambulation is inversely related to the hours of regular use of a neuroprosthesis (129). Therefore, direct comparisons between different systems on the same volunteers would require them to have the comparable amounts of practice with each device, which is often impractical. In addition, methodologies vary and almost uniformly require subjects to achieve a steady-state metabolic response for validity, which is not always possible with FNS-assisted ambulation. Nevertheless, several small-scale studies of the metabolic costs of walking with transcutaneous stimulation systems such as Parastep and hybrid orthosis systems such as the LSU-RGO have been reported.

The energy expenditure required for experienced users to walk distances up to 200 feet with the Parastep system has been reported to be about equivalent to a 1.5-mile walk at 3 mph for an able-bodied adult (130). The physiologic cost index (PCI), which is the ratio of change in heart rate from baseline (beats/min) to steady-state velocity (m/min), has been used as a measure of energy costs during normal walking as well as ambulating with transcutaneous stimulation (131). The PCI has been shown to be an indicator of energy costs in disabled individuals and applied as a measure of gait efficiency with different assistive devices after SCI (132,133). A wide range of walking performances was observed when PCI was applied to five fully trained Parastep users with mid- to low-thoracic level injuries (to avoid compromise of the sympathetic contribution to the cardiac plexus with injuries above T4). Winchester and associates reported PCIs ranging from 2.3 to 6.3 beats/m and walking velocities ranging from about 5 to over 24 m/min (129). These values are comparable to those reported for patients with paraplegia walking in an RGO (134). Just as with other upright mobility devices for individuals with SCI, walking with the Parastep system is slower and less energy efficient than normal walking, which exhibits a PCI ranging between 0.11 and 0.51 beats/m (mean, 0.21 beats/m) at self-selected speeds. However, it provides reasonable upright mobility at velocities and energy costs that appear to be within the physiologic capacities of people with paraplegia (135). With energy costs similar to long leg braces, transcutaneous FNS systems may be better suited as a means of providing the documented physical benefits of exercise than as a daily mode of personal transportation (136–139).

Oxygen consumption ($\dot{V}O_2$), heart rate, and velocity during walking with an RGO alone and with a hybrid FNS-RGO system have also been documented. In a single-subject case study, Isakov and colleagues reported lower PCI values and slightly faster velocities with a hybrid FNS-RGO system than with the brace alone (133). The addition of FNS to the reciprocating orthosis appeared to decrease mean PCI from 2.55 beats/m to 1.54 beats/m at average self-selected velocities of about 24 and 25 m/min, respectively. These results are at the upper limits of performance observed by Winchester and coworkers for the Parastep system and Bowker and associates for the RGO alone, but the statistical significance of any apparent differences can not be determined, and care should be taken when comparing the results (129,134,135).

Hirokawa and colleagues performed a well-controlled study of oxygen consumption during ambulation with the LSU-RGO and the hybrid FNS-RGO system involving six subjects with comparable experience with each device (140). Rate of energy expenditure (kcal/kg/min) and energy costs per meter walked (kcal/kg/m) were derived from net oxygen consumption during repeated 30-meter walks at self-selected speeds and at preset velocities ranging from 0.1 to 0.4 m/s as controlled by a metronome. Rate of energy consumption increased with walking velocity in a similar manner for both RGO-only and hybrid systems. However, a 16% reduction in rate of energy consumption was observed at all walking speeds with the hybrid FNS-RGO system as compared with the orthosis alone. Rate of energy consumption increased at the same rate under both conditions. When expressed in terms of energy consumed per meter walked, a similar 16% to 18% reduction in energy costs was observed with the hybrid system at velocities slower than the self-selected pace of 21 m/s, although these advantages diminished rapidly with increasing walking speed (118). As with reports of the Parastep system, these values are still considerably larger than those reported for able-bodied ambulation, indicating that hybrid systems may also be most useful as an effective mode of exercise for individuals with SCI rather than a means of transportation (124,141).

The true value of lower extremity FNS systems in their current forms lies in their ability to facilitate or provide options for short-duration mobility-related tasks, such as overcoming physical obstacles or architectural barriers in the vicinity of the wheelchair. Exercise, standing, standing transfers, and one-handed reaching are all possible with relatively simple transcutaneous or surgically implanted FNS systems without extensive external bracing. The functional impact of lower extremity neuroprosthetic applications of FNS on the ability to complete activities of daily living is still an active area of research. It is clear from preliminary work, however, that exercise and standing with FNS can improve tissue viability and overall health, facilitate standing transfers by eliminating the heavy lifting and lowering required by an assistant, and allow selected individuals with SCI to regain access to objects, places, and opportunities impossible or exceedingly difficult from the wheelchair. FNS can augment and extend the function of the wheelchair and may prove to be a valuable option to enhance the well being and independence of patients with disabilities. All this can be achieved with reliable implanted components that maximize cosmesis, personal convenience, and long-term use. From the reports in the literature to date, walking with FNS appears to be a promising form of exercise, rather than an alternative to wheelchair locomotion. The metabolic energy currently required to walk with FNS is too high to make it a truly practical alternative to the wheelchair for long-distance transportation over level surfaces, although this remains a worthwhile and achievable long-term goal.

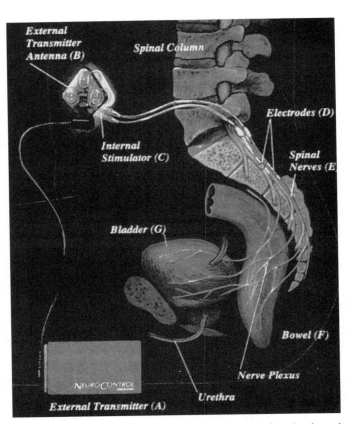

FIGURE 25.10. The Vocare system, which consists of an implanted stimulator and electrodes, and an external power and control unit.

BLADDER NEUROPROSTHESES

Normal function of the lower urinary tract requires alternation between micturition and continence. Patients with suprasacral cord lesions can have electrical stimulation applied to the surviving sacral nerves or nerve roots to improve bladder and bowel function. An implantable device is now clinically available for this purpose (Fig. 25.10). The technique has been used by more than 1,500 patients in at least 20 countries since the 1980s to produce effective micturition and to improve bowel function (142–149).

Operating Principles

Micturition

Contraction of the detrusor muscle of the bladder can be produced by electrical activation of the parasympathetic preganglionic efferent neurons, whose cell bodies are in the sacral segments of the spinal cord and whose axons usually travel in the S3 and sometimes S4 or S2 anterior roots and nerves. These axons are closely accompanied for much of their course by somatic efferent axons to the external sphincter and pelvic floor. The latter axons, being of larger diameter than the parasympathetic axons, have a lower threshold for electrical activation, and it is therefore difficult to produce contraction of the detrusor without contrac-

tion of the external sphincter. However, micturition can be produced by the technique of poststimulus voiding, which uses the fact that the detrusor muscle of the bladder relaxes more slowly than the striated muscle of the external sphincter. Bladder pressure can be built up by a series of bursts of electrical stimulation, each lasting a few seconds, and is maintained between the bursts; the external sphincter contracts strongly during bursts but relaxes rapidly for a few seconds between bursts, allowing urine to flow. It was initially thought by some that the intermittent contraction of the sphincter during voiding might produce harmful pressures in the bladder, leading to ureteric reflux or hydronephrosis, but these fears have not been borne out in long-term follow-up.

Continence

The major cause of incontinence in subjects with suprasacral SCI continues to be detrusor hyperreflexia. Research is in progress evaluating reflex inhibition of the detrusor by electrical stimulation of large afferent neurons in the sacral dermatomes, a process known as *neuromodulation*, which shows some benefit in able-bodied subjects with urge incontinence (150,151). However, the most dramatic abolition of reflex incontinence can be produced by surgical division of the sacral sensory nerve roots, and since the mid-1980s, this procedure, known as *posterior rhizotomy*, has increasingly been combined with implantation of an electrical stimulator intended to stimulate the motor roots for micturition.

The rhizotomy also reduces the risk for damage to the upper urinary tracts by lowering the pressure at which urine is stored in the bladder, and may result in some improvement in reflux or hydronephrosis if these have already occurred. It also abolishes spasticity of the external urethral and anal sphincters and abolishes the autonomic hyperreflexia and potentially dangerous increases in blood pressure that can otherwise result from sacral afferent input when the bladder or bowel is distended. However, it also abolishes other potentially useful sacral reflexes, such as reflex erection and reflex ejaculation, as well as sacral sensation and orgasm from sacral stimulation if these were preserved after the injury.

Reflex ejaculation too is not always effective, but seminal emission can now be produced from a high proportion of men with SCI by rectal probe electrostimulation, and other techniques for obtaining viable sperm are available. These alternative techniques for assisting with erectile function or fertility can still be used after posterior rhizotomy, and the implant itself may produce erection when S2 roots are stimulated, an effect that appears to be potentiated by oral administration of sildenafil. A decision about posterior rhizotomy should therefore be made on a case-by-case basis. However, the advantages of posterior rhizotomy are such that it is generally carried out when a bladder stimulator is implanted, thereby improving both micturition and continence.

Candidate Selection

Micturition by electrical stimulation requires intact parasympathetic efferent neurons to the detrusor. The function of these neurons can be demonstrated by the presence of reflex detrusor contractions when performing a cystometrogram. It is desirable to show a pressure rise of at least 35 cm H_2O in a woman and 50 cm H_2O in a man. Other sacral reflexes, such as ankle tendon reflexes, the bulbocavernosus reflex, anal skin reflex, and reflex erection, are confirmatory. In the United States, the procedure is approved by the FDA as a Humanitarian Use Device (Vocare, NeuroControl Corporation, Cleveland, Ohio) for subjects with complete SCI, although subjects with incomplete lesions have received the implant in other countries. Device implantation can occur at any time after the subject reaches neurologic stability. Candidates should also have a degree of emotional and social stability. Frequent urinary tract infection and problems with catheters or anticholinergic medication are further indications, and it is wise to evaluate the urogenital system for any other complications, such as stones, strictures, or diverticula, and to treat these concurrently.

Female patients with paraplegia and persistent reflex incontinence are often particularly grateful for posterior rhizotomy because of the lack of satisfactory urine-collecting devices. Male patients with paraplegia and low tetraplegia often wish to dispense with a urine-collection bag, whereas male patients with higher tetraplegia may choose to continue to wear a condom collection device. If a tetraplegic man plans to use condom drainage with electrical stimulation, it is wise to check preoperatively that the condom can be retained satisfactorily. It is also advisable to discuss options for sexual function and to offer a trial of various techniques for erectile function.

Technique

Electrodes may be placed either intradurally on the sacral anterior nerve roots in the cauda equina through a lower lumbar laminectomy or extradurally on the mixed sacral nerves in the sacral canal through a laminectomy of S1 to S3. The intradural approach has been more widely used in Europe, but extradural electrodes are usually used in the United States because the technique of implanting them carries less risk for trauma to the nerves or cerebrospinal fluid leakage. Intraoperative electrical stimulation and recording of bladder pressure are used to confirm the identity of the nerves supplying the bladder. Leads from the electrodes are tunneled subcutaneously to a radio receiver-stimulator placed under the skin of the abdomen or chest and are powered and controlled by a battery-powered remote control operated by the patient.

The posterior rhizotomy is best done intradurally where the sensory and motor roots can be more easily separated. If intradural electrodes are being implanted, the rhizotomy can be done at the cauda equina. If extradural electrodes are used, the rhizotomy is usually done at the conus medullaris through a separate laminectomy, although it can also be done within the lower end of the dural sac.

Postoperatively, urodynamic studies are used to guide the setting of stimulus parameters to give an acceptable voiding pressure and rate and pattern of flow. The patient can usually be discharged within 1 week of surgery with a working device. The stimulus program should be checked between 1 and 3 months after the operation because the response of the bladder may change with repeated use; thereafter, review is recommended at least annually, monitoring lower and upper urinary tract function.

Clinical Outcomes

Most patients with an implanted bladder stimulator use it routinely for producing micturition four to six times per day. Residual volume in the bladder after implant-driven micturition is usually less than 60 mL and often less than 30 mL (148). A substantial decrease in symptomatic urine infection with or without pyrexia has been reported by many groups following the use of the implant (143,148,152,153). In our initial series of 20 subjects in Cleveland, the average postvoid residual volume with the stimulator was 22 ± 14 mL, and the median number of urine infections decreased from 7 to 1 per year (154).

Continence is achieved in more than 85% of patients (155–157). This is largely attributable to abolishing the detrusor hyperreflexia and increase in bladder compliance, which follow posterior sacral rhizotomy and which persist long term provided the rhizotomy is complete from S2 caudally. About 10% to 15% of patients report some stress incontinence of urine after implantation of the stimulator and posterior rhizotomy (158). It is not always clear whether this stress incontinence was formerly masked by more profound reflex incontinence or whether it results from the abolition of spasticity in the external urethral sphincter. However, being of small volumes, it is usually more manageable than reflex incontinence, which may require a change of clothing, and is managed in some subjects by low-level stimulation of the external urethral sphincter. Urodynamic studies show that there are substantial increases in bladder capacity and compliance after the abolition of reflex bladder contraction by posterior rhizotomy (158,159). Typically, bladder capacity is greater than 400 mL, with a storage pressure of less than 40 cm H_2O. Voiding pressure can be controlled by adjusting the parameters of electrical stimulation, and although it is sometimes greater than in non-SCI subjects, this does not appear to be harmful to the upper tracts (142,143,152,159,160).

Several centers in Europe have followed patients long term, particularly with regard to the upper tracts (144,148,159). This experience indicates that trabeculation, ureteric reflux, and hydronephrosis tend to decrease in patients who undergo implantation and posterior rhizotomy. It appears likely in these patients that any harmful effects from transient high pressure during micturition are outweighed by the beneficial effects of low-pressure storage of urine, during the majority of each day. There is also a reduction in the incidence of autonomic dysreflexia because of the interruption of afferent fibers from the bladder, lower bowel, and perineum by posterior sacral rhizotomy. This outcome is particularly beneficial to tetraplegic male patients formerly dependent on an indwelling catheter prone to blockage from frequent infection. The ability to micturate on demand and improved continence of urine both contribute to a reduction in use of intermittent and indwelling catheterization. In our series in Cleveland, 18 of 20 subjects became catheter-free (154). Most users become free of urine-collection bags, but some male tetraplegic patients with impaired ability to handle clothing or a urine bottle choose to continue to wear a condom drainage system for convenience. Reduction of urinary tract infection results in substantially less use of antibiotics. The abolition of detrusor hyperreflexia by posterior rhizotomy allows patients to discontinue anticholinergic medication, which in turn reduces constipation and other side effects, such as a dry mouth, blurred vision, and drowsiness.

Regular stimulation of the sacral parasympathetic nerves contributes to transport of stool through the distal colon into the rectum, and most users report a reduction in constipation and reduced need for laxatives and stool softeners. Some users are able to defecate by a pattern of intermittent stimulation similar to that used for micturition but with longer intervals between bursts of stimulation to allow passage of stool. However, most patients also check with a finger in the rectum whether there is stool remaining after this procedure and, if so, remove it manually. The frequency of bowel emptying increases toward the preinjury pattern, and the overall time spent on bowel management is greatly reduced. In the Cleveland series, the time spent on bowel emptying was reduced by 75% (154).

Studies in Europe indicate that the use of the implanted stimulator together with posterior sacral rhizotomy results in substantial savings in the cost of bladder and bowel care, particularly from reduction in supplies needed for bladder care, medications, and visits to physicians for management of complications (161). In the United States, interviews by a life care plan analyst with patients between 6 months and 6 years after implantation in Cleveland indicated that savings in bladder and bowel care equaled the cost of purchasing and implanting the stimulator after about 5 years, and thereafter are expected to result in pro-gressive savings to the health care payer (162). Although loss of reflex erection is an important consequence of posterior rhizotomy, the implant itself may produce erection when S2 roots are stimulated.

Complications

Infection of these implants is rare, occurring in 1% of the first 500 implants. Infection is usually introduced at surgery or through a subsequent break in the skin. A technique of coating the implants with antibiotics was introduced in 1982 and reduces the infection rate (163). Technical faults in the implanted equipment are uncommon, occurring on average once every 19.6 implant-years (149). The most common site for faults are in cables, which are sometimes mechanically damaged by compression against a rib but which can usually be repaired under local anesthesia.

RESPIRATORY MUSCLE STIMULATION

Fifteen to 20 percent of patients with acute cervical SCI suffer from respiratory insufficiency on initial presentation (164). Although a significant number of these patients are eventually able to breath spontaneously, 4.2% develop chronic respiratory insufficiency and require some form of mechanical ventilatory support (165). Because the average age at time of injury is 32 years, these patients are generally maintained on mechanical ventilation for 20 to 25 years or longer (166–168).

Unfortunately, mechanical ventilation is associated with substantial morbidity, mortality, inconvenience, and social stigma, including significant patient and caregiver anxiety associated with machine dependence, physical discomfort, fear of disconnection, difficulty with speech, reduced mobility, and embarrassment associated with the ventilator and attached tubing. Artificial respiration by phrenic nerve pacing, in contrast, eliminates many of these problems and provides a more natural form of artificial ventilation, more closely mimicking spontaneous breathing.

Phrenic nerve pacing has now been applied in more than 1,000 patients worldwide and has become a clinically accepted technique to provide artificial ventilatory support in patients with trauma-induced ventilator-dependent tetraplegia (169–174). Although there may be significant patient variability, most patients describe much better speech, improved level of comfort, reduced anxiety and embarrassment, increased mobility, and greater sense of well-being and overall health as most important benefits compared to mechanical ventilation (168, 173,175–178) (Table 25.2).

Stimulation Devices

Available phrenic nerve stimulation systems have similar basic configurations. The stimulating electrodes, radiofrequency receivers, and attached wiring compose the internal components. A radiofrequency transmitter, wires, and antenna constitute the external components. The stimulating electrodes are implanted

TABLE 25.2. POTENTIAL BENEFITS OF PHRENIC NERVE PACING

Increased mobility
  Easier bed-to-chair transfers
  Easier transport outside the home, including occupational and recreational activities

Improved speech

Improved sense of well-being and overall health
  More normal breathing and, in some individuals, tracheostomy closure
  Reduced volume of respiratory secretion
  Reduced incidence of respiratory tract infections

Reduced anxiety and embarrassment
  Elimination of fear of ventilator disconnection by individual and caregiver
  Elimination of ventilator tubing
  Elimination of ventilator noise
  Possible closure of tracheostomy

Improved comfort level
  Elimination of pull of ventilator tubing and positive-pressure breathing

Reduced level of required nursing care

Reduced overall costs
  Reduction and/or elimination of ventilator supplies

on each phrenic nerve either in the cervical or thoracic regions. Small wires tunneled subcutaneously connect the electrodes to radiofrequency receivers, which are implanted in an easily accessible area over the anterior portion of the thorax. External antennas connect to the transmitter. The transmitter generates a radiofrequency signal, which is inductively coupled to the implanted receivers. The signal is demodulated by the receivers, converting it to electrical signals, which are delivered to the stimulating electrodes in contact with the phrenic nerves.

Bilateral phrenic nerve stimulation results in descent of the diaphragm and a fall in intrathoracic pressure, resulting in inspiratory airflow. Diaphragm contraction also results in an expansion of the lower rib cage through a direct insertional action and outward movement of the abdominal wall through an increase in intraabdominal pressure. In fact, palpation of the lower rib cage and abdominal wall provides useful physical findings, which can be used to assess both the presence and extent of diaphragm contraction. Cessation of stimulation results in diaphragm relaxation, an increase in intrathoracic pressure, and exhalation. To provide a normal level of ventilation, this pattern is repeated 8 to 14 times/min. Stimulus amplitude and frequency and train rate can be adjusted by the operator to alter tidal volume and respiratory rate, respectively. Inspiratory time and inspiratory flow rate can be varied, in tandem, by changing the duration of stimulation.

There are three commercially available systems. The technical characteristics are presented in Table 25.3. The Avery system (Avery Laboratories Inc., Commack, New York) has full FDA approval and is the mostly widely used system worldwide. Monopolar electrodes are used most commonly, but bipolar electrodes are also available and are recommended in patients with cardiac pacemakers. The Atrotech system (Atrotech OY, Tampere, Finland) is commercially available in most developed countries and is currently being used under an Investigational Device Exemption from the FDA in the United States. The four-pole electrode system and stimulation paradigm reduces the stimulation frequency of individual axons to about one fourth of that with unipolar stimulation. This technique allows for greater time for recovery, lessens the risk for fatigue, enhances transformation of muscle fibers to more fatigue-resistant type I fibers, and shortens the reconditioning process (179). The MedImplant system (MedImplant Biotechnisches Labor, Vienna, Austria) has limited availability, predominantly in Austria and Germany. It is not available in the United States. This system

TABLE 25.3. TECHNICAL FEATURES OF PHRENIC NERVE STIMULATION SYSTEMS

	Manufacturer			
Device	Avery Laboratories Inc., USA		Atrotech OY, Finland	MedImplant Inc., Austria
Transmitter (stimulus generator)	S-232G	Mark IV	PX 244	MedImplant
Size (mm)	179 × 114 × 97	146 × 140 × 25	185 × 88 × 28	170 × 130 × 51
Transmitter/battery Weight (kg)	3.6	0.54	0.45 + 0.6 (12 V) 0.45 + 0.045 (9 V)	1.42
Rate (breaths/min)	10–50	6–24	8–35	5–60
Pulse width (µs)	150	150	200	100–1,000
Battery life (hr)	160	400	160–320 (12 V) 8 (9 V)	24
Sigh possible	Yes	Yes	Yes	Yes
Antenna receiver	902A Model I-107A	902A Model I-110A	TC 27-250/80 RX 44-27-2	RF transmission cell Implantable receiver
Size (mm)	46 (diam) × 16	30 (diam) × 8	49 (diam) × 8.5	56 × 53 × 14
Electrodes	Monopolar, bipolar	Monopolar, bipolar	Quadripolar	Quadripolar
No. of receivers to stimulate both hemidiaphragms	2	2	2	1

uses a four-electrode array positioned around each nerve. As with the Atrotech device, only a portion of the nerve is stimulated, and consequently, only a portion of the diaphragm is activated at any given time. This form of sequential stimulation is also thought to reduce the incidence of fatigue compared with conventional monopolar stimulation.

Patient Evaluation and Assessment

The degree of respiratory insufficiency consequent to cervical SCI is related to the exact location and degree of spinal cord damage. Injuries above the C3 level result in complete paralysis of the major inspiratory muscles and acute respiratory failure. Injuries involving the C3 to C5 level often result in acute respiratory failure, as well, owing to damage of the phrenic motor neuron pools or phrenic nerves directly. Damage to the spinal cord below the C6 level does not result in injury to the phrenic motor neurons or phrenic nerves. In patients who remain ventilator dependent, the success of phrenic nerve pacing is highly dependent on bilateral intact phrenic nerve and diaphragm function, as determined by phrenic nerve conduction studies.

Candidates for phrenic nerve pacing must be free of significant lung disease or primary muscle disease because these factors also preclude successful pacing. Candidates must be fully informed of all the risks and potential benefits. Implantation of the device requires a major surgical procedure with associated potential complications. After careful evaluation, some patients with sufficient inspiratory muscle strength may be better suited for noninvasive means of ventilatory assistance. In these patients, intermittent mouth positive-pressure ventilation may be an effective alternative to conventional mechanical ventilation.

Bilateral measurements of phrenic nerve function by experienced personnel are mandatory for all potential candidates of phrenic nerve pacing. Phrenic nerve integrity can be assessed by measurements of nerve conduction time. In adults (age range, 18 to 74 years), mean onset latency is 7.5 ± 0.6 ms with an upper limit of 9.0 ms (180,181). Successful pacing in adults has been achieved with mild prolongation of conduction velocity up to 14 ms. Other indicators of adequate phrenic nerve function include diaphragm descent of at least 3 to 4 cm during supramaximal tetanic stimulation and transdiaphragmatic pressures of about 10 cm H_2O with single-shock stimulation to either phrenic nerve.

Although the success of phrenic nerve pacing depends on technical considerations, patient psychosocial conditions are equally important. Before any technical assessment, therefore, a critical evaluation of the motivation of both the patient and family members is mandatory. Phrenic nerve pacing is most likely to be successful in home situations in which the patient and family members are anxious to improve the overall health, mobility, social interaction, and occupational potential of the patient. The patient should also have a clear understanding of the potential benefits to be achieved (Table 25.2).

Surgical Implantation

Phrenic nerve electrodes may be positioned either in the cervical region or within the thorax (169,171,182). The thoracic ap-

proach requires a thoracotomy, which has significant associated risks including hemothorax and pneumothorax, and which requires chest tube placement and intensive postoperative care. The cervical approach is simpler from a surgical point of view. However, the cervical approach is limited by incomplete phrenic nerves in the cervical region, activation of other nerves, and risk for mechanical stress resulting from movement of the neck. The thoracic approach, therefore, is the preferred method of electrode placement (183,184). Although there are a number of acceptable surgical approaches for thoracic electrode placement, the second intercostal space is most commonly used (182,185). At the discretion of the thoracic surgeon, the third interspace through an axillary incision or median sternotomy may be preferred. Iatrogenic injury to the phrenic nerve has been a common cause of pacemaker failure in the past (186). Therefore, it is critical that the electrodes are manipulated with extreme care to avoid mechanical trauma to the nerve and its blood supply. A radiofrequency receiver is positioned in a subcutaneous pocket on the anterior chest wall; wires from the electrode are passed through the third or fourth interspace and connected to the receiver.

The pacing system should be tested before closure of the surgical incisions. Threshold currents of each electrode should be determined by gradually increasing stimulus amplitude until a diaphragm twitch is observed. Threshold current should range between 0.1 and 2.0 mA. Suprathreshold current should result in a forceful, smooth diaphragm contraction. If threshold values are high or the difference between the lowest and highest thresholds among leads exceeds 1 mA, the electrode leads may need to be repositioned around the phrenic nerve. We prefer to place the receivers over the lower anterior rib cage just above the costal margin. In thin people, however, the anterior abdominal wall may be preferable to avoid pressure injury. The receivers in the Avery and Atrotech systems, both of which require two receivers, should be placed at least 15 cm apart.

Pacing Schedules

Pacing is usually started about 2 weeks after surgery to allow adequate time for all surgical wounds to begin healing and inflammation and for edema around the electrode site to resolve (185). The diaphragm must be gradually reconditioned to improve strength and endurance. During the initial trials of phrenic nerve pacing, minute ventilation necessary to maintain normal values of PCO_2 (35 to 45 mm Hg) over 5- to 10-minute periods should be determined. Respiratory rate is usually set at 8 to 12 breaths/min; tidal volume is adjusted by altering stimulation frequency to maintain the desired level of ventilation.

There are no definitive guidelines in terms of pacing schedules to achieve full-time ventilatory support. General recommendations are to provide phrenic nerve pacing for 10 to 15 minutes each hour initially and to increase this time gradually, as tolerated. Although the conditioning phase may take 8 to 10 weeks or longer, it is possible to bring some patients up to full-time support within 4 weeks. After full-time pacing is achieved during waking hours, pacing is provided during sleep and gradually increased until full-time pacing is achieved. During the conditioning phase, the patient must be carefully monitored for signs of fatigue, which is usually manifested by the patient's complaint of shortness of breath or reduction in inspired volume. Higher levels of stimulation may be required in the sitting compared with supine posture as a result of the shorter diaphragm length during sitting. This can be alleviated to a significant degree, however, by the use of a snug-fitting abdominal binder, which reduces the change in abdominal girth.

Complications

Although a number of complications have been reported since phrenic nerve pacing was first introduced, technical developments and patient experience have markedly reduced their incidence (176,186). With careful patient selection, appropriate use of stimulus parameters, adequate patient monitoring, and involvement of experienced professionals, the incidence of complications should be very low. Nonetheless, complications do arise, and appropriate precautions must be taken and remedial action instituted promptly, when necessary. All patients require a backup mechanical ventilator in the event of pacemaker failure.

Phrenic nerve pacing systems may fail to provide adequate ventilatory support as a result of a variety of factors. Battery failure is one of the most common causes of failure, which is easily prevented by regular battery changes or recharging schedules. Breakage of antenna wires at connection points is also a common cause of failure. Receiver failure was a common occurrence with older systems but is much less common with current systems owing to improvement in housing materials. Iatrogenic injury to the phrenic nerve may occur during implantation but can be prevented by meticulous dissection technique. After implantation, adverse tissue reaction and scar tissue formation can lead to gradual reduction in inspired volume and may require surgical intervention. Increases in airway resistance due to increased secretion or decrements in respiratory system compliance due to atelectasis also result in reductions in inspired volume generation. Removal of secretions either by suctioning or other means usually results in prompt improvement in respiratory system mechanics. A more serious, but fortunately less common, complication is the development of infection of the implanted materials, which necessitates removal of all implanted components (177,182,187). Diaphragm contraction without coincident contraction of the upper airway muscles results in collapse of the upper airway or obstructive apneas. This complication is completely preventable by maintaining a patent tracheostomy, especially nocturnally when risk is the highest. Exposure of the system to strong magnetic fields can lead to phrenic nerve injury. Thus, magnetic resonance imaging is contraindicated in these patients. Electrotherapeutic devices that generate strong radio-frequency fields could interfere with the pacing device and should also be avoided.

In children, paradoxical motion of the rib cage may be substantial because of its high compliance, resulting in reduced inspired volume generation. Because compliance gradually decreases between 10 and 15 years of age, the performance of the pacing system can be expected to improve over time (186). Because the diaphragm has a very small percentage of type I, fatigue-resistant fibers in small children, a much longer period of conditioning may be required to achieve full-time ventilatory support compared with adults (171).

Patient Outcomes

In patients with ventilator-dependent tetraplegia with intact phrenic nerve function, phrenic nerve pacing is clearly an effective means of providing ventilatory support with significant advantages over mechanical ventilation (171). However, earlier analyses of large patient groups describe significant numbers of individuals in whom successful ventilatory support could not be achieved. A large number of patients were implanted before 1985, and data were available only for 165 of 477 patients (171). In a retrospective analysis, about half of the patients who were deemed failures should not have been selected for phrenic nerve pacing. It is important to note that this study and others were performed at a time when the technology of phrenic nerve pacing and patient selection methods were not fully developed. Unfortunately, there are few recent analyses of modern-day success rates and incidence of side effects and complications. Long-term follow-up of 14 tetraplegic patients who used bilateral low-frequency stimulation recorded using the device successfully for as long as 15 years with a mean use of 7.6 years (186).

There is some evidence that improved electrode and receiver design is associated with a low incidence of pacer malfunction and high success rates when applied in appropriate candidates. The outcome of 64 patients (45 tetraplegic patients) who underwent phrenic nerve pacing with the Atrotech system since 1990 was recently evaluated (187). The duration of pacing averaged 2 years. The incidence of electrode and receiver failure was quite low at 3.1% and 5.9%, respectively. These values are lower than those previously reported with monopolar and bipolar systems. In this group, four patients developed infections, but none occurred in the tetraplegic group. Ongoing analyses, perhaps in the form of an international registry, are needed to track the incidence of side effects, complications, and true successes of this technique.

Although there are no controlled studies, it is conceivable that phrenic nerve pacing may improve life expectancy in patients with tetraplegia. Carter, for example, reported only 63% survival at 9 years in patients on positive-pressure ventilation (165). In contrast, all 12 tetraplegic patients who completed the Yale phrenic nerve pacing protocol were alive after 9 years. It is possible that mechanical ventilation is associated with a higher incidence of respiratory tract infections and mechanical problems related to the mechanical ventilator, tubing, and tracheostomy.

Future Directions

Diaphragmatic pacing devices can provide important health and lifestyle benefits compared with mechanical ventilation (173, 188,189). However, existing systems continue to have limitations and require further refinement. Many patients with ventilator-dependent tetraplegia cannot be offered phrenic nerve pacing owing to partial or complete injury of one of the phrenic nerves. Electrical stimulation of intercostal muscles may be an important alternative to phrenic pacing (190,191). Although this method alone is not likely to support adequate ventilation in humans, combining intercostal stimulation with unilateral phrenic pacing may generate sufficient volumes to maintain long-term ventila-

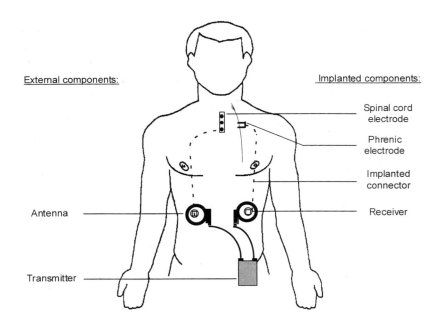

External components:

Antenna

Transmitter

Implanted components:

Spinal cord
electrode

Phrenic
electrode

Implanted
connector

Receiver

FIGURE 25.11. Combined intercostals and diaphragm pacing system.

tion (192–194) (Fig. 25.11). Conventional placement of phrenic nerve electrodes carries the risk for phrenic nerve injury and generally requires a thoracotomy, which is a major surgical procedure with associated risk, inpatient hospital stay, and high cost. Preliminary results suggest that intramuscular diaphragm pacing can provide similar benefits as conventional phrenic nerve pacing without the need for an invasive surgical procedure and less risk for phrenic nerve injury (195). The laparoscopy-guided procedure can be performed on an outpatient basis and therefore at much lower overall cost. Ongoing investigations will need to coordinate paced breaths with the patient's respiratory drive, which would improve speech cadence, match ventilation with metabolic demand, and eliminate the need for tracheostomy in many patients. The development of a fully implantable system would eliminate the need for the application of devices on the body surface and the risk for decoupling between the transmitter and receiver.

THERAPEUTIC EFFECTS OF NEUROMUSCULAR ELECTRICAL STIMULATION

Persons with SCI are at risk for multiple complications of immobility, including cardiovascular deconditioning, muscle atrophy, joint contractures, decubitus ulcers, osteoporosis, and thromboembolic disease. With the commercial development and availability of NMES-mediated exercise equipments (ERGYS and REGYS, Therapeutic Alliances, Inc., Fairborn, Ohio; StimMaster, Electrologic of America Inc., Beaver Creek, Ohio), a number of these conditions may be prevented or treated. This section reviews the efficacy of NMES-mediated exercises in preventing and treating cardiovascular deconditioning, muscle atrophy, osteoporosis, and deep venous thrombosis.

Cardiovascular Deconditioning

Heart disease is a leading cause of death after SCI (196). Alterations in cardiovascular physiology after SCI include substantial

decrease in oxygen uptake, overall impaired autonomic response to exercise, and ventricular wall atrophy (197–200). These abnormalities lead to lower physical work capacity and, in conjunction with a sedentary lifestyle, may contribute to lower levels of high-density lipoprotein (HDL) and higher risk for cardiovascular disease. However, as in able-bodied people, exercise for those with SCI can increase the level of HDL and decrease serum total cholesterol and low-density lipoprotein (LDL) levels (141,202). Among wheelchair athletes, indices of cardiovascular function, such as oxygen uptake, cardiac output, and stroke volume, are significantly higher than those of sedentary SCI patients (203, 204). Thus, in view of the aging population of patients with SCI, the increasing incidence of SCI among older individuals, and positive benefits of exercise among able-bodied individuals, an aggressive cardiac prevention program is appropriate for patients with SCI.

Until recently, exercise options for patients with SCI were limited to upper extremity ergometry. However, the therapeutic effects of upper extremity ergometry are limited by venous pooling in the lower extremities and abdomen, which may result in upper extremity ischemia, the potential for upper extremity musculoskeletal injury, and inefficient energy expenditure. With the development of lower extremity NMES-mediated exercise systems, improved exercise performance as reflected by acute changes and training effects on cardiovascular indices can be achieved.

Acute cardiovascular effects of NMES therapy can be demonstrated with lower extremity NMES-mediated exercises alone or in combination with upper extremity exercises. NMES-mediated nonergometry lower extremity exercises increase stroke volume and cardiac output and decrease total peripheral resistance in patients with paraplegia (205–207). NMES of the lower extremities in combination with rowing is associated with higher oxygen consumption than rowing alone (208). Similarly, NMES-mediated leg cycle ergometry in combination with arm ergometry is associated with significantly higher peak oxygen consumption and stroke volume compared with arm ergometry alone (209–212). These acute cardiovascular effects in response to NMES-mediated exercises of the lower extremity are likely mediated by increase in venous return associated with skeletal muscle pump as well as decrease in total peripheral resistance (206, 207,213).

The cardiovascular training effects can be achieved with NMES-mediated leg cycle ergometry, leg cycle ergometry in combination with arm crank ergometry, and lower extremity neuroprosthesis systems. Lower extremity stress testing after training with NMES-mediated leg cycle ergometry demonstrates significant increases in peak oxygen uptake, pulmonary ventilation, heart rate, and cardiac output and significant decreases in total peripheral resistance compared with pretraining status (214,215). Hybrid training protocols that combine leg cycle and arm crank ergometry are associated with even higher posttraining peak oxygen consumption than leg cycle ergometry training alone (216,217). Similarly, training programs with ambulation neuroprostheses systems increase peak oxygen consumption and reduce total cholesterol and LDL compared with pretraining levels (138,141). Training with NMES-mediated leg cycle ergometry is also associated with reversal of left ventricular atrophy (201).

With the aging of the spinal cord population and increasing incidence of SCI among older Americans, cardiovascular fitness is becoming more relevant in the long-term rehabilitation management of patients with SCI. As in able-bodied people, exercise among those with SCI is associated with acute changes in cardiovascular indices that translate into substantial training effect. These training effects include increased peak oxygen consumption, stroke volume, and cardiac output in response to stress testing; improvements in serum total cholesterol, HDL, and LDL levels; and reversal of left ventricular atrophy. It is likely that these training effects, if maintained, will lead to prevention of cardiovascular disease in the long term, with concomitant decreases in associated morbidity and mortality and overall improvements in quality of life. Although these postulated long-term benefits remain to be demonstrated in future controlled trials, it appears prudent to include cardiovascular fitness programs for patients with SCI as part of their ongoing rehabilitation management.

Muscle Atrophy

A major complication of immobility from SCI is muscle atrophy. The sequelae of muscle atrophy, including decreased strength and endurance, formation of contractures due to impaired muscle balance, weakening of myotendinous junction, decreased strength of tendons and ligaments and their insertions on bone, increased risk for decubiti from exposure of bony prominences, and altered cosmesis, have significant rehabilitation ramifications. Disuse atrophy develops over weeks and predominantly affects type I muscle fibers leading to conversion to easily fatigable type II muscle fibers (218,219). This section reviews the affects of NMES on the physiology of paralyzed muscles after SCI and its efficacy in reversing and preventing muscle atrophy and improving performance.

Chronic NMES produces characteristic histochemical and morphologic changes in paralyzed muscles after SCI. Chronic low-frequency (10-Hz) intramuscular NMES converts type II fiber to more fatigue-resistant type I fiber with concomitant increases in strength and endurance (7,8,220,221). At higher frequencies of stimulation employed by most commercially available transcutaneous NMES systems, fiber conversion from type II to type I is modest or minimal (222,223). However, further evaluation of the type II muscle fibers with ATPase technique demonstrates significant increase in the number of type IIa fibers, which are characterized by fast-twitch contractility and intermediate fatigability (224). Consistent with this observation, evaluation of myosin heavy-chain (MHC) composition of single fibers by sodium dodecyl sulfate–polyacrylamide gel electrophoresis before and after NMES training demonstrates significant increase in the expression of MHC of the type seen in type IIa fibers (225). Although studies generally report increases in the population of more fatigue-resistant fiber types after NMES therapy, observations on change in fiber size are inconsistent. Some studies report significant increases in the size of all fiber types, whereas others report no changes (222,223,226).

With the induction of these histochemical and morphologic changes, training with NMES partially reverses muscle atrophy among chronic SCI survivors, prevents atrophy among subacute survivors, and increases muscle performance. Computed tomography evaluations demonstrate significant increases in the cross-sectional area of lower extremity muscles after NMES-mediated ergometry and nonergometry training programs (226–230). Magnetic resonance imaging evaluation of patients with tetraplegia within 1 year of injury also demonstrates significant increases in cross-sectional area of the quadriceps femoris muscles after NMES nonergometry training. This increase is comparable to cross-sectional area 6 weeks after injury (231). In recognition of the likelihood that total reversal of muscle atrophy is not achievable, prevention of atrophy is a reasonable strategy. In a controlled study, 26 SCI survivors were assigned to control, NMES-mediated isometric contractions, or NMES-mediated cycle ergometry. After 3 and 6 months of training, only NMES-mediated ergometry prevented loss of lower limb and gluteal lean body mass. After 6 months of training, NMES-mediated ergometry also prevented loss of total body lean body mass (232). Corresponding to the changes in muscle bulk, significant improvements in muscle strength and endurance are observed after NMES-mediated ergometry and nonergometry training programs (228,229,233,234).

In summary, NMES-mediated lower extremity exercise programs facilitate the conversion of type IIa fibers to more fatigue-resistant type IIb or type I fibers, partially reverse muscle atrophy among chronic SCI survivors, prevent atrophy among acute SCI survivors, and increase overall stimulated muscle strength and endurance. The histochemical changes and improvements in muscle performance have significant ramifications on the candidacy of SCI survivors for the various neuroprostheses programs. With respect to secondary complications, it remains uncertain whether partial reversal of muscle atrophy is sufficient to be clinically useful. In view of the inherent difficulty in completely reversing muscle atrophy, the efficacy of NMES-mediated exercises in preventing atrophy should be further investigated in controlled trials before formulating recommendations.

Osteoporosis

The onset of osteoporosis due to nonuse and unloading occurs within a few weeks or months of SCI, with bone loss occurring below the level of the lesion (235). Pathologic fractures follow the progression of osteoporosis, with the annual incidence of long-bone fracture in the lower extremity estimated to be 4% to 7% (236). Electrical stimulation of the sciatic nerve of rats prevents suspension-induced osteopenia (237). In humans, a program of weightbearing and strengthening appears to decrease hypercalciuria (238). However, the effect on osteoporosis is uncertain.

In view of the relationship between loading and loss of bone mass, exploration of NMES-mediated exercises for reversal or prevention of osteoporosis is reasonable. Initial experience with NMES-mediated leg cycle ergometry and leg extension exercises demonstrated no evidence of reversal of osteoporosis (227,234, 239). However, significant decreases were also not reported. In view of the dynamic nature of bone loss after SCI, a possibility that NMES-mediated exercises decrease the rate of bone loss was proposed (234). Consistent with this hypothesis, the rate of bone loss during NMES-mediated leg cycle ergometry is lower than expected (240). The evolving data now suggest that leg cycle ergometry has the potential to reverse disuse osteoporosis (241–243). The phenomenon appears to be dose dependent, with reversal of osteoporosis observed at higher-intensity regimens and loss of effect at lower intensities (242,243).

Deep Venous Thrombosis

The incidence of deep vein thrombosis in SCI varies from 49% to 100% in the first 12 weeks, with the first 2 weeks having the highest incidence (244). Stasis and hypercoagulability are the two major factors contributing to the development of deep venous thrombosis in this high-risk population. NMES of the lower extremity is associated with increased venous flow and enhanced systemic fibrinolytic activity in patients with SCI (206, 207,213,245). NMES with low-dose subcutaneous heparin is associated with significantly lower incidence of deep venous thrombosis among acute SCI patients compared with low-dose subcutaneous heparin alone or saline placebo (246). A similar study with low-molecular-weight heparin in conjunction with external pneumatic compression or NMES suggested superior outcomes with the combination therapy using NMES (244). However, these studies had small sample sizes, and results should be confirmed in larger studies involving multiple centers. Furthermore, the stimulation can be painful for those with incomplete lesions, and autonomic dysreflexia may occur for those with lesions above T6.

CONCLUSIONS

The principal goal of the rehabilitation management of patients with SCI is to maximize quality of life. Although quality of life is clearly influenced by a wide range of variables, including social, emotional, psychological, vocational, and educational factors, the persistent neurologic impairment after injury to the central motor system remains a powerful reminder and determinant of one's physical disability and handicap. NMES systems bypass the injured central circuitry to activate neural tissue and contract muscles to provide function to what is otherwise a nonfunctioning limb or structure and provide therapeutic benefit to address the complications of immobility. Recent advances in clinical medicine and biomedical engineering have made the clinical implementation of NMES systems to enhance the mobility and function of a paralyzed person more feasible. Hand neuprosthesis systems can significantly enhance the upper extremity activities of daily living of patients with tetraplegia. Several lower extremity systems with and without bracing are being investigated for the purpose of functional transfers and standing and to a lesser degree for ambulation for patients with paraplegia. Bladder FNS system can provide catheter-free micturition for patients with either paraplegia or tetraplegia. Phrenic pacing systems can provide artificial ventilatory support for patients with ventilator-dependent tetraplegia. Computer-mediated NMES cycle ergometry systems are available to prevent or treat various complications of immobility, including cardiovascular deconditioning, muscle atrophy, osteoporosis, and deep venous thrombosis.

After decades of development, the clinical utility of NMES systems is finally becoming realized. However, in view of the dynamic nature of the present health care environment, the future of NMES technology is still difficult to predict. By necessity, scientists and clinicians must continue to explore new ideas and improve on the present systems. Components will be smaller, more durable, and more reliable. The issues of cosmesis and ease of donning and doffing will require systems to be fully implantable. Consumers will direct future developments. In the present health care environment, in which cost has become an overwhelming factor in the development and implementation of new technology, the consumer will become one of technology's greatest advocates. The usual drive toward greater complexity will be tempered by the practical issues of clinical implementation, whereby patient acceptance is often a function of a tenuous balance between the burden or cost associated with using a system and the system's impact on the user's life. Finally, NMES will be become available to those with paralysis secondary to cerebral dysfunction, such as stroke, cerebral palsy, traumatic brain injury, and multiple sclerosis.

ACKNOWLEDGEMENTS

This work was supported in part by grants from the National Center for Medical Rehabilitation Research of the National Institutes of Child Health and Human Development, Neuprosthesis Program of the National Institutes of Neurological Diseases and Strokes, U.S. Food and Drug Administration, and Veterans Affairs Functional Electrical Stimulation Center of Excellence.

CONFLICT OF INTEREST

Drs. Chae, Triolo, Kilgore, and Creasey serve as consultants to NeuroControl Corporation, which has a direct financial interest in the subject matter or materials discussed in this chapter. Dr. Creasey is also a minor stockholder in NeuroControl Corporation.

REFERENCES

1. McNeal R. Analysis of a model for excitation of myelinated nerve. *IEEE Trans Biomed Eng* 1976;23:329–337.
2. Mortimer JT. Motor prostheses. In: Brookhart JM, Mountcastle VB, eds. *Handbook of physiology: the nervous system II.* Bethesda, MD: American Physiological Society, 1981:155–187.
3. Henneman E. Relation between size of neurons and their susceptibility to discharge. *Science* 1957;126:1345–1347.
4. Burke RE. Motor units: anatomy, physiology, and functional organization. In: Brookhart JM, Mountcastle VB, eds. *Handbook of physiology: the nervous system II.* Bethesda, MD: American Physiological Society, 1981:345–422.
5. Sweeney JD. Skeletal muscle response to electrical stimulation. In: Reilly JP, ed. *Electrical stimulation and electropathology.* New York: Cambridge University Press, 1992:391–398.
6. Riley DA, Allin EF. The effects of inactivity, programmed stimulation, and denervation of the histochemistry of skeletal muscle fiber types. *Exp Neurol* 1973;40:391–398.
7. Peckham PH, Mortimer JT, Marsolais EB. Alteration in the force and fatigability of skeletal muscle in quadriplegic humans following exercise induced by chronic electrical stimulation. *Clin Orthop* 1976;114:326–334.
8. Marsolais E, Kobetic R. Functional walking in paralyzed patients by means of electrical stimulation. *Clin Orthop* 1983;175:39–36.
9. Kagaya H, Shimada Y, Sato K, et al. Changes in muscle force following therapeutic electrical stimulation in patients with complete paraplegia. *Paraplegia* 1996;34:24–29.
10. Peckham PH, Mortimer JT, Marsolais EB. Upper and lower motor neuron lesions in the upper extremity muscles of tetraplegics. *Paraplegia* 1976;14:115–121.
11. Grandjean PA, Mortimer JT. Recruitment properties of monopolar and bipolar epimysial electrodes. *Ann Biomed Eng* 1986;14:53–66.
12. Kilgore KL, Peckham PH, Keith MW, et al. Electrode characterization for functional application to upper extremity FNS. *IEEE Trans Biomed Eng* 1990;37:12–21.
13. Keith MW, Peckham PH, Thrope GB, et al. Implantable functional neuromuscular stimulation in the tetraplegic hand. *J Hand Surg [Am]* 1989;14:524–530.
14. Naples GG, Mortimer JT, Scheiner A, et al. A spiral nerve cuff electrode for peripheral nerve stimulation [see Comments]. *IEEE Trans Biomed Eng* 1988;35:905–916.
15. Glenn WWL, Phelps ML. Diaphragm pacing by electrical stimulation of the phrenic nerve. *Neurosurgery* 1985;14:53–66.
16. Kim JH, Manuelidis EE, Glen WW, et al. Diaphragm pacing: histopathological changes in the phrenic nerve following long-term electrical stimulation. *J Thorac Cardiovasc Surg* 1976;72:602–608.
17. Waters R, McNeal D, Faloon W, et al. Functional electrical stimulation of peroneal nerve for hemiplegia. *J Bone Joint Surg* 1985;67:792–793.
18. Kralj A, Bajd T. *Functional electrical stimulation: standing and walking after spinal cord injury.* Boca Raton: CRC Press, 1989.
19. Graupe D. EMG pattern analysis for patient-responsive control of FES in paraplegics for walker-supported walking. *IEEE Trans Biomed Eng* 1989;36:711–719.
20. Chizeck HJ, Kobetic R, Marsolais EB, et al. Control of functional neuromuscular stimulation systems for standing and locomotion in paraplegics. *Proc IEEE* 1988;76:1155–1165.
21. Crago PE, Chizeck HJ, Neuman MR, et al. Sensors for use with functional neuromuscular stimulation. *IEEE Trans Biomed Eng* 1986;33:256–268.
22. Kilgore KL, Peckham PH, Keith MW, et al. An implanted upper-extremity neuroprosthesis: follow-up of five patients. *J Bone Joint Surg Am* 1997;79:533–541.
23. Benton LA, Baker LL, Bowman BR, et al. *Functional electrical stimulation: a practical clinical guide.* Downey, CA: Ranchos Los Amigos Medical Center, 1981.
24. Bajd T, Kralj A, Turk R, et al. The use of a four channel electrical stimulator as an ambulatory aid for paraplegic patients. *Phys Ther* 1983;63:1116.
25. Graupe D, Kohn K. *Functional electrical stimulation for ambulation by paraplegics.* Malabar, FL: Krieger, 1994.
26. Gallien P, Brissot R, Eyssette M, et al. Restoration of gait by functional electrical stimulation for spinal cord injured patients. *Paraplegia* 1995;33:660–664.
27. Handa Y, Hoshimiya N, Iguchi Y, et al. Development of percutaneous intramuscular electrode for multichannel FES system. *IEEE Trans Biomed Eng* 1989;36:706–710.
28. Memberg W, Peckham PH, Keith MH. A surgically implanted intramuscular electrode for an implantable neuromuscular stimulation system. *IEEE Trans Rehabil Eng* 1994;2:80–91.
29. Scheiner A, Polando G, Marsolais EB. Design and clinical application of a double helix electrode for functional electrical stimulation. *IEEE Trans Biomed Eng* 1994;41:425–431.
30. Waters RL, Campbell JM, Nakai R. Therapeutic electrical stimulation of the lower limb by epimysial electrodes. *Clin Orthop* 1988;233:44–52.
31. Holle J, Frey M, Gruber H, et al. Functional electrostimulation of paraplegics: experimental investigations and first clinical experience with an implantable stimulation device. *Orthopaedics* 1984;7:1145–1160.
32. Haugland MK, Hoffer JA, Sinkjaer T. Skin contact force information in sensory nerve signals recorded by implanted cuff electrodes. *IEEE Trans Rehabil Eng* 1994;2:18–28.
33. Memberg WD, Peckham PH, Thorpe GB, et al. An analysis of the reliability of percutaneous intramuscular electrodes in upper extremity FNS applications. *IEEE Trans Rehabil Eng* 1993;1:126–132.
34. Smith BT, Betz RR, Mulcahey MJ, et al. Reliability of percutaneous intramuscular electrodes for upper extremity functional neuromuscular stimulation in adolescents with C5 tetraplegia. *Arch Phys Med Rehabil* 1994;75:939–945.
35. Letechipia JE, Peckham PH, Gazdik M, et al. In-line lead connector for use with implanted neuroprosthesis. *IEEE Trans Biomed Eng* 1991;38:707–709.
36. Handa Y, Hoshimiya N. Functional electrical stimulation for the control of the upper extremities. *Med Prog Technol* 1987;12:51–63.
37. Nathan RH, Ohry A. Upper limb functions regained in quadriplegia: a hybrid computerized FNS system. *Arch Phys Med Rehabil* 1990;71:415–421.
38. Snoek GJ, Ijzerman MJ, in't Groen FA, et al. Use of the NESS Handmaster to restore hand function in tetraplegia. *Spinal Cord* 2000;38:244–249.
39. Peckham PH, Keith MW. Motor prostheses for restoration of upper extremity function. In: Stein RB, Peckham PH, Popovic DB, eds. *Neural prostheses: replacing motor function after disease or disability.* New York: Oxford University Press, 1992:162–190.
40. Keith MW, Kilgore KL, Peckham PH, et al. Tendon transfers and functional electrical stimulation for restoration of hand function in spinal cord injury. *J Hand Surg [Am]* 1996;21:89–99.
41. Buckett JR, Peckham PH, Thrope GB, et al. A flexible, portable system for neuromuscular stimulation in the paralyzed upper extremity. *IEEE Trans Biomed Eng* 1988;35:897–904.
42. Johnson MW, Peckham PH. Evaluation of shoulder movement as a command control source. *IEEE Trans Biomed Eng* 1990;37:876–885.
43. Perkins TA, Brindley GS, Donaldson ND, et al. Implant provision of key, pinch and power grips in a C6 tetraplegic. *Med Biol Eng Comput* 1994;32:367–372.
44. Scott TR, Peckham PH, Keith MW. Upper extremity neuroprostheses

using functional electrical stimulation. In: Brindley GS, Rushton DN, eds. *Baillieres Clin Neurol* 1995;4:57–75.

45. Hart RL, Kilgore KL, Peckham PH. A comparison between control methods for implanted FES hand-grasp systems. *IEEE Trans Rehabil Eng* 1998;6:208–218.

46. Vodovnik L, Long C, Reswick JB, et al. Myo-electric control of paralyzed muscles. *IEEE Trans Biomed Eng* 1965;12:169–172.

47. Peckham PH, Mortimer JT, Marsolais EB. Controlled prehension and release in the C5 quadriplegic elicited by functional electrical stimulation of the paralyzed forearm musculature. *Ann Biomed Eng* 1980;8:369–388.

48. Saxena S, Nikolic S, Popovic D. An EMG-controlled grasping system for tetraplegics. *J Rehabil Res Dev* 1995;32:17–24.

49. Solomonow M, Barrata R, Shoji H, et al. The myoelectric signal of electrically stimulated muscle during recruitment: an inherent feedback parameter for a closed-loop control scheme. *IEEE Trans Biomed Eng* 1986;33:735–745.

50. Hoshimiya N, Naito A, Yajima M, et al. A multichannel FES system for the restoration of motor functions in high spinal cord injury patients: a respiration-controlled system for multijoint upper extremity. *IEEE Trans Biomed Eng* 1989;36:754–760.

51. Handa Y, Handa T, Nakatsuchi Y, et al. [A voice-controlled functional electrical stimulation system for the paralyzed hand]. *Iyodenshi To Seitai Kogaku* 1985;23:292–298.

52. Peckham PH, Thrope G, Buckett JR, et al. Coordinated two mode grasp in the quadriplegic initiated by functional neuromuscular stimulation. In: Campell RM, ed. *IFAC control aspects of prosthetics and orthotics*. Oxford, UK: Pergamon Press, 1983.

53. Nathan RH. Control strategies in FNS systems for the upper extremities. *Critical reviews in biomedical engineering*. 1993;21:485–568.

54. Handa Y, Handa T, Ichie M, et al. Functional electrical stimulation (FES) systems for restoration of motor function of paralyzed muscles: versatile systems and a portable system. *Front Med Biol Eng* 1992;4: 241–255.

55. Triolo R, Nathan R, Handa Y, et al. Challenges to clinical deployment of upper limb neuroprostheses. *J Rehabil Res Dev* 1996;33:111–122.

56. Popovic D, Stojanovic A, Pjanovic A, et al. Clinical evaluation of the bionic glove. *Arch Phys Med Rehabil* 1999;80:299–304.

57. Peckham PH, Mortimer JT. Restoration of hand function in the quadriplegic through electrical stimulation. In: Reswick JB, Hambrecht FT, eds. *Functional electrical stimulation: applications in neural prosthesis*. New York: Marcel Dekker, 1977:83–95.

58. Peckham PH, Marsolais EB, Mortimer JT. Restoration of key grip and release in the C6 tetraplegic patient through functional electrical stimulation. *J Hand Surg [Am]* 1980;5:462–469.

59. Smith B, Peckham PH, Keith MW, et al. An externally powered, multichannel implantable stimulator for versatile control of paralyzed muscle. *IEEE Trans Biomed Eng* 1987;34:499–508.

60. Peckham PH, Keith MW, Kilgore KL, et al. Efficacy of an implanted neuroprosthesis for restoring hand grasp in tetraplegia: a multicenter study. *Arch Phys Med Rehabil* (in press).

61. Wuolle KS, Van Doren CL, Thrope GB, et al. Development of a quantitative hand grasp and release test for patients with tetraplegia using a hand neuroprosthesis. *J Hand Surg [Am]* 1994;19:209–218.

62. Smith BT, Mulcahey MJ, Betz RR. Quantitative comparison of grasp and release abilities with and without functional neuromuscular stimulation in adolescents with tetraplegia. *Paraplegia* 1996;34:16–23.

63. Wuolle KS, Van Doren CL, Bryden AM, et al. Satisfaction and usage of a hand neuroprosthesis. *Arch Phys Med Rehabil* 1999;80:206–213.

64. Grill JH, Peckham PH. Functional neuromuscular stimulation for combined control of elbow extension and hand grasp in C5 and C6 quadriplegics. *IEEE Trans Rehabil Eng* 1998;6:190–199.

65. Bryden AM, Memberg WD, Crago PE. Electrically stimulated elbow extension in persons with C5/C6 tetraplegia: a functional and physiological evaluation. *Arch Phys Med Rehabil* 2000;81:80–88.

66. Crago PE, Memberg WD, Usey MK, et al. An elbow extension neuroprosthesis for individuals with tetraplegia. *IEEE Trans Rehabil Eng* 1998;6:1–6.

67. Lemay MA, Crago PE, Keith MW. Restoration of pronosupination

68. Lauer RT, Kilgore KL, Peckham PH, et al. The function of the finger intrinsic muscles in response to electrical stimulation. *IEEE Trans Rehabil Eng* 1999;7:19–26.

69. Johnson MW, Peckham PH, Bhadra N, et al. Implantable transducer for two-degree freedom joint angle sensing. *IEEE Trans Rehabil Eng* 1999;7:349–359.

70. Smith B, Tang Z, Johnson MW, et al. An externally powered, multichannel, implantable stimulator-telemeter for control of paralyzed muscle. *IEEE Trans Biomed Eng* 1998;45:463–475.

71. Grill WM Jr, Mortimer JT. Quantification of recruitment properties of multiple contact cuff electrodes. *IEEE Trans Rehabil Eng* 1996;4: 49–62.

72. Loeb GE, Zamin CJ, Schulman JH, et al. Injectable microstimulator for functional electrical stimulation. *Med Biol Eng* 1991;29: NS13–NS19.

73. Bhadra N, Kilgore KL, Peckham PH. Implanted stimulator for restoration of hand function in spinal cord injury. *Med Eng Phys* 2001; 23:19–26.

74. Betz RR, Mulcahey MJ, Smith BT, et al. Bipolar latissimus dorsi transposition and functional neuromuscular stimulation to restore elbow flexion in an individual with C4 quadriplegia and C5 denervation. *J Am Paraplegia Soc* 1992;15:220–228.

75. Jaeger RJ. Lower extremity applications of functional neuromuscular stimulation. *Assist Technol* 1992;4:19–30.

76. Marsolais EB, Kobetic R. Functional electrical stimulation for walking in paraplegia. *J Bone Joint Surg [Am]* 1987;69:728–733.

77. Marsolais EB, Kobetic R, Chizeck HJ, et al. Orthoses and electrical stimulation for walking in complete paraplegics. *J Neurol Rehab* 1991; 5:13–22.

78. Moynahan M, Mullin C, Cohn J, et al. Home use of a functional electrical stimulation system for standing and mobility in adolescents with spinal cord injury. *Arch Phys Med Rehabil* 1996;77:1005–1013.

79. Triolo RJ, Reilley B, Freedman W, et al. Development and standardization of a clinical evaluation of standing function. *IEEE Trans Rehab Eng* 1993;1:18–25.

80. Triolo RJ, Eisenhower G, Stabinski T, et al. Inter-rater reliability of a clinical test of standing function. *J Spinal Cord Med* 1995;18:13–21.

81. Jaeger RJ, Yarkony GM, Roth EJ. Rehabilitation technology for standing and walking after spinal cord injury. *Am J Phys Med Rehabil* 1989; 68:128–133.

82. Yarkony GM, Roth EJ, Cybulski GR, et al. Neuromuscular stimulation in spinal cord injury: restoration of functional movement of the extremities. *Arch Phys Med Rehabil* 1992;73:78–86.

83. Jaeger RJ, Yarkony GM, Smith RM. Standing the spinal cord injured patient by electrical stimulation: refinement of a protocol for clinical use. *IEEE Trans Biomed Eng* 1989;36:720–728.

84. Yarkony GM, Jaeger RJ, Roth E, et al. Functional neuromuscular stimulation for standing after spinal cord injury. *Arch Phys Med Rehabil* 1990;71:201–206.

85. Kobetic R, Marsolais EB. Synthesis of paraplegic gait with multichannel functional neuromuscular stimulation. *IEEE Trans Biomed Eng* 1994;2:66–67.

86. Triolo RJ, Bieri C, Uhlir J, et al. Implanted FNS systems for assisted standing and transfers for individuals with cervical spinal cord injuries. *Arch Phys Med Rehabil* 1996;7:1119–1128.

87. Marsolais EB, Kobetic R. Implantation technique and experience with percutaneous intramuscular electrodes in the lower extremities. *J Rehabil Res Dev* 1986;23:1–8.

88. Davis R, Eckhouse R, Patrick JF, et al. Computer-controlled 22-channel stimulator for limb movement. *Acta Neurochir* 1987;39S: 117–120.

89. Donaldson N, Rushton D, Tromans T. Neuroprostheses for leg function after spinal cord injury. *Lancet* 1997;350:711.

90. Akers JM, Peckham PH, Keith MW, et al. Tissue response to chronically stimulated implanted epimysial and intramuscular electrodes. *IEEE Trans Rehabil Eng* 1997;5:207–220.

91. Buckett J, Triolo R, Ferencz D, et al. A wearable controller for clinical

control by FNS in tetraplegia: experimental and biomechanical evaluation of feasibility. *J Biomech* 1996;29:435–442.

studies involving multi-implant FNS systems. *J Spinal Cord Injury* 1998;21:179.

92. Vrabec T, Triolo R, Uhlir J, et al. *A clinical interface for control and evaluation of FNS systems.* Proceedings of the Second National Meeting VA Rehabilitation Research and Development Service, Washington, DC, 2000.

93. Triolo RJ, Bogie K. Lower extremity applications of functional neuromuscular stimulation after spinal cord injury. *Top Spinal Cord Injury Rehabil* 1999;5:44–65.

94. Sharma M, Marsolais EB, Polando G, et al. Implantation of a 16-channel functional electrical stimulation walking system. *Clin Orthop* 1998:236–242.

95. Kobetic R, Triolo RJ, Uhlir JP, et al. Implanted functional electrical stimulation system for mobility in paraplegia: a follow-up case report. *IEEE Trans Rehabil Eng* 1999;7:390–398.

96. Davis JA, Triolo RJ, Uhlir JP, et al. Clinical performance of a surgically implanted neuroprostheses for exercise, standing, transfers and upright mobility. *J Spinal Cord Med* 2000;23:3(abst).

97. Uhlir JP. *Performance of implanted epimysial electrodes in the lower extremities of individuals with spinal cord injury.* Proceedings of the Second National Meeting VA Rehabilitation Research and Development Service, Washington, DC, 2000.

98. Davis JA, Triolo RJ, Uhlir JP, et al. *Performance of a surgically implanted neuroprosthesis for standing and transfers.* Proceedings of the Fifth Annual Conference of the International Functional Electrical Stimulation Society Meeting, Aalborg, Denmark, 2000.

99. Barnette N, Lamitie H. *A comparison of energy expenditure between KAFO and FNS standing in adolescents with spinal cord injuries.* Department of Physical Therapy. Glenside, PA: Beaver College, 1991.

100. Moynahan M. Postural responses during standing in subjects with spinal-cord injury. *Gait and Posture* 1995;3:156–165.

101. Bieri C, Triolo RJ, Danford GS, et al. A functional performance measure for effort and assistance required for sit-to-stand and standing pivot transfer maneuvers. *J Spinal Cord Injury Med* 2000;23:4(abst).

102. Wibowo MA. *Selection and activation of hip extensor muscles for standing with FNS.* Department of Biomedical Engineering. Cleveland, OH: Case Western Reserve University, 1998.

103. Wibowo MA, Triolo RJ, Uhlir JP, et al. *The effect of stimulated hip extensor moment on the loads imposed on the arms during standing with FES.* Proceedings of the 1998 Annual RESNA Conference, Washington, DC, 1998.

104. Miller P, Kobetic R, Lew R. *Energy costs of walking and standing using functional electrical stimulation.* Proceedings of the Thirteenth Annual RESNA Conference, Washington, DC, 1990.

105. Glaser RM. Physiologic aspects of spinal cord injury and functional neuromuscular stimulation. *Cent Nerv Syst Trauma* 1986;3:49–61.

106. Bajd T, Kralj A, Turk R. Standing up of a healthy subject and a paraplegic patient. *J Biomech* 1982;15:1–10.

107. Isakov E, Mizrahi J, Najenson T. Biomechanical and physiological evaluation of FES-activated paraplegic patients. *J Rehabil Res Dev* 1986;23:9–19.

108. Bedbrook GM. A balanced viewpoint in the early management of patients with spinal injuries who have neurological damage. *Paraplegia* 1985;23:8–15.

109. Bajd T, Kralj A, Turk R, et al. *FES rehabilitative approach in incomplete SCI patients.* Proceedings of the Ninth Annual RESNA Conference, Minneapolis, MN, 1986.

110. Bajd T, Kralj A, Stefancic M, et al. Use of functional electrical stimulation in the lower extremities of incomplete spinal cord injured patients. *Artif Organs* 1999;23:403–409.

111. Kralj A, Bajd T, Kvesic Z, et al. *Electrical stimulation of incomplete paraplegic patients.* Proceedings of the Fourth Annual RESNA Conference, Washington, DC, 1981.

112. Granat MH, Ferguson AC, Andrews BJ, et al. The role of functional electrical stimulation in the rehabilitation of patients with incomplete spinal cord injury: observed benefits during gait studies. *Paraplegia* 1993;31:207–215.

113. Borges G, Ferguson K, Kobetic R. Development and operations of portable and laboratory electrical stimulation systems for walking in paraplegic subjects. *IEEE Trans Biomed Eng* 1989;36:798–800.

114. Kobetic R, Marsolais EB, Samane P, et al. The next step: artificial walking. In: Rose J, Ganble JG, eds. *Human walking.* Baltimore, MD: Williams & Wilkins, 1994:225–252.

115. Brindley GS, Polkey CE, Rushton DN. Electrical splinting of the knee in paraplegia. *Paraplegia* 1979;16:428–437.

116. Granat MH, Heller BW, Nicol DJ, et al. Improving limb flexion in FES gait using the flexion withdrawal response for the spinal cord injured person. *J Biomed Eng* 1993;15:51–56.

117. Solomonow M, Baratta RV, Hirokawa S. The RGO generation II: muscle stimulation powered orthosis as a practical walking system for paraplegics. *Orthopaedics* 1989;12:1309–1315.

118. Solomonow M. Biomechanics and physiology of a practical functional neuromuscular stimulation powered walking orthosis for paraplegics. In: Stein RB, Peckham PH, Popovic DP, eds. *Neural prostheses: replacing motor function after disease or disability.* New York: Oxford University Press, 1992:202–232.

119. Kantor C, Andrews BJ, Marsolais EB, et al. Report on a conference on motor prostheses for workplace mobility of paraplegic patients in North America. *Paraplegia* 1993;31:439–456.

120. Schwirlich L, Popovich D. *Hybrid orthoses for deficient locomotion.* Proceedings of the seventh symposium, Advances in External Control of Human Extremities, Dubrovnik, Yugoslavia, 1984.

121. Andrews BJ, Baxendale RH, Barnett R, et al. Hybrid FES orthosis incorporating closed loop control and sensory feedback. *J Biomed Eng* 1988;10:189–195.

122. McClelland M, Andrews BJ, Patrick JH, et al. Augmentation of the Oswestry Parawalker orthosis by means of surface electrical stimulation: gait analysis of three patients. *Paraplegia* 1987;25:32–38.

123. Franceschini M, Baratta S, Zampolini M, et al. Reciprocating gait orthosis: a multicenter study of their use by spinal cord injured patients. *Arch Phys Med Rehabil* 1997;78:582–586.

124. Solomonow M, Aguilar E, Reisin E, et al. Reciprocating gait orthosis powered with electrical muscle stimulation (RGO II). I. Performance evaluation of 70 paraplegic patients. *Orthopedics* 1997;20:315–324.

125. Petrofsky JS, Phillips CA, Douglas R, et al. A computer-controlled walking system: the combination of an orthosis with functional electrical stimulation. *J Clin Eng* 1986;11:121–133.

126. Andrews BJ, Baxendale RH, Barnett R, et al. *A hybrid orthosis for paraplegics incorporating feedback control.* Proceedings of the Ninth Symposium, External Control of Human Extremities, Dubrovnik, Yugoslavia, 1987.

127. Popovic DB, Schwirtlich L. Design and evaluation of the self-fitting modular orthosis (SFMO). *IEEE Trans Rehabil Eng* 1993;1:165–174.

128. Popovic DB. Functional electrical stimulation for lower extremities. In: Stein RB, Peckham PH, Popovic DB, eds. *Neural prostheses, replacing motor function after disease or disability.* New York: Oxford University Press, 1992:233–251.

129. Winchester P, Carollo JJ, Habasevich R. Physiologic costs of reciprocal gait in FES assisted walking. *Paraplegia* 1994;32:680–686.

130. Graupe D, Kohn K. Clinical results and observations over 12 years of FES-based ambulation. *Functional electrical stimulation for ambulation by paraplegics.* Malabar, FL: Kreiger, 1994:136.

131. MacGregor J. The evaluation of patient performance using long-term ambulatory monitoring technique in the domiciliary environment. *Physiotherapy* 1981;67:30–33.

132. Rose J, Gamble JG, Medeiros JM. Energy cost of walking in normal children and those with cerebral palsy: comparison of heart rate and oxygen uptake. *J Pediatr Orthop* 1989;9:276–279.

133. Isakov E, Douglas R, Berns P. Ambulation using the reciprocating gait orthosis and functional electrical stimulation. *Paraplegia* 1992;30:239–245.

134. Bowker P, Messenger N, Ogilvie C, et al. Engergetics of paraplegic walking. *J Biomed Eng* 1992;14:344–350.

135. Chaplin E. Functional neuromuscular stimulation for mobility in people with spinal cord injuries: the Parastep I System. *J Spinal Cord Med* 1996;19:99–105.

136. Klose KJ, Jacobs PL, Nash MS, et al. Evaluation of training program for persons with SCI paraplegia using the Parastep 1 ambulation system. 1. Ambulation performance and anthropometric measures. *Arch Phys Med Rehabil* 1997;78(8):808-814.

137. Guest RS, Klose KJ, Needham-Shropshire BM, et al. Evaluation of a training program for persons with SCI paraplegia using the Parastep 1 ambulation system. 4. Effect on physical self-concept and depression. *Arch Phys Med Rehabil* 1997;78:804–807.

138. Jacobs PL, Nash MS, Klose KJ, et al. Evaluation of a training program for persons with SCI paraplegia using the Parastep 1 ambulation system. 2. Effects on physiological responses to peak arm ergometry. *Arch Phys Med Rehabil* 1997;78:794–798.

139. Nash MS, Jacobs PL, Montalveo BM, et al. Evaluation of a training program for persons with SCI paraplegia using the Parastep 1 ambulation system. 5. Lower extremity blood flow and hyperemic responses to occlusion are augmented by ambulation training. *Arch Phys Med Rehabil* 1997;78:806–814.

140. Hirokawa S, Grimm M, Le T, et al. Energy consumption in paraplegic ambulation using the reciprocating gait orthosis and electrical stimulation of the thigh muscles. *Arch Phys Med Rehabil* 1990;71:687–694.

141. Solomonow M, Reisin E, Aguilar E, et al. Reciprocating gait orthosis powered with electrical muscle stimulation (RGO II). II. Medical evaluation of 70 paraplegic patients. *Orthopedics* 1997;20:411–418.

142. Arnold EP, Gowland SP, MacFarlane MR, et al. Sacral anterior root stimulation of the bladder in paraplegia. *Aust N Z J Surg* 1986;56:319–324.

143. Brindley GS, Polkey CE, Rushton DN, et al. Sacral anterior root stimulators for bladder control in paraplegia: the first 50 cases. *J Neurol Neurosurg Psychiatry* 1986;49:1104–1114.

144. Robinson LQ, Grant A, Weston P, et al. Experience with the Brindley anterior sacral root stimulator. *Br J Urol* 1988;62:553–557.

145. Brindley GS, Rushton DN. Long-term follow-up of patients with sacral anterior root stimulator implants. *Paraplegia* 1990;28:469–475.

146. Madersbacher H, Fischer J. Sacral anterior root stimulation: prerequisites and indications. *Neurourol Urodyn* 1993;12:489–494.

147. Creasey GH. Electrical stimulation of sacral roots for micturition after spinal cord injury. *Urol Clin North Am* 1993;20:505–515.

148. Van Kerrebroeck PE, Koldewijn EL, Debruyne FM. Worldwide experience with the Finetech-Brindley sacral anterior root stimulator. *Neurourol Urodyn* 1993;12:497–503.

149. Brindley GS. The first 500 patients with sacral anterior root stimulator implants: general description. *Paraplegia* 1994;32:795–805.

150. Bosch JL, Groen J. Sacral (S3) segmental nerve stimulation as a treatment for urge incontinence in patients with detrusor instability: results of chronic electrical stimulation using an implantable neural prosthesis. *J Urol* 1995;154:504–507.

151. Ishigooka M, Hashimoto T, Hayami S, et al. Electrical pelvic floor stimulation: a possible alternative treatment for reflex urinary incontinence in patients with spinal cord injury. *Spinal Cord* 1996;34:411–415.

152. Madersbacher H, Fischer J, Ebner A. Anterior sacral root stimulator (Brindley): experience especially in women with neurogenic urinary incontinence. *Neurourol Urodyn* 1988;7:593–601.

153. Colombel P, Egon G. Electrostimulation of the anterior sacral nerve roots. *Ann Urol Paris* 1991;25:48–52.

154. Creasey G. Restoration of bladder, bowel, and sexual function. *Top Spinal Cord Rehabil* 1999;5:21–32.

155. Madersbacher H, Fischer J. Anterior sacral root stimulation and posterior scaral root rhizotomy. *Aktuelle Urol* 1993;24[Suppl]:32–35.

156. Van Kerrebroeck PE, Koldewijn EL, Rosier PF, et al. Results of the treatment of neurogenic bladder dysfunction in spinal cord injury by sacral posterior root rhizotomy and anterior sacral root stimulation. *J Urol* 1996;155:1378–1381.

157. Egon G, Barat M, Colombel P, et al. Implantation of anterior sacral root stimulators combined with posterior sacral rhizotomy in spinal injury patients. *World J Urol* 1998;16:342–349.

158. MacDonagh RP, Forster DM, Thomas DG. Urinary continence in spinal injury patients following complete sacral posterior rhizotomy. *Br J Urol* 1990;66:618–622.

159. Van Kerrebroeck PEV, Kolewijn EL, Wijkstra H, et al. Urodynamic evaluation before and after intradural posterior sacral rhizotomies and implantation of the Finetech-Brindley anterior sacral root stimulator. *Urodinamica* 1992;1:7–12.

160. Cardozo L, Krishnan KR, Polkey CE, et al. Urodynamic observations on patients with sacral anterior root stimulators. *Paraplegia* 1984;22:201–209.

161. Wielink G, Essink-Bot ML, Van Kerrebroeck PE, et al. Sacral rhizotomies and electrical bladder stimulation in spinal cord injury. 2. Cost-effectiveness and quality of life analysis. Dutch Study Group on Sacral Anterior Root Stimulation. *Eur Urol* 1997;31:441–446.

162. Creasey GH, Kilgore KL, Brown-Triolo DL, et al. Reduction of costs of disability using neuroprostheses. *Assist Technol* 2000;12(1):67–75.

163. Rushton DN, Brindley GS, Polkey CE, et al. Implant infections and antibiotic-impregnated silicone rubber coating. *J Neurol Neurosurg Psychiatry* 1989;52:223–229.

164. National Spinal Cord Injury Statistical Center, University of Alabama at Birmingham. *Annual statistical report 1997.* Birmingham: University of Alabama, 1997.

165. Carter RE, Donovan WH, Halstead L, et al. Comparative study of electrophrenic nerve stimulation and mechanical ventilatory support in traumatic spinal cord injury. *Paraplegia* 1987;25:86–91.

166. DeVivo MJ, Ivie CS 3rd. Life expectancy of ventilator-dependent persons with spinal cord injuries. *Chest* 1995;108:226–232.

167. Esclarin A, Bravo P, Arroyo O, et al. Tracheostomy ventilation versus diaphragmatic pacemaker ventilation in high spinal cord injury. *Paraplegia* 1994;32:687–693.

168. Whiteneck GG, Charlifue SW, Frankel HL, et al. Mortality, morbidity, and psychosocial outcomes of persons spinal cord injured more than 20 years ago. *Paraplegia* 1992;30:617–630.

169. Glenn WW, Hogan JF, Loke JS, et al. Ventilatory support by pacing of the conditioned diaphragm in quadriplegia. *N Engl J Med* 1984;310:1150–1155.

170. Glenn WW, Hogan JF, Phelps ML. Ventilatory support of the quadriplegic patient with respiratory paralysis by diaphragm pacing. *Surg Clin North Am* 1980;60:1055–1078.

171. Glenn WW, Sairenji H. Diaphragm pacing in the treatment of chronic ventilatory isufficiency. In: Roussos C, Macklem PT, eds. *The thorax: lung biology in health and disease,* Vol. 29. New York: Marcel Dekker, 1985:1407.

172. Hunt CE, Brouillette RT, Weese-Mayer DE, et al. Diaphragm pacing in infants: technique and results. *Pacing Clin Electrophysiol* 1988;11:2135–2141.

173. Ilbawi MN, Idriss FS, Hunt CE, et al. Diaphragmatic pacing in infants: techniques and results. *Ann Thorac Surg* 1985;40:323–329.

174. Thoma H, Gerner H, Holle J, et al. The phrenic pacemaker: substitution of paralyzed functions in tetraplegia. *Trans Am Soc Artif Intern Organs* 1987;33:472–479.

175. Chen CF, Lien IN. Spinal cord injuries in Taipei, Taiwan, 1978–1981. *Paraplegia* 1985;23:364–370.

176. Dobelle WH, D'Angelo MS, Goetz BF, et al. 200 Cases with a new breathing pacemaker dispel myths about diaphragm pacing. *Trans Am Soc Artif Intern Organs* 1994;40:244–252.

177. Glenn WW, Phelps ML, Elefteriades JA, et al. Twenty years of experience in phrenic nerve stimulation to pace the diaphragm. *Pacing Clin Electrophysiol* 1986;9:780–784.

178. Hackler RH. A 25-year prospective mortality study in the spinal cord injured patient: comparison with the long-term living paraplegic. *J Urol* 1977;117:486–488.

179. Oda T, Glenn WW, Fukuda Y, et al. Evaluation of electrical parameters for diaphragm pacing: an experimental study. *J Surg Res* 1981;30:142–153.

180. McKenzie DK, Gandevia SC. Phrenic nerve conduction times and twitch pressures of the human diaphragm. *J Appl Physiol* 1985;58:1496–1504.

181. McLean IC, Mattoni TA. Phrenic nerve conduction studies: a new technique and its application in quadriplegic patients. *Arch Phys Med Rehabil* 1981;62:70–73.

182. Glenn WW, Holcomb WG, Hogan J, et al. Diaphragm pacing by radiofrequency transmission in the treatment of chronic ventilatory insufficiency: present status. *J Thorac Cardiovasc Surg* 1973;66:505–520.

183. Fodstad H. The Swedish experience in phrenic nerve stimulation. *Pacing Clin Electrophysiol* 1987;10:246–251.

184. Vanderlinden RG, Epstein SW, Hyland RH, et al. Management of

chronic ventilatory insufficiency with electrical diaphragm pacing. *Can J Neurol Sci* 1988;15:63–67.

185. Glenn WW, Phelps ML. Diaphragm pacing by electrical stimulation of the phrenic nerve. *Neurosurgery* 1985;17:974–984.

186. Glenn WW, Brouillette RT, Dentz B, et al. Fundamental considerations in pacing of the diaphragm for chronic ventilatory insufficiency: a multi-center study. *Pacing Clin Electrophysiol* 1988;11:2121–2127.

187. Weese-Mayer DE, Silvestri JM, Kenny AS, et al. Diaphragm pacing with a quadripolar phrenic nerve electrode: an international study. *Pacing Clin Electrophysiol* 1996;19:1311–1319.

188. Biering-Sorensen F, Jacobsen E, Hjelms E, et al. [Diaphragm pacing by electric stimulation of the phrenic nerves]. *Ugeskr Laeger* 1990; 152:1143–1145.

189. Marcus CL, Jansen MT, Pousen MK, et al. Medical and psychosocial outcome of children with congenital central hypoventilation syndrome. *J Pediatr* 1991;119:888–895.

190. DiMarco AF, Altose MD, Cropp A, et al. Activation of the inspiratory intercostal muscles by electrical stimulation of the spinal cord. *Am Rev Respir Dis* 1987;136:1385–1390.

191. DiMarco AF, Budzinska K, Supinski GS. Artificial ventilation by means of electrical activation of the intercostal/accessory muscles alone in anesthetized dogs. *Am Rev Respir Dis* 1989;139:961–967.

192. DiMarco AF, Supinski GS, Petro J, et al. Artificial respiration via combined intercostal and diaphragm pacing in a quadriplegic patient. *Am Rev Respir Dis* 1994;149:A135.

193. DiMarco AF, Supinski GS, Petro JA, et al. Evaluation of intercostal pacing to provide artificial ventilation in quadriplegics. *Am J Respir Crit Care Med* 1994;150:934–940.

194. DiMarco AF, Kowalski KE, Petro JA, et al. *Evaluation of intercostal and diaphragm pacing to provide ventilatory support in tetraplegic patients.* Proceedings of the ATS International Conference, San Francisco, 2001.

195. DiMarco AF, Mortimer JT, Stellato T, et al. *Bilateral phrenic nerve pacing via intramuscular electrodes in tetraplegic patients.* Proceedings of the ATS International Conference, San Francisco, 2001.

196. DeVivo MJ, Stover SL. Long-term survival and causes of death. In: Stover SL, DeLisa JA, Whiteneck GG, eds. *Spinal cord injury.* Gaithersburg, MD: Aspen, 1995:289–316.

197. Coutts KD, Rhodes EC, McKenzie DC. Maximal exercise responses of tetraplegics and paraplegics. *J Appl Physiol* 1983;55:479–482.

198. Ellenberg M, MacRitchie M, Franklin B, et al. Aerobic capacity in early paraplegia: implications for rehabilitation. *Paraplegia* 1989;27: 261–268.

199. Drory Y, Ohry A, Brooks ME, et al. Arm crank ergometry in chronic spinal cord injured patients. *Arch Phys Med Rehabil* 1990;71: 389–392.

200. Figoni SF. Exercise responses and quadriplegia. *Med Sci Sports Exerc* 1993;25:433–441.

201. Nash MS, Bilsker S, Marcillo AE, et al. Reversal of adaptive left ventricular atrophy following electrically-stimulated exercise training in human tetraplegics. *Paraplegia* 1991;29:590–599.

202. Brenes G, Dearwater S, Shapera R, et al. High density lipoprotein cholesterol concentrations in physically active and sedentary spinal cord injured patients. *Arch Phys Med Rehabil* 1986;67:445–450.

203. Okuma H, Ogata H, Hatada K. Transition of physical fitness in wheelchair marathon competitors over several years. *Paraplegia* 1989; 27:237–243.

204. Zwiren LD, Bar-Or O. Responses to exercise of paraplegics who differ in conditioning level. *Med Sci Sports* 1975;7:94–98.

205. Figoni SF. Perspectives on cardiovascular fitness and SCI [published erratum appears in *J Am Paraplegia Soc* 1991;14(1):21]. *J Am Paraplegia Soc* 1990;13:63–71.

206. Thomas AJ, Davis GM, Sutton JR. Cardiovascular and metabolic responses to electrical stimulation-induced leg exercise in spinal cord injury. *Methods Inf Med* 1997;36:372–375.

207. Raymond J, Davis GM, Bryant G, et al. Cardiovascular responses to an orthostatic challenge and electrical-stimulation-induced leg muscle contractions in individuals with paraplegia. *Eur J Appl Physiol* 1999; 80:205–212.

208. Laskin JJ, Ashley EA, Olenik LM, et al. Electrical stimulation-assisted rowing exercise in spinal cord injured people: a pilot study. *Paraplegia* 1993;31:534–541.

209. Raymond J, Davis GM, Fahey A, et al. Oxygen uptake and heart rate responses during arm vs combined arm/electrically stimulated leg exercise in people with paraplegia. *Spinal Cord* 1997;35:680–685.

210. Phillips WT, Burkett LN. Augmented upper body contribution to oxygen uptake during upper body exercise with concurrent leg functional electrical stimulation in persons with spinal cord injury. *Spinal Cord* 1998;36:750–755.

211. Raymond J, Davis GM, Climstein M, et al. Cardiorespiratory responses to arm cranking and electrical stimulation leg cycling in people with paraplegia. *Med Sci Sports Exerc* 1999;31:822–828.

212. Hooker SP, Figoni SF, Rodgers MM, et al. Metabolic and hemodynamic responses to concurrent voluntary arm crank and electrical stimulation leg cycle exercise in quadriplegics. *J Rehabil Res Dev* 1992; 29:1–11.

213. Phillips W, Burkett LN, Munro R, et al. Relative changes in blood flow with functional electrical stimulation during exercise of the paralyzed lower limbs. *Paraplegia* 1995;33:90–93.

214. Hooker SP, Figoni SF, Rodgers MM, et al. Physiologic effects of electrical stimulation leg cycle exercise training in spinal cord injured persons. *Arch Phys Med Rehabil* 1992;73:470–476.

215. Hooker SP, Scremin AM, Mutton DL, et al. Peak and submaximal physiologic responses following electrical stimulation leg cycle ergometer training. *J Rehabil Res Dev* 1995;32:361–366.

216. Krauss JC, Robergs RA, Depaepe JL, et al. Effects of electrical stimulation and upper body training after spinal cord injury. *Med Sci Sports Exerc* 1993;25:1054–1061.

217. Mutton DL, Scremin AM, Barstow TJ, et al. Physiologic responses during functional electrical stimulation leg cycling and hybrid exercise in spinal cord injured subjects. *Arch Phys Med Rehabil* 1997;78: 712–718.

218. Burnham R, Dearwater S, Stein R, et al. Skeletal muscle fibre type transformation following spinal cord injury. *Spinal Cord* 1997;35: 86–91.

219. Thomas CK, Zaidner EY, Calancie B, et al. Muscle weakness, paralysis, and atrophy after human cervical spinal cord injury. *Exp Neurol* 1997;148:414–423.

220. Peckham PH, Mortimer JT, Van Der Meulen JP. Physiologic and metabolic changes in white muscle of cat following induced exercise. *Brain Res* 1973;50:424–429.

221. Pette D, Muller W, Leisner E, et al. Time dependent effects on contractile properties, fibre population, myosin light chains and enzymes of energy metabolism in intermittently and continuously stimulated fast twitch muscles of the rabbit. *Pflugers Arch* 1976;364:103–112.

222. Martin TP, Stein RB, Hoeppner PH, et al. Influence of electrical stimulation on the morphological and metabolic properties of paralyzed muscle. *J Appl Physiol* 1992;72:1401–1406.

223. Chilibeck PD, Jeon J, Weiss C, et al. Histochemical changes in muscle of individuals with spinal cord injury following functional electrical stimulated exercise training. *Spinal Cord* 1999;37:264–268.

224. Greve JM, Muszkat R, Schmidt B, et al. Functional electrical stimulation (FES): muscle histochemical analysis. *Paraplegia* 1993;31: 764–770.

225. Andersen JL, Mohr T, Biering-Sorensen F, et al. Myosin heavy chain isoform transformation in single fibres from m. vastus lateralis in spinal cord injured individuals: effects of long-term functional electrical stimulation (FES). *Pflugers Arch* 1996;431:513–518.

226. Neumayer C, Happak W, Kern H, et al. Hypertrophy and transformation of muscle fibers in paraplegic patients. *Artif Organs* 1997;21: 188–190.

227. Pacy PJ, Hesp R, Halliday DA, et al. Muscle and bone in paraplegic patients, and the effect of functional electrical stimulation. *Clin Sci* 1988;75:481–487.

228. Ragnarsson KT. Physiologic effects of functional electrical stimulation-induced exercises in spinal cord-injured individuals. *Clin Orthop* 1988:53–63.

229. Sloan KE, Bremner LA, Byrne J, et al. Musculoskeletal effects of an

electrical stimulation induced cycling programme in the spinal injured. *Paraplegia* 1994;32:407–415.

230. Scremin AM, Kurta L, Gentili A, et al. Increasing muscle mass in spinal cord injured persons with a functional electrical stimulation exercise program. *Arch Phys Med Rehabil* 1999;80:1531–1536.

231. Dudley GA, Castro MJ, Rogers S, et al. A simple means of increasing muscle size after spinal cord injury: a pilot study. *Eur J Appl Physiol* 1999;80:394–396.

232. Baldi JC, Jackson RD, Moraille R, et al. Muscle atrophy is prevented in patients with acute spinal cord injury using functional electrical stimulation. *Spinal Cord* 1998;36:463–469.

233. Gerrits HL, Haan A, Sargeant AJ, et al. Altered contractile properties of the quadriceps muscle in people with spinal cord injury following functional electrical stimulated cycle training. *Spinal cord* 2000;38:214–223.

234. Rodgers MM, Glaser RM, Figoni SF, et al. Musculoskeletal responses of spinal cord injured individuals to functional neuromuscular stimulation-induced knee extension exercise training. *J Rehabil Res Dev* 1991;28:19–26.

235. Garland DE, Stewart CA, Adkins RH, et al. Osteoporosis after spinal cord injury. *J Orthop Res* 1992;10:371–378.

236. Ragnarsson KT, Sell GH. Lower extremity fractures after SCI: a retrospective study. *Arch Phys Med Rehabil* 1981;62:418–423.

237. Wei CN. Does electrical stimulation of the sciatic nerve prevent suspension-induced changes in rat hindlimb bones? *Jpn J Physiol* 1998;48:33–37.

238. Kaplan RE, Roden W, Gilbert E, et al. Reduction of hypercalciuria in tetraplegia after weight-bearing and strengthening. *Paraplegia* 1981;19:289–293.

239. Leeds EM, Klose KJ, Ganz W, et al. Bone mineral density after bicycle ergometry training. *Arch Phys Med Rehabil* 1990;71:207–209.

240. Hangartner TN, Rodgers MM, Glaser RM, et al. Tibial bone density loss in spinal cord injured patients: effects of FES exercise. *J Rehabil Res Dev* 1994;31:50–61.

241. BeDell KK, Scremin AME, Perell KL, et al. Effects of functional electrical stimulation-induced lower extremity cycling on bone density of spinal cord-injured patients. *Am J Phys Med Rehabil* 1996;75:29–34.

242. Bloomfield SA, Mysiw WJ, Jackson RD. Bone mass and endocrine adaptations to training in spinal cord injured individuals. *Bone* 1996;19:61–68.

243. Mohr T, Podenphant J, Biering-Sorensen F, et al. Increased bone mineral density after prolonged electrically induced cycle training of paralyzed limbs in spinal cord injured man. *Calcif Tissue Int* 1997;61:22–25.

244. Merli GJ, Crabbe S, Paluzzi RG, et al. Etiology, incidence, and prevention of deep vein thrombosis in acute spinal cord injury. *Arch Phys Med Rehabil* 1993;74:1199–1205.

245. Katz RT, Green D, Sullivan T, et al. Functional electrical stimulation to enhance systemic fibrinolytic activity in spinal cord injury patients. *Arch Phys Med Rehabil* 1987;68:423–426.

246. Merli GJ, Herbison GJ, Ditunno JF, et al. Deep vein thrombosis: prophylaxis in acute spinal cord injured patients. *Arch Phys Med Rehabil* 1988;69:661–664.

PAIN IN PATIENTS WITH SPINAL CORD INJURY

WILLIAM L. BOCKENEK
PAULA J.B. STEWART

One of the most difficult issues in the care of patients with spinal cord injury (SCI) is the management of acute and chronic pain. The etiology of the pain is often poorly understood and the selection of treatment anecdotal. The onset can occur immediately after injury and may persist for the lifetime of the patient. Even with the best available medical and surgical care, severe pain syndromes often develop. The functional and socioeconomic implications of pain in patients with SCI are often overshadowed by the loss of mobility, employability, and bowel and bladder function, both in the lay and medical press. However, pain itself often has a great effect on the ability of the person with SCI to regain ambulatory function, return to work, or become independent in bowel and bladder function. This chapter addresses the issues surrounding pain management in the population with SCI, with the greatest emphasis on the topic of chronic pain.

SCOPE OF THE PROBLEM

The initial description of pain in patients with SCI dates back to the early twentieth century beginning with World War I veterans and has been followed by many additional reports (1–14). In a recent review of the literature that included studies from 1947 to 1988, the presence of pain was noted by 69% of patients with SCI, with about one third of those describing pain as severe (15). In another sample of eight studies published from 1979 to 1995 that included more than 2,100 patients with SCI, the prevalence of pain ranged from 47% to 96%, with an average of 66% (16). An additional report, which emphasized the variation in classification schemes used to describe pain in patients with SCI, noted a prevalence of 64% in a sample of 353 patients with SCI. Within this group of patients, neurogenic pain was noted to represent 30%, non-neurogenic pain 17%, and both neurogenic and non-neurogenic pain 17% of cases (17). In two series, it has been estimated that chronic pain occurs in up to 94% of patients with SCI, with 30% to 40% of them experiencing severe, disabling pain (18,19).

Even with the numerous reports in the literature reflecting such a high incidence of pain in SCI, the issue remains a comparatively neglected one (20). The International Association for the Study of Pain (IASP) recently published a comprehensive

taxonomy of pain conditions; however, no attempt was made to define or categorize the various types of pain that occur following SCI (21). Out of more than 2,400 articles that have been published in the journal *Pain* over a period of 20 years (1977 to 1997), only 19 were specifically related to SCI pain. Similarly, of nearly 1,700 articles published in *Paraplegia* in a 30-year period (1967 to 1997), only 16 were specifically related to the problem of SCI pain (20).

The impact of pain on quality of life and function in patients with SCI has been addressed in several publications. In a study by Nepomuceno and colleagues, 23% to 37% (depending on level of injury) of patients with SCI were willing to trade the possibility of recovery of bladder, bowel, or sexual function for pain relief (22). Several studies have revealed the association of pain in SCI with interference in daily activities and with a poorer quality of life (23–25). The presence of severe and disabling pain secondary to SCI that compromises quality of life has been reported to range widely, from as low as 5% to as high as 45% (4,22,26).

PHYSICAL FACTORS

Numerous physical factors have been associated with development of pain in patients with SCI and have been described in a recent review (27). Specific etiologies of SCI have been associated with an increased incidence of post-injury pain. People who sustain a SCI secondary to a gunshot wound report more pain; however, it has also been noted that surgical removal of the bullet has not been helpful in reducing subsequent pain either early in the rehabilitation process or 1 year after injury (11,28). Injuries related to violence in general have also been associated with a greater incidence of pain (29,30). Pain and spasticity have been found to have a strong interrelationship (4,31). These two factors influence one another in a number of ways. For example, although significant spasticity may exacerbate musculoskeletal pain, pain of any kind (i.e., neuropathic or musculoskeletal) often aggravates spasticity.

The effect of surgical intervention on the incidence of pain has not been clearly defined in the literature. Laminectomy has been suggested to increase the incidence of pain due to the scarring of ligaments and muscles after surgery (5). In another study, it was found that patients who have dysesthetic pain (i.e., neuropathic pain below the level of the injury) were less likely to have had surgical stabilization (11). On the other hand, two additional reports found that there was no difference in the severity of pain between those treated with instrumentation or spinal fusion and those who did not have surgery (19,32). In a more recent study, patients who underwent surgery after SCI were more likely to experience musculoskeletal pain 2 weeks after injury (33). However, from 4 weeks until 12 months after injury, surgically managed patients did not appear to experience pain more frequently than patients who did not have surgery. In addition, there were no apparent differences in the prevalence of visceral pain, neuropathic pain at level of injury, or neuropathic pain below level of injury in the surgical and nonsurgical groups at any stage.

The incidence of pain in patients with complete versus incomplete lesions is also controversial. Numerous reports have noted a higher incidence of neuropathic pain in those with incomplete lesions (11,12,22,34–36). However, other investigators have found no significant difference in the prevalence or severity of pain in those with a complete lesion, as opposed to those with an incomplete lesion (19,23,26,32,37,38). Three of these reports emphasized that psychosocial factors, rather than completeness of injury, were more closely associated with the experience of pain (19,23,32).

Numerous authors have noted that the level of cord lesion is a significant factor in the development of pain. Overall, it is noted that the lower the level of injury, the greater the incidence of severe pain (2,3,5,11,14,22). Based on the above reports, the incidence of severe pain in patients with lesions of the cauda equina approximate 42% to 51%; in those with lesions of the thoracic cord, 25%; and in those with injuries to the cervical cord, 10% to 15%. One author, however, has indicated a higher incidence of pain in patients with cervical cord injuries, whereas others have noted a higher incidence in those with thoracolumbar cord injuries (1,2,36).

Upper limb pain occurring in the acute phase of rehabilitation after SCI has received significant attention in the literature and even more so with chronic SCI and the effects of aging (38–60). As a result of the increased reliance on the use of the upper limbs for wheelchair mobility and transfers, as patients with SCI age, the prevalence of degenerative changes associated with aging is expected. In earlier studies, Nichols and associates noted a prevalence of shoulder pain in SCI patients of 51% (39), whereas Bayley and colleagues found a 30% incidence of persistent and chronic shoulder pain during transfers in a sample of 94 patients with complete paraplegia (42). In another group of patients with paraplegia, the prevalence of pain in the upper limbs increased with time since injury (43). Fifty-two percent of patients complained of pain within the first 5 years after injury, whereas by 20 years after injury, all patients had upper limb pain or paresthesia. An additional report of 60 SCI patients studied within the first 18 months after injury revealed that 78% of patients with tetraplegia and 35% of patients with paraplegia had shoulder pain in the first 6 months (46). When reexamined 6 to 18 months after SCI, 33% of the patients with tetraplegia and 35% of the patients with paraplegia continued to have pain. Early on, the functional disability resulting from shoulder pain

was not a significant problem for patients with paraplegia; however, 84% of the patients with tetraplegia having pain described severe to moderate functional disability during the first 6 months after SCI. Impairments persisted in those with shoulder spasticity at follow-up evaluation between 6 and 18 months after injury. Although the shoulder is the primary focus of most of the literature, carpal tunnel syndrome has been noted to increase in prevalence with time as well (41,43).

The etiology and pathophysiology of pain in SCI are discussed later in this chapter; however, a mention of the degenerative changes that occur in the upper limbs that is associated with subsequent occurrence of pain is briefly noted here. There are numerous reports in the literature describing the radiologic changes in the upper limbs that occur in patients with SCI (42, 45,48,49). On the contrary, Wing and Tredwell found little evidence of radiographic degenerative shoulder changes in a group of ambulatory crutch users with a mean duration of 8.7 years since injury (40). In addition, Wylie and Chakera demonstrated greater radiographic degenerative changes in 12 of 38 inactive patients with SCI than in active patients with injuries of 20 years' duration (44). Because of these discrepancies in the literature, Lal performed radiologic evaluations of 53 patients with SCI ranging from the onset of injury until 15 years after injury (49). In this study, 72% of patients demonstrated radiologic evidence of degenerative changes in the shoulder, with only 11% complaining of pain in the shoulders. High-risk factors for degenerative changes included a higher level of wheelchair activity, higher age (>30 years), and female gender. The acromioclavicular joint was universally involved in all affected patients, with common findings including spur formation, necrosis, and impingement. Further study was recommended to help understand the clinical relevance of the above data, pathophysiology, and effective management techniques.

As noted previously, upper limb pain in SCI has been well described in the literature. However, a subset of upper limb pain, reflex sympathetic dystrophy (RSD) (now often referred to as *complex regional pain syndrome*), deserves some individual attention because it has been reported by numerous investigators as well (52–60). RSD is a syndrome of pain, vasomotor and other autonomic disturbances, soft tissue swelling, and trophic changes such as hair loss and osteoporosis initiated by nerve or soft tissue injury (61). Steinbrocker and associates (62) and Kozin and colleagues (63) have described three similar stages in the progression of RSD. The first stage is characterized by pain, hyperesthesia, edema, and tenderness. Stage 2 is characterized by decrease in pain, increased edema, and trophic changes. Atrophy and resolution of the vasomotor changes characterizes stage 3. Triple-phase bone scan is recommended as the most sensitive and specific diagnostic test to confirm the clinical diagnosis (64). There are few reports of RSD in patients with SCI, although the condition is well recognized in the population with hemiplegia (52). Most of the published cases of RSD in SCI indicated upper limb involvement, although one report described lower limb involvement in a patient with tetraplegia (52–59,65). Gellman and colleagues studied 60 consecutive patients (average time after injury, 9 months) admitted to a spinal cord unit and found 7 (11.7%) with complaints of diffuse hand pain, swelling, and stiffness (52). Six of the seven were found to have positive triple-phase bone scans (overall incidence, 10%). This report recognized a higher incidence than previously reported. Lefkoe and coworkers suggested that the diagnosis of RSD may actually be underestimated in the population with SCI owing to the early use of systemic steroids that may be protective, the natural course and treatment of SCI (aggressive mobilization may be protective as well), the frequent presence of autonomic dysfunction, the relatively low incidence of SCI compared with neurologic insults such as stroke, and the diagnostic uncertainty often surrounding the presence of pain syndromes in SCI (65). Wainapel concludes that the reported incidence of RSD in SCI is low because it is misdiagnosed as pain of alternate etiology (55).

PSYCHOLOGICAL AND SOCIAL FACTORS

Numerous psychological and social factors have been found to influence the development, intensity, duration, and successful management of post-SCI pain (19,22,23,25–27,30,32,66–74). As noted previously, several authors have noted that psychosocial issues are often found to be more prognostic than many of the recognized physical factors (22,23,32). In addition, people with SCI and chronic pain are more likely to suffer more psychological distress than those without pain (30). Depression and adjustment disorder after SCI have been frequently cited in the literature to be closely linked to the pain experience (19,22,23,26, 66). Cairns and associates studied 68 patients with acute traumatic SCI with a pain assessment rating scale and a depression assessment scale and noted that pain and depression were independent at the time of admission; however, by discharge, they were found to be closely related (23). Changes in pain affected depression more than changes in depression affected pain. These authors concluded that the relationship between pain and depression tended to develop over time. Improvements in pain management were noted to have a greater effect on reducing depression than reduced depression had on pain. Stormer and colleagues, in a multicenter study of 901 patients with SCI, found a highly significant correlation between chronic pain and depressed mood (70). Increases in chronic pain significantly correlated with those patients having difficulty coping after SCI, those who felt their paralysis was a significant burden, and those who experienced a great loss after injury (e.g., home, work, or social relationships). Kennedy and colleagues studied 76 patients with SCI 6 weeks after injury and 45 of these same patients 1 year after discharge (74). They found that at 6 weeks, increases in anxiety correlated well with pain, whereas at 1 year, both depression and anxiety were highly correlated with pain intensity.

Ragnarsson noted that the perception of pain intensity tends to vary based on the individual's level of physical and intellectual activity (27). Greater activity results in fewer pain complaints, whereas those that are inactive or on bed rest tend to report pain more frequently. Similarly, activity levels tend to be reduced in patients with depression or difficulty adjusting to their disability, which then sets the stage for increased pain perception. Additional psychosocial factors that have been associated with increased incidence of pain in SCI include increased anger, poorer adjustment, inadequate social support systems, greater anxiety,

and as noted previously, a perception of decreased quality of life (9,22–25,32).

CLASSIFICATION OF PAIN IN PATIENTS WITH SPINAL CORD INJURY

Despite the fact that pain in SCI has been described and discussed in the literature since the early twentieth century, there remains little consensus regarding the definition and classification of the various types of pain typically seen (20). Numerous authors have noted this lack of consensus and have indicated that the wide variation in the reported prevalence of pain in SCI is partly a consequence of this controversy (4,11,13,15,26,75, 76). An understanding of the various definitions and classification schema is essential in interpreting the literature, performing new research, developing a treatment plan for individual patients, and communicating with colleagues and patients.

Pain, as defined by the IASP, is an unpleasant sensory and emotional experience associated with actual or potential tissue damage (21). Although pain most often has a proximate physical cause, activity induced in the nociceptor and nociceptive pathways by a noxious stimulus is not, by itself, pain. Pain is a psychological state that is individualized and subjective (77). Pain can be subdivided into acute, subacute, and chronic phases. This differentiation is important in the classification of pain and to ensure appropriate management. Multiple authors have proposed definition schemes differentiating these three phases (78–82). A summary of these schemes is as follows (77):

Acute pain phase. This phase is provoked by various forms of nociceptive stimuli. It focuses on the "sensory-discriminative dimension" of pain. This phase is episodic, recurrent, and self-limiting; and cognitive and affective components of the pain perception are less prominent. It can usually be treated effectively. This phase lasts from less than 1 day to 3 months, but has the potential to become chronic (83).

Subacute pain phase. This phase involves pain that is ill defined; is a transitional phase between the acute and chronic phase; involves nociceptive stimuli that are apparent; follows the acute pain phase; and can last as long as 6 months.

Chronic pain phase. This phase is provoked by nociceptive stimuli that are often unknown. It involves enduring pain that was not responsive to appropriate medical or surgical treatment. This phase lasts longer than the usual course of an acute injury or disease, usually with pain lasting for more than 3 to 6 months. It may develop into a chronic pain syndrome.

It is important to understand the difference between chronic pain and a *chronic pain syndrome* (77). In patients with chronic pain, the experience of pain is present, but the person manifests function and behavior appropriate to the degree of tissue injury. During the chronic pain phase, if functional limitations and reduced productivity result from pain and pain-related behaviors, then a chronic pain syndrome may have developed (77). Associated with the chronic pain syndrome are a myriad of complicating factors, including increased psychological distress, depression, and social and vocational handicaps (83). Therefore, although patients may have chronically painful conditions and be in the chronic pain phase, chronic pain behaviors and associated disability may not develop.

There have been numerous attempts in the literature to provide pain classification systems; however, none has been universally accepted. In general, most systems have used criteria based on location or region of pain (e.g., above lesion, below lesion), on source of presumed stimulus (e.g., musculoskeletal or somatic, visceral, radicular), or on descriptors of the perception of the pain (e.g., epicritic-sharp, stabbing, localized versus protopathic-diffuse, burning) (20,84). The numerous problems inherent in these earlier classification systems were extensively reviewed and reported by Siddall and associates (20). To summarize, in those systems that rely on classification based on location or region of pain, problems arise owing to a lack of specificity (85,86). This type of classification is overly simplified because it does not differentiate between the types of pain that may occur above, at, or below a lesion. Further clarification is needed because musculoskeletal and visceral pain, as well as pain arising from nervous structures, can occur at any of these levels.

Those systems that attempt to classify pain by source of presumed stimulus may provide more accuracy but are also fraught with problems. Numerous terms have been used to describe the source of painful stimuli: musculoskeletal, visceral, root, sympathetic, and psychic; musculoskeletal, radicular, border reaction, and central; root, visceral and central; neurologic, central or psychological; segmental nerve, spinal cord, visceral, mechanical, and psychogenic; central, root, visceral, and musculoskeletal (4, 5,8–10,15). The authors argue that because the pathophysiology of most types of SCI pain is poorly understood and controversial, it is inappropriate to base a classification system on terms that imply etiology. Similarly, using a classification system based on descriptors such as epicritic or protopathic is also less than optimal. To illustrate the difficulty, epicritic is often used interchangeably with radicular pain, and protopathic is thought of as a more central (spinal cord) lesion.

Many authors have attempted to classify pain using one criterion; however, most have used systems that combine several criteria. Included within these mixed classification systems is location or level of pain, origin of pain, and pain descriptors. Siddall and associates contended that mixed classification systems not only have some of the same problems noted previously with the single classification systems but also introduce new problems associated with the different discriminating criteria that are used within the same classification system (20). One additional issue is the lack of consensus among authors on the number, types, and terminology used to describe pain in SCI. Discussed earlier were the most commonly used terms in the various classification schemes; however, some authors include less commonly used pain terms, such as syringomyelia pain and anterior spinal artery syndrome pain, both of which are included in "central dysesthesia syndrome" (10,12,14,87–89). Others have included the categories of headache pain (as seen in autonomic dysreflexia), RSD, phantom pain, and pain associated with spasticity and compressive neuropathies (4,6,14,15). Another term rarely included in classification systems is the *double lesion syndrome*, which has been described by Beric to be one of the more complex causes of post-SCI pain (90). It is a slowly progressive condition occurring months after SCI with charac-

teristic neurologic, neurophysiologic, and urodynamic findings (91,92). It generally is thought to represent an occult cauda equina dysfunction in cervical and thoracic SCI patients (93). This syndrome features conversion of an upper motor neuron lesion of the distal lower limbs and bladder into a lower motor neuron lesion, often with associated pain (93).

Any attempt to introduce a new classification system is likely to be met with similar difficulties as well as additional criticism and lack of consensus. Several recent publications have also proposed a mixed classification schema that attempts to integrate the efforts of prior authors. However, one must realize that any classification is likely to be artificial until the pathophysiology of pain is better elucidated (20,27,94) (Fig. 26.1). The following is a brief summary of pain classification based on origin of stimulus combined with location of stimulus with respect to level of injury.

Mechanical, Musculoskeletal, and Nociceptive Pain

The term *musculoskeletal pain* (MP) refers to pain that arises from normally or partially innervated tissues. This type of pain is most commonly seen above or at the level of the lesion but can also be seen below the level of injury in neurologically incomplete SCI or within the zone of partial preservation (95). MP can be seen acutely or chronically and is the only type of SCI pain for which the pathophysiology and etiology are usually easily identifiable. Examples of MP include pain arising from damage to the spinal column and associated structures (i.e., ligaments, surrounding musculature, and soft tissues), from an acute traumatic injury, or postoperatively. After injury and during the rehabilitation phase, pain can be generated by overuse of intact structures (e.g., upper limb activities), leading to acute bursitis or tendonitis (see chapter 16 for details). Incisional pain, persistent postoperative spinal instability or fracture pain, and pain due to infection are also common. MP is most commonly found in close proximity to the insult and is easily localized. It can be characterized by a sharp pain (radiating or non-radiating) or a dull aching pain (typically non-radiating). It is usually relieved with rest, bracing such as with a thoracolumbosacral orthosis (TLSO), and treatment of the underlying cause, such as with antibiotics and drainage for an infection or surgery in the case of vertebral instability. Chronic upper limb MP pain is commonly seen in people with SCI as well and is associated with degenerative joint disease and overuse (38–59).

Neuropathic Pain

Neuropathic pain (NP) is a term used to describe pain that follows damage to the central or peripheral nervous system and is difficult to categorize (21). NP above the level of injury is most easily defined because its pathophysiology is more obvious. Compression neuropathies in chronic SCI have been reported in the upper limbs, involving both the median nerve in patients with carpal tunnel syndrome and the ulnar nerve; at Guyon's canal; and at the cubital tunnel (20,41,43). Overuse and excessive local compression over the route of the nerve at sites typically

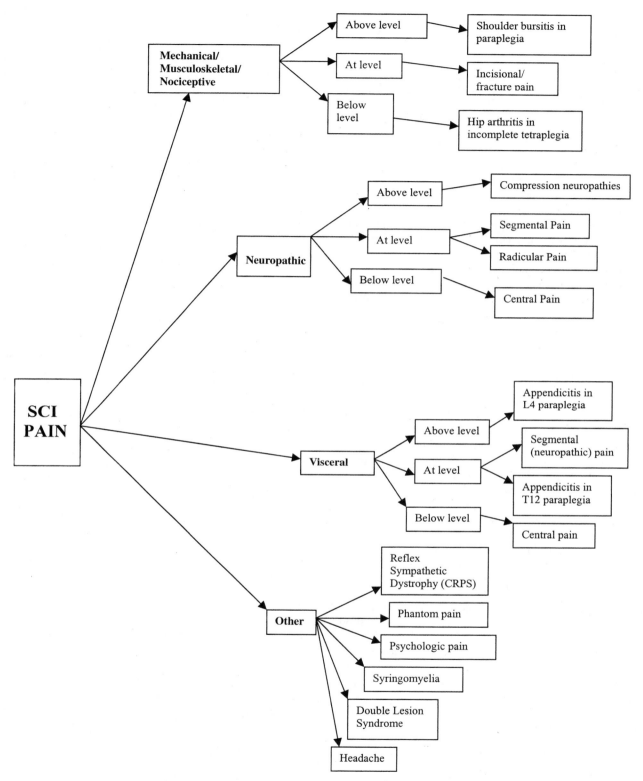

FIGURE 26.1. Classification of pain in patients with spinal cord injury.

associated with compression neuropathies, such as wrist and elbow, is a common occurrence in active patients with SCI. Use of assistive devices, such as crutches and canes; routine pressure relief; and weight shifts using the upper limbs, transfers, and wheelchair mobility may increase the risk for these neuropathies.

NP occurring at the level of injury has been typically subdivided into two major types: radicular or nerve root pain, and pain at the level of injury not associated with nerve root damage (2,4,5,10,13–15). This second type of pain not associated with nerve root damage has been described by various terms, including *segmental pain, end-zone pain, hyperalgesic border reaction,* and *neuropathic at level central pain* (6,9,10,14,20,27,85). Pain derived from root involvement usually occurs early after initial injury arising from direct root damage, spinal column instability after spinal fracture or ligamentous injury, impingement by loose bone fragments or disk material, or inflammation. A less common cause for radicular pain that occurs later after SCI includes the previously mentioned and controversial double lesion syndrome (92). Radicular pain is described as burning, stabbing, shooting, or electric-shock–like and is often paroxysmal and associated with allodynia (pain evoked by non-noxious stimuli) or hyperesthesia (increased sensitivity to stimuli) (6,9,20).

Segmental pain occurs in the absence of root damage and is believed to be associated with pathology within the spinal cord or other parts of the central nervous system (9,14,20,27,85). It has been proposed that injury to the gray matter of the dorsal horn and subsequent hyperactivity of nociceptor cells located in the gray matter are the likely source of this pain (96–98). Although usually described in terms similar to those for radicular pain, segmental pain can be distinguished by its typically bilateral distribution through one or more adjacent dermatomes (6, 27,85). Its presentation, however, can vary depending on the level of injury (27,94). In cervical cord injuries, the pain is usually bilateral and described as hot, cold, tingling, or numbness involving multiple adjacent dermatomes spanning the shoulders, arms, and hands. In thoracic cord injuries, it is typically described as a tightness or circumferential burning around the chest or abdomen in a dermatomal distribution. In lumbar lesions, a similar dermatomal distribution is noted, with spread into the groin and lower limbs (94).

The "burning-hands syndrome" described in patients with central cord syndrome, as well as in football players with "stingers," is another form of segmental pain (27,95,99). It is our experience that although this pain presents early as severe, it often diminishes with time as neurologic recovery occurs. Burning-hands syndrome and the other segmental and radicular pain presentations often mimic the clinical findings seen in RSD (27). It is important to differentiate the two because there are often different treatment options.

Pain that follows injury to the cauda equina or conus medullaris is considered radicular pain or segmental pain, respectively (22). When lesions involve both the cauda equina and conus medullaris, a combination of pain types is seen. In these cases, the characteristics of the pain are similar to the descriptions given earlier but are often of greater severity (2,3,22). Likewise, the typical distribution is bilateral and symmetric, affecting the sacral dermatomes primarily.

NP below the level of injury has been recently referred to as *deafferentation central pain,* but in previous reports had also been described as *remote, central, diffuse burning, phantom, central dysesthetic,* and *dysesthetic* pain (2,4–6,8–15,27,85,100). It has been even more recently suggested that the term deafferentation has fallen out of favor owing to reports that deafferentation alone is not sufficient for the development of central pain (CP) in patients with SCI (16,97,101). Amongst the numerous terms in the literature, the term CP appears to be most quoted and is therefore used in the remainder of this chapter.

CP is most commonly characterized as burning or aching but also as tingling, shooting, stabbing, pressure, cold, numbness, pins and needles, electric sensations, or a nonspecific uncomfortable feeling such as with a muscle cramp (2,3,11,20,23, 27,70,97). It is typically diffuse (as opposed to dermatomal), asymmetric, and patchy and may be perceived as coming from a specific body part or region below the level of injury (27,97). It is often noted to be continuous and only relieved by sleep (31). Although chronic, CP may vary in intensity as well as location and is often influenced by noxious stimuli below the level of injury, stress (physical and psychological), boredom, and fatigue (27,97). CP may develop immediately after injury, gradually over the course of weeks to months after injury, or years after injury (6,100).

Central dysesthesia syndrome deserves special note among the various types of central pain because it is unique in several ways (19,23). It is found almost exclusively in patients with an incomplete SCI syndrome that includes absence of spinothalamic and anterolateral functions, with relative dorsal column function preservation. It typically occurs late (weeks to months after injury) and often at the time of partial recovery of function. As further recovery occurs, the dysesthetic pain often diminishes.

Visceral Pain

Visceral pain (VP) can occur above, at, or below the level of injury (2,4–6,9,14,15,20,27,97). It can be nociceptive at all three levels and neuropathic at the level or below the level of injury. Nociceptive VP above or at the level of injury occurs primarily in those with a neurologic lesion below the mid-thoracic level, where the splanchnic innervation is left intact. Nociceptive VP at or near the level of injury may be poorly localized and vague because the sensation from the abdominal and pelvic organs is not segmentally innervated. However, if the pleural or parietal peritoneum is involved, greater localization is possible because it is segmentally innervated and correlates with the trunk dermatomes (10).

Nociceptive VP below the level of injury is also poorly localized and vague. It is not clear how this vague pain is perceived, especially in those with complete lesions; however, it is thought that the vagus nerve may convey painful sensations arising from abdominal pathology (102). In any person with tetraplegia or high-level paraplegia suspected of abdominal pathology, monitoring for other signs of acute illness, such as nausea and vomiting, anorexia, autonomic dysreflexia, and fever, is strongly recommended because this type of pain is most often nonspecific and nonlocalized (10,102). Occasionally, VP is perceived at or below the level of injury and is not associated with abdominal pathology. This type of pain is believed to be of neuropathic origin and can present similarly to the radicular, segmental, or central pains described previously (27).

PATHOPHYSIOLOGY OF PAIN

To comprehend the treatment options available for the management of pain syndromes in patients with SCI, a basic understanding of the anatomy and physiology of normal pain pathways is beneficial. Following this discussion is a review of the pathophysiology behind the development of pain, with an emphasis on neuropathic pain. A brief review of the mechanisms of pain secondary to SCI is also presented. Those interested in further information and detail involving proposed pain mechanisms should refer to the extensive literature on this topic (7,9, 10,12,13,16,78,88,101,103–108).

Any discussion of current concepts involving pain pathways and pain physiology should include recognition of the literature that has paved the way for our current understanding. One of the most commonly discussed theories was based on the early work of Melzack and Wall (109). Their original gate-control theory describes the ability of nonpainful sensory input to inhibit nociceptive activity. Nonpainful sensation, such as touch and vibration, result in increased activation of large nerve fibers that subsequently modify the activity of smaller (pain-mediating) fibers located in the dorsal horn of the spinal cord. The balance of large-fiber and small-fiber activity determines the level of pain transmission. A predominance of large-fiber input (e.g., rubbing a painful "funny bone") closes the "gate" in the dorsal horn of the spinal cord and relieves the pain. On the other hand, a reduction in large-fiber activity, whereby painful stimuli are allowed to be transmitted through active small fibers, opens the gate and increases painful sensations. This theory, based on counterirritant stimuli, also allows for the attenuation or promotion of pain through central control mechanisms. Psychological factors (e.g., depression, anxiety), arousal, motivation, level of activity, and circumstances that alter the perception of pain can all participate in modulation of the pain experience through higher centers in the brain (103).

Considerable research in the area of pain neurophysiology followed the introduction of the original gate-control theory. Although the essential concepts remain the same, using data from more recent literature, Melzack introduced an updated theory in 1991 (110). It is still believed that low-threshold touch fibers can inhibit nociceptive fiber pain production. In addition, it is now thought that nociceptive afferents, when stimulated, can also modulate pain perception. This new knowledge helps to explain the effectiveness of noxious counterirritant stimuli (e.g., acupuncture and transcutaneous electrical nerve stimulation [TENS]) in decreasing pain. The contribution of higher centers in the brain and their input at the level of the dorsal horn have been further elucidated and confirmed. Now, increased emphasis is placed on the involvement of neurons within the thalamus, cortex, and limbic systems. Although the original theory was based on peripheral pain modulation, it is now thought that a much more complex interaction occurs between the peripheral afferents and brain centers. Whereas pain modulation normally occurs with involvement of peripheral afferent input,

it is suggested that the peripheral input is not required and that pain may be maintained or attenuated by independent central mechanisms. The presence of a central modulating system that enhances pain has also been suggested by others (111). This updated version lends further support to the contribution of the cognitive and psychological aspects of pain perception.

Similar to the evolution of the principles introduced by Melzack and Wall in the gate-control theory, our understanding of the neuroanatomy and neurophysiology of pain has also undergone significant revision and updating through the years (103). Initial thoughts (112) focused on two major nociceptive systems: the spinothalamic system and the spinoreticulothalamic system. The spinothalamic system was thought to be responsible for the transmission of localized, sharp pain that ascends contralaterally to the lateral thalamus and somatosensory cortex somatotopically. The overall functions of this system are to transmit pain impulses associated with trauma or disease of the peripheral tissues and to assist in minimizing the ultimate tissue damage through a withdrawal reflex. The spinoreticulothalamic system transmits diffuse, poorly localized pain stimuli through both ipsilateral and contralateral tracts to the reticular system of the brain stem (medulla and pons) and midbrain, ending its initial travels within the medial thalamus. Much less organized than the spinothalamic system, diffuse projections ascend to the limbic system, including the hippocampus and amygdala, the hypothalamus, and pituitary gland. This second system lends to the arousal, avoidance, emotional, and defensive responses seen with pain perception.

Although these initial thoughts were appropriate for the available research at the time, they are now thought to be grossly oversimplified (103). More recent reports have provided an updated and more detailed version of these initial general observations (106–108). As a result of the work of investigators such as Berkley, it is now believed that there are multiple neural mechanisms, each responsible for the many different types of pain sensations and the many types of peripheral tissues innervated (113). The interested reader is referred to the previously cited publications for an extensive study; however, a brief review follows.

Primary (first-order) afferent neurons begin at the level of the peripheral organ (e.g., skin, viscera) and subsequently terminate in the dorsal horn of the spinal cord (Fig. 26.2). The three primary afferent neurons, A-beta, A-delta, and C fibers, are differentiated by their diameters, presence or absence of myelin, speed of conduction, and type of afferent information they transmit. The A-beta (non-nociceptive) fibers respond to low-intensity, nonpainful, proprioceptive-vibratory, and light-touch stimuli. They have a thick myelin sheath and are fast conducting. The A-delta nociceptive fibers respond to well-localized sharp pain and assist in rapid withdrawal from painful stimuli. They are thinly myelinated and are relatively fast conducting yet much slower that the A-beta fibers. The final main type of afferent neuron is the C nociceptive fiber. These fibers tend to be polymodal (i.e., respond to a variety of noxious stimuli) and transmit poorly localized, dull pain. They are of smaller diameter and are unmyelinated and therefore conduct very slowly. Most nociceptive afferents are of this type and are further classified into afferents specific for thermal, mechanical, or chemical noxious stim-

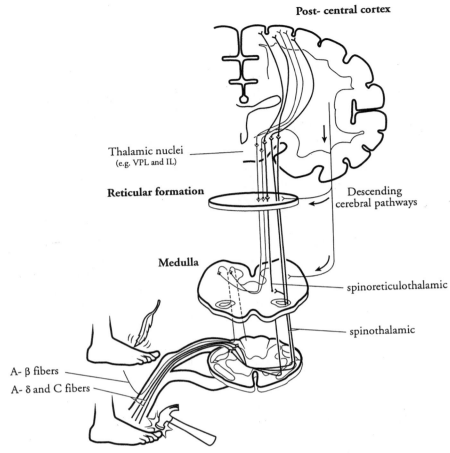

FIGURE 26.2. The main somatosensory pathways, beginning at the level of the peripheral organ and eventually terminating in the somatosensory cortex (post–central cortex). VPL, ventral posterolateral thalamic nuclei; IL, intralaminar thalamic nuclei.

uli. The A-delta nociceptive afferents are similarly sub-classified, whereas the A-beta afferents respond only to innocuous mechanical stimuli.

The primary afferents (A-beta, A-delta, and C fibers) project from the peripheral organ to the spinal cord gray matter. This gray matter, located in the dorsal horn, is organized into anatomically distinct layers identified by Rexed (Rexed laminae) (114). It is at this level that significant integration occurs involving input from the autonomic and somatomotor systems and cerebral centers and resulting in modulation of both nociceptive and innocuous stimuli. These secondary (second-order) afferent neurons travel from the Rexed laminae of the dorsal horn to cerebral structures, including the thalamus (especially the ventral posterolateral nucleus) and reticular formation of the brain stem. The axons transmitting nociceptive and temperature stimuli cross over in the spinal cord at about the level of entry and travel up the cord (contralateral to the site of entry) through the anterolateral white-matter columns while those axons transmitting non-nociceptive stimuli (touch and proprioception) travel through the ipsilateral dorsal columns. The final pathway travels from the nuclei of the thalamus to the somatosensory areas of the cerebral cortex.

The tertiary (third-order) afferent neurons carry the somatotopically-organized information from the thalamus to the somatosensory cortex (areas I and II). In the past, it was thought that the cortex had little involvement in pain perception; however, recent work (115) involving brain imaging has found increased activity in the somatosensory cortex following noxious stimuli applied to the a peripheral limb. Additional evidence for involvement of these higher centers comes from the neurosurgical literature, where it has been noted that both neoplastic and nonneoplastic pain sensations have been diminished with certain destructive procedures of the cerebrum (lobotomy, leukotomy, and cingulotomy) (103,116).

This already complex system of peripheral afferents, spinal interneurons, and central processing mechanisms is made even more complex by the neurochemical (neurotransmitters) and neuromodulatory substances involved in pain mediation (Fig. 26.3). Brief noxious stimuli are often followed by persistent pain that lasts longer than would be expected from the stimulus alone. Substances thought to be associated with increased and persistent pain perception, hyperalgesia, and the associated inflammation include neuropeptides, such as substance P, vasoactive intestinal peptide, somatostatin, and cholecystokinin; amino acids, such

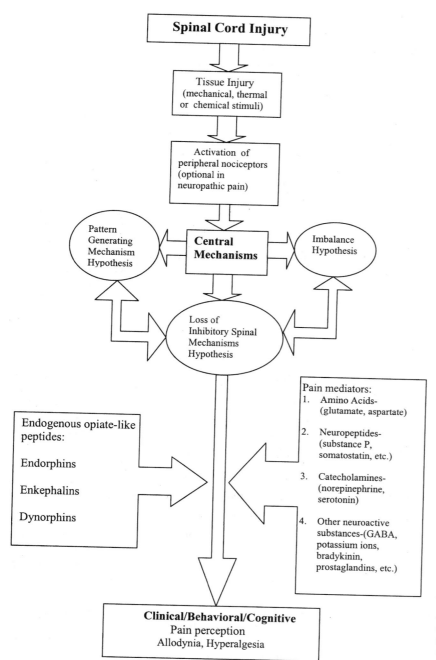

FIGURE 26.3. Diagram of the complex system of proposed central processing mechanisms and the various neurochemical and neuromodulatory substances involved in pain mediation after spinal cord injury. The end result is the perception of pain and its associated behaviors. GABA, γ-aminobutyric acid. (Adapted in part from Yezierski RP. Pain following spinal cord injury: the clinical problem and experimental studies. *Pain* 1996; 68:190; and Eide PK. Pathophysiological mechanisms of central neuropathic pain after spinal cord injury. *Spinal Cord* 1998;36:605.)

as glutamate or aspartate; nucleotides, such as adenosine triphosphate; catecholamines, such as norepinephrine and serotonin; and other neuroactive substances, such as potassium ions, bradykinin, histamine, and prostaglandins (103,106).

Whereas the previously listed substances are known to mediate pain, the endogenous opiate-like peptides, endorphins, enkephalins, and dynorphins act to produce analgesia. Their mode of action is similar to opiates such as morphine, and they use similar receptor sites in the brain and spinal cord. The four opiate receptor sites most commonly recognized are mu (mor-

phine), delta (enkephalin), kappa (ketocyclazocine), and epsilon (B-endorphin). Naloxone, a synthetic narcotic antagonist, blocks both endogenous opioids and morphine by binding preferentially to opioid receptor sites. Long-term use of narcotics in patients with chronic pain results in a decreased number of these receptors or a reduction in their binding affinity (down-regulation). Therefore, to achieve the same level of analgesia, increased narcotic doses are required (103).

Having provided a general overview on the pathophysiology and anatomy of normal pain pathways, we will now review several proposed mechanisms for the development of pain in SCI. Although most of this discussion will deal with mechanisms leading to NP, a brief mention of MP mechanisms is included as well. It is essential to differentiate these two types of pain because the management options typically differ. MP originates from the activation of peripheral nociceptors after tissue injury. Many types of high-intensity stimuli, such as mechanical, thermal, or chemical, can elicit activation of these high-threshold free nerve endings (101,117). Induction of peripheral nociceptor stimulation in patients with SCI could include fracture pain, postoperative incisional pain, ligamentous or soft tissue injury, or overuse injuries during the rehabilitation or post-rehabilitation phase. Management of MP is a much easier task than that of NP because it is often responsive to analgesics such as nonsteroidal antiinflammatory drugs (NSAIDs), acetaminophen, or mild narcotics (see Treatment).

NP is much more complex both in its proposed mechanisms and pathophysiology and in its treatment options. Peripheral nociceptor activation is not required for the development of NP but may be present. It is unlikely that any one mechanism is responsible for the many clinical representations of NP. Several proposed mechanisms have been reported in the literature, and the following discussion includes three of the most accepted postulates.

Several authors have described an "imbalance hypothesis" (12,88,104). This hypothesis is based on the premise that an imbalance in afferent information conveyed by the dorsal columns and anterolateral (spinothalamic) tracts may lead to the development of post-injury CP. Support for this hypothesis comes from both the spinal cord and stroke literature (118–120). Patients with more severe spinal cord involvement with total absence of all sensory modalities below the level of injury (i.e., complete injuries) usually do not present with as severe pain syndromes as those with partial or complete disruptions of the spinothalamic pathways but preservation of the dorsal columns (88). Similarly, NP in patients with stroke invariably has deficits attributable to the absence of anterolateral sensory modalities coupled with relatively intact dorsal column functioning (120).

Two additional postulates for the development of chronic pain in SCI involve the presence of a "pattern-generating mechanism" within the injured spinal cord and the closely related "loss of spinal inhibitory mechanisms" (7,105). These hypotheses are based on the belief that not all post-injury pain is due to noxious input, but instead may be due to deafferentation or loss of inhibitory control and changes in firing patterns, including burst activity and discharges on neurons adjacent to the site on injury (7). The loss of spinal and supraspinal inhibitory control may allow for recruitment of surrounding neurons, with subsequent exacerbation and spread of pain. Significant support for these two hypotheses can be found in the literature, including the existence of abnormal focal hyperactivity in the spinal cord and thalamus of patients with spinal injury (100,121) and the presence of abnormal responses and after-discharges of spinal sensory neurons after experimental SCI (122,123). Evidence for the loss of inhibitory control in the development of pattern generators is also described in the literature involving the inhibitory neurotransmitter γ-aminobutyric acid (GABA) (124–127). The previ-

ously mentioned experimental studies and several similar clinical observations support the hypothesis that changes in the physiologic properties of spinal neurons and the development of focal pattern generators occur as a result of anatomic and neurochemical changes that ultimately lead to clinical symptoms, including allodynia, hyperalgesia, and pain (3,10,11,16,98,100,105) (Fig. 26.3).

TREATMENT

The purpose of a pain classification system for SCI is to reflect the underlying pathophysiology of SCI-associated pain and secondarily to suggest treatment strategies (24,25). The reality of SCI-associated pain is that it often presents as multiple but separate painful conditions and may evolve over time (128). For example, in the immediate post-injury phase, the pain is primarily nociceptive and related to musculoskeletal trauma. Although neuropathic pain can develop immediately, it often occurs months to years after injury. Thus, the practitioner is challenged to be thorough in investigating pain complaints and to shift treatment modalities over time.

In considering MP, NP, and VP, it is useful to determine not only whether the pain is above, at, or below the level of injury but also whether the pain is acute or chronic. Thus, in the following overview of treatment approaches for SCI-related pain, options for each of these categories of pain are presented with some discussion of these factors. There is also an effort to present typical SCI pain syndromes in an order that reflects the evolution of pain that can be seen in a patient with traumatic SCI.

Mechanical, Musculoskeletal, and Nociceptive Pain

Those medications most useful in MP include narcotics, tramadol, muscle relaxants, NSAIDs, and acetaminophen (129). The choice of medication is determined by the severity and acuity of pain. These medications are often used in combination to maximize effectiveness.

Early after injury, there is usually severe, acute pain related to fractures, lacerations, and surgical wounds, which is best treated with narcotics (129). Narcotics are classified as agonist, agonist-antagonist, or antagonist based on their interaction with central (brain) receptors. Multiple factors influence the choice of one narcotic over another. The most common considerations are potency, duration of effect, route of administration, tolerability and availability, and side-effect profile. All narcotics share the side effects of constipation, sedation, respiratory depression, and urinary retention and can lead to dependency. Long-term use can result in tolerance as the receptor sites upregulate and more medication is required for the same effect. Addiction can occur, rarely (129,130).

As the pain from the acute trauma associated with SCI subsides, strong narcotics are usually weaned, and milder narcotics, such as codeine, hydrocodone, and propoxyphene, are substituted. Many of these agents have a synergistic effect with NSAIDs and acetaminophen and are available in combination

TABLE 26.1. SUMMARY OF THE MORE COMMONLY PRESCRIBED NARCOTICS

Generic Name (Brand Name)	Dose (mg)/Route/Frequency (hr)	Other Properties and Side Effects
Codeine	15–60/p.o., s.c., i.m./every 4–5	Combination preparations include acetaminophen, carisprodol, and aspirin
Propoxyphene (Darvon)	65–130/p.o./every 4	Combination preparations include aspirin, caffeine, and acetaminophen.
Hydrocodone (Vicodin)	5–10/p.o./every 4–5	Combination preparations include acetaminophen and ibuprofen.
Oxycodone (Roxicodone, OxyContin-CR)	5–10/p.o./every 4–5 10–40/p.o./every 8–12 (CR)	Combination preparations include acetaminophen and aspirin. Decreased euphoria CR.
Morphine (MS Contin, Oramorph SR)	10–30/p.o., s.c., i.m./every 4 15–60/p.o./every 8–12 (SR)	Intravenous form available for drip or frequent dosing. Intrathecal dosing available. Decreased euphoria with SR. Lower abuse potential.
Hydromorphone (Dilaudid)	2–4 p.o., i.m., s.c., i.v./every 4–6 3/p.o./every 6–8	Also comes in suppository form (p.r.).
Meperidine (Demerol)	25–75/p.o., s.c., i.m., i.v./every 3–4	Intravenous form should be given slowly. Prolonged use may result in seizures (toxic metabolite). High abuse potential.
Methadone (Dolophine)	25–1.0/p.o., s.c., i.m./every 3–4	Can be used for detoxification. Decreased euphoria, lower abuse potential.
Fentanyl (Duragesic)	25–200 µg/hr (patch) every 3 d 200–1,600 µg (lozenge) every 6 hr	Comes in patch and lozenge form.

CR, controlled release; SR, sustained release; PO, oral; IM, intramuscular; SQ, subcutaneous; IV, intravenous; PR, per rectum; mg, milligrams; mcg, micrograms; CR, controlled release; SR, sustained release.
Adapted from *Tarascon Pocket Pharmacopoeia 2000.* Loma Linda, CA: Tarascon Publishing, 2000.

formulations. Care must be taken not to exceed more than 4 g of acetaminophen daily because liver toxicity can result (129). See Table 26.1 for a summary of the more commonly prescribed narcotics.

An additional nonnarcotic medication for moderate to moderately severe pain is tramadol, a synthetic analgesic that binds to the µ-receptor and blocks reuptake of serotonin and norepinephrine. It shares the side effects of the narcotic analgesics but to a lesser degree. It can cause dizziness and can lower the seizure threshold in combination with certain medications. Addiction potential is somewhat less than with the narcotic medications (129,131,132).

Early after SCI, painful and intense muscle spasm may develop at the level of the vertebral fracture or postsurgical incision site, especially in the cervical region. These spasms can be overwhelming. Physical interventions can be employed, such as heat, ice, massage, and stretching and positioning, but often the patient is not physically able to participate in these interventions in the acute post-injury phase (133–137). Muscle relaxants can be effective and allow for a reduction in the dosing of narcotic medications by diminishing muscle excitability and reducing the pain that accompanies tense muscles (138). Almost all of these medications affect the central nervous system, resulting in sedation. Long-term use of many of these agents may be associated with addiction and withdrawal (139). The use of these drugs should be limited to no more than 2 to 3 weeks. If muscle spasm related to the acute trauma persists beyond this time frame, alternative methods should be employed and the muscle spasm reevaluated. See Table 26.2 for a summary of the commonly used muscle relaxants.

There are five classes of traditional NSAIDs: the salicylates, propionic acids, acetic acids, fenamates, and oxicams. These medications share a common mechanism of action of inhibiting

prostaglandin synthesis, which results in the key actions of the drugs: mild to moderate analgesia, antipyresis, antithrombosis, and anti-inflammation. They all differ in their side-effect profile and duration of effect, but each of the NSAIDs can cause some gastric distress and renal or hepatic impairment. The choice of one class over the other often depends on the side-effect profile. The indications for NSAIDs would seemingly make them ideal for use in the acute phase of injury; however, caution must be exercised when prescribing these medications. Most patients with traumatic SCI received methylprednisolone at the time of acute care admission, which, in combination with NSAIDs, can potentiate gastric bleeding. Additionally, most patients with SCI are placed on deep venous thrombosis prophylaxis, which can further increase bleeding risk. Using the lowest effective doses of the NSAIDs with the least amount of enterohepatic recirculation and adding gastrointestinal (GI) cytoprotectants, such as misoprostol, may reduce the risk for GI bleeding (129). There is also controversy about the use of NSAIDs in patients receiving surgical repair and fusion of vertebral fractures because they may reduce the healing potential of bone (140).

The Cox-2 inhibitors are a relatively new class of NSAIDs that are thought to have fewer side effects related to GI bleeding and hepatic and renal impairment. Meloxicam (Mobic) has been available in Europe for more than a decade and is similar to drugs in the oxicam class but has far more Cox-2–inhibitor action than other oxicams. Celecoxib (Celebrex) and rofecoxib (Vioxx) are the most selective Cox-2 inhibitors and as a consequence greatly reduce GI and renal side effects (141). See Table 26.3 for a summary of the commonly used NSAIDs.

TENS can be a useful adjunctive agent in the treatment of acute MP and NP (142–145). This modality may have a counterirritant effect that reduces the pain perception, and it may increase endorphins, enkephalins, and dynorphins in the cere-

TABLE 26.2. SUMMARY OF COMMONLY USED MUSCLE RELAXANTS

Generic Name (Brand Name)	Dose (mg)/Route/Frequency	Other Properties and Side Effects
Carisprodol (Soma, Rela)	350/p.o./t.i.d.–q.i.d.	Combination preparation with aspirin with or without codiene. Contraindicated in acute intermittent porphyria.
Chlorzoxazone (Parafon Forte, Paraflex)	250–500/p.o./t.i.d.–q.i.d.	Rare GI side effects. Bleeding, hepatotoxicity.
Cyclobenzaprine (Flexeril)	10/p.o./t.i.d.–q.i.d.	Anticholinergic side effects.
Diazepam (Valium)	2–10/p.o., i.m., i.v./t.i.d.–q.i.d.	Sustained release formulation available but not recommended. Cardiovascular and respiratory dysfunction.
Metaxalone (Skelaxin)	800/p.o./t.i.d.–q.i.d.	Paradoxic CNS excitation. Hematologic toxicity. Hemolytic anemia. Avoid if hepatic dysfunction.
Methocarbamol (Robaxin)	750–1,500/p.o., i.m., i.v./t.i.d.–q.i.d.	Can be given a loading dose followed by maintenance dose. Combination preparation with aspirin.
Orphenadrine (Norflex)	100/p.o./b.i.d. 60/i.m., i.v./b.i.d.	Rare anaphylaxis in asthmatics given i.m./i.v. dosing. Works more as analgesic with secondary muscle relaxation. Combination preparation with aspirin and caffeine.

CNS, central nervous system; GI, gastrointestinal; PO, oral; IM, intramuscular; IV, intravenous; mg, milligram; CNS, central nervous system; GI, gastrointestinal; bid, every 12 hours; tid, every 8 hours; qid, every 6 hours.
Adapted from *Tarascon Pocket Pharmacopoeia 2000*. Loma Linda, CA: Tarascon Publishing, 2000.

TABLE 26.3. SUMMARY OF COMMONLY USED NONSTEROIDAL ANTIINFLAMMATORY MEDICATIONS

Generic Name (Brand Name)	Dosage (mg)/Route/Frequency	Other Properties and Side Effects
Salicylates, acetylated Aspirin (Ecotrin, Empirin, Bayer)	650/p.o./q.i.d.	Antipyretic, antiinflammatory, platelet inhibition, often used in combination preparation with narcotics and muscle relaxants, severe allergic reactions, enteric-coated and buffered available.
Salicylates, nonacetylated Diflunisal (Dolobid)	250–500/p.o./b.i.d.–t.i.d.	Weak antiinflammatory effect; lacks antipyretic activity.
Salsalate (Disalcid, Salflex)	1,000–1,500/p.o./t.i.d.–q.i.d.	Weak antiinflammatory effect; no platelet inhibition.
Proprionic Acid Ibuprofen (Motrin)	400–800/p.o./t.i.d.–q.i.d.	OTC forms include Advil, Nuprin, Rufen; transdermal form available.
Naproxen (Naprosyn, Naprosyn EC)	250–500/p.o./b.i.d.	High incidence of GI side effects. OTC form is Alleve; controlled release available.
Acetic acids Diclofenac (Cataflam, Voltaren, Voltaren XR)	50/p.o./b.i.d.–t.i.d. XR-100/p.o./q.d.	LFT monitoring suggested if use is prolonged; side effects in up to 20%, extended release (XR) available.
Etodolac (Lodine, Lodine XL)	200–400/t.i.d.–q.i.d. XL-400–1200/p.o./q.d.	Short half-life necessitates frequent dosing, possible gastric-sparing properties; extended release (XL) available.
Indomethacin (Indocin, Indocin SR)	25–50/p.o., p.r./t.i.d. SR-75/p.o./b.i.d.–q.d.	Most potent and toxic NSAID, dose-related side effects in up to 25%–50%, CNS/hematologic toxicity, extended release (SR) available.
Ketorolac (Toradol)	10/p.o./q.i.d. 15–60/i.v., i.m./q.i.d.	FDA-approved for only five consecutive days; GI bleeding at higher doses; rapid analgesia with i.m. form.
Nabumetone (Relafen)	500–750/p.o./q.d.-b.i.d.	Long half-life allows q.d. or b.i.d. dosing; nonacidic prodrug.
Oxicams Piroxicam (Feldene)	20/p.o./q.d.	Long half-life permits q.d. dosing; accumulation in elderly people may result from enterohepatic recirculation; dermatologic side effects.
Cox-2 inhibitors Celecoxib (Celebrex)	20/p.o./b.i.d.	Contraindicated with sulfonamide allergy.
Rofecoxib (Vioxx)	12.5–5.0/p.o./q.d.	

FDA, U.S. Food and Drug Administration; OTC, over the counter; GI, gastrointestinal; LFT, liver function tests; PO, oral; mg, milligram; IV, intravenous; IM, intramuscular; qd, every 24 hours; bid, every 12 hours; tid, every 8 hours; qid, every 6 hours; FDA, Food and Drug Administration; OTC, over the counter; GI, gastrointestinal.
Adapted from *Tarascon Pocket Pharmacopoeia 2000*. Loma Linda, CA: Tarascon Publishing, 2000.

brospinal fluid (142). It has the advantage of being noninvasive and having few side effects (146). An additional adjunctive pharmacologic agent, calcitonin (an anti-resorptive agent used in osteoporosis treatment), has been shown to have a primary analgesic effect in MP but appears to be less useful for NP (140, 147,148).

More chronic MP may originate from the shoulder, elbow, or wrist as a result of overuse in an imbalanced shoulder or upper limb (149,150). Relieving pain with rest, ice, compression, and the use of acetaminophen or NSAIDs is the recommended first step (151). Once the acute pain has resolved, gentle range-of-motion exercises and strengthening can be initiated (150). Pain can often be effectively reduced and possibly prevented by the use of appropriate adaptive equipment and modifications to existing equipment.

After these conservative measures have been exhausted, injection of a local anesthetic or steroid can be considered. Local anesthetic will provide immediate relief of pain, can help diagnostically, and will provide a prognosis of the effectiveness of additional injections (152,153). Typically, a long-acting anesthetic such as bupivacaine (Marcaine) is combined with an injectable steroid (153). Injectable steroids result in fewer systemic effects than those administered orally but can lead to tendon rupture if injected inappropriately (129).

Neck and upper back pain due to poor posture in the wheelchair are common in SCI patients (154,155). The normal lordotic curves of the lumbar and cervical spines are often lost, and kyphosis results, with the weight of the head being supported in front of the spine by the musculature of the upper back and neck. The constant strain from the poor biomechanics of this posture results in chronic upper back and neck pain and can also lead to chronic tension and vascular headaches (156). Treatment begins with maximizing optimal posture in the wheelchair with seating system interventions (157). Occasionally, a thoracolumbar orthosis is prescribed to support the trunk, or anti-spasticity medications are used to reduce truncal tone. In addition to positioning, the patient may benefit from therapy modalities, such as heat, ice, and soft tissue mobilization or massage (158). Care must be taken not to cause tissue injury when using heat or ice over insensate areas.

On occasion, chiropractic interventions have been found to be helpful. These interventions are often classified as *complementary* or *alternative*. There is a growing interest in and use of therapeutic interventions that are not a part of traditional Western medicine, including acupuncture, magnets, homeopathy, ultraviolet light, herbs, and others. Federal funding is currently aiding in research efforts to establish the efficacy and safety of these therapies, but in general, their use is far greater than the evidence available and is being driven by consumer demand (159).

MP can also be seen below the level of injury in patients with incomplete SCI. Typical etiologies include heterotopic ossification, pressure sores, fractures, and degenerative joint disease. Prevention is often the key to treatment in many of these disorders but is not always successful. As discussed previously, interventions may include therapy modalities, adaptive equipment, medications, and possibly surgery.

Neuropathic Pain

NP occurring above the level of injury is most commonly associated with a compressive peripheral neuropathy (e.g., carpal tunnel syndrome and ulnar neuropathy) or radiculopathy (160–162). It is more likely attributable to a defined etiology and thus more easily treatable. These conditions can be treated similarly to MP with therapy modalities, adaptive equipment, medications, and anesthetic or steroid injections, but with failure of more conservative therapy, surgery is more likely an option in NP (163,164). Medication choices may differ slightly as well, with the introduction of medications more directed toward pain of nerve origin (see below).

With segmental or radicular pain at the level of injury or central pain below the level of injury, the exact mechanism of pain is often unclear, and the pain is more difficult to treat (165). Radicular pain at the level of injury due to directed compression of unstable spinal fragments typically occurs at the time of initial injury. Treatment should be directed toward decompression and spine stabilization. Despite these efforts, however, the pain may persist. Nonsurgical treatments of persistent radicular pain and segmental pain are similar and may include medications and therapy modalities such as TENS (166). Anticonvulsant medications are often efficacious in NP (167), and carbamazepine has long been the drug of choice (168). Its mechanism of action appears to hinge on its modulation of sodium channels, and it is especially effective in lacinating-type pain. Because of a potential for hepatitis, heptocellular or cholestatic jaundice, and blood dyscrasias, the use of this medication must be carefully monitored with hematologic and liver function testing. Gabapentin has replaced carbamazepine as the first-line drug for this pain because of its lower side-effect profile, its high efficacy, and the need for minimal laboratory surveillance. Its exact mechanism of action is not understood, but studies have demonstrated that it binds to calcium channels, which may play a role in central sensitization after peripheral deafferentation (129,169,170). See Table 26.4 for a summary of anticonvulsants commonly used for neuropathic pain.

If anticonvulsant medications fail to control the NP, other adjunctive medications with reported efficacy include anti-spasticity agents (baclofen, tizanidine, clonidine) and anti-arrthymic agents (mexiletine and lidocaine) (129,171,172). Although mexiletine has been used successfully in phantom limb pain, diabetic neuropathy, and thalamic pain, there is debate about its efficacy and safety in the SCI population with NP (173–176). Capsaicin cream, a chili-pepper derivative that is thought to deplete substance P from the dorsal horn, has also been used successfully in the treatment of segmental and radicular pain and may play a role in the management of MP as well (129).

Tricyclic antidepressant medications are the first choice for central pain below the level of injury (177–180). These agents have multiple side effects, including anticholinergic effects (dry mouth, constipation, urinary retention), sedation (which can be helpful when used at bedtime), cardiac arrhythmias, and exacerbation of spasticity (181). Amitryptiline is often prescribed first because of its strong sedative effects; however, in patients with cardiac disease, the nontricyclic trazodone is recommended be-

TABLE 26.4. SUMMARY OF ANTICONVULSANTS COMMONLY USED IN THE MANAGEMENT OF PAIN

Generic Name (Brand Name)	Dose (mg)/Route/Frequency	Other Properties and Side Effects
Carbamazepine (Tegretol)	100–200/p.o./t.i.d.–q.i.d.	Modulates sodium channels. Hepatotoxicity, aplastic anemia, monitor CBC, LFT.
Gabapentin (Neurontin)	100–900/p.o./t.i.d.–q.i.d.	May modulate calcium channels.
Topiramate (Topamax)	25–50/p.o./q.d.–b.i.d.	
Clonazepam (Klonopin)	0.5–1/p.o./t.i.d.	Potentiates inhibitory effects of GABA. Similar side effects as other benzodiazepenes.
Lamotrigine (Lamictal)		Hepatotoxicity, drug interactions.
Divalproex (Depakote)	250/p.o./b.i.d.–t.i.d.	Modulates sodium channels. Rashes, gingival hyperplasia,
Phenytoin (Dilantin)	100/p.o./t.i.d.	hepatic toxicity, drug interactions.

CBC, complete blood count; LFT, liver function test; mg, milligram; PO, oral; GABA, gamma amino-butyric acid; bid, every 12 hours; tid, every 8 hours; qid, every 6 hours.
Adapted from *Tarascon Pocket Pharmacopoeia 2000*. Loma Linda, CA: Tarascon Publishing, 2000.

cause of its reduced incidence of arrhythmias (129). Nortriptyline may substitute for amitryptiline in patients with orthostatic hypotension (129). Results have been disappointing with the use of the newer selective serotonin reuptake inhibitors (129). See Table 26.5 for a summary of commonly utilized antidepressants.

Central pain is more easily modulated by emotional influences than the other types of pain already discussed, and biofeedback training, meditation, hypnosis, or other similar approaches that utilize a team-based pain management program may be effective (128,182–185). This was recently highlighted by a National Institutes of Health consensus panel, which studied the effectiveness of behavioral intervention on chronic pain (186). It was determined that in patients with chronic pain, relaxation techniques are often effective forms of management. Moderate benefit was assigned to cognitive-behavioral interventions and biofeedback. These findings can be generalized to central pain conditions, which tend to be chronic in nature.

Visceral Pain

The etiology of VP can be nociceptive or neuropathic. All visceral complaints deserve a thorough evaluation in the population with SCI because the presentation is often not typical. Above the level of spinal injury, VP is usually nociceptive secondary to visceral injury or inflammation. This nociceptive VP is easier to localize than pain below the level of injury and is best treated by identifying the cause. Below the level of injury, the pain can be nociceptive or neuropathic and is often very difficult to localize. A celiac plexus block can sometimes be helpful in differentiating nociceptive pain from neuropathic pain and may assist in treatment (187). If the pain is completely relieved with the block, there is greater certainty that the origin of the pain was visceral (nociceptive) rather than musculoskeletal or radicular. If nociceptive, the approach is similar to that outlined for visceral pain occurring above the level of injury. If neuropathic, management is often similar to NP as previously discussed, depending on whether it presents as segmental, radicular, or central.

TABLE 26.5. SUMMARY OF ANTIDEPRESSANTS COMMONLY USED IN PAIN MANAGEMENT

Generic Name (Brand Name)	Dose (mg)—Pain Management	Inhibition of Serotonin	Inhibition of Norepinephrine	Anticholinergic	Sedative
Tertiary amines					
Amitriptyline (Elavil)	10–75	Strong	Mild	Strong	Strong
Imipramine (Tofranil)	25–75	Strong	Mild	Mild	Mild
Doxepin (Sinequan)	25–75	Mild	Slight	Mild	Moderate
Secondary amines					
Nortriptyline (Pamelor)	25–75	Moderate	Moderate	Mild	Mild
Protriptyline (Vivactil)	15–25	Mild	Strong	Moderate	Slight
Desipramine (Norpramin)	50–75	Mild	Strong	Slight	Slight
Triazolopyridine					
Trazodone (Desyrel)	50–150	Moderate	None	Slight	Mild
Bicyclic (SSRI)					
Fluoxetine (Prozac)	10–40	Strong	Slight	Slight	Slight

SSRI, selective serotonin reuptake inhibitor.
Adapted from *Merck Manual*, 15th edition. Rahway, NJ; Merck and Co., Inc., 1988; and Gilman AG, Goodman LS, Gilman A, eds. *The Pharmacologic Basis of Therapeutics*, 6th ed. Macmillan, New York: 1980.

CHRONIC PAIN SYNDROME

Chronic pain syndrome has been described by some authors as epidemic in our culture and results from a complex interplay of physical and psychosocial factors (184). In postacute SCI, chronic pain has been characterized as more disabling than the SCI (188). Further, those with SCI who have chronic pain are psychologically more similar to able-bodied patients with chronic pain than to those with SCI without pain (188). Chronic pain can develop above, at, and below the level of injury and can be associated with MP, NP, or both.

When the pain is associated with sleep disturbance, fatigue, anxiety, social withdrawal, and anger, the syndrome is best managed with a multidimensional approach (182,184,189,190). The hallmarks of this approach are an emphasis on increasing physical activity, improving sleep, treating depression, and treating the pain (191). Most of the cognitive-behavioral interventions for chronic pain today have as their foundation Fordyce's behavioral theories of pain (150,192). Interventions such as biofeedback, visualization, behavior modification, and hypnosis can be effective (190). Narcotic pain medications are not usually initially chosen for long-term pain management. However, if efforts to treat the pain with nonnarcotic medications or therapy interventions are unsuccessful, there is a growing literature supporting the use of narcotics for chronic nonmalignant pain (193,194).

SPECIAL TOPICS
Invasive Procedures
Intrathecal Baclofen and Morphine

Most of the time, pain in patients with SCI can be managed adequately by the previously discussed methods. In situations in which the pain remains and is severe or is interfering with function, a therapeutic trial with intrathecal medications can be offered. Intrathecal baclofen, clonidine, and morphine have all been reported to have efficacy either as a single agent (171, 195–197) or in combination (198). Drug tolerance is less with intrathecal medications, but withdrawal is still possible.

Dorsal Root Entry Zone

The dorsal root entry zone is the site of initial integration of sensory information within the spinal cord. It is often damaged in SCI at the level of the injury, and it appears that these damaged neurons, through constant abnormal neuroelectrical activity, may contribute to zone of injury pain. By lesioning this area, these damaged neurons are destroyed, and the NP is reduced (199). This procedure is done by exposing the spinal cord at the level of injury, and two to three levels above and below, and then using a thermocouple to destroy the Rexed layers I through V bilaterally. About half of paraplegic patients experience good relief of pain for at least 5 years (200). This procedure is most effective for localized NP at or just below the level of injury but ineffective in diffuse NP below the level of injury. It also is not performed on dermatomes innervating the limbs because the resulting loss of proprioception may significantly impair function.

Spinal Cord Stimulators

Spinal cord stimulation, which was developed in the 1970s, has been used successfully to treat vasculopathic pain, postherpetic neuralgia, pain in multiple sclerosis, and phantom limb pain and has helped decrease spasticity and improve bladder function (201,202). Given the successful application of this intervention in other deafferentation syndromes, several investigators have tested the technique in patients with SCI (201,203–209). None of the investigators found spinal cord stimulation to be effective in the treatment of SCI-associated pain, except for Buchhaas and colleagues, who found good relief of pain in six of seven patients with cauda equina syndrome (210).

Deep Brain Stimulation

Implantation of electrodes into the periaqueductal gray area or the sensory thalamic area for the purpose of relieving pain was first done in 1954 (211). Since then, this technique has been shown to provide lasting pain relief in 47% of patients with intractable deafferentation pain and in 60% of patients with nociceptive pain. The benefits appear to be mediated by the release of endogenous opioids. Despite the successful application of this technique in several pain syndromes, there is no documented long-term benefit in the population with SCI (212).

Cordotomy

Generally, cordotomy is not indicated for the patient with SCI because of the occurrence of deafferentation pain months to years after the procedure. However, in the SCI patient with end-stage cancer, there may be a role for anterolateral cordotomy. Patients experiencing severe intractable pain unilaterally in the lower portion of the body may also be candidates. The procedure can be performed as an open procedure or percutaneously with radiofrequency ablation of the spinothalamic tract using computed tomography localization. Usually, the procedure is performed at the T2 level on the side contralateral to the pain, thus producing a mid-thoracic sensory level to pinprick and temperature ipsilateral to the pain. The technique is less effective for bilateral lower limb pain. In the setting of chest or thoracic pain, the technique can be technically challenging, with serious potential complications due to respiratory depression and progression of weakness above the level of injury (150).

Other Conditions
Complex Regional Pain Syndrome

Complex regional pain syndrome (CRPS) types I and II, formerly known as RSD and causalgia, respectively, have been discussed previously. Treatment is controversial; there are numerous reports in the literature of successful treatment methods, but few of the methods have been studied rigorously (213). Tricyclic antidepressants, steroids, NSAIDs, narcotics, and anticonvulsants have all been tried with varying degrees of success (213). Propranolol, prazosin, phenoxybenzamine, and guanethidine have all been reported to benefit CRPS type II, possibly by modulating the vasomotor components of the disease (213). TENS and sympathetic blockade in conjunction with physical therapy for range-of-motion exercises have also been reported as beneficial (213). If all other therapeutic interventions fail, sympathectomy may be considered, but the literature supports only variable results (213). Side effects can include post-sympathectomy dysesthesias and neuralgia. A recent report noted success with the use of spinal cord stimulation in intractable CRPS (214).

Syringomyelia

Late onset of pain in SCI can be associated with a syrinx. It has been reported to be present in about 65% of patients with paraplegia who develop late-onset NP (154). Pain is often relieved by draining the syrinx using a shunt (154). If the pain persists, the dorsal root entry zone procedure has been shown to result in pain relief in 77% of patients in whom shunting fails (200).

CONCLUSIONS

In this chapter, a summary of previous pain classification systems has been presented as well as a new mixed classification schema based on these previous systems. The basis of the classification has been supported, with a discussion of the pathophysiology of pain in SCI. Using this classification as a foundation, a detailed discussion of pain syndromes and treatment options has been presented. It is important to keep in mind the complexity and evolving nature of pain in the population with SCI in order to identify correctly the underlying cause and choose an appropriate pain intervention. As our understanding of pain mechanisms evolves at a molecular level, newer and more precise applications of pain interventions will be developed.

REFERENCES

1. Holmes G. *Pain of central origin: contributions to medical and biological research.* New York: Hober, 1919:235-245.
2. Davis L, Martin J. Studies upon spinal cord injuries. *J Neurosurg* 1947;4:483-491.
3. Botterell EH, Callaghan JC, Jousse AT. Pain in paraplegia: clinical management and surgical treatment. *Proc R Soc Med* 1954;47:281-288.
4. Kaplan LI, Grynbaum VB, Lloyd KE, et al. Pain and spasticity in patients with spinal cord dysfunction: results of a follow-up study. *JAMA* 1962;182:918-925.
5. Burke DC. Pain in paraplegia. *Paraplegia* 1973;10:297-313.
6. Burke DC, Woodward JM. Pain and phantom sensation in spinal paralysis. In: Vinken PJ, Bruyn GW, eds. *Handbook of clinical neurology.* New York: Elsevier, 1976:115-113.
7. Melzack R, Loeser JD. Phantom body pain in paraplegics: evidence for a central "pain generating mechanism" for pain. *Pain* 1978;4:195-210.
8. Bedbrook GM. Pain and phantom sensation. In: Bedbrook GM, ed. *The care and management of spinal cord injuries.* New York: Springer-Verlag, 1981:180-211.
9. Donovan WH, Dimitrijevic MR, Dahm L, et al. Neurophysiologic approaches to chronic pain following spinal cord injury. *Paraplegia* 1982;20:135-146.
10. Tunks E. Pain in spinal cord injured patients. In: Bloch RF, Basbaum M, eds. *Management of spinal cord injuries.* Baltimore: Williams & Wilkins, 1986:180-211.
11. Davidoff G, Roth E, Guarracini M, et al. Function-limiting dysesthetic pain syndrome among traumatic spinal cord injury patients: a cross-sectional study. *Pain* 1987;29:39-48.
12. Beric A, Dimitrijevic MR, Lindblom U. Central dysesthesia syndrome in spinal cord injury patients. *Pain* 1988;34:109-116.
13. Britell CW, Mariano AJ. Chronic pain in spinal cord injury. *Physical and Medical Rehabilitation: State of the Art Reviews* 1991;5:71-82.
14. Nashold BS. Paraplegia and pain. In: Nashold BS, Ovelmen-Levitt J, eds. *Deafferentiation pain syndromes: pathophysiology and treatment.* New York: Raven Press, 1991:301-319.
15. Bonica JJ. Introduction: semantic, epidemiologic, and educational issues. In: Casey KL, ed. *Pain and central nervous system disease: the central pain syndromes.* New York: Raven Press, 1991:13-29.
16. Yezierski RP. Pain following spinal cord injury: the clinical problem and experimental studies. *Pain* 1996;68:185-194.
17. Levi R, Hultling C, Nash MS, et al. The Stockholm spinal cord injury study. 1. Medical problems in a regional SCI population. *Paraplegia* 1995;33:308-315.
18. Loubser PG, Donovan WH. Chronic pain associated with spinal cord injury. In: Narayan RK, Wilberger JE, Povlishock JT, eds. *Neurotrauma.* New York: McGraw-Hill, 1996:1311-1322.
19. Summers JD, Rapoff MA, Varghese G, et al. Psychosocial factors in chronic spinal cord injury pain. *Pain* 1991;47:183-189.
20. Siddall PJ, Taylor DA, Cousins MJ. Classification of pain following spinal cord injury. *Spinal Cord* 1997;35:69-75.
21. Merkskey H, Bogduk N, eds. *Classification of chronic pain: descriptions of chronic pain syndromes and definitions of pain terms,* 2nd ed. Task Force on Taxonomy of the International Association for the Study of Pain. Seattle: IASP Press, 1994.
22. Nepomuceno C, Fine PR, Richards JS, et al. Pain in patients with spinal cord injury. *Arch Phys Med Rehabil* 1979;60:605-609.
23. Cairns DM, Adkins RH, Scott MD. Pain and depression in acute traumatic spinal cord injury: origins of chronic problematic pain? *Arch Phys Med Rehabil* 1996;77:329-335.
24. Rose M, Robinson JE, Ells P, et al. Pain following spinal cord surgery: results from a postal survey [Letter]. *Pain* 1988;34:101-102.
25. Lundqvist C, Siosteen A, Blomstrand C, et al. Spinal cord injuries: clinical, functional, and emotional status. *Spine* 1991;16:78-83.
26. Mariano AJ. Chronic pain and spinal cord injury. *Clin J Pain* 1992;8:87-92.
27. Ragnarsson KT. Management of pain in persons with spinal cord injury. *J Spinal Cord Med* 1997;20:186-199.
28. Richards JS, Stover SL, Jaworski T. Effect of bullet removal on subsequent pain in persons with spinal cord injury secondary to gunshot wound. *J Neurosurg* 1990;73:401-404.
29. Rintala DH, Loubser PG, Castro J, et al. Chronic pain in a community-based sample of men with spinal cord injury: prevalence, severity, and relationship with impairment, disability, handicap, and subjective well-being. *Arch Phys Med Rehabil* 1998;79:604-614.
30. Rintala DH, Hart KA, Fuhrer MJ. Self-reported pain in persons with chronic spinal cord injury. *J Am Paraplegia Soc* 1991;14:83(abst).
31. Fenellosa P, Pallares J, Cervera J, et al. Chronic pain in the spinal cord injured: statistical approach and pharmacological treatment. *Paraplegia* 1993;31:722-729.
32. Richards JS, Meredith RL, Nepomuceno C, et al. Psycho-social aspects of chronic pain in spinal cord injury. *Pain* 1980;8:355-366.
33. Sved P, Siddall PJ, McClelland J, et al. Relationship between surgery and pain following spinal cord injury. *Spinal Cord* 1997;35:526-530.
34. Kakulas BA, Gaekwad U, Smith E, et al. The neuropathology of pain and abnormal sensations in human spinal cord injury derived from the clinicopathological data base at the Royal Perth Hospital. In: Dimitrijevic MR, Wall PD, Lindblom U, eds. *Recent achievements in restorative neurology. 3. altered sensation and pain.* Karger: Basal, 1990:37-41.
35. Davidoff G, Guarracini M, Roth E, et al. Trazodone hydrochloride in the treatment of dysesthetic pain in traumatic myelopathy: a ran-

domized, double-blind placebo-controlled study. *Pain* 1987:29: 151–161.

36. Demirel G, Yllmaz H, Gencosmanoglu B, et al. Pain following spinal cord injury. *Spinal Cord* 1998;36:25–28.

37. Wagner Anke AG, Stenehjem AE, Kvalvik SJ. Pain and life quality within 2 years of spinal cord injury. *Paraplegia* 1995;33:555–569.

38. Subbarao JU, Klopfstein J, Turpin R. Prevalence and impact of wrist and shoulder pains in patients with spinal cord injury. *J Spinal Cord Med* 1995;18:9–13.

39. Nichols PJR, Norman PA, Ennis JR. Wheelchair user's shoulder? shoulder pain in patients with spinal cord injuries. *Scand J Rehabil Med* 1979;11:29–32.

40. Wing PC, Tredwell SJ. The weight bearing shoulder. *Paraplegia* 1983; 21:107–113.

41. Alijure J, Eltorai I, Bradley WE, et al. Carpal tunnel syndrome in paraplegics. *Paraplegia* 1985;23:182.

42. Bayley JC, Cochrant TP, Sledge CB. The impingement syndrome in paraplegics. *J Bone Joint Surg [Am]* 1987;69:676–678.

43. Gellman H, Chandler DR, Petrasek J, et al. Carpal tunnel syndrome in paraplegic patients. *J Bone Joint Surg [Am]* 1988;70:517–519.

44. Wylie EJ, Chakera TM. Degenerative joint abnormalities in patients with paraplegia of duration greater than 20 years. *Paraplegia* 1988; 26:101–106.

45. Barber DB, Gail NG. Osteonecrosis: an overuse injury of the shoulder in paraplegia: a case report. *Paraplegia* 1991;29:423–426.

46. Silfverskiold J, Waters RL. Shoulder pain and functional disability in spinal cord injury patients. *Clin Orthop* 1991;272:141–145.

47. Sie IH, Waters RL, Adkins RH, et al. Upper extremity pain in the postrehabilitation spinal cord injured patient. *Arch Phys Med Rehabil* 1992;73:44–48.

48. Pentland WE, Twomey LT. Upper limb function in persons with long term paraplegia and implications for independence: part II. *Paraplegia* 1994;32:219–224.

49. Lal S. Premature degenerative shoulder changes in spinal cord injury patients. *Spinal Cord* 1998;36:186–189.

50. Dalyan M, Cardenas DD, Gerard B. Upper extremity pain after spinal cord injury. *Spinal Cord* 1999;37(3):191–195.

51. Curtis KA, Drysdale GA, Lanza RD, et al. Shoulder pain in wheelchair users with tetraplegia and paraplegia. *Arch Phys Med Rehabil* 1999; 80:453–457.

52. Gellman H, Eckert RR, Botte MJ, et al. Reflex sympathetic dystrophy in cervical spinal cord injury patients. *Clin Orthopaed Rel Res* 1998; 233:126–131.

53. Aisen PS, Aisen ML. Shoulder-hand syndrome in cervical spinal cord injury. *Paraplegia* 1994;32:588–592.

54. Gallien P, Nicolas B, Robineau S, et al. The reflex sympathetic dystrophy syndrome in patients who have a spinal cord injury. *Paraplegia* 1995;33(12):715–720.

55. Wainapel SF. Reflex sympathetic dystrophy following traumatic myelopathy. *Pain* 1984;18:345–349.

56. Cremer SA, Maynard F, Davidoff G. The reflex sympathetic dystrophy syndrome associated with traumatic myelopathy: report of 5 cases. *Pain* 1989;37:187–192.

57. Philip PA, Philip M, Monga TN. Reflex sympathetic dystrophy in central cord syndrome: case report and review of the literature. *Paraplegia* 1990;28:48–54.

58. Levy CE, Lorch F. Recovery of upper limb motor function in tetraplegia with stellate ganglion block treatment of reflex sympathetic dystrophy: a case report. *Am J Phys Med Rehabil* 1996;75:479–482.

59. Andrews LG, Armitage KJ. Sudek's atrophy in traumatic quadriplegia. *Paraplegia* 1971;9:159.

60. Janig W, Stanton-Hicks M, eds. *Reflex sympathetic dystrophy: a reappraisal. Progress in pain research and management*. Seattle: IASP press, 1996:93–105.

61. Dotson RM. Causalgia-reflex sympathetic dystrophy-sympathetically maintained pain: myth and reality. *Muscle Nerve* 1993;16: 1049–1055.

62. Steinbrocker O, Spitzer N, Friedman HH. The shoulder-hand syndrome in reflex dystrophy of the upper extremity. *Ann Intern Med* 1947;92:22–49.

63. Kozin F, McCarty DJ, Sims J, et al. The reflex sympathetic dystrophy syndrome. I. Clinical and histologic studies: evidence for bilaterality, response to corticosteroids and articular involvement. *Am J Med* 1976; 60:321–331.

64. McKinnon SE, Holder LE. The use of three-phase radionuclide bone scanning in the diagnosis of reflex sympathetic dystrophy. *J Hand Surg* 1984;9:556.

65. Lefkoe TP, Cardenas DD. Reflex sympathetic dystrophy of the lower extremity in tetraplegia: case report. *Spinal Cord* 1996;4:239–242.

66. Elliot T, Harkins SW. Psychosocial concomitants of persistent pain among persons with spinal cord injuries. *J Neurorehabil* 1991;1:7–16.

67. Lipton JA, Marbach JJ. Ethnicity and the pain experience. *Soc Sci Med* 1984;19:1279–1298.

68. Zatzick DF, Dimsdale JE. Cultural variations in the response to painful stimuli. *Psychosom Med* 1990;52:544–557.

69. Dew MA, Lynch KA, Ernst J, et al. A causal analysis of factors affecting adjustment to spinal cord injury. *Rehabil Psychol* 1985;30:39–46.

70. Stormer S, Gerner HJ, Gruninger W, et al. Chronic pain/dysesthesia in spinal cord injury patients: results of a multicentre study. *Spinal Cord* 1997;35(7):446–455.

71. Wegener ST, Elliot TR. Pain assessment in spinal cord injury. *Clin J Pain* 1992;8(2):93–101.

72. Umlauf RL. Psychological interventions for chronic pain following spinal cord injury. *Clin J Pain* 1992;8(2):111–118.

73. Richards JS. Chronic pain and spinal cord injury: review and comment. *Clin J Pain* 1992;8(2):119–122.

74. Kennedy P, Frankel H, Gardner B, et al. Factors associated with acute and chronic pain following traumatic spinal cord injuries. *Spinal Cord* 1997;35:814–817.

75. Bedbrook GM. Pain in paraplegia and tetraplegia. In: Bedbrook GM, ed. *Lifetime care of the paraplegic patient*. Edinburgh: Churchill-Livingstone, 1985:245–256.

76. Siddall PJ, Taylor DA, Cousins MJ. Pain associated with spinal cord injury. *Curr Opin Neurol* 1995;8:447–450.

77. Taub NS, Worsowicz GM, Gnatz SM, et al. Pain rehabilitation. 1. Definitions and diagnosis of pain. *Arch Phys Med Rehabil* 1998;79: S49–S53.

78. Bonica JJ. *Management of pain*, 2nd ed. Philadelphia: Lea & Febiger, 1990.

79. Walsh NE, Dumitru D, Schoenfeld LS, et al. Treatment of the patient with chronic pain. In: Delisa JA, Gans BM, eds. *Rehabilitation medicine: principles and practice*. Philadelphia: Lippincott Williams & Wilkins, 1988.

80. Rosner H. The pharmacologic management of acute postoperative pain. In: Lefkowitz M, Lebovits AH, eds. *A practical approach to pain management*. Boston: Little, Brown, 1996:5–14.

81. Schmidt KM, Aaron WS, eds. *St. Anthony's ICD.9.CM. code book*, Vols, 1–3. Reston, VA: St. Anthony's, 1996.

82. Scheer SJ, Watanabe TK, Radack KL. Randomized controlled trials in industrial low back pain. 3. Subacute/chronic pain interventions. *Arch Phys Med Rehabil* 1997;78:414–423.

83. Chaplin ER. Chronic pain: a sociobiological problem. *Physical Medicine and Rehabilitation: State of the Art Reviews* 1991;5(1):1–47.

84. Goddard MJ, Dean BZ, King JC. Pain rehabilitation. 1. Basic science, acute pain, and neuropathic pain. *Arch Phys Med Rehabil* 1994;75: S4–S8.

85. Riddoch G. The clinical features of central pain. *Lancet* 1938;234: 1150–1156.

86. Maury M. About pain and its treatments in paraplegics. *Paraplegia* 1978;15:349–352.

87. Frisbie J, Aguilera E. Chronic pain after spinal cord injury: an expedient diagnostic approach. *Paraplegia* 1990;28:465–469.

88. Beric A. Central pain: "new" syndromes and their evaluation. *Muscle Nerve* 1993;16:1017–1024.

89. Triggs WJ, Beric A. Sensory abnormalities and dysesthesias in the anterior spinal artery syndrome. *Brain* 1992;115:189–198.

90. Beric A. Post-spinal cord injury pain states. In: Wallace M, Dunn J, Yaksh T, eds. *Pain: nociceptive and neuropathic mechanisms with clinical correlates*. Anesthesiology Clinics of North America; Philadelphia: WB Saunders, 1997.

91. Beric A, Dimitijevic MR, Light JK. A clinical syndrome of rostral and caudal spinal injury: neurological, neurophysiological, and urodynamic evidence for occult sacral lesions. *J Neurol Neurosurg Psychiatr* 1987;50:600–606.

92. Beric A. Altered sensation and pain in spinal cord injury. In: Dimitrijevic MR, Wall PD, Lindblom U, eds. *Recent achievements in restorative neurology. 3. Altered sensation and pain.* Basel: S. Karger, 1990: 27–36.

93. Beric A. Post-spinal cord injury pain states. *Pain* 1997;72:295–298.

94. Bryce TN, Ragnarsson KT. Pain after spinal cord injury. *Phy Med Rehabil Clin North Am Top Spinal Cord Med* 2000;11:157–168.

95. Maynard F, Bracken M, Creasy G, et al. *International standards for neurological classification of spinal cord injury.* Chicago: American Spinal Injury Association, 1996.

96. Woosley RM. Pain in spinal cord disorder. In: Young RR, Woosley RM, eds. *Diagnosis and management of disorders of the spinal cord.* Philadelphia: WB Saunders 1995:354–362.

97. Nashold BS, Bullitt E. Dorsal root entry zone lesions to control central pain in paraplegics. *J Neurosurg* 1981;55:414–419.

98. Nashold BS, Ostdahl RH. Dorsal root entry zone lesions for pain relief. *J Neurosurg* 1979;51:59–69.

99. Maroon JC. Burning hands in football spinal cord injuries. *JAMA* 1977;238:2049–2051.

100. Edgar RE, Best CG, Qual PA, et al. Computer assisted DREZ microcoagulation: post-traumatic spinal deafferentiation pain. *J Spinal Disord* 1993;6:48–56.

101. Eide PK. Pathophysiological mechanisms of central neuropathic pain after spinal cord injury. *Spinal Cord* 1998;36,601–612.

102. Charney K, Juler G, Comarr A. General surgery problems in patients with spinal cord injuries. *Arch Surg* 1975;110:1083–1085.

103. Clark WC. Pain and suffering. In: Downey JA, Myer SJ, Gonzalez EG, et al., eds. *The physiological basis of rehabilitation medicine*, 2nd ed. Boston: Butterworth-Heinemann, 1994;705–737.

104. Botterel EH, Callaghan HC, Jousse AT. Pain in paraplegia: clinical management and surgical treatment. *Proc R Soc Med* 1953;47: 281–288.

105. Wiesenfeld-Hallin Z, Hao JX, Alskogius H, et al. Allodynia-like symptoms in rats after spinal cord ischemia: an animal model of central pain. In: Boivie J, Hansson P, Linblom U, eds. *Touch, temperature, and pain in health and disease. 3. Mechanisms and assessments. Progress in pain research and management.* Seattle: IASP Press, 1994:355–372.

106. Price DD. *Psychological and neural mechanisms of pain.* New York: Raven Press, 1988.

107. Fields HL. *Pain.* New York: McGraw-Hill, 1987.

108. Fields HL. *Pain syndromes in neurology.* London: Butterworths, 1990.

109. Melzack R, Wall PD. Pain mechanisms: a new theory. *Science* 1965; 150:971–979.

110. Melzack R. The gate control theory 25 years later: new perspectives in phantom limb pain. In: Bond MR, Charlton JE, Woolf CJ, eds. *Proceedings of the VIth World Congress on Pain*, Vol. 1. Amsterdam: Elsevier, 1991:9–21.

111. Fields HL. Is there a facilitating component to central pain modulation? *Am Pain Soc J* 1992;1:71–74.

112. Clark WC, Hunt HF. Pain. In: Darling RC, Downey JA, eds. *Physiological basis of rehabilitation medicine.* Philadelphia: WB Saunders, 1971:373–401.

113. Berkley KJ. Suspension of neural pathways for pain and nociception. *J Cardiovasc Electrophysiol* 1991;2[Suppl]:S13–S17.

114. Rexed B. A cytoarchitechtonic atlas of the spinal cord of the cat. *J Comp Neurol* 1954:110:297–390.

115. Talbot JD, Marrett S, Evans AC, et al. Multiple representations of pain in the human cerebral cortex. *Science* 1991;251:1355–1358.

116. Corkin S, Twitchell TE, Sullivan EV. Safety and efficacy of cingulotomy for pain and psychiatric disorder. In: Hitchcock E, ed. *Alteration in brain function.* Amsterdam: Elsevier, 1979.

117. Meyer RA, Campbell JN, Raja SN. Peripheral neural mechanisms of nociception. In: Wall PD, Melzack R, eds. *Textbook of pain.* Edingburgh: Churchill Livingstone, 1994;13–44.

118. White JC, Sweet WH. *Pain: its mechanisms and neurosurgical control.* Springfield: Thomas, 1955.

119. Cassinari V, Pagni CA. *Central pain.* Cambridge, MA: Harvard University Press, 1969.

120. Leijon G. Clinical findings in patients with central post-stroke pain. In: Boivie J, Casey KL, eds. *Pain and central nervous system disease: the central pain syndromes.* New York: Raven Press, 1991:65–75.

121. Lentz FA, Tasker RR, Dostrovsky JO. Abnormal single unit activity recorded in the somatosensory thalamus of a quadriplegic patient with central pain. *Pain* 1987;31:225–236.

122. Yezierski RP, Park SH. The mechanosensitivity of spinal sensory neurons following intraspinal injections of quisqualic acid in the rat. *Neurosci Lett* 1993;157:115–119.

123. Hao JX, Xu XJ, Yu YX, et al. Transient spinal cord ischemia induces temporary hypersensitivity of dorsal horn wide dynamic range neurons to myelinated, but not unmyelinated fiber input. *Exp Neurol* 1992b;68:384–391.

124. Hao JX, Xu XJ, Yu YX, et al. Baclofen reverses the hypersensitivity of dorsal horn wide dynamic range neurons to mechanical stimulation after transient spinal cord ischemia: implications for a tonic GABAergic inhibitory control of myelinated fiber input. *Neurophysiology* 1992c;68:392–396.

125. Yaksh TL. Behavioral and autonomic correlates of the tactile evoked allodynia produced by spinal glycine inhibition: effects of modulatory receptor systems and excitatory amino acid antagonists. *Pain* 1989; 37:111–123.

126. Hao JX, Xu XJ, Wiesenfeld-Hallin Z. Intrathecal gamma-aminobutyric acid (GABA-b) receptor antagonist CGP 35348 induces hypersensitivity to mechanical stimuli in the rat. *Neurosci Lett* 1994;182: 299–302.

127. Zhang AI, Hao JX, Seiger A, et al. Decreased GABA immunoreactivity in spinal cord dorsal horn neurons after transient spinal cord ischemia in the rat. *Brain Res* 1994;656:187–190.

128. Balazy TE. Clinical management of chronic pain in spinal cord injury. *Clin J Pain* 1992;8(2):102–110.

129. Stitik TP, Klecz R, Zafonte RO, et al. Pharmacotherapy of disability. In: DeLisa JA, Gans BM, ed. *Rehabilitation medicine: principles and practice*, 3rd ed. Philadelphia: Lippincott Williams & Wilkins, 1998: 789–828.

130. *Principles of analgesic use in the treatment of acute pain and cancer pain.* Chicago: American Pain Society, 1993.

131. Houmes RJM, Voets MA, Verkaaik A, et al. Efficacy and safety of tramadol versus morphine for moderate and severe postoperative pain with special regard to respiratory depression. *Anesth Analg* 1992;74: 514–520.

132. Lee CR, McTavish D, Sorkin EM. Tramadol: a preliminary review of its pharmacodynamic and pharmacokinetic properties, and therapeutic potential in acute and chronic pain states. *Drugs* 1993;46(2): 313–340.

133. Lehmann JF, DeLateur BJ. Ultrasound, shortwave, superficial heat and cold in the treatment of pain. In: Wall PD, Melzack R, ed. *Textbook of pain*, 3rd ed. New York: Churchill-Livingstone, 1994: 1237–1250.

134. Lehmann JF, DeLateur RJ. *Therapeutic heat and cold.* Baltimore: Williams & Wilkins, 1990.

135. Haldeman S. Manipulation and massage for the relief of pain. In: Wall PD, Melzack R, ed. *Textbook of pain.* Edinburgh: Churchill-Livingstone, 1989:942–951.

136. Kanemetz HL. History of massage. In: Basmajian JV, ed. *Manipulation, traction and massage*, 3rd ed. Baltimore: William & Wilkins, 1985:985.

137. Atchison JW, Stroll ST, Gilliar WG. Manipulation, traction and massage. In: Braddom RL, ed. *Physical medicine and rehabilitation.* Philadelphia: WB Saunders, 1996:421–429.

138. Cioni B, Meglio M, Pentimalli L, et al. Spinal cord stimulation in the treatment of paraplegic pain. *J Pain Symptom Manage* 1995;82(1): 35–39.

139. *Physicians' desk reference.* Montvale: Medical Economics Company, 2000.

140. Chesnut C, Baylink D, Doyle H, et al. Salmon-calcitonin nasal spray prevents vertebral fractures in established osteoporosis. Further interim trials of the "PROOF" study. *ECO abstract, OP Int* 1998:813.

141. Buttar NS, Wang KK. The "aspirin" of the new millenium: cyclooxygenase-2 inhibitors. *Mayo Clin Proc* 2000;75:1027–1038.

142. Richardson RR, Meyer PR Jr, Cerullo LJ. Transcutaneous electrical neurostimulation in musculoskeletal pain of acute spinal cord injuries. *Spine* 1980;5(1):42–45.

143. Deyo RA, Walsh NE, Martin DC, et al. A controlled trial of transcutaneous electrical nerve stimulation (TENS) and exercise for chronic low back pain. *N Engl J Med* 1990;322:1627–1634.

144. Woolf CF, Thompson JW. Stimulation fibre-induced analgesia: transcutaneous electrical nerve stimulation (TENS) and vibration. In: Wall PD, Melzack R, eds. *Textbook of pain*, 3rd ed. New York: Churchill Livingstone, 1994:1191–1208.

145. Finsen V, Person L, Lovlien M, et al. Transcutaneous electrical nerve stimulation after major amputation. *J Bone Joint Surg Br.* 1988;70:109–112.

146. Cheing GLY, Hui-Chan CWY. Transcutaneous electrical nerve stimulation: nonparallel antinociceptive effects on chronic clinical pain and acute experimental pain. *Arch Phys Med Rehabil* 1999;80:305–312.

147. Kotaniemi A, Piiramen H, Paimela L, et al. Is continuous intranasal salmon calcitonin effective in treating axial bone loss in patients with active rheumatoid arthritis after receiving low dose glucocorticosteroid therapy? *J Rheumatol* 1996;23:1875–1879.

148. Jaeger H, Maier C. Calcitonin in phantom limb pain: a double-blind study. *Pain* 1992;48:21–27.

149. Strawkowski JA, Wiand JW, Johnson EW. Upper limb musculoskeletal pain syndromes. In: Braddon RL, ed. *Physical Medicine and Rehabilitation*. Philadelphia: WB Saunders, 1996:756–783.

150. Curtis KA, Tyner TM, Zachary L, et al. Effect of a standard exercise protocol on shoulder pain in long-term wheelchair users. *Spinal Cord* 1999;37:421–429.

151. Cooney WPI. Sports injuries to the upper extremity. *Postgrad Med* 1984;76(4):45–50.

152. Tucker GT, Mather LE. Properties, absorption, disposition of local anesthetic agents. In: Cousins MF, Bridenbaugh PO, ed. *Neural blockade in clinical anesthesia and management of pain*, 2nd ed. Philadelphia: Lippincott Williams & Wilkins, 1988:47–110.

153. Tollison CD, ed. *Handbook of pain management*. Baltimore: Williams & Wilkins, 1994:51–67.

154. Janssen TW, van Oers CA, van der Woude LH, et al. Physical strain in daily life of wheelchair users with spinal cord injuries. *Med Sci Sports Exerc* 1994;26:661–670.

155. Koo TK, Mak AF, Lee YL. Posture effect on seating interface biomechanics: comparison between two seating cushions. *Arch Phys Med Rehabil* 1996;77:40–47.

156. Watson DH, Trott PH. Cervical headache: an investigation of neutral head posture and upper cervical flexor muscle performance. *Cephalgia* 1993;13(4):272–284.

157. Britell CW. Wheelchair prescription. In: Kottke FJ, Lehmann JF, eds. *Krusen's handbook of physical medicine and rehabilitation*, 4th ed. Philadelphia: WB Saunders, 1990:548–563.

158. Travell JG, Simons DG. *Myofascial pain and dysfunction: the trigger point manual*. Baltimore: Williams & Wilkins, 1983.

159. Spencer JW, Jacobs JJ. *Complementary alternative medicine: an evidence based approach*. St Louis; Mosby, 1999.

160. Dozono K, Hachisuka K, Hatada K, et al. Peripheral neuropathies in the upper extremities of paraplegic wheelchair marathon racers. *Paraplegia* 1995;33:208–211.

161. Nakano KK. Entrapment neuropathies. *Muscle Nerve* 1978;1:264–279.

162. Hartz CR, Linscheid RL, Gramse RR, et al. Pronator teres syndrome: compressive neuropathy of the median nerve. *J Bone Joint Surg [Am]* 1981;63:885–890.

163. Gianini F, Passero S, Cioni R, et al. Electrophysiologic evaluation of local steroid injection in carpal tunnel syndrome. *Arch Phys Med Rehabil* 1991;72:738–742.

164. Gelberman RH, Aronson D, Weisman MH. Carpal tunnel syndrome: results of a prospective trial of steroid injection in carpal tunnel syndrome. *J Bone Joint Surg* 1980;62:1181–1184.

165. O'Brien JP. Mechanisms of spinal pain. In: Wall PD, Melzack R, ed. *Textbook of pain*, 3rd ed. New York: Churchill Livingstone, 1994:240–251.

166. McQuay H, Carroll D, Jadad AR, et al. Anticonvulsant drugs for management of pain: a systematic review. *Br Med J* 1995;311:1047–1052.

167. Swerdlow M. Anticonvulsant drugs in chronic pain. *Clin Neuropharmacol* 1984;7:51–82.

168. Sanford PR, Lindblom LB, Haddox JD. Amitriptyline and carbamazepine in the treatment of dysesthetic pain in spinal cord injury. *Arch Phys Med Rehabil* 1992;73(3):300–301.

169. Backonja M, Beydoun A, Edwards KR, et al. Gabapentin for the symptomatic treatment of painful neuropathy in patients with diabetes mellitus: a randomized controlled trial. *JAMA* 1998;280(21):1831–1836.

170. Rowbotham, M, Harden N, Stacey B, et al. Gabapentin for the treatment of postherpetic neuralgia. *JAMA* 1998;280(21):1837–1842.

171. Nakamura M, Ferreira SH. Peripheral analgesic action of clonidine: mediation by release of endogenous enkephalin-like substances. *Eur J Pharmacol* 1988;146:223–228.

172. Cambpell RWF. Drug therapy: mexiletine. *Med Intel* 1987;316(1):29–34.

173. Davis RW. Successful treatment for phantom pain. *Orthopedics* 1993;16(6):691–695.

174. Dejgard A, Petersen P, Kastrup J. Mexiletine for treatment of chronic painful diabetic neuropathy. *Lancet* 1988;1(8575-8576):9–11.

175. Awerbuch GI, Sandyk R. Mexiletine for thalmic pain syndrome. *Int J Neurosci* 1990;5(2–4):129–133.

176. Chiou-Tan FY, Tuel SM, Johnson JC, et al. Effect of mexiletine on spinal cord injury dysesthetic pain. *Am J Phys Med Rehabil* 1996;75(2):84–87.

177. Mitchell BM, Lynch SA, Muir J, et al. Effects of desipramine, amitriptyline, and fluoxetine on pain in diabetic neuropathy. *N Engl J Med* 1992;326(19):1250–1256.

178. Magni G. The use of antidepressants in the treatment of chronic pain: a review of the current evidence. *Drugs* 1991;42(5):730–748.

179. Loubser PG, Akman NM. Effects of intrathecal baclofen on chronic spinal cord injury pain. *J Pain Symptom Manage* 1996;12(4):241–247.

180. McQuay HJ, Tramer M, Nye BA, et al. A systematic review of antidepressants in neuropathic pain. *Pain* 1997;68:217–228.

181. Anghene P, van Houdenkove B. Antidepressant-induced analgesia in chronic non-malignant pain: a meta-analysis of 39 placebo controlled studies. *Headache* 1994;34:44–49.

182. Turner JA, Cardenas DD. Chronic pain problems in individuals with spinal cord injuries. *Semin Clin Neuropsychiatry* 1999;4(3):186–194.

183. Segatore M. Understanding chronic pain after spinal cord injury. *J Neurosci Nurs* 1994;26(4):230–236.

184. Grabois M. Pain clinics: role in the rehabilitation of patients with chronic pain. *Ann Acad Med* 1983;12:428–433.

185. Woolsey RM. Chronic pain following spinal cord injury. *J Am Paraplegia Soc* 1986;9:51–53.

186. NIH Technology Assessment Panel. Integration of behavioral and relaxation approaches into the treatment of chronic pain and insomnia. *JAMA* 1996;276(4):313–318.

187. Bonica JJ, Buckley FP. Regional analgesia with local anesthetics. In: Bonica JJ, ed. *Management of pain*, 2nd ed. Philadelphia: Lea & Febiger, 1990:1883–1979.

188. Cohen MJ, McArthur DL, Vulpe M, et al. Comparing chronic pain from spinal cord injury to chronic pain of other origins. *Pain* 1988;35(1):57–63.

189. Loeser JD, Seres JL, Newman RI. Interdisciplinary, multimodal management of chronic pain. In: Bonica JJ, ed. *Management of pain*, 2nd ed. Philadelphia: Lea & Febiger, 1990:2107–2120.

190. King JC, Kelleher WJ. The chronic pain syndrome: the in-patient interdisciplinary rehabilitative behavioral modification approach. *Physical Medicine and Rehabilitation: State of the Art Reviews* 1991;5:165–186.

191. Bonica JJ. General considerations of chronic pain. In: Bonica JJ, ed. *Management of pain*, 2nd ed. Philadelphia: Lea & Febiger, 1990:180–196.

192. Fordyce WE. *Behavioral methods for chronic pain and illness*. St. Louis: CV Mosby, 1976.

193. Jamison RM, Anderson KO, et al. Survey of opioid use in chronic nonmalignant pain patients. *Arch Phys Med Rehabil* 1994;19:225–230.

194. Portenoy R. Opioid therapy for chronic nonmalignant pain: current status. In: Fields HL, ed. *Progress in pain research and management*. Seattle: IASP Press, 1994:247–282.

195. Loubser PG, Clearman RR. Case reports: evaluation of central spinal cord injury pain with diagnostic spinal anesthesia. *Anesthesiology* 1993;79:376–378.

196. Herman RM, D'Luzansky SC, Ippolito R. Intrathecal baclofen suppresses central pain in patients with spinal lesions: a pilot study. *Clin J Pain* 1992;8(4):338–345.

197. Kroin JS, Ali A, York M, et al. The distribution of medication along the spinal canal after chronic intrathecal administration. *Neurosurgery* 1993;33(2):226–230.

198. Siddall PJ, Gray M, Rutkowski S, et al. Intrathecal morphine and clonidine in the management of spinal cord injury pain: a case report. *Pain* 1994;59(1):147–148.

199. Friedman AH, Bullitt E. Dorsal root entry zone lesions in the treatment of pain following brachial plexus avulsion, spinal cord injury and herpes zoster. *Appl Neurophysiol* 1988;51(2–5):164–169.

200. Friedman AH, Nashold BS. DREZ lesions for relief of pain related to spinal cord injury. *J Neurosurg* 1986;65:465–469.

201. Cole JD, Sedgwick EM. Intractable central pain in spinal cord injury is not relieved by spinal cord stimulation. *Paraplegia* 1991;29:167–172.

202. North RB, Kidd DH, Zahurak M, et al. Spinal cord stimulation for chronic intractable pain: experience over two decades. *Neurosurgery* 1993;32(3):384–394.

203. Cioni B, Meglio M, Pentimalli L, et al. Spinal cord stimulation in the treatment of paraplegic pain. *J Pain Symptom Manage* 1995;82(1):35–39.

204. North RB, Long DM. Spinal cord stimulation for intractable pain: eight year followup. *Pain* 1994;29[Suppl 2]:79.

205. ten Vaarwerk IAM, Staal MJ. Spinal cord stimulation in chronic pain syndromes. *Spinal Cord* 1998;36:671–682.

206. Bajd T, Gregoric M, Vodovnik L, et al. Electrical stimulation in treating spasticity resulting from spinal cord injury. *Arch Phys Med Rehabil* 1985;66:515–517.

207. Richardson RR, Meyer PR, Cerullo LJ. Neurostimulation in the modulation of intractable paraplegic and traumatic neuroma pains. *Pain* 1980;8:75–84.

208. Meglio M, Cioni B, Rossi GF. Spinal cord stimulation in management of chronic pain. *J Neurosurg* 1989;70:519–524.

209. Meglio M, Cioni B, Prezioso A, et al. Spinal cord stimulation (SCS) in deafferentation pain. *PACE* 1989;12(Pt II):709–712.

210. Buchhaas U, Koulousakis A, Nittner K. Experience with spinal cord stimulation (SCS) in the management of chronic pain in a traumatic transverse lesion syndrome. *Neurosurg Rev* 1985;12[Suppl]:582–587.

211. Schvarcz JR. Chronic self-stimulation of the medial posterior inferior thalamus for the alleviation of deafferentation pain. *Acta Neurochir Suppl* 1980;30:295–301.

212. Levy RM, Lamb S, Adams JE. Treatment of chronic pain by deep brain stimulation: long term follow-up and review of the literature. *Neurosurgery* 1987;21(6):885–893.

213. Naveira FA, Snell JA, Rauck RL. Blocks of the sympathetic nervous system. In: Tollison DC, Satterthwaite JR, eds. *Sympathetic pain syndromes: reflex sympathetic dystrophy and causalgia*. Physical Medicine and Rehabilitation: state of the art reviews. Philadelphia: Hanley & Belfus, 1996:245–336.

214. Kemler MA, Barendse GAM, van Kleef M, et al. Spinal cord stimulation in patients with chronic reflex sympathetic dystrophy. *N Engl J Med* 2000;343(9):618–624.

AGING IN SPINAL CORD INJURY

SUSAN W. CHARLIFUE
DANIEL P. LAMMERTSE

Since the 1970s, on-the-scene emergency, acute, and rehabilitation treatments have improved, allowing more people with spinal cord injury (SCI) to survive the early years after trauma (1). In addition, because of advances in the availability of long-term health interventions, as well as the monitoring, and even prevention of secondary conditions in the later postinjury years, more and more people with SCI survive and thrive, often living into their 60s, 70s, and beyond. With the benefits of long, productive lives, however, come the problems faced by all aging individuals. These include not only the physical deterioration that naturally occurs but also issues related to psychological changes with age, alterations in living situations and family structure, and the potential depletion of many social and economic resources. Adding SCI-specific issues to these has the potential to further complicate the aging process.

This chapter describes aging with SCI and offers suggestions for minimizing the effects of aging in people with SCI. First, an update of SCI mortality and life expectancy is discussed, demonstrating the growing numbers of people facing the various consequences of the aging process. This is followed by a brief discussion of aging theory, in order to describe what scientists believe happens as we age. Next, within this general theoretic framework, the impact of SCI and aging on both physical and psychosocial health is discussed, and specific aging research in SCI is reviewed by body system. To conclude, some thoughts on the future of SCI and aging are presented.

MORTALITY AND LIFE EXPECTANCY

Patterns in causes of deaths after SCI have undergone substantial change, as reported by a variety of studies. Whereas renal failure and urinary tract complications were once reported to be the leading causes of death (2–7), this is no longer the case. In recent years, respiratory complications are more frequently contributing to deaths in people with tetraplegia, and heart disease and cancer are contributors to mortality among those with paraplegia (8–17). It is important to note these changing patterns in cause of death because many of the more recent causes are often the culmination of chronic conditions encountered by individuals with SCI who are living longer and have a greater risk for exposure to the consequences of normal human aging.

Not only have causes of death been changing, but survival after injury has also improved substantially. In an extensive overview of the SCI survival and mortality literature, DeVivo and Stover identified numerous studies demonstrating these improvements in life expectancy (18). They note, however, that life expectancy for the person with SCI is still much lower than that of the general population. Specifically, several studies clearly demonstrate that survival is influenced by level and severity of injury as well as by age at injury and decade of injury (19–24). Individuals with higher-level, more neurologically complete lesions and those who are injured at older ages have higher mortality rates, in general. With improvements in emergency and rehabilitative services, as well as ongoing medical management of health issues many years after injury, life expectancy in the more recent decades has also improved (25). Even taking the demographic factors into account, findings on survival tend to be fairly consistent from one study to another, with life expectancies often extending into the sixth and seventh decades of life. The data appear to indicate that individuals with SCI potentially live many years with and may be at greater risk to encounter chronic health conditions typically associated with aging. In addition, many of these conditions, especially when complicated by SCI, may lead to death. With these factors in mind, it is critical that clinicians understand the theoretic and practical issues of human aging in order to address better the consequences of these processes in this unique population.

AGING THEORY

Why and how people age are intriguing and, as yet, unresolved questions. It has been suggested that there are more than 300 theories to explain aging, and no single theory has been generally accepted as sufficient to explain this complex phenomenon (26, 27). The basic concept of aging is loss of adaptability with time (28). According to Shock, it is likely that human aging is "the result of the interplay of many specific characteristics rather than a single process that regulates physiological and psychological functions" (29). The variety of aging theories that have been suggested may, taken individually, seem reasonable explanations of what happens as we grow older. Although each possibility that is put forward may be a necessary component of aging, none is singularly sufficient to explain the process. Significant to an understanding of aging is the underlying finding of biogerontologists that all biologic systems decline constantly as a result of cell death (30). This can occur through any number of mechanisms and has been described in the context of differing theories, including cellular, genetic, endocrine, neurologic, immunologic, and metabolic theories, to name only a few. The overlap among these theories is substantial; however, the general message is that there are limited internal resources or limited defenses against external forces that eventually lead to the decline and ultimate death of an organism (31). Some of the more popular theories of aging are discussed below.

In recent years, there has been wider acceptance of the free radical theory of aging. First described by Harman in the 1950s, this theory hypothesizes that free radicals are produced during normal metabolism and subsequently react with biologic molecules. The accumulated damage due to free radicals relates to decreased function; however, the degree to which these reactions may contribute to cell damage and to pathology and senescence is yet to be determined (32). In acute SCI, it has been demonstrated that oxygen free radicals and lipid peroxides have been implicated in postischemic cell injury and death, whereas free radical scavengers are associated with an amelioration of ischemic injury (33–38). Somewhat related to the free radical theory of aging is the concept of somatic mutation. This is basically a DNA damage theory and postulates that aging results from the accumulation of mutations in somatic cells (that may or may not be caused by accumulation of free radicals) (39). However, this theory is flawed in that cells that divide rapidly tend to eliminate defective mutations relatively quickly. Therefore, these cells do not survive to contribute to the aging process (39).

There are a variety of evolutionary theories that attempt to explain aging. One such theory is that of the "disposable soma" (also called *optimality theory*). This describes a process that results in failure of the cells either to survive, proliferate, or function at complete efficiency (40). In essence, cellular damage happens because maintenance and repair become increasingly less effective at older ages, when the body is disposable (41). Because this theory is based in evolutionary biology, the described age-related inefficiency will have developed over centuries of adaptation. Therefore, applying this theory, there is no reason to believe that individuals with SCI would age differently from anyone else, and even the trauma and resultant altered organ system function would be unlikely to accelerate or otherwise modify the aging process. Similarly, spinal cord trauma and its sequelae would have little effect on any genetically "programmed" aging processes in an individual.

The various biologic theories of aging that address the intrinsic or organism issues rarely consider the extrinsic or environmental stresses on individuals. Such stressors are often accounted for in theories addressing "wear and tear." These theories suggest that aging is caused by some kind of wear or damage to the various body components, either by the use of the parts or by injuries to the genetic mechanisms (39). A person with SCI may age more quickly because of added stresses that push some physical systems beyond their ability to repair themselves, and thus, become symptomatic. This may be seen first in tissues that undergo heavy or unusual use, such as the shoulders or urinary tract. For example, for people using wheelchairs, the upper extremities are subject to more frequent and more demanding use, which may lead to overuse and pain (42).

With regard to the genitourinary system, the function of the lower urinary tract has been noted to decline with age in terms of bladder capacity, the ability to postpone voiding, urethral and bladder compliance, and an increase in voluntary bladder contractions (43). In the individual with SCI, these lower urinary tract changes may be aggravated or even accelerated by such things as years of trauma to the urethra through catheterization, bladder hypertrophy due to chronic sphincter–detrusor dyssynergia, and even chronic infections. These factors, in addition to aging, may alter a previously effective program of urinary management.

In light of these possibilities, the wear-and-tear theory seems to lend itself well to aging in SCI. The examples typify one of the main issues with aging in SCI: that is, while the actual wear and tear on an aging body structure may be relatively minor, the functional consequences of even a small change for the person with SCI can be life-altering. The following sections describe many of the aging-related changes encountered by people with SCI and how these changes affect both physical and psychosocial function and health.

ORGAN SYSTEM EFFECTS OF AGING IN SPINAL CORD INJURY PATIENTS

Just as SCI can have a major effect on organ system functioning in the acute injury phase, evolving postinjury physiology leaves SCI survivors with autonomic and somatic nervous system dysfunction, which results in lasting impairment of many organ systems. It is reasonable to suspect that the cumulative affect of this pathophysiology over many years of survival will result in the development of secondary complications, which will become increasingly prevalent with longer duration of impairment. A number of reports have described the health complications associated with aging and SCI (2,44).

Gastrointestinal System

A number of studies have described the consequences of the aging process on gastrointestinal physiology in the general population (45–47). These studies show that there is a generalized decline in gut motility and diminished acid secretion that accompany the aging process. The esophagus appears to be less affected by these changes than the remainder of the gut. The stomach exhibits diminished emptying of fluid meals but relatively unimpaired emptying of solid food. Acid secretion in the stomach is also diminished with increasing years. Although the small bowel shows little, if any, specific change related to aging, the colon and rectum exhibit diminished motility and an increase in diverticular disease (48). Surveys of SCI individuals have documented a variety of secondary complications and functional changes that accompany the aging process. Although some have speculated on an increased incidence of gastroesophageal reflux disease in persons with SCI, a recent report showed no significant difference in the overall incidence of reflux disease but a higher prevalence of more severe esophagitis in the SCI subjects

(49). Although some have suggested that gastric motility changes may be implicated in chronic abdominal distention in long-term SCI, others have noted that the underlying cause of gastric dilatation remains poorly understood (50). It is now appreciated that gallstone disease is about seven times more prevalent in the SCI population than in the general population, having been found at autopsy in 29% of a group of SCI subjects compared with a 4% incidence in nondisabled matched controls (51). The added risk for gallstone disease appears to be restricted to individuals with lesions above T10, with the increased incidence of stones generally occurring within the first year after injury. For this reason, it does not appear as though the risk for gallstones is related to aging in SCI, but clinicians should be aware of the increased incidence of this condition when evaluating abdominal complaints in the long-term follow-up population. A recent report examining the prevalence and natural history of gallstones in SCI patients concluded that, although there was an increased risk for gallstones, the risk for biliary complications was not of sufficient magnitude in this group to warrant prophylactic cholecystectomy (52).

In the gastrointestinal system, colorectal function is most significantly altered by SCI and would be expected to be a prominent source of problems in the aging SCI survivor population. Indeed, the British study of patients more than 20 years after injury showed that 42% of the subjects had difficulties with constipation, whereas 27% reported problems with fecal incontinence, and 35% had gastrointestinal pain (2,53). Constipation was more likely to be reported by people with paraplegia and those who used digital stimulation, manual evacuation, or Valsalva maneuver for their bowel routines. Those with tetraplegia were more likely to report fecal incontinence. Colonic transit time is prolonged in patients with SCI, especially in the left colon and rectum (54,55). This slowing of distal gut motility correlates with the common report of constipation in this population. The most profound alteration in gastrointestinal physiology resulting from SCI is the loss of volitional control over bowel emptying. This requires the application of a specific, individualized bowel evacuation regimen that uses a variety of reflex-stimulation maneuvers, laxatives, and dietary interventions. It is thought that constipation manifested by difficulties in producing reflex bowel evacuation is commonly the result of anorectal dyssynergia or inadequate rectal expulsive force due to SCI gut motility impairment (55). The primary treatment approach is founded on an assessment of the bowel routine with suggestions for alterations based on commonsense "return to basics." Many patients may have chosen excessively long intervals between bowel programs for their convenience. These individuals should be encouraged to maintain a bowel program frequency of daily or every other day. Laxative and enema use should be avoided or kept to a minimum. Suppository use should be supplemental to digital stimulation and evacuation when necessary. In persons with refractory bowel dysfunction characterized by excessively long duration of bowel program or frequent fecal incontinence, the performance of an elective colostomy may significantly improve quality of life (56,57).

Hemorrhoids are also a common accompaniment to chronic SCI with most survivors reporting the condition and accompanying periodic rectal bleeding (58). Topical therapy may suffice for minor symptomatic lesions, but banding is commonly required on more severe hemorrhoids. Although operative hemorrhoidectomy can generally be avoided, it may be necessary in the most severe refractory cases with abundant hemorrhoid tissue and recurrent major bleeding.

Although there is no evidence to date to suggest that persons with SCI are at added risk for colon cancer, it would be safe to assume that this population is at equal risk to the general population for this common cancer. For that reason, periodic SCI follow-up should include screening for colorectal cancer (50). Because of the frequent presence of hemorrhoids, rectal prolapse, and other distal rectal pathology in the SCI group, fecal occult blood may not be a reliable screening tool. SCI survivors in the at-risk age group should therefore be screened periodically by endoscopic means. Because of the high frequency of gastrointestinal problems in the aging SCI population, specific attention to bowel symptoms should be incorporated into routine follow-up procedures and education regarding bowel program performance, and a bowel-friendly diet should be emphasized.

Genitourinary System

Normal aging in the general population is accompanied by diminished bladder capacity and urethral compliance as well as an increase in uninhibited detrusor contractions and residual bladder volumes (59). Aging is also associated with a gradual decline in kidney function characterized by a decrease in glomerular filtration rate and renal plasma flow (60). At the same time, age-related changes in the diurnal output of urine result in an increase in nocturia. Furthermore, elderly individuals appear to be at increased risk for urinary tract infections, presumably related to the decline in immune function, postmenopausal changes, and the effects of prostatism (61). The physiologic disruption of genitourinary function following SCI is characterized by the loss of volitional control over micturition as well as the loss of coordination of detrusor and sphincter reflexes. In the long-term, after these reflexes have recovered, there is a tendency for sphincter–detrusor dyssynergia and elevated lower urinary tract pressure. This ultimately leads to hypertrophy of the detrusor muscle and decreased bladder compliance. Over time, the cumulative effect of these changes can lead to hydronephrosis and upper tract deterioration as well (61).

Although these SCI-related alterations in urinary tract physiology pose significant risks to health, urinary tract complications, which were formerly one of the leading causes of death in SCI, now account for only 2.3% of deaths in this population (62). This improvement in urinary tract–related mortality is probably a result of advances in urologic management and modern antibiotic treatment. It should be noted, however, that urologic complications continue to be common in the SCI survivor group (63). Data from the SCI Model Systems in the United States show that the incidence of abnormal renal function testing increases with both duration of injury and age. These data also show that removal of urinary tract stones increased from 3.1% at 5 years to 10.8% at 20 years after injury and was most common in persons managed with an indwelling catheter. Urinary tract infections remain a common complication in the U.S. follow-up population, ranging from 1.5 to 2.2 infections per year throughout the 20 years of follow-up.

Certain urinary complications appear to be associated with the method of bladder management. Most studies have documented higher rates of urinary tract infection, bladder stones, and bladder cancer associated with the use of indwelling catheter management. In patients who are managed with an indwelling catheter, the routine use of anticholinergic medication may improve health outcomes (64). Persons on long-term intermittent catheterization may be at added risk for urethral stricture and epididymitis, two complications that have been found to increase with the number of years on intermittent catherization (65). Bladder cancer appears to be one of the few neoplasms for which the incidence is unequivocally increased by the presence of SCI (66–69). Risk factors for the development of this cancer that derive from SCI and its management include recurrent urinary tract infection as well as the use of indwelling catheters (70,71). The latency from injury to the time of cancer diagnosis is typically about 20 years. It does appear as though malignant degeneration requires the cumulative effects of various risk factor exposures (e.g., recurrent infections, indwelling catheter management, urinary tract stones, and cigarette smoking) over a long period of time. A recent study showed that indwelling catheter management resulted in a fourfold higher risk for the development of bladder cancer than nonindwelling catheter methods of management (70). SCI survivors who develop bladder carcinoma typically present with hematuria. Unfortunately, because hematuria commonly occurs with urinary tract infection, bladder stones, and catheter changes, this sign is not a reliable indicator of bladder cancer in the SCI population. The clinical approach should be based on prevention and early detection. The patient should be educated regarding the fundamentals of bladder management in an effort to reduce the risk for recurrent urinary tract infection. Adequate hydration, hygienic bladder management technique, and routine urologic follow-up should be stressed. Individuals choosing indwelling catheter methods of bladder management should receive adequate informed consent regarding the accompanying risk for bladder cancer. Smoking cessation programs should also be strongly encouraged for those who smoke because cigarette smoking has also been identified as a significant risk factor for bladder cancer.

These tumors are commonly metastatic and invasive at the time of diagnosis in persons with SCI, highlighting the importance of the development of effective screening methods. Urine cytology and biochemical markers of urinary tract malignancy do not appear to be appropriate screening tools at present, owing to their high false-positive rate, which can be due to concomitant urinary tract infection and related hematuria. Although some have questioned the effectiveness of screening cystoscopy to detect these tumors in chronically catheterized SCI patients, most clinicians feel that this method remains the best option for early detection of bladder cancer in this population (71,72). Because of the risk for chronic prostatitis related to recurrent urinary tract infection, it is reasonable to speculate that there may be some added risk for prostate cancer in men with chronic SCI. To date, there is no compelling evidence that such an association exists. In fact, one recent study found that there was a lower incidence of carcinoma of the prostate in those SCI individuals

who were more disabled, suggesting that, at the very least, there is no added risk for this cancer in this population (73). Nonetheless, men aging with SCI should be considered at risk and be provided with age-specific prostate cancer screening that would be recommended for their general population counterparts (74). Guided by an awareness of these issues, the long-term follow-up of persons with SCI should include attention to the potential for functional deterioration and the development of urinary tract cancers.

Nervous System

Studies of general population aging have documented a number of changes referable to the nervous system, including diminished strength and reaction time, loss of vibratory sense, decreased fine coordination and agility, loss of muscle mass, diminished deep tendon reflexes, and a deterioration of station and gait (75). Histologic investigation of the aging spinal cord has documented loss of myelinated tracts as well as a loss of anterior horn cells, although these changes may not occur to a significant degree until after the fifth decade (76). The British aging study of persons with SCI of more than 20 years' duration showed that 12% of the subjects reported some sensory loss, whereas 21% complained of increasing motor deficits over the years (77). Although it is tempting to speculate that age-related dropout of anterior horn cells and loss of myelinated tracts may contribute to these reported symptoms, verification of this mechanism awaits further study.

Surveys of chronic SCI survivors have shown a high incidence of upper extremity entrapment neuropathies, with up to 63% of people with paraplegia showing evidence of this problem on electrodiagnostic testing and symptom survey (78,79). SCI individuals are at risk for nerve entrapments in the upper extremities by virtue of their repetitive hand contact with the wheelchair rim. Positioning of the wrist during critical transfer and pressure relief maneuvers may also be contributory. Although most clinicians have thought that the incidence of significant entrapment increases with duration of injury, this association has not been conclusively proved. The most frequent site of involvement is the median nerve at the wrist, but ulnar nerve entrapments at the elbow and wrist are also common. The treatment approach should include an assessment of the mechanics of activities of daily living and mobility activities to determine the underlying sources of repetitive trauma. Activity modification may result in a resolution of symptoms in some cases. Although many individuals may not be able to eliminate offending activities completely from their daily routines, education regarding wrist conservation can have a beneficial effect for some. Wrist splinting should also be offered as a means of reducing repetitive trauma and the extremes of wrist flexion and extension, which are known to contribute to carpal tunnel symptoms. Corticosteroid injection therapy has been tried as an additional conservative measure for persons with carpal tunnel syndrome but has commonly been of only temporary benefit. When conservative measures have failed to produce symptomatic relief in people with significant entrapments, surgical release of the transverse carpal ligament is commonly recommended. Patients undergoing this surgery should anticipate a period of activity restriction after the surgery, which may necessitate a temporary increase in personal care assistance. More recently, advances in surgical technique, including the percutaneous endoscopic approach to transverse carpal ligament section, have reduced the duration of postoperative activity restriction. Although ulnar entrapments at the wrist may prompt consideration of surgical treatment, SCI survivors with these neuropathies are usually successfully treated with activity and equipment modification and, as such, rarely require surgical intervention.

Neurologic deterioration in chronic SCI is most commonly the result of progressive posttraumatic cystic myelopathy (80). This condition, also referred to as *posttraumatic syringomyelia*, is characterized by the progressive enlargement of a cystic cavity originating at the site of injury and extending in either a cephalad or caudal direction in the spinal cord. More recently, this concept of progressive cystic myelopathy has been expanded to include progressive noncystic or myelomalacic myelopathies, which are thought to be a part of a pathophysiologic continuum. The signs and symptoms of this late progressive neurologic deterioration include loss of motor and sensory function, increased spasticity, late-onset neurologic pain, increased autonomic dysreflexia, increased sweating, and the development of a variable, positional Horner syndrome. The diagnosis is confirmed by the combination of the typical history and physical findings and the magnetic resonance imaging abnormality of an enlarging syrinx cavity or myelomalacic spinal cord. The onset of this neurologic complication may vary from several months to several decades after injury but most commonly occurs within the first 5 to 10 years after injury. The underlying mechanism of the progressive spinal cord pathology appears to be related to arachnoid scarring, which interferes with spinal fluid flow and spinal cord mobility. When neurologic deterioration is progressive, surgical treatment, including untethering of the arachnoid scar and, in some cases, shunting of cyst cavity fluid, is indicated (81). Because of the potential for late neurologic change in all patients with SCI, periodic assessment of motor and sensory function as well as a neurologic review of systems should be included in periodic follow-up. Signs or symptoms of neurologic deterioration should result in appropriate electrodiagnostic and imaging studies (81, 82).

Musculoskeletal System

Musculoskeletal system aging in the general population is characterized by a deterioration of articular cartilage function, which ultimately leads to degenerative arthritic changes, both in the spine and in joints of the appendicular skeleton (42). Osteoporosis is also a common accompaniment to the aging process, most commonly seen in postmenopausal elderly women but also occurring in aging men as well (83). Considering the unique physical stresses required of a SCI person during mobility activities, it is not surprising that overuse syndromes of the upper extremities are common in this population. Likewise, with paralysis and disuse being known risk factors for osteoporosis in the disabled population, it should be expected that these individuals have added risk for fracture as they age with their injuries.

Surveys have documented that upper extremity pain is reported by more than 50% of SCI survivors (84,85). Shoulder discomfort is the most frequent complaint, followed by pain at the wrist. Upper extremity discomfort is most commonly produced by transfers, wheelchair propulsion, and pressure relief maneuvers. Acromioclavicular degenerative changes may be seen on x-ray films, but plain radiographs are commonly of little value in the assessment of shoulder pain in these individuals. Arthrography and, more recently, magnetic resonance imaging have better diagnostic yield and commonly show impingement syndrome and rotator cuff tears in symptomatic individuals with SCI reporting shoulder pain (86,87). Most authors agree that the prevalence and severity of upper extremity overuse problems are correlated with age and duration of injury. Conservative management should include a review of daily activities and mobility mechanics that may result in suggestions for activity modification in an effort to avoid pain-causing maneuvers. Many individuals with overuse syndrome at the shoulders have a muscular imbalance across the glenohumeral joint, with anterior musculature development significantly greater than that posterior to the shoulder. An exercise regimen specifically designed to address the posterior shoulder girdle may reestablish muscular balance across the joint and restore optimal glenohumeral geometric relationships (88). When conservative measures fail, surgery for impingement or rotator cuff tears has been suggested. Although operative treatment has produced successful outcome in some patients, postoperative rehabilitation may be difficult and prolonged, considering the shoulder activity restrictions commonly used after such procedures. Patients contemplating operative treatment for impingement or rotator cuff tears should also anticipate a prolonged but temporary impact on independence, with additional personal care assistance commonly required (89,90).

Osteoporosis due to paralysis and disuse is commonly thought to be the underlying risk factor for pathologic fractures after SCI. Recent surveys have documented an extremity fracture rate of more than 30% for individuals followed for several decades (91). It has been shown that lower extremity osteoporosis develops rapidly in the first postinjury year, with about one third of the original bone mass being lost by 16 months after injury, before relative stability is achieved (92). Although a number of interventions have been proposed, including standing, functional electrical stimulation, and treatment with biphosphonates, no treatment has yet been shown to provide long-term prevention of osteoporosis and protection from fracture risk. With at least one preliminary trial of pamidronate showing some promise, however, it is hoped that continued investigation in this area yields effective treatment in the future (93). Because of the frequency of musculoskeletal complaints in this population, SCI clinicians should incorporate a thorough symptom review and examination as a part of periodic reassessment. The contribution of suboptimal posture to chronic back pain has also been noted by a number of authors and may be amenable to equipment and seating system interventions (42).

Integument

Normal aging of the skin results in atrophy and changes in the histologic structures that make up the dermis (94). Collagen content and elasticity and vascularity of the dermis are diminished, predisposing aging skin to injury. Thinning of the epidermis and flattening of the dermoepidermal junction results in less tolerance to shear and greater likelihood of epidermal detachment and blister formation. Decreased vascularity and sweating may also add to the risk for thermal injury. Persons with SCI are known to be at risk for skin trauma that results in pressure ulcers. Immobility, lack of sensory protection, and spasticity all contribute to the common occurrence of skin sores in this population. A recent analysis of SCI Model Systems data from the United States showed that the incidence of pressure ulcers increases from 15% at 1 year of follow-up to nearly 30% at year 20 (63). This risk is highest in those who are most disabled, with complete tetraplegia persons having a 40% prevalence of pressure ulcers at the 20-year follow-up. The clinical approach to skin sores in SCI is primarily prevention through patient education regarding skin protection, pressure relief, hygiene, and routine surveillance. Conservative treatment of pressure sores is commonly effective if initiated promptly and performed diligently. The basic principles of pressure relief, debridement, and asepsis are still the foundation of successful conservative management (95). Large and deep skin sores commonly require myocutaneous flap closure. Local infection requires treatment with appropriate antibiotics, and deep wounds should raise the suspicion of contiguous osteomyelitis. In such cases, a bone biopsy should be performed for the purposes of diagnosis and identification of the causative organisms in order to guide antibiotic therapy. Chronic open skin sores of long duration have been associated with the development of Marjolin ulcers and of squamous carcinoma in the sore. Because of the high frequency of skin sore occurrence in the chronic SCI population, periodic assessment should include a thorough evaluation of the integument and reinforcement of skin sore prevention education.

Immune System

Research on normal aging in the immune system has shown age-related decline of immune function with increased risk for infection (96–98). Recent studies in SCI individuals have shown evidence of diminished immune function in those with tetraplegia manifested as impaired phagocytosis of *Staphylococcus aureus*, whereas those with paraplegia with lesions at or below T10 showed no loss of phagocytic function (99). The British study of SCI survivors injured more than 20 years ago showed a dramatic increase in urinary tract infections among those aged 60 years and older and a slight increase in frequency of infection between the tenth and thirtieth postinjury years (2). Immune system function is influenced by a variety of factors, including chronic pain, depression, deterioration of psychosocial supports, neuroendocrine changes, and the influence of various medications (100). Because many of these factors may coexist in persons with SCI, precise attribution of their relative contribution in any one individual is impossible. Nonetheless, it would appear safe to assume that persons aging with SCI will have more likelihood of immune impairment when compared with their nondisabled counterparts. Recently, several studies have suggested that exercise and rehabilitation therapies have been associated with improved cellular immunity in persons with SCI (101,102). Although research in this important area is still in its infancy, it is hoped that further research advances in immunologic assessment and treatment will yield therapies that can improve immune defenses in persons with chronic SCI.

Respiratory System

Studies of aging in the general population have shown a number of changes that result in a gradual loss of respiratory system function with advancing years (103,104). Loss of lung and chest wall compliance is accompanied by a decrease in the number of alveoli. There is a progressive loss of vital capacity as well as centrally mediated respiratory drive. SCI is associated with respiratory complications, both in the immediate postinjury period and during long-term follow-up (63). Persons with complete tetraplegia are at the highest risk, followed by those with incomplete tetraplegia and paraplegia. Older age at the time of injury is also associated with a higher risk for respiratory complications. In persons aging with SCI, the combined effects of these changes are likely to pose a significant risk for respiratory tract complications, such as pneumonia and atelectasis. Indeed, in an analysis of Model Systems mortality statistics in persons with SCI who survived at least 24 hours, pneumonia was found to be the leading cause of death, accounting for nearly 18% of the total (18). Furthermore, pneumonia is the leading cause of death in all age groups and in all postinjury time periods.

Several studies have investigated the incidence of respiratory tract morbidity in persons aging with SCI. In a study of 834 persons followed at one of two British SCI centers at least 20 years after injury, the incidences of pneumonia and atelectasis were found to increase with age (going from 1.6% in the group less than 30 years of age to 5.4% in the group older than 60 years of age), but not with years after injury (2). U.S. Model Systems data reveal similar findings, with pneumonia incidence increasing from 1.5% per year in the 16- to 30-year-old age group to 8.2% in the group older than 76 years of age (105). Thus, it would appear that within the time frames studied, the risk for respiratory complications is associated with the age of the patient rather than duration of injury.

What should these findings mean to clinicians? An appreciation of the respiratory risk in aging SCI patients should lead to heightened surveillance for changes in function. Periodic assessments should include measurement of vital capacity, especially in those with cervical levels of injury who are at the highest risk (106). Persons with SCI who have respiratory disability should receive pneumococcal vaccination as well as yearly influenza immunization. Obese individuals should be encouraged to lose weight in order to reduce the risk for further respiratory compromise that may accompany overweight. Smoking cessation programs should be offered to all smokers as a means to lessen the risk for respiratory complications. Despite these efforts, those with borderline respiratory reserve may face the prospect of aging-related respiratory failure due to the combined effects of the gradual decline in function and the development of respiratory complications such as pneumonia. In these circumstances, difficult choices regarding the acceptance of mechanical ventilatory support will need to be made.

Cardiovascular System

According to the Centers for Disease Control and Prevention, cardiovascular diseases are the most common causes of death in the United States among both men and women of all racial and ethnic groups (107). Age is the most important risk factor for ischemic heart disease, but the contribution of other risk factors is significant and can result in severe forms of the disease at any age (108). Atherosclerosis in humans appears to develop gradually, usually in the absence of any known disease, and is often exacerbated by genetic and environmental factors (109). In addition to these changes, there are a number of age-related alterations in the structure and function of the heart and blood vessels. Physical inactivity, common in older individuals, is also associated with cardiovascular deconditioning (109).

Heart disease is now known to be one of the leading causes of death in long-term SCI, causing more than 20% of deaths in the time period from 1993 to 1998 (62). A number of studies have documented abnormalities of glucose and lipid metabolism as well as other risk factors for the development of cardiovascular disease (110–112). People with SCI tend to have a lipid profile characterized by low high-density lipoprotein levels, with levels of less than 35 mg/dL being up to four times more common when compared with those in the general population. This effect is related to the degree of neurologic impairment and is more pronounced in people with tetraplegia and those with complete injuries (113). Serum low-density lipoprotein levels in those with SCI are not significantly different from those in the general population.

With regard to insulin resistance, a study of male veterans with SCI found 22% to have diabetes on oral glucose tolerance testing, compared with only 6% of nondisabled control subjects (111). Although 82% of the control subjects had normal glucose tolerance, only 50% of those with paraplegia and 38% of those with tetraplegia had normal testing. It has been suggested that changes in body composition, which are common in SCI, contribute to impaired glucose metabolism (112). SCI individuals typically have a reduction of lean muscle mass and a corresponding increase of fat mass. In addition, the diminished activity level of those with SCI may also contribute to insulin resistance.

These alterations in lipid and glucose metabolism indicate that people with SCI have an elevated risk for coronary heart disease and other manifestations of cardiovascular disease. Therefore, interventions should include periodic assessment of risk factors such as blood lipids, glucose, weight, blood pressure, dietary habits, smoking, activity level, and alcohol consumption. Prevention efforts can first be directed at modifiable risk factors. Individuals should be encouraged to follow a "heart-healthy" diet that limits intake of saturated fats and cholesterol. Weight management should be promoted and incorporated into nutritional counseling. When adverse lipid profiles require pharmacologic management, compliance with medication regimens should be encouraged. Exercise and a general increase in physical activity should also be encouraged, and smoking cessation programs should be promoted strongly. With a combination of these efforts, individuals aging with SCI can lessen their risk for cardiovascular diseases.

SPINAL CORD INJURY AND AGING: PSYCHOSOCIAL ASPECTS

The physical changes of aging in people with SCI are often accompanied by changes in an individual's satisfaction with life, perceived well-being, living situation, and degree of community integration. Unlike physical aging, however, these aspects of a person's life may actually improve. In addition, when potential problems do arise, much can be done to intervene and either delay, modify, or eliminate potential negative consequences. Investigating these issues provides a complex, often confusing picture because so many interrelated factors are involved. Consideration must be given not only to the physical and potential cognitive changes associated with aging but also to the highly individualized psychological adjustment to these changes. Economic factors, environmental barriers and facilitators, cultural issues, and changes in the intimate and more remote social network may also affect, or be affected by, physiologic aging. Consideration of these multiple factors in the evaluation of individuals aging with SCI is critical to understand the thorough contextual basis that underlies this complex phenomenon.

Independence

Declining function is one of the many consequences of aging (114). As people grow older, many experience a loss of physical independence resulting from diminished muscle strength, decreased sensory acuity, slowed reflexes, decreased coordination, and lower energy levels (115). Other health conditions that significantly affect older people include incontinence, chronic pain, arthritis, osteoporosis, and hypertension (116). These and other chronic conditions, as well as injuries, can limit an individual's ability to carry out the predominant social role expected of a person at a given age, whether that role involves attending school, working, or living independently. Data from the 1996 National Health Interview Survey showed that more than 22% of the civilian community-dwelling population of the United States aged 45 to 64 years and more than 36% of those aged 65 years and older reported some degree of activity limitation (117).

With SCI, the presence of some form of activity limitation is almost inevitable from the onset of the injury. This is not a static condition, however, and aging may magnify issues of dependency as needs, abilities, and limitations change over time. Three main issues appear to be of concern to people aging with SCI: their overall health, their ability to remain independent, and their ability to sustain a satisfying lifestyle (118). Research has indicated that some of these concerns may be well founded. In a study of British individuals with SCI of 20 or more years' duration, increasing age was a significant predictor of functional decline. The average age when additional functional assistance was first needed was 49 years for those with tetraplegia or tetraparesis and 54 years for those with paraplegia or paraparesis (115). Functional decline or decreasing physical independence has been identified as an adverse outcome of long-term SCI, with one study showing 22% of participants reporting a decline over a 3-year time span (119). Another investigation demonstrated both cross-sectional and longitudinal significant increases in the need for assistance among older individuals (120). In addition to chronologic age, increasing duration of time since injury has been shown to be related to decreased levels of activity (121).

Fortunately, preserving functional ability and maintaining independence are areas that are amenable to intervention, either through changing the manner in which certain activities are accomplished, such as transfers, or by using adaptive equipment. Even when assistance from others is necessary, this can be incorporated into an individual's life in such a way that optimizes independence for the person with SCI.

Stress, Depression, and Perceived Quality of Life

A change in the level of independence is one component that appears to accompany the aging process and has been shown to be consistently related to reports of health, stress, depression, and declining quality of life both in the general population and in people with SCI (115,122,123). Life stressors may include financial worries, employment difficulties, declining health, loss of independence (124), erosion in the quality of one's social network, or the death of loved ones (125,126). Although there is evidence that chronic stressors can be detrimental to health (127), it is important to acknowledge that not all stressors are negative. Events such as marriage, the birth of children or grandchildren, or planning a vacation may also be stressful. Research has shown that to assume older people experience more stress than younger individuals may not be entirely accurate (128). Aldwin and colleagues evaluated stress and coping using a sample of 1,065 men who participated in the longitudinal Normative Aging Study (128). They found age differences in the types of problems reported, with health and "general hassles" being reported as problems more often with increasing age, but there was also a trend for the older groups to rate their problems as less stressful (128).

Stress and poor health also have been linked with depression in older individuals (129). Depressive symptoms in older adults may include feelings of sadness, guilt, or worthlessness; loss of interest in daily activities; difficulty concentrating; appetite and weight changes; difficulty sleeping; and fatigue (130). The consequences of depression in later life can be quite serious, the mental health and physical health of older individuals are often inseparable (131). Specifically, prospective cohort studies have demonstrated compelling evidence that psychosocial factors, such as depression, are independent, etiologic, and prognostic factors for coronary heart disease (132–134). Unfortunately, depression is often underdiagnosed or undiagnosed, particularly when depressive symptoms are attributed to other medical problems (135). In addition, it may be difficult to separate depressive symptoms from cognitive decline in elderly individuals, or to determine whether these conditions are interrelated (136,137).

Despite the many reports of increasing depression with age, there is evidence that perceived quality of life is not necessarily worse for older people, even those with chronic illnesses (138). Part of the misconception is possibly due to a lack of understanding of what "quality of life" actually means. Often used interchangeably with concepts such as life satisfaction, happiness, and well being, quality of life is multidimensional and includes

biologic, psychological, interpersonal, social, economic, and cultural dimensions (139). Because of its complex nature, it is important to understand what factors have an impact on a person's perceived quality of life (140). For some, it may be determined by financial security; for others, maintaining health and having good relationships with others are determinants of life satisfaction. Often, it is not aging, in and of itself, that is associated with lower perceived quality of life. Income level, social support, and participation in activities have been found to more predictive of higher quality of life, and a person's sense of contentment has been suggested as an underlying factor of life satisfaction (141,142). In addition, elderly people may have developed expectations that are more commensurate with adaptation to illness than younger individuals and may be more able to cope with life stresses (138).

Studies of stress, depression, and quality of life in people aging with SCI tend to support what is found in the general aging literature, although there is a tendency for baseline stress and depression to be greater for people with SCI compared to what is reported in the general population (143). Gerhart and colleagues found no significant differences in perceived stress by age, duration of injury, gender, or severity of impairment among a group of British individuals aging with SCI (144). In fact, there was a tendency toward less stress in older people. Although there was no evidence of a strong relationship between stress and medical outcomes, there was a clear relationship between stress and other psychosocial outcomes, particularly depressive symptoms, life satisfaction, and quality of life. Similarly, findings from the Baylor College of Medicine Life Status Study showed no relationship between age and stress in a sample of community-dwelling people with SCI, and a relationship between stress with depressive symptoms and life satisfaction (145).

Of all the possible psychosocial outcomes, depression has tended to garner more attention by researchers studying SCI. Unfortunately, most studies address this topic in terms of immediate and early postinjury adjustment and response to SCI. Few of these studies analyze depressive symptoms by age, and even fewer address this topic in people aging with SCI. Those that do explore the relationship of depressive symptoms and age in the years after injury show varying results, but in general, older age has not been found to be correlated with current age, age when injured, or duration of injury (119,146). Preliminary analysis of data from an investigation of ours shows outcomes 3 years after injury, with individuals injured at age 55 and older having considerably lower scores on measures of depressive symptoms than individuals injured between the ages of 18 and 34 years (unpublished data).

In contrast to the scarce information on long-term stress and depression as they relate to aging with SCI, the literature on the quality of life with SCI provides far more insight into long-term outcomes. It has been suggested, not surprisingly, that quality of life among people with SCI is generally lower than among those without disabilities (147,148). Although several studies support the finding that life satisfaction for people with SCI is not necessarily negatively impacted by aging, others find significant differences in self-perceived quality of life, with younger individuals and those injured for shorter periods of time rating their quality of life better than older individuals (2,114,120,121,

149,150). The variation in these findings may best be explained by the differences in how older and younger individuals assess quality of life. In a study of priority shifting among men with SCI, more of the younger men placed a high focus on health, work, learning, and family, whereas more of the older individuals placed higher priority on socializing or spending time in passive leisure activities (150). More telling, however, was not how these groups differed from each other, but how men with SCI differed overall from men without disabilities. In fact, much of the evidence relating to life satisfaction after SCI is related more to level of injury, expectations about functional abilities, health, social support, participation in activities, and other personal and environmental factors than to aging (21,149–154).

Clearly, identifying the potential multitude of underlying factors that might contribute to declines in perceived quality of life, increased stress, or depressive symptoms is a difficult task. To understand these phenomena effectively, health care providers must assess not only the physical health and well-being of the individual aging with SCI but also the psychological status, social situation, and environment because all have an impact on successful aging.

Family Issues

SCI can have a far-reaching impact on family members, friends, and even others in the community close to the individual, particularly when that person requires physical assistance from others. Overall, about one third of SCI survivors require assistance from others (155). In one recent study, people with SCI were seven times more likely to need personal care services than individuals in a comparable nondisabled sample (156). In addition, evidence suggests that SCI survivors' need for help increases as they age (115). This, coupled with the fact that 40% of all SCI survivors are now older than 45 years of age and one fourth have been injured for 20 or more years, makes it clear that the number of personal assistance users will only increase in the coming years (157). Related to this issue is the fact that many SCI caregivers are also aging and are faced with their own age-related health issues.

Caregiving

Pearlin and colleagues describe *caregiving* as the behavioral expression of one's commitment to the welfare of another, whereby caring is the affective component (158). Using this definition, all caring relationships include some degree of assisting one another. However, when serious or prolonged impairment figures into the relationship, caregiving may become the dominant component of the interactions and may, under some circumstances, "expand to the point where it occupies virtually the entirety of the relationship" (158). *Caregiver stress* refers to the ongoing problems within the caregiving role that cause disruptions or changes that have potential for taxing or exceeding the caregiver's resources (159). Often, outcomes of this imbalance in behavioral expression include stress or depression. Studies of depression are pervasive in the literature and span all illnesses and disabilities, and these rates are especially high among women (160).

A particular concern for caregivers is the risk for injury incurred while performing caregiving tasks. It can reasonably be predicted that caregivers should have higher rates of physical illness because they are continuously exposed to high levels of stress (161). Even in the absence of actual bodily injury or illness, perceived health may be affected by caregiving, often as a manifestation of role strain, stress, or depression. Symptoms and health problems include hypertension, arthritis, back pain, stomach upset or indigestion, and cardiac problems (162). In addition, caregivers also tend to ignore their own health and are more apt to forego health-promoting behaviors if those behaviors conflict with caregiving; thus, they end up in a cycle of neglect (163). The potentially resulting poor health of the caregiver can have negative consequences for the recipient of that assistance, and with the advancing age of both, these consequences are likely to be magnified. Therefore, the physical and emotional health of family members, particularly if they provide personal assistance services to their loved one with SCI, also need to be addressed during routine follow-up. Detecting potential difficulties as early as possible and offering appropriate interventions, such as seeking occasional respite care or using home health agency assistance, can help families maintain a positive focus on issues other than caregiving.

Another aspect of caregiving relates to the SCI person's willingness and ability to adapt to needing more assistance. There is evidence that assistance provided by a caregiving spouse is not always perceived positively by the recipient, and increasing age is a significant predictor of negative reactions to receiving assistance (164). This may be of particular concern for those with SCI who, having been independent when younger, begin to need assistance as they age. The new need for help can be a difficult dilemma because maintaining some semblance of independence can be of paramount importance to people aging with SCI. Beneficial strategies include encouraging people with SCI to prioritize those activities that are most time consuming, difficult, or tedious as those that can be delegated to others, such as dressing, tub transfers, or bowel programs. This can enable them to preserve their energy and use it to engage in more gratifying pursuits.

Role Changes

SCI often requires that families make adjustments in what home and work activities are done by whom. Differences between men's and women's caregiving participation are often attributed to gender role norms, and caregiving is often viewed as an extension of women's social roles, whereas for men, it is a new, unfamiliar role (165–168). In addition, the differential distribution of day-to-day tasks after injury may add to an imbalance in perceived equality of family members, causing greater difficulty in maintaining family relationships (160). Role functions that may have changed early after injury are not likely to be static. As people with SCI age and forfeit some degree of independence, further adjustments in the distribution of tasks undoubtedly need to be made. This particularly affects those who previously had been able to assume larger proportions of familial responsibility after their injuries and find themselves becoming more dependent with age. It is advisable that clinicians be aware that this type of role-related stress in a relationship can ultimately have a detrimental impact on the health of both the caregiver and care recipient.

Environmental Issues

Not all issues for the person aging with SCI are focused on physical or psychosocial changes that may occur as time passes. An important and often overlooked factor is the environment. The primary tenet of the disability rights movement and a new paradigm on disability has been that environmental factors place important restrictions on the degree to which people with disabilities can fully participate in society. Furthermore, the physical, attitudinal, and policy barriers in the environment are viewed as equally causal as (or more causal than) the underlying organ system impairments in determining activity limitation and participation restrictions.

The three most frequently cited current conceptual models of disability recognize the importance of the environment as a cause of disability. The Quebec Classification, published in 1995, was the first to prominently articulate the role of environmental factors influencing societal participation among people with disabilities (169). In this schema, the three primary determinants of participation include the following:

1. Internal factors related to disability, such as impairments of body structure and function, activity limitations, and compensatory abilities
2. Internal factors not related to disability, such as demographic characteristics and life experiences
3. Environmental factors, defined as all external factors influencing participation

The Institute of Medicine updated its conceptual model of disability in 1997, explicitly identifying the role of the environment, and shows disability more clearly as the interaction of the person with the environment (170). Finally, in the World Health Organization's (WHO's) most recent draft of the International Classification of Functioning and Disability, environmental factors are depicted as one of two contextual factors interacting with health conditions to produce impairments of body structure and function, activity limitations, and participation restrictions (171). Not only are environmental factors clearly identified in the current WHO model as the context in which disability occurs, but they are also classified as one of four equally prominent domains (along with impairments, activity limitations, and participation restrictions).

Studies in the general population have suggested that environmental, as well as personal, factors have significant effects on health behaviors of older individuals living independently in the community, particularly for those in low-resource areas (172). Access to resources, the ability to move around in the community, attitudes of others, and the impact of public policies may all be altered for people as they age. This can be even more pronounced in those aging with a disability such as SCI. Recent research has shown that significant differences exist between people with and without disabilities in terms of the frequency with which they encounter environmental barriers and the magnitude of the problems those barriers create (173). Of interest, however,

is that SCI patients aged 55 years and older report encountering fewer environmental barriers than younger patients and also report fewer problems encountered with those barriers that are present (unpublished data). Different factors may account for this finding. First, older individuals with SCI, who might have encountered a variety of environmental barriers when younger or more newly injured, may have made adjustments to their lives in order to avoid or minimize such barriers. Thus, as they age, they are less likely to encounter some of the environmental barriers that older people without disabilities may face. Second, older individuals with SCI may be less likely to be as mobile in their communities and may spend more time at home, thus not encountering external barriers as often. Whether these adjustments to avoid environmental barriers are enhancements to quality of life is unclear. It is recommended, therefore, that exploration of perceived and real environmental barriers be included as part of long-term follow-up. If, in fact, identified barriers are perceived as minimally limiting to both activity and quality of life, they are unlikely to have an overall negative impact for the individual aging with SCI. If identified barriers do, however, act to diminish a person's perceived health, quality of life, or life satisfaction, then addressing these barriers and seeking ways to eliminate or minimize their impact is warranted.

LOOKING TO THE FUTURE

As more people with SCI survive into their later years, the community of health care providers will be faced with new challenges in order to facilitate the successful aging of these individuals. Increasing contacts with and liaisons to gerontologists and other professionals with an expertise in aging will become increasingly important to the SCI rehabilitation community.

It has been suggested that if aging with SCI is to be effectively managed, strategies to minimize conditions and complications that occur with aging must be identified and implemented (174). This is a multifaceted process involving clinical follow-up, continuing education for both clinicians and individuals aging with SCI, and further research. The first critical component involves systematic surveillance by an experienced SCI team in order to identify potential problems at their earliest onset. A recommended follow-up regimen is shown in Table 27.1.

Ongoing education for the clinician involves learning about the physical, psychological, social, and environmental consequences of aging and their potential impact on people with SCI. Education for the person with SCI, already enhanced through an ever-changing electronic world of information, can be further improved through the dissemination of pertinent and timely information about aging. Stressing the need for continued rehabilitation or equipment modifications will also be valuable. Research efforts to understand the complexity of aging with SCI will need to continue with larger, more representative study samples.

Aging needs to be viewed without prejudice as simply another step along the continuum of life with SCI—equal in importance to initial rehabilitation, returning to work, developing relationships, and engaging in other life activities. In doing so, the likelihood of successfully managing the myriad changes that will be

TABLE 27.1. FOLLOW-UP GUIDELINES FOR HEALTHY SPINAL CORD INJURY SURVIVORS

General Health Maintenance	Spinal Cord Injury (SCI) Specific
Things to do monthly	**Things to do daily**
Women: breast self-examination	Self skin checks
Men: testicular self-examination	
Things to do every year	**Things to do every year**
Check-up with health care provider	Check weight and blood pressure
Gynecologic exam and Pap smear[a]	Flu immunization, especially T8 and higher-
Clinical breast cancer exam,	level injuries
beginning at age 40[a]	
Mammography, beginning at age	
40–50[b]	
Digital rectal exam, beginning at age 40	
Digital prostate exam and PSA, beginning at	
age 50[c]	
Fecal occult blood, beginning at age 50	
Things to do every 2–3 years	**Things to do at least every 2–3 years with SCI specialist/team[d]**
Complete blood count with biochemistry survey	Full history and physical review with
Cardiac risk assessment, beginning at age 40	physician[d]
	Urologic assessment—upper and lower
	tracts[d,e]
	Assess equipment and posture[d]
	Assess range of motion, contractures, and
	functional status[d]
	Full skin evaluation[d]
Things to do every 5 years	**Things to do at least every 5 years with SCI specialist/team**
Vital capacity (lung test)	Motor and sensory testing
Lipid panel (cholesterol)	Review changes in life situation, including
Eye evaluation, beginning at age 40	coping, adjustment, life satisfaction
Screening sigmoidoscopy or colonoscopy,	
after age 50	
Things to do every 10 years	**Things to do every 10 years**
Tetanus booster	Pneumococcal pneumonia vaccination at
	earliest opportunity, especially for T8 and
	higher level injuries

[a]In women.
[b]In addition to baseline mammogram between age 30 and 40, or between age 40 and 50. (Note: a number of guidelines conflict on the age at which yearly mammography should begin, with some specifying age 40 yr others age 50)
[c]In men. Age 40 if black, or if grandfather, father or brother has or had prostate cancer.
[d]Assessments done annually for the first 3–5 yrs after injury, until health established.
[e]Do annually for the first 3 yrs after any major change in urologic management.
Adapted with permission from Craig Hospital, Denver, Co.

encountered by both the clinician and the person with SCI will be greatly enhanced.

REFERENCES

1. Waters RL, Apple DF, Meyer PR, et al. Emergency and acute management of spine trauma. In: Stover SL, DeLisa JA, Whiteneck GG, eds. *Spinal cord injury: clinical outcomes from the Model Systems.* Gaithersburg, MD: Aspen, 1995:56–78.
2. Whiteneck GG, Charlifue SW, Frankel HL, et al. Mortality, morbidity, and psychosocial outcomes of persons spinal cord injured more than 20 years ago. *Paraplegia* 1992;30:617–630.
3. Barber KE, Cross RR Jr. The urinary tract as a cause of death in paraplegia. *J Urol* 1952;67:494–502.
4. Bunts RC. Preservation of renal function in the paraplegic. *J Urol* 1959;81:720–727.
5. Dietrick RB, Russi S. Tabulation and review of autopsy findings in fifty five paraplegics. *JAMA* 1958;166:41–44.
6. Nyquist RH, Bors E. Mortality and survival in traumatic myelopathy during nineteen years, from 1946 to 1965. *Paraplegia* 1967;5:22–48.
7. Tribe CR. Causes of death in the early and late stages of paraplegia. *Paraplegia* 1963;1:19–47.
8. Frisbie JH, Kache A. Increasing survival and changing causes of death in myelopathy patients. *J Am Paraplegia Soc* 1983;6:51–56.
9. Carter RE. Experiences with high tetraplegics. *Paraplegia* 1979;17:140–146.

10. Kiwerski J, Weiss M, Chrostowska T. Analysis of mortality of patients after cervical spine trauma. *Paraplegia* 1981;19:347–351.

11. DeVivo MJ, Kartus PL, Stover SL, et al. Cause of death for patients with spinal cord injuries. *Arch Intern Med* 1989;149:1761–1766.

12. DeVivo MJ, Black KJ, Stover SL. Causes of death during the first 12 years after spinal cord injury. *Arch Phys Med Rehabil* 1993;74:248–254.

13. Samsa GP, Patrick CH, Feussner JR. Long-term survival of veterans with traumatic spinal cord injury. *Arch Neurol* 1993;50:909–914.

14. Le CT, Price M. Survival from spinal cord injury. *J Chronic Dis* 1982;35:487–492.

15. Ducharme SH, Freed MM, Oates C, et al. The role of self-destruction in spinal cord injury mortality. *Model Systems' SCI Digest* 1981;2:29–38.

16. Charlifue SW, Gerhart KA. Behavioral and demographic predictors of suicide after traumatic spinal cord injury. *Arch Phys Med Rehabil* 1991;72:488–492.

17. DeVivo MJ, Black KJ, Richards JS, et al. Suicide following spinal cord injury. *Paraplegia* 1991;29:620–627.

18. DeVivo MD, Stover SL. Long-term survival and causes of death. In: Stover SL, DeLisa JA, Whiteneck GG, eds. *Spinal cord injury: clinical outcomes from the Model Systems.* Gaithersburg, MD: Aspen, 1995:289–316.

19. Vaidyanathan S, Soni BM, Gopalan L, et al. A review of the readmissions of patients with tetraplegia to the Regional Spinal Injuries Centre, Southport, United Kingdom, between January 1994 and December 1995. *Spinal Cord* 1998;36:838–846.

20. Yeo JD, Walsh J, Rutkowski S, et al. Mortality following spinal cord injury. *Spinal Cord* 1998;36:329–336.

21. McColl MA, Walker J, Stirling P, et al. Expectations of life and health among spinal cord injured individuals. *Spinal Cord* 1997;35:818–828.

22. Alander DH, Parker J, Stauffer ES. Intermediate-term outcome of cervical spinal cord-injured patients older than 50 years of age. *Spine* 1997;22:1189–1192.

23. DeVivo MJ, Ivie CS. Life expectancy of ventilator-dependent persons with spinal cord injuries. *Chest* 1995;108:226–232.

24. Frankel HL, Coll JR, Charlifue SW, et al. Long-term survival in spinal cord injury: a fifty year investigation. *Spinal Cord* 1998;36:266–274.

25. Hartkopp A, Brønnum-Hansen H, Seidenschnur AM, et al. Survival and cause of death after traumatic spinal cord injury: a long-term epidemiological survey from Denmark. *Spinal Cord* 1997;35:76–85.

26. Ashok BT, Ali R. The aging paradox: free radical theory of aging. *Exp Gerontol* 1999;34:293–303.

27. Harman D. Aging: phenomena and theories. *Ann N Y Acad Sci* 1998;854:1–7.

28. Evans, JG. Ageing and disease. In: *Research and the Ageing Population.* Ciba Foundation Symposium. Chichester, UK: Wiley, 1988;134:38–57.

29. Shock NW. *Normal human aging: the Baltimore Longitudinal Study of Aging.* Washington, DC: U.S. Department of Health and Human Services, NIH Publication No. 84-2450, 1984.

30. Smith EL. Age: the interaction of nature and nurture. In: Smith EL, Serfass RC, eds. *Exercise and ageing: the scientific basis.* Hillside, NJ: Enslow, 1981:11–17.

31. Charlifue SW. Research into the aging process. In: Whiteneck GG, Charlifue SW, Gerhart KA, et al., eds. *Aging with spinal cord injury.* New York: Demos, 1993:9–21.

32. Schneider EL, Reed JD. Modulations of aging processes. In: Finch CE, Schneider, EL eds. *Handbook of the biology of aging,* 2nd ed. New York: Van Nostrand Reinhold, 1985:45–76.

33. Braughler JM, Hall ED. Involvement of lipid peroxidation in CNS injury. *J Neurotrauma* 1992;9:S1–7.

34. Hall ED, Yonkers PA, Andrus P, et al. Biochemistry and pharmacology of lipid antioxidants in acute brain and spinal cord injury. *J Neurotrauma* 1992;9:S425–442.

35. Xu J, Beckman JS, Hogan EL, et al. Xanthine oxidase in experimental spinal cord injury. *J Neurotrauma* 1991;8:11–18.

36. Nockels R, Young W. Pharmacologic strategies in the treatment of experimental spinal cord injury. *J Neurotrauma* 1992;9:S211–217.

37. Sampath D, Holets V, Perez Polo JR. Effect of a spinal cord photolesion injury on catalase. *Int J Dev Neurosci* 1995;13:645–654.

38. Amar AP, Levy ML. Pathogenesis and pharmacological strategies for mitigating secondary damage in acute spinal cord injury. *Neurosurgery* 1999;44:1027–1039.

39. Morse DR, Rabinowitz H. A unified theory of aging. *Int J Psychosom* 1990;37:5–24.

40. Morley A. Somatic mutation and aging. *Ann N Y Acad Sci* 1998;854:20–22.

41. Bonneux L, Barendregt JJ, Van der Maas PJ. The expiry date of man: a synthesis of evolutionary biology and public health. *J Epidemiol Commun Health* 1998;52:619–623.

42. Waters RL, Sie IH, Adkins RH. The musculoskeletal system. In: Whiteneck GG, Charlifue SW, Gerhart KA, et al., eds. *Aging with spinal cord injury.* New York: Demos, 1993:53–71.

43. Resnick NM. Urinary incontinence in the elderly. *Hosp Pract* 1986;21(11):80C–80L,80Q passim.

44. Whiteneck GG, Charlifue SW, Gerhart KA, et al, eds. *Aging with spinal cord injury.* New York: Demos, 1993.

45. Moore JG, Tweedy C, Christian PE, et al. Effects of age on gastric emptying of liquid-solid meals in man. *Dig Dis Sci* 1983;28:340–344.

46. James OF. Gastrointestinal and liver function in old age. *Clin Gastroenterol* 1983;12:671–691.

47. Kupfer RM, Heppell M, Haggith JW, et al. Gastric emptying and small bowel transit rate in the elderly. *J Am Geriatr Soc* 1985;33:340–343.

48. Whiteway J, Morson BC. Pathology of aging: diverticular disease. *Clin Gastroenterol* 1985;14:829–846.

49. Singh G, Triadafilopoulos G. Gastroesophageal reflux disease in patients with spinal cord injury. *J Spinal Cord Med* 2000;23:23–27.

50. Cosman BC, Stone JM, Perkash I. The gastrointestinal system. In: Whiteneck GG, Charlifue SW, Gerhart KA, et al., eds. *Aging with spinal cord injury.* New York: Demos, 1993:117–127.

51. Apstein MD, Dalecki-Chipperfield K. Spinal cord injury is a risk factor for gallstone disease. *Gastroenterology* 1987;92:966–968.

52. Moonka R, Stiens SA, Resnick WJ, et al. The prevalence and natural history of gallstones in spinal cord injured patients. *J Am Coll Surg* 1999;189:274–281.

53. Menter RR, Weitzenkamp D, Cooper D, et al. Bowel management outcomes in individuals with long-term spinal cord injuries. *Spinal Cord* 1997;35:608–612.

54. Menardo G, Bausano G, Corazziari E, et al. Large-bowel transit in paraplegic patients. *Dis Colon Rectum* 1987;30:924–928.

55. Nino-Murcia M, Stone JM, Chang PJ, et al. Colonic transit in spinal cord injured patients. *Invest Radiol* 1990;25:109–112.

56. Stone JM, Wolfe VA, Nino-Murcia M, et al. Colostomy as treatment for complications of spinal cord injury. *Arch Phys Med Rehabil* 1990;71:514–518.

57. Frisbie JH, Tuh CG, Nguyen CH. Effect of enterostomy on quality of life in spinal cord injury patient. *J Am Paraplegia Soc* 1986;9:3–5.

58. Stone JM, Nino-Murcia M, Wolfe VA, et al. Chronic gastrointestinal problems in spinal cord injury patients: a prospective analysis. *Am J Gastroenterol* 1990;85:1114—1119.

59. Resnick NM, Yalla SV. Aging and its affect on the bladder. *Semin Urol* 1987;5:82–86.

60. Lanig IS. The genitourinary system. In: Whiteneck GG, Charlifue SW, Gerhart KA, et al., eds. *Aging with spinal cord injury.* New York: Demos, 1993:105–115.

61. Madersbacher G, Oberwalder M. The elderly para- and tetraplegic: special aspects of the urological care. *Paraplegia* 1987;4:318–323.

62. DeVivo MJ, Krause JS, Lammertse DP. Recent trends in mortality and causes of death in persons with spinal cord injury. *Arch Phys Med Rehabil* 1999;80:1411–1419.

63. McKinley WO, Jackson AB, Cardenas DD, et al. Long-term medical complications after traumatic spinal cord injury: a regional Model Systems analysis. *Arch Phys Med Rehabil* 1999;80:1402–1410.

64. Kim YH, Bird ET, Priebe M, et al. The role of oxybutynin in spinal cord injured patients with indwelling catheters. *J Urol* 1997;158:2083–2086.

65. Perrouin-Verbe B, Labat JJ, Richard I, et al. Clean intermittent cathe-

terization from the acute period in spinal cord injury patients: long-term evaluation of urethral and genital tolerance. *Paraplegia* 1995; 33:619–624.

66. Stonehill WH, Dmochowski RR, Patterson AL, et al. Risk factors for bladder tumors in spinal cord injury patients. *J Urol* 1996;155: 1248–1250.

67. Melzak J. The incidence of bladder cancer in paraplegia. *Paraplegia* 1966;4:85–96.

68. El-Masri WS, Fellows G. Bladder cancer after spinal cord injury. *Paraplegia* 1981;19:265–270.

69. Kaufman J, Fam B, Jacobs S, et al. Bladder cancer and squamous metaplasia in spinal cord injury patients. *J Urol* 1977;118:967–971.

70. Groah SL, Weitzenkamp D, Lammertse DP, et al. The risk of bladder cancer in spinal cord injury. In press.

71. Yang CC, Clowers DE. Screening cystoscopy in chronically catheterized spinal cord injury patients. *Spinal Cord* 1999;37:204–207.

72. Navon JD, Soliman H, Khonsari F, et al. Screening cystoscopy and survival of spinal cord injured patients with squamous cell cancer of the bladder. *J Urol* 1997;157:2109–2111.

73. Frisbie JH, Binard J. Low prevalence of prostatic cancer among myelopathy patients. *J Am Paraplegia Soc* 1994;17:148–149.

74. Wyndaele JJ, Iwatsubo E, Perkash I, et al. Prostate cancer: a hazard also to be considered in the aging male patient with spinal cord injury. *Spinal Cord* 1998;36:299–302.

75. Pathy M. The central nervous system: clinical presentation and management of neurologic disorders in old age. In: Brocklehurst JC, ed. *Textbook of geriatric medicine and gerontology*, 2nd ed. Edinburgh: Churchill Livingstone, 1985.

76. Morrison LR. *The effect of advancing age upon the human spinal cord*. Cambridge, MA: Harvard University Press, 1959.

77. Lammertse DP. The nervous system. In: Whiteneck GG, Charlifue SW, Gerhart KA, et al., eds. *Aging with spinal cord injury*. New York: Demos, 1993:129–137.

78. Gellman H, Sie I, Waters RL. Late complications of the weight-bearing upper extremity in the paraplegic patient. *Clin Orthop* 1988; 233:132–135.

79. Davidoff G, Werner R, Waring W. Compressive mononeuropathies in the upper extremity in chronic paraplegia. *Paraplegia* 1991;29: 17–24.

80. Edgar R, Quail P. Progressive post-traumatic cystic and non-cystic myelopathy. *Br J Neurosurg* 1994;8:7–22.

81. Falci SP, Lammertse DP, Best L, et al. Surgical treatment of posttraumatic cystic and tethered spinal cords. *J Spinal Cord Med* 1999;22: 173–181.

82. Bursell JP, Little JW, Stiens SA. Electrodiagnosis in spinal cord injured persons with new weakness or sensory loss: central and peripheral etiologies. *Arch Phys Med Rehabil* 1999;80:904–909.

83. Riggs BL, Melton LJ. Involutional osteoporosis. *N Engl J Med* 1986; 314:1676–1684.

84. Dalyan M, Cardenas D, Gerard B. Upper extremity pain after spinal cord injury. *Spinal Cord* 1999;37:191–195.

85. Subbarao JV, Klopfstein J, Turpin R. Prevalence and impact of wrist and shoulder pain in patients with spinal cord injury. *J Spinal Cord Med* 1995;18:9–13.

86. Escobedo DM, Hunter JC, Hollister MC, et al. Imaging of rotator cuff tears in individuals with paraplegia. *Am J Roentgenol* 1997;168: 919–923.

87. Bayley JC, Cochran TP, Sledge CB. The weight-bearing shoulder: the impingement syndrome in paraplegics. *J Bone Joint Surg* 1987; 69:676–678.

88. Olenik LN, Laskin JJ, Burnham R, et al. Efficacy of rowing, backward wheeling and isolated scapular retractor exercise as remedial strength activities for wheelchair users: complication of electromyography. *Paraplegia* 1995;33:148–152.

89. Goldstein B, Young J, Escobedo EN. Rotator cuff repairs in individuals with paraplegia. *Am J Phys Med Rehabil* 1997;76:316–322.

90. Robinson MD, Hussey RW, Ha CY. Surgical decompression of impingement in the weightbearing shoulder. *Arch Phys Med Rehabil* 1993;74:324–327.

91. Frisbie JH. Fractures after myelopathy: the risk quantified. *J Spinal Cord Med* 1997;20:66–69.

92. Garland DE, Stewart CA, Adkins RH, et al. Osteoporosis after spinal cord injury. *J Orthopaed Res* 1992;10:371–378.

93. Nance PW, Schryvers O, Leslie W, et al. Intravenous pamidronate attenuates bone density loss after acute spinal cord injury. *Arch Phys Med Rehabil* 1999;80:243–251.

94. Fenske NA, Lober CW. Structural and functional changes of normal aging skin. *J Am Acad Dermatol* 1986;15:571–585.

95. Yarkony GM. Aging skin, pressure ulcerations, and spinal cord injury. In: Whiteneck GG, Charlifue SW, Gerhart KA, et al., eds. *Aging with spinal cord injury*. New York: Demos, 1993:39–52.

96. Weksler ME. Senescence of the immune system. *Med Clin North Am* 1983;67:263–272.

97. Ershler WD. Biomarkers of aging: immunological events. *Exp Gerontol* 1988;23:387–389.

98. Gardner ID. The effect of aging on susceptibility to infection. *Rev Infect Dis* 1980;2:801–810.

99. Campagnolo DI, Bartlett JA, Chatterton R, et al. Adrenal and pituitary hormone patterns after spinal cord injury. *Am J Phy Med Rehabil* 1999;78:361–366.

100. Nash MS, Fletcher MA. The immune system. In: Whiteneck GG, Charlifue SW, Gerhart KA, et al., eds. *Aging with spinal cord injury*. New York: Demos, 1993:159–181.

101. Kliesch WF, Cruse JN, Lewis RE, et al. Restoration of depressed immune function in spinal cord injury patients receiving rehabilitation therapy. *Paraplegia* 1996;34:82–90.

102. Nash MS. Immune responses to nervous system decentralization and exercise in quadriplegia. *Med Sci Sports Exerc* 1994;26:164–171.

103. Caird FI, Aktar AJ. Chronic respiratory diseases in the elderly. *Thorax* 1972;27:764–768.

104. Wilmot CB, Hall KM. The respiratory system. In: Whiteneck GG, Charlifue SW, Gerhart KA, et al., eds. *Aging with spinal cord injury*. New York: Demos, 1993:93–104.

105. Menter RR, Hudson LM. Effects of age at injury and the aging process. In: Stover SL, DeLisa JA, Whiteneck GG, eds. *Spinal cord injury: clinical outcomes from the Model Systems*. Gaithersburg, MD: Aspen, 1995:272–288.

106. Lanig IS, Lammertse DP. The respiratory system in spinal cord injury. *Phys Med Rehabil Clin North Am* 1992;3:725–740.

107. US Department of Health and Human Services, Centers for Disease Control and Prevention, National Center for Chronic Disease Prevention and Health Promotion. Chronic diseases and their risk factors: the nation's leading causes of death. 1999;December:6.

108. Weisfeldt ML, Gerstenblith G. Cardiovascular aging and adaptation to disease. In: Hurst JW, Schlant RC, Rackley CE, et al., eds. *The heart, arteries and veins*, 7th ed. New York: McGraw-Hill Information Services Company, 1990:1488–1496.

109. Ragnarsson KT. The cardiovascular system. In: Whiteneck GG, Charlifue SW, Gerhart KA, et al., eds. *Aging with spinal cord injury*. New York: Demos, 1993:73–92.

110. Brenes G, Dearwater S, Shapera R, et al. High-density lipoprotein cholesterol concentrations in physically active and sedentary spinal cord injured patients. *Arch Phys Med Rehabil* 1986;67:445–450.

111. Bauman WA, Spungen AM. Disorders of carbohydrate and lipid metabolism in veterans with paraplegia or quadriplegia: a model of premature aging. *Metabolism* 1994;43:949–956.

112. Bauman WA, Kahn NN, Grimm DR, et al. Risk factors for atherogenesis and cardiovascular autonomic function in persons with spinal cord injury. *Spinal Cord* 1999;37:601–616.

113. Bauman WA, Adkins RH, Spungen AM, et al. The effect of residual neurological deficit on serum lipoproteins in individuals with chronic spinal cord injury. *Spinal Cord* 1998;36:13–17.

114. Charlifue SW, Gerhart KA, Whiteneck GG. Conceptualizing and quantifying functional change: an examination of aging with spinal cord injury. *Top Geriatr Rehabil* 1998;13:35–48.

115. Gerhart KA, Bergstrom E, Charlifue SW, et al. Long-term spinal cord injury: functional changes over time. *Arch Phys Med Rehabil* 1993; 74:1030–1034.

116. Darnton-Hill I. Healthy aging and the quality of life. *World Health Forum* 1995;16:335–343.

117. Adams PF, Hendershot GE, Marano MA. *Current estimates from the National Health Interview Survey, 1996.* National Center for Health Statistics. Vital and Health Statistics, 1999;10:105.

118. McColl MA, Rosenthal C. A model of resource needs of aging spinal cord injured men. *Paraplegia* 1994;32:261–270.

119. Gerhart KA, Charlifue SW, Menter RR, et al. Aging with spinal cord injury. *Am Rehabil* 1997;23:19–25.

120. Charlifue SW, Weitzenkamp DA, Whiteneck GG. Longitudinal outcomes in spinal cord injury: aging, secondary conditions, and well-being. *Arch Phys Med Rehabil* 1999;80:1429–1434.

121. Krause JS, Crewe NM. Chronologic age, time since injury, and time of measurement: effect on adjustment after spinal cord injury. *Arch Phys Med Rehabil* 1991;72:91–100.

122. Idler EL, Kasl SV. Self-ratings of health: do they also predict change in functional ability? *J Gerontol* 1995;50B:S344–S353.

123. George LK. Social factors and illness. In: Binstock RH, George LK, eds. *Handbook of aging and the social sciences,* 4th ed. San Diego: Academic Press, 1996:229–252.

124. Zautra AJ. Investigations of the ongoing stressful situations among those with chronic illness. *Am J Commun Psychol* 1996;24:697–717.

125. Samuels SC. Midlife crisis: helping patients cope with stress, anxiety, and depression. *Geriatrics* 1997;52:55–64.

126. Pearlin LI, McKean Skaff M. Stress and the life course: a paradigmatic alliance. *Gerontologist* 1996;36:239–247.

127. Cohen S, Frank E, Doyle E, et al. Types of stressors that increase susceptibility to the common cold in healthy adults. *Health Psychol* 1998;17:214–223.

128. Aldwin CM, Sutton KJ, Chiara G, et al. Age differences in stress, coping, and appraisal: findings from the Normative Aging Study. *J Gerontol* 1996;51B:179–188.

129. Musil CM, Haug MR, Warner CD. Stress, health, and depressive symptoms in older adults at three time points over 18 months. *Issues in Mental Health Nursing* 1998;19:207–224.

130. George LK. Depressive disorders and symptoms in later life. *Generations* 1993;17:35–38.

131. Reynolds CF, Kupfer DJ. Depression an aging: a look to the future. *Psychiatric Services* 1999;50:1167–1172.

132. Ford DE, Mead LA, Chang PP, et al. Depression is a risk factor for coronary artery disease in men: the precursors study. *Arch Intern Med* 1998;158:1422–1426.

133. Sesso HD, Kawachi I, Vokonas PS, et al. Depression and the risk of coronary heart disease in the Normative Aging Study. *Am J Cardiol* 1998;82:851–856.

134. Hemingway H, Marmot M. Evidence based cardiology: psychosocial factors in the aetiology and prognosis of coronary heart disease. Systematic review of prospective cohort studies. *Br Med J* 1999;318:1460–1467.

135. Koenig HG. Late-life depression: how to treat patients with comorbid chronic illness. *Geriatrics* 1999;54:56–61.

136. Bassuk SS, Berkman LF, Wypij D. Depressive symptomatology and incident cognitive decline in an elderly community sample. *Arch Gen Psychiatry* 1998;55:1073–1081.

137. Gottfries CG. Is there a difference between elderly and younger patients with regard to the symptomatology and aetiology of depression? *Int Clin Psychopharmacol* 1998;13:S13–S18.

138. Cassileth BR. Psychosocial status in cancer patients. In: Abeles RP, Gift HC, Ory MG, eds. *Aging and quality of life.* New York: Springer, 1994:133–144.

139. Flanagan JC. A research approach to improving our quality of life. *American Psychologist* 1978;33:138–147.

140. Keister KJ, Blixen CE. Quality of life and aging. *J Gerontol Nursing* 1988;24:22–28.

141. Baxter J, Shetterly SM, Eby C, et al. Social network factors associated with perceived quality of life: the San Luis Valley Health and Aging Study. *J Aging Health* 1998;10:287–310.

142. Fisher BJ. Successful aging, life satisfaction, and generativity in later life. *Int J Aging Hum Dev* 1995;41:239–250.

143. Kemp BJ, Krause JS. Depression and life satisfaction among people ageing with post-polio and spinal cord injury. *Disabil Rehabil* 1999;21:241–249.

144. Gerhart KA, Weitzenkamp DA, Kennedy P, et al. Correlates of stress in long-term spinal cord injury. *Spinal Cord* 1999;37:183–190.

145. Rintala DH, Hart KA, Fuhrer MJ. Perceived stress in individuals with spinal cord injury. In: Krotoski DM, Nosek MA, Turk MA, eds. *Women with physical disabilities: achieving and maintaining health and well-being.* Baltimore: Paul H. Brookes, 1996:223–242.

146. Fuhrer MJ, Rintala DH, Hart KA, et al. Depressive symptomatology in persons with spinal cord injury who reside in the community. *Arch Phys Med Rehabil* 1993;74:255–260.

147. Westgren N, Levi R. Quality of life and traumatic spinal cord injury. *Arch Phys Med Rehabil* 1998;79:1433–1439.

148. Post MW, van Dijk AJ, van Asbeck FW, et al. Life satisfaction of persons with spinal cord injury compared to a population group. *Scand J Rehabil Med* 1998;30:23–30.

149. Post MWM, de Witte LP, van Asbeck FWA, et al. Predictors of health status and life satisfaction in spinal cord injury. *Arch Phys Med Rehabil* 1998;79:395–402.

150. Weitzenkamp DA, Gerhart KA, Charlifue SW, et al. Ranking the criteria for assessing quality of life after disability: evidence for priority-shifting among long-term spinal cord injury survivors. *Br J Health Psychol* 2000;5:57–69.

151. McColl MA, Stirling P, Walker J, et al. Expectations of independence and life satisfaction among ageing spinal cord injured adults. *Disabil Rehabil* 1999;21:231–240.

152. Richards JS, Bombardier CH, Tate D, et al. Access to the environment and life satisfaction after spinal cord injury. *Arch Phys Med Rehabil* 1999;80:1501–1506.

153. Fuhrer MJ, Rintala DM, Hart KA, et al. Relationship of life satisfaction to impairment, disability, and handicap among persons with spinal cord injury living in the community. *Arch Phys Med Rehabil* 1992;73:552–557.

154. Clayton KS, Chubon RA. Factors associated with quality of life of long-term spinal cord injured persons. *Arch Phys Med Rehabil* 1994;75:633–638.

155. Dew MA, Lynch K, Ernst J, et al. Reaction and adjustment to spinal cord injury: a descriptive study. *J Appl Rehabil Counseling* 1983;14:31–39.

156. Eisenberg MG, Saltz CC. Quality of life among spinal cord injured persons: long term rehabilitation outcomes. *Paraplegia* 1991;29:514–520.

157. Menter RR. Spinal cord injury and aging: exploring the unknown. 1993 Heiner Sell Lecture of the American Spinal Injury Association. *J Am Paraplegia Assoc* 1993;16:179–189.

158. Pearlin LI, Mullan JT, Semple SJ, et al. Caregiving and the stress process: an overview of concepts and their measures. *Gerontologist* 1990;30:583–594.

159. O'Brien MT. Multiple sclerosis: stressors and coping strategies in spousal caregivers. *J Commun Health Nursing* 1993;10:123–135.

160. Holicky R. Caring for the caregivers: the hidden victims of illness and disability. *Rehabil Nursing* 1996;21:247–252.

161. Schulz R, Visintainer P, Williamson GM. Psychiatric and physical morbidity effects of caregiving. *J Gerontol* 1990;45:181–191.

162. Bush HA, Job SA. Stressors of providing care to the elderly. *AORN J* 1993;57:938–946.

163. Gaynor S. The long haul: the effects of home care on caregivers. *J Nurs Scholarship* 1990;4:208–212.

164. Newsom JT, Schulz R. Caregiving from the recipient's perspective: negative reactions to being helped. *Health Psychology* 1998;17:172–181.

165. Allen SM, Goldscheider F, Ciambrone DA. Gender roles, marital intimacy, and nomination of spouse as primary caregiver. *Gerontologist* 1999;39:150–158.

166. Stoller EP. Gender and the organization of lay health care: a socialist-feminist perspective. *J Aging Studies* 1993;7:151–170.

167. Miller B, Cafasso L. Gender differences in caregiving: fact or artifact? *Gerontologist* 1992;32:498–507.

168. Revenson TA. Social support and marital coping with chronic illness. *Ann Behav Med* 1994;16:122–130.

169. Fougeyrollas P. Documenting environmental factors for preventing the handicap creation process. Quebec contributions relating to ICIDH and social participation of people with functional differences. *Disabil Rehabil* 1995;17:145–153.

170. Brandt EN, Pope AM, eds. *Enabling America: assessing the role of rehabilitation science and engineering.* Washington, DC: National Academy Press, 1997.

171. World Health Organization (WHO). *International classification of functioning and disability: ICIDH-2. Beta-2 draft: full version, July 1999.* Document # WHO/HSC/ACE/99.1.

172. Seigley L. The effects of personal and environmental factors on health behaviors of older adults. *Nurs Connect* 1998;11:47–58.

173. Craig Hospital Research Department. *Craig Hospital inventory of environmental factors (CHIEF) manual.* Englewood, CO: Craig Hospital, 2000.

174. Whiteneck GG, Menter RR. Where do we go from here? In: Whiteneck GG, Charlifue SW, Gerhart KA, et al., eds. *Aging with spinal cord injury.* New York: Demos, 1993:361–369.

TENDON TRANSFERS TO IMPROVE FUNCTION OF PATIENTS WITH TETRAPLEGIA

ROBERT L. WATERS
LINDA MARIE MUCCITELLI

One of the greatest potentials for improving the quality of life in an individual who has suffered a spinal cord injury (SCI) resulting in tetraplegia is through rehabilitation and surgical restoration of upper extremity function. Hanson found that 75% of male patients with tetraplegia preferred restoration of hand function to restoration of bowel, bladder, or sexual function (1). Reconstructive surgery after tetraplegia can often improve the patient's motor function by one level. Careful selection and evaluation of surgical candidates, in combination with an experienced surgeon and hand rehabilitation team, are critical for success. This chapter covers the history of hand surgery related to restoring function after cervical level injury as well as current and innovative surgical procedures; evaluations that provide the surgeon and the hand rehabilitation team with information to choose appropriate candidates for surgical intervention; postoperative care of patients undergoing common surgical procedures; and functional outcomes.

HISTORY

Early trials of surgery to improve paralytic hand function in the SCI population began after World War II. These attempts to improve hand function were often based on experience with hand reconstruction developed for peripheral nerve injuries and commonly failed.

In 1949, Bunnell recommended flexor tenodesis of the thumb and finger flexors (2). This procedure never found favor because of the difficulty in controlling the many joints of the fingers and thumb (3). In 1957, Nickel developed the flexor hinge hand surgical procedure to control the finger and thumb positions (4). In this procedure, all joints of the thumb and fingers are fused with the exception of the metacarpophalangeal (MP) joints of the index and long fingers. The thumb metacarpal is fused to the index metacarpal in a position of abduction opposite the long and index fingers. The flexor digitorum profundus (FDP) or flexor digitorum sublimis (FDS) to the index and long fingers is tenodesed to the radius, and the joints are fused in precise positions. This causes the index and long finger to flex at the MP joints, opposing the palmar surface of their fingertips against the palmar surface of the tip of the thumb in a "three-jaw chuck," when the wrist is actively extended. Although this procedure enabled precise control of pinch, it did not prove practical for SCI patients because the position of the rigidly fused thumb interfered with transfers and manual wheelchair propulsion.

In 1975, Moberg observed that rather than restoring pinch between the tips of the thumb and the fingers, which requires complex reconstruction and precise control of finger position, useful pinch could be obtained by a much simpler method (5). He demonstrated that functional pinch could be easily achieved between the thumb and side of the index finger because this often occurred naturally in patients with C6 tetraplegia if spasticity or contracture in the flexor pollicis longus (FPL) was present. Moberg's key-pinch procedure is the simplest type of hand reconstruction in patients with C6 tetraplegia. The genius of this approach is that by focusing on pinch between the thumb and the side of the index finger, rather than palmar prehension between the pads of the fingers and thumb, it is not necessary to control the exact position of the finger because any point on the side of the middle phalanx of the index finger is adequate for thumb opposition. Moberg's demonstration that a simple procedure could reliably and predictably improve function popularized hand surgery for patients with tetraplegia and generated interest in hand surgery programs, as evidenced by the number of articles published in recent literature (5–24).

PRINCIPLES OF HAND SURGERY AS APPLIED TO TETRAPLEGIA

Tenodesis

Tenodesis action is a fundamental mechanism of hand function that increases the strength of pinch and grasp. In the paralyzed hand, "passive tenodesis" action at the thumb and fingers can allow grasp and release, even in the absence of voluntary motor control. If spasticity or myostatic contracture shortens a paralyzed muscle, the thumb and fingers flex if the wrist is extended. It is a common clinical observation that many patients with C6 tetraplegia, without any active finger or thumb flexion, can pinch or grasp objects by extending the wrist.

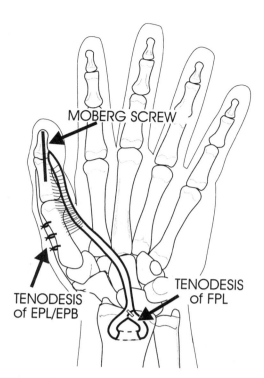

FIGURE 28.1. Moberg's key-grip procedure. (Courtesy of Lydia Cabico.), FPL, flexor pollicis longus; EPL, extensor pollicis longus; EPB, extensor pollicis brevis.

Moberg observed that lateral, or key, pinch between the thumb and side of the index finger was often present in patients having a natural tenodesis of the FPL owing to spasticity or contracture (6). The procedure he devised replicates what he observed as often occurring naturally. In Moberg's procedure, the FPL is sutured to the volar aspect of the radius so that, as the wrist is extended, the thumb opposes the side of the index finger (Fig. 28.1).

Tendon Transfer

The basic principle in reconstructive surgery of this type is to use functioning proximal musculature to control distal parts. For example, the extensor carpi radialis longus (ECRL), which is partially innervated at the C6 level, is transferred to the FDP to enable grasp (function at the C8 motor level). The two tendons are anastomosed under sufficient tension so that maximal force is generated with the wrist in an extended position.

Because patients with tetraplegia have limited muscle function, one of the basic tenets is that the procedures minimize risk for loss of function. Thus, in the example cited previously, the ECRL can only be transferred if the extensor carpi radialis brevis (ECRB) is also strong and can provide wrist extension if the ECRL is transferred to restore finger flexion.

It is generally not possible to perform tendon transfers simultaneously to restore both active opening and closing in one surgical procedure because, in the healing phase, the joints must be held in a position of flexion or extension to avoid tension on the

tendon anastomosis until adequate tendon healing has occurred. Consequently, providing both finger and thumb opening as well as pinch and grasp requires two separately staged procedures.

Arthrodesis

Stabilization of a joint can be achieved by surgical arthrodesis. Surgical arthrodesis is performed by removing the cartilage on either side of the joint and fusing the exposed ends together. The joint is immobilized until bony fusion occurs. Commonly, arthrodesis of the interphalangeal (IP) joint of the thumb is performed with tendon transfer procedures to restore active lateral thumb opposition. In this case, motion is blocked at the IP joint, so that the forces generated by the transferred tendon act at the carpometacarpal or MP joint.

Wrist fusion is generally contraindicated in patients with tetraplegia. Loss of passive wrist extension interferes with manual wheelchair propulsion and transfers.

CANDIDATE SELECTION AND EVALUATION

Timing

Upper extremity surgery should not be performed before patients have completed a program of rehabilitation. This includes functional skills training, proper positioning by means of splints, and active and passive range-of-motion (ROM) programs.

It is recommended that surgery be performed at least 1 year after the injury and that candidates demonstrate neurologic stability for at least 6 months. Serial neurologic examinations should be performed every 3 months to determine when neurologic recovery has plateaued. VandenBerghe and associates stated that if recovery has plateaued, surgery can be considered 6 months after injury (25). Although Ditunno and colleagues (26) reported that recovery in some muscles in tetraplegia could occur up to 24 months after injury, Waters and associates demonstrated that most recovery occurs within 9 months after injury (27,28). As a general rule, delay of surgery for 1 year allows adequate time for neurologic stabilization. Once the timing is appropriate, a detailed assessment of the candidate is necessary to achieve a successful surgical outcome (Table 28.1).

Physical Assessment

Assessments of occupational performance, upper extremity muscle strength, sensation, ROM, and spasticity are performed.

Occupational Performance Assessment

Occupational performance is a term used in occupational therapy that refers to the physical and mental abilities and skills required for satisfactory engagement in a given occupation (29). *Occupation* refers to any activity that occupies a person's time and gives meaning to his or her life. Occupations have multiple dimensions, including performance, contextual, temporal, psychological, social, symbolic, and spiritual. Occupational performance areas include activities of daily living (ADLs), work or productive activities, and play or leisure activities (30). These areas must

TABLE 28.1. CRITERIA FOR CANDIDATE SELECTION AND EVALUATION

Timing
    Functional status maximized
    One year after injury
    Neurologic stability for at least 6 months

Clinical assessment
    Occupational performance status: present status and potential for improvement with surgery
    Manual muscle test: muscle must have 4/5 strength for transfer
    Sensory exam: two-point discrimination
    Range of motion
    Spasticity in hand: must be absent or minimal

Behavioral assessment
    Motivation
    History of compliance and follow-through
    Understanding of expected surgical and functional outcomes
    Commitment to postoperative rehabilitation
    Psychological adjustment
    Social support

be assessed, and the type and degree of functional gains and their impact on occupational performance discussed with the individual before surgical intervention.

Occupational performance is assessed using both informal and standardized evaluations, which may be performance-based, self-assessments, or interview. Performance-based assessments require the therapist to observe the patient performing an activity and rate the patient's ability to accomplish the task. Self-assessment tools are evaluations that are completed by patients regarding their ability to perform certain activities. Informal interviews help to establish a therapeutic relationship and allow the therapist to understand what is meaningful in a patient's life. The purpose of any of these assessments is to provide functional baseline data and patient-identified goals. Standardized measures used to compare preoperative status to follow-up changes are needed to evaluate cost efficiency and effectiveness of surgical intervention, which are of increasing importance in clinical care, quality assurance, and national health care planning. It is therefore imperative that occupational performance and patient-identified goals are measured preoperatively and postoperatively.

Functional assessments provide information regarding the performance dimension of occupation. Among the tools that can be used for patients with SCI are the modified Barthel index, the Functional Independence Measure (FIM), the Self-Care Assessment Tool, the PULSES profile, the Kenny Self Care Evaluation, and the Quadriplegia Index of Function (QIF) (31). Studies have shown that the QIF is more sensitive in detecting changes in the SCI population than the FIM (32) and the Kenny Self Care Evaluation (33).

Evaluating the other components of occupational performance can be achieved through obtaining a patient's occupational history and administering the Canadian Occupational Performance Measure (COPM) (34). During an informal interview, the patient is asked to provide a detailed account of his or her activities for a typical day before onset of disability and how he or she is currently spending time. This allows the thera-

pist to understand what the patient's life was like before the disability and how the disability has interrupted and changed the patient's life. In addition, it provides information regarding a patient's balance of work-rest-leisure, habits and routines, values, role involvement, and the need for further education or equipment. Information gathered during this and other informal assessments will assist the therapist to individualize patient treatment.

The COPM also allows patients to identify occupational performance goals that they either want to, need to, or are expected to perform. Patients are asked to rate their performance and satisfaction for each activity based on a scale between 1 (most negative) and 10 (most positive). When this assessment is performed before surgical intervention, and again after the postoperative rehabilitation process, it provides outcome data that can show change in a patient's perception of performance and satisfaction. This measure has been shown to be sensitive to change in patients' perception of their occupational performance over time (34). Studies reflecting patient performance and satisfaction are needed to justify surgical intervention in today's health care system, where resources for health care are becoming increasingly limited.

The COPM is also helpful in determining appropriate timing for introducing the possibility of surgical intervention during the rehabilitation process. If, for example, a patient identifies on an initial COPM an activity that he or she would like to perform, the therapist first assesses whether the patient can perform the activity with the use of adaptive equipment. If the patient may benefit from the use of equipment, a trial period of training is initiated. After intervention, the COPM can be administered again to evaluate the patient's perception of performance and satisfaction in relation to the activity now performed with equipment. If the patient's performance and satisfaction scores have not improved significantly and the therapist feels that surgical intervention could improve the patient's performance of this activity, the patient is educated regarding the potential benefits of surgery.

Manual Muscle Test

Testing of upper extremity motor groups is performed using the standard six (0 to 5) manual muscle test (MMT) advocated by the American Spinal Injury Association (ASIA) (35). MMT of all upper extremity muscles is important, including the muscles of the shoulder girdle (36). It is important to assess the strength of the shoulder musculature because successful hand function depends on precise placement of the hand as well as function of the musculature of the hand. The results of the MMT provide information regarding the availability of muscles for transfers. If indicated, the patient is seen preoperatively to strengthen muscles that have been selected for tendon transfers. If surgical intervention of both extremities is indicated, the strongest extremity is usually operated on first. If both extremities are of equal strength, the dominant one should be reconstructed first. This affords the patient the maximal functional benefit.

Sensory Examination

In addition to the standard sensory examination performed in SCI (35), Moberg advocates the Weber two-point discrimination test as the most valuable test of sensation (37). There is a correlation between two-point discrimination and accuracy of proprioception at the MP and IP joints. In tetraplegia, two-point discrimination of 10 mm or less at the pulp of the thumb was found to be predictive of proprioception and gnosis adequate for control of hand function without visual cues (37). This sensibility allows the patient greater ease when performing ADLs.

Patient Classification

Both Zancolli (38) and Moberg (39) made significant contributions to the development of tetraplegia hand surgery and patient classification. Zancolli classified patients based on the residual motor function present in the upper extremity. Moberg emphasized the importance of evaluation of sensation in addition to motor function.

To facilitate communication among professionals, a classification based on the segmental innervation of individual muscles of the upper limb was developed at an international conference in Edinburgh, Scotland, in 1978 and later modified to its present form of nine groups in 1984 (40). This International Classification takes into account the motor groups that are functioning and available for transfer, as well as sensibility, and includes the presence or absence of afferent impulses, either visual or cutaneous sensibility or both. Sensibility is tested by measuring two-point discrimination. If only visual or ocular clues are available to control hand function, the patient is classified in the "O" (ocular) group. Individuals in this group have two-point discrimination of greater than 10 mm at the pulp of the thumb. Patients who have both visual clues and cutaneous afferents present (two-point discrimination is less than 10 mm) are classified as "O-Cu" (ocular-cutaneous). Each of these two main groups is further subdivided into 10 subgroups based on the residual motor function present below the elbow (Table 28.2). If only visual afferents are present in an individual with bilateral C5

TABLE 28.2. MODIFIED INTERNATIONAL CLASSIFICATION FOR INDIVIDUALS WITH TETRAPLEGIA

Motor

Group	Functional muscles[a]
0	Weak or absent BR (grade 3 or less)
1	BR
2	BR, ECRL
3	BR, ECRL, ECRB
4	BR, ECRL, ECRB, PT
5	BR, ECRL, ECRB, PT, FCR
6	BR, ECRL, ECRB, PT, FCR, finger extensors
7	BR, ECRL, ECRB, PT, FCR, finger extensors, thumb extensors
8	BR, ECRL, ECRB, PT, FCR, finger extensors, thumb extensors, finger flexors
9	Lacks intrinsics only

Sensory

O:	Two-point discrimination in thumb >10 mm
Cu:	Two-point discrimination I thumb <10 mm

[a]Functional muscle: grade 4 or 5.
BR, brachioradialis; ECRL, extensor carpi radialis longus; ECRB, extensor carpi radialis brevis; PT, pronator teres; FCR, flexor carpi radialis.

TABLE 28.3. RANCHO LOS AMIGOS NEUROLOGIC CLASSIFICATION FOR HAND FUNCTION[a]

Functional Level	Key Muscles[b]	Muscles Functioning
C5	Elbow flexors	Biceps brachialis
		Deltoid
C6	Wrist extensors	ECRL
		ECRB
		Brachioradialis
		Pronator teres
C7	Elbow extensors	Triceps
		EDC
		FCR
C8	Finger flexors	FDP (middle finger)
T1	Small finger abductor	Hand intrinsics

[a]Modified from American Spinal Injury Association standards.
[b]Strength must be at least 4/5.
ECRL, extensor carpi radialis longus; ECRB, extensor carpi radialis brevis; EDC, extensor digitorum communis; FCR, flexor carpi radialis; FDP, flexor digitorum profundus.

motor levels and no digital sensation, Moberg recommends limiting reconstruction to one extremity (5). If cutaneous afferents are also present, both extremities may undergo surgical reconstruction, but it is advisable to perform surgery on only one extremity at a time. However, most patients desire only one hand reconstruction unless they wish to perform a unique task that can only be performed if both hands undergo reconstruction.

The classification system for motor level recommended by ASIA has become widely accepted (35). In this classification system, the motor level is determined by the highest neurologic segment having at least grade 3/5 muscle with the postural muscles having a grade 5/5 (35). However, strength of only 3/5 is insufficient to perform activities that require the muscle to stabilize for more than extremely light loads, and most routine functional demands necessitate greater strength and endurance (8). Thus, a muscle of only grade 3/5 has insufficient strength to meet functional demands, and in our experience, grade 3/5 strength in a muscle is inadequate for tendon transfer.

According to the International Classification, a muscle should have 4/5 strength to be considered functional (8). Therefore, in evaluating muscle strength for consideration of tendon transfer, muscles should be at least grade 4/5. For these reasons, we have modified the ASIA system in our hand clinic for classifying patients into different functional categories for hand reconstruction. The modification consists of defining functional level as the lowest motor segment having 4/5 strength, based on the same key muscle groups and neurologic segments as in the ASIA classification (Table 28.3). This system provides easier communication with rehabilitation providers who are not familiar with the International Classification system but who are familiar with the ASIA system.

Range of Motion

The ROM of all upper extremity joints is assessed. Joints must have sufficient motion to allow for functional use of the extremity after reconstruction. Although each patient must be evaluated individually according to the intended use of the extremity, in general, we have found the following guidelines helpful in achieving maximal functional benefits. For all procedures involving the hand, there must be full ROM at the wrist and the MP joints as well as full perpendicular abduction of the thumb. For the posterior deltoid or biceps-to-triceps transfer, there must be functional ROM at the shoulder and no more than a 30-degree elbow flexion contracture. In the biceps rerouting procedure, there must be at least 0 to 45 degrees of passive pronation and supination. If the procedure is performed to increase function, the elbow range should be within functional limits. If the purpose of the procedure is to correct a supination deformity, an elbow flexion contracture of up to 90 degrees is acceptable.

Spasticity

Spasticity in a muscle should be absent or minimal if it is to be used for tendon transfer because the lack of normal motor function interferes with precise motor recruitment.

Behavioral Assessment

Motivation, History of Compliance, and Follow-through

It is important to evaluate not only potential candidates' motivational level but also their ability to comply and follow-through with a postoperative program. These are critical factors and are extremely important in achieving an optimal outcome (41). The patient's history of adherence with therapeutic measures in the past should be reviewed. Poor history of compliance and follow-through does not necessarily preclude a patient from undergoing surgery; however, it should be considered when making a surgical decision. In some cases, surgery may be deferred while the occupational therapist works with the patient to become more actively engaged in daily occupations.

Understanding Expected Surgical and Functional Outcomes

Candidates must understand the expected outcome of surgery. The surgical procedure for which the patient is being considered and the goals of the surgery are reviewed. It is recommended that candidates observe postoperative rehabilitation and speak with individuals who have undergone the procedure to familiarize themselves with the process and to avoid any unrealistic expectations regarding surgical outcomes. Patients often expect that surgery will provide them with nearly normal upper extremity function. It is important for candidates to understand that surgery may improve their function but will not restore it to preinjury status.

Commitment to Postoperative Rehabilitation

Patients also need to be aware of the commitment to the postoperative rehabilitation process. Education is provided regarding the type and time of immobilization and restrictions, the rehabilitation program, and how these will affect the patient's lifestyle. Special attention needs to be given to individuals who anticipate returning to roles as caretakers or full-time employees because more extensive planning may be necessary to accommodate the relatively long postoperative recovery and rehabilitation time. Additional assistance or equipment is also necessary during recovery for many ADLs, such as weight shifts, transfers, toileting, hygiene, bathing, dressing, feeding, telephone use, and possibly, work. During the postoperative period, patients who use manual wheelchairs need to rely on power wheelchairs or assistance from an attendant. An assessment of possible assistive technology for mobility and ADLs is necessary. The hand control of a power wheelchair may need to be switched, depending on which extremity is undergoing surgery. Equipment needed to enhance the patient's postoperative functional status is ordered, and the patient or caregiver is trained in its use before surgical intervention. The patient must understand that the need for additional physical assistance as a result of postoperative restrictions will last at least 3 months.

Psychological Status and Social Support

Psychological status needs to be assessed before selecting the patient as a candidate for surgery. During the initial phase postoperatively, patients will return to a state of dependency similar to their status immediately after their injury. The ability to adjust to these changes in loss of functional independence and the need for additional assistance after some level of independence has been achieved can be challenging. Providing education that reflects what the patient can expect in the postoperative period is one step toward preparing the patient to face these changes. In addition, the candidate must be able to state a specific plan that demonstrates the ability to meet his or her changing needs. The candidate must have access to additional attendant care and support of family or friends. It is recommended that the candidate be able to direct others in his or her care personally, or to arrange for attendant care training preoperatively.

Decision Making

Based on information gathered during the assessments, a decision is made with the candidate regarding appropriate intervention. If all the physical and behavioral criteria are met and expected functional gains meet the goals of the candidate, surgery is indicated. If the physical or behavioral criteria have not been met, further treatment may be indicated to prepare the patient for potential future therapy or surgical intervention.

If a patient is not performing at his or her maximum functional capacity, functional skills training can be initiated. This includes teaching a patient to use adaptive equipment or techniques to allow performance of certain activities. For example, an individual who has strong wrist extensors but is not self-feeding may be able to accomplish this task with a U-cuff or a wrist-driven wrist-hand orthosis. The patient may have had weakness that prevented him or her from using this equipment effectively during rehabilitation or may have never been educated about its availability. Effective performance of an activity with equipment does not necessarily preclude the patient from having surgery because performing the activity without the use of equipment may still be a goal. However, if there is any potential to improve a patient's function, training should be performed with equipment first because this may be satisfactory to the patient, serving to maximize function without surgical intervention.

Treatment programs can be designed to improve upper extremity muscle strength and ROM if these criteria were not met. If the patient lacks the strength required in a muscle to make it a viable option for transfer (4/5), but has at least a grade 3 + / 5, a strengthening program can be initiated. Patients lacking the ROM required to undergo surgery may be candidates for various methods to gain the needed motion. This can include exercise, serial splinting, or casting.

If the patient has not met the behavioral criteria, a trial outpatient therapy program may be indicated. The purpose of the program is to provide further education, and it allows ongoing assessment of patient readiness. The program is designed based on the problem areas identified during the evaluation process. If poor history of compliance and follow-through was noted, the therapist can design a program consisting of functional skills training, upper extremity exercises, or both. This allows the therapist to reevaluate the patient's motivation and ability to follow through with a program. If the patient demonstrates a lack of understanding in regard to the expected outcome of the procedure or the rehabilitation process, further education should be provided to reinforce the information. In addition, further intervention may be needed to assist the patient in devising a postoperative plan to meet his or her changing functional needs. This may include exploration of adaptive equipment, functional skills training, or caregiver training. Referrals to a case manager, social worker, or psychologist may be indicated. It is extremely important to postpone surgery until the behavioral criteria are met because these elements are just as important as the physical criteria in achieving successful surgical and functional outcomes.

COMMON SURGICAL PROCEDURES
C5 Functional Level (IC 0, 1)

Patients with C5 functional level have functional use of deltoids, elbow flexors (biceps, brachialis, and brachioradialis [BR] mus-

cles), and possibly minimal wrist and hand motion and elbow extension. At the C5 level, the muscles generally available for transfer are the deltoid and BR. In this group, the most helpful procedures are transfer of the BR to the ECRB to restore wrist extension (C6 function) and transfer of the deltoid to triceps to provide elbow extension.

Brachioradialis–to–Extensor Carpi Radialis Brevis Transfer

The BR tendon is released distally from the radius and is dissected proximally until at least 3 cm of excursion from the resting position of the muscle is obtained (Fig. 28.2). To achieve this excursion, it usually is necessary to mobilize the BR tendon and muscle proximally to the level of the elbow joint. The BR tendon is inserted into the ECRB tendon. The tendon is sutured together with the elbow in 90 degrees of flexion, the forearm in neutral rotation, and the wrist in 45 degrees of extension. The tension of the BR should be sufficient to hold the wrist in neutral flexion-extension.

It is difficult to determine the strength of the BR by MMT because it is not possible to isolate its contribution to elbow flexion from the biceps and brachialis. Moberg recommended performing surgery under local anesthesia, detaching the tendinous insertion of the BR and connecting it to a tensiometer (9). The strength of the BR is measured at surgery to determine whether it is suitable for transfer. Although not reported in the literature, we have found that patients with grade 1/5 or 2/5 wrist extension strength preoperatively have adequate strength for BR-to-ECRB transfer.

Freehafer demonstrated that active wrist extension could be provided in patients with wrist extensors lacking strength for tenodesis grasp by transfer of the BR to the ECRB; however, he did not report the percentage of patients with successful results (42).

Johnson and associates reported in a study of nine patients that after BR-to-ECRB transfer, the strength of the wrist extensors improved to a grade of 4/5 in six patients and to a grade of 3 + /5 in three patients. Function of the hand improved markedly in seven patients, and no patient had loss of function. The patients had improvement in the ability to pick up objects, to

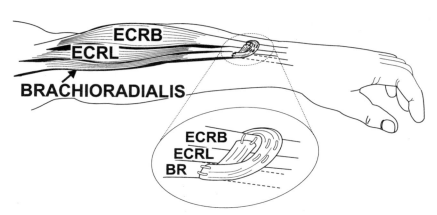

FIGURE 28.2. Transfer of the brachioradialis to the extensor carpi radialis brevis. (Courtesy of Lydia Cabico.), ECRB, extensor carpi radialis brevis; ECRL, extensor carpi radialis longus; BR, brachioradialis.

feed and groom themselves, to tend to personal hygiene, to write and type, and to use a telephone (43).

After surgery, it is easier for patients to use hand orthoses because precision of hand placement is enhanced by the restoration of active motion at the wrist (6). Although wrist extensor strength after BR-to-ECRB transfer is sufficient to provide some wrist control (3 + /5—active movement against gravity with slight resistance), it may not provide sufficient strength (4/5—active movement against gravity with moderate resistance) to obtain strong lateral pinch (6,24).

Posterior Deltoid–to–Triceps Transfer

If patients have 4/5 posterior deltoid strength, a posterior deltoid-to-triceps transfer can be performed. This procedure allows for active elbow extension, enabling patients to stabilize themselves for sitting and transferring and to reach overhead against gravity. At surgery, the interval between the posterior and middle deltoid is identified by the oblique orientation of the fibers of the posterior deltoid in contrast to the vertical fibers of the middle deltoid. The distal end of the deltoid is attached to a free tendon graft from the leg (anterior tibialis tendon or flexor hallucis longus) and to the triceps tendon (Fig. 28.3).

Raczka and associates found that 14 of 22 patients who had undergone posterior deltoid-to-triceps transfer self-reported functional improvement after surgery, whereas 13 patients reported an overall increase in independence (13). The ability to stabilize the arm and reach overhead was the most commonly reported benefit of the surgery. Patients reported functional improvements in the areas of grooming and personal hygiene, pressure relief, writing speed and clarity, and self-feeding (13).

Raczka and associates also found that the ability to transfer was unaffected by unilateral deltoid-to-triceps transfer (13). The reason may be in part related to the fact that the latissimus dorsi is the prime shoulder depressor muscle and plays an important role in wheelchair transfers. Because it is innervated at the same levels as the triceps, patients lacking adequate triceps strength usually have impaired latissimus function, so that restoration of unilateral elbow extension alone may be insufficient to restore independent transfer capability. Nevertheless, these investigators found that two of four patients who underwent bilateral deltoid-to-triceps transfer reported significantly improved transfer ability (13).

Biceps-to-Triceps Transfer

Surgical transfer is performed by transferring the biceps tendon medially instead of laterally to avoid compression of the radial nerve. The tendon of the biceps is sutured to the triceps (44, 45).

Several investigators have reported results of biceps-to-triceps tendon transfer. In a series of 13 such procedures, Revol and coauthors reported that active elbow extension was obtained in each case and the mean torque of the elbow was 3.7 Nm (44). Although elbow flexion strength declined 47% because of the loss of the biceps as a flexor, no patients complained about the reduction.

Kuz and associates reviewed four biceps-to-triceps transfers for active elbow extension in three patients with tetraplegia using medial routing technique (45). All three patients had marked functional improvement in activities that involve active elbow extension, and no loss of function was noted in any activities. No patient achieved less than grade 4 extension strength; none had an extension lag greater than eight degrees. Supination and flexion strength after transfer were rated as at least grade 4 in each limb.

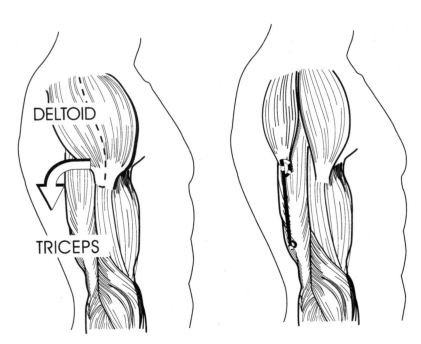

FIGURE 28.3. Transfer of the posterior deltoid to the triceps. (Courtesy of Lydia Cabico.)

C6 Functional Level (IC 2, 3, 4)

Moberg's Key-grip Procedure: Passive Flexor Pollicis Longus Tenodesis

To restore the lateral, or key, grip in patients without a natural tenodesis, Moberg surgically created FPL tenodesis by securing the proximal end of the tendon to the distal radius (9). To prevent thumb IP joint flexion, an intermedullary screw is percutaneously inserted through the distal tip of the thumb and placed across the IP joint. The extensor pollicis longus (EPL) and extensor pollicis brevis (EPB) tendons are secured proximal to the MP joint to prevent excess flexion. It is necessary that the fingers be positioned in flexion to provide lateral support for thumb opposition (5). If the patient lacks a natural tenodesis of the finger flexors, this can be created surgically. Because the force of thumb opposition is generated by wrist dorsiflexion, pinch force is directly related to wrist extensor torque (6).

Colyer and Kappelman reported that six of eight patients who had undergone FPL tenodesis to restore lateral pinch were pleased with postoperative results. Three individuals were able to perform postoperative self-catheterization, and one was able to handle papers, which led to self-employment. Ease and speed of performing manual tasks improved after surgery, as did scores on the Jebsen hand function test (17).

Reiser and Waters reported on the long-term follow-up of patients who underwent the Moberg procedure (24). Seven of the nine patients who had undergone the Moberg procedure an average of 7.4 years earlier continued to report enhancement of function. Functional activities most commonly improved were grooming, eating, writing, and desktop skills. Function in the early postoperative period was not compared with functional status at the follow-up time of the study.

Active Tendon Transfers for Lateral Pinch

Most surgeons now agree that, when possible, transfer of an active motor (muscle) to the FPL to provide lateral pinch and to the finger flexors to provide grasp provides better function and is preferable to Moberg's simple FPL tenodesis (6,7,10,11, 15,46,47). With passive tenodesis, control of distal function by proximal joint movement eliminates a degree of freedom of hand placement and precision of movement because wrist motion must simultaneously accompany pinch. Because pinch can be obtained independently of wrist position after active tendon transfer, the precision, versatility, and usefulness of pinch is enhanced in comparison to FPL tenodesis. Additionally, we have found that active tendon transfers are generally preferable to passive tenodesis; the latter procedures may stretch because the hands are used for weightbearing, transfers, and manual wheelchair propulsion (6). Patients who have grade 4/5 wrist extension strength suitable for Moberg's FPL tenodesis have sufficient BR strength to perform BR-to-FPL transfer. Therefore, for the reasons cited previously, we no longer perform FPL tenodesis to achieve lateral pinch. To provide lateral pinch, tendon transfer of the BR to the FPL has been our procedure of choice (6) (Fig. 28.4).

The BR is released and sutured into the FPL tendon in the forearm. A Moberg screw is inserted into the thumb to provide

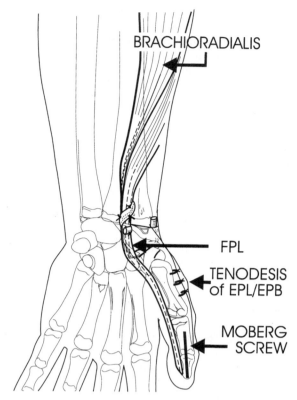

FIGURE 28.4. Transfer of the brachioradialis to the flexor pollicis longus for active lateral pinch. (Courtesy of Lydia Cabico.), FPL, flexor pollicis longus; EPL, extensor pollicis longus; EPB, extensor pollicis brevis.

IP stabilization. The thumb extensors are tenodesed to the first metacarpal unless they are volitional. A K-wire is inserted across the MP joint.

Brachioradialis to Flexor Pollicis Longus

Waters and associates reported functional improvement in 15 of 17 hands after transfer of the BR to FPL (6). Twelve patients reported at least four functional activities (hygiene, grooming, mobility, and writing) that they were able to perform more efficiently after surgery. Nine patients were able to pick up a pen and write, and the five patients who required a wrist-hand orthosis preoperatively were able to grasp objects without it after surgery.

Brachioradialis to Flexor Pollicis Longus Combined with Posterior Deltoid to Triceps

Paul and associates evaluated the outcome in 10 arms of nine patients who had posttraumatic tetraplegia at the fifth or sixth cervical level after combined transfer of the BR to the FPL and the posterior deltoid to the triceps tendon to restore key pinch and extension of the elbow (48). Key pinch improved from essentially none preoperatively to an average of 2 pounds postoperatively: an average of 3 pounds for the patients who had tetraplegia at the sixth cervical level and an average of 0.9 pound for those who had tetraplegia at the fifth cervical level. There was an improvement in the performance of ADLs, including wheelchair use, and most of the patients discontinued use of special equipment for the upper extremity. The results of this study, when compared with those of each procedure performed separately, suggested that a combination of the operations improves function of the upper extremity and shortens the duration of dependence because there is only one rehabilitation phase (48).

Transfer to Flexor Digitorum Profundus to Provide Finger Flexion

To provide finger flexion, tendon transfer to the FDP has been the procedure of choice because it provides grasp and a firm surface for lateral or palmar thumb pinch. The flexor carpi radialis, pronator teres (PT), and ECRL have all been used as motors for lateral pinch and for finger flexion.

Both one-stage and two-stage reconstructive procedures have been advocated (49). In the first stage, tendon transfers and surgical tenodeses are performed to enable finger extension in response to active wrist flexion. Tendon transfer to obtain active finger or thumb flexion is then performed as a second-stage procedure.

Lamb and Chan argued that restoration of active flexion and extension of the fingers is too ambitious (15). Their recommendation was to provide grasp by active finger flexion and allow release to be accomplished by wrist flexion, relaxing the flexors and using the natural tenodesis effect of the extensors. We have confirmed these observations (6,50).

We prefer transfer of the BR to the FPL but prefer PT to the FDP. In agreement with Lamb and Chan, we found that surgical procedures to restore thumb and finger opening were unnecessary and that adequate finger and thumb opening could be obtained by volar flexion of the wrist (6). The strength of lateral pinch after active tendon transfer of the BR is about the same as after passive tenodesis of the FPL (Moberg's procedure) when patient groups are controlled for wrist extensor torque (3,24). However, precision, versatility, and utility of pinch are enhanced after active transfer.

Although Lamb and others report good results after transfer of the ECRL to the tendons of the FDP, some patients with good ECRL function may not have equally good ECRB function. Lamb and Chan reported weakness of wrist dorsiflexion postoperatively in 6 of 45 hands after transfer of the ECRL to the FDP (15). Surgery can be performed under local anesthesia, and the strength of the ECRB can be directly determined at the time of surgery after detachment of the ECRL.

In our experience, it is possible to differentiate ECRB and ECRL strength by MMT preoperatively. The ECRL has a higher innervation than the ECRB, and motor recovery occurs before recovery in the ECRB. Patients who have strong ECRL function and weak ECRB strength are unable to dorsiflex the wrist without marked radial wrist deviation. Patients who also have strong ECRB function are able to achieve strong wrist dorsiflexion without maximal radial wrist deviation.

The PT has been our choice to serve as an active motor for the FDP tendons and for restoring finger flexion rather than transfer of the ECRL (50). Of all the available motors, we think that the PT is the most expendable and results in the least functional deficit.

Brachioradialis to Flexor Pollicis Longus Combined with Extensor Carpi Radialis Longus to Flexor Digitorum Profundus

Lamb and Chan used the BR tendon as a motor for the FPL tendon and the ECRL to power the FDP, leaving the ECRB to provide wrist extension. Eighty-three percent of patients undergoing these transfers were assessed to have excellent or good results, and none reported impairment of hand function as a result of surgery (15).

Lo and associates reviewed eight patients with C6 tetraplegia who underwent 12 procedures at an average of 3.8 years of follow-up (51). There were three bilateral procedures. All patients had BR-to-FPL and ECRL-to-FDP transfers to improve grasp strength and key pinch. Subjective improvement in quality of life, ADLs, and patient-identified goals were reported in all patients. Objective tests showed mild improvement in key pinch and grip strength.

Brachioradialis to Flexor Pollicis Longus Combined with Pronator Teres to Flexor Digitorum Profundus

Waters and associates reported the results after PT-to-FDP transfer in conjunction with BR transfer to the FPL. Ten of 11 patients reported significant improvement in their ability to control a manual wheelchair. Patients reported improved ability to dress themselves because they could grasp the loops on their pants. They could also hold a glass more firmly and open a jar. Independence in bowel and bladder care, however, is related more to the restoration of lateral pinch than to active finger flexion (50).

Ainsley and associates reported on patient satisfaction after tenodesis transfers for opening and active transfers for gross grasp and lateral pinch (41). Twenty-one of 23 patients stated they were satisfied with their gains and glad that they had undergone the surgical procedures. They reported gains in self-care activities and decreased need for attendants. Grasp strength in these individuals was not measurable preoperatively, but 1 year after surgery, it averaged 13 pounds. Lateral pinch strength averaged 5 pounds.

Posterior Deltoid–to–Triceps Transfer

Functional C6 patients may also lack triceps function. Unlike most functional C5 patients, functional C6 patients lacking triceps function usually have grade 4 posterior deltoid strength sufficient to achieve adequate motor elbow extension. Moberg recommended that the deltoid-to-triceps transfer to restore elbow extension be performed before hand reconstruction (9). We have found that both deltoid-to-triceps transfer and hand surgery can be done simultaneously without diminishing outcomes (48).

Biceps Brachii Rerouting

Paralytic supination contracture of the forearm may be seen in patients with absent or minimal neurologic function caudal to the fifth cervical nerve root. Patients with active elbow flexion

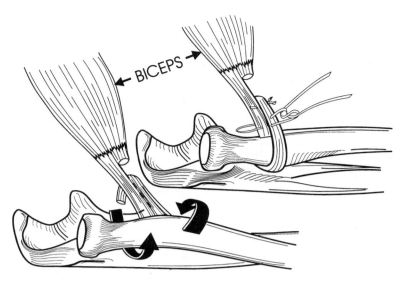

FIGURE 28.5. Rerouting of the biceps to correct paralytic supination deformity. (Courtesy of Lydia Cabico.)

and wrist extension may also have supination deformity and are unable to benefit from active wrist motion. When the forearm is supinated, unopposed gravity maintains the wrist in dorsiflexion, eliminating the functional usefulness of active wrist dorsiflexion. The contracture is the result of unopposed supination by the biceps and the supinator, with concomitant paralysis of the pronator teres. Therefore, these patients have difficulty performing ADLs such as grooming, feeding, and writing, as well as wheelchair propulsion using a joystick, owing to lack of forearm pronation, which is necessary for successful use of splints, orthoses, and effective wrist extension.

Paralytic supination contracture can be corrected by rerouting of the biceps brachii dorsally and laterally around the radial neck (52–54) (Fig. 28.5). The interosseous membrane may be divided, as recommended by Zancolli (54), or left intact (52). This procedure is performed in 75% of our patients with this deformity. It is a simple procedure with no need for reeducation of the muscles and is therefore less problematic.

Gellman and associates studied six patients with traumatic tetraplegia who had undergone lengthening and rerouting of the biceps brachii (52). A total of eight arms were surgically treated. They concluded that patient satisfaction could be predicted based on a postoperative functional ROM. Performance of ADLs was enhanced when the procedure was performed on the dominant extremity. Patients who underwent surgical correction of their supination deformity on the dominant extremity reported improvement in the ability to feed and groom themselves, perform personal hygiene, and write and type. These investigators did not find any decrease in elbow flexion strength postoperatively. Maximal gains in ROM were noted after 3 months, whereas maximal functional gain occurred after 6 months. Passive pronation of 90 degrees was obtained in seven of eight forearms postoperatively. At an average postoperative follow-up of 27 months, all patients had retained at least 80 degrees of pronation.

C7 Functional Level (IC 5, 6, 7)

Patients with a C7 motor level have functional wrist extensors, PT, finger extensors, and triceps. Because both the triceps and latissimus dorsi are innervated by C7 and C8, they lack normal strength at the C7 level. They also lack finger and thumb flexion and intrinsic musculature of the hand. The goals of hand surgery at this functional level are to restore active grasp and to improve hand control. Because patients with C7 tetraplegia may have active finger and thumb extension, they do not develop a natural tenodesis of the finger flexor tendons and, paradoxically, may be less functional preoperatively than individuals with C6 tetraplegia lacking active finger extension. Those patients having active thumb extension through the EPL may be able to pinch. However, the thumb is supinated, and pinch is usually in the plane of the palm. Restoration of the thumb flexion can be achieved by transfer of the BR to FPL. Restoration of finger flexion is achieved through transfer of ECRL, flexor carpi ulnaris, or PT to the FDP (6,17,46).

C8 Functional Level (IC 8)

Patients with function at this level lack intrinsic hand musculature. They are able to flex and extend the fingers because of intact extrinsic muscle function; however, the resulting muscle imbalance from the unopposed extrinsic finger flexors and extensors usually results in an intrinsic minus or "claw-hand" posture. Because patients with finger intrinsic musculature generally have good hand function despite diminished grip strength and an intrinsic minus posture, surgery is rarely indicated. A lumbrical bar splint, which prevents hyperextension of the MPs, may improve a patient's function.

Tendon transfers to restore finger intrinsic function after peripheral nerve injuries or leprosy are technically complicated and have yielded inconsistent results in our experience when applied to tetraplegia. If the transfer is set at sufficient tension to improve grip strength significantly, simultaneous wrist and MP extension may be restricted, interfering with mobility, which usually requires placement of the hand in a flat position with the wrist dorsiflexed to get in and out of a wheelchair. Also, we do not recommend capsulodesis of the MP joints to correct intrinsic minus deformity because this procedure also prevents MP extension to the neutral position.

In contrast to the fingers, many patients benefit from restoration of intrinsic thumb function. Freehafer devised a simple and innovative procedure using the FDS of the ring finger tendon as an *in situ* vascularized graft (42). The tendon of the FDS is detached proximally and anastomosed to the distal end of the PT, which is detached from the radius. The sublimis tendon is cut distally at the level of the MP joint of the ring finger and retrieved in the palm at the distal end of the transverse carpal ligament. It is then rerouted and inserted into the tendon of the abductor pollicis brevis at the thumb MP joint. This tendon transfer substitutes for paralysis of the adductor pollicis and improves pinch strength against the side of the index finger. Additionally, it exerts a counterclockwise rotational force on the thumb to balance the clockwise rotational force exerted by the EPL, improving the precision of thumb control.

Postoperative Rehabilitation

Postoperative care is based on the type of surgery performed. Protocols are determined through collaboration of surgeons and therapists. This does not preclude the need for close communication among the physician, therapist, and patient to ensure individualized patient care. Deviations from the protocol may be required depending on the surgical result and the patient's progress. The ultimate goal during the rehabilitative phase is that all treatment be both safe and effective.

Immobilization

Immobilization of the extremity in a plaster cast is the first step after surgery. The period of immobilization will vary depending on the surgery and the protocol established between the surgeon and therapist. After placement of the cast, the extremity is evaluated to assess for areas of constriction, discoloration, or poor circulation. Immobilization is the first step that influences adhesion formation. The position of the extremity in the cast allows adhesions to form that hold the extremity in the desired position. Early passive motion that is recommended for prevention of adhesions after a tendon repair is not as critical with tendon transfers because the approach used by the surgeon during a tendon transfer procedure is usually through tissue that has not been injured or has minimal scar. Therefore, problems with adhesions are lessened.

During the immobilization period, the therapist provides intervention to address patients' functional needs. This includes training in the use of adaptive equipment or compensatory techniques to allow the patients to maximize their level of independence. In addition, caregiver training may be needed for activities patients are unable to perform by themselves.

Edema Management

The patient is instructed in proper positioning techniques to control edema. The extremity is elevated after surgery to avoid dependent edema. Problem solving with the patient to determine the most appropriate position while the patient is sitting and sleeping is important. The use of pillows, wedges, or other devices may be needed to achieve the desired position. It is helpful to tell the patient the extremity must always be higher than the heart. Active ROM of the uninvolved joints is also encouraged at this time, not only to control edema, but also to maintain range and strength. Instruction in retrograde massage to reduce swelling may be indicated.

Scar Management

Management of scars can begin after the cast is removed. The extremity is soaked in water, and the scar is massaged with a lotion. The scars and adjacent tissue can be massaged by applying deep, slow, circular pressure with the finger pads to stimulate circulation and help break down adhesions. The goal is to soften the subcutaneous scar, which is often thick and attenuated to the skin and deeper soft tissue structures. Some form of a compressive device, such as a silicone gel pad, can be incorporated into the program to minimize the scar.

Occasionally, the patient's scars are hypersensitive. Treatment of these hypersensitive scars includes desensitization techniques. Rubbing progressively coarser fabrics and materials over the scar helps to reduce sensitivity. Transcutaneous electrical nerve stimulation can be used if conventional desensitization techniques are not effective (55).

Mobilization

The goals of therapy during the mobilization period are to protect the transfer, reeducate the muscle, improve ROM and strength, and incorporate the tendon transfer into functional activities. After the patient is cleared for motion, a removable thermoplastic splint, which places the extremity in the same position as the postsurgical cast, is fabricated to protect the transfers from overstretching. During the initial stages of the mobilization period, the splint is removed during the exercise periods and when the patient is bathing or dressing. As light functional activities are introduced into the therapy program, the time in the splint is gradually reduced. The splint may be used for protection at night for as long as 3 months.

Gentle active exercise is initiated within restrictions, and reeducation of the transferred muscle begins. Facilitation techniques, which provide visual and tactile cues, can be used. This includes tapping over the tendon insertion or stroking or applying pressure over the muscle belly. The patient gradually progresses from active assistive motions to active and resistive ones. Initially, short periods of 20 minutes of exercise should be performed six to eight times a day, with adequate rest periods between sessions because the muscle may fatigue.

If contraction of the rerouted muscle is not obtained volitionally and if strengthening is needed, modalities such as biofeedback and therapeutic electrical stimulation can help reeducate muscles after tendon transfers (6,56). During rehabilitation, the transferred muscles undergo motor reeducation and develop the recruitment pattern of a primary motor. A study evaluating motor reeducation using electromyograms in patients after tendon transfer demonstrated that motor reeducation occurs after surgery (57). Success after tendon transfer depends on reeducating the pattern of motor recruitment so that the muscle of the transferred tendon fires appropriately to its new function rather than the old function. We have found biofeedback and other training techniques to be valuable adjuncts to sensorimotor reeducation in some patients.

Functional Skills Training

Once voluntary contraction of the transferred muscles is obtained, light ADLs are incorporated into the treatment program. This allows the patient to begin to associate the transfer with function, which helps effective activation of the transfer. Activities are graded progressively by performance time and resistance applied, eliminating any that create heavy resistance to the tendons until after 3 months. Activities should focus on the desired functional outcomes as stated by the patient during the preoperative evaluation process.

Strengthening

The mobilization phase progresses toward full ROM and strength when resistance can be applied. Resistance exercises that isolate the transferred muscle can be developed with the use of putty or free weights. However, because the surgery is designed to restore function rather than a particular motion, resistive exercises should be presented in the form of functional activities whenever possible. Craft activities, such as woodworking, copper tooling, and macramé, are often used because they can be graded and are repetitious.

INNOVATIVE PROCEDURES

Many research centers are using neuromuscular electrical stimulation (NMES) systems with patients who have C4, C5, and C6 tetraplegia. Devices have been developed that allow NMES to provide upper extremity function through the use of surface electrodes, percutaneous electrodes, and implanted systems. In addition, some of these procedures have been performed in combination with surgical reconstruction. The goals of these procedures include providing grasp and release (58) and lateral and palmar prehension (59) for those individuals who cannot achieve this by tendon transfers alone.

Functional Outcomes

Bionic Glove

The bionic glove, developed by Prochazka and colleagues at the University of Alberta, uses NMES coupled with an orthotic glove for grasp (60). These investigators reviewed nine patients with C6 to C7 tetraplegia who had used the bionic glove for at least 1 year. Results showed that active force of tenodesis grasp was significantly greater than passive grasp and that most manual tasks improved significantly. In a study by Popovic and associates, 12 patients with C5 to C7 tetraplegia who had used the device for 6 months or longer were reviewed (61). Results showed that the bionic glove could significantly improve independence in this population if their initial FIM and QIF scores are 20% to 50% of the maximum values.

Neuromuscular Electrical Stimulation Combined with Orthoses

Nathan and Ohry reported results in two patients with C4 tetraplegia who used a computerized NMES system combined with an orthosis for reaching and grasping (62). Improvements were noted in writing, drinking, and picking up and replacing the pen or cup.

Smith and associates reviewed the results of the application of NMES combined with a suspended sling to provide upper extremity function in a patient with C4 tetraplegia (63). The patient demonstrated the ability to perform hand-to-mouth activities once the item was placed in his hand.

Hand Neuroprosthesis

Stroh and associates reviewed 34 patients from eight different centers with C5 or C6 motor level who underwent procedures for an implantable hand neuroprosthesis (64). Results indicated that 87% of the patients were very satisfied with the neuroprosthesis, 88% reported a positive impact on their life, 87% reported improvements in ADLs, and 81% reported improved independence. Patients reported using the device a median of 5.5 days per week. Fifteen patients reported using the neuroprosthesis 7 days per week, and five reported not using the device at all.

A follow-up study by Mulcahey and associates reviewed five patients with C5 or C6 tetraplegia who underwent surgical reconstruction and implantation of the NMES system (58). Results showed improvement in pinch and grasp force, improved ability to manipulate six standard objects, and increased independence in six ADLs. All participants reported that they were generally satisfied with the NMES for performing most of the ADLs tested.

Davis and associates reported improvement in an adolescent with C5 tetraplegia who underwent bilateral tendon transfers and implantation of the FreeHand system in the right dominant extremity (65). Tendon transfers consisted of bilateral posterior deltoid to triceps and BR to ECRB, and on the left upper extremity, the FPL tendon was tied into the radius and the thumb IP was tenodesed using the distal end of the FPL. Improvements were noted in occupational performance with all activities the patient identified as important during the administration of the COPM. These activities included shaving independently after setup, eating soup without adaptive splints, performing upper-body dressing, accessing personal belongings in drawers and closets, and preparing a sandwich. The COPM performance score of these goals increased from 17.6 to 40.2, and satisfaction scores increased from 12.8 to 38.2. The total FIM score increased 6 points after right upper extremity tendon transfers and NMES and a total of 18 points after left upper extremity tendon transfers. These scores demonstrate improvement in both patient performance and satisfaction. After surgery, right pinch strength improved from 0 to mean scores of 1.89 pounds for lateral pinch and 2.30 pounds for palmar pinch. The left pinch force improved from a mean score of 0.33 pounds to 1.33 pounds (65).

SUMMARY

Upper extremity surgical intervention for individuals who have sustained a SCI resulting in tetraplegia has evolved over the years. These procedures can improve function, adding to the quality of life. Careful patient selection, combined with an experienced hand surgeon and therapist, is essential for a successful outcome. Studies demonstrating functional outcomes and patient satisfaction are critical during these times of limited health care resources.

REFERENCES

1. Hanson RW, Franklin WR. Sexual loss in relation to other functional losses for spinal cord injured males. *Arch Phys Med Rehabil* 1976;57:291–293.
2. Bunnell S. *Tendon transfers in the hand and forearm.* American Academy of Orthopaedic Surgeons, Instructional Course Lectures, No. 6. St. Louis: CV Mosby, 1949.
3. Street DM, Stambaugh HD. Finger flexor tenodesis. *Clin Orthop* 1959;13:155–163.
4. Nickel VL, Perry J, Garrett AL. Development of useful function in the severely paralyzed hand. *J Bone Joint Surg* 1963;45A:933–952.
5. Moberg EA. The present state of surgical rehabilitation for the upper limb in tetraplegia. *Paraplegia* 1987;25:351–356.
6. Waters R, Moore K, Graboff S, et al. Brachioradialis to flexor pollicis longus tendon transfer for active lateral pinch in the tetraplegic. *J Hand Surg [Am]* 1985;10(3):385–391.
7. Hentz VR, Brown M, Keoshian LA. Upper limb reconstruction in quadriplegia: functional assessment and proposed treatment modification. *J Hand Surg [AM]* 1983;8:119–131.
8. Moberg E, Freehafer AA, Lamb DK, et al. International federation of societies for surgery of the hand: a report from the committee on spinal injuries 1980. *Scand J Rehab Med* 1982;14:3–5.
9. Moberg E. *The upper limb in tetraplegia, a "new approach" to surgical rehabilitation.* Stuttgart: George Thieme, 1978.
10. House JH, Gwathmey FW, Lundsgaard DK. Restoration of strong grasp and lateral pinch in tetraplegia due to cervical spinal cord injury. *J Hand Surg [AM]* 1976;1:152–159.
11. House JH, Shannon M. Restoration of strong grasp and lateral pinch in tetraplegia: a comparison of two methods of thumb control in each patient. *J Hand Surg [Am]* 1985;10(1):22–29.
12. Brys D, Waters RL. Effect of triceps function on the brachioradialis transfer in quadriplegia. *J Hand Surg [Am]* 1987;12:237–239.
13. Raczka R, Braun R, Waters RL. Posterior deltoid-to-triceps transfer in quadriplegia. *Clin Orthop* 1984;187:163–167.
14. Hiersche DL, Waters RL. Interphalangeal fixation of the thumb in Moberg's key grip procedure. *J Hand Surg [Am]* 1985;10:30–32.
15. Lamb DW, Chan KM. Surgical reconstruction of the upper limb in traumatic tetraplegia. *J Bone Joint Surg [Br]* 1983;65:291–298.
16. Zancolli E. Functional restoration for the upper limb in traumatic quadriplegia. *Structural and dynamic basis of hand surgery*, 2nd ed. Philadelphia: JB Lippincott, 1979.
17. Colyer R, Kappelman B. Flexor pollicis longus tenodesis in tetraplegia at the sixth cervical level. *J Bone Joint Surg [Am]* 1981;63:376–379.
18. Freehafer AA, Kelly CM, Peckham PH. Tendon transfer for the restoration of upper limb function after a cervical spinal cord injury. *J Hand Surg [Am]* 1984;9:887–893.
19. Freehafer AA, Kelly CM, Peckham PH. Planning tendon transfers in tetraplegia: "Cleveland technique." In: Hunter J, Schneider L, Mackin E, eds. *Tendon surgery in the hand.* St. Louis: CV Mosby, 1987.
20. House J. Reconstruction of the thumb in tetraplegia following spinal cord injury. *Clin Orthop* 1985;195:117–128.
21. Kelly C, Freehafer A, Peckham P, et al. Postoperative results of opponensplasty and flexor tendon transfer in patients with spinal cord injuries. *J Hand Surg [Am]* 1985;10:890–894.
22. Lacey SH, Wilber RG, Peckham PH, et al. The posterior deltoid to triceps transfer: a clinical and biomechanical assessment. *J Hand Surg [Am]* 1986;11:542–547.
23. Smith AG. Early complications of key grip hand surgery for tetraplegia. *Paraplegia* 1981;19:123–126.
24. Reiser T, Waters RL. Long term follow up of the Moberg key grip procedure. *J Hand Surg [Am]* 1986;11:724–728.
25. VandenBerghe A, VanLaere M, Hellings S, et al. Reconstruction of the upper extremity in tetraplegia: functional assessment, surgical procedures and rehabilitation. *Paraplegia* 1991;29(2):103–112.
26. Ditunno JF, Stover SL, Freed MM, et al. Motor recovery of the upper extremities in traumatic quadriplegia: a multicenter study. *Arch Phys Med Rehabil* 1992;73:431–436.
27. Waters RL, Adkins RH, Yakura JS, et al. Motor and sensory recovery following incomplete tetraplegia. *Arch Phys Med Rehabil* 1994;75:306–311.
28. Waters RL, Adkins RH, Yakura JS, et al. Motor and sensory recovery following complete tetraplegia. *Arch Phys Med Rehabil* 1993;74:242–247.
29. American Occupational Therapy Association. Uniform terminology for occupational therapy, 3rd ed. *Am J Occup Ther* 1994;48:1047–1054.
30. Pedretti LW. Occupational performance: a model for practice in physical dysfunction. In: Pedretti LW, ed. *Occupational therapy practice skills for physical dysfunction*, 4th ed. St. Louis: CV Mosby, 1996:3–12.
31. Yavuz N, Tezyurek M, Akyuz, M. A comparison of two functional tests in quadriplegia: the quadriplegia index of function and the functional independence measure. *Spinal Cord* 1998;36:832–837.
32. Marino RJ, Huang M, Knight P, et al. Assessing self care status in quadriplegia: comparison of the quadriplegia index of function (QIF) and the functional independence measure (FIM). *Paraplegia* 1993;31:225–233.
33. Gresham GE, Labi MLC, Dittmar SS, et al. The quadriplegia index of function (QIF): sensitivity and reliability demonstrated in a study of thirty quadriplegic patients. *Paraplegia* 1986;24:38–44.
34. Law M, Baptiste S, Carswell A, et al. *Canadian occupational performance measure*, 2nd ed. Ottawa: Canadian Association of Occupational Therapists, 1994.
35. American Spinal Injury Association. *Standards for neurological and functional classification of spinal cord injury (revised).* Chicago: Author, 1996.
36. Murphy C, Chuinard R. Management of the upper extremity in traumatic tetraplegia. *Hand Clin* 1988;4:201–209.
37. Moberg E. Surgical rehabilitation of the upper limb in tetraplegia. *Paraplegia* 1990;28:330–334.
38. Zancolli EA. Surgery for the quadriplegic hand with active, strong wrist extension preserved: a study of 97 cases. *Clin Orthop* 1975;112:101–113.
39. Moberg E. Criticism and study of methods for examining sensibility in the hand. *Neurology* 1962;12:8–19.
40. McDowell CL, Moberg EA, House JH. The Second International Conference on Surgical Rehabilitation of the Upper Limb in Traumatic Quadriplegia. *J Hand Surg [Am]* 1986;11:604–608.
41. Ainsley J, Voorhees C, Drake E. Reconstructive hand surgery for quadriplegic persons. *Am J Occup Ther* 1985;39:715–721.
42. Freehafer AA. Tendon transfers in patients with cervical spinal cord injury. *J Hand Surg [Am]* 1991;16:804–809.
43. Johnson DL, Gellman H, Waters RL, et al. Brachioradialis transfer for wrist extension in tetraplegic patients who have fifth-cervical-level neurological function. *J Bone Joint Surg [Am]* 1996;78:1063–1067.

44. Revol M, Briand E, Servant JM, Biceps-to-triceps transfer in tetraplegia: the medial route. *J Hand Surg [Br]* 1999;24(2):235–237.

45. Kuz JE, Van Heest AE, House JH. Biceps-to-triceps transfer in tetraplegic patients: report of the medial routing technique and follow-up of three cases. *J Hand Surg [AM]* 1999;24(1):161–172.

46. Freehafer AA, Von Hamm E, Allen V. Tendon transfers to improve grasp after injuries of the cervical spinal core. *J Bone Joint Surg [Am]* 1974;56(6):951–959.

47. Lamb DW, Landry RM. The hand in quadriplegia. *Paraplegia* 1971; 9:204–212.

48. Paul SD, Gellman H, Waters R, et al. Single-stage reconstruction of key pinch and extension of the elbow in tetraplegic patients. *J Bone Joint Surg [Am]* 1994;76(10):1451–1456.

49. Lipscomb P, Elkins E, Henderson E. Tendon transfers to restore function of hands in tetraplegia, especially after fracture-dislocation of the sixth cervical vertebra on the seventh. *J Bone Joint Surg [Am]* 1958; 40(5):1071–1080.

50. Gansel J, Waters RL, Gellman H. Pronator teres to flexor digitorum profundus transfer in quadriplegia. *J Bone Joint Surg [Am]* 1990;72(3): 427–432.

51. Lo IK, Turner R, Connolly S, et al. The outcome of tendon transfers for C6-spared quadriplegics. *J Hand Surg [BR]* 1998;23(2):156–161.

52. Gellman H, Kan D, Waters RL, et al. Rerouting of the biceps brachii for paralytic supination contracture of the forearm in tetraplegia due to trauma. *J Bone Joint Surg [Am]* 1994;76:398–402.

53. Owings R, Wickstrom J, Perry J, et al. Biceps rerouting in treatment of paralytic supination contracture of the forearm. *J Bone Joint Surg [Am]* 1971;53:137–142.

54. Zancolli E. Paralytic supination contracture of the forearm. *J Bone Joint Surg [Am]* 1967;49:1275–1284.

55. Waylett-Rendall J. Desensitization of the traumatized hand. In: Hunter JM, Mackin EJ, Callahan AD, eds. *Rehabilitation of the hand: surgery and therapy*, 4th ed. St. Louis: CV Mosby, 1995:693–700.

56. Gellman H. The hand and upper limb in tetraplegia. *Curr Orthop* 1991;5:233–238.

57. Waters RL, Stark LZ, Gubernick I, et al. Electromyographic analysis of brachioradialis to flexor pollicis longus tendon transfer in quadriplegia. *J Hand Surg [AM]* 1990;15:335–339.

58. Mulcahay MJ, Betz RR, Smith BT, et al. Implanted functional electrical stimulation hand system in adolescents with spinal injuries: an evaluation. *Arch Phys Med Rehabil* 1997;78:597–607.

59. Lamb DW. The current state of the management of the upper limb in tetraplegia. *Paraplegia* 1992;30:65–67.

60. Prochazka A, Gauthier M, Wieler M, et al. The bionic glove: an electrical stimulator garment that provides controlled grasp and hand opening in quadriplegia. *Arch Phys Med Rehabil* 1997;78(6):608–614.

61. Popovic D, Stojanovic A, Pjanovic A, et al. Clinical evaluation of the bionic glove. *Arch Phys Med Rehabil* 1999;80(3):299–304.

62. Nathan RH, Ohry A. Upper limb functions regained in quadriplegia: a hybrid computerized neuromuscular stimulation system. *Arch Phys Med Rehabil* 1990;71:415–421.

63. Smith BT, Mulcahey MJ, Betz RR. Development of an upper extremity FES system for individuals with C4 tetraplegia. *IEEE Trans Rehabil Eng* 1996;4(4):264–270.

64. Stroh WK, Van Doren CL, Bryden AM, et al. Satisfaction with and usage of a hand neuroprosthesis. *Arch Phys Med Rehabil* 1999;80(2): 206–213.

65. Davis SE, Mulcahey MJ, Betz RR, et al. Outcomes of upper-extremity tendon transfers and functional electrical stimulation in an adolescent with C-5 tetraplegia. *Am J Occup Ther* 1997;51:307–312.

29

PEDIATRIC SPINAL CORD DISORDERS

LAWRENCE C. VOGEL
RANDAL R. BETZ
MARY JANE MULCAHEY

This chapter reviews spinal cord disorders in children and adolescents, including spinal cord injury (SCI), myelomeningocele, and hydrosyringomyelia. Although these disorders are not limited to the pediatric population, the clinical presentation and management of children and adolescents with these spinal cord disorders are unique because of the impact of growth and development. Both SCI and myelomeningocele share many of the same manifestations related to spinal cord dysfunction, namely paralysis, sensory loss, and bladder, bowel, and sexual dysfunction. Children with these disorders also experience similar complications as a result of growth, such as scoliosis and hip dysplasia. However, myelomeningocele has many distinguishing features because of associated brain abnormalities and its onset *in utero*, resulting in cognitive and behavioral abnormalities and congenital malformations, such as clubfeet, respectively.

GENERAL PRINCIPLES

The general principles in caring for children and adolescents with spinal cord disorders are fundamentally different than those in adults with similar impairments. Care for pediatric spinal cord disorders must be family centered because of the central role of parents and family for a child or adolescent (1–3). In view of the growth and development inherent in childhood, care must be developmentally based and should be responsive to the dynamic changes that occur with growth. Children and young adolescents need developmentally appropriate care with compatible physical and philosophical characteristics, including recreation therapy and child-life activities. In contrast, older adolescents benefit from an adolescent approach rather than a more traditional pediatric or adult setting.

Anticipatory guidance for children or adolescents and their families is critical. It must be provided in a developmentally sensitive manner to prepare them for potential complications and transitions, such as sexual development and functioning or progression from ambulation in the young and energetic child to wheelchair mobility in the older child or adolescent.

Transition into adulthood is a major goal in caring for children and adolescents with spinal cord disorders (4,5). Transition planning must be initiated early in childhood and intensify as they become adolescents. A preeminent goal for children and

adolescents with spinal cord disorders is that they have satisfying and productive lives as independently functioning adults in society. Transition encompasses many spheres of functioning, including independent living, employment, financial resources, socialization, and health care (4–8). From the time of diagnosis, even if present at birth, parents need to be reassured that their child has the potential to be an independently functioning adult. Parents, health care providers, and other adults significantly involved with the child must foster these expectations for the child's future. As a result, these expectations will become ingrained into the child and adolescent's life, assuring a more successful transition into adulthood.

An example of the importance for transition planning to begin at an early age for children is the central role that employment has in adult life, including life satisfaction. Adults with childhood-onset SCI are employed less frequently compared with the general population, and employment is significantly associated with life satisfaction. Compared with their able-bodied peers, children and adolescents with SCI have significantly less prevocational experiences (9). The fact that young adults with pediatric-onset SCI are employed less often than their able-bodied peers emphasizes the need to address transitional issues more aggressively and at younger ages. Children with spinal cord disorders should be expected to have age-appropriate chores, similar to their peers (9). As they grow older, they must be involved in developmentally appropriate prevocational and vocational activities that will prepare them for adult employment (9–11).

Provision of comprehensive primary care, including preventive medicine, health care maintenance, and management of intercurrent illnesses for children and adolescents with spinal cord disorders is frequently neglected and overshadowed by tertiary care needs (12–15). In addition to the standard childhood immunizations, children and adolescents with spinal cord disorders should receive the pneumococcal vaccine when they are 2 years of age or older and yearly influenza vaccination beginning at 6 months of age (16). For influenza vaccination, the split virus preparation should be used in children until they are 13 years of age, and children 8 years and younger should receive 2 doses of the vaccine 1 month apart the first time they are immunized against influenza (16).

Psychosocial and sexuality issues must be addressed in a developmentally appropriate manner. Sexuality is often overlooked in children and adolescents with spinal cord disorders. Sexuality issues common to all children and adolescents, as well as spinal cord disorder–specific areas, must be addressed. This is particularly important because children and adolescents with disabilities tend to be "infantalized" or treated as asexual beings.

SPINAL CORD INJURIES

The manifestations and complications of pediatric SCI are unique because of distinctive anatomic and physiologic features of children and adolescents and growth and development (17–20). Unique aspects of pediatric SCI include spinal cord injury without radiologic abnormalities (SCIWORA), upper cervical injuries, birth injuries, lap-belt injuries, and delayed onset of neurologic deficits. The interaction between growth and development and the manifestations and complications of SCI are responsible for many of the unique features of pediatric SCI. As a result of growth, there is a high incidence of scoliosis and hip dislocation in patients who sustained their SCI before 8 to 10 years of age. Development helps to explain why the untrainable toddler becomes the model patient during the early years of school and then the noncompliant adolescent with pressure ulcers, urinary tract infections (UTIs), and substance abuse. SCI can impact growth, as reflected by failure of paralyzed limbs to grow normally. Impaired mobility resulting from the SCI limits the ability of children and adolescents to explore their environment, resulting in psychosocial, educational, and vocational disadvantages and delays.

Epidemiology

Among the SCIs that occur each year in the United States, about 3% to 5% occur in individuals younger than 15 years of age, and about 20% occur in those younger than 20 years of age (21–25). Similar to adults with SCI, boys more commonly sustain SCI than girls during adolescence. However, the preponderance of male patients becomes less marked as age of injury decreases, such that female SCI patients equal male SCI patients in those 3 years of age and younger (22,23,26,27). The life expectancy of children and adolescents with SCI is a function of neurologic level and category (26,28). The less severe the SCI, in respect to both neurologic level and classification, the longer the expected survival. Compared with the general population, life expectancy ranges from 59% to 64% for individuals with C1 to C4 injuries, 70% to 73% for those with C5 to C8 lesions, 80% to 84% for those with paraplegia, and 88% to 89% for those with Frankel D incomplete SCI (28).

Neurologic level and degree of completeness vary as a function of age (26,28). Among children who sustained their SCI when they were 8 years of age or younger, 70% were paraplegic, and about two thirds had complete lesions. In contrast, about half of older children, adolescents, or adults were paraplegic, and about half had complete lesions. In addition, younger children are more likely to have upper cervical injuries (above C4) and less likely to have C4 to C6 injuries, which is the more typical level for tetraplegia in individuals older than 8 years of age, including adults (22,26–28). The higher risk for upper cervical injuries is probably due to a proportionately larger head and underdeveloped neck musculature in infants and younger children.

Motor vehicle crashes are the most common cause of SCI in children and adolescents, with violence and sports being the next most common etiologies (26,28,29). Violence causes SCI in children in all age ranges but is a particularly important cause in adolescents, especially among African Americans and Hispanics (26,28). Although violence remains a significant cause of SCI in the pediatric population, in the recent past, there has been a decrease in the percentage of SCI due to violence in children and adolescents similar to that in adults (21,30). Unique etiologies of SCI in children and adolescents include lap-belt injuries, birth injuries, child abuse (31–36), C1 to C2 subluxation due to tonsillophayrngitis (37), and transverse myelitis (38,39). Additionally, children with skeletal dysplasias, juvenile rheumatoid arthritis, and Down syndrome are susceptible to cervical SCI.

Lap-belt injuries usually occur in children weighing between 40 and 60 pounds (40–44). In these children, the lap belt rises above the pelvic brim and acts as a fixed anterior fulcrum, resulting in flexion-distraction forces in the mid-lumbar spine. The three components of lap-belt injuries are abdominal wall bruising, intraabdominal injuries, and spinal cord damage. The abdominal wall bruising is caused by trauma from the lap belt and ranges from abrasions and contusions to full-thickness skin loss. The most common intraabdominal injuries include tears or perforations of the small or large intestines, with injuries less frequently occurring to the kidneys, liver, spleen, pancreas, bladder, or uterus. Although the injury forces are localized to the mid-lumbar spine, the neurologic level varies from a conus or cauda equina lesion to mid-thoracic levels. The most common location for vertebral damage is between L2 and L4, with distraction-type injuries (Fig. 29.1). However, 23% to 30% of patients with SCI related to lap-belt injuries have SCIWORA (Fig. 29.2). Computed tomography (CT) scans for trauma routinely miss the fracture, especially if it goes through the ligaments and spontaneously reduces. To reduce the incidence of lap belt injuries, children who weigh more than 40 pounds and who are 4 to 8 years of age should travel in motor vehicles with approved belt-positioning booster seats (45).

Neonatal SCIs are relatively uncommon, with an incidence of about 1 per 60,000 births (46–52). Upper cervical lesions are most common and are related to torsional forces during delivery. In contrast, SCIs related to breech deliveries most commonly result in lower cervical or upper thoracic injuries and are related to traction forces that occur during delivery. Thoracic or lumbar lesions are uncommon and may result from vascular occlusion associated with umbilical artery catheters or paradoxical air embolism through transitional cardiovascular shunts. Brachial plexus or phrenic nerve injuries and hypoxic encephalopathy may be associated with neonatal SCI. Because affected neonates present with a flaccid-type paralysis, the differential diagnosis includes spinal muscular atrophy, amyotonia congenita, congenital myotonic dystrophy, and neural tube defects.

In children and adolescents with Down syndrome, atlantoaxial instability is related to ligamentous laxity (53–56). An atlanto–dens interval (ADI) greater than 4.5 mm is considered

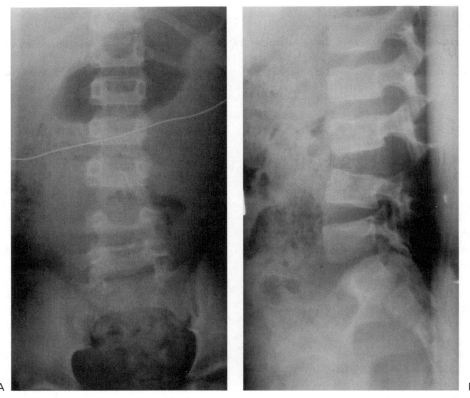

FIGURE 29.1. A,B; Spine radiograph of a 7-year-old boy who sustained a complete L2 to L3 spinal cord injury as a result of a lap-belt injury. The radiograph demonstrates a flexion-distraction injury at L3 to L4.

abnormal and occurs in about 15% to 20% of individuals with Down syndrome, with the majority being asymptomatic. Only neurologically symptomatic patients require a C1-to-C2 fusion; however, restriction of asymptomatic patients with an increased ADI from high-risk activities remains controversial. Additionally, occipitoatlantal instability occurs commonly in children with Down syndrome and must be carefully sought (55).

Children and adolescents with juvenile rheumatoid arthritis (JRA) may develop C1 to C2 instability as a result of synovitis of the facet and synovial joints surrounding the odontoid process, as well as from destruction of the odontoid process as a result of the inflammatory process (57) (Fig. 29.3). In addition, individuals with polyarticular JRA may experience fusion of the cervical vertebra, particularly C2 to C3. This may progress to eventual fusion of a significant portion of the cervical spine, placing the patient at risk for a cervical fracture and possible tetraplegic SCI from relatively minor trauma (58) (Fig. 29.4).

Cervical myelopathy may be associated with skeletal dysplasias, such as achondroplasia and Morquio syndrome (59–61). Infants with achondroplasia may experience compression of the upper cervical cord and the caudal medulla as a result of a small foramen magnum (61). In addition, individuals with achondroplasia, primarily boys, are at risk for developing spastic paraplegia related to spinal stenosis (59). Children with dwarfing syndromes with odontoid dysplasia, such as Morquio mucopolysac-

charidosis IV, may develop atlantoaxial instability, and of those with instability, more than half will develop a myelopathy (59, 60).

Pathophysiology

Anatomic and physiologic characteristics of children, particularly those who are 10 years of age and younger, are responsible for SCIWORA and delayed onset of neurologic findings. Among children 10 years of age or younger at the time of sustaining a SCI, about 60% have SCIWORA (62,63). In contrast, SCIWORA is found in about 20% of children injured after 10 years of age. The high incidence of SCIWORA in younger children with SCI is a result of unique anatomic and biomechanical characteristics of the spine (63,64). This includes increased elasticity of the spine in relation to a less flexible spinal cord, shallow and horizontally oriented facet joints, anterior wedging of the vertebral bodies, vulnerability of the growth zone of vertebral endplates, and poorly developed uncinate processes.

Despite the benign radiologic picture of SCIWORA, affected individuals are more likely to have complete lesions (27,62,63, 65). Although plain radiographs, tomography, CT, myelography, and dynamic flexion-extension studies are normal, magnetic resonance imaging (MRI) abnormalities are frequently seen in patients with SCIWORA (63,66–68) (Fig. 29.2). Both ex-

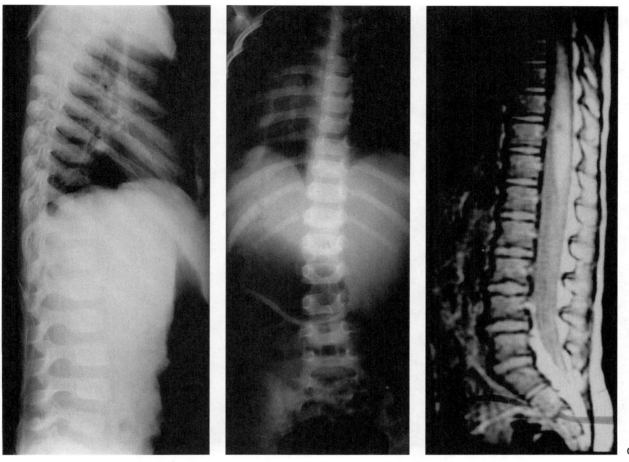

FIGURE 29.2. A–C; Spine radiographs and magnetic resonance imaging (MRI) study of a 2½-year-old boy who sustained a complete L2 spinal cord injury as a result of a lap-belt injury. There are no abnormalities on the plain radiographs; thus, the patient has a spinal cord injury without radiologic abnormalities (SCIWORA). However, the MRI demonstrates a lucent area in the lumbar spinal cord (**C**).

traneural and neural abnormalities may be identified. The primary extraneural MRI findings include rupture of the anterior or posterior longitudinal ligaments, intradiskal abnormalities, and endplate fractures. Neural abnormalities include cord disruption, hemorrhage, and edema. The MRI abnormalities correlate with the severity of the neurologic deficit and the prognosis for recovery (67). Complete neurologic deficits are generally associated with cord disruption and extensive cord hemorrhage, minor cord hemorrhage or edema is more likely associated with incomplete lesions, and no cord abnormalities on MRI correlate with mild partial cord syndromes.

In about 25% to 50% of children who sustain a SCI, there is a delay in onset of neurologic abnormalities that ranges from 30 minutes to 4 days (23,61,64,69–71). Many of these children with delayed onset of neurologic findings experience transient and subtle neurologic symptoms, such as paresthesias or subjective weakness. The mechanisms that may be responsible for this phenomenon include natural expansion of the cord injury by inflammation, posttraumatic occlusion of radicular arteries, and

repeated trauma to the spinal cord as a result of occult spinal instability.

Medical Issues

Urology

Clean intermittent catheterization is the standard bladder management for children and adolescents with SCI (12,72–77). Intermittent catheterization is initiated when the child is about 3 years old, or earlier if the child is experiencing recurrent UTIs or exhibits renal impairment. Children with adequate hand function begin self-catheterization when they are developmentally 5 to 7 years old (75).

The issues of using prophylactic antibiotics to prevent UTIs and the treatment of asymptomatic bacteriuria in children are no different from those in adults with SCI (78). Prophylactic antibiotics should be limited to patients who experience recurrent and severe UTIs and those with obstructive uropathy or compromised renal function, including vesicoureteral reflux and

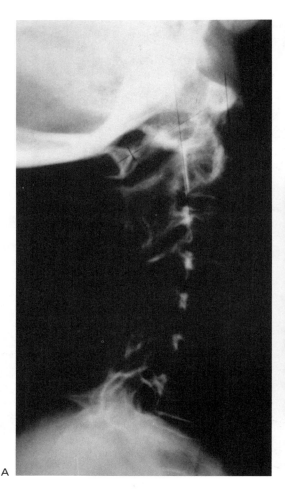

A

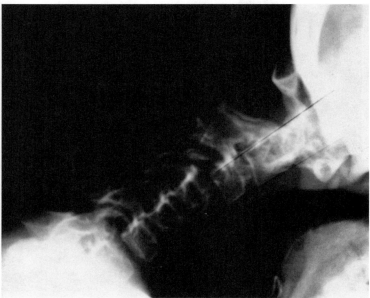

B

FIGURE 29.3. A,B; Extension and flexion cervical spine radiographs of a 14-year-old girl with severe polyarticular juvenile rheumatoid arthritis. The radiographs demonstrate erosion of the odontoid process and marked narrowing of the spinal canal on the flexion view (**B**) compared with the extension view (**A**).

hydronephrosis. Patients with asymptomatic bacteriuria are generally not treated unless they have compromised renal function. Treatment should be limited to those with symptomatic UTIs as reflected by systemic toxicity (fever, chills, dysreflexia, or exacerbation of spasticity), incontinence, or cloudy and foul-smelling urine. The use of fluoroquinolones may be contraindicated in children younger than 18 years of age because of theoretic adverse cartilage events (79). However, fluoroquinolones may be used in the pediatric population if alternative safe and effective antimicrobials are not suitable (80).

Similar to adults, continence and independence are important aspects of bladder management for children and adolescents with SCI. Interventions that may be beneficial in managing incontinence include anticholinergics, modification of fluid intake and catheterization schedule, and treatment of urologic complications, such as UTIs and urolithiasis. For patients with persistent incontinence, urodynamics should be performed (72,81). Patients with limited bladder capacity unresponsive to anticholinergics may be candidates for a bladder augmentation (76, 82–86).

For individuals who are not independent in performing intermittent catheterization, continent catheterizable conduits and functional electrical stimulation (FES) are potential alternatives

(76,83,87). A continent catheterizable conduit, the Mitrofanoff procedure, consists of creating a catheterizable conduit using the appendix or a segment of small bowel that connects the bladder to a stoma either in the umbilicus or on the lower abdominal wall (88,89). This may allow individuals with limited upper extremity function, such as those with C6 or C7 injuries, to catheterize themselves (90,91). In addition, continent catheterizable conduits may facilitate independence in bladder management for individuals who have difficulty accessing their native urethra, such as girls who cannot actively abduct their legs or those who have difficulty transferring to a commode or toilet.

The Vocare system is an FES system that assists in both bladder and bowel management (92–95). Candidates for the Vocare system include those who have recurrent UTIs or abnormal sensation related to catheterization and those who are incontinent despite medications. Candidates must have a spastic bladder. The Vocare system is most appropriate for patients who can independently transfer to a toilet and pull their pants down (chapter 25 discusses this in greater depth).

Bowel Management

Similar to the adult SCI population, the critical issues for bowel management in pediatric SCI include complete and regular emp-

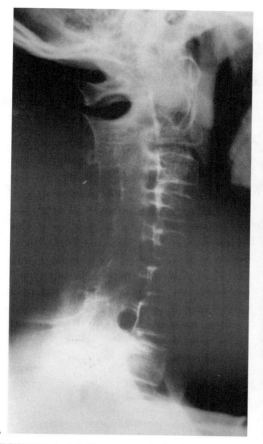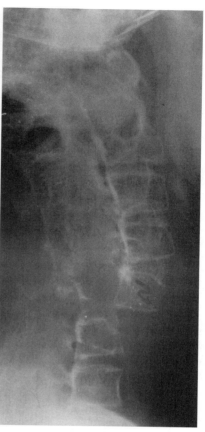

FIGURE 29.4. A,B; These are cervical radiographs of a boy with polyarticular juvenile rheumatoid arthritis. At 12 years of age, there was fusion of his cervical spine from C2 to C7 (**A**). At 17 years of age, he was involved in a motor vehicle crash and sustained a C5 to C6 fracture-dislocation, resulting in complete C5 to C6 tetraplegia (**B**).

tying, short duration of the bowel program, continence, aesthetics, and prevention of constipation or diarrhea (77,96–101). The need for regularity in the performance of bowel programs is frequently in conflict with the lack of conformity of children and adolescents. However, anxiety regarding fecal incontinence is a strong incentive for compliance with bowel program scheduling. Bowel programs are initiated when children are 2 to 4 years of age, which is a developmentally appropriate age, or earlier if they are experiencing diarrhea or constipation (102). By 5 to 7 years of age, children should be responsible for maintaining their bowel program schedule and be independent in performing the bowel program commensurate with their neurologic function.

The essential ingredients for a bowel program include privacy, independence, and a regular schedule with respect to frequency and time of the day. The bowel program should take place on a toilet or a commode. A sitting position facilitates defecation, and if neurologically capable, the child should be taught and encouraged to increase intraabdominal pressure. It is important that these basic principles be initiated once a bowel program is initiated, regardless of the age of the child or adolescent.

Options for bowel programs include the antegrade conti-

nence enema, enema continence catheters, pulsed irrigation enemas (103), and the Vocare system (104). The antegrade continence enema procedure allows antegrade evacuation of the bowel by administering an enema directly into the cecum through the appendix, which is accessible through an abdominal wall stoma (105). Management of bowel dysfunction with an enema continence catheter has been reported to be beneficial in improving continence and decreasing constipation (106).

Deep Venous Thrombosis

The literature available about thromboembolic complications in pediatric SCI is limited (107,108). The incidence of deep venous thrombosis (DVT) in children and adolescents with SCI is less than in the adult population and ranges from 2.5% to 17.5%, and the incidence of pulmonary emboli ranges from 0% to 2.3%. Postphlebitic syndrome develops in about 25% of children and adolescents with SCI who have developed DVT (109). In addition to the risk for DVT in the acute phase of a SCI, children and adolescents are at risk for DVT after surgical procedures, such as after spine fusions (110).

Both treatment and prophylaxis for DVT in children and

adolescents who have sustained a SCI are similar to those for adults (111,112). DVT prophylaxis should include graduated elastic stockings for older children and adolescents as well as anticoagulation. For children who are too small to wear commercially available graduated elastic stockings, use of custom-made lower extremity garments, such as Jobst stockings, may be a consideration. Using elastic wraps to wrap the legs is limited because unevenness of wrapping may result in constrictions with venous obstruction, increasing the risk for DVT. Additionally, some elastic wraps contain latex, which is contraindicated because of the risk for latex allergy in this patient population. Alternatives for prophylactic anticoagulation are the same as for adults, except that low-molecular-weight heparin (LMWH) is not specifically approved for use in children. Nonetheless, it is common practice to use LMWH in this situation because of the ease of administration and the fact that laboratory monitoring is not needed. The dosage of LMWH for children would be 0.5 mg/kg administered subcutaneously every 12 hours (0.75 mg/kg every 12 hours for infants younger than 2 months old) (113, 114).

Management of DVT includes anticoagulation with intravenous heparin, initiated with a bolus of 75 U/kg over 10 minutes (5,000 to 10,000 units in adults), followed by continuous infusion of 28 U/kg/hr for infants or 20 U/kg/hr for children older than 1 year (20,000 to 40,000 U/day in adults) (115,116). The heparin infusion is adjusted to maintain the activated partial thromboplastin time between 60 and 85 seconds. Oral anticoagulation with warfarin sodium, 0.2 mg/kg, is initiated concurrently with heparinization. Dosage adjustments are made to maintain a prothrombin time of 2 to 3 INR (international normalized ratio). Alternatively, DVT in children can be managed with LMWH.

Hypercalcemia

Hypercalcemia affects 10% to 23% of individuals with SCI and most commonly involves adolescent and young adult males during the first 3 months after injury (117–120). Hypercalcemia results from increased bone resorption as a result of the immobilization associated with a SCI. The increased bone turnover characteristic of growing children and adolescents and the large and active bone mass, particularly in adolescent boys, is the basis for the increased incidence of hypercalcemia in the pediatric SCI population. The excessive calcium load is not adequately excreted by the kidneys because hypercalcemia depresses renal function, resulting in decreased calcium excretion and impairment in renal concentrating ability. Parathyroid hormone is usually depressed because of the hypercalcemia.

Patients with hypercalcemia typically present with an insidious onset of abdominal pain, nausea, vomiting, lethargy, malaise, polydipsia, polyuria, and dehydration. Affected patients may exhibit behavioral changes or an acute psychosis. In a series of 87 individuals younger than 16 years old, 18 (24%) experienced hypercalcemia (120). Five of the patients with hypercalcemia had a clinical presentation consistent with an acute abdomen, and two of them actually underwent exploratory laparotomies. Patients with hypercalcemia can also be asymptomatic.

Serum calcium levels are elevated above age-applicable norms,

which are 10.8 mg/dL in children and 10.2 mg/dL in adolescents. In addition, ionized calcium is elevated above its upper limit of 1.23 mmol/L. Serum phosphorus is normal, and alkaline phosphatase is either normal or slightly elevated above age-appropriate norms.

Management includes hydration with intravenous normal saline at about 1.5 to 2 times the maintenance rate. Furosemide (Lasix, 0.5 to 1 mg/kg per dose once or twice daily) is administered to hasten renal excretion of calcium (121). In addition, pamidronate is very effective in managing hypercalcemia and should be administered intravenously at a dose of 1 mg/kg, with a usual adult dose of 60 mg administered over 4 hours (18, 122–125). Usually a single dose of pamidronate is adequate for resolution of the hypercalcemia.

Complications of hypercalcemia include nephrocalcinosis, urolithiasis, and renal failure. Tori and Hill found that 10 of their 18 (55%) pediatric patients with hypercalcemia experienced urinary stones, compared to an 18% incidence of stones in patients without hypercalcemia (120). In addition, 2 of their 18 patients developed renal failure and nephrocalcinosis. In the future, use of bisphosphonates, such as alendronate, may prevent this entity.

Autonomic Dysreflexia

The pathophysiology, clinical presentation, and management of autonomic dysreflexia in children and adolescents with SCI are similar to those in the adult SCI population (126,127). Differences between the pediatric and adult SCI population relate to developmental variations of blood pressure in children and adolescents, appropriate blood pressure cuff sizes, their ability to communicate, and varying dependency on their parents or guardians.

For children and adolescents, blood pressure is a function of age and body size. Blood pressure increases as children grow older, with older adolescents reaching adult norms (128). For children and adolescents without SCI, median systolic blood pressure can be estimated by the following formula: 90 mm Hg + (2 × age in years) (129). Similar to adults with SCI, children and adolescents with cervical and upper thoracic SCI have lower baseline blood pressures compared with the general population. Because of lower blood pressures in children and adolescents with SCI as a consequence of both their age and their neurologic level, it is important that baseline blood pressures be determined on a regular basis. Blood pressure elevations of 20 to 40 mm Hg above baseline may be considered a sign of autonomic dysreflexia. Blood pressure measurement in children and adolescents is confounded by the need to use appropriately sized blood pressure cuffs and anxiety that children may experience with health care professionals (130). Anxiety associated with obtaining blood pressures may make it difficult to obtain accurate measurements both for baseline determinations and during an episode of autonomic dysreflexia. A calm and reassuring environment for the child or the adolescent in the presence of their parents may be helpful.

Because of varying cognitive and verbal communication abilities of children as they progress through infancy, childhood, and adolescence, symptoms of autonomic dysreflexia may not be expressed or may be communicated less clearly compared with those in adults. For example, in preschool-aged children, even though they are verbal, autonomic dysreflexia may present with vague symptoms rather than complaints of a pounding headache. Medical alert identification should be used and appropriate education provided for those adults who have significant interactions and responsibility for children with SCI, such as teachers, school nurses, coaches, and community-based health care providers. Education about autonomic dysreflexia should include diagnosis as well as emergency management.

Children and adolescents should assume increasing responsibility for their care as they grow older, including prevention, diagnosis, and treatment of autonomic dysreflexia. This would include consistently wearing medical alert identification, maintaining an information sheet or card about autonomic dysreflexia, and taking responsibility for educating health care providers or other supervising adults about its diagnosis and management.

Management of children and adolescents experiencing autonomic dysreflexia should be conducted efficiently in a calm and reassuring atmosphere. Symptomatic measures are successful in managing most episodes of autonomic dysreflexia. For those who do not respond to conservative measures, nifedipine (Procardia, Adalat, 0.25 mg/kg or 10 mg in adolescents weighing 40 or more kg) should be administered by chew and swallow for those who can follow directions or sublingually for younger children and infants. Patients with recurrent autonomic dysreflexia may be managed with prazosin (Minipress, 25 to 150 mcg/kg per 24 hours ÷ every 6 hours) or terazosin (Hytrin, 1 to 5 mg daily).

Hyperhidrosis

Hyperhidrosis is excessive sweating that is primarily seen in individuals with tetraplegia or thoracic paraplegia (131–134). In a series of 154 individuals with SCI, 27% were affected by hyperhidrosis (131). The exact pathogenesis of hyperhidrosis has not been elucidated. It is probably the result of sympathetic overactivity of the rostral portion of the spinal cord immediately below the zone of injury (131). Similar to autonomic dysreflexia, the increased sympathetic output may be a response to noxious stimuli below the zone of the SCI. Noxious stimuli may include bladder irritation from a UTI or urolithiasis (132); postinjury myelopathic changes, including posttraumatic syringomyelia (135–138) and tethering of the spinal cord at the injury site (139); or unexplained stimuli.

Sweat glands are innervated by the sympathetic nervous system (sympathetic cholinergics). The sympathetics that innervate the sweat glands of the face and neck originate from T1 to T7, those for the trunk from T4 to T12, and those for the legs from T9 to L2 (134). This pattern of sympathetic innervation of the sweat glands is the basis for excessive sweating in the face and neck, which are above the zone of injury, as a result of noxious stimuli occurring below the zone of injury.

Hyperhidrosis should be treated if it is embarrassing, impairs function, or increases the risk for pressure ulcers. The mainstay of management is avoidance and alleviation of precipitating factors. If conservative measures are unsuccessful, medications that inhibit sympathetic overactivity, such as propantheline (140) or transdermal scopolamine (134), should be considered.

Temperature Regulation

The severity of temperature regulation defects is dependent on the level and completeness of the SCI (127,133,141). Spinal cord injuries at T6 or above interfere with the central control of the major splanchnic sympathetics and voluntary muscles of the lower body, producing a poikilothermic state. The patient is unable to increase core temperature by vasoconstriction and shivering below the zone of the SCI. Similarly, the patient is unable to decrease core body temperature by vasodilation and sweating below the zone of injury. Therefore, these patients are at risk for hypothermia or hyperthermia as a result of exogenous stresses, such as environmental temperatures, and endogenous factors, such as exercise (142). Infants and young children with SCI are particularly vulnerable to the extremes of environmental temperatures because of their relatively large surface area and their variable communication, cognitive, and problem-solving abilities. At the other extreme are adolescents with SCI who may be susceptible to hypothermia or hyperthermia because of erratic judgment that they may demonstrate.

Rarely, children with SCI are seen who cannot engage in summertime outdoor activities because the inability to sweat causes heat exhaustion symptoms. Functional cooling suits are commercially available for children with this problem (1).

Fever

Fever frequently occurs during the first 3 months after a SCI and is problematic because of multiple causes and loss of sensation (127,143,144). Although fever in the acute SCI period is not unique to children with SCI, children tend to become febrile more readily and with higher temperature elevations compared with adults. UTIs are responsible for most episodes of fever, with other common causes being pressure ulcers, surgical site infections, DVT, heterotopic ossification, pathologic fractures, pulmonary disorders, and epididymitis. Patients with intraabdominal disorders may present with subtle signs and symptoms, necessitating a high index of suspicion in the presence of fever, anorexia, abdominal distention, and nausea and vomiting (145). Multiple sources of fever are seen in 15% of febrile patients, whereas no etiology is found for 8% to 11% of febrile episodes, which may reflect thermoregulatory abnormalities (143,144).

Evaluation of a febrile child with SCI must encompass a thorough history and physical examination as well as appropriate laboratory and imaging studies guided by the clinical evaluation. The history should include recent blood transfusions and surgical procedures. The physical examination must encompass a general evaluation to identify problems such as otitis media or pneumonia. The evaluation must also be geared to SCI-specific problems, such as identifying a swollen extremity with limited range consistent with a fracture or heterotopic ossification or a swollen scrotum due to epididymitis.

The choice of laboratory and imaging studies must be based on clinical findings, but studies typically include urinalysis and culture, complete blood count with differential, erythrocyte sedimentation rate, and C-reactive protein. Liver function tests, serum amylase and lipase, plain abdominal radiographs, abdominal and pelvic ultrasound, gallium scan, and CT may be helpful in evaluating the patient for potential intraabdominal disorders.

Cardiovascular Disease

Coronary artery and cerebrovascular diseases and hypertension are significant causes of morbidity and mortality in adults with SCI (146). In general, patients with SCI lead relatively sedentary lifestyles because of mobility impairments, which presumably increases their risk for cardiovascular disease (147). Irrespective of whether individuals with SCI are at greater risk for cardiovascular disease than the general population, they should be encouraged to adopt a lifestyle and pursue preventive measures that reduce their risk for cardiovascular complications. This becomes especially important for children and adolescents with SCI because of their relatively long lifespan and the need to make significant adaptations to the normally practiced preventive measures, such as exercise, diet, stress reduction, and avoidance of tobacco.

Exercise is a key element in the prevention of cardiovascular complications. A regular exercise program becomes a major challenge in children and adolescents with SCI because of their motor limitations superimposed on developmentally based compliance issues and preferences (148,149). Because of their size and motivation, younger children with paraplegia are physically active by crawling and by ambulating with a variety of orthotics. With this exception, the pediatric SCI population shares significant limitations of exercise options with the adult SCI population. Children and adolescents with SCI, especially those with lesions at T6 and higher, have decreased cardiovascular adaptations to exercise, which may manifest as decreased cardiac output, exertional hypotension, and hyperthermia (142,150–153). Additionally, children and adolescents must take special precautions when exercising; one of the authors' patients with a T1 level injury died of a crush injury and suffocation at home during unsupervised weightlifting.

Various exercise programs are available for children and adolescents with SCI, including therapeutic recreational activities and adapted physical education (154–157). Exercise programs should concentrate on cardiovascular fitness and on increasing aerobic capacity, muscle strength, and endurance (158). Exercise programs must be developmentally based, compatible with age-appropriate and contemporary activities, congruent with preinjury interests, and incorporated into the family and community (155,156). Exercise programs should facilitate independence, be integrated into the child or adolescent's lifestyle and routine, and most important, be fun.

Children and adolescents with SCI should be assessed for their risk for cardiovascular disorders, which includes factors such as obesity, sedentary lifestyle, smoking, hyperlipidemia, hypertension, and family history. Screening for hyperlipidemia after 2 years of age should be undertaken in children and adolescents with a high-risk family history.

Pain

Similar to the adult SCI population, chronic pain is a significant problem among children and adolescents with SCI (159,160).

Pain can be very disabling and negatively affect school, work, and social interactions. Pain may originate from the area of trauma in a radicular pattern (compression of a nerve root at the level of injury) or from mechanical instability of an unhealed fracture, or it may consist of central pain or dysesthesia (160–163). Evaluation of all the different types of pain in infants and younger children may be complicated by their variable communication abilities.

Self-abusive behavior, or self-mutilation, is occasionally seen in infants, children, adolescents, and adults with SCI and may be a manifestation of dysesthesia (164–166). Self-abusive behavior most commonly presents with biting of fingertips, which can result in finger amputations.

Management of dysesthesia, as well as self-mutilation, should incorporate physical modalities, psychological interventions, and medications (167,168). Physical modalities may include physical therapy, hydrotherapy, and transcutaneous electrical neural stimulation. Children and parents need to be reassured that dysesthesia generally resolves within 3 to 6 months. The medications primarily used in the pediatric SCI population include amitriptyline (Elavil, 0.1 mg/kg per dose at night), carbamazepine (Tegretol, 10 to 20 mg/kg/day given in two to four divided doses), and gabapentin (Neurontin), which can be used in children older than 12 years of age (900 to 1,800 mg/day in three divided doses) (161,169,170). Other medications that may be beneficial include phenytoin (Dilantin, 3 to 5 mg/kg/day in one or two divided doses), oral clonidine (Catapres, 5 to 7 µg/kg/day in divided doses every 6 to 12 hours) or transdermal clonidine (0.1- to 0.3-mg patch weekly).

Latex Allergy

Immediate-type, immunoglobulin E–mediated allergic reactions to latex have been identified with increasing frequency (171–173). They are seen in children with myelomeningocele, SCI, and congenital genitourinary anomalies and in health care workers (127,174,175). About 6% to 18% of children and adolescents with SCI have evidence of latex allergies (175). Among adults with SCI who had chronic indwelling catheters, 7 of 15 (47%) had evidence of latex allergy (176).

Latex allergy is presumably the result of frequent and extensive contact with latex-containing products, especially medical supplies and equipment. Additional risk factors may include young age of initial exposure and longer duration of exposure to latex-containing products. Reactions can be elicited by direct contact with latex through cutaneous, mucosal, intravenous, or serosal routes or by airborne dissemination of latex antigens that have adhered to glove powder. Allergic reactions to latex may manifest as localized or generalized urticaria, wheezing, angioedema, or anaphylaxis. Intraoperative allergic reactions to latex may be life threatening, and they may be difficult to diagnose because of surgical drapes covering the patient's skin, which may exhibit an urticarial rash.

Diagnosis of latex allergy is established by a history consistent with an immediate-type allergic reaction or with *in vitro* assays or skin tests. Individuals with either a positive history or a positive laboratory or skin test should be considered allergic to latex. Clinical manifestations may be subtle, such as the child who develops a blotchy facial rash when he or she blows up a balloon. Latex allergy should be suspected in individuals who have unexplained intraoperative allergic reactions and in individuals allergic to kiwi, bananas, avocados, or chestnuts (177). Skin tests are probably the most sensitive method of identifying latex allergy but are limited by the lack of availability of standardized preparations and the potential for precipitating a severe allergic reaction (172). Laboratory tests exhibit varying sensitivity and specificity, depending on the specific antigens and assay used.

Because of the potential severity of latex allergy, individuals at risk, such as those with SCI or myelomeningocele, should be cared for in a latex-free environment. This approach should minimize the risk for sensitizing patients in addition to preventing allergic reactions in patients with known as well as those with undiagnosed latex allergies. Patients and their families and caregivers must be educated about the potential for latex allergy and the necessity to avoid all latex-containing products. Individuals allergic to latex should wear a medical alert identification and carry autoinjectable epinephrine.

Pulmonary Disease

Pulmonary complications are major problems during both the acute and chronic phase of SCI (18,146,178–180). Children with high cervical injuries require aggressive and early ventilatory support and generally require lifelong ventilatory support, phrenic nerve pacing, or both (181–183). Candidates for a phrenic nerve pacemaker are those with a SCI at C3 or higher (184, 185). In children, bilateral phrenic nerve stimulation must be performed to avoid excessive mediastinal shifts. Tracheostomies are needed because of upper airway obstruction that occurs in young children during phrenic nerve pacing. In addition, some children may fail to thrive when they are entirely dependent on phrenic nerve pacing; therefore, supplemental nighttime ventilation through the tracheostomy may be required (185). Noninvasive ventilatory support systems, such as biphasic positive airway pressure and airway secretion management, may be applicable in the pediatric SCI population (186,187).

Children who sustained cervical SCI as newborns or infants may be at risk for incipient respiratory failure. This may be manifested as sleep-disordered breathing, with sleep apnea, headache, restless sleep, snoring, morning confusion, daytime sleeping, and mental dullness (179,188–190). A high index of suspicion must be maintained in these young children with tetraplegia, and sleep studies should be considered. Risk factors for sleep-induced respiratory failure include intercostal and diaphragmatic paralysis, use of medications such as baclofen or diazepam, and obesity (190).

Spasticity

Compared with the adult SCI population, a smaller percentage of children with SCI experience spasticity, which may reflect the higher percentage of paraplegic children with SCI (191). Nonetheless, spasticity remains a major problem for a significant number of children with SCI (192–194). The general principles of managing spasticity in children with SCI are no different than those for the adult SCI population (191). Clinical evaluation must include a thorough history and physical examination, with special attention paid to potential inciting factors. Factors that exacerbate or perpetuate spasticity include noxious stimuli below the zone of injury and frequently are not clinically apparent. Therefore, a high index of suspicion and a thorough evaluation are necessary, particularly in view of the age-dependent variability in the ability to communicate. Hip subluxation is an example of a noxious stimulus that may exacerbate spasticity and that is more common in the pediatric SCI population.

The goals of managing spasticity are to improve function, prevent complications, and alleviate pain, inconvenience, and embarrassment (191,195). In treating spasticity, both its advantages and disadvantages must be taken into account. Prevention is the foundation of a therapeutic program and encompasses avoidance of precipitating factors and establishment of good bladder, bowel, and skin programs. Nonpharmacologic interventions include relief of inciting factors and a basic program of stretching, range-of-motion, and positioning exercises.

For spasticity that is unresponsive to conservative management and that affects the child's functioning, medications are indicated. Orally administered baclofen (Lioresal) is the initial drug of choice and is initiated at 0.125 mg/kg/dose given two to three times daily (5 mg two to three times daily in children 12 years and older) (196). Doses are increased every 3 to 5 days in increments of 0.125 mg/kg/dose (5 mg/dose in children 12 years and older). The usual maximum daily dose is 1 to 2 mg/kg/day administered four times daily (80 mg/day in children 12 years and older). Although baclofen remains the drug of choice for managing spasticity in adolescents, the potential for drug experimentation must be considered (197).

Other drugs that may be beneficial include diazepam, clonidine, dantrolene, gabapentin, and tizanidine. The second drug of choice is diazepam (valium, 0.1 mg/kg/dose every night to four times daily), which may be used in combination with baclofen or as a single drug for patients who do not tolerate baclofen. Clonidine (5 to 7 μg/kg/day divided every 6 to 12 hours) may be effective as a single agent or in combination with other drugs (198). Transdermal administration of clonidine (0.1- to 0.3 mg patch weekly) may be used in adolescents (199,200). Dantrolene (Dantrium) is generally not used to manage spasticity in children and adolescents with SCI. Although not approved for use for spasticity, gabapentin (Neurontin, 900 to 1,800 mg/day in three divided doses for children older than 12 years of age) may help to control spasticity. Although tizanidine (Zanaflex) is not approved for use in pediatrics, in clinical practice, it is used by some clinicians and demonstrates efficacy similar to that in adults with SCI (201). Because of the potential for hepatotoxicity, liver function studies should be performed, particularly during the first 6 months of therapy.

For spasticity unresponsive to standard management, therapeutic options include intrathecal baclofen, selective dorsal root rhizotomies, epidural spinal cord stimulation, and localized injection of botulinum toxin (202–207). Baclofen can be administered intrathecally by a pump that is implanted in a subcutaneous pocket in the anterior abdominal wall. Intrathecal baclofen has been used increasingly in children and adolescents with SCI with encouraging results (208). In addition to SCI, experience with intrathecal baclofen in the pediatric population has been expanded to children and adolescents with cerebral palsy (209). Disadvantages of intrathecal baclofen are cost of both the initial implantation and pump refills and the rare occurrence of serious adverse reactions (210,211). Motor point blocks may be performed for localized spasticity. The usual dose of botulinum toxin is 4 U/kg for injection into a single muscle, with a maximum of 10 U/kg (maximum of 400 units) if botulinum toxin is injected into more than one muscle.

Pressure Ulcers

Similar to the adult population, pressure ulcers are one of the most common complications for children and adolescents with SCI (212,213). The true incidence of pressure ulcers in either the pediatric or adult SCI population is not known. In a retrospective study of individuals who sustained their SCI when they were younger than 13 years of age, 55% developed at least one pressure ulcer during a mean follow-up period of 10.3 years (212). The peak age for prevalence of pressure ulcers was 8 years of age. Issues that are unique to the pediatric population include variable degrees of compliance in both preventive and therapeutic endeavors associated with different developmental stages of children and adolescents (212,214). Toddlers and younger children may be at risk for skin breakdown as a result of inadvertent trauma from careless activities and play characteristic of these age groups. These younger patients have limited cognitive abilities to follow the usual preventive measures that older individuals follow, such as pressure relief measures. Preventive measures may include wristwatches with automatic resetting timers to remind children to perform pressure relief measures. Additionally, pressure ulcer prevention activities must be developmentally based, and responsibility must be progressively shifted from the parents to the children as they grow up. In addition, new equipment must be appropriately matched to the child's increasing size. Properly fitting wheelchairs and adequate cushions must be prescribed with pressure mapping to reduce the risk for pressure ulcer development.

Rehabilitation

Rehabilitation must be developmentally based, and as a consequence, goals must respond to the dynamic evolutionary forces that accompany growing patients into adulthood (1,215–222). Goals of rehabilitation should be to maintain health and restore productivity with the ultimate goal of life satisfaction. The challenge in caring for children and adolescents with SCI is to address the changing objectives of each developmental stage, with the ultimate goal being that the patient becomes an adult with a high quality of life (223). Pediatric-focused care must establish a solid foundation from which satisfactory quality of life flourishes throughout childhood and into adulthood.

Traditional interventions include mobility; activities of daily living; bowel, bladder, and skin programs; recreation; psychological and vocational counseling; and social services.

Conventional rehabilitation must be expanded to encompass effective mobility and access in the community as well as recreational, educational, and vocational interventions that facilitate a productive and satisfying life. As children and adolescents

grow, new equipment is needed because of both increasing size and changing needs. Using mobility as an example, infants and young toddlers may crawl, progress to parapodia, and use strollers for wheeled mobility. Preschool-aged and early school-aged children may crawl at home but use a variety of orthotics for ambulation or standing in school; they should be independent in appropriate types of wheelchairs. Except for individuals who have less severe neurologic impairments allowing community ambulation, older children and adolescents primarily, if not exclusively, use wheelchairs for all their mobility. These older patients may have needs for standing or sports-specific wheelchairs, with older adolescents needing access to motor vehicles for community mobility.

Ambulation

Long-term community ambulation is dependent on several factors, including neurologic level and category, age, body size, compliance, and preferences. Individuals who are most likely to be community ambulators are those who are young, have L3 or lower lesions, or have an American Spinal Injury Association (ASIA) Impairment Scale score of D (224,225). Although individuals of all ages with SCI want to walk, children are more likely to be active ambulators compared with adolescents and adults because of their smaller size, increased energy level, and less concern for cosmetics (225–230).

Parapodia allow children with SCI to stand without the need for upper extremity weightbearing, so that they can perform activities with both hands (225,231). Parapodia may also allow children to ambulate. The requirements for using parapodia include the absence of significant contractures of the lower extremities and head control; thus, children with neurologic levels as high as C4 who have head control can use parapodia. Patients who use parapodia are either therapeutic or household ambulators; nonetheless, parapodia provide users with some independence in mobility as well as an opportunity to be upright and face their peers at eye level. Parapodia can be initiated in children as young as 9 to 12 months of age, which is the developmentally appropriate time to initiate standing, and they are useful in providing young children with the opportunity to be upright, before the use of other orthotics. Parapodia also have the advantage of not requiring intensive therapy. Although parapodia are accepted by preschool-aged and early school-aged children, most children elect to stop using parapodia by 7 to 10 years of age.

Two of the more commonly used parapodia are the Rochester parapodium and swivel walkers. The Rochester parapodium has hip and knee joints that facilitate donning and doffing. They allow the patient to sit while wearing the brace, and also assists the patient in transferring from the floor or chair to standing (231,232) (Fig. 29.5). Using the Rochester parapodium, a child can ambulate by swiveling their upper trunk and swinging their arms. Alternatively, with walkers or forearm crutches, they can perform a swing-to or a swing-through gait.

The ORLAU (Orthotic Research and Locomotion Assessment Unit) swivel walker allows for a reciprocal-like movement of paired foot plates (233) (Fig. 29.6). Advantages of the ORLAU swivel walker include the reciprocal-like gait, the plastic chute that facilitates donning, and the sturdy construction that

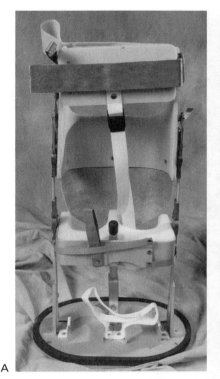
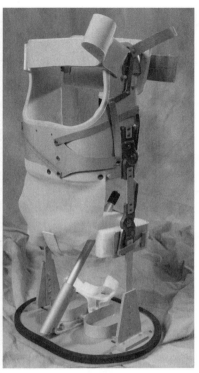

A   B

FIGURE 29.5. **A,B**; Rochester parapodium; front (**A**) and back (**B**) views.

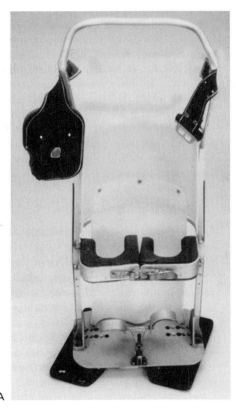
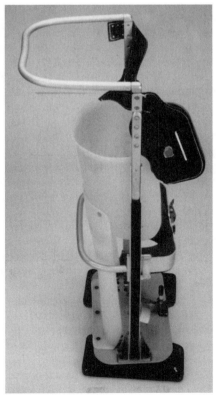

A   B

FIGURE 29.6. **A,B**; The ORLAU (Orthotic Research and Locomotion Assessment Unit) swivel walker; front (**A**) and side (**B**) views.

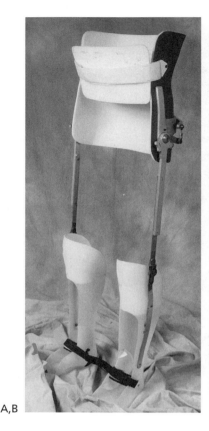
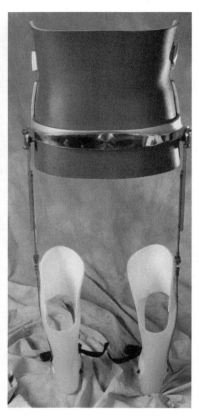

A,B

FIGURE 29.7. A,B; Reciprocating gait orthosis (RGO); front (**A**) and back (**B**) views.

allows use by adolescents. However, the ORLAU swivel walker, because it has no joints, does not allow the wearer to sit.

Reciprocating gait orthoses (RGOs) are used by paraplegic patients with L2 or higher-level lesions (225,230,231) (Fig. 29.7). In comparison to other orthotics, such as hip-knee-ankle-foot orthoses (HKAFOs) or knee-ankle-foot orthoses (KAFOs), that may be used in this group of patients, RGOs provide a reciprocating gait and are more energy efficient (234). RGOs may be initiated in children as young as 15 to 18 months old. Patients with active hip flexors and those who are young and well motivated are most likely to be community ambulators (230,231). However, most RGO users are therapeutic or household ambulators.

Standing, with or without ambulation, may have immense psychological and functional benefits for children and adolescents with SCI (230,235). In addition to parapodia, there are a variety of static and mobile standing devices that are suitable for children, including standing wheelchairs, standing frames, and mobile standing devices (230). Because of their size, standing wheelchairs are appropriate only for older children and adolescents. Mobile standing devices, such as the Standing Dani and the Rifton standing walker, are most acceptable for preschool-aged to preadolescent children. They are primarily used for household, school, or vocational activities.

Use of FES systems for upright mobility in children and adolescents has been demonstrated to be feasible as well as practical (1,236). Using implanted FES systems, adolescents stood at home two to four times a week; common activities while stand-

ing included reaching high places, accessing environments, and exercise (237). In another study, an implanted FES system was compared with KAFOs (238). FES was comparable or better than orthotics in facilitating independence and was preferred over braces for most activities. Contraindications to the use of FES for upright mobility include hip dislocation, lower extremity contractures, severe scoliosis, and myocutaneous flaps that have been surgically created to treat pressure ulcers. Therefore, prevention of these complications is critical for children and adolescents with SCI who may one day benefit from innovative treatments such as FES.

Upper Extremity Function

A variety of both static and dynamic orthotics are available to improve hand function of individuals with tetraplegia (239,240). However, children and adolescents typically abandon use of these braces because of cosmesis, the added stigma, and the burden of carrying equipment around to different activities. In contrast, surgical reconstruction, including tendon transfers, of the upper extremities to restore hand function has been shown to be beneficial in the pediatric SCI population (241,242). Surgical reconstruction of the upper extremities has been performed to restore elbow extension, wrist extension, finger flexion, and thumb pinch. Children as young as 5 to 6 years of age have undergone tendon transfers, with the ability to cooperate in rehabilitation being the key factor.

Implantable FES systems have been successfully used in adolescents with C5 or weak C6 tetraplegic injuries to restore grasp and release in those who would not be candidates for reconstructive surgeries (243,244). Similar to adults with SCI, use of the Freehand system in adolescents has resulted in increased independence in activities and improved satisfaction (240,245). Findings in animal studies and U.S. Food and Drug Administration clinical trials in humans suggest that children as young as 6 years of age may benefit from this technology (246).

Psychosocial Issues and Sexuality

Both general and SCI-specific sexuality issues need to be addressed with the patient and family (247–249). From the onset of the SCI, parents and patients, as developmentally appropriate, need to be informed in an optimistic fashion about future sexuality issues, including fertility. Sexuality counseling needs to be addressed progressiviely with older children and adolescents without parents being present. Finally, girls who have sustained SCI and their parents can be reassured that the SCI will result in minor or no abnormalities or delays in onset or resumption of menstruation (250).

As for all children with special needs, federal laws protect the educational rights of children and adolescents with SCI (251). The public laws, the Education for All Handicapped Children Act (EAHCA, 1975) and the Individuals with Disabilities Education Act (IDEA, 1990), require that they be educated in the least restrictive environment (252). Education plays a critical role in the lives of children and adolescents with SCI in several ways (11,223,247,248). Along with play, education is the main occupation for children and adolescents. It is very important that they return to school as soon as possible after injury, and ideally, they should return to the school that they had attended before their injury. Returning to school permits the individual with a SCI to reestablish friendships and peer interactions. In addition, education is a major determinant for adult employment, which in turn is a crucial ingredient of life satisfaction for adults with SCI. Returning to school can be a traumatic event for the patient as well as the teachers and students. From the patient's perspective, this transition back into school may be greatly facilitated by visiting the school and classrooms before discharge from SCI rehabilitation. From the students' and teachers' perspectives, the previously described visit may be very beneficial. If that is not possible, the teachers and students may benefit from viewing a video of the patient as well as educational materials about SCI. A teaching manual about SCI designed for teachers and nurses may also be useful (247,248).

Children and adolescents with SCI should receive psychological evaluation and counseling in an ongoing manner, appropriate for their developmental stage (253). Because of the significant impact that families have on their children or adolescents with SCI, counseling and support must be provided for parents, siblings, and other significant family members (247,248). Support and peer groups are also beneficial for patients, parents, and other family members.

Attendant care should be considered for children with tetraplegia even though family members are available for daily care. Availability of attendant care allows the parents to maintain their parental role, including use of limit setting and provision of support and guidance for their children. It is frequently difficult for parents to fulfill both roles of parent and caregiver, and parents can easily become stressed if they are required to "wear both hats." At a minimum, parents need respite care, particularly if their children have high-level tetraplegia with complicated and intense needs.

Play and recreation must be an integral component of the rehabilitation program for children and adolescents with SCI (155–157). Play and recreation-based therapy should be consistent with preinjury interests of the patient. Play is critical for young children in rehabilitation because it is their primary activity of daily living. Recreation and play provide older children and adolescents with time away from rehabilitation staff. They need to be provided appropriate outlets and access to typical childhood and adolescent activities, such as television, movies, music, talk, and sports. They need to be educated about and exposed to community activities and wheelchair sports that are available in their community.

Similar to the adult SCI population, substance abuse and psychological problems are major issues for children and adolescents with SCI (254). Adolescents with SCI may be at greater risk for suicide because of the tremendous impact of a SCI superimposed upon the usual turbulence of adolescence.

Surgical Treatment
Halo Fixators

Proper halo ring application is crucial in preventing pin loosening and pin tract infections. Children 12 years of age and younger present unique issues with halo fixation. Multiple pins (10, as compared with 4 in adults) with low torque (2 inchpounds) have been demonstrated to be safe in infants (255). For children between 2 and 12 years old, torque may range from 4 to 6 inch-pounds. For patients older than 12 years of age, pins should be torqued to 8 inch-pounds. For children younger than 6 years of age, CT scanning of the skull is recommended for pin placement because of the variability in skull thickness (256, 257). If halo fixation fails because of loosening or infection, a Minerva-type cervicothoracolumbosacral orthosis is effective. Because use of Crutchfield tongs in patients younger than 12 years old may be associated with skull penetration and dural fluid leaks, a halo ring for traction is effective and is the preferred alternative.

Spine Boards

In children younger than 8 to 10 years of age, the head is proportionately larger than the body. As a consequence, when children of this age group are immobilized on a standard spine board, their neck will be inadvertently flexed (Fig. 29.8B). Therefore, when spinal stabilization is needed in an emergency situation, younger children should be immobilized on child-specific spine boards (258) (Fig. 29.8C). However, if a standard spine board must be used in a younger child, excessive cervical flexion can be avoided by raising the torso 2 to 4 cm, leaving the head at the board level (Fig. 29.8D).

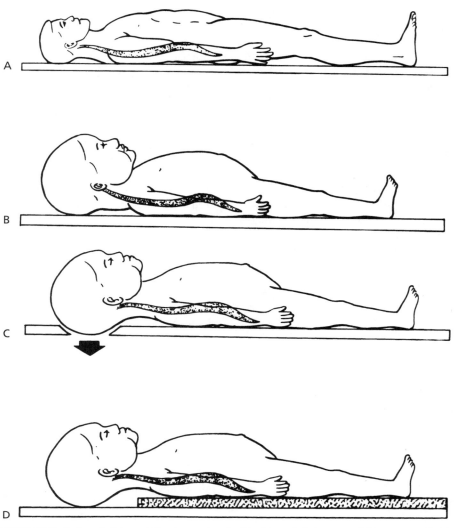

FIGURE 29.8. **A**; An adult immobilized on a standard backboard. **B**; A young child on a standard backboard; the relatively large head results in a kyphotic position of the neck. **C**; The child is on a modified backboard with a cut-out to recess the occiput, providing safe cervical positioning. **D**; The double mattress pad raises the chest, providing for safe cervical positioning. (From Herzenberg JE, Hensinger RN, Dedrick DK, et al. Emergency transport and positioning of young children who have an injury of the cervical spine: the standard backboard may be hazardous. *J Bone Joint Surg [Am]*, 1989;71:15–22, with permission.)

Spine Deformities

Spine deformities are common in pediatric SCI, particularly if the injury is sustained before skeletal maturity (259–262) (Fig. 29.9). Among children injured before puberty, 98% developed scoliosis, with 67% requiring surgical correction (260). In contrast, when the injury occurred after skeletal maturity, the risk for scoliosis was 20%, with 5% requiring surgery. The spine deformity may be caused by muscle weakness or imbalance or residual deformity, or it can be iatrogenic, as a result, for example, of a laminectomy (263). Problems that can complicate spine deformities include pelvic obliquity, impaired use of the upper extremities secondary to poor sitting balance, pressure ulcers, pain, poor fitting of lower extremity orthotics, and gastrointesti-

nal and cardiopulmonary abnormalities. Because of the high incidence of scoliosis, radiographs of the thoracolumbosacral spine should be obtained every 6 months before skeletal maturity and every 12 months thereafter.

Although controversial, prophylactic bracing with a lightweight thoracolumbosacral orthosis (TLSO) may be effective in delaying surgery. Among 24 children with SCI who were braced prophylactically, 80% maintained their curvatures, and 20% had curve progression over 50 degrees, necessitating surgery (264). In contrast, of the five children who were never braced, four experienced curve progressions beyond 50 degrees and required surgery. The greatest benefits were seen when prophylactic bracing was initiated before the spine curvature exceeded 20 degrees or within 1 year of the SCI. Major disadvantages of routine

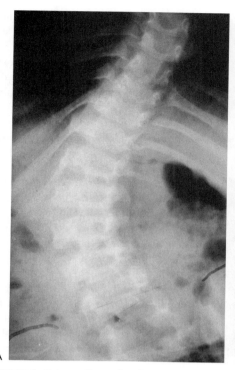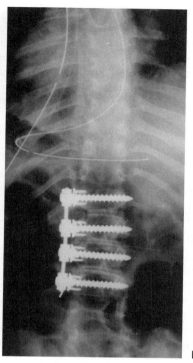

FIGURE 29.9. Spine radiographs of an 8-year-old boy who sustained an incomplete T4 spinal cord injury (ASIA impairment scale score of D) when he was 2 years old. **A;** A 52-degree thoracolumbar curve. **B;** Radiograph obtained after the patient underwent an anterior spine fusion with instrumentation when he was 8½ years old.

bracing include interference with mobility and independent functioning, such as self-catheterization. Bracing with a TLSO should be prescribed for patients with poor trunk support to facilitate upper extremity function and sitting. Bracing with a TLSO would also be indicated for immature children with curves greater than 20 to 45 degrees (265).

Surgical correction for spine deformities should be undertaken when the curve progresses beyond 40 degrees in children older than 10 years of age (1). For younger children, curves up to 80 degrees are tolerated if they are somewhat flexible and temporarily decrease while in a TLSO; otherwise, surgery would be indicated regardless of age.

Hip Deformities

Hip dislocation, subluxation, and contractures are extremely common in pediatric SCI, especially among children injured at younger ages (1,263,266,267). In one series, hip instability was observed in 100% of children injured when they were younger than 5 years of age and in 83% of those injured when they were younger than 10 years of age (1). In another series, hip instability was found in 60% of children injured when they were 8 years of age or younger (268). Hip instability developed in patients with tetraplegia or paraplegia, in boys and girls, and in patients with flaccid as well as spastic SCI (269).

Indications for surgical management of hip instability are not entirely clear. With the development of FES systems for standing and walking and the future possibility of spinal cord regeneration, aggressive prophylactic surgical treatment of hip instability should be considered (1,270). Management of hip instability may include surgical release of hip contractures, a capsulorrhaphy, varus osteotomies, and acetabular augmentations (anterior or posterior) (263,271).

Prophylactic bracing from the time of sustaining the SCI should be considered in children injured when they were younger than 5 years old. Prophylactic bracing could be an abduction-flexion orthosis with free, unrestricted flexion, maintaining 20 degrees of abduction bilaterally.

Heterotopic Ossification

The incidence of heterotopic ossification (HO) in pediatric SCI is about 3%, compared with about 20% in adults with SCI (263,272). Similar to adults, the hip is most commonly involved in children and adolescents with SCI. The average onset of HO is reported as 14 months for pediatric SCI, as compared with onset in adults with SCI, which is typically 1 to 4 months after injury (273). Prophylaxis for HO using etidronate disodium (Didronel) (274) is not routinely used in the pediatric SCI population because of the relatively low risk for HO. In addition, etidronate disodium may be contraindicated in prepubertal children because of the potential development of rachitic-like changes (275–277). Management of HO in children with SCI is equivalent to that in adults. Indications for surgical interventions include significant functional deficits. Resection of HO probably should be undertaken about 1 to 1.5 years after its onset to avoid progression of femoral neck osteoporosis and intraarticular fibrosis if surgery is postponed until the bone scan and alkaline phosphatase level are normal (272,278). Postoperative use of radiation therapy may be contraindicated in younger children because of long-term consequences of radiation. However, indomethacin (Indocin, 1 to 3 mg/kg/day in three or four divided doses, with a maximum dose of 200 mg/day) is used in the postoperative period (279).

Osteopenia and Pathologic Fractures

Osteopenia begins immediately after sustaining a SCI and plateaus 6 to 12 months later. Children and adolescents with SCI have bone densities of about 60% of normal age- and sex-matched controls (280). A combination of standing, stepping, and FES may increase bone mineral density by about 25%.

Pathologic long bone fractures occur as a consequence of loss of bone mineral density. Pathologic fractures occur in about 14% of children and adolescents with SCI (1,263). The etiology in 40% of patients includes gait training, range of motion, and minor trauma. The etiology of the pathologic fractures in the remaining 60% of the patients was not identified. Patients with pathologic fractures typically present with fever and a swollen extremity. The most common sites of fracture are the supracondylar region of the femur and the proximal tibia. Initial radiologic findings may be subtle, and the diagnosis of a pathologic fracture in growing children may require a high index of suspicion (263) (Fig. 29.10).

Treatment of pathologic fractures should consist of removable splints (1,263,281). If casts are necessary, they must be well padded over all bony prominences and bivalved to enable inspection to prevent pressure ulcers. Because the bone is osteoporotic, it generally will not hold internal or external fixation very well. Fortunately, exuberant callous develops within 3 to 4 weeks, at which time the splinting or casting can be minimized with resumption of range of motion. Ambulation with orthotics should be postponed for 6 to 8 weeks after sustaining a fracture.

Prevention is critical but may be particularly challenging in the pediatric SCI population because of risk-taking behavior observed in children and adolescents of different ages. Caretakers must focus on safety in risky activities. Bone mineral loss should be minimized by encouraging weightbearing with orthotics or FES. Good nutrition and adequate sunlight are essential. Appropriate training and adequate equipment for transfers are essential

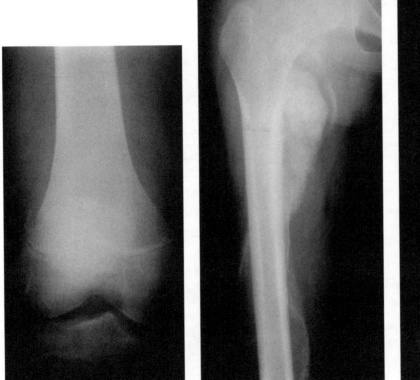
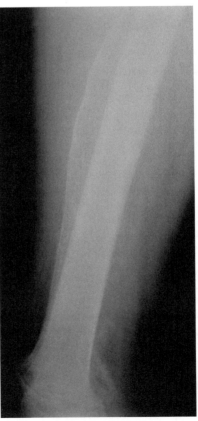

A,B

C

FIGURE 29.10. This 15-year-old boy with a T10 complete spinal cord injury sustained a supracondylar femoral fracture 9 months after his injury. There was no apparent cause of the fracture. **A**; A slight defect of the medial aspect of the femoral metaphysis. **B,C**; Radiographs taken 2 months later demonstrate exuberant callus formation of the entire femur.

components of pediatric SCI rehabilitation. In the future, bisphosphonates, such as alendronate, may have a role in preventing pathologic fractures.

NEURAL TUBE DEFECTS

Spina bifida and anencephaly are the two most common forms of neural tube defects, also referred to as *spinal dysraphism* (282–286). Spina bifida can be classified based on whether neural tissue is exposed (283,284). Myelomeningoceles are open lesions that either have absent skin covering or are covered only by a thin membrane. Spina bifida lesions with intact skin covering, referred to as *occult spinal dysraphism*, include lipomeningocele, diastematomyelia, dermal sinus, meningocele, tight filum terminale, and myelocystocele. The diagnosis of spina bifida occulta should be reserved for the common spinal abnormality that is only identified on plain radiographs as a failure of fusion of the spinous processes of the lower lumbar or sacral spine without neurologic abnormalities.

Myelomeningoceles are the most common form of nonfatal neural tube defects, and they are characterized by significant defects of both the brain and the spinal cord. This section reviews the epidemiology, etiology, pathogenesis, clinical manifestations, management, and prevention of myelomeningoceles.

Epidemiology

In 1990, the incidence of myelomeningocele in the United States was 3.2 per 10,000 live births (287). The incidence of myelomeningocele has demonstrated trends in respect to time, geography, and race and ethnicity. These trends may be related to changing nutritional status, periconceptual use of folic acid, availability of prenatal diagnosis, and elective pregnancy termination (288,289). In the United States, the incidence of myelomeningocele has decreased form 5.9 cases per 10,000 births in 1984 to 3.2 cases per 10,000 births in 1990 (287). In the United States from 1983 through 1990, the rates of myelomeningocele varied among racial and ethnic groups, with the lowest incidence in Asians and Pacific Islanders (2.3 per 10,000) and the highest rates for Hispanics (6.0 per 10,000) (287). However, by 1990, the rates for myelomeningocele were nearly identical for blacks, Hispanics, and whites. There appears to be a higher incidence of neural tube defects in lower socioeconomic populations (290). Worldwide, there have also been significant differences in the incidence of neural tube defects, with higher rates in certain countries, such as China (291).

Mortality is highest during infancy and is primarily related to problems with hindbrain function, central nervous system infection, and hydrocephalus (292,293). Analysis of survival data is complicated by different treatment approaches used since the 1960s. In a recent report, 56% of patients survived to their twentieth birthday (294).

Etiology

The etiology of myelomeningocele is unknown, although presumably it involves both genetic and environmental factors (295). Maternal diabetes mellitus (296) and maternal use of valproic acid (297) and carbamazepine (298) are associated with an increased risk for neural tube defects. Other factors that may be associated with the development of neural tube defects include maternal obesity (299–301), fever (302), and hyperthermia (303). The increased incidence of neural tube defects in lower socioeconomic groups suggests that nutritional deficiencies, including folic acid, may play a role in their etiology (290). The risk for neural-tube defects is increased in individuals homozygous for a common mutation in the gene for methylenetetrahydrofolate reductase (MTHFR) (304). These observations support the potential role of folic acid deficiency in the etiology of neural tube defects.

The role of genetic factors in the etiology of neural tube defects is supported by the observed increased risk in individuals who have previously had an affected baby, first-degree relatives, and individuals who have neural tube defects themselves (283). The recurrence risk ranges from 1% to 5% in a family with one affected child and up to 10% in families with two affected children (286,295,305–307).

Pathophysiology

Neural tube defects are caused by failure of the neural tube to close between the third and fourth weeks of gestation, resulting in abnormalities of the brain and spinal cord (308). The major abnormalities of the brain include hydrocephalus in 80% to 90% of children with myelomeningoceles and Chiari II malformation in virtually all affected individuals (309). The main characteristics of Chiari II malformation are a small posterior fossa, caudal displacement of the cerebellar vermis and brain stem into the cervical spinal canal, kinking of the cervicomedullary junction, and beaking of the tectum. The hydrocephalus is caused primarily by obstruction of cerebrospinal fluid (CSF) movement as a result of the complex deformities of the posterior fossa and brain stem, related to the Chiari II malformation.

The defect of the spine and spinal cord can occur from the thoracic to the sacral levels, with the lumbosacral region involved in about 66% to 75% of cases (310). At the level of the defect, the spinal canal is open dorsally with defects of the posterior elements of several contiguous vertebrae (311). At the level of the myelomeningocele defect, the spinal cord exhibits varying degrees of dysplasia, is present as a flat neural plate, and is covered by a thin membrane. Damage to the spinal cord and resulting neurologic abnormalities are probably a result of several factors. These include spinal cord dysplasia; tethering of the spinal cord at the myelomeningocele defect; toxicity of amniotic fluid; mechanical trauma from the uterine wall during later gestation, labor, and delivery; and damage to the neural plate during its surgical repair (312,313).

Clinical Presentation

An affected neonate should undergo repair of the myelomeningocele shortly after birth to reduce the risk for infection and ventriculitis (314). If the myelomeningocele sac is leaking, closure should be undertaken within the first 24 hours of life; otherwise, the closure can be performed within the first 2 to 3 days of life (311,314,315). The goals of the initial closure are to cover the defect with skin, untether the spinal cord, and reconstruct the neural tube and dura. After closure of the myelomeningocele defect, the patient needs to be monitored closely for the development of hydrocephalus. This eventually develops in 80% to 90% of cases, necessitating a ventriculoperitoneal shunt (284,285, 316,317).

The primary manifestations of myelomeningocele are a result of the brain and spinal cord abnormalities. Children with myelomeningocele exhibit a variety of cognitive defects (318). Prior episodes of meningitis or ventriculitis adversely affect cognition (319). About 30% of individuals with myelomeningocele have below-normal intelligence, primarily perceptual motor abnormalities with normal verbal skills. They frequently have disorders of visuospatial organization and may experience learning disabilities, hearing and visual impairments, and seizures (320). Individuals with myelomeningocele may exhibit "cocktail chatter," which is characterized by excessive talking and superficiality of content (321). Children with myelomeningocele frequently demonstrate defects in coordination and dexterity of hand function (322–324).

Because most individuals with myelomeningocele have hydrocephalus and require ventriculoperitoneal shunts, they are at risk for shunt infections and shunt malfunction. In younger children, shunt malfunction is manifest by symptoms of increased intracranial pressure, including nausea, vomiting, and severe headache. In contrast, the symptoms of shunt malfunction in adolescents and young adults may be subtler. They may present with indolent symptoms of irritability, decreased perceptual motor function, shortened attention span, intermittent headaches, poor school performance, weakness, or worsening scoliosis.

Chiari II malformation may result in hindbrain dysfunction (309). In infants and younger children, symptoms may include feeding and swallowing abnormalities, stridor, vocal cord paralysis, weak cry, apnea, sleep-disordered breathing (325–328), nystagmus, opisthotonos, and weakness and spasticity of the upper extremities. Older children and adolescents are more likely to present with progressive scoliosis, decreased upper extremity function, neck pain, and depressed respiratory function. Symptoms of Chiari II malformation usually resolve with adequate shunting of the hydrocephalus; however, some patients may require a posterior fossa decompression (309,329).

Hydrosyringomyelia in association with Chiari II malformation is a common finding in individuals with myelomeningocele (309,329). The clinical manifestations are similar to those of developmental hydrosyringomyelia associated with Chiari I malformation, which is discussed later in this chapter.

The main manifestations of spinal cord dysfunction are motor paralysis, sensory loss, spasticity, and bladder, bowel, and sexual dysfunction. The extent of the neurologic deficit is dependent on the location of the myelomeningocele. In contrast to spinal cord injuries in which the degree of motor deficits either approximate or exceed the sensory deficits, individuals with myelomeningocele have sensory deficits that are generally more severe than the motor deficits. The nature of the spinal cord abnormality in myelomeningocele is more severe involvement of the dorsal aspect of the spinal cord, including the posterior spinal nerve roots, with relative sparing of the anterior spinal nerve roots. In the absence of normal sensation, the function of muscles under voluntary control is limited. Although most patients with myelomeningocele have flaccid paralysis, about 10% to 30% exhibit spasticity (330,331).

Several classification systems are used to characterize spinal cord dysfunction in individuals with myelomeningocele (330, 332,333). These classification systems are generally used to predict ambulation potential. It is important to document accurately and serially the motor and sensory levels and the presence and degree of spasticity. This is particularly important for early identification of complications such as retethering of the spinal cord, hydrosyringomyelia, and hydrocephalus.

A major aspect of the myelomeningocele abnormality at birth is tethering of the spinal cord at the site of the defect. One of the major goals of the initial surgical correction in the neonate is to untether the spinal cord. However, there is a tendency for the spinal cord to become adherent to the myelomeningocele repair site (311). This results in retethering of the spinal cord and a low-lying spinal cord, which is found in most patients with myelomeningocele (285,334). During growth, the retethered spinal cord cannot migrate cephalad as it normally would. In some patients, the retethered spinal cord may impair remaining spinal cord function, manifest by the onset or worsening of weakness, sensory loss, spasticity, progressive scoliosis, changes in bowel or bladder function, pain, or orthopedic deformities in the lower extremities. Because most patients with low-lying spinal cords are asymptomatic, the decision to untether the spinal cord surgically must be based on the presence of well-documented clinical changes.

The clinical manifestations and management of the neurogenic bladder and bowel in patients with myelomeningocele are not significantly different from those in children and adolescents with SCI. However, individuals with myelomeningocele may have congenital anomalies of the genitourinary system that require additional monitoring or treatment (335). Male patients with myelomeningocele are at increased risk for cryptorchidism (336,337).

Urodynamic testing should be performed during the neonatal period, once the baby has been stabilized after repairing the myelomeningocele defect (338–342). Newborns at risk for urinary tract deterioration demonstrate high bladder pressures (leak point pressure of 40 cm H_2O or higher) or detrusor–sphincter dyssynergia. These high-risk neonates should be managed with intermittent catheterization and anticholinergics as soon as they are identified by urodynamic testing. Compared with SCI patients, another major difference in individuals with myelomeningocele is that they have neurogenic bladder dysfunction from conception. This may significantly retard the growth of the bladder, especially in children with high-pressure, low-volume bladders. Bladder augmentation may be required if the bladder capacity is inadequate despite anticholinergic therapy (342).

Intermittent catheterization is standard management of the neurogenic bladder in patients with myelomeningocele (74,75, 338,342,343). However, the ability to perform self-catheterization may be complicated by visuomotor deficits that are commonly found in patients with myelomeningocele and developmental delays that may also be present (75,344).

Bowel incontinence is a major problem for children with myelomeningocele, particularly those without bulbocavernosus or anocutaneous reflexes (345). Aggressive interventions, including education and regular, consistently timed reflex-triggered bowel evacuations, are effective (345). Patients with bowel program complications unresponsive to more conservative measures may be candidates for antegrade continence enemas (105), pulsed irrigation enemas (104), enema continence catheters (106,346), or biofeedback (347–349).

Secondary manifestations or complications may be present at birth and may be considered congenital defects, or they may be acquired postnatally. Congenital defects, such as clubfeet, dislocated hips, or extension contractures of the knees, are secondary complications of the primary spinal cord defect with resulting *in utero* paralysis. Postnatally acquired secondary complications result in significant morbidity and occasionally mortality. Prevention and early management of secondary complications are integral in the overall management of children and adolescents with myelomeningocele. Meningitis, ventriculitis, tethered cord, and shunt malfunction have already been discussed.

Orthopedic Issues

Children and adolescents with myelomeningocele experience a variety of orthopedic complications, particularly disorders of the lower extremities and spine (310,350). Orthopedic deformities are the result of several factors, including paralysis, unopposed muscle function, congenital malformation, and spasticity (350). Orthopedic deformities may be present at birth and result from paralysis present *in utero*, affecting the position of the fetus. Examples of this include clubfeet, dislocated hips, and extension contractures of the knees (310). Other orthopedic abnormalities, such as congenital vertebral and rib anomalies, present in as many as 15% of patients, may be present at birth and are primary defects associated with myelomeningocele. Postnatally acquired orthopedic complications, such as dislocated hips, hip and knee contractures, and pathologic fractures, may develop as a consequence of the neuromuscular defects associated with myelomeningocele. Finally, scoliosis, kyphosis, and lordosis may be a consequence of both congenital vertebral anomalies and neuromuscular defects (351). The management of these orthopedic complications is generally complicated and should be directed by clinicians experienced in caring for children and adolescents with myelomeningocele. Depending on the neurologic level, many children and adolescents with myelomeningocele ambulate to varying degrees, so that management of the lower extremity deformities must take this into account.

Contractures and dislocation of hips are common in children with myelomeningocele, particularly in patients with thoracic and upper lumbar to mid-lumbar lesions, of which up to 90% may be affected (285,352). In thoracic level lesions, the hip dislocation occurs because all of the hip musculature is denervated (350). In contrast, for lumbar level lesions, hip dysplasia results from muscle imbalance with active hip flexors and adductors but paralyzed extensors and abductors. Management of hip dysplasia in the myelomeningocele population is controversial, particularly because hip dysplasia is usually not painful and may not significantly affect the ability to walk (353). In patients with thoracic and upper lumber to mid-lumbar lesions, treatment of the hip dysplasia is usually reserved for those with pelvic obliquity, who would be at higher risk for pressure ulcers. Children with lower lumbar lesions have good ambulation potential. Their dislocated hips should be surgically corrected by 4 years of age, including both skeletal corrections and muscle transfers, to prevent recurrent dislocation.

Hip contractures are common complications in patients with myelomeningocele and can interfere with ambulation, particularly if they exceed 30 to 40 degrees. Surgical releases are frequently complicated by recurrences (285). Management of hip contractures must be individualized and based on the neurologic level, presence of hip dysplasia, and ambulation status. Hip contractures in patients with thoracic and upper lumbar levels are generally managed by surgical releases and aggressive postoperative bracing and physical therapy. For individuals with mid-lumbar to lower lumbar lesions, contractures are managed by a combination of surgical releases and appropriate tendon transfers.

The major abnormalities of the knees are extension and flexion contractures and a valgus rotation deformity (285,350). Extension contractures are relatively uncommon and are usually the result of breech delivery. They may also be seen in patients with mid-lumbar level lesions who have strong quadriceps without strong knee flexors. Most of these cases can be managed with physical therapy and splinting. For extension knee contractures that are resistant to conservative management, a modified V-Y quadricepsplasty should be performed. Knee flexion contractures of less than 20 degrees are generally well tolerated, but more severe contractures may limit ambulation potential. Physical therapy and splinting may be effective in children younger than 2 years of age; otherwise, surgical correction is indicated. Valgus rotation deformities of the knee result from iliotibial band tightness and the forces of ambulation. For younger children, treatment includes muscle transfers, distal iliotibial band sectioning, and KAFOs. Distal femoral osteotomies may be necessary if the deformity becomes fixed.

Deformities of the ankle and feet are common in children and adolescents with myelomeningocele, and they tend to be resistant to conservative measures and generally require surgical correction (285,350). About half of patients with myelomeningocele have clubfeet, as a result of muscle paralysis and *in utero* positioning. These clubfeet tend to be rigid, are resistant to casting, and usually require surgical repair (350). In patients with low lumbar lesions, calcaneovalgus deformities result from unopposed contraction of the anterior tibial muscle, toe extensors, or the peroneal muscles. The deformity is usually progressive, results in a crouch gait, and predisposes to pressure ulcers of the feet from shoe or brace wear. Surgical correction consists of transferring the anterior tibial tendon to the os calcis (350). Cavus deformities of the foot are frequently accompanied by claw-toe deformities in individuals with sacral level lesions, predisposing to pressure ulcers under the toes or metatarsal heads.

Pathologic fractures are most prevalent in children 3 to 7 years of age and are particularly common after cast immobilization or during skeletal traction (285). The fractures are usually in an epiphyseal or metaphyseal location. They can present with exuberant callus formation, raising concerns of a tumor to the inexperienced clinician. The fractures typically present with a swollen, warm, erythematous extremity in a febrile child. They should be managed with splinting and weightbearing initiated within 2 to 3 weeks to prevent further osteoporosis and to reduce the risk for further fractures (350).

Scoliosis is a common complication of myelomeningocele, affecting most patients (285,351,354). It may be caused by a number of factors, including congenital vertebral anomalies, neuromuscular weakness, pelvic obliquity, and hip contractures (317,351). Almost all patients with thoracic level lesions develop scoliosis, with a decreased incidence in lower level lesions (351, 355). Progressive scoliosis may be associated with uncompensated hydrocephalus, hydrosyringomyelia, or retethered spinal cord (356,357). Surgical correction of hydrocephalus, hydrosyringomyelia, and a retethered spinal cord may slow or halt progression of the scoliosis in patients with less severe curvatures (less than 40 degrees) but generally do not have an effect on more severe curves (356–358).

Management of scoliosis should include close monitoring of the motor and sensory examination, degree of spasticity, and deep tendon reflexes of both the upper and lower extremities. Serial radiographs should be performed at least annually. Imaging studies to exclude hydocephalus, hydrosyringomyelia, and retethered cord should be performed in patients with progressive scoliosis, especially if associated with progressive weakness or spasticity. Patients with curves greater than 25 degrees and those with unbalanced curves should wear bivalved molded body jackets when they are awake and sitting, standing, or walking. Particular care must be taken to avoid development of pressure ulcers under the body jacket. Timing of the surgical repair and the extent and type of spine fusion depend on the child's age (preferably performed after 10 years of age), location and flexibility of the curve, neurologic level, and ambulation status. The lumbosacral joint should generally not be fused in children who are ambulatory. Hip contractures should be corrected before spine surgery to avoid excessive torque to the spine fusion after surgery (285).

Kyphosis affects 8% to 15% of patients with myelomeningocele, particularly those with thoracic level lesions, and is commonly severe (>90 degrees) (310,311,354) (Fig. 29.11). The kyphosis may interfere with sitting or wearing orthotics and is a common cause of skin breakdown. Progression of the kyphosis may also compromise ventilation because abdominal contents are pushed up into the thorax. Surgical correction of kyphotic deformities is complex and technically demanding and is associated with significant morbidity and mortality (311,354). Surgical correction usually requires the resection of a portion of the spine and dural sac. It is critical that adequate functioning of the ventriculoperitoneal shunt be ensured in the preoperative evaluation.

Medical Issues

Individuals with myelomeningocele frequently have reduced stature that may be caused by a variety of factors (359,360). These include spine and other orthopedic deformities, decreased growth in paralyzed extremities, nutritional deficiencies, preco-

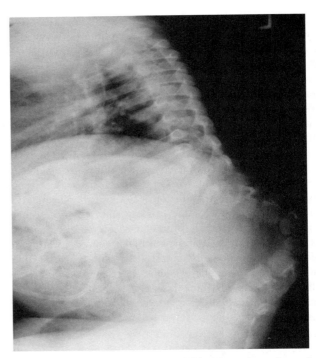

FIGURE 29.11. Severe kyphosis in a child with myelomeningocele.

cious puberty, and growth hormone deficiency. About 10% to 20% of individuals with myelomeningocele experience precocious puberty (361–363). Precocious puberty is presumably related to brain abnormalities and more commonly affects girls and those with hydrocephalus (361). Children with myelomeningocele frequently become obese, particularly as they become adolescents (331,362,364–368).

Individuals with myelomeningocele are at particularly high risk for latex allergy, with 18% to 64.5% being affected (369–371). The high incidence of latex allergy in the myelomeningocele population may be related to the multiple surgeries beginning at a young age that these children undergo (372–374). Sensitization to latex may be reduced in the myelomeningocele population by minimizing exposure to latex (375–378).

Similar to individuals with SCI, children and adolescents with myelomeningocele are susceptible to developing pressure ulcers (379,380). Prevention and management of pressure ulcers in patients with myelomeningocele may be complicated by associated cognitive and behavioral disturbances.

Psychosocial Issues and Sexuality

In addition to the psychosocial and sexuality issues that are integral to the development of all children and adolescents, individuals with myelomeningocele face additional burdens because of their chronic physical, psychological, and cognitive deficits (364, 381,382). This is compounded by the onset of disability at birth and the varying expectations that parents have for their child's future (383). Sexuality and reproductive health issues must be addressed in a developmentally appropriate fashion for children and adolescents as well as for their parents (384,385). This should include sexual abuse and exploitation, fertility, and sexual functioning.

Although most children with myelomeningocele should be educated in a regular school setting, their psychosocial and sexuality development may be limited by cognitive defects, visuomotor disturbances, learning disabilities, and frequent absences related to health care needs (317). Adult outcomes, including employment and independence, are areas that must be an integral component of the comprehensive care for this population of children (386,387).

Prevention

Folic acid has been demonstrated to be effective in preventing neural tube defects if taken in the periconceptual period (388–391). It has been estimated that periconceptual use of folic acid can reduce the risk for neural tube defects by 50% in the general population and 72% in high-risk women who have previously had an affected pregnancy (390,391). The U.S. Public Health Service recommends that all women of childbearing age consume 0.4 mg of folic acid daily, but care should be taken to keep total folate consumption to less than 1 mg/day (390). Women who have had a prior neural tube defect–affected pregnancy should consume 4.0 mg of folic acid daily from at least 1 month before conception through the first 3 months of the pregnancy (390,391).

Prenatal Diagnosis and Management

Prenatal screening for myelomeningocele is accomplished by maternal serum alpha-fetoprotein testing between 16 and 18 weeks of gestation (392–394). Confirmation of the diagnosis can be established with high-resolution ultrasound or elevated levels of alpha-fetoprotein or acetylcholinesterase in the amniotic fluid (393,395). Prenatal diagnosis provides the parents the opportunity to consider termination of the pregnancy. It alternatively assists parents and health care providers in planning the most appropriate prenatal and postnatal care, such as *in utero* surgery, elective cesarean section, and delivery in a medical center that is experienced in caring for newborns with myelomeningocele (394).

Experimental evidence suggests that some of the neurologic deficits associated with myelomeningocele may be caused by prolonged exposure of the dysplastic spinal cord to the intrauterine environment, as a result of toxicity of the amniotic fluid or physical trauma (312,313,396). *In utero* repair of the myelomeningocele sac has been performed on fetuses at 22 to 28 weeks of gestation, and a preliminary report has demonstrated a decreased incidence of hydrocephalus (397–400). However, current reports are insufficient at this time to assess the long-term neurologic benefit of this intervention.

Elective prelabor cesarean section has been advocated as a means to prevent further damage to the dysplastic spinal cord as a result of uterine contractions and passage through the birth canal (286,401). The most appropriate circumstances for this approach may be fetuses with lower extremity movement noted on ultrasound, minimal to no hydrocephalus, and neural ele-

ments that protrude dorsally (286). However, currently there is insufficient evidence to support prophylactic cesarean delivery of infants with myelomeningocele (402,403).

Lipomeningocele

Lipomeningoceles are a form of occult spinal dysraphism with intact skin covering the defect (283,404). In lipomeningocele, the spinal cord remains within the spinal canal, with the junction between the cord and the lipoma also residing within the canal (Fig. 29.12). Individuals with lipomeningoceles are generally normal at birth. Neurologic symptoms first appear during the second year of life, and most patients exhibit some neurologic deficits by early childhood. The typical presenting complaint is that of a cosmetic deformity, a subcutaneous fat collection in the lower back and upper buttocks. About half of affected children have cutaneous markings, such as a midline dimple, hairy patch, or a hemangiomatous nevus. Surgery is performed with the goal of untethering the spinal cord. Removal of the entire lipoma is generally not performed because the neural tissue extends into the lipoma, and aggressive surgical excision of the lipoma may result in a significantly greater neurologic deficit.

Sacral Agenesis

Sacral agenesis is not a neural tube defect. It is a relatively uncommon, congenital anomaly, with varying degrees of deficien-

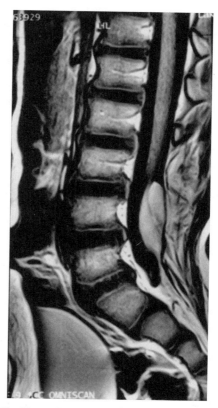

FIGURE 29.12. Magnetic resonance image of a child with a lipomeningocele, demonstrating tethering of the spinal cord and an intraspinal lipoma.

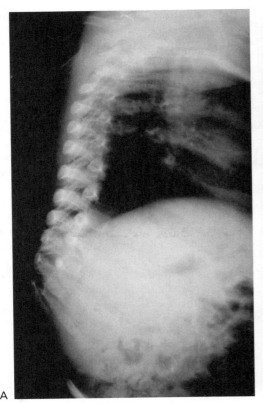
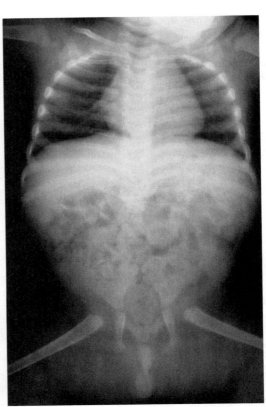

FIGURE 29.13. A,B; Radiographs of a child with sacral agenesis demonstrating abrupt loss of the vertebral column at T12 to L1.

cies of the sacrum, and associated neurologic abnormalities (405–407) (Fig. 29.13). Sacral agenesis is associated with maternal diabetes mellitus, with 1% of infants born to diabetic mothers having sacral agenesis (408). About 12% to 16% of infants with sacral agenesis are born to mothers with diabetes mellitus. Patients generally present either during infancy or between 4 and 5 years of age with persistent urinary incontinence and chronic constipation (407). Most affected children also have neurologic deficits of their lower extremities; 40% had weakness, and 86% had decreased muscle stretch reflexes. Interestingly, sensation was usually intact caudally for several segments below the motor level in most individuals with sacral agenesis (405,406). About two thirds of affected patients have severe orthopedic deformities of their lower extremities, including webbed knees requiring amputation, with clubfeet being the most common problem (Fig. 29.13).

HYDROSYRINGOMYELIA

Hydrosyringomyelia, or cystic formation in the spinal cord, may also be referred to as *syringomyelia*, *hydromyelia*, or *syrinx* (409–411). Although hydrosyringomyelia may be associated with spinal cord trauma, tumors, or arachnoiditis, this section is limited to developmental hydrosyringomyelia. Hydromyelia refers to a dilated central canal communicating with the fourth

ventricle and lined by ependyma. In contrast, syringomyelia refers to tubular cavitation within the spinal cord, which is lined by glial cells. From a clinical perspective, there is no clear distinction between syringomyelia and hydromyelia, and in this section, they are discussed as one entity and referred to as hydrosyringomyelia or syrinx.

Developmental hydrosyringomyelia is frequently associated with Chiari I malformation, in which there is caudal displacement of the cerebellar tonsils below the foramen magnum (410, 411) (Fig. 29.14). It is postulated that the syrinx is caused by altered CSF dynamics at the craniospinal junction, as a result of the Chiari I abnormality. The syrinx is most commonly located in the cervical or cervicothoracic spinal cord but may involve the entire spinal cord. The syrinx may also extend into the brain stem, in which case it is referred to as *syringobulbia*.

Although hydrosyringomyelia may become symptomatic at any age, it typically does not become clinically apparent until adulthood (410,412). Nonetheless, many affected patients develop symptoms during childhood or adolescence, and with the ready availability of MRI, diagnosis at an earlier age is facilitated (409). The classic presentation of hydrosyringomyelia includes occipital or neck pain, suspended and dissociated sensory loss in a cape distribution, hypotonic weakness of the upper extremities, and spastic weakness in the lower extremities. The occipital and cervical pain may be caused by compression or stretching of upper cervical roots by the Chiari I malformation or distortion

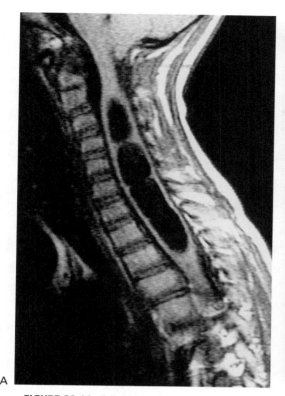
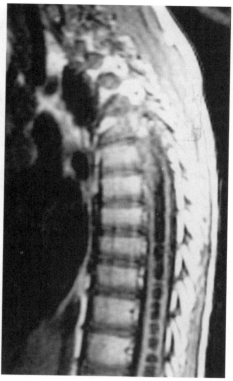

A

B

FIGURE 29.14. **A,B;** Magnetic resonance imaging study of a child with hydrosyringomyelia involving the cervical and the thoracic spinal cord. This figure also demonstrates the Chiari I malformation with caudal displacement of the cerebellar tonsils below the foramen magnum.

of descending fibers of the trigeminal nerves. The usual location of a syrinx in the central part of the spinal cord preferentially affects fibers crossing through the central white matter, compromising temperature and pain sensation, with relative sparing of the posterior columns. As the syrinx expands, anterior horn cells, corticospinal tracts, and the posterior columns become affected. The typical location of the syrinx in the cervical or cervicothoracic spinal cord is responsible for the flaccid upper extremity weakness and spastic lower extremity weakness.

Other symptoms of hydrosyringomyelia include dysesthesia in the peripheral dermatomes of the sensory or motor dysfunction. Symptoms related to posterior column dysfunction are relatively common. In one series of 58 patients with hydrosyringomyelia, 76% had abnormalities of proprioception, with involvement of the arms alone in 25%, legs alone in 25%, and both the arms and legs in 50% (413). In this same series of 58 patients, 32 (55%) had nystagmus, 50 (86%) had ataxia or limb incoordination primarily due to proprioceptive defects, 5 (9%) had bladder dysfunction, and 2 experienced erectile dysfunction. Eighteen of the 58 patients had symptoms referable to syringobulbia, including swallowing problems, nystagmus, tongue fibrillation, and impaired pharyngeal sensation. Other symptoms referable to brain-stem involvement and impingement on the dorsal nuclei of the vagus nerve include either episodic or chronic stridor.

Orthopedic abnormalities associated with hydrosyringomyelia include scoliosis, pes cavus, and Charcot joints (409,414,

415). In children and adolescents, scoliosis is a relatively common manifestation of hydrosyringomyelia and frequently is progressive, necessitating bracing and surgical intervention (409, 414,416–418). For patients with scoliosis, characteristics that may indicate an underlying hydrosyringomyelia include a left thoracic curve, progressive curves in male patients, and an abnormal neurological examination such as asymmetric or absent umbilical reflexes.

MRI is the most appropriate imaging technique to diagnose hydrosyringomyelia and associated neurologic abnormalities, such as Chiari I malformation (410,419). The use of MRI with gadolinium contrast is indicated to exclude intraspinal tumors. Conventional metrizamide myelography with delayed CT imaging can also be used to diagnose hydrosyringomyelia, although MRI is the preferred imaging modality. Plain radiographs of the head, neck, and spine should also be obtained to identify associated abnormalities, such as scoliosis, a shallow posterior fossa, widening of the spinal canal, basilar invagination, or Klippel-Feil anomaly (411).

In general, hydrosyringomyelia is a neurodegenerative process with relentless progression that is usually protracted over time (411). It is imperative that a patient's clinical course be followed closely in a serial fashion to identify progression of neurologic findings. Management of hydrosyringomyelia, including indications, timing of interventions, and the specific treatment modality, is not entirely clearcut (411). For the occasional patient with hydrocephalus, a ventriculoperitoneal shunt should be performed initially. For patients who are asymptomatic, careful clinical observation is essential. However, the decision to observe without surgical interventions must be weighed against the natural history of hydrosyringomyelia, which is one of progressive loss of neurologic function and recovery of neurologic deficits, which is variable after surgical interventions. Currently, the treatment of choice is posterior fossa decompression with the goal of restoring adequate CSF dynamics at the craniospinal junction (410,411,413,418–420). Among patients undergoing posterior fossa decompression, about 70% demonstrate either improvement or stabilization of their neurologic status; whereas complete resolution of neurologic deficits is rarely observed. Another treatment option is direct decompression of the syrinx using either a one-time aspiration of the syrinx or a shunt from the syrinx to the subarachnoid space, pleura, or peritoneum (418,420–422). Close clinical follow-up is essential after surgical interventions have been performed, and MRI is useful in monitoring the progression of the syrinx.

ACKNOWLEDGMENTS

We would like to acknowledge the assistance of Carol Paulus-Kalis and Jim Cockerill.

REFERENCES

1. Betz RR, Mulcahey MJ. *Spinal cord injury rehabilitation.* In: Weinstein SL, ed. The Pediatric Spine: Principles and Practice. New York: Raven Press, 1994:781–810.
2. Bray GP. Rehabilitation of the spinal cord injured: a family approach. *J Appl Rehabil Counseling* 1978;9:70–78.
3. Shelton T, Jeppson E, Johnson B. Facilitation of parent/professional collaboration at all levels of health care. In: *Family centered care: an early intervention resource manual.* Rockville, MD: American Occupational Therapy Association, 1989;2:3–8.
4. Anderson CJ, Johnson KA, Klaas SJ, et al. Pediatric spinal cord injury: transition to adulthood. *J Voc Rehabil* 1998;10:103–113.
5. Smith QW, Frieden L, Nelson MR, et al. Transition to adulthood for young people with spinal cord injury. In: Betz RR, Mulcahey MJ, eds. *The child with a spinal cord injury.* Rosemont, Illinois: American Academy of Orthopaedic Surgeons, 1996:601–612.
6. Vogel LC, Klaas SJ, Lubicky, JP, et al. Long-term outcomes and life satisfaction of adults with pediatric spinal cord injuries. *Arch Phys Med Rehabil* 1998;79:1496–1503.
7. American Academy of Pediatrics Committee on Children With Disabilities and Committee on Adolescence. Transition of care provided for adolescents with special health care needs. *Pediatrics* 1996;98:1203–1206.
8. Johnson CP. Transition into adulthood. *Pediatr Ann* 1995;24:268–273.
9. Anderson CJ, Vogel LC. Decreased work experience in adolescents with spinal cord injuries compared with peers: implications for adult employment. *Dev Med Child Neurol* (in press).
10. White PH. Resilience in children with disability: transition to adulthood. *J Rheumatol* 1996;23:960–962.
11. Massagli, TL, Dudgeon, BJ, Ross, BW. Educational performance and vocational participation after spinal cord injury in childhood. *Arch Phys Med Rehabil* 1996;77:995–999.
12. Vogel LC. Long-term prophylactic medical care. In: Betz RR, Mulcahey MJ, eds. *The child with a spinal cord injury.* Rosemont: American Academy of Orthopaedic Surgeons, 1996:679–688.
13. Bernardez SJ, Brown LT, Nora J, et al. Primary care for the spinal cord injured patient. *J Am Acad Phys Assist* 1994;8:526–531.
14. Massagli TL, Jaffe KM. Pediatric spinal cord injury: treatment and outcome. *Pediatrician* 1990;17:244–254.
15. Tepperman PS. Primary care after spinal cord injury: what every physician should know. *Postgrad Med* 1989;86:211–218.
16. American Academy of Pediatrics Committee on Infectious Diseases. Active immunization. In: Peter G, ed. *1997 Red book: report of the committee on infectious diseases,* 24th ed. Elk Grove Village, Illinois: American Academy of Pediatrics, 1997:4–36.
17. Betz RR, Mulcahey MJ, eds. *The child with a spinal cord injury.* Rosemont, Illinois: American Academy of Orthopaedic Surgeons, 1996.
18. Massagli TL. Medical and rehabilitation issues in the care of children with spinal cord injury. *Phys Med Rehabil Clin N Am* 2000;11:169–182.
19. Vogel LC, Betz RR, Mulcahey MJ. The child with a spinal cord injury. *Dev Med Child Neurol* 1997;39;202–207.
20. Vogel LC, ed. Pediatric issues. *Top Spinal Cord Inj Rehabil* 1997;3(2).
21. Nobunaga AI, Go BK, Karunas RB. Recent demographic and injury trends in people served by the Model Spinal Cord Injury Care Systems. *Arch Phys Med Rehabil* 1999;80:1372–1382.
22. Hadley MN, Zabramski JM, Browner CM, et al. Pediatric spinal trauma: review of 122 cases of spinal cord and vertebral column injuries. *J Neurosurg* 1988;68:18–24.
23. Hamilton MG, Myles ST. Pediatric spinal injury: review of 174 hospital admissions. *J Neurosurg* 1992;77:700–704.
24. Kewalramani LS, Kraus JF, Sterling HM. Acute spinal-cord lesions in a pediatric population: epidemiological and clinical features. *Paraplegia* 1980;18:206–219.
25. Osenbach RK, Menezes AH. Pediatric spinal cord and vertebral column injury. *Neurosurgery* 1992;30:385–390.
26. Vogel LC, DeVivo MJ. Etiology and demographics. In: Betz RR, Mulcahey MJ, eds. *The child with a spinal cord injury.* Rosemont, Illinois: American Academy of Orthopaedic Surgeons, 1996:3–12.
27. Ruge JR, Sinson GP, McLone DG, et al. Pediatric spinal injury: the very young. *J Neurosurg* 1988;68:25–30.
28. Vogel LC, DeVivo MJ. Pediatric spinal cord injury issues: etiology, demographics, and pathophysiology. *Top Spinal Cord Inj Rehabil* 1997;3:1–8.
29. Haffner DL, Hoffer MM, Wiedbusch R. Etiology of children's spinal injuries at Rancho Los Amigos. *Spine* 1993;18:679–684.
30. Rovinsky D, Haskell A, Huffman GR, et al. Firearm related spinal cord injuries in children and adolescents: a fifteen year experience. *Top Spinal Cord Inj Rehabil* 2000;6:1–6.
31. Gabos PG. Tuten HR, Leet A, et al. Fracture-dislocation of the lumbar spine in an abused child. *Pediatrics* 1998;101:473–477.
32. Gosnold JK, Sivaloganathan S. Spinal cord damage in a case of nonaccidental injury in children. *Med Sci Law* 1980;20:54–57.
33. Feldman KW, Weinberger E, Milstein JM, et al. Cervical spine MRI in abused infants. *Child Abuse Neglect* 1997;21:199–205.
34. Piatt JH, Steinberg M. Isolated spinal cord injury as a presentation of child abuse. *Pediatrics* 1995;96:780–781.
35. Shannon P, Smith CR, Deck J, et al. Axonal injury and the neuropathology of shaken baby syndrome. *Acta Neuropathol* 1998;95:625–631.
36. Swischuk LE. Spine and spinal cord trauma in the battered child syndrome. *Radiology* 1969;92:733–738.
37. Wilberger JE Jr. Clinical aspects of specific spinal injuries. In: Wilberger JE Jr ed. *Spinal cord injuries in children.* Mount Kisco, NY: Futura, 1986;69–95.
38. Dunne K, Hopkins IJ, Shield LK. Acute transverse myelopathy in childhood. *Dev Med Child Neurol* 1986;28:198–204.
39. Knebusch M, Strassburg HM, Reiners K. Acute transverse myelitis in childhood: nine cases and review of the literature. *Dev Med Child Neurol* 1998;40:631–639.
40. Shoemaker BL, Ose M. Pediatric lap belt injuries: care and prevention. *Orthop Nurs* 1997:16;15–23.
41. Apple DF, Murray HH. Lap belt injuries in children. In: Betz RR, Mulcahey MJ, eds. *The child with a spinal cord injury.* Rosemont, Illinois: American Academy of Orthopaedic Surgeons, 1996:169–177.

42. Garrett JW, Braunstein PW. The seat belt syndrome. *J Trauma* 1962; 2:220-238.

43. Johnson DL, Falci S. The diagnosis and treatment of pediatric lumbar spine injuries caused by rear seat lap belts. *Neurosurgery* 1990;26: 434-441.

44. Statter MB, Vargish T. The spectrum of lap belt injuries sustained by two cousins in the same motor vehicle crash. *J Trauma* 1998:45; 835-837.

45. Centers for Disease Control. Motor-vehicle occupant fatalities and restraint use among children aged 4-8 Years—United States, 1994-1998. *MMWR Morb Mortal Wkly Rep* 2000;49:135-137.

46. Bresnan MJ, Abroms IF. Neonatal spinal cord transection secondary to intrauterine hyperextension of the neck in breech presentation. *J Pediatr* 1974;84:734-737.

47. Hankins GDV. Lower thoracic spinal cord injury: a severe complication of shoulder dystocia. *Am J Perinatol* 1998;15:443-444.

48. Lanska MJ, Roessmann U, Wiznitzer M. Magnetic resonance imaging in cervical cord birth injury. *Pediatrics* 1990;85:760-764.

49. MacKinnon JA, Perlman M, Kirpalani H, et al. Spinal cord injury at birth: diagnostic and prognostic data in twenty-two patients. *J Pediatr* 1993;122:431-437.

50. Perlman M. Neonatal spinal cord injury in the infant: etiology, diagnosis, treatment and outcome. In: Betz RR, Mulcahey MJ, eds. *The child with a spinal cord injury.* Rosemont, Illinois: American Academy of Orthopaedic Surgeons, 1996:161-167.

51. Rossitch E, Oakes WJ. Perinatal spinal cord injury: clinical, radiographic and pathologic features. *Pediatr Neurosurg* 1992;18:149-152.

52. Ruggieri M, Smarason AK, Pike M. Spinal cord insults in the prenatal, perinatal, and neonatal periods. *Dev Med Child Neurol* 1999;41: 311-317.

53. American Academy of Pediatrics Committee on Sports Medicine. Atlantoaxial instability in Down syndrome. *Pediatrics* 1984;74: 152-154.

54. Loder RT, Hensinger RN. Developmental abnormalities of the cervical spine. In: Weinstein SL, ed. *The pediatric spine: principles and practice.* New York: Raven, 1994;397-420.

55. Tredwell SJ, Newman DE, Lockith G. Instability of the upper cervical spine in Down syndrome. *J Pediatr Orthop* 1990;10:602-606.

56. Ward WT. Atlanto-axial instability in children with Down syndrome. In: Betz RR, Mulcahey MJ, eds. *The child with a spinal cord injury.* Rosemont, Illinois: American Academy of Orthopaedic Surgeons, 1996:89-96.

57. Nathan FF, Bickel WH. Spontaneous axial subluxation in a child as the first sign of juvenile rheumatoid arthritis. *J Bone Joint Surg [Am]* 1968;50:1675-1678.

58. Vogel LC, Lubicky JP. Cervical spine fusion not protective of cervical spine injury and tetraplegia. *Am J Orthop* 1997;26:636-640.

59. Goldberg MJ. Orthopedic aspects of bone dysplasias. *Orthop Clin North Am* 1976;7:445-455.

60. Gulati MS, Agin MA. Morquio syndrome: a rehabilitative perspective. *J Spinal Cord Med* 1996;19:12-16.

61. Yang SS, Corbett DP, Brough AJ, et al. Upper cervical myelopathy in achondroplasia. *Am J Clin Pathol* 1977;68:68-72.

62. Pang D, Wilberger JE. Spinal cord injury without radiographic abnormalities in children. *J Neurosurg* 1982;57:114-129.

63. Pang D. Spinal cord injury without radiographic abnormality (SCIWORA) in children. In: Betz RR, Mulcahey MJ, eds. *The child with a spinal cord injury.* Rosemont, Illinois: American Academy of Orthopaedic Surgeons, 1996:139-160.

64. Osenbach RK, Menezes AH. Spinal cord injury without radiographic abnormality in children. *Pediatr Neurosci* 1989;15:168-175.

65. Dickman CA, Zambramski JM, Hadley MN, et al. Pediatric spinal cord injury without radiographic abnormalities: report of 26 cases and review of the literature. *J Spinal Disord* 1991;4:296-305.

66. Felsberg GJ, Tien RD, Osumi AK, et al. Utility of MR imaging in pediatric spinal cord injury. *Pediatr Radiol* 1995;25:131-135.

67. Grabb PA, Pang D. Magnetic resonance imaging in the evaluation of spinal cord injury without radiographic abnormality in children. *Neurosurgery* 1994;35:406-413.

68. Shimada K, Tokioka T. Sequential MRI studies in patients with cervical cord injury but without bony injury. *Paraplegia* 1995;33:573-578.

69. Schwartz GR, Wright SW, Fein JA, et al. Pediatric cervical spine injury sustained in falls from low heights. *Ann Emerg Med* 1997;30: 249-252.

70. Choi JU, Hoffman HJ, Hendrick EB, et al. Traumatic infarction of the spinal cord in children. *J Neurosurg* 1986;65:608-610.

71. Hamilton MG, Myles ST. Pediatric spinal injury: review of 174 hospital admissions. *J Neurosurg* 1992;77:700-704.

72. Chao R, Mayo ME. Long-term urodynamic follow up in pediatric spinal cord injury. *Paraplegia* 1994;32:806-809.

73. Fernandes ET, Reinberg Y, Vernier R, et al. Neurogenic bladder dysfunction in children: review of pathophysiology and current management. *J Pediatr* 1994;124:1-7.

74. Lapides J, Diokno AC, Silber SJ, et al. Clean intermittent self-catheterization in the treatment of urinary tract disease. *J Urol* 1972;107: 458-461.

75. McLaughlin JF, Murray M, Van Zandt K, et al. Clean intermittent catheterization. *Dev Med Child Neurol* 1996;38:446-454.

76. Pontari MA, Bauer SB. Urologic issues in spinal cord injury: assessment, management, outcome, and research needs. In: Betz RR, Mulcahey MJ, eds. *The child with a spinal cord injury.* Rosemont, Illinois: American Academy of Orthopaedic Surgeons, 1996:213-231.

77. Vogel LC, Pontari M. Pediatric spinal cord injury issues: medical issues. *Top Spinal Cord Inj Rehabil* 1997;3:20-30.

78. National Institute on Disability and Rehabilitation Research Consensus Statement. The prevention and management of urinary tract infections among people with spinal cord injuries. *J Am Paraplegia Soc* 1992;15:194-204.

79. Christ W, Lehnert T, Ulbrich B. Specific toxicologic aspects of the quinolones. *Rev Infect Dis* 1988;10:S141-146.

80. Schaad UB. Pediatric use of quinolones. *Pediatr Infect Dis J* 1999; 18:469-470.

81. Pannek J, Diederichs W, Botel U. Urodynamically controlled management of spinal cord injury in children. *Neurourol Urodyn* 1997; 16:285-292.

82. Gearhart JP, Albertsen PC, Marshall FF, et al. Pediatric applications of augmentation cystoplasty: the Johns Hopkins experience. *J Urol* 1986;136:430-432.

83. Gray GJ, Yang C. Surgical procedures of the bladder after spinal cord injury. *Phys Med Rehabil Clin N Am* 2000;11:57-72.

84. Kass EJ, Koff SA. Bladder augmentation in the pediatric neuropathic bladder. *J Urol* 1983;129:552-555.

85. Linder A, Leach GE, Raz S. Augmentation cystoplasty in the treatment of neurogenic bladder dysfunction. *J Urol* 1983;129:491-493.

86. Sidi AA, Aliabadi H, Gonzalez R. Enterocystoplasty in the management and reconstruction of the pediatric neurogenic bladder. *J Pediatr Surg* 1987;22:153-157.

87. Vogel LC. Unique management needs of pediatric spinal cord injury patients. *J Spinal Cord Med* 1997;20:17-20.

88. Duckett JW, Snyder HM. Continent urinary diversion: variations on the Mitrofanoff principle. *J Urol* 1986;136:58-62.

89. Mitrofanoff P. Trans-appendicular continent cystotomy in the management of the neurogenic bladder. *Chir Pediatr* 1980;21:297-305.

90. Chaviano AC, Anderson CJ, Matkov TG, et al. Mitrofanoff continent catheterizable stoma for pediatric patients. *Top Spinal Cord Inj Rehabil* 2000;6:30-35.

91. Pontari MA, Weibel B, Morales V, et al. Improved quality of life after continent urinary diversion in pediatric patients with quadriplegia after spinal cord injury. *Top Spinal Cord Inj Rehabil* 2000;6: 25-29.

92. Brindley GS, Polkey CE, Rushton DN. Sacral anterior root stimulators for bladder control in paraplegia. *Paraplegia* 1982;20:365-381.

93. Chancellor MB, Rivas DA. Neuromodulation and neurostimulation in urology. *Top Spinal Cord Inj Rehabil* 1996;1(3):18-35.

94. Creasey GH. Implications of implantation of bladder stimulation systems in children and adolescents. *Top Spinal Cord Inj Rehabil* 2000; 6:36-41.

95. Smith BT. Functional electrical stimulation. *Top Spinal Cord Inj Rehabil* 1997;3:56-69.

96. Branwell JG, Creasey GH, Aggarwal AM, et al. Management of the neurogenic bowel in patients with spinal cord injury. *Urol Clin North Am* 1993;20:517–526.

97. Chen D, Nussbaum SB. The gastrointestinal system and bowel management following spinal cord injury. *Phys Med Rehabil Clin N Am* 2000;11:45–56.

98. Consortium for Spinal Cord Medicine. *Neurogenic bowel management in adults with spinal cord injury.* Washington DC: Paralyzed Veterans of America, 1998.

99. Goetz LL, Hurvitz EA, Nelson VS, et al. Bowel management in children and adolescents with spinal cord injury. *J Spinal Cord Med* 1998; 21:335–341.

100. Kirshblum SC, Gulati M, O'Connor KC, et al. Bowel care practices in chronic spinal cord injury patients. *Arch Phys Med Rehabil* 1998; 79:20–23.

101. Stiens SA, Bergman SB, Goetz LL. Neurogenic bowel dysfunction after spinal cord injury: clinical evaluation and rehabilitative management. *Arch Phys Med Rehabil* 1997;78:S86–S102.

102. Gleeson RM. Bowel continence for the child with a neurogenic bowel. *Rehabil Nurs* 1990;15:319–321.

103. Puet TA, Jackson H, Amy S. Use of pulsed irrigation evacuation in the management of the neuropathic bowel. *Spinal Cord* 1997;35: 694–699.

104. Frost F, Hartwig D, Jaeger R, et al. Electrical stimulation of the sacral dermatomes in spinal cord injury: effect on rectal manometry and bowel emptying. *Arch Phys Med Rehabil* 1993;74:696–701.

105. Ellsworth PI, Webb HW, Crump JM, et al. The Malone antegrade colonic enema enhances the quality of life in children undergoing urological incontinence procedures. *J Urol* 1996;155:1416–1418.

106. Liptak GS, Revell GM. Management of bowel dysfunction in children with spinal cord disease or injury by means of the enema continence catheter. *J Pediatr* 1992;120:190–194.

107. Radecki RT, Gaebler-Spira D. Deep vein thrombosis in the disabled pediatric population. *Arch Phys Med Rehabil* 1994;75:248–250.

108. Waring WP, Karunas RS. Acute spinal cord injuries and the incidence of clinically occurring thromboembolic disease. *Paraplegia* 1991;29: 8–16.

109. David M, Andrew M. Venous thromboembolic complications in children. *J Pediatr* 1993;123:337–346.

110. Vogel LC, Lubicky JP. Deep vein thrombosis complicating scoliosis surgery in pediatric spinal cord injury. *J Spinal Cord Med* 1995;18: 272.

111. Consortium for Spinal Cord Medicine. Prevention of thromboembolism in spinal cord injury. *J Spinal Cord Med* 1997;20:259–283.

112. Ginsberg JS. Management of venous thromboembolism. *N Engl J Med* 1996;335:1816–1828.

113. Massicotte P, Adams M, Marzinotto V, et al. Low-molecular-weight heparin in pediatric patients with thrombotic disease: a dose finding study. *J Pediatr* 1996;128:313–318.

114. Dix D, Andrew M, Marzinotti V, et al. The use of low molecular weight heparin in pediatric patients: a prospective cohort study. *J Pediatr* 2000;136:439–445.

115. Andrew M, Michelson AD, Bovill E, et al. Guidelines for antithrombotic therapy in pediatric patients. *J Pediatr* 1998;132:575–588.

116. Michelson AD, Bovill E, Andrew M. Antithrombotic therapy in children. *Chest* 1995;108:506S–522S.

117. Maynard FM. Immobilization hypercalcemia following spinal cord injury. *Arch Phys Med Rehabil* 1986;67:41–44.

118. Nand S, Goldschmidt JW. Hypercalcemia and hyperuricemia in young patients with spinal cord injury. *Arch Phys Med Rehabil* 1976; 57:553.

119. Steinberg FU, Birge SJ, Cooke NE. Hypercalcemia in adolescent tetraplegia patients: case report and review. *Paraplegia* 1978;16:60–67.

120. Tori JA, Hill LL. Hypercalcemia in children with spinal cord injury. *Arch Phys Med Rehabil* 1978;59:443–447.

121. Bilezikian JP. Management of acute hypercalcemia. *N Engl J Med* 1992;326:1196–1203.

122. Gallacher SJ, Ralston SH, Dryburgh FJ, et al. Immobilization-related hypercalcaemia: a possible novel mechanism and response to pamidronate. *Postgrad Med J* 1990;66:918–922.

123. Kedlaya D, Branstater ME, Lee JK. Immobilization hypercalcemia in incomplete paraplegia: successful treatment with pamidronate. *Arch Phys Med Rehabil* 1998;79:222–225.

124. Lteif AN, Zimmerman D. Bisphosphonates for treatment of childhood hypercalcemia. *Pediatrics* 1998;102:990–993.

125. Tamion F, Bonmarchand F, Girault C, et al. Intravenous pamidronate sodium therapy in immobilization-related hypercalcemia. *Clin Nephrol* 1995;43:138–139.

126. Consortium for Spinal Cord Medicine. Acute management of autonomic dysreflexia: adults with spinal cord injury presenting to healthcare facilities. *J Spinal Cord Med* 1997;20:284–309.

127. Vogel LC. Management of medical issues. In: Betz RR, Mulcahey MJ, eds. *The child with a spinal cord injury.* Rosemont, Illinois: American Academy of Orthopaedic Surgeons, 1996:189–212.

128. National High Blood Pressure Education Program Working Group on Hypertension Control in Children and Adolescents. Update on the 1987 Task Force Report on High Blood Pressure in Children and Adolescents: a working group report from the National High Blood Pressure Education Program. *Pediatrics* 1996;98:649–658.

129. Chameides L, Hazinski MF, eds. *Pediatric advanced life support.* Dallas: American Heart Association, 1997:2–5.

130. Perloff D, Grim C, Flack J, et al. Human blood pressure determination by sphygmomanometry. *Circulation* 1993;88:2460–2470.

131. Anderson, LS, Biering-Sorensen F, Muller PG, et al. The prevalence of hyperhidrosis in patients with spinal cord injuries and an evaluation of the effect of dextropropoxyphene hydrochloride in therapy. *Paraplegia* 1992;30:184–191.

132. Fast A. Reflex sweating in patients with spinal cord injury: a review. *Arch Phys Med Rehabil* 1977;58:435–437.

133. Guttmann L, ed. *Spinal cord injuries: comprehensive management and research,* 2nd ed. Oxford, UK: Blackwell Scientific, 1976:295–330.

134. Staas WE, Nemunaitis G. Management of reflex sweating in spinal cord injured patients. *Arch Phys Med Rehabil* 1989;70:544–546.

135. Glasauer FE, Czyrny JJ. Hyperhidrosis as the presenting symptom in post-traumatic syringomyelia. *Paraplegia* 1994;32:423–429.

136. Ottomo M, Heimburger RF. Alternating Horner's syndrome and hyperhidrosis due to dural adhesions following cervical spinal cord injury. *J Neurosurg* 1980;53:97–100.

137. Rossier AB, Foo D, Shillito J, et al. Posttraumatic cervical syringomyelia: incidence, clinical presentation, electrophysiological studies, syrinx protein and results of conservative and operative treatment. *Brain* 1985;108:439–461.

138. Stanworth PA. The significance of hyperhidrosis in patients with posttraumatic syringomyelia. *Paraplegia* 1982;20:282–287.

139. Falci SP, Lammertse DP, Best L, et al. Surgical treatment of posttraumatic cystic and tethered spinal cords. *J Spinal Cord Med* 1999;22: 173–181.

140. Canaday BR, Stanford RH. Propantheline bromide in the management of hyperhidrosis association with spinal cord injury. *Ann Pharmcother* 1995;29:489–492.

141. Formal C. Metabolic and neurologic changes after spinal cord injury. *Phys Med Rehabil Clin N Am* 1992;3:783–796.

142. Petrofsky JS. Thermoregulatory stress during rest and exercise in heat in patients with a spinal cord injury. *Eur J Appl Physiol* 1992;64: 503–507.

143. Beraldo PSS, Neves EGC, Alves CMF, et al. Pyrexia in hospitalized spinal cord injury patients. *Paraplegia* 1993;31:186–191.

144. Sugarman B, Brown D, Musher D. Fever and infection in spinal cord injury patients. *JAMA* 1982;248:66–70.

145. Sheridan R. Diagnosis of the acute abdomen in the neurologically stable spinal cord-injured patient: a case study. *J Clin Gastroenterol* 1992;15:325–328.

146. DeVivo MJ, Krause JS, Lammertse DP. Recent trends in mortality and causes of death among persons with spinal cord injury. *Arch Phys Med Rehabil* 1999;80:1411–1419.

147. Yekutiel M, Brooks ME, Ohry A, et al. The prevalence of hypertension, ischaemic heart disease and diabetes in traumatic spinal cord injured patients and amputees. *Paraplegia* 1989;27:58–62.

148. Figoni SF. Perspectives on cardiovascular fitness and SCI. *J Am Paraplegia Soc* 1990;13:63–71.

149. Pentland B. Quadriplegia and cardiorespiratory fitness. *Lancet* 1993; 341:413–414.

150. Ben-Ari E, Fisman EZ, Pines A, et al. Significance of exertional hypotension in apparently healthy men: an 8.9-year follow-up. *J Cardiopulm Rehabil* 1990;10:92–97.

151. Hopman MT, Oeseburg B, Binkhorst RA. Cardiovascular responses in persons with paraplegia to prolonged arm exercise and thermal stress. *Med Sci Sports Exerc* 1993;25:577–583.

152. King ML, Freeman DM, Pellicone JT, et al. Exertional hypotension in thoracic spinal cord injury: case report. *Paraplegia* 1992;30:261–266.

153. Sawka MN, Latzka WA, Pandolf KB. Temperature regulation during upper body exercise: able-bodied and spinal cord injured. *Med Sci Sports Exerc* 1989;21:S132–140.

154. Hoffman MD. Cardiorespiratory fitness and training in quadriplegics and paraplegics. *Sports Med* 1986;3;312–330.

155. Johnson, KA, Klaas SJ. Recreation therapy. In: Betz RR, Mulcahey MJ, eds. *The child with a spinal cord injury.* Rosemont, Illinois: American Academy of Orthopaedic Surgeons, 1996:619–624.

156. Johnson KA, Klaas SJ. Recreation issues and trends in pediatric spinal cord injury. *Top Spinal Cord Inj Rehabil* 1997;3(2)79–84.

157. Johnson KA, Klaas SJ. Recreation involvement and play in pediatric spinal cord injury. *Top Spinal Cord Inj Rehabil* 2000;6:105–109.

158. Cowell LL, Squires WG, Raven PB. Benefits of aerobic exercise for the paraplegic: a brief review. *Med Sci Sports Exerc* 1986;18:501–508.

159. Anderson JM, Schutt AH. Spinal cord injury in children: a review of 156 cases seen from 1950 through 1978. *Mayo Clin Proc* 1980; 55:499–504.

160. Lau C, McCormack G. Chronic pain management in pediatric spinal cord injury. In: Betz RR, Mulcahey MJ, eds. *The child with a spinal cord injury.* Rosemont, Illinois: American Academy of Orthopaedic Surgeons, 1996:653–670.

161. Bryce TN, Ragnarsson KT. Pain after spinal cord injury. *Phys Med Rehabil Clin N Am* 2000;11:157–168.

162. Richards JS. Chronic pain and spinal cord injury: review and comment. *Clin J Pain* 1992;8:119–122.

163. Siddall PJ, Taylor DA, Cousins MJ. Classification of pain following spinal cord injury. *Spinal Cord* 1997;35:69–75.

164. Anderson CJ, Vogel LC. Self-injurious behavior in pediatric spinal cord injury. *J Spinal Cord Med* 1999;22:15.

165. Dahlin, PA, Van Buskirk NE, Novotny RW, et al. Self-biting with multiple finger amputations following spinal cord injury. *Paraplegia* 1985;23:306–318.

166. Marmolya G, Yagan R, Freehafer A. Acro-osteolysis of the fingers in a spinal cord injury patient. *Spine* 1989;14:137–139.

167. Balazy TE. Clinical management of chronic pain in spinal cord injury. *Clin J Pain* 1992;8:102–110.

168. Umlauf RL. Psychological interventions for chronic pain following spinal cord injury. *Clin J Pain* 1992;8:111–118.

169. Bowsher D. Central pain following spinal and supraspinal lesions. *Spinal Cord* 1999;37:235–238.

170. Sandford PR, Lindblom LB, Haddox JD. Amitriptyline and carbamazepine in the treatment of dysesthetic pain in spinal cord injury. *Arch Phys Med Rehabil* 1992;73:300–301.

171. Kwittken PL, Sweinberg SK, Campbell DE, et al. Latex hypersensitivity in children: clinical presentation and detection of latex-specific immunoglobulin E. *Pediatrics* 1995;95:693–699.

172. Landwehr LP, Boguniewicz M. Current perspectives on latex allergy. *J Pediatr* 1996;128:305–312.

173. Slater JE. Latex allergy. *J Allergy Clin Immunol* 1994;94:139–149.

174. Konz KR, Chia JK, Kurup VP, et al. Comparison of latex hypersensitivity among patients with neurologic defects. *J Allergy Clin Immunol* 1995;95:950–954.

175. Vogel LC, Schrader T, Lubicky JP. Latex allergy in children and adolescents with spinal cord injuries. *J Pediatr Orthop* 1995;15: 517–520.

176. Monasterio EA, Barber DB, Rogers SJ, et al. Latex allergy in adults with spinal cord injury: a pilot investigation. *J Spinal Cord Med* 2000; 23:6–9.

177. Fisher AA. Association of latex and food allergy. *Cutis* 1993;52:70–71.

178. Jackson AB, Groomes TE. Incidence of respiratory complications following spinal cord injury. *Arch Phys Med Rehabil* 1994;75:270–275.

179. Lanig IS, Peterson WP. The respiratory system in spinal cord injury. *Phys Med Rehabil Clin N Am* 2000;11:29–43.

180. McKinley WO, Jackson AB, Cardena D, et al. Long-term medical complications after traumatic spinal cord injury: a regional model systems analysis. *Arch Phys Med Rehabil* 1999;80:1402–1410.

181. Carter RE. Experience with ventilator dependent patients. *Paraplegia* 1993;31:150–153.

182. Frates RC, Splaingard ML, Smith EO, et al. Outcome of home mechanical ventilation in children. *J Pediatr* 1985;106:850–856.

183. Nelson VS, Lewis CC. Ventilatory support: preparing for discharge. *Top Spinal Cord Inj Rehabil* (in press).

184. Phrenic nerve pacing in quadriplegia [Editorial]. *Lancet* 1990;336: 88–90.

185. Weese-Mayer DE, Hunt CE, Brouillette RT, et al. Diaphragm pacing in infants and children. *J Pediatr* 1992;120:1–8.

186. Nelson VS. Non-invasive mechanical ventilation for children and adolescents with spinal cord injuries. *Top Spinal Cord Inj Rehabil* 2000; 6:12–15.

187. Tromans AM, Mecci M, Barrett FH, et al. The use of the BiPAP biphasic positive airway pressure system in acute spinal cord injury. *Spinal Cord* 1998;36:481–484.

188. Bach JR. Inappropriate weaning and late onset ventilatory failure of individuals with traumatic spinal cord injury. *Paraplegia* 1993;31: 430–438.

189. Bonekat HW, Andersen G, Squires J. Obstructive disordered breathing during sleep in patients with spinal cord injury. *Paraplegia* 1990; 28:392–398.

190. Flavell H, Marshall R, Thornton AT, et al. Hypoxia episodes during sleep in high tetraplegia. *Arch Phys Med Rehabil* 1992;73:623–627.

191. Vogel LC. Spasticity: diagnostic workup and medical management. In: Betz RR, Mulcahey MJ, eds. *The child with a spinal cord injury.* Rosemont, Illinois: American Academy of Orthopaedic Surgeons, 1996:261–268.

192. Alpiner NM. Spasticity: pathophysiology and objective assessments. In: Betz RR, Mulcahey MJ, eds. *The child with a spinal cord injury.* Rosemont, Illinois: American Academy of Orthopaedic Surgeons, 1996:233–253.

193. Hurvitz EA, Nelson VS. Functional evaluation of spasticity and its effect on rehabilitation. In: Betz RR, Mulcahey MJ, eds. *The child with a spinal cord injury.* Rosemont, Illinois: American Academy of Orthopaedic Surgeons, 1996:255–260.

194. Little JW, Micklesen P, Umlauf R, et al. Lower extremity manifestations of spasticity in chronic spinal cord injury. *Am J Phys Med Rehabil* 1989;68:32–36.

195. Barnes MP. Local treatment of spasticity. *Clin Neurol* 1993;2:55–71.

196. Rice GPA. Pharmacotherapy of spasticity: some theoretical and practical considerations. *Can J Neurol Sci* 1987;14:510–512.

197. Perry HE, Wright RO, Shannon MW, et al. Baclofen overdose: drug experimentation in a group of adolescents. *Pediatrics* 1998;101: 1045–1048.

198. Donovan WH, Carter RE, Rossi CD, et al. Clonidine effect on spasticity: a clinical trial. *Arch Phys Med Rehabil* 1988;69:193–194.

199. Weingarden SI, Belen JG. Clonidine transdermal system for treatment of spasticity in spinal cord injury. *Arch Phys Med Rehabil* 1992;73: 876–877.

200. Yablon SA, Sipski ML. Effect of transdermal clonidine on spinal spasticity. *Am J Phys Med Rehabil* 1993;72:154–157.

201. Mathias CJ, Luckitt J, Desai P, et al. Pharmacodynamics and pharmacokinetics of the oral antispastic agent tizanidine in patients with spinal cord injury. *J Rehabil Res Dev* 1989;26:9–16.

202. Apple DF, Murray HH. Spasticity: surgical management. In: Betz RR, Mulcahey MJ, eds. *The child with a spinal cord injury.* Rosemont, Illinois: American Academy of Orthopaedic Surgeons, 1996: 269–283.

203. Hambleton P. Therapeutic application of botulinum toxin. *J Med Microbiol* 1993;39:243–245.

204. Jankovic J, Brin MF. Therapeutic uses of botulinum toxin. *N Engl J Med* 1991;324:1186–1194.

205. Ochs GA. Intrathecal baclofen. *Bailliere's Clin Neurol* 1993;2:73–86.

206. Penn RD, Savoy SM, Corcos D, et al. Intrathecal baclofen for severe spinal spasticity. *N Engl J Med* 1989;320:1517–1521.

207. Snow BJ, Tsui JKC, Bhatt MH, et al. Treatment of spasticity with botulinum toxin: a double-blind study. *Ann Neurol* 1990;28: 512–515.

208. Armstrong RW, Steinbok P, Farrell K, et al. Continuous intrathecal baclofen treatment of severe spasms in two children with spinal cord injury. *Dev Med Child Neurol* 1992;34:731–738.

209. Albright AL, Barron WB, Fasick MP, et al. Continuous intrathecal baclofen infusion for spasticity of cerebral origin. *JAMA* 1993;270: 2475–2477.

210. Delhaas EM, Brouwers JRBJ. Intrthecal baclofen overdose: report of 7 events in 5 patients and review of the literature. *Int J Clin Pharmacol* 1991;29:274–280.

211. Teddy P, Jamous A, Gardner B, et al. Complications of intrathecal baclofen delivery. *Br J Neurosurg* 1992;6:115–118.

212. Hickey KJ, Anderson CJ, Vogel LC. Pressure ulcers in pediatric spinal cord injury. *Top Spinal Cord Inj Rehabil* 2000;6:85–90.

213. Yarkony GM, Heinemann AW. Pressure ulcers. In: Stover SL, DeLisa JA, Whiteneck GG, eds. *Spinal cord injury: systems.* Gaithersburg, MD: Aspen, 1995:100–119.

214. Bonner L. Pressure ulcer prevention. In: Betz RR, Mulcahey MJ, eds. *The child with a spinal cord injury.* Rosemont, Illinois: American Academy of Orthopaedic Surgeons, 1996:285–292.

215. Banta JV. Rehabilitation of pediatric spinal cord injury: the Newington Children's Hospital experience. *Conn Med* 1984;48:14–18.

216. Flett PJ. The rehabilitation of children with spinal cord injury. *J Paediatr Child Health* 1992;28:141–146.

217. Jarosz DA. Pediatric spinal cord injuries: a case presentation. *Crit Care Nurs Q* 1999;22(2):8–13.

218. Mulcahey MJ. Unique management needs of pediatric spinal cord injury patients: rehabilitation. *J Spinal Cord Med* 1997;20:25–30.

219. Mulcahey MJ, Betz RR. Considerations in the rehabilitation of children with spinal cord injuries. *Top Spinal Cord Inj Rehabil* 1997;3: 31–36.

220. Nelson MR, Tilbor, AG, Frieden L, et al. Introduction to pediatric rehabilitation. In: Betz RR, Mulcahey MJ, eds. *The child with a spinal cord injury.* Rosemont, Illinois: American Academy of Orthopaedic Surgeons, 1996:461–470.

221. Spoltore TA, O'Brien AM. Rehabilitation of the spinal cord injured patient. *Orthop Nurs* 1995;14:7–14.

222. Zager RP, Marquette CH. Developmental considerations in children and early adolescents with spinal cord injury. *Arch Phys Med Rehabil* 1981;62:427–431.

223. Jaffe KM, McDonald CM. Rehabilitation following childhood injury. *Pediatr Ann* 1992;21:438–447.

224. Hussey RW, Stauffer ES. Spinal cord injury: requirements for ambulation. *Arch Phys Med Rehabil* 1973;54:544–547.

225. Vogel LC, Lubicky JP. Ambulation in children and adolescents with spinal cord injuries. *J Pediatr Orthop* 1995;15:510–516.

226. Creitz L, Nelson VS, Haubenstricker L, et al. Orthotic prescriptions. In: Betz RR, Mulcahey MJ, eds. *The child with a spinal cord injury.* Rosemont, Illinois: American Academy of Orthopaedic Surgeons, 1996:537–553.

227. Kelly MA, Stokes KS. Standing and ambulation for the child with paraplegia or tetraplegia. In: Betz RR, Mulcahey MJ, eds. *The child with a spinal cord injury.* Rosemont, Illinois: American Academy of Orthopaedic Surgeons, 1996:519–532.

228. Moynahan M, Hunt M, Halden E. Evaluation of standing and ambulation: needs and outcomes. In: Betz RR, Mulcahey MJ, eds. *The child with a spinal cord injury.* Rosemont, Illinois: American Academy of Orthopaedic Surgeons, 1996:503–517.

229. Rheault S, Dagenais T. Standing and ambulation: an overview. In: Betz RR, Mulcahey MJ, eds. *The child with a spinal cord injury.* Rosemont: American Academy of Orthopaedic Surgeons, 1996: 501–502.

230. Vogel LC, Lubicky JP. Pediatric spinal cord injury issues: ambulation. *Top Spinal Cord Inj Rehabil* 1997;3:37–47.

231. Vogel LC, Lubicky JP. Ambulation with parapodia and reciprocating gait orthoses in pediatric spinal cord injury. *Dev Med Child Neurol* 1995;37:957–964.

232. Kinnen E, Gram M, Jackman KV, et al. Rochester parapodium. *Clin Prosthet Orthot* 1987;8:24–25.

233. Stallard J, Rose GK, Farmer IR. The Orlau swivel walker. *Prosthet Orthot Int* 1978;2(1):35–42.

234. Katz DE, Haideri N, Song K, et al. Comparative study of conventional hip-knee-ankle-foot orthoses versus reciprocating-gait orthoses for children with high-level paraparesis. *J Pediatr Orthop* 1997;17: 377–386.

235. Fitzsimmons AS. The physiologic benefits of standing. In: Betz RR, Mulcahey MJ, eds. *The child with a spinal cord injury.* Rosemont, Illinois: American Academy of Orthopaedic Surgeons, 1996: 533–535.

236. Cybulski GR, Penn RD, Jaeger RJ. Lower extremity functional neuromuscular stimulation in cases of spinal cord injury. *Neurosurgery* 1984; 15:132–146.

237. Moynahan MA, Mullin C, Cohn J, et al. Home uses of a FES system for standing and mobility in adolescents with spinal cord injury. *Arch Phys Med Rehabil* 1996;77:1005–1013.

238. Bonaroti D, Akers J, Smith BT, et al. Comparison of functional electrical stimulation to long leg braces for upright mobility in children with complete thoracic level spinal injuries. *Arch Phys Med Rehabil* 1999;80:1047–1053.

239. Krajnik S, Bridle M. Hand splinting in tetraplegia: current practice. *Am J Occup Ther* 1992;46:149–156.

240. Mulcahey MJ. Upper extremity orthoses and splints. In: Betz RR, Mulcahey MJ, eds. *The child with a spinal cord injury.* Rosemont, Illinois: American Academy of Orthopaedic Surgeons, 1996: 375–392.

241. Mulcahey MJ. Rehabilitation and outcomes of upper extremity tendon transfer surgery. In: Betz RR, Mulcahey MJ, eds. *The child with a spinal cord injury.* Rosemont, Illinois: American Academy of Orthopaedic Surgeons, 1996:419–448.

242. Mulcahey MJ, Betz RR, Smith BT, et al. A prospective evaluation of upper extremity tendon transfers in children with cervical spinal cord injury. *J Pediatr Orthop* 1999;19:319–328.

243. Mulcahey MJ, Betz RR, Smith BT, et al. Implanted FES hand system in adolescents with SCI: an evaluation. *Arch Phys Med Rehabil* 1997; 78:597–607.

244. Peckham PH, Marsolais EB, Mortimer JT. Restoration of key grip and release in the C6 tetraplegic patient through functional neuromuscular stimulation. *J Hand Surg* 1980;5:462–469.

245. Kilgore KL, Peckham PH, Keith MW, et al. An implanted upper-extremity neuroprosthesis: follow-up of five patients. *J Bone Joint Surg [Am]* 1997;79:533–541.

246. Akers JM, Smith BT, Betz RR. Implantable electrode lead in a growing limb. *IEEE Trans Rehabil Eng* 1999;7:35–45.

247. Anderson CJ. Unique management needs of pediatric spinal cord injury patients: psychological issues. *J Spinal Cord Med* 1997;20: 21–24.

248. Anderson CJ. Psychosocial and sexuality issues in pediatric spinal cord injury. *Top Spinal Cord Inj Rehabil* 1997;3:70–78.

249. Yarkony GM, Anderson CJ. Sexuality. In: Betz RR, Mulcahey MJ, eds. *The child with a spinal cord injury.* Rosemont, Illinois: American Academy of Orthopaedic Surgeons, 1996:625–637.

250. Anderson CJ, Mulcahey MJ, Vogel LC. Menstruation and pediatric spinal cord injury. *J Spinal Cord Med* 1997;20:56–59.

251. American Academy of Pediatrics Committee on Children With Disabilities. Provision of educationally-related services for children and adolescents with chronic diseases and disabling conditions. *Pediatrics* 2000;105:448–451.

252. The Individuals With Disabilities Education Act (IDEA). 20 USC B 1400 et seq, June 4, 1997.

253. Sammallahti P, Kannisto M, Aalberg V. Psychological defenses and psychiatric symptoms in adults with pediatric spinal cord injuries. *Spinal Cord* 1996;34:669–672.

254. Callen L. Substance use and abuse. In: Betz RR, Mulcahey MJ, eds. *The child with a spinal cord injury.* Rosemont, Illinois: American Academy of Orthopaedic Surgeons, 1996:671–677.

255. Mubarak SJ, Camp JF, Vuletich W, et al. Halo application in the infant. *J Pediatr Orthop* 1989;9:612–614.

256. Garfin SR, Roux R, Botte MJ, et al. Skull osteology as it affects halo pin placement in children. *J Pediatr Orthop* 1986;6:434–436.

257. Letts M, Kaylor D, Gouw G. A biomechanical analysis of halo fixation in children. *J Bone Joint Surg [Br]* 1988;70:277–279.

258. Herzenberg JK, Hensinger RN, Dedrick DK, et al. Emergency transport and positioning of young children who have an injury of the cervical spine: the standard backboard may be hazardous. *J Bone Joint Surg [Am]* 1989;71:15–22.

259. Bergstrom EMK, Short DJ, Frankel HL, et al. The effect of childhood spinal cord injury on skeletal development: a retrospective study. *Spinal Cord* 1999;37:838–846.

260. Dearolf WW III, Betz RR, Vogel LC, et al. Scoliosis in pediatric spinal cord-injured patients. *J Pediatr Orthop* 1990;10:214–218.

261. Lancourt JE, Dickson JH, Carter RE. Paralytic spinal deformity following traumatic spinal-cord injury in children and adolescents. *J Bone Joint Surg [Am]* 1981;63:47–53.

262. Mayfield JK, Erkkila JC, Winter RB. Spine deformity subsequent to acquired childhood spinal cord injury. *J Bone Joint Surg [Am]* 1981; 63:1401–1411.

263. Betz RR, Orthopaedic problems in the child with spinal injury. *Top Spinal Cord Inj Rehabil* 1997;3:9–19.

264. Lieberman GS, Betz RR. Bracing for delaying the progression of scoliosis in the immature patient with spinal cord injury. *J Spinal Cord Med* 1998;21:193.

265. Lubicky JP, Betz RR. Spinal deformity in children and adolescents after spinal cord injury. In: Betz RR, Mulcahey MJ, eds. *The child with a spinal cord injury.* Rosemont, Illinois: American Academy of Orthopaedic Surgeons, 1996:363–370.

266. Miller F, Betz RR. Hip joint instability. In: Betz RR, Mulcahey MJ, eds. *The child with a spinal cord injury.* Rosemont, Illinois: American Academy of Orthopaedic Surgeons, 1996:353–361.

267. Rink P, Miller F. Hip instability in spinal cord injury patients. *J Pediatr Orthop* 1990;10:583–587.

268. Vogel LC, Gogia RS, Lubicky JP. Hip abnormalities in children with spinal cord injuries. *J Spinal Cord Med* 1995;18:172.

269. Betz RR, Beck T, Huss GK, et al. Hip instability in children with spinal cord injury. *J Am Paraplegia Soc* 1999;17:119.

270. Betz RR, Mulcahey MJ, Smith BT, et al. Implications of hip subluxation for FES-assisted mobility in patients with spinal cord injury. *Orthopedics* 2001;24:181–184.

271. McCarthy JJ, Weibel B, Betz RR. Results of pelvic osteotomies for hip subluxation or dislocation in children with spinal cord injury. *Top Spinal Cord Inj Rehabil* 2000;6:48–53.

272. Garland DE. A clinical perspective on common forms of acquired heterotopic ossification. *Clin Orthop* 1991;263:13–29.

273. Garland DE, Shimoya ST, Lugo C, et al. Spinal cord insults and heterotopic ossification in the pediatric population. *Clin Orthop* 1989; 245:303–310.

274. Banovac K, Gonzalez F, Renfree KJ. Treatment of heterotopic ossification after spinal cord injury. *J Spinal Cord Med* 1997;20:60–65.

275. Bellah RD, Zawodniak L, Librizzi RJ, et al. Idiopathic arterial calcification of infancy: prenatal and postnatal effects of therapy in an infant. *J Pediatr* 1992;121:930–933.

276. Pazzaglia UE, Beluff G, Ravelli A, et al. Chronic intoxication by ethane-1-hydroxy-1,1-diphosphonate (EHDP) in a child with myositis ossificans progressiva. *Pediatr Radiol* 1993;23:459–462.

277. Silverman SL, Hurvitz EA, Nelson VS, et al. Rachitic syndrome after disodium etidronate therapy in an adolescent. *Arch Phys Med Rehabil* 1994;75:118–120.

278. Freebourn TM, Barber DB, Able AC. The treatment of immature heterotopic ossification in spinal cord injuries with combination surgery, radiation therapy and NSAID. *Spinal Cord* 1999;37:50–53.

279. Wick M, Muller EJ, Hahn MP, et al. Surgical excision of heterotopic bone after hip surgery followed by oral indomethicin application: is there a clinical benefit for the patient? *Arch Orthop Trauma Surg* 1999;119:151–155.

280. Betz RR, Triolo RJ, Hermida VM, et al. The effects of functional neuromuscular stimulation on the bone mineral content in the lower limbs of spinal cord injured children. *J Am Paraplegia Soc* 1991;14: 65–66.

281. Miller F. Pathologic long-bone fractures: diagnosis, etiology, management, and prevention. In: Betz RR, Mulcahey MJ, eds. *The child with a spinal cord injury.* Rosemont, Illinois: American Academy of Orthopaedic Surgeons, 1996:331–338.

282. Botto LD, Moore CA, Khoury MJ, et al. Neural-tube defects. *N Engl J Med* 1999;341:1509–1519.

283. Kaufman BA. Congenital intraspinal anomalies: spinal dysraphism—embryology, pathology, and treatment. In: Bridwell KH, DeWald RL, eds. *The textbook of spinal surgery,* 2nd ed. Philadelphia: Lippincott-Raven, 1997:365–399.

284. Lemire RJ. Neural tube defects. *JAMA* 1988;259:558–562.

285. Lindseth RE. Myelomeningocele. In: Morrissy RT, Weinstein SL, eds. *Lovell & Winter's pediatric orthopaedics,* 4th ed. Philadelphia: Lippincott-Raven, 1996:503–535.

286. Shurtleff DB, Lemire RJ. Epidemiology, etiologic factors, and prenatal diagnosis of open spinal dysraphism. *Neurosurg Clin N Am* 1995;6: 183–193.

287. Centers for Disease Control. Spina bifida incidence at birth: United States, 1983–1990. *MMWR Morb Mortal Wkly Rep* 1992;40: 497–500.

288. Yen IH, Khoury MJ, Erickson JD, et al. The changing epidemiology of neural tube defects, United States 1968–1989. *Am J Dis Child* 1992;146:857–861.

289. Shurtleff DB, Luthy DA, Nyberg DA, et al. Meningomyelocele: management in utero and post natum. *Ciba Found Symp* 1994;181: 270–286.

290. Wasserman CR, Shaw GM, Selvin S, et al. Socioeconomic status, neighborhood social conditions, and neural tube defects. *Am J Public Health* 1998;88:1674–1680.

291. Lian ZH, Yang HY, Li Z. Neural tube defects in Beijing-Tianjin area of China: urban-rural distribution and some other epidemiologic characteristics *J Epidemiol Commun Health* 1987;41:259–262.

292. Hunt GM. A study of deaths and handicap in a consecutive series of spina bifida treated unselectively from birth. *Z Kinderchir* 1983; 38[Suppl II]:100–102.

293. McLone DG. Continuing concepts in the management of spina bifida. *Pediatr Neurosurg* 1992;18:254–256.

294. Hunt GM. The median survival time in open spina bifida. *Dev Med Child Neurol* 1997;39:568.

295. Hall JG, Solehdin F. Genetics of neural tube defects. *Ment Retard Dev Disab Res Rev* 1998;4:269–281.

296. Becerra JE, Khoury MJ, Cordero JF, et al. Diabetes mellitus during pregnancy and the risks for specific birth defects: a population based case-control study. *Pediatrics* 1990;85:1–9.

297. Lammer EJ, Sever LE, Oakley GP. Teratogen update: valproic acid. *Teratology* 1987;35:465–473.

298. Rosa FW. Spina bifida in infants of women treated with carbamazepine during pregnancy. *N Engl J Med* 1991;324:674–677.

299. Shaw GM, Velie EM, Schaffer D. Risk of neural tube defect-affected pregnancies among obese women. *JAMA* 1996;275:1093–1096.

300. Waller DK, Mills JL, Simpson JL, et al. Are obese women at higher risk for producing malformed offspring? *Am J Obstet Gynecol* 1994; 170:541–548.

301. Watkins ML, Scanlon KS, Mulinare J, et al. Is maternal obesity a risk factor for anencephaly and spina bifida? *Epidemiology* 1996;7: 507–512.

302. Graham JM, Edwards MJ, Edwards MJ. Teratogen update: gestational effects of maternal hyperthermia due to febrile illnesses and resultant patterns of defects in humans. *Teratology* 1998;58:209–221.

303. Edwards MJ, Shiota K, Smith MSR, et al. Hyperthermia and birth defects. *Reprod Toxicol* 1995;9:411–425.

304. Christensen B, Arbour L, Tran P, et al. Genetic polymorphisms in methylenetetrahydrofolate reductase and methionine synthase, folate levels in red blood cells, and risk of neural tube defects. *Am J Med Genet* 1999;84:151–157.

305. McBride ML. Sib risks of anencephaly and spina bifida in British Columbia. *Am J Med Genet* 1979;3:377–387.

306. Myers GJ. Myelomeningocele: the medical aspects. *Pediatr Clin North Am* 1984;31:165–175.

307. Toriello HV, Higgins JV. Occurrence of neural tube defects among first-, second-, and third-degree relatives of probands: results of a United States study. *Am J Med Genet* 1983;15:601–606.

308. Urui S, Oi S. Experimental study of the embryogenesis of open spinal dysraphism. *Neurosurg Clin North Am* 1995;6:195–202.

309. Rauzzino M, Oakes WJ. Chiari II malformation and syringomyelia. *Neurosurg Clin North Am* 1995;6:293–309.

310. Swank M, Dias L. Myelomeningocele: a review of the orthopaedic aspects of 206 patients treated from birth with no selection criteria. *Dev Med Child Neurol* 1992;34:1047–1052.

311. Pang D. Surgical complications of open dysraphism. *Neurosurg Clin N Am* 1995;6:243–257.

312. Drewek MJ, Bruner JP, Whetsell WO, et al. Quantitative analysis of the toxicity of human amniotic fluid to cultured rat spinal cord. *Pediatr Neurosurg* 1997;27:190–193.

313. Heffez DS, Aryanpur J, Hutchins GM, et al. The paralysis associated with myelomeningocele: clinical and experimental data implicating a preventable spinal cord injury. *Neurosurgery* 1990;26:987–992.

314. Hahn YS, Open myelomeningocele. *Neurosurg Clin North Am* 1995;6:231–241.

315. Charney EB, Weller SC, Sutton LN, et al. Management of the newborn with myelomeningocele: time for a decision-making process. *Pediatrics* 1985;75:58–64.

316. Stein SC, Schut L. Hydrocephalus in myelomeningocele. *Childs Brain* 1979;5:413–419.

317. Steinbok P, Irvine B, Cochrane DD, et al. Long-term outcome and complications of children born with meningomyelocele. *Childs Nerv Syst* 1992;8:92–96.

318. Hunt GM, Poulton A. Open spina bifida: a complete cohort reviewed 25 years after closure. *Dev Med Child Neurol* 1995;37:19–29.

319. McLone DG, Czyzewski D. Raimondi AJ, et al. Central nervous system infections as a limiting factor in the intelligence of children with myelomeningocele. *Pediatrics* 1982;70:338–342.

320. Cull C, Wyke MA. Memory functions of children with spina bifida and shunted hydrocephalus. *Dev Med Child Neurol* 1984;26:177–183.

321. Swisher LP, Pinsker EJ. The language characteristics of hyperverbal, hydrocephalic children. *Dev Med Child Neurol* 1971;13:746–755.

322. Grimm RA. Children with myelomeningocele. *Am J Occup Ther* 1976;30:234–240.

323. Jansen J, Taudorf K, Pedersen H, et al. Upper extremity function in spina bifida. *Childs Nerv Syst* 1991;7:67–71.

324. Turner A. Hand function in children with myelomeningocle. *J Bone Joint Surg [Br]* 1985;67:268–272.

325. Kirk VG, Morielli A, Brouillette RT. Sleep-disordered breathing in patients with myelomeningocele: the missed diagnosis. *Dev Med Child Neurol* 1999;41:40–43.

326. Petersen MC, Wolraich M, Sherbondy, et al. Abnormalities in control of ventilation in newborn infants with myelomeningocele. *J Pediatr* 1995;126:1011–1015.

327. Swaminathan S, Paton JY, Davidson SL, et al. Abnormal control of ventilation in adolescents with myelodysplasia. *J Pediatr* 1989;115:898–903.

328. Waters K, Forbes P, Morielli A, et al. Sleep-disordered breathing in children with myelomeningocele. *J Pediatr* 1998;132:672–681.

329. Park TS, Cail WS, Maggio WM, et al. Progressive spasticity and scoliosis in children with myelomeningocele. *J Neurosurg* 1985;62:367–374.

330. Bartonek A, Saraste H, Knutson LM. Comparison of different systems to classify the neurological level of lesion in patients with myelomeningocele. *Dev Med Child Neurol* 1999;41:796–805.

331. Curtis BH, Brightman, E. Spina bifida: a follow-up of ninety cases. *Conn Med* 1961;26:145–150.

332. McDonald CM, Jaffe KM, Shurtleff DB, et al. Modifications to the traditional description of neurosegmental innervation in myelomeningocele. *Dev Med Child Neurol* 1991;33:473–481.

333. McDonald CM. Rehabilitatioin of children with spinal dysraphism. *Neurosurg Clin North Am* 1995;6:393–412.

334. Shurtleff DB, Duguay S, Duguay G, et al. Epidemiology of tethered cord with meningomyelocele. *Eur J Pediatr Surg* 1997;7[Suppl I]:7–11.

335. Shurtleff DB. Selection process for the care of congenitally malformed infants. In: Shurtleff DB, ed. *Myelodysplasias and exstrophies: significance, prevention and treatment.* Orlando, FL: Grune & Stratton, 1986:89–115.

336. Jutson JM, Beasley SW, Bryan AD. Cryptorchidism in spina bifida and spinal cord transection: a clue to the mechanism of transinguinal descent of the testis. *J Pediatr Surg* 1988;23:275–277.

337. Kropp KA, Voeller KKS. Cryptorchidism in meningomyelocele. *J Pediatr* 1981;99:110–113.

338. Joseph DB, Bauer SB, Colodny AH, et al. Clean, intermittent catheterization of infants with neurogenic bladder. *Pediatrics* 1989;84:78–82.

339. Kasabian NG, Bauer SB, Dyro FM, et al. The prophylactic value of clean intermittent catheterization and anticholinergic medication in newborns and infants with myelodysplasia at risk of developing urinary tract deterioration. *Am J Dis Child* 1992;146:840–843.

340. Roach MB, Switters DM, Stone AR. The changing urodynamic pattern in infants with myelomeningocele. *J Urol* 1993;150:944–947.

341. Sidi AA, Dykstra DD, Gonzalez R. The value of urodynamic testing in the management of neonates with myelodysplasia: a prospective study. *J Urol* 1986;135:90–93.

342. Stone AR. Neurologic evaluation and urologic management of spinal dysraphism. *Neurosurg Clin N Am* 1995;6:269–277.

343. Uehling DT, Smith J, Meyer J, et al. Impact of an intermittent catheterization program on children with myelomeningocele. *Pediatrics* 1985;76:892–895.

344. Hannigan KF. Teaching intermittent self-catheterization to young children with myelodysplasia. *Dev Med Child Neurol* 1979;21:365–368.

345. King JC, Currie DM, Wright E. Bowel training in spina bifida: importance of education, patient compliance, age, and anal reflexes. *Arch Phys Med Rehabil* 1994;75:243–247.

346. Shandling B, Gilmour RF. The enema continence catheter in spina bifida: successful bowel management. *J Pediatr Surg* 1987;22:271–273.

347. Loening-Baucke V, Desch L, Wolraich M. Biofeedback training for patients with myelomeningocele and fecal incontinence. *Dev Med Child Neurol* 1988;30:781–790.

348. Wald A. Use of biofeedback in treatment of fecal incontinence in patients with meningomyelocele. *Pediatrics* 1981;68:45–49.

349. Whitehead WE, Parker L, Bosmajian L, et al. Treatment of fecal incontinence in children with spina bifida: comparison of biofeedback and behavior modification. *Arch Phys Med Rehabil* 1986;67:218–224.

350. Karol LA. Orthopedic management in myelomeningocele. *Neurosurg Clin N Am* 1995;6:259–268.

351. Piggott H. The natural history of scoliosis in myelodysplasia. *J Bone Joint Surg [Br]* 1980;62:54–58.

352. Shurtleff DB. Mobility. In: Shurtleff DB ed. *Myelodysplasias and exstrophies: significance, prevention and treatment.* Orlando, FL: Grune & Stratton, 1986:313–356.

353. Feiwell E, Downey DS, Blatt T. The effect of hip reduction on function in patients with myelomeningocele. *J Bone Joint Surg [Am]* 1978;60:169–173.

354. Lubicky JP. Spinal deformity in myelomeningocele. In: Bridwell KH, DeWald RL, ed. *The textbook of spinal surgery,* 2nd ed. Philadelphia: Lippincott-Raven, 1997:903–931.

355. Mackel JL, Lindseth RE. Scoliosis in myelodysplasia. *J Bone Joint Surg [Am]* 1975;57:1031.

356. Hall PV, Lindseth RE, Campbell RL, et al. Myelodysplasia and developmental scoliosis. *Spine* 1976;1:48–56.

357. Tomlinson RJ, Wolfe MW, Nadall JM, et al. Syringomyelia and developmental scoliosis. *J Pediatr Orthop* 1994;14:580–585.

358. Hall P, Lindseth R, Campbell R, et al. Scoliosis and hydrocephalus in myelocele patients. *J Neurosurg* 1979;50:174–178.

359. Rosenblum MF, Rinegold DN, Charney EB. Assessment of stature of children with myelomeningocele, and usefulness of arm-span measurement. *Dev Med Child Neurol* 1983;25:338–342.

360. Rotenstein D, Reigel DH. Growth hormone treatment of children with neural tube defects: results from 6 months to 6 years. *J Pediatr* 1996;128:184–189.

361. Elias ER, Sadeghi-Nead A. Precocious puberty in girl with myelodysplasia. *Pediatrics* 1994;93:521–522.

362. Hunt GM. Open spina bifida: outcome for a complete cohort treated unselectively and followed into adulthood. *Dev Med Child Neurol* 1990;32:108–118.

363. Trollman R, Strehl E, Dorr HG. Precocious puberty in children with myelomeningocele: treatment with gonadotropin-releasing hormone analogues. *Dev Med Child Neurol* 1998;40:38–43.

364. Hayden PW. Adolescents with meningomyelocele. *Pediatr Rev* 1985;6:245–252.

365. Hayes-Allen MC. Obesity and short stature in children with myelomeningocele. *Dev Med Child Neurol* 1972;4[Suppl 27]:59–64.

366. Hunt GM. Spina bifida: implications for 100 children at school. *Dev Med Child Neurol* 1981;23:160–172.

367. Roberts D, Shepherd RW, Shepherd K. Anthropometry and obesity in myelomeningocele. *J Paediatr Child Health* 1991;27:83–90.

368. Shurtleff DB. Dietary management. In: Shurtleff DB ed. *Myelodysplasia and extrophies: significance, prevention and treatment.* Orlando, FL: Grune & Stratton, 1986:285–298.

369. Kelly KJ, Pearson ML, Kurup VP, et al. A cluster of anaphylactic reactions in children with spina bifida during general anesthesia: epidemiologic features, risk factors, and latex hypersensitivity. *J Allergy Clin Immunol* 1994;94(1):53–61.

370. Meeropol E, Kelleher R, Bell S, et al. Allergic reactions to rubber in patients with myelodysplasia. *N Engl J Med* 1990;323:1072.

371. Yassin MS, Sanyurah S, Lierl MB, et al. Evaluation of latex allergy in patients with meningomyelocele. *Ann Allergy* 1992;69:207–211.

372. Mazon A, Nieto A, Estornell F, et al. Factors that influence the presence of symptoms caused by latex allergy in children with spina bifida. *J Allergy Clin Immunol* 1997;99:600–604.

373. Michael T, Niggemann, B, Moers A, et al. Risk factors for latex allergy in patients with spina bifida. *Clin Exp Allergy* 1996;26:934–939.

374. Niggemann B, Kulig M, Bergmann R, et al. Development of latex allergy in children up to 5 years of age: a retrospective analysis of risk factors. *Pediatr Allergy Immunol* 1998;9:36–39.

375. Cremer R, Kleine-Diepenbruck U, Hoppe A, et al. Latex allergy in spina bifida patients: prevention by primary prophylaxis. *Allergy* 1998;53:709–711.

376. Cremer R, Hoppe A, Keine-Diepenbruck U, et al. Longitudinal study on latex sensitization in children with spina bifida. *Pediatr Allergy Immunol* 1998;9:40–43.

377. De Swert LFA, Van Laer KMIA, Verpoorten CMA, et al. Determination of independent risk factors and comparative analysis of diagnostic methods for immediate type latex allergy in spina bifida patients. *Clin Exp Allergy* 1997;27:1067–1076.

378. Szepfatusi Z, Seidl R, Bernert G, et al. Latex sensitization in spina bifida appears disease-associated. *J Pediatr* 1999;134:344–348.

379. Harris MB, Banta JV. Cost of skin care in the myelomeningocele population. *J Pediatr Orthop* 1990;10:355–361.

380. Okamoto GA, Lamers JV, Shurtleff DB. Skin breakdown in patients with myelomeningocele. *Arch Phys Med Rehabil* 1983;64:20–23.

381. Hayden PW, Davenport SLH, Campbell MM. Adolescents with myelodysplasia: impact of physical disability on emotional maturation. *Pediatrics* 1979;64:53–59.

382. Zurmohle UM, Homann T, Schroeter C, et al. Psychosocial adjustment of children with spina bifida. *J Child Neurol* 1998;13:64–70.

383. Loomis JW, Javornisky JG, Monahan JJ, et al. Relations between family environment and adjustment outcomes in young adults with spina bifida. *Dev Med Child Neurol* 1997;39:620–627.

384. Joyner BD, McLorie GA, Khoury AE. Sexuality and reproductive issues in children with myelomeningocele. *Eur J Pediatr Surg* 1998;8:29–34.

385. Sawyer SM, Roberts KV. Sexual and reproductive health in young people with spina bifida. *Dev Med Child Neurol* 1999;41:671–675.

386. Bodzioch J, Roach JW, Schkade J. Promoting independence in adolescent paraplegics: a 2-week "camping" experience. *J Pediatr Orthop* 1986;6:198–201.

387. Tew B, Laurence KM, Jenkins V. Factors affecting employability among young adults with spina bifida and hydrocephalus. *Z Kinderchir* 1990;45:34–36.

388. American Academy of Pediatrics Committee on Genetics. Folic acid for the prevention of neural tube defects. *Pediatrics* 1999;104:325–327.

389. Berry RJ, Li Z, Erickson JD, et al. Prevention of neural-tube defects with folic aid in China. *N Engl J Med* 1999;341:1485–1490.

390. Centers for Disease Control. Recommendations for the use of folic acid to reduce the number of cases of spina bifida and other neural tube defects. *MMWR Morb Mortal Wkly Rep* 1992;41(RR-14):1–7.

391. MRC Vitamin Study Research Group. Prevention of neural tube defects: results of the Medical Research Council vitamin study. *Lancet* 1991;338:131–137.

392. American Academy of Pediatrics Committee on Genetics. Maternal serum α-fetoprotein screening. *Pediatrics* 1991;88:1282–1283.

393. Burton BK. α-Fetoprotein screening. *Adv Pediatr* 1986;33:181–196.

394. Hobbins JC. Diagnosis and management of neural tube defects. *N Engl J Med* 1991;324:690–691.

395. Babcook CJ. Ultrasound evaluation of prenatal and neonatal spina bifida. *Neurosurg Clin North Am* 1995;6:203–218.

396. Meuli M, Meuli-Simmen C, Hutchins GM, et al. The spinal cord lesion in human fetuses with myelomeningocele: implications for fetal surgery. *J Pediatr Surg* 1997;32:448–452.

397. Adzick NS, Sutton LN, Crombleholme TM, et al. Successful fetal surgery for spina bifida. *Lancet* 1998;352:1675–1676.

398. Bruner JP, Tulipan N, Paschall RL, et al. Fetal surgery for myelomeningocele and the incidence of shunt-dependent hydrocephalus. *JAMA* 1999;282:1819–1825.

399. Bruner JP, Richards WO, Tulipan NB, et al. Endoscopic coverage of fetal myelomeningocele in utero. *Am J Obstet Gynecol* 1999;180:153–158.

400. Tulipan N, Bruner JP. Myelomeningocele repair in utero: a report of three cases. *Pediatr Neurosurg* 1998;28:177–180.

401. Luthy DA, Wardinsky T, Shurtleff DB, et al. Cesarean section before the onset of labor and subsequent motor function in infants with meningomyelocele diagnosed antenatally. *N Engl J Med* 1991;324:662–666.

402. Merrill DC, Goodwin P, Burson J, et al. The optimal route of delivery for fetal meningomyelocele. *Am J Obstet Gynecol* 1998;179:235–240.

403. Owen J. Prophylactic cesarean for prenatally diagnosed malformations. *Clin Obstet Gynecol* 1998;41:393–404.

404. Sutton LN. Lipomyelomeningocele. *Neurosurg Clin North Am* 1995;6:325–338.

405. Estin D, Cohen AR. Caudal agenesis and associated caudal spinal cord malformations. *Neurosurg Clin North Am* 1995;6:377–391.

406. Renshaw TS. Sacral agenesis. *J Bone Joint Surg [Am]* 1978;60:373–383.

407. Wilmshurst JM, Kelly R, Borzyskowski M. Presentation and outcome of sacral agenesis: 20 years' experience. *Dev Med Child Neurol* 1999;41:806–812.

408. Guzman L, Bauer SB, Hallett M, et al. Evaluation and management of children with sacral agenesis. *Urology* 1983;22:506–510.

409. Isu T, Iwasaki Y, Akino M, et al. Hydrosyringomyelia associated with a Chiari I malformation in children and adolescents. *Neurosurgery* 1990;26:591–597.

410. Menkes JH, Till K. Malformations of the central nervous system. In Menkes JH, ed. *Textbook of child neurology*, 5th ed. Baltimore: Williams & Wilkins, 1995:240–324.

411. Nohria V, Oakes WJ. Chiari malformations, hydrosyringomyelia, and the tethered cord syndrome. In: Weinstein SL, ed. *The pediatric spine: principles and practice.* New York: Raven, 1994:685–705.

412. Cahan LD, Bentson JR. Considerations in the diagnosis and treatment of syringomyelia and the Chiari malformation. *J Neurosurg* 1982;57:24–31.

413. Logue V, Edwards MR. Syringomyelia and its surgical treatment— an analysis of 75 patients. *J Neurol Neurosurg Psychiatry* 1981;44: 273–284.

414. Isu T, Chono Y, Iwasaki Y, et al. Scoliosis associated with syringomyelia presenting in children. *Childs Nerv Syst* 1992;8:97–100.

415. Williams B. Orthopaedic features in the presentation of syringomyelia. *J Bone Joint Surg [Br]* 1979;61:314–323.

416. Farley FA, Song KM, Birch JG, et al. Syringomyelia and scoliosis in children. *J Pediatr Orthop* 1995;15:187–192.

417. Phillips WA, Hensinger RN, Kling TK. Management of scoliosis due to syringomyelia in childhood and adolescence. *J Pediatr Orthop* 1990; 10:351–354.

418. Schlesinger EB, Antunes JL, Michelsen WJ, et al. Hydromyelia: clinical presentation and comparison of modalities of treatment. *Neurosurgery* 1981;9:356–365.

419. Batzdorf U. Syringomyelia related to abnormalities at the level of the craniovertebral junction. In: Batzdorf U, ed. *Syringomyelia: current concepts in diagnosis and treatment.* Baltimore: Williams & Wilkins, 1991:163–182.

420. Williams B, Page N. Surgical treatment of syringomyelia with syringopleural shunting. *Br J Neurosurg* 1987;1:63–80.

421. Barbaro NM. Surgery for primarily spinal syringomyelia. In: Batzdorf U, ed. *Syringomyelia: current concepts in diagnosis and treatment.* Baltimore: Williams & Wilkins, 1991:183–198.

422. Barbaro NM, Wilson CB, Gutin PH, et al. Surgical treatment of syringomyelia. *J Neurosurg* 1984;61:531–538.

NONTRAUMATIC SPINAL CORD INJURY: ETIOLOGY, INCIDENCE, AND OUTCOME

WILLIAM O. MCKINLEY

The pathogenesis of nontraumatic spinal cord injury (SCI) includes such etiologies as vertebral spondylosis (spinal stenosis), tumorous compression, and vascular ischemia (1–4). Although nontraumatic cases make up a significant percentage of hospital admissions for SCI, the incidence, demographics, clinical presentations, and outcomes for the nontraumatic SCI population have not been well studied. Most studies of SCI are based on individuals with traumatic (e.g., motor vehicle collision, acts of violence, falls) rather than nontraumatic SCI. Epidemiologic data, frequently cited from the National SCI Statistical Database, reveal that individuals with SCI have a mean age of 31 years, 81% are male, 54% are single, and 62% are employed (5). Although this dataset documents 38 causes of SCI, nearly all are of traumatic etiology. The objectives of this chapter are to review the literature pertaining to nontraumatic SCI incidence, demographics, clinical presentation, and functional outcome. A better understanding of these issues will assist in the medical management, rehabilitation, and long-term follow-up of these patients.

INCIDENCE AND DEMOGRAPHICS

Unlike those with acute traumatic SCI, patients with nontraumatic SCI do not necessarily enter major trauma centers and are not as easily tracked in SCI databases. Nonetheless, several studies have revealed a significant incidence of nontraumatic SCI. Kurtzke reported that the annual incidence rate for nontraumatic SCI may be as high as 8 per 100,000, but he noted that this could not be validly estimated because of incomplete or nonrepresentative reporting (6). McKinley and colleagues, in a 5-year study performed at a Level I Regional SCI Model System, reported a 39% incidence of individuals with nontraumatic SCI primarily due to myelopathy, resulting from spinal stenosis and neoplastic spinal cord compression (SCC) who were admitted to SCI inpatient rehabilitation (7–9) (Fig. 30.1). These and other studies revealed that spinal stenosis accounted for 16% to 21% of SCI admissions, whereas neoplastic SCC has been reported in as many as 10% to 14% of those with SCI (7–11).

Guttman and associates, in a study of 3,000 SCI admissions, reported that nearly one third were the result of nontraumatic

etiology (12). Myelitis and poliomyelitis each occurred at a rate of about 5%, with less than 5% attributed to such etiologies as multiple sclerosis, spondylosis, and congenital and vascular insults. Buchan and coworkers reviewed SCI etiology and demographics in both first-time admissions and readmissions in pediatric and adult populations (13). Of the 310 SCI admissions, 79% were of nontraumatic etiology, with 44% congenital (primarily spina bifida), 13% intervertebral disk disease, 9% spinal neoplasm, 9% myelitis (including multiple sclerosis, transverse myelitis, and encephalomyelitis), and a 4% miscellaneous group (including infection and vascular lesions). Wide variations in ages were noted within these different etiologies. As expected, spina bifida was much more prevalent within the pediatric population, neoplasm was commonly seen in teenagers and individuals in the fifth through seventh decades, and intervertebral disk disease was most prominent in those older than fifty years of age.

The demographic comparison between nontraumatic and traumatic SCI reveals several differences that may be of importance when considering functional outcome and discharge issues. Studies have revealed that individuals in the nontraumatic SCI group are more likely to be significantly older, female, married, and retired when compared with those with traumatic SCI (7–10) (Table 30.1). Murray reported that nontraumatic SCI made up only 31% of patients younger than 40 years old. On the other hand, he showed that 87% of those older than 40 years of age presented with nontraumatic SCI, neoplasm (53%) and spondylosis (25%), as the leading cause (14). The etiologic presentation of nontraumatic SCI may assist in explaining these differences. Spinal stenosis and tumorous invasion of the spinal cord are leading categories of nontraumatic SCI and more commonly involve individuals in their fifth decade and beyond. These individuals are also more likely to be married and retired (15). Neoplastic SCC has a peak incidence between 50 and 70 years of age (8,10,16–18). SCI in those younger than 50 years of age is more commonly due to traumatic, rather than nontraumatic, etiology.

Older age has been shown to affect rehabilitation outcome after SCI. DeVivo and associates reported a higher prevalence of comorbidities and poorer outcomes (increased medical com-

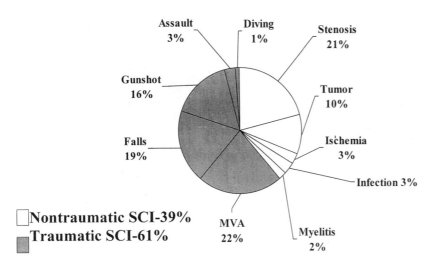

FIGURE 30.1. Etiology of SCI rehabilitation admissions: nontraumatic vs. traumatic SCI. Multiple Sclerosis and Guillain Barré syndrome are not included.

plications, rehospitalization, discharge to nursing homes, and need for attendant assistance) in traumatic SCI patients with older age (19). Others have reported shorter hospital length of stay (LOS), lower hospital charges, decreased likelihood of divorce and separation, and decreased return to work for those of older age with new-onset SCI (20–23). Given the likelihood of nontraumatic SCI to affect older individuals, factors such as demographics, neurologic presentation, concomitant illness, and rehabilitation functional outcome become important issues for consideration. Individuals with nontraumatic SCI may present with associated medical complications, such as cardiopulmonary disease or diabetes, which could adversely affect medical and functional progress during rehabilitation and lead to decreased functional outcomes. Additionally, the use of medications, such as those used to control spasticity or pain after SCI, must be closely monitored to prevent sedative side effects, especially in

elderly patients who may have decreased tolerance. Memory and retention may be poor in older patients, which could result in diminished rehabilitation efficiency and long-term functional improvement.

PATHOPHYSIOLOGY

There are numerous potential etiologies of nontraumatic SCI. The more common pathophysiologies include SCI resulting from spinal stenosis, cancerous compression, vascular ischemia, and multiple sclerosis. Other etiologies include inflammatory diseases of both infectious (viral, bacterial, fungal, parasitic) and noninfectious (transverse myelitis and poliomyelitis) nature, motor neuron diseases, radiation myelopathy, syringomyelia, paraneoplastic syndrome, vitamin B_{12} deficiency, Friedreich ataxia, and compression secondary to rheumatoid arthritis.

Spinal stenosis is a common cause of pain and disability in individuals older than 50 years of age and a common diagnosis in patients older than 65 years of age undergoing lumbar surgery (15,24–26). The degenerative changes that cause progressive narrowing of the spinal canal and the vertebral foramina may give rise to spondylotic myelopathy, cauda equina syndrome (CES), or radiculopathy. Spinal cord compression secondary to stenosis can occur anteriorly (vertebral body osteophytes), posteriorly (ligamentum flavum), and laterally (intervertebral foramen), and the lower cervical (C4 to C7) and lumbar (L2 to L4) regions of the vertebral column are more commonly involved, partly owing to their propensity for increased mobility. Anteroposterior canal diameters of 17 to 18 mm are normal; however, diameters of less than 14 mm increase the risk for myelopathy or radiculopathy (27). The chronic nature of onset for spinal stenosis–induced myelopathy often gives rise to a stepwise period of clinical deterioration with periods of stability.

SCI as a result of *neoplastic SCC* involves several complex medical and quality-of-life issues stemming from both the neoplastic effects and the neurologic sequelae of the spinal cord involvement. These functional impairments contribute to ongo-

TABLE 30.1. DEMOGRAPHICS: NONTRAUMATIC AND TRAUMATIC SPINAL CORD INJURY

	Nontraumatic (n = 86)	Traumatic (n = 134)	Significance
Age (yr)	61.2	38.6	$p < 0.01$
Gender			
Male	50%	84%	$p < 0.01$
Female	50%	16%	
Ethnicity			
White	47%	35%	NS
Nonwhite	54%	65%	
Marital status			
Married	57%	38%	$p < 0.01$
Not married	23%	17%	
Never married	12%	45%	
Work Status			
Working/student	24%	67%	$p < 0.01$
Not working	76%	33%	

ing psychosocial problems surrounding disposition, care and assistance, financial resources, and patient quality of life. Neoplastic SCC is often classified according to its proximity to the spinal cord and its surrounding meninges. Extramedullary neoplastic SCC accounts for more than 90%, with the majority being epidural (primarily metastatic from the breast, lung, or prostate) and the remainder, intradural (most often neurofibromas and meningiomas) (28,29). Intramedullary neoplastic SCC accounts for less than 5% of spinal cord tumors and consists primarily of gliomas, with ependymomas and astrocytomas seen most commonly. Ependymomas represent a primarily benign tumor involving the ependymal cells, which line the central nervous system. Astrocytomas (the most common intramedullary spinal cord tumors in children) are often graded 1 through 4 (30). Grades 1 and 2 carry the best clinical prognosis for 5-year survival (greater than 80%) and are seen most commonly (25% of the time) (31). One-year survival rate for grades 3 and 4 astrocytomas are poor.

Vertebral metastasis is seen in 15% to 40% of individuals with cancer (4). The pathogenesis is usually hemodynamic spread to bone marrow through the Batson epidural venous plexus through the pelvic, abdominal, and thoracic veins (32). This type of spread is thought to be exacerbated by increased thoracic pressure, such as with Valsalva maneuver or coughing. The primary cancer sites for spinal metastases are usually breast, lung, and prostate in greater than half of patients, although nearly 10% have an unknown primary tumor site (18). In children, the common primary metastases include lymphoma, sarcoma, and neuroblastomas (33). Spinal cord metastasis causes epidural SCC in up to 5% of those with systemic cancer (34). The pathophysiology of SCI includes cord compression and ischemia with subsequent edema, demyelination, hemorrhage, and cystic necrosis. Clinical onset is usually days to weeks and is accompanied by pain (present in 95% and worse when supine) and paresis, which is a rare initial clinical finding but is present in up to 75% of patients at the time of diagnosis. The thoracic region is the most common site of metastatic epidural SCC (18).

Cancer-related etiologies for SCI include paraneoplastic syndrome and radiation myelopathy. *Paraneoplastic myelitis* represents the remote effects of systemic cancer that is not due to direct invasion or compression of the spinal cord. Pathologically, subacute necrosis of the gray or white matter is seen with no evidence of infection, inflammation, or ischemia and is often associated with bronchogenic cancer (35). *Radiation myelopathy* has an incidence of less than 3% and involves delayed necrosis of the spinal cord gray or white matter. Its onset is anytime from 6 to 48 months (most commonly, 12 to 15 months) after radiation therapy to the vertebral or surrounding region and occurs after a total radiation dose of 2,500 to 6,000 cGy (36). This has helped to demonstrate the importance of the timing and location of radiation treatments and has lead to recommendations for sites for radiation along with daily, weekly, and total radiation quantities.

Vascular-associated myelopathy includes a number of potential etiologies for SCI, including aortic dissection, postsurgical ischemia, vascular embolism, arteriovenous malformation, systemic ischemic hypotension, and hemorrhage. The incidence of vascular strokes involving the spinal cord is less than 1% of all central nervous system strokes (37). Of significance, regarding vascular injury to the spinal cord, are the blood supply and tissue vulnerability surrounding the spinal cord. Spinal arteries form an anastomotic chain along the length of the spinal cord, with potential vulnerability in various watershed regions, primarily in the thoracolumbar region, supplied by the great spinal artery of Adamkiewicz (38,39). The spinal cord is less vulnerable to ischemia than the brain and can withstand permanent damage with up to 30 minutes of interrupted blood supply (e.g., with aortic clamping) (40). The gray matter is more susceptible to injuries than the white matter, in part owing to its higher metabolic rate. The brain is more vulnerable than the spinal cord, in part because of its greater total blood flow need (41).

The most common cause of vascular SCI are those related to aortic aneurysms, involving either intraoperative ischemia, systemic hypotension, or spinal artery occlusion by the aortic dissection (42–45). They commonly involve the thoracic region because of common aneurysm sites and regions of vascular spinal cord anastomotic vulnerability. Embolic ischemia with atheromatous emboli to the spinal cord is rare (46). One embolic phenomenon involves that of caisson disease, or decompression sickness, seen with embolic occlusion of the venous plexus by nitrogen bubbles during decompression (47). Spinal hemorrhage is most often seen as a result of anticoagulation (25% to 35%), arteriovenous malformation, or coagulopathy (48–50). It is often found in the cervical spinal cord region and necessitates prompt evaluation for surgical clot evacuation. Prognosis after spinal cord decompression is greater if undertaken within 24 hours.

Rheumatoid arthritis can give rise to SCC secondary to atlantoaxial subluxation after loosening of the transverse ligament of the odontoid process, leading to displacement of the atlas. There are hosts of *motor system disorders* that may give rise to spinal cord injury. The most common motor neuron disease is that of amyotrophic lateral sclerosis involving degeneration of motor neurons in the spinal cord, brain stem, or both. Life expectancy in patients with ALS is usually 4 to 7 years, and important considerations are given to consequences of bulbar multiple involvement, such as impairment of respiration or swallowing. *Syringomyelia* is seen with posttraumatic and sometimes idiopathic longitudinal spinal canal cavitation, which is commonly located near the anterior commissure and can lead to alterations of pain and temperature sensation along with other sensory and motor abnormalities. Surgical management, if applicable, involves decompression and consideration of shunting of cerebrospinal fluid into the subarachnoid space or peritoneal cavity.

Inflammatory myelitis can give rise to SCI of infectious (viral, bacterial, fungal, and parasitic) or noninfectious etiology. Human immunodeficiency virus and *acquired immunodeficiency syndrome* (AIDS) can lead to spinal cord involvement in various ways, including compression by associated neoplasms (e.g., Kaposi sarcoma or lymphoma), direct infection by opportunistic organisms, or vacuolar degeneration of the white matter (seen in up to 30% of AIDS patients on autopsy) (51). *Herpes simplex virus* can gives rise to an acute viral infection involving the dorsal root ganglion or posterior cord. *Poliomyelitis* involving the spinal cord is now quite rare and involves enterovirus involvement of the anterior horn cells. Individuals diagnosed with polio may be at risk for postpolio syndrome (fatigue, weakness, and pain) decades later, which may represent late muscle denervation (52).

Bacterial spinal cord infections usually manifest as spinal epidural abscess, which, although rare, is seen more frequently with increased numbers in immunosuppressed patients. The pathophysiology involves the extension of adjacent vertebral osteomyelitis (most common) or hematogenous spread from distant infectious sites (perinephric, pharyngeal, and paraspinal) through the arterial supply or Batson plexus (53,54). *Staphylococcus aureus* represents the most common organism for bacterial spinal cord infection, and prognosis is good if treatment is begun before weakness is present or within 24 hours of diagnosis (55, 56). *Mycobacterium tuberculosis* represents the most common cause of chronic spinal cord abscess (57). Pathophysiology includes hematogenous seeding of the paravertebral epidural area, with vertebral body destruction and SCC or ischemia (53). Neurologic compromise of patients with vertebral tuberculosis is known as *Pott disease*.

Syphilis represents a rare spinal cord insult by the *Treponema* species parasite in the tertiary stages of syphilis. Pathophysiology is that of a chronic inflammatory process involving the dorsal root ganglion and posterior column (tabes dorsalis) or syphilitic meningitis (58). *Acute transverse myelitis* represents the occurrence of inflammatory legions of the spinal cord not due to viral invasion. Diagnosis often includes the exclusion of vascular, infectious, or multiple sclerosis as an etiology, which may be seen in the postviral or postvaccinal setting. SCI is due to perivascular demyelination and spinal cord necrosis or edema. The prognosis is worse when accompanied by legions seen on magnetic resonance imaging, severe weakness, and electrodiagnostic evidence of denervation (59,60).

Multiple sclerosis of the spinal cord involves multifocal spinal demyelative lesions. The usual presentation of chronic spinal multiple sclerosis is that of a slowly progressive, asymmetric spastic paraparesis with variable sensory ataxia (61). Associated lesions in the cerebrum, brain stem, and optic nerves often complicate diagnosis and clinical outcome. *Vitamin B₁₂ deficiencies* can lead to subacute combined degeneration of the spinal cord with posterior and lateral column changes. The pathophysiology involves the inability to transport vitamin B_{12} across the intestinal mucosa. *Friedreich ataxia* also leads to posterior column degeneration (61).

CLINICAL PRESENTATION

As with any type of SCI, nontraumatic SCI is associated with muscle weakness, sensory impairment, and bladder, bowel, and sexual dysfunction. The clinical presentation of individuals with nontraumatic SCI, however, reveals a pattern of less severe neurologic impairment than those with traumatic SCI. They are much more likely to present with paraplegia (as opposed to tetraplegia) and with motor incomplete (as opposed to complete) lesions (Table 30.2). This can most likely be related to both etiology and to the location of spinal involvement, along with the insidious onset of nontraumatic SCI. Neoplastic SCC tends to involve the thoracic and lumbar regions more than the cervical region and, thus, weakness to the lower extremities only (17,

TABLE 30.2. INJURY CHARACTERISTICS: NONTRAUMATIC AND TRAUMATIC SPINAL CORD INJURY

	Nontraumatic (n = 86)	Traumatic (n = 134)	Significance
Impairment			
Tetraplegia	27%	46%	$p < 0.05$
Paraplegia	73%	54%	
Level of injury			
Cervical	27%	46%	$p < 0.05$
Thoracic	38%	41%	
Lumbosacral	35%	13%	
Complete or incomplete			
Complete	42%	9%	$p < 0.05$
Incomplete	58%	91%	

62,63). Significantly more incomplete injuries are seen with neoplastic and spondylitic SCC. Epidural compression is the most common presentation for spinal cord tumors. Most patients present with the insidious onset of weakness or with bowel or bladder symptoms, and treatment with radiation or surgery and chemotherapy may improve their potential to maintain an incomplete neurologic status.

Medical complications in individuals with nontraumatic SCI can present as a consequence of the SCI or as commonly seen secondary complications. Both admission and follow-up issues represent areas for potential complications after SCI. Weakness, numbness, bladder incontinence, and pain are commonly seen presenting symptoms and follow-up complaints. Secondary medical complications related to SCI (such as urinary tract infections, spasticity, orthostatic hypotension, pressure sores, wound complications, and deep venous thrombosis) can affect hospital LOS, mortality, and rehospitalization. It is recommended that intensive interdisciplinary efforts be used in the medical management and rehabilitation of these patients. Preventative efforts and education should be directed toward those areas of greatest risk, including bladder management, recurrent urinary tract infections, spasticity, orthostasis, deep venous thrombosis, and prevention of pressure sores. A comparison of 116 patients with SCI (32% nontraumatic SCI) admitted to our SCI Model System revealed a significantly lower incidence in nontraumatic SCI (compared with traumatic SCI) for spasticity, orthostasis, deep venous thrombosis, autonomic dysreflexia, and pneumonia. Our suspicion is that many of these differences can be related to the prevalence of paraplegia (as opposed to tetraplegia) and lower motor unit (as opposed to upper motor unit) dysfunction seen in nontraumatic SCI.

FUNCTIONAL OUTCOME

Patients with SCI often experience changes in functional abilities in mobility (such as transfers and ambulation) and basic self-care tasks (such as dressing, bathing, grooming, and toileting). Previous studies in patients with SCI of traumatic etiology have

TABLE 30.3. LENGTH OF STAY AND FUNCTIONAL OUTCOME COMPARISONS: NONTRAUMATIC AND TRAUMATIC SPINAL CORD INJURY

	Tetraplegia—Incomplete			Paraplegia—Complete			Paraplegia—Incomplete		
	(N) Mean	SD	p	(N) Mean	SD	p	(N) Mean	SD	p
Acute care LOS (d)			0.364			0.775			0.429
Nontraumatic	(23) 13.70	10.78		(8) 14.75	9.71		(55) 11.82	8.45	
Traumatic	(46) 18.59	24.45		(41) 16.32	14.76		(32) 13.59	12.35	
Rehabilitation LOS			0.022			0.227			0.881
Nontraumatic	(23) 31.00	17.98		(8) 30.63	14.38		(55) 26.44	10.68	
Traumatic	(46) 46.17	28.11		(41) 40.61	22.05		(32) 26.06	12.09	
FIM motor, admission			0.008			0.397			0.675
Nontraumatic	(23) 35.74	15.92		(8) 29.25	6.34		(55) 42.20	11.59	
Traumatic	(46) 25.20	14.55		(41) 32.10	8.96		(32) 43.38	14.07	
FIM motor, discharge			0.436			0.003			0.008
Nontraumatic	(23) 59.22	20.87		(8) 44.13	19.20		(55) 61.24	14.84	
Traumatic	(46) 54.33	26.00		(41) 0.02	11.49		(32) 69.25	10.08	
FIM motor, efficiency			0.671			0.015			0.015
Nontraumatic	(23) 0.89	0.57		(8) 0.42	0.39		(55) 0.79	0.52	
Traumatic	(46) 0.97	0.85		(41) 0.86	0.46		(32) 1.07	0.50	

LOS, Length of stay; FIM, functional independence measure; d, days.

shown rehabilitative functional outcomes to be associated with level of injury, completeness of injury, and age (19,20,64). However, there have been only a limited number of studies addressing functional benefits after nontraumatic SCI (7–10,14,65,66). Given the significant demographic and clinical variations between the two groups, outcome comparison is somewhat difficult.

Studies of individuals with nontraumatic SCI have revealed significant Functional Independence Measure (FIM) changes during rehabilitation and similar FIM efficiencies (FIM change/day) when compared with those with traumatic SCI (7,9,10,66) (Table 30.3). Although there was greater FIM change in the traumatic SCI patient subgroups, a longer rehabilitation LOS may have allowed trauma patients more time for neurologic and functional gains. This is supported by the fact that the FIM efficiencies were comparable between two groups, indicating similar rates of functional gains. The intensity of therapy has been shown to affect outcome, and the LOS may affect outcome as a result by allowing more exposure to the various therapies (67).

Outcome after spinal stenosis management has been the subject of numerous studies. Despite the widespread surgical treatment of spinal stenosis, uncertainties remain concerning diagnostic criteria, indications for surgery, optimal surgical procedures, and patient characteristics associated with favorable surgical outcome. Indications for surgical and conservative management of spinal stenosis have not been well defined, in part as a result of poorly delineated outcome criteria, a lack of randomized studies, and an uncertainty regarding the natural progression of spinal stenosis. Conservative approaches to symptomatic spondylosis, including rest, traction, physical therapy, and medication, have been used with some success; however, much of the information concerning outcomes has centered on post-

surgical patients (68,69). Surgery is indicated if signs of progressive neurologic deterioration develop or progress despite conservative management, and is intended to relieve the compression of the cauda equina seen on magnetic resonance imaging or computed tomographic scans. Interestingly, studies of decompressive laminectomy for degenerative lumbar stenosis have found the outcome to be less favorable than had been previously reported (26,70–77).

Postoperative parameters found to be significantly correlated with surgical outcome after myelopathy due to spinal stenosis include clinical examination, radiographic findings, walking capacity, decreases in postoperative pain, and satisfaction with the results of surgery; however, these may not accurately define a patient's functional status. Studies have indicated a considerable variation of reported success rates, from 26% to 100%, although some long-term studies indicate progressive deterioration and a reoperation rate of 18% within 5 years (26,70–77). Favorable prognostic factors have been shown to include a preoperative duration of symptoms of less than 4 years, no preoperative back pain, a pronounced constriction of the spinal canal, no concomitant disease affecting walking ability, no prior surgical intervention, no comorbidity of diabetes, no hip joint arthrosis, and no preoperative fracture of the lumbar spine. Postoperative radiographic stenosis was common in patients operated on for lumbar spinal stenosis, and this did not correlate with clinical outcome. Capacity to return to work, a commonly used indicator of outcome after spinal surgery for other diagnoses, was not found to be overly useful in lumbar spinal stenosis because most patients with this condition are retired. No significant relationships were found between surgical outcome and patient age, gender, presence of pseudo-claudication, history of prior back surgery, duration of symptoms, or the number of levels decompressed. Significant mobility, self-care, and sphincter control functional improvements have been noted in individuals with myelopathy or CES resulting from spinal stenosis (7). Despite a significantly older group, patients with spondylotic myelopathy or CES had similar discharge FIM and discharge to community rates as those with traumatic SCI.

Treatment of individuals with neoplastic SCC has been somewhat controversial, and the relative merits of interventions, such as surgery, radiation therapy, chemotherapy, and steroids, have been studied (78–81). A review of the literature has identified the following determinants of prognosis and treatment choice in patients with SCI secondary to neoplasm: early recognition of SCC, tumor biology and cell type, neurologic status at the time of surgical intervention, completeness of the spinal cord insult, progression of neurologic symptoms, general medical status of the patient, bowel control at admission, and ambulatory ability (65,82–85). The potential for ambulation is 80% in patients who are ambulating at the initiation of radiation therapy but 50% or less if they are unable or paraplegic at that time. The more radiosensitive tumors, such as breast, prostate, and lymphoma, may have better outcomes.

There are many important considerations for rehabilitation of individuals with neoplastic SCC. Rehabilitation management of these patients combines factors involved with both SCI and cancer rehabilitation principles along with an emphasis on pain management.

Again, there is a paucity of literature reviewing the rehabilitation outcome of neoplastic SCI with respect to functional changes in mobility, bowel and bladder function, and self-care skills (8,10,14,65,66). This lack of data may, somewhat, reflect a hesitancy to rehabilitate patients whose life expectancy may be shortened. Patients with metastatic SCC have a reported life expectancy of between 2 and 16 months after treatment; therefore, inpatient rehabilitation goals may vary compared with that in patients with traumatic SCI (17,62,86–88). Although the 1-year mortality in patients with neoplastic invasion of the spinal cord has been estimated to be more than 80%, select patients may survive for extended periods, sometimes as long as 4 to 9 years (78,81,89).

Previous studies have noted the importance of inpatient rehabilitation in the general SCI population and in patients with cancer (8,10,66,90–94). Studies assessing metastatic disease of the spinal cord demonstrated functional improvement in the ability (or inability) to ambulate, rectal sphincter control and bladder function, back pain, and motor strength (18,78–81). Marciniak and colleagues compared admission to discharge functional abilities and demonstrated significant functional gains in the four major diagnostic categories studied, including SCI (92). Yoshioka and colleagues found rehabilitation to be an effective component of care in the terminal cancer patient (94). They implemented a basic rehabilitation program for patients with terminal cancer and surveyed the patients' caregivers about the utility of the rehabilitation program. Of the respondents, 78% were satisfied with rehabilitation in the terminal stage, and 63% found the rehabilitation program to be effective.

Functional improvements have been reported, by McKinley and colleagues, during the rehabilitation stay for patients with neoplastic SCC, not only in wheelchair mobility and ambulation, but also in self-care and transfer abilities (8). Patients demonstrated significant functional FIM gains during rehabilitation, and 84% returned home after rehabilitation. Follow-up surveys indicated that most patients, 3 months after discharge, maintained or improved on their discharge level of function for both mobility (either ambulation or wheelchair) and dressing. These results may help validate the importance of a concentrated inpatient rehabilitation program.

Disabling pain has been noted to occur in 64% to 90% of patients with neoplastic SCC, and successful management of pain is important in the overall treatment of these patients (9, 16,62). Most studies of neoplastic SCC have focused on the outcomes of decreased pain and ambulation after treatment with steroids, radiation, and surgery (16–18,62,63,82,86–88). Studies revealed that pain improved in 78% to 91%, whereas 18% to 100% of patients studied remained nonambulatory after treatment (17,63,72,82,87,88). Overall, less than half of patients regain lost functional capacity (95). The most significant factor for functional prognosis and survival appears to be pretreatment motor function, emphasizing the importance of early diagnosis and treatment (5,8,10,11). Socially acceptable bowel and bladder maintenance is an essential issue surrounding care for those with SCI because successful bladder management can lead to decreased morbidity (skin breakdown or further urologic or renal compromise) and increased quality of life. Careful bladder assessment and treatment of the patients in this study lead to improved patient continence with self-voiding, intermittent catheterization or indwelling catheter, as necessary.

LOS and functional outcome are important considerations when comparing the possible benefits of inpatient rehabilitation. The inpatient rehabilitation unit offers an interdisciplinary team approach for treatment, rehabilitation, and education for patients, family, and caregivers. Family members are encouraged to become directly involved in the rehabilitation process. The goals of the educational efforts include prevention of further morbidity with a thorough understanding of the medical disease process, bladder and skin care, proper techniques for physical assistance to the patients, and general emotional support. McKinley and colleagues reported length-of-stay differences between nontraumatic SCI and traumatic SCI comparison groups (7–10,66). Individuals with tetraplegic incomplete nontraumatic SCI had shorter LOS than their traumatic SCI counterparts. This may reflect an earlier FIM plateau resulting from higher admission motor FIM scores seen in the nontraumatic SCI group. One might expect to find increased LOS in the traumatic SCI group secondary to initial spinal instability and associated injuries. Patients with spondylotic myelopathy or CES secondary to spinal stenosis do not usually present with spinal instability requiring surgical or orthotic intervention or short-term immobilization. Additionally, associated injuries commonly seen in traumatic SCI (concomitant brain injury, thoracopulmonary trauma, abdominal visceral injury, and nonspinal fractures) are not typically present in this population.

Patients with neoplastic SCC have been noted to have a shorter rehabilitation LOS compared with patients with traumatic SCI. Factors that may have influenced the shorter rehabilitation LOS include differing patterns of neurologic recovery and bias toward early discharge in patients with potentially terminal cancer. Neoplasms of the spinal cord are primarily epidural in origin, causing compression resulting from a space-occupying lesion rather than actual spinal cord invasion. There is some potential for resolution of symptoms if the tumor is treated with surgical excision or radiation therapy or if concomitant edema responds to treatment with steroids. Conversely, traumatic SCI patients present with primary SCI secondary to contusion, hemorrhage, or other forms of secondary SCI injury that may require longer LOS for neurologic and functional improvement.

Another factor in the shorter-rehabilitation LOS in tumor patients may be the rehabilitation team's and patient's family's desire for earlier discharge given the patient's potential limited life expectancy. This is especially pertinent given that spinal cord tumors often present secondary to metastasis and may represent terminal illness. The shorter LOS allows patients to have more time at home with family and friends, enhancing quality of life. Cancer rehabilitation, in general, focuses on brief inpatient stays because of limited life expectancy. On the other hand, traumatic SCI patients are expected to have longer life expectancies than patients with tumors, and the rehabilitation team's goals are to maximize long-term functional gains achieved in an intensive setting.

No statistical significance was found in acute care LOS. The comparable acute care LOS in the tumor and traumatic SCI groups was an interesting finding given their differing etiologies. The traumatic SCI patients may have had acute medical issues arising from the trauma itself, including spinal and hemodynamic stabilization, assessment for concomitant abdominal injuries, multiple fractures, electrolyte imbalances, and concomitant head injury that may affect LOS. Similarly, tumor SCC patients may have undergone an oncology workup for the tumor, assessment of spine stabilization, and adjuvant therapy, including radiation and chemotherapy. Additional issues affecting their acute care LOS include monitoring for paraneoplastic complications such as hypercalcemia and immunosuppression.

CONCLUSIONS

Patients with nontraumatic SCI appear to represent a significant proportion of individuals with SCI admitted to rehabilitation settings, and it is important to evaluate their demographics, neurologic and clinical presentation, and functional outcomes. These individuals tend to be older and have a greater incidence of incomplete and paraplegic injuries than their traumatic SCI counterparts. During patient rehabilitation, they have been shown to achieve comparable rates of functional gains, have a shorter rehabilitation LOS, and achieve similar discharge to community rates. The information revealed in this chapter will assist with making decisions regarding inpatient rehabilitation for this patient population and should encourage future investigations in this area.

This chapter adds to the growing body of literature reviewing the incidence, demographics, clinical presentation, and functional outcome of individuals with nontraumatic SCI. Many of the studies reported here have limitations, which suggest areas for future research. Individuals younger than 18 years of age are not admitted to many adult inpatient rehabilitation units. Therefore, the incidence of congenital or pediatric tumor-related

SCI may not been adequately assessed. Multicenter database studies and national databases including both urban and rural hospital settings could lend themselves to a greater number of study patients and would have assisted in the analysis of individuals within the different nontraumatic SCI and traumatic SCI subgroups (i.e., tetraplegic complete and incomplete and paraplegic complete and incomplete injuries). A comparison of associated medical complications between nontraumatic and traumatic SCI would have been beneficial when assessing LOS and functional outcomes. Cost of care remains an important issue and may be underappreciated for nontraumatic SCI when estimating overall costs. Additionally, studies are necessary to address more fully functional outcome and quality-of-life issues, to access prognostic factors predictive of functional improvement during rehabilitation, to compare potential benefits of alternative therapeutic delivery systems such as outpatient and home health rehabilitation, and to address the maintenance of functional improvements.

REFERENCES

1. Adams RD, Salam-Adams M. Chronic nontraumatic diseases of the spinal cord. *Neurol Clin* 1991;9:605–623.
2. Dawson DM, Potts F. Acute nontraumatic myelopathies. *Neurol Clin* 1991;9:585–602.
3. Schmidt RD, Markovchick V. Nontraumatic spinal cord compression. *J Emerg Med* 1992;10:189–199.
4. Byrne TN, Waxman SG. *Spinal cord compression: diagnosis and principles of treatment. Contemporary neurology series.* Philadelphia, FA Davis, 1990.
5. Stover SL, DeLisa JA, Whiteneck GG. *Spinal cord injury: clinical outcomes from the Model Systems.* Gaithersburg, MD: Aspen, 1995.
6. Kurtzke JF. Epidemiology of spinal cord injury. *Exp Neurol* 1975;48:163–236.
7. McKinley W, Tellis A, Cifu D, et al. Rehabilitation outcome of individuals with nontraumatic myelopathy resulting from spinal stenosis. *J Spinal Cord Med* 1998;21:131–136.
8. McKinley WO, Conti-Wyneken A, Vokac C, et al. Rehabilitative functional outcome of patients with neoplastic spinal cord compression. *Arch Phys Med Rehabil* 1996;77:892–895.
9. McKinley WO, Hardman J, Seel R. Nontraumatic spinal cord injury: incidence, epidemiology and functional outcome. *Arch Phys Med Rehabil* 1998;79:1186–1187.
10. McKinley WO, Tewksbury MA. Neoplastic vs. traumatic spinal cord injury: an inpatient rehabilitation comparison. *Am J Phys Med Rehabil* 2000;79:138–144.
11. Gibson CJ. *Final report of the Rochester Regional Model Spinal Cord Injury System, 9-30-85 to 7-29-90.* Rochester, NY: Rochester Regional Model Spinal Cord Injury System, 1991.
12. Guttman L. *Spinal cord injuries: comprehensive management and research.* Oxford, UK: Blackwell, 1973.
13. Buchan AC, Fulford GE, Jellinek E, et al. A preliminary survey of the incidence and etiology of spinal paralysis. *Parplegia* 1972;10:23–28.
14. Murray P. Functional outcome and survival in spinal cord injury secondary to neoplasia. *Cancer* 1985;55:197–201.
15. Nurick S. The pathogenesis of the spinal cord disorder associated with cervical spondylosis. *Brain* 1972;95:87–100.
16. Sundaresan N, Galicich J, Bains M, et al. Vertebral body resection in the treatment of cancer involving the spine. *Cancer* 1984;53:1393–1396.
17. Helweg-Larsen S. Clinical outcome in metastatic spinal cord compression: a prospective study of 153 patients. *Acta Neurol Scand* 1996;94:269–275.
18. Gilbert RW, Kim JH, Posner JB. Epidural spinal cord compression

from metastatic tumor: diagnosis and treatment. *Ann Neurol* 1978;3:
40–51.

19. DeVivo MJ, Kartus PL, Rutt RD, et al. The influence of age at time
of spinal cord injury on rehabilitation outcome. *Arch Neurol* 1990;47:
687–691.

20. Yarkony GM, Roth EJ, Heinemann AW, et al. Spinal cord injury
rehabilitation outcome: the impact of age. *J Clin Epidemiol* 1988;41:
173–177.

21. Charles ED, Fine PR, Stover SL, et al. The costs of spinal cord injury.
Paraplegia 1978;15:302–310.

22. Meyer AR, Feltin M, Master RJ. Re-hospitalization and spinal cord
injury: a cross-sectional survey of adults living independently. *Arch Phys
Med Rehabil* 1985;66:704–708.

23. Devivo MJ, Fine PR. Spinal cord injury: its short-term impact on
martial status. *Arch Phys Med Rehabil* 1985;66:501–504.

24. Lees F, Turner J. Natural history and prognosis of cervical spondylosis.
Br Med J 1963;2:1607–1610.

25. Katz J, Dalgas M, Stucki G, et al. Diagnosis of lumbar stenosis. *Rheum
Dis Clin North Am* 1994;20:471–483.

26. Turner JA, Ersek M, Herron L, et al. Surgery for lumbar spinal stenosis:
attempted meta-analysis of the literature. *Spine* 1992;17:1–8.

27. Payne EE, Spillane JD. The cervical spine: an anatomicopathological
study of 70 specimens (using a special technique) with particular reference to the problems of cervical spondylosis. *Brain* 1957;80:571–596.

28. Alter M. Statistical aspects of spinal tumors. In: Vinken PJ, Bruyn GS,
eds. *Handbook of clinical neurology*, Vol 19. Amsterdam: North Holland
Publishing, 1975:1–22.

29. Levy WJ, Bay J, Dohn D. Spinal cord meningioma. *J Neurosurg* 1982;
57:804–812.

30. Epstein F, Epstein N. Intramedullary tumors of the spinal cord. In
Shillito J, Matsoin DD, eds: *Pediatric neurosurgery: surgery of the developing nervous system*. New York: Grune & Stratton, 1982:529–539.

31. Reimer R, Onofrio BM. Astrocytomas of the spinal cord in children
and adolescents. *J Neurosurg* 1985;63:669–675.

32. Batson OV. The function of the vertebral veins and their role in the
spread of metastases. 1940. *Clin Orthop* 1995;(312)4–9.

33. Lewis DW, Packer RJ, Raney B, et al. Incidence, presentation, and
outcome of spinal cord disease in children with systemic cancer. *Pediatrics* 1986;78:438–442.

34. Barron KD, Hirano A, Araki S, et al. Experiences with metastatic neoplasms involving the spinal cord. *Neurology* 1959;9:91–106.

35. Henson RA, Urich H. *Cancer and the nervous system*. Oxford, UK:
Blackwell, 1982.

36. Burns BJ, Jones AN, Robertson JS. Pathology of radiation myelopathy.
J Neurol Neurosurg Psychiatry 1972;35:888.

37. Sandson TA, Friedman JH. Spinal cord infarction: report of 8 cases
and review of the literature. *Medicine* 1989;68:228–298.

38. Jellinger K. Circulation disorders of the spinal cord. *Acta Neurochir
(Wien)* 1972;26:327.

39. Lazorthes G. Blood supply and vascular pathology of the spinal cord.
In: Pia HW, Djindijan R, eds. *Spinal angiomas*. Berlin: Springer-Verlag,
1978:10.

40. Otomo E, VanBuskirk C, Workman JB. Circulation of the spinal cord
studied by autoradiography. *Neurology* 1960;10:112.

41. Nystrom B, Stjernschantz J, Smedegard G. Regional spinal cord blood
flow in the rabbit, cat, and monkey. *Acta Neurol Scand* 1984;19:63.

42. Adams HD, VanGeertruyden HH. Neurologic complications of aortic
surgery. *Ann Surg* 1956;144:574.

43. Blumbergs PC, Byrne E. Hypotensive central infarction of the spinal
cord. *J Neurol* 1980;43:751.

44. Foo D, Rosier AB. Anterior spinal artery syndrome and its natural
history. *Paraplegia* 1983;21:1.

45. Slater EE, DeSantis RW. The clinical recognition of dissecting aortic
aneurysm. *Am J Med* 1976;600:625.

46. Slavin RE, Gonzalez-Vitale JC, Marin OSM. Atheromatous emboli to
the lumbosacral spinal cord. *Stroke* 1975;6:411.

47. Hellenback JM, Bove AA, Elliott DH. Mechanisms underlying spinal
cord damage in decompression sickness. *Neurology* 1975;25:308–316.

48. Mattle H, Sieb JP, Rohner M, et al. Nontraumatic spinal epidural and
subdural hematomas. *Neurology* 1987;37:1351–1358.

49. Beatty RM, Winston KR. Spontaneous cervical epidural hematomas:
a consideration of etiology. *J Neurosurg* 1984;61:143–148.

50. Foo D, Chang YC, Rossier AB. Spontaneous cervical epidural hemorrhage, anterior cord syndrome and familial vascular malformations:
case report. *Neurology* 1980;30:308–311.

51. Petito CK, Navio BA, Cho ES, et al. Vacuolar myelopathy pathologically resembling subacute combined degeneration in patients with acquired immunodeficiency syndrome. *N Engl J Med* 1985;312:
874–879.

52. Dalakas MC, Hallett M. The post-polio syndrome. In: Plum F, ed.
Advances in contemporary neurology. Philadelphia: FA Davis, 1988:
51–94.

53. Baker AS, Ojemann RJ, Swartz NM, et al. Spinal epidural abscess. *N
Engl J Med* 1975;293:463–468.

54. Danner RL, Hartman BJ. Update of spinal epidural abscess: 35 cases
and review of the literature. *Rev Infect Dis* 1987;9:265–274.

55. Kaufman DM, Kaplan JG, Litman N. Infectious agents in spinal epidural abscesses. *Neurology* 1980;30:844–850.

56. Verner EF, Musher DM. Spinal epidural abscesses. *Med Clin North
Am* 1985;69(2):375–384.

57. Mann JS, Cole RB. Tuberculous spondylitis in the elderly: a potential
diagnostic pitfall. *Br Med J* 1987;294:1149–1150.

58. Merritt HH, Adams RD, Solomon HC. Neurosyphilis. New York:
Oxford University Press, 1946.

59. Misra UK, Kalita J, Kumar S. A clinical MRI and neurophysiological
study of acute transverse myelitis. *J Neurol Sci* 1996;138:150–156.

60. Kalita J, Misra UK, Mandal SK. Prognostic predictors of acute transverse myelitis. *Acta Neurol Scand* 1998;98:60–63.

61. Adams RD, Victor M. *Principles of neurology*, 4th ed. New York:
McGraw-Hill, 1989.

62. Kim R, Spencer S, Meredith R, et al. Extradural spinal cord compression: analysis of factors determining functional prognosis. Prospective
study. *Radiology* 1990;176:279–282.

63. Sundaresan N, Galicich J, Lane J, et al. Treatment of neoplastic epidural cord compression by vertebral body resection and stabilization.
J Neurosurg 1985;63:676–684.

64. Ditunno JF Jr, Cohen ME, Formal C, et al. Functional outcomes. In:
Stover SL, DeLisa JA, Whiteneck GG, eds. *Spinal cord injury: clinical
outcomes from the Model Systems*. Gaithersburg, MD: Aspen, 1995:
1170–1184.

65. Hacking HGA, Van As HHJ, Lankhorst GJ. Factors related to the
outcome of inpatient rehabilitation in patients with neoplastic epidural
spinal cord compression. *Paraplegia* 1993;31:367–374.

66. McKinley WO, Huang ME, Brunsvold KT. Neoplastic vs traumatic
spinal cord injury: an outcome comparison after inpatient rehabilitation. *Arch Phys Med Rehabil* 1999;80(10):1253–1257.

67. Spivak G, Spettell CM, Ellis DW, et al. Effects of intensity of treatment
and length of stay on rehabilitation outcomes. *Brain Inj* 1992;6:
419–434.

68. Onel D, Sari H, Donmez C. Lumbar spinal stenosis: clinical/radiologic
therapeutic evaluation in 145 patients. Conservative treatment or surgical intervention? *Spine* 1993;18:291–298.

69. Porter RW, Hibbert C, Evans C. The natural history of root entrapment syndrome. *Spine* 1984;9:418–421.

70. Verbiest H. Results of surgical treatment of idiopathic developmental
stenosis of the lumbar vertebral canal: a review of twenty-seven years
experience. *J Bone Joint Surg* 1977;59:181–188.

71. Epstein JA, Janin Y, Carras R, et al. A comparative study of the treatment of cervical spondylotic myeloradiculopathy: experience with 50
cases treated by means of extensive laminectamy, foraminotomy, and
excision of osteophytes during the past 10 years. *Acta Neurochir* 1982;
61:89–104.

72. Hall S, Bartleson JD, Ontorio BM, et al. Lumbar spinal stenosis: clinical features, diagnostic procedures, and results of surgical treatment in
68 patients. *Ann Intern Med* 1985;103:271–275.

73. Caputy A, Lussenhop AJ. Long-term evaluation of decompressive surgery for degenerative lumbar stenosis. *J Neurosurg* 1992;77:669–676.

74. Herno A, Airaksinen O, Saari T. Long-term results of surgical treatment of lumbar spinal stenosis. *Spine* 1993;18:1471–1474.

75. Herron LD, Mangelsdorf C. Lumbar spinal stenosis: results of surgical treatment. *J Spinal Disord* 1991;4:26–33.

76. Weir B, de Leo R. Lumbar stenosis: analysis of factors affecting outcome in 81 surgical cases. *Can J Neurol Sci* 1981;8:295–298.

77. Paine KW. Results of decompression for lumbar spinal stenosis. *Clin Orthop Relat Res* 1976;115:96–100.

78. Dunn RC, Kelly WA, Wohns RNW, et al. Spinal epidural neoplasia: a 15-year review of the results of surgical therapy. *J Neurosurg* 1980;52:47-51.

79. Livingston KE, Perrin RG. The Neurosurgical Management of Spinal Metastases Causing Cord and Cauda Equina Compression. *J Neurosurg* 1978;49:839–843.

80. Siegal T, Siegal T. Current considerations in the management of neoplastic spinal cord compression. *Spine* 1989;14:2:223–228.

81. Young RF, Post EM, King GA. Treatment of spinal epidural metastases: randomized prospective comparison of laminectomy and radiotherapy. *J Neurosurg* 1980;53:741–748.

82. Greenburg HS, Kim J, Posner J. Epidural spinal cord compression from metastatic tumor: results with a new treatment protocol. *Ann Neurol* 1980;8:361–366.

83. Barcena A, Lobato R, Coirdobes F, et al. Spinal metastatic disease: analysis of factors determining functional prognosis and the choice of treatment. *Neurosurgery* 1984;15:6:820–827.

84. Brice J, McKissock W. Surgical treatment of malignant extradural spinal tumors. *Br Med J* 1965;2:1341–1344.

85. Fundlay GFG. Adverse effects of the management of malignant spinal cord compression. *J Neurol Neurosurg Psychiatry* 1984;47:761–768.

86. Leviov M, Dale J, Stein M, et al. The management of metastatic spinal cord compression: a radiotherapeutic success ceiling. *Int J Radiat Oncol Biol Phys* 1993;27:231–234.

87. Maranzano E, Latini P. Effectiveness of radiation therapy without surgery in metastatic spinal cord compression: final results from a prospective trial. *Int J Radiat Oncol Biol Phys* 1995;32:959–967.

88. Sundaresan N, Sachdev VP, Holland J, et al. Surgical treatment of spinal cord compression from epidural metastasis. *J Clin Oncol* 1995;9:2330–2335.

89. Bach F, Larsen B, Rohde K, et al. Metastatic spinal cord compression: occurrence, symptoms, clinical presentations and prognosis in 398 patients with spinal cord compression. *Acta Neurochir* 1990;107:37–43.

90. DeLisa JA. Rehabilitation of the patient with cancer or human immunodeficiency virus. In: DeLisa JA, ed. *Rehabilitation medicine: principles and practice.* Philadelphia: JB Lippincott, 1993:916–933.

91. DeVivo M, Rutt R, Black K. Trends in spinal cord demographics and treatment outcomes between 1973 and 1986. *Arch Phys Med Rehabil* 1996;77:45–47.

92. Marciniak C, Sliwa J, Spill G, et al. Functional outcome following rehabilitation of the cancer patient. *Arch Phys Med Rehabil* 1996;77:54–57.

93. LaBan MM. Rehabilitation of patients with cancer. In: Kottke FJ, Lehman JF, eds. *Krusen's handbook of physical medicine and rehabilitation*, 4th ed. Philadelphia: WB Saunders, 1990:1102–1112.

94. Yoshioka H. Rehabilitation for the terminal cancer patient. *Am Phys Med Rehabil* 1994;73:199–206.

95. Byrne TN. Spinal cord compression from epidural metastases. *N Engl J Med* 1992;327:614–619.

31

TUMORS OF THE SPINE AND SPINAL CORD

ROBERT F. HEARY
ROSEMARIE FILART

In this chapter, tumors are divided into those that primarily involve the spine bony substance, i.e. spine tumors, and those that primarily involve the structures within the spinal canal, i.e. tumors of the spinal cord. Primary tumors are the most common spinal cord tumor; while secondary tumors (tumors that originate from a different location and metastasize) are the most common spine tumor.

Secondary tumors are 25 times more common than primary tumors. Overall, for 30–70% of patients with disseminated metastatic disease, spinal involvement is identified. Reportedly, 10–40% of patients that were later diagnosed with occult tumors had symptoms suggestive of spine involvement as their initial presentation (1–5).

Back pain is the most common presenting symptom of spine and spinal cord tumors causing spinal cord compression (SCC) (1,4,6,7). SCC is the second most common neurologic complication in cancer after brain metastases. The most common cause of SCC is from impingement of the spinal cord by an expanding secondary spine tumor (1,4–8).

Spine tumors are dramatically different from spinal cord tumors in presentation, treatment, and prognosis. Overall treatment success for all tumors of the spine and spinal cord depends upon the tumor biology, presenting neurologic impairment, and the medical condition of the patient. Treatment requires thoughtful discussion between the patient and their medical, surgical, and cancer rehabilitation team. When all risks, benefits, and alternatives to treatment have been explained, the optimal treatment plan can be determined. This chapter provides an overview of the classification, evaluation, and treatment of patients with spine and spinal cord tumors, with an emphasis on the surgical and cancer rehabilitation management.

CLASSIFICATION

There are numerous classification schemes for spine and spinal cord tumors. The anatomic location of tumor destruction and site of origin are two clinically relevant classifications. Moreover, because of a different general clinical presentation and natural history, the anatomically based classification further delineates spine from spinal cord tumors. Specifically, spine tumors refer to tumors that are extradural and exert their deleterious effects by compression of the spinal cord and/or spinal nerve roots. Spinal cord tumors refer to tumors that are either (1) intradural extramedullary that exert their deleterious effects by compression of the spinal cord parenchyma and/or spinal nerve roots; or (2) intramedullary that exert their deleterious effects by compression or direct invasion of the spinal cord parenchyma (9,10) (Figure 1).

In a cross sectional view, this classification scheme defines tumors in relation to the dural sheath, where outside the dura is referred to the extradural space and inside the dura is known as the intradural space. The extradural section lies outside of both the dural sheath and spinal cord and includes the vertebral bodies and epidural tissues. Within the confines of the dura, or the intradural space, there is the intramedullary space that comprises solely of the spinal cord parenchyma, and the extramedullary space, which is the substance outside of the spinal cord and includes the nerve roots and leptomeninges (9,10).

Overall, 55% of tumors are found in the extradural space, i.e. spine tumors, and the remaining percentage are comprised of spinal cord tumors; 40% in the intradural extramedullary space and 5% in the intramedullary space. Primary tumors are the most common tumor in the intradural space; whereas, secondary tumors are the most common tumors of the extradural space (9,10,11).

Spine Extradural Tumors

Spine tumors exert their deleterious neurologic effects by compression of the spinal nerve roots and/or spinal cord. In the extradural space, tumor involvement occurs primarily within the bony substance with fewer occurring from the soft tissues. The vertebral body (VB) is most commonly affected, although the posterior elements including the pedicles and laminae may also be involved. Metastatic secondary lesions are the most common spine tumor and affect predominantly the vertebral body. Primary tumors and extensions of intradural tumors occur less frequently (1,6,7,12,13).

Primary spine tumors are most commonly malignant in the adult population. The most common malignant primary spine tumor is multiple myeloma. This tumor most commonly arises

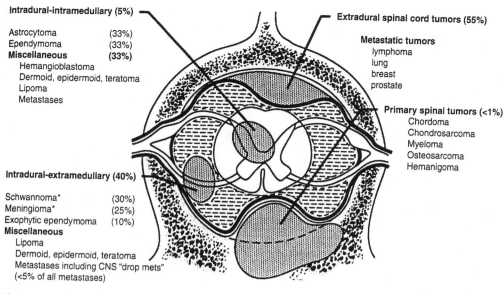

FIGURE 31.1. Intraspinal location and relative incidence of spinal tumors. Primary and metastatic tumors of the spine and spinal cord. Adapted from Tumors of the Central Nervous System. In: *American Cancer Society of Clinical Oncology*; 2nd edition. Atlanta: ACS, 1995:400–410.

from the vertebral bodies, and later, invades the surrounding epidural tissues. Osteogenic sarcoma may also develop from a malignant conversion of other tumors or from radiation treatment (14). The most common benign primary spine tumor is the vertebral hemangioma (1–12% of spine tumors), which commonly arises in the thoracic and lumbar levels (15).

The most common primary sources of secondary tumors in the spine are metastatic lung, breast, and prostate carcinomas (1,5,7). These metastatic carcinomas carry epidemiologic implications; as prostate (29%) and lung/bronchus (14%) carcinoma lead the list of the estimated annual new cancer cases for men, while breast (30%) and lung/bronchus (12%) lead the list for women (16). Despite the large volume of published studies regarding the type of metastatic carcinoma causing SCC, there is great variability in epidemiologic profiles with enormous differences in the composition of patients studied. Various studies published have reported on the primary sources of secondary spine tumors that presented with spinal cord compression (Table

31.1) (5,17–21). In addition to lung, breast, and prostate; other sources of secondary spine tumors include kidney, lymphoma, malignant melanoma, thyroid, soft tissue sarcoma, gastrointestinal tract (GI), or from an unknown primary source (17–21). Osteogenic sarcoma can be classified as a secondary spine tumor when spine involvement results from metastases from other involved bones; although, it is also classified a primary malignant spine tumor when the first involved site is the spine (14).

Spinal Cord Intradural Extramedullary and Intramedullary Tumors

Spinal cord tumors originate from the intradural extramedullary space, or intramedullary space, and exert their deleterious neurologic effects by compression of the spinal cord and/or spinal nerve roots. Intradural extramedullary spinal cord tumors arise within the confines of the dura, but outside the spinal cord parenchyma. They impinge the spinal nerve root or displace the

TABLE 31.1. EPIDEMIOLOGIC PROFILES OF CARCINOMAS CAUSING METASTATIC EPIDURAL SPINAL CORD COMPRESSION IN VARIOUS STUDIES [NUMBER(PERCENTAGES)]

	Lung	Breast	Prostate	Kidney	GI	Myeloma	Unknown	Other	N
Gilbert, et al (18)	30(13)	48(20)	21(9)	17(7)	9(4)	9(4)	4(2)	97(41)	235
Greenberg, et al (19)	11(13)	21(25)	12(14)	3(4)	6(7)	1(1)	3(4)	26(31)	83
Rodichok, et al (20)	31(33)	21(23)	4(4)	2(2)	6(6)	3(3)	3(3)	23(25)	93
Hacking, et al (21)	8(11)	14(19)	15(20)	7(9)	N/L^	11(15)	5(7)	14(19)	74
Sioutos, et al (17)	45(41)	19(17)	21(19)	15(13)	9(10)	N/L^	N/L^	N/L^	109
Total	125(21)	123(21)	73(12)	44(7)	30(5)	24(4)	15(3)	160(27)	594

*Percentages do not add up to 100% due to rounding.
^Not listed.
N = total sample.

spinal cord. Also within the confines of the dura, intramedullary spinal cord tumors arise within the parenchyma of the spinal cord tissue proper and directly damage spinal cord tissue.

Primary tumors are the most common spinal cord tumor. In general, the reported primary tumors include ependymoma, astrocytoma, dermoid, malignant glioblastoma, epidermoid, teratoma, hemangioblastoma, hemangioma, primary lymphoma, oligodendroglioma, and cholestoma. Secondary spinal cord tumors are rare (9,11). The following will expound on the two sites of spinal cord tumors.

Compared with spine tumors, the tumor biology of primary intradural extramedullary spinal cord tumors tends to be more favorable. The majority of these tumors are benign. Greater than 75% of intradural extramedullary spinal cord tumors are primary tumors. The most common among them are meningiomas and nerve sheath tumors, i.e. schwannomas and neurofibromas. Also, encroachment of lipomas can be seen. Metastatic secondary tumors make up less than 4% of the intradural extramedullary tumors. They arise either by hematogenous spread, or by direct extension from the CSF as a "drop metastases" from malignant brain tumors (i.e. medullablastoma, ependymoma), perineural tumor growth from the nerve roots, or through the dura from an extradural tumor (9–11,22). The most common intramedullary spinal cord tumors are primary ependymomas (40%), and astrocytomas (35%). Intramedullary spinal cord tumors have a variable degree of tumor aggressiveness that spans from malignant astrocytomas to ependymomas, which have a clinically benign course. The majority of intramedullary tumors are malignant (9-11,22). Intramedullary ependymomas are the most common gliomas in the filum terminale in the lumbar spine, of which myxopapillary ependymomas are the most common histological subtype (23). Of note, myxopapillary ependymomas will present with signs and symptoms of cauda equina compression. Because it is usually amenable to a complete surgical excision and cure, it has a more favorable prognosis than other intramedullary ependymomas. Intramedullary ependymomas are also found in all spine levels and the conus medullaris. Astrocytomas are the most common primary intramedullary tumor arising outside of the filum terminale and are usually found in the cervical spine, followed by the thoracic spine (10,23).

Secondary tumors among intramedullary spinal cord tumors are rare (1–2%), and have been reported to originate from small cell lung cancer, breast cancer, GI tract (colon cancer), malignant melanoma, and lymphoma (24,25). They arise by hematogenous spread or by direct extension from tumor invasion along the nerve roots into the intramedullary space (22,24,25).

PATHOGENESIS OF METASTASES TO THE SPINAL BONY SUBSTANCE

With a secondary tumor being the most commonly encountered spine tumor, it is prudent to discuss its pathogenesis of metastases. There are several theories of metastatic spread from the primary site to the bony spine substance. Hematogenous and direct extension are two main theories.

Hematogenous spread has been reported primarily through the vertebral venous plexus that was described by Batson and others. This venous plexus is a valveless system for the thoracic, abdominal, and pelvic viscera; draining each time the intrabdominal pressure increases, as in straining and coughing. With the flow of blood, malignant cells from respective viscera are deposited into the vertebrae and epidural tissues (12,26,27). Classically, prostate cancer metastasizes through hematogenous spread via the Batson's plexus. Hematogenous spread can also be facilitated through the hematopoietic bone marrow of the vertebral column that maintains a fertile area for tumor cell deposition from a complex arteriolar sinusoidal system.

There are other mechanisms theorized in metastatic tumor growth in the spine including the production of humoral factors, chemotactic migration of tumor cells, and the "seed and soil hypothesis," where the vascular blood flow through bone deposits tumor cells and extravasation occurs through the vessel membrane. Tumor specific growth factors are released by the tumor and become adhered to the vascular epithelium. It is hypothesized that malignant cells then seed into these areas (12,28,29).

Direct extension is the second reported mechanism of metastases to the spine. This mechanical invasion into the bony substance can occur from adjacent vertebrae, leptomeninges, or paravertebral structures (9,22). Pancoast tumor of the lung and retroperitoneal sarcomas are among those that invade in this manner.

PATHOGENESIS OF NEUROLOGIC INJURY OF THE SPINAL CORD

The pathogenesis of injury to the spinal cord that leads to neurologic changes from spinal cord compression have been investigated among patients with newly detected tumors. Under gross pathology, direct mechanical injury of the spinal cord occurs from one or a combination of the following: (1) impairment of the vascular integrity of the spinal cord, (2) an extradural or intradural extramedullary mass; such as tumor laden soft tissue or bony structures, bony fragments from a collapsed vertebral body, hemorrhage, or edema invading through the intervertebral foramina into the spinal cord parenchyma or directly compressing the spinal cord; (3) an extradural or less commonly, an intradural extramedullary mass, causing spinal instability often with subluxation, and eventual collapse with obligatory disruption of the spinal cord; and (4) intramedullary spinal cord tumor, hemorrhage, or edema directly invading the spinal cord parenchyma and vascular structures (12,28,29). Tumor invasion from the VB or paravertebral epidural spaces is most commonly seen causing anterior spinal cord compression (12,28,29).

Micropathologic changes, adapted from animal models, suggest that early events of tumor related spinal cord damage involve impingement of vascular flow, resulting in the development of vasogenic cord edema and neurologic damage. Vasogenic edema causes further vascular flow impairment and direct cord displacement. The compilation of events results in cord ischemia. Specifically, direct mechanical compression increases prostaglandins. Prostaglandin estradiol 2 (PGE2) leads to inflammatory changes including increased vascular permeability and vasogenic cord edema and disrupts artery and arteriolar membrane integrity. This leads to extravasation of blood and impaired blood flow. Additionally, occlusion of the venous drainage causes interstitial and parenchymal hypoxia that stimulates vascular endothelial growth factors, which perpetuate inflammatory changes and vasogenic edema (13,28–32). Subsequent ischemic damage occurs in the spinal cord substance and demyelination may follow.

In late stages, ischemic areas may become infarcted. Further damage is seen with subsequent necrosis and gliosis. In summary, tumor compression causes decreased blood flow and a cascade of inflammatory changes. Therefore, initial conservative management consists of steroids and intravascular hydration (12, 28–32).

Other theories such as the role of released of excitatory transmitters, serotonin and glutamate, and cytokines are under investigation. Osteoclastic activating factors, stimulated by prostaglandins, are theorized to lead to bony destruction (3,13,32). Osteoblastic destruction may occur, stimulating periosteal reactions and inflammatory changes which may obscure the tumor. Therefore, the detection of the spinal tumor becomes more difficult (32).

The thoracic spine is the most common site for tumor related SCC. It is theorized that the spinal canal has the smallest diameter at this level and therefore, is at greatest risk for compromise from external tumor compression (2,9).

The rate and duration of compression impacts on the ability of the spinal cord to maintain its integrity. The spinal cord demonstrates adjustment, to an extent, from gradual compression of weeks to months, as seen with less aggressive tumors. This is in sharp contrast to the rapid neurologic decline following a rapid spinal cord compression at a rate of hours to days, as seen with rapidly growing tumors. In animal studies, Tarlov et al, demonstrated that with an alteration in the rate and duration of compression, there was a correlative neurologic outcome. Specifically, when compression was rapid, reversibility of an incomplete lesion was more likely if decompression was performed within 9 hours. Conversely, when compression was gradual between 20–48 hours, incomplete lesions were reversed if decompression was performed within 7 days (33,34). Clinical studies have produced similar findings (13). Therefore, early identification and management of SCC impacts favorably on neurologic recovery.

PRESENTATION AND EVALUATION OF SPINE AND SPINAL CORD TUMORS

Spine Extradural Tumors

The history taking may extract red flags that suggests cancer including back pain, unexplained weight loss, prior history of cancer, chronic fatigue, fevers, night sweats, bowel and bladder disturbances, and a family history of cancer. Other more focused items for cancer include the presence of enlarged lymph nodes, breast masses, hematuria, dysuria, neck masses, chronic cough, smoking, and toxin or radiation exposure. Pain is the most common presenting symptom for spinal tumors. Therefore, a pain history is important in identifying the location of the lesion. Pain caused by spine tumors is frequently worsened with the recumbent position, whereas spine pain frequently found in degenerative conditions will be worsened in the upright position.

Pain is typically axial pain and if nerve root impingement occurs, radicular pain is present (5, 7,35).

The physical exam is extremely important. This involves a general medical and comprehensive exam to document motor, sensory, and reflex function. An inspection of the vertebral column may reveal evidence of kyphoscoliosis, a finding that suggests significant bony architectural destruction. Pain with percussion of the vertebrae or with range of motion suggests pain sensitive elements are affected. Neurologic deficits may include evidence of nerve root impingement with radicular signs, and a positive straight leg raising test. Determining a sensory level of preserved function is essential for medical and surgical management and prognosis. Because metastases are the most common type of spine tumor, attention is given towards cancer evaluation measures, for example: breast, lung, and skin exams for women, and prostate, lung, and skin exams for men (1,4,6,13). In addition, chronic signs or symptoms of spine tumors, those that have been present for more than three months, have been reported. Gradual development of overt myelopathy has been reported in less aggressive spine tumors, with the onset of symptoms to be as long as two years (14,36,37).

Spinal Cord Intradural Extramedullary and Intramedullary Tumors

History and physical exam is performed as previously discussed with spine tumors. Spinal cord tumors usually present with pain and neurologic deficits. The degree and progression of neurologic signs and symptoms depend on the aggressiveness of the tumor. As a general rule, intradural extramedullary tumors more frequently present with a prolonged history of pain and radicular symptoms; then later develop spinal cord dysfunction, such as motor and sensory deficits, and bowel and bladder dysfunction. Intramedullary tumors present usually with spinal cord dysfunction, which is in contrast to extradural tumors that more frequently present with pain prior to the onset of neurologic abnormalities.

Diagnostic Evaluation of Patients without Myelopathic Symptoms

Once tumor is suspected in a patient with no myelopathic symptoms, i.e. spinal cord dysfunction, investigational studies are performed patient specific and focused on the most common etiology of the tumor. An in depth review is beyond the scope of this text, however, a general overview is discussed. Preliminary laboratory studies may guide further evaluation including the erythrocyte sedimentation rate (ESR) and complete blood count. Cancer screening measures in men include prostate specific antigen (PSA) and in women, a mammogram. Serum tumor markers are available but are non-specific (7,32). If lung cancer is suspected, a chest x-ray is warranted as the initial radiological exam. Colorectal cancer screening can be achieved with a flexible sigmoidoscopy or colonoscopy depending on the suspected area. Thyroid function tests may be the initial screening for a thyroid mass, followed by more advanced serologic exams and appropriate diagnostic imaging tools. Serum calcium, uric acid, and serum protein electrophoresis and urine protein electrophoresis may be the initial laboratory evaluations for multiple myeloma. Cerebrospinal fluid (CSF) for protein, leukocytosis, biochemical markers, and cell count can assess leptomeningeal carcinomatosis seen associated with intradural extramedullary involvement, but will not reliably distinguish between spine and spinal cord tumors. Otherwise, a CSF fluid examination is not essential in the initial standard evaluation, unless a concomitant CNS infection is suspected. Biopsy of the mass lesion prior to intervention is performed when the diagnosis is unclear or there is a metastatic tumor of unknown primary source (7,13,22,37).

An efficient use of diagnostic imaging is indicated in the evaluation of back pain that is strongly suspected of being tumor related. The choice of imaging relies heavily on the tumor biology and clinical presentation. The following will review the spectrum of imaging techniques utilized to detect spine and spinal cord tumors.

Plain radiographs are of low cost and are able to identify gross abnormalities; however, in isolation, they do not rule-in or rule-out tumors. In a tumor related back pain evaluation, an initial evaluation may include plain radiographs of the symptomatic areas to assess for bony destruction, scoliosis, kyphosis, and paravertebral soft tissue changes.

According to the Recommendations from the NIH panel on Acute Low Back Problems in Adults; for acute low back pain, plain x-rays are not recommended within the first month of symptoms unless the following risk factors are present: age over 70, high clinical suspicion for tumor or infection, history of recent trauma, cancer, unexplained weight loss, fever >100°F, low back pain worse at night, IV drug use, prolonged use of steroids, or osteoporosis. Thereafter, plain x-rays are indicated for persistent symptoms of over 30 days or based on the development of any of above risk factors (38). Plain radiographs provide adjunctive information and help guide further imaging studies. Unfortunately, plain radiographic findings commonly detect gross abnormalities that occur only in later stages of tumor involvement within the spinal column (10,38). There are classic radiological signs for bony destruction due to tumor. A common sign is erosion of the pedicle. In unilateral destruction, the pedicle appears as a "winking owl", whereas in bilateral destruction, it appears as a "blinking owl" (39). Other signs suggestive of bony destruction due to tumor include interpedicular widening and vertebral body collapse. Vertebral body collapse and therefore, spinal instability, occurs most commonly when there is greater than 50% destruction of the vertebral body (VB), which is the most common plain radiographic sign of tumor involvement (38). Loss or diminished anterior column support may lead to subluxation, which can be detected prior to overt VB collapse.

Osteoblastic destruction is most characteristic of prostate cancer, but can be seen also in myeloma and lymphoma. In children, osteoblastic changes occur with medulloblastoma, osteosarcoma, lymphoma, carcinoid tumors, and retinoblastoma. Osteolytic changes have been seen with lung, breast, gastrointestinal, lymphoma, melanoma, renal, and thyroid cancers. Breast and lung cancer can also have mixed osteoblastic and osteolytic changes (10,32,38,40).

Bone scintigraphy may be performed to evaluate the presenting bony spine lesion and locate lesions outside of the spine. In the appropriate clinical setting, positive spine findings suggest either primary or metastatic spine tumors. For either acute or chronic low back pain, bone scans are indicated when tumor is suspected based on the medical history, physical examination, and collaborative data (38).

Bone scans utilize isotopes such as 99m Technecium for planar imaging or single photon emission computed tomography (SPECT). If there is increased isotope uptake in the blood pool phase, then that area has increased blood flow due to proliferation of small vessels suggesting granulation tissue or tumor. If there is increased uptake in the delayed phase, that area has increased bone turnover with increased osteoblastic activity. In comparison to planar bone scans alone, a SPECT scan is advantageous because of the increased ability to anatomically locate the tumor with the added computed tomography. In general, the findings of increased uptake of radionuclide tracers correlate to an area of increased blood flow, and the amount of osteoid synthesized by osteoblasts from the tumor itself or from reactive bone (41–43).

Bone scans are moderately sensitive for detecting spine tumor in comparison to plain x-rays, and may help identify other areas of tumor involvement (10,38,41,42). The disadvantages of bone scans are that they are not specific, in that other inflammatory conditions appear similarly. Also, it is difficult to differentiate acute from chronic conditions. For increased tracer uptake and subsequent detection, the affected area needs to have increased blood flow or osteoid synthesis; otherwise the findings may be interpreted as negative. Therefore, in highly destructive lesions and lytic lesions, which do not have significant increased blood flow or osteoid synthesis, bone scans may be interpreted as negative. This is seen with myeloma, previously irradiated areas, neuroblastomas, and cancers of the lung, breast, and kidney. Additionally, if the bony spinal substance has metastatic lesions that are uniform with minimal normal areas present, the differential uptakes may not be evident in standard bone scans. Therefore, the uniform areas may be interpreted as normal. Bone scans are contraindicated in pregnancy (10,41–43).

Computerized tomographic (CT) scans historically provided the most efficient and rapid means of screening for tumors, and are useful for surgical planning. However, it has been replaced by MRI in most centers. For acute low back pain conditions, the NIH panel does not recommend a CT scan unless there are neurological changes, a strong suspicion for tumor, infection, fracture, other space occupying lesions, or for surgical intervention. For those with more than one-month duration of symptoms or when surgical intervention is being considered, a CT scan may be performed (38).

CT findings suggestive of a tumor mass include spinal canal widening, neural foramina enlargement, bony cortical destruction, and herniated discs. Calcified lesions may suggest a meningioma (10). CT is also best for evaluating bony non-marrow replacing lesions and acute hemorrhage. When a MRI is contraindicated, then CT is the alternative. The disadvantages are that it is expensive in comparison to plain x-rays, it lacks specificity, and it is poor for identifying soft tissue abnormalities in comparison to MRI (10,38).

Although historically, a CT myelogram had been reported to be better in detecting small epidural lesions or root compressions than MRI, more recent studies found MRI to be equal to or better than a CT myelogram (38, 44). Subsequently, MRI has replaced CT myelogram in clinical practice for the evaluation of spinal cord compromise. Additionally, CT myelogram carries the risk of contrast dye induced nephrotoxicity, worsening neurologic function due to positioning for the procedure, and bleeding complications from the lumbar puncture. CT myelogram is more recently only utilized when MRI is either contraindicated, not readily available, or in order to confirm equivocal MRI findings (10,38,44).

MRI has replaced CT scans in many medical centers in the evaluation of a patient with a suspected tumor causing neurologic deficits. The advantages for MRI are multifold in the radiological evaluation for spine and spinal cord tumors. In comparison to a CT scan, it has a higher sensitivity for detecting lesions and soft tissue abnormalities, and has greater tissue contrast capability. In addition, MRI better identifies lesions for radiotherapy or surgical interventions, and better differentiates extradural and intradural lesions. In comparison to CT myelogram, MRI overcomes blocks in imaging more easily by visualizing areas above and between blocks, in a non-invasive manner. The disadvantages of MRI include that it is less sensitive than CT in detecting calcification, bony cortical abnormalities, and acute hemorrhage. The image quality is more affected by motion than a CT scan. Contraindications to MRI include persons with pacemakers, non-compatible metallic implants, and severe claustrophobia (10,38,44).

MRI signs of tumor involvement include a widened spinal canal, and an irregular spinal cord margin. Vertebral metastases are usually hyperdense in T2 and post-T1 weighted images. With the addition of Gadolinium, the enhanced MRI demonstrates tumor enhancement, as well as, differentiation between extradural and intradural regions (10,38,45).

SPINAL CORD COMPRESSION RESULTING FROM SPINAL AND SPINAL CORD TUMORS

The oncologic medical emergency presenting as an acute neurologic decline with disabling myelopathic changes at a definable level in motor, sensory, or bowel or bladder function from a spinal cord lesion is spinal cord compression (SCC). SCC is the second most common neurologic complication in cancer, after brain metastases, and can be caused by either spine or spinal cord tumors. SCC results from the compression of the spinal cord by either extradural or intradural extramedullary encroachment into the spinal cord, or from intramedullary sources (1,7, 8,9). The most common etiology is a spine tumor from the extradural space compressing the spinal cord parenchyma (1, 13). The following sections will expound on the presentation, evaluation, and medical interventions for spinal cord compression.

Retrospectively, prior to myelopathic changes, the most common subjective and objective finding is back pain. Pain may be local, referred, or radiating pain. Pain may be exacerbated with Valsalva maneuvers or recumbency, which may be due to trac-

tion on the spinal cord when lumbar lordosis is reduced (1,7, 13,36).

Upon inspection of the vertebral column, scoliosis or kyphosis may be evident. Percussion over the affected vertebral levels may be tender. Loss of motor function is the second most common complaint followed closely by sensory deficits below the spinal level of the lesion. Affected spinal levels of spinal cord involvement are identified based on the sensory and motor exam. Acutely, deep tendon reflexes are lost and muscle tone is reduced. With provocative testing, straight leg raising may be positive if concomitant lumbar root compression is present. Bowel and bladder retention or incontinence occurs.

Spasticity and autonomic dysfunction is seen less commonly at the time of diagnosis. If the spinal cord compression is not treated immediately, severe spinal cord damage progresses within hours to days and depending on the location of the lesion, paraplegia or tetraplegia results (1,6,7,13,36,37).

Because of the rapid neurologic decline, evaluation for SCC relies on the rapid identification of the lesion through diagnostic imaging studies. Extensive laboratory evaluation and a biopsy are performed after the patient is medically stabilized. Preliminary and preoperative studies may be performed in preparation for immediate medical and surgical intervention. The imaging techniques are chosen for their rapid accessibility and ability to identify the spinal cord lesion for emergent medical and/or surgical intervention. Commonly this includes plain radiography to identify the general architecture and gross lesions, and MRI to identify the area of compression (1,7,10,13). In plain radiographs, the classic radiological signs for bony destruction due to tumor are important to determine. In a study of patients with known epidural SCC from metastases, 87% had greater than 50% VB collapse, 66% had pedicle destruction, 23% had VB involvement without collapse, and 6% had normal radiographs (46).

Computerized tomographic (CT) scans are useful for surgical planning and may assist in the diagnosis. CT myelogram is less utilized when the capability to perform a MRI is available. When a MRI is contraindicated, it provides for a rapid peri-operative evaluation (10,38). MRI is the procedure of choice in the initial radiological evaluation of spinal cord compression. Axial and sagittal views are useful. With the addition of Gadolinium, the enhanced MRI demonstrates tumor enhancement, as well as, differentiation between extradural and intradural regions (10, 38,44,45).

Management of Spinal Cord Compression

The mainstay of SCC management includes hydration, steroids, radiation treatment, and surgery. Intravenous (IV) hydration is administered to achieve adequate blood pressure, which maintains spinal cord blood flow in order to reduce the risk of cord ischemia. Intravascular volume can be monitored through non-invasive or invasive techniques, such as a central venous pressure monitor, depending on the severity of the patient's presentation. The addition of pharmacologic pressor support is considered (13,22).

Corticosteroids are indicated in acute spinal cord compression. The theoretical rationale is based on the fact that when there are efforts to reduce the tumor related inflammatory changes and prostaglandin production; there is subsequent increase in spinal cord blood flow. The dose, however, is controversial. Most commonly, the loading dose for Decadron (dexamethasone) is 100mg IV, followed by 24mg qid (IV or oral) for the first 48–72hrs. A tapering dose schedule follows over 7–10days (2,4,9,13). Alternatively, a 10mg IV loading dose is given, followed by oral 4–24mg qid for the first 48–72hrs. Tapered dose schedule is prescribed with concomitant radiation therapy (4, 13). The major steroid complications are the increased risk of infection and the decreased fusion rates if a surgical spinal fusion were subsequently performed. Timing after steroid therapy, and similarly, after radiation treatment is important if surgical intervention is later planned.

Radiation treatment (RT) is indicated for patients with SCC due to soft tissue encroachment. RT can be employed as monotherapy in cases of spinal stability with or without neurologic changes and as an adjunctive therapy to surgery for patients with spinal instability. In persons with spinal cord tumors, radiation therapy is less frequently utilized, except for residual or unresectable tumors. In the postoperative management, RT may be employed after wounds have healed which is approximately 3–6 weeks post-operatively. The basis of radiation treatment is to provide decompression of neural structures and it is often the first line therapy for SCC through cytoreduction of the tumor, prevention of neurologic progression, prevention of local recurrences, and relief of pain. Radiosensitive tumors include lymphoma, small cell lung cancer, and multiple myeloma. Less radiosensitive tumors include prostate, breast, non-small cell lung, and renal cancer. The usual treatment levels are towards two vertebral spaces above and below the lesion (11,13,22). Major complications include the development of radiation myelopathy, radiation plexopathy, and tumor recurrence. Other less frequent complications includes pericarditis, fibrosis and contractures, postradiation necrosis, sarcomatous degeneration of certain tumors, i.e. giant cell tumors, and cognitive deficits (47,48).

In SCC, indications for chemotherapy include an adjuvant to radiation therapy or surgery for chemosensitive primary or secondary spine tumors: lymphoma, myeloma, breast, prostate, and germ cell tumors. Pediatric tumors are usually chemosensitive (13,47,48). Complications are dependent on the chemotherapeutic drug profile. Peripheral neuropathy is seen with vinca alkaloids and cisplatin. Cognitive effects are seen with cytokines. Vocal cord paralysis has been noted with vinca alkaloids. Vinca alkaloids and cylophosphamide may produce a syndrome of inappropriate antidiuretic hormone (SIADH). Pancytopenia due to bone marrow toxicity may occur (13,47,48).

Hormonal therapy is used as an adjuvant only. It is considered in metastasis from tumors such as thyroid, breast, and prostate. Conservative treatment with no intervention is considered in cases with poor prognosis, i.e. late stage cancer, or when the patient prefers it (22,48).

In SCC, the goal of surgical intervention is primarily to relieve the pressure on the spinal cord through surgical decompression in hopes to preserve or recover neurologic function. Although consensus may vary among centers, conditions with clear surgical indications for intervention include: (1) spinal instability, (2) neural elements impingement with spinal deformity due to fractured bone, (3) failure to respond to radiation, (4) persistent symptoms from radiosensitive tumors, despite reaching the maximal allowable radiation dose for spinal cord tolerance, (5) radiation treatment is contraindicated, and (6) tissue diagnosis is needed (2,13).

SURGICAL MANAGEMENT OF SPINE AND SPINAL CORD TUMORS

The surgical management of tumors of the spine and spinal cord is a complex decision making process. Numerous factors must be weighed in the initial evaluation to determine which patients would benefit from surgical intervention. The three main determinants for surgical candidacy are tumor biology, neurologic condition, and general medical condition.

Tumor biology refers to the aggressiveness of the spine or spinal cord tumor. This factor is becoming increasingly difficult to determine as medical oncologists improve their success rates with prolonging the lifespan of patients afflicted with these tumors. As a general rule, most surgeons will not entertain surgical intervention if the patient has a prognosis of less than three months survival (49). It is oftentimes difficult for the surgeon, working in conjunction with the oncology team, to determine the exact long-term prognosis. As a result, a determination of the relative risks versus benefits will be made by the surgeon and communicated to the patient. Following this detailed discussion, a decision regarding surgical intervention will be made.

With respect to neurologic status, an important determination will be whether the patient's neurologic examination is stable or deteriorating. If the examination is both stable and normal, a detailed diagnostic work-up is frequently indicated. However, if the patient is undergoing a progressive neurologic deterioration; frequently, urgent surgery will be required prior to completion of a comprehensive preoperative diagnostic work-up.

The patient's general medical systemic condition can provide clues as to whether spinal surgery should be performed. A history of a significant weight loss, cachexia, or numerous other factors suggestive of an immunocompromised state may all lead the surgeon away from surgical treatment of these patients. The rationale behind this line of thinking is that a major spinal surgery is a significant metabolic insult and the patient must be strong enough to tolerate the surgical procedure in order for benefit to be achieved.

Spine Extradural Tumors

Spine tumors originate in the extradural space. The actual surgical procedures are quite similar in the management of primary and metastatic tumors. One difference in the surgical treatment is that a more aggressive surgical procedure may be entertained in patients with primary tumors, as long-term survival is more likely.

Preoperative Considerations

The preoperative work-up for a patient with a spine tumor assess the patient's overall systemic health. Patients debilitated by malnutrition resulting from disseminated cancer, will tend to be poor surgical candidates with a decreased chance of surgical success (50). A detailed physical examination will determine if the patient is neurologically intact, has an incomplete neurologic deficit, or a complete spinal cord lesion. As the postoperative results are dramatically superior in patients with better neurologic condition preoperatively, determination of any existing neurologic abnormalities prior to surgery is critical. Patients with primary tumors of the spine are oftentimes a diagnosis of exclusion. As metastatic lesions are far more common, frequently a metastatic work-up would be negative prior to the determination that the patient has a primary tumor of the spine. In these situations, a percutaneous needle biopsy of the involved vertebra is frequently helpful (51). This biopsy may determine if the lesion is benign or malignant. It will also aid the surgeon in planning whether surgery should be performed and if so, which specific surgical procedure would be optimal.

Primary bone tumors tend to involve a single vertebra with sparing of the adjacent intervertebral disc spaces. A clinical pearl is that spinal infections will frequently involve adjacent vertebra with involvement of the intervening intervertebral disc, this will be readily diagnosed on MRI. While the intervertebral disc space is ordinarily spared with any spine tumors, with metastatic disease, multiple vertebrae may be involved and either a MRI or a bone scan is useful preoperatively to determine if it is a single lesion,or multiple lesions are present.

Surgical Considerations

The actual surgical technique utilized to treat either primary or metastatic spine tumors is similar. Occasionally, a focal "lesionectomy" may be possible. This involves merely resecting the lesion, if only a small portion of the vertebra is involved and removing the lesion will not impart instability to the vertebral segment. This is quite uncommon and rarely utilized. Much more commonly, a corpectomy will be performed. A typical corpectomy will involve excision of the majority of the involved vertebral body as well as the intervertebral disc above and below the involved vertebra. All gross tumors are resected to the greatest extent possible. As the majority of corpectomies for spine tumors involve metastatic disease, the goal of surgery is palliation rather than surgical cure (53). As such, subtotal tumor resection, which leaves a minimal amount of residual tumor, is acceptable in this procedure. In the thoracic and lumbar spines, the goal of surgery is a "pedicle-to-pedicle" decompression, where the thecal sac is decompressed from the vertebra above to the vertebra below the involved segment, and the width of decompression allows for a complete decompression of the spinal cord (53). In the cervical spine, the width of the corpectomy defect is a minimum of 15 mm (54). This allows for a complete decompression of the spinal cord which measures approximately 13 mm or less in the coronal dimension, in the cervical spine.

After resection of the involved tumor and vertebral body, the corpectomy is completed. Next, reconstruction of the anterior column of the spine is performed (55). This process typically involves placement of a "spacer" into the space between the vertebra above and below. Different materials have been utilized to function as spacers. The gold standard is use of autologous

bone graft products (49). This is particularly useful in primary tumors of the bone where a longer survival may be anticipated. Potential sources for autologous tissue to be utilized as spacers include the iliac crest, the fibula, and rib grafts. Alternative choices for spacers may include use of allograft bone, which will typically involve fibula grafts in the cervical spine and either fibula, tibia, or humerus bone in the thoracic or lumbar spines (56). Additional spacers more recently developed include the use of cages that may be filled with autologous bone products. Likewise, polymethylmethacrylate (PMMA) has been utilized to function as a spacer in patients with metastatic tumors with a limited prognosis for survival (49,57,58).

Following placement of the spacer, and radiographic confirmation intraoperatively of adequate positioning, instrumentation will typically be utilized to provide immediate stability to the construct. In the cervical spine, the most commonly utilized instrumentation construct will include an anterior cervical plate with screws inserted into the vertebral bodies of the adjacent normal vertebrae, above and below the spacer (49,59). In the thoracolumbar spine, anterior instrumentation constructs will typically also utilize screws placed in the normal vertebrae above and below the involved segment (58). The screws are secured to one another utilizing either rods or a plate construct. In the majority of tumor corpectomies, the posterior elements are not involved, and as such, the anterior column reconstruction/stabilization fusion procedure will be adequate with no posterior surgery necessary. If significant involvement of the posterior elements is present, then consideration of a posterior stabilization procedure will also be entertained.

The usual indications for performing both an anterior and posterior (AP) decompression stabilization procedure include circumferential involvement of the vertebral body with both anterior and posterior column disruptions (60). Other indications for combined AP surgery include the presence of significant instability on preoperative diagnostic studies, involvement of multiple levels, or involvement of anatomically unfavorable positions (61). Anatomically unfavorable locations are areas where anterior decompression and stabilization is not feasible as a stand-alone procedure. These locations typically involve the occipital-cervical junction, the cervical-thoracic junction, and the lower lumbar spine. For technical reasons beyond the scope of this chapter, anterior surgery alone in these anatomically unfavorable positions is inadequate to completely stabilize the spine.

Two surgical approaches are rarely utilized for radical resection of spinal tumors. These are the lateral extracavitary approach performed via a posterior spinal approach, and the "enbloc" corpectomy approach. In the former procedure, both an anterior decompression, as well as a simultaneous posterior stabilization procedure is able to be performed from a single dorsal approach (62). This technique is most frequently utilized when a patient is unable to tolerate an anterior transthoracic or retroperitoneal approach to a spine tumor. Criticisms of this procedure include difficulty achieving an adequate decompression of the neural elements anteriorly, prolonged operative times, and frequent high blood loss. The surgical indications for the lateral extracavitary approach will most frequently include patients with metastatic disease, or patients with significant pulmonary insufficiency that are unable to tolerate an anterior thoracotomy approach (61). In the "en-bloc" corpectomy, the entire vertebral body is removed "en-bloc" in order to attempt to achieve a gross total resection of a tumor. This radical procedure requires both an anterior and posterior operation to be performed and is indicated in patients with a primary tumor of the bone where a surgical cure is the goal (63). Like the extracavitary approach, this radical procedure is rarely indicated and would not be performed for metastatic lesions of the vertebra.

Significant differences do exist between surgery performed for primary and metastatic spine tumors. As a general rule, attempts are made to keep surgery for metastatic lesions to a more limited procedure when possible. In addition, metastatic tumors have surgery for palliative, and not curative, indications (60). As such, greater reliance may be placed on the use of hardware, cages, or PMMA. With metastatic lesions, fusions are usually not necessary. As the medical oncologists are becoming increasingly successful prolonging survival with certain biologically favorable forms of spine tumors, such as breast and prostate carcinomas; increased attempts at obtaining spinal fusion in these favorable tumor types should be considered.

Postoperative Considerations

Following surgical resection of a spine tumor, the postoperative period includes careful monitoring of hemodynamic stability, monitoring for signs of infection, and assuring adequate circulating red blood cell volume with the use of blood transfusions as needed. In addition, avoidance of postoperative complications such as deep venous thrombosis (DVT), pulmonary embolus (PE), atelectasis, pneumonia, and urinary tract infection is important. When radiation therapy (RT) is indicated, a three week period is usually required following surgery to ensure that adequate wound healing has occurred. If RT is initiated prior to three weeks, an increased incidence of wound breakdown and/or wound infection may be seen. Likewise, if chemotherapy is to be utilized, this adjuvant treatment is withheld until the patient is metabolically stabilized, which usually requires a minimum of two weeks from the time of the index surgical procedure.

The postoperative results following spine tumor surgery are typically evaluated with respect to the neurologic function as well as the short-term and long-term spinal stability. As a general rule, patients with spine tumors who are neurologically intact prior to surgery will remain neurologically intact postoperatively. In patients with incomplete spinal cord injuries or nerve root compression, frequent improvement in the neurologic condition is noted in the postoperative period. In patients who have a complete spinal cord injury, neurologic improvement is rarely, if ever, seen. With respect to pain relief, good to excellent results are commonly seen following stable instrumented fusion constructs (58,60). As has been previously stated, another goal of spine tumor surgery is to achieve spinal stability. This is necessary to prevent neurologic worsening in the postoperative period, as well as eventual vertebral body collapse. Failures of spinal stability may occur in either the early or late postoperative periods (50). Early spinal instability is ordinarily the result of either graft or hardware failure, or may be the direct result of intraoperative events. If a patient has a worsened neurologic exam follow-

ing surgery, immediate neuroimaging studies (either a MRI or a CT-myelogram) is indicated to confirm that the neurologic elements are free of active neural compression. In the early postoperative period, a graft may dislodge due to an inadequate fusion/stabilization construct, or due to a lack of recognition of the degree of spinal instability initially present.

In the late postoperative period, defined as greater than two weeks from the index surgical procedure, neurologic demise and/or spinal instability may result. This may be the result of hardware failure or may be the result of recurrent disease. Recurrent tumor may present at the operative level or at the levels above or below the operated area. The work-up for late postoperative problems would be similar to the work-up performed prior to the index surgical procedure including plain film radiographs, and possibly the use of CT scans and/or MR imaging. The goal of surgery for patients with primary tumors of the spine is a stable fusion. The best fusion results have been reported with the use of autologous bone grafts. The use of surgical hardware has become increasingly widespread. With steady improvements in the instrumentation constructs, it is possible for spinal stability to be imparted for greater than two years, even in the absence of a documented fusion. For most metastatic tumors, currently utilized instrumentation constructs will maintain spinal stability beyond the expected lifespan of these patients (57).

In patients with primary tumors of the spine, long-term survival is frequent, and as such, it is essential to achieve a long-term bony fusion. Eventually, all hardware constructs will fail if a bony arthrodesis is unable to be achieved. As such, if the adequacy of the anterior fusion procedure, in patients with primary bone tumors of the spine, is in any way questionable, then a posterior stabilization/fusion procedure to augment the anterior procedure should be considered (53). Patients with spine tumors are particularly prone to troubles with postoperative wound infections. Specific factors that increase the risks of postoperative wound infections include the institution of radiation therapy, the use of perioperative corticosteroid medications, the presence of immune compromised states, and poor nutritional status. Postoperative wound infections are classified as either superficial or deep. Superficial wound infections are superficial to the deep fascia of the spine and may be treated with local drainage. This drainage procedure may be accomplished at the bedside utilizing local anesthesia. With adequate drainage, antibiotic medication is not necessary. In deep wound infections, the infection is deep to the fascial layer and will require surgical revision in the operating room. Deep wound infections classically present with pain and an elevated ESR. The presence of fever and leukocytosis may also be present; however, deep wound infections have also frequently been seen in patients who are afebrile with no leukocytosis. As such, a high index of suspicion for wound infection must be maintained in patients with spine tumors. Following operative revision of a deep wound infection, intravenous antibiotics directed toward the causative organism would be required. The usual antibiotic treatment regimen would be carried out for a minimum of two to six weeks. The use of spinal orthotics will be discussed in a separate section of this chapter.

Spinal Cord Intradural Extramedullary and Intramedullary Tumors

Typically, surgery for spinal cord tumors is performed from a dorsal approach via a laminectomy. In addition, spinal stability is rarely compromised, and as such, stabilization procedures are infrequently necessary. Spinal cord tumors are typically resected with the aid of the operating microscope and microneurosurgical techniques (64–68). This section will focus on four tumors as representative examples for the management of spinal cord tumors.

Preoperative Considerations

The preoperative neuroradiographic imaging evaluation centers on advanced imaging studies (64,65). Plain film radiographs are usually normal. An exception is seen in patients with neurofibromas who often have enlargement of the neuroforamina seen on plain radiographs and best visualized with enlargement of the neuroforamen on oblique view films.

Intradural extramedullary tumors, neurofibromas and meningiomas, demonstrate uniform enhancement on MRI with gadolinium. These lesions will frequently displace the spinal cord. Intramedullary spinal cord tumors, ependymomas and astrocytomas, may demonstrate irregular enhancement with gadolinium and may have both solid and cystic components (67,68). A myelogram, with a post-myelogram CT scan, is utilized less frequently than MR imaging (65). On myelography, intramedullary tumors will widen the spinal cord whereas extramedullary tumors will displace the spinal cord.

Intraoperative Considerations

Intramedullary spinal cord tumors are usually approached from a dorsal approach utilizing multilevel laminectomies. Evoked potential monitoring may be utilized; however, the benefit of this intraoperative adjunct is debatable (65). The limited value of intraoperative monitoring is the result of frequent abnormal baseline studies prior to surgery, as well as the perceived need to proceed with the surgical procedure, despite the abnormal monitoring. As such, many surgeons do not utilize evoke potential monitoring for intramedullary spinal cord tumors. The mainstay of surgical treatment of intramedullary spinal cord tumors is microneurosurgical technique (65–68). The operating microscope is essential for adequate magnification, illumination, and visualization of tissue planes. Frequently, a small biopsy specimen is sent for frozen section pathologic diagnosis during the early stage of the procedure. Unfortunately, these frozen section diagnoses may be unreliable, and as such, the information gained from the frozen section diagnosis must be used in conjunction with the clinical appearance, under the operating microscope, to determine if an aggressive tumor removal is possible (65,67). The usual surgical approach for an intramedullary spinal cord tumor will include a midline myelotomy. This involves splitting of the dorsal columns of the spinal cord. As a result of this myelotomy, frequent sensory deficits, which may be permanent, will occur.

With an intramedullary ependymoma, it is often possible to develop a plane between the tumor and the surrounding spinal cord (65,66,68,69). This allows the tumor to be "shelled out," and in so doing, allows for a gross total resection of the tumor, as well as the walls of any cysts present (66). Ependymomas tend to displace the neighboring spinal cord and significantly narrow the involved spinal cord segment (68). Despite significant compression from intramedullary ependymomas, a remarkable degree of preservation of neurologic function may be present in this spinal cord tissue (65). As such, the potential for neurologic improvement postoperatively is significant.

Unlike ependymomas, intramedullary astrocytomas rarely have a clear plane between the neoplastic tissue and the surrounding spinal cord. By definition, astrocytomas are invasive tumors, which cause symptoms both by invading and displacing spinal cord tissue. At the time of surgery, no clear plane of demarcation will be identified. As a result, the surgical goal is either a simple biopsy for diagnosis, or a subtotal resection of the clearly abnormal tissue (69). Any cystic component may also be drained at this time. With intramedullary astrocytomas, most neurosurgeons prefer a limited resection with maximal preservation of neurologic function for this surgically incurable tumor (65). Depending on the extent of the bony removal required to accomplish tumor resection, spinal stability may be adversely affected. This problem most frequently occurs in the pediatric population, where children have an increased incidence of delayed post-laminectomy kyphotic deformity following resection of intradural tumors (70). If concern for postoperative instability is present, then an instrumented fusion may be performed at the time of the initial surgery. This is infrequently necessary in the adult population.

Intradural extramedullary spinal cord tumors are typically meningiomas, or nerve sheath tumors. Evoked potential monitoring is more valuable with intradural extramedullary tumors than with intramedullary tumors. This is particularly true in the cervical and lumbar regions where decisions regarding sacrifice of a nerve root may have functional significance. The surgical approach to intradural extramedullary tumors will generally be multilevel laminectomies. The dura is routinely opened over the dorsal root entry zone on the side of the lesion, or in the midline if a centrally located lesion is present (64). Neurofibromas, a nerve sheath tumor, ordinarily arise from sensory nerve rootlets in the intradural space. These tumors may be entirely intradural or may extend through an enlarged neuroforamen into the extradural space. In these instances, the neurofibroma is referred to as a "dumbbell" tumor (71). Chronic pressure from these slow growing tumors will lead to the enlargement of the neuroforamen (64). With an isolated neurofibroma lesion, the decision to totally resect the tumor, and therefore sacrifice nerve rootlets, may be assisted by the use of evoked potential monitoring or electromyographic (EMG) monitoring. Depending on the level of the lesion, this may or may not have clinical significance. In the cervical and lumbar regions, a detailed discussion between the surgeon and patient must be entertained preoperatively to determine whether a gross total removal, with potential neurologic deficit, is preferable to an incomplete surgical debulking (71). In patients with neurofibromatosis Type 2 (NF-2), extensive involvement throughout the spinal cord may be present. In these circumstances, surgery is ordinarily performed to internally debulk the tumor and decrease spinal cord compression. No attempt is made for gross total removal as significant disabling neurologic dysfunction may occur if this were performed. The neurofibroma arises directly from the nerve root and removal of multiple nerve roots may result in loss of both motor and sensory functions.

If spinal stability is compromised via the bony resection for neurofibroma resection, then a simultaneous stabilization procedure may be necessary (71). Due to the frequent thinning and morphologic changes in the involved bone, the stabilization construct will often times require extension to levels rostral and caudal to the excised area, in order for adequate stability to be achieved (64).

Intradural extramedullary meningiomas typically arise from the spinal dura. These tumors are usually accessible via a laminectomy with a midline dural opening. Intradural extramedullary meningiomas usually attach either dorsally or laterally to the dura, and as such, they may be resected from a posterior approach. The tumor is resected, along with the adjacent involved dura. Either a partial thickness of dura is resected or a complete dural resection, with use of a dura graft, is performed.

Postoperative Considerations

Unlike spine tumors, which frequently require extensive reconstruction/fusion procedures, spinal cord tumors usually are treated with a simple decompression procedure. As a result, the general medical management postoperatively is considerably more simple and is similar to patients undergoing a routine decompressive laminectomy. Specific concern must be raised regarding the possibility of cerebral spinal fluid (CSF) leak. At the time of surgical intervention, the spinal dura may be either closed primarily, or a dural graft may be utilized. Depending on the adequacy of the dural closure and the preference of the operating surgeon, a lumbar subarachnoid drain may be utilized at the time of surgery. These lumbar drains are used to divert CSF and assist with definitive dural closure. If a CSF leak is determined postoperatively, which usually occurs within the first week of surgery, then a lumbar subarachnoid drain may be placed at that time. CSF diversion for a five to seven day period of time will frequently be adequate to resolve the leak. If CSF diversion via a lumbar drain is not adequate, then surgical re-exploration and closure of the dura may be necessary (64,65).

Postoperatively, radiation therapy and/or chemotherapy are rarely necessary for spinal cord tumors (65,67). With aggressive intramedullary astrocytomas or the rare glioblastoma multiforme of the spinal cord, adjuvant therapy may be utilized (67). Neither radiation nor chemotherapy is utilized for intradural extramedullary spinal cord tumors. The current trend with respect to spinal cord tumors is to follow patients radiographically in the postoperative period. Rather than administer adjuvant therapy, most surgeons prefer to repeat surgical exploration and tumor excision (64,67).

Following surgery, the sensory exam will usually be worse than the preoperative evaluation. This may be the result of either disruption of the posterior columns via the myelotomy (68), or the result of sacrifice of a nerve root for intradural extramedullary tumors (71). There is frequently some degree of permanence of the sensory deficit (65). Motor weakness may be present preoperatively. Frequently, there will be a transient deterioration in motor power in the acute postoperative period. Over the course of the first few months postoperatively, motor power generally improves to a level greater than the preoperative status (65,66). Because the presence of abnormalities of bowel or bladder function preoperatively is variable with spinal cord tumors, no generalizations regarding postoperative recovery of bowel and bladder function may be made accurately.

Tumor recurrence may occur following spinal cord tumor surgery and is inevitable when a subtotal resection has been performed. The presence of a residual or recurrent tumor may or may not be associated with neurologic abnormalities (67). If a recurrent or residual tumor is detected on postoperative imaging studies, and the patient remains clinically stable, then the normal routine would be to follow serial neurologic exams and neuroimaging studies until worsening of the neurologic exam occurs. At that time, decisions regarding further surgery and/or adjuvant therapy may be made (65,67). This situation with a recurrent or residual tumor will occur with astrocytomas, which are biopsied, or subtotally resected extensive neurofibromas where debulking was performed (71). With neurofibromas, these tend to be slow growing tumors unless sarcomatomous degeneration has occurred. When a neurofibroma undergoes transformation into a neurofibrosarcoma, the end result is invariably rapid tumor progression with eventual death within one year.

Gross total tumor resection for spinal cord tumors is frequently feasible with meningiomas. Likewise, many ependymomas can be completely resected. This is particularly true with the myxopapillary variant ependymomas of the filum terminale. The presence of residual or recurrent tumors of either ependymomas or meningiomas is an indication for repeat surgical intervention to attempt a gross total resection.

Spinal Orthotics

The use of spinal orthotics is very individualized. The type of orthotic, the duration of use, and the need for the device are all dependent upon the preference of the treating surgeon, the comfort level of the treating surgeon with respect to spinal stability, the risk of neurologic demise, and the degree of inherent bony instability. In patients with tumors of the spine or spinal cord, the goal of a spinal orthosis is to diminish motion at the pathologic motion segment. This will improve patient comfort, diminish pain, and ideally, improve function. The orthotic must immobilize the patient above and below the unstable region. Spinal orthoses are frequently utilized in patients with spine tumors; however, they are rarely necessary for patients with spinal cord tumors (72).

Spinal orthoses may occasionally be utilized in lieu of spinal surgery. This may occur in a patient with diffuse metastatic disease and a poor prognosis, or for a patient with severe systemic disease who would be unable to survive a spinal surgical procedure. In these instances, the brace is utilized to diminish pain, and to potentially provide a stabilizing force, to limit the possibility of vertebral body collapse with neurologic compromise (72).

In patients who will undergo spinal surgery for a spine tumor, an orthosis may be prescribed preoperatively to improve patient comfort and to provide a degree of spinal stability until the surgical procedure is performed. Following the surgical procedure, the need for an orthosis is dependent upon the surgeon's level of comfort with the final stabilization construct. If the surgeon is completely comfortable that a stable instrumented fusion is present, he may opt to avoid an orthosis altogether. This will most frequently be the case when a combined anterior/posterior major spinal reconstruction is performed. When either an anterior or posterior approach is performed, the spinal orthosis may be utilized to assist in providing additional stability. As a general rule, a spinal fusion will require a minimum of twelve weeks to occur after the index surgical procedure. In patients with spine tumors, this duration of time may be significantly longer. This is particularly the case if allograft bone is used rather than autograft. An orthosis may be necessary for six months or greater until either radiographic fusion is confirmed, or the surgeon's level of comfort allows for discontinuance of the device. Of note, long-term use of spinal orthoses is associated with a diminished compliance.

Different orthoses impart varying degrees of spinal stability. In addition, an orthosis may be designed for comfort only, or for both comfort and stability. Soft cervical collars are designed for patient comfort. They impart no appreciable biomechanical stability. Likewise, a Knight brace may be used to provide comfort for patients with thoracolumbar spine pathology. These braces also do not impart biomechanical stability (72).

In the cervical spine, if immobilization is necessary, as well as comfort, then a rigid head-cervical orthosis may be utilized. Even greater stability can be achieved with a halo/vest orthosis (73). Halo/vests are particularly beneficial in the upper cervical spine and have the added benefit of assuring patient compliance. In the thoracolumbar spine region, a molded thoracolumbosacral orthosis (TLSO) brace may be utilized for both comfort and stability. Similarly, a body cast may be fitted which will have the added benefit of assuring patient compliance (72).

Spinal orthoses do not replace the need for a biomechanically stable construct. Orthoses have been found to hinder some efforts toward rehabilitation. As such, in patients with limited life expectancy, it is the goal to perform more aggressive internal stabilization procedures, which will lessen or eliminate the need for external spinal orthoses.

CANCER REHABILITATION IN SPINE AND SPINAL CORD TUMORS

Cancer rehabilitation utilizes a comprehensive team approach that employs both physical medicine and rehabilitation management. Goals are discussed with the patient and caregivers. Important considerations in setting the cancer rehabilitation goals are survival prognosis, desired discharge disposition, and quality of life. Adjustments in the intensity and duration of the patient's rehabilitation program are made according to the changes in the patient's medical status, survival prognosis, and functional gains

(74,75). Cancer rehabilitation of patients with spine and spinal cord tumors aims to relieve their symptoms, improve their quality of life, enhance their functional independence, and prevent further complications. Rehabilitation is particularly important as the survival rate of these patients increases. Rehabilitation provides complementary medical care to the oncology and surgical management. The medical aspects of rehabilitation require the knowledge of both the tumor related and spinal cord dysfunction issues. When the impairment is primarily back pain without myelopathic changes, cancer rehabilitation management may begin in the acute medical and surgical setting and be followed in outpatient rehabilitation. Cancer rehabilitation for those with SCC and subsequent spinal cord dysfunction may begin in the acute medical and surgical care setting; be continued in acute inpatient rehabilitation ward; and then, followed in an outpatient setting.

The specific techniques for rehabilitation, for persons who developed spinal cord dysfunction as a result of tumor related SCC, are similar to those with traumatic SCI as detailed in Chapter 19. The rehabilitation program encompasses issues relating to mobility (ambulation, wheelchair training, and transfers); activities of daily living (ADL), including dressing, grooming and hygiene skills; neuropathic bowel and bladder management, skin care, pain management, neuromuscular dysfunction management, patient and family education, psychological support, a full equipment evaluation, and patient and family training in preparation for a home discharge. Modifications in the treatment goals are coordinated based on the patient goals, medical co-morbidities, age, and patient survival prognosis. The following are specific medical issues that are present in tumor related spinal cord dysfunction that should be kept in mind during the rehabilitation program.

Pain

Pain is a major issue among cancer patients and affects a person's quality of life (4). The pain may be caused by bony metastases, by compression of the spinal cord, or by encroachment of the tumor around nerve roots resulting in radicular pain. The pain caused by compression of the spinal cord is often worse in the recumbent position, due to the tumor increasing epidural venous congestion, and as a result, producing pressure on the spinal cord. Radicular pain is often dysesthetic in nature, radiating to the arm in cervical lesions, leg in the lumbosacral lesions, and around the trunk in thoracic lesions. The clinician's focus is to relieve the patient's pain in an effort to improve the patient's quality of life. Surgical stabilization of involved vertebral levels can greatly reduce pain (76). Spinal orthotics can reduce pain by limiting the rotational forces that may precipitate nerve irritation over the braced vertebral levels. Medications include tricyclic depressants, anticonvulsants, and narcotic analgesics (See chapter 26). For bone pain, other pharmacologic agents such as calcitonin nasal spray and bisphosphonates may be used. Radiopharmacology agents such as strontium and samarian have been used specifically for bone pain related to osteoblastic metastatic lesions (4). Bone marrow toxicity is a limiting factor for the radiopharmacology agents (47,48). Modalities for neuropathic and nociceptive pain that have been used with variable results include cold and heat modalities, transcutaneous electrical nerve stimulation (TENs), and biofeedback. Interventional procedures include intrathecal morphine, and ganglion blocks (4,38).

Neurologic

Spasticity is seen with upper motor neuron injuries after spinal shock resolves. When it interrupts with the patient's function, treatment is indicated (See chapter 14). Neoplastic plexopathies occur with the tumor invasion into the brachial plexus, as seen with lung and breast cancer, and into the lumbosacral plexus, as seen with breast cancer and lymphoma. Treatment for pain is difficult with limited results from radiotherapy, TENS, and dorsal rhizotomies (4). Radiation induced plexopathies reportedly produce less pain and can be further differentiated from neoplastic plexopathies by the presence of myokymic discharges on EMG studies, more frequently seen in the former. Both types of plexopathies have poor recovery rates (47,77,78).

Paraneoplastic syndromes involving neuropathies have included demyelinating and axonal peripheral neuropathies. They have been associated with small cell lung cancer, multiple myeloma, and lymphoma (78–80). Chemotherapy induced neuropathies; however, have better recovery rates, which are related to the withdrawal of the offending agent. Chemotherapeutic agents associated with neuropathies include the vinca alkaloids, cisplatin, taxol, procarbazine, suramin, misonidazole, and hexamethylamine (47,48,77). Other paraneoplastic syndromes seen include amyotrophic lateral sclerosis (ALS), Eaton-Lambert myasthenic syndrome, myasthenia gravis, and inflammatory myopathy (47,48,77). EMG and repetitive stimulation studies may be useful for further evaluation of these syndromes.

Myelopathic changes may be seen with cancer treatments. Therefore, a workup is needed to assess neoplastic induced myelopathic changes from treatment induced changes. Evaluation may include CSF studies, MRI or CT scan of the affected spinal levels, and electrophysiologic studies. Radiation treatment of spinal tumors or for systemic tumor involvement with spinal radiation ports may produce radiation myelopathy. Acute effects of radiation treatment may present with myelopathic deterioration during radiation treatment. If no other cause for the deterioration is found, corticosteroid treatment may be given with continued radiation treatment. Subacute myelopathy, following radiation treatment, may occur between weeks to months of radiation treatment with a positive Lhermitte sign. When no other cause is found and somatosensory evoked potentials are normal, then the cause may be due to a subacute transient radiation-induced myelopathy, which carries a favorable prognosis and is reversible. On the other hand, chronic radiation myelopathy (CRM) carries a poor prognosis due to the progressive neurologic decline and occurs with variable onsets from 1 month to 28 months post radiation. If no other cause is found for the myelopathic decline with no new MRI findings or a negative myelography, and a Brown Sequard syndrome is present, CRM may be the etiology (47,78–82).

Vague neurologic symptoms including muscle weakness, lethargy, hyporeflexia, progressive altered mentation, and seizures may be indicative of hypercalcemia. Hypercalcemia associated with cancer may be due to the malignancy or hormonal therapy. Hypercalcemia is the most common metabolic oncologic emergency and rapid identification is imperative. A prolonged condition may present with renal tubular abnormalities, cardiac arrhythmias, coma, and/or death. The mechanism is not completely understood but the tumor production of osteoclast activators such as parathyroid hormone (PTH) related protein (PTH-rP), osteolytic cytokines, and osteotrophic factors is proposed. Rapid evaluation involves serology, i.e. albumin-corrected calcium, PTH, PTH-rP, other appropriate chemistries, and an electrocardiogram. For mild conditions, intravenous (IV) normal saline to increase urinary calcium excretion is indicated. For moderate and severe cases, furosemide is added to the IV fluid administration to decrease renal absorption of calcium, along with continuous cardiac monitoring to assess for arrhythmias. A bisphosphonate such as pamidronate at doses of 60–90mg may be administered. Hormonal therapy and calcium supplements are withheld. A preventive rehabilitation strategy is mobility, to prevent osteolysis and therefore, reduce the risk for hypercalcemia (83–85).

Cardiovascular

With prescription writing, attention is given to the pertinent cardiac history, amount and location of radiation treatment, medications, and previous cardiac surgeries. Chemotherapeutic agents may cause cardiac side effects. A common late effect of doxorubicin, mitomycin C, vincristine, and etopside is cardiomyopathy. Possible late effects of plant derivatives and 5-fluorouracil are cardiac ischemia and infarction (47,48). Energy conservation techniques are taught to reduce the development of fatigue and complications. Cardiac complications from the carcinoma itself may occur. Pericardial effusions and subsequent cardiac tamponade from cardiac compression from large pericardial effusions may occur. Pericardium metastases may occur from extension or hematogenous spread, from lung or esophageal tumors. Malignant pericardial effusions are seen with lung, breast, lymphoma, leukemias, GI cancers, melanoma, and sarcomas. Overall, up to 20–30% of patients develop cardiac complications. The patient may present with dyspnea, cough, or retrosternal pain when supine and with symptoms relieved when they lean forward. Circulatory collapse may occur. Pericarditis and pericardial fibrosis may occur after radiation or chemotherapy (48,83,86).

Superior vena cava (SVC) syndrome is the compression of the SVC by adjacent masses. Obstruction produces pleural effusions and tachypnea, plethora of the face, cyanosis, and tracheal, arm, and facial edema. Severe cases produce cerebral edema and diminished cardiac function with subsequent neurologic changes. SVC syndrome in the cancer patient is caused most commonly by mediastinal tumors, i.e. small cell or squamous cell lung cancer. This is a medical emergency requiring airway protection and immediate consideration of chemotherapy or radiation (83).

Pulmonary

Components of pulmonary rehabilitation are indicated for reducing the cycle of dyspnea and deconditioning, the optimization of pulmonary toilet, respiratory secretion management, and evaluation for non-invasive ventilatory techniques. Pulmonary parameters such as vital capacity, peak cough flows, and oxygen saturation by pulse oximetry guide the patient's progress.

In addition to prolonged bedrest, the diminished pulmonary function may occur from specific cancer related conditions such as respiratory infections; radiation-induced pneumonitis or fibrotic changes; chemotherapy-induced pneumonitis, fibrosis, and pulmonary edema; diaphragmatic paralysis; or kyphoscoliosis from vertebral body destruction (47,48). Identification and management of these conditions emphasizes an initial order for low-level rehabilitation therapies with a gradual increase when tolerated.

When a patient develops kyphoscoliosis, a restrictive pattern of pulmonary impairment may occur. A spinal orthosis specific for the affected spinal levels is prescribed to maintain an upright posture for improved daily function, for patients with kyphoscoliosis and decreased pain (72). If the long term prognosis is favorable, surgical correction of the spinal deformity may be considered.

Gastrointestinal

Neurogenic bowel results from neural lesions at the spinal cord, parasympathetic system, and sympathetic chain. Neurogenic bowel program goals are to prevent GI complications, regulate bowel evacuation, and maintain social continence (87). Among cancer patients, GI complications may be more frequently encountered. Constipation and impaction are increased due to the frequent need for narcotic analgesic medications. Other risk factors include electrolyte abnormalities, immobility, and dietary and nutritional factors. Ileus may occur following spinal shock, post-surgery, radiation treatment, or pharmacologic side effects. Enteritis and obstruction may occur due to tumor involvement or radiation therapy (47,48). Bowel programs with digital stimulation can be instituted, but with attention to mucosal fragility (See chapter 10). The use of digital stimulation in a bowel program is not instituted among patients with neutropenia, or ostomies with non-functional rectal vaults.

Patients may have enteric gastrostomy tubes or ostomy sites. Therapy precautions are written for these sites. Unless a caregiver is present, the patient is trained to maintain these sites with the use of adaptive devices, if needed.

Genitourinary

Neurogenic bladder results from neural lesions of the spinal cord, somatic, parasympathetic system, and/ or sympathetic system. Neurogenic bladder program goals are to effectively drain the bladder, maintain adequate bladder pressures to prevent reflux, maintain social continence, and to decrease risk of renal disease and infections with approaches such as timed voids, intermittent catheterization, or indwelling catheters, with attention to mucosal fragility. Among GU cancer patients, modes of bladder drainage may be indicated such as suprapubic tubes. Training for the patient or caregiver is performed. Nephrotoxicity may occur and present as renal insufficiency or renal failure with hypertension. This is due to damage of tubular cells from chemo-

therapy or endothelial cell damage due to radiation. The patient is managed accordingly with diet adjustments, antihypertensive medication, and supplementation. When severe renal failure occurs, patients may eventually undergo dialysis and, later, possibly renal transplantation (47,48). Rehabilitation may be performed with added precautions for blood pressure parameters and for dialysis arteriovenous fistulas, ports, and surgical sites.

Musculoskeletal

If vertebral bodies are involved, both plain x-rays and a MRI are obtained in the initial evaluation as baseline studies. Follow-up evaluations include both clinical and plain radiographic exams. If the condition worsens, a MRI is warranted. Vertebral body compression fractures may be treated with a spinal orthosis if the area is stable, with a retained vertebral body height > 50% and with no neurologic symptoms (72). Prior to instituting therapies, the clinician may assess sites of other known or suspected bony metastases with radiological studies. The humerus and femur are the most frequent long bone sites. Bony weakness due to pathologic changes or osteoporosis is noted. Avoidance of aggressive exercise, passive range of motion (ROM), active assisted ROM, and weight bearing activities over those affected areas with cortex involvement of >50% are considered. However, gentle active ROM may be performed in those affected areas with cortex involvement of <50%. Range of motion, weight-bearing activities, stretching exercises, and functional activities may be tolerated over stable affected areas with cortex involvement <25%. With an exercise prescription, it is important to monitor cortical bone involvement and stability of the affected bony areas, and the aggressiveness and natural history of the tumor. A consideration of early surgical referral for metastatic lesions in functionally active limbs may be indicated. This is elucidated by the example of the benefit with prophylactic stabilization for humeral metastases in a paraplegic patient using the upper extremities for mobility and weight bearing activities. Also, osteoporosis identification and management is instituted (40,88).

Skin

Increased skin fragility is seen following radiation treatment, and, therefore, special attention is given over the radiated areas. Pressure sore prevention is performed with daily skin checks, weight shifts when sitting, and every 2–3 hour turns when in the supine position. Nutrition plays a significant role in maintaining the integrity of the skin. The rehabilitation team assesses for the appropriate bed, wheelchair cushion, and transfer training technique.

Lymphedema is a common condition. The etiology of the lymphedema is evaluated before treatment. If an etiology such as venous thrombosis, tumor bulk causing impairment of lymphatic drainage, or infection is detected, appropriate medical intervention is indicated. For residual lymphedema where there is no further evaluation indicated, the goal is the reduction of lymphedema to improve functional mobility, skin care, quality of life, and cosmesis. This is managed with mechanisms that mobilize and promote lymphatic and vascular circulation such as decongestive lymphatic therapy, elastic stockings, ace wraps, and pressure garments (75,89).

Hematologic Issues

For anemia, in symptomatic cases or when the hemoglobin is less than 8g/dL, transfusion is considered to improve exercise tolerance, unless otherwise contraindicated. When transfusion is indicated, premedication, and irradiated and/or leukocyte poor filters are utilized accordingly. For thrombocytopenia, there are proposed exercise guidelines; for example, for a platelet count of <20,000 per microliter, no exercise is recommended, for platelet count of 25,000–50,000 per microliter, exercise may be modified with no heavy resistive activities or prolonged stretching. For platelet count of >50,000 per microliter, the program is modified to the patient's toleration (88).

Pharmacologic DVT prophylaxis is indicated. However, the duration of deep vein thrombosis (DVT) prophylaxis remains controversial. Due to a possible prolonged hypercoagulable state, patients may require prolonged anticoagulation. Inferior vena caval filters are considered depending on patient prognosis.

Nutrition

Dysphagia is a common symptom and hinders oral feedings. This may result from tumor involvement, esophageal dysfunction and mucosal damage due to infection, anterior approach in cervical spine surgery, chemotherapy effects, radiation treatment effects, fibrosis, and stricture due to radiation treatment (47). A swallowing evaluation performed at the bedside, by videofluoroscopy, or by direct fiberoptic visualization ascertains the presence of aspiration with oral feeds, and subsequently, the appropriate food consistency. Cachexia is a frequent complication of the cancer and its treatment. Nutritional feedings should be optimized with supplementation by nasogastric tube, enteral feeding, or parenteral route. The use of the gut with enteral feedings is preferable to parenteral nutrition. Calorie counts and nutritional labs are monitored. Other supplements to consider are appetite stimulants including progestational agents, such as megestrol acetate or an anabolic steroid such as oxandrolone. Patient or caregiver training is performed for the use of feeding devices (75).

Sexual Dysfunction

Sexual dysfunction management is complex involving the psychosocial and medical impact of spinal cord dysfunction, cancer, cancer treatments, neurologic damage, and general functional condition. The goals of intimacy and family among cancer survivors with sexual dysfunction should be addressed. When the patient is medically stable and prepared to address these issues, the clinician reviews with the patient available options in medical intervention, counseling, and marital therapy (85).

Psychologic

Patients with cancer and spinal cord dysfunction have evidently two major medical conditions to adjust to. Psychologic assessment and strategies are made for adjustment counseling and strategies for coping with their medical conditions and level of function. Social integration is facilitated through the involvement of the patient's own social support system with the rehabilitation team, as well as, formal support groups such as education groups, behavior training groups, and support groups for cancer patients or spinal cord injury patients. Clinicians should monitor for symptoms of depression. Exercise and rehabilitation therapies have added benefit to improve mood disturbances and perceived quality of life (1,75).

Mobility

Mobility allows for independence, performance of daily function, improved mental health, and avoidance of complications of immobility such as decreased skin integrity, physical deconditioning, hypercalcemia, precipitation of osteoporosis, and diminished pulmonary function (84,90,91). Mobility training is instituted with transfers, bed mobility, and regular weight shifts to prevent skin breakdown. If the patient is ambulatory, an assistive device such as a walker, cane, or crutches are tried. Fall prevention techniques such as balance, optimal body mechanics, and environmental modification are important to teach patients and care givers. Wheelchair mobility facilitates ambulatory patients for community distances, as well as, for non-ambulatory patients. Power and manual wheelchair training is essential for the appropriate patient. Seating systems may require custom molding.

Goals with those for specific neurologic levels are similar to that noted in chapter 19. Unlike the patient who suffered a traumatic SCI, the patient with tumor related spinal cord dysfunction may be more limited by fatigue and underlying medical issues. Therefore, the use of a power wheelchair may become more useful for those patients.

Vocational Rehabilitation

A patient's goal to return to school, work, or productive avocations is facilitated for the cancer survivors. Vocational rehabilitation ultimately re-integrates cancer survivors back into the workforce. Computer access programs and ergonomic restructuring of the home and work place allow patients to become more independent.

DIFFERENCES FROM TRAUMATIC SPINAL CORD INJURY

Patients following a non-traumatic spinal cord dysfunction carry a different patient profile. Non-traumatic injured patients are more commonly in an older age group and include a higher percentage of women. They are also more commonly married and retired from work. There is a higher percentage of motor incomplete injury and paraplegia. The length of stay in an acute rehabilitation unit varies, but is notably shorter. This may reflect the differences in the patterns of neurologic recovery with the bias towards early discharge in patients with terminal cancer.

Additionally, prognostic indicators for neurologic recovery such as the ASIA exam is not as useful, possibly due to the nature of the lesion, the patient's general medical condition, and the duration and extent of neurological damage by the neoplastic lesion (92).

REHABILITATION OUTCOMES

Cancer rehabilitation is well established (74,89). However, there are few small studies providing outcome data for tumor related spinal cord dysfunction (93). Overall survival of patients with tumor related SCC depends on the natural history of the cancer and the patient's medical condition. Patients may survive a year or more following spinal cord compression (18). Hacking et al, surmised from a 1993 study that there are 6 prognostic indicators for survival greater than one year after discharge. These included tumor biology, spinal cord dysfunction as the presenting symptom, slow progression of symptoms, tumor treated with combination surgery and radiation therapy, partial bowel control upon admission, and partial independence with transfers upon admission. Each indicator is worth 1 point; the greater the number of points, the greater the individual's chances are of survival past one year. Therefore, a score of 5–6 had a 77% chance of survival. These findings, however, are controversial (21).

Ambulation following spinal cord compression is most notably dependent on the degree of ambulation on initial presentation. Reports of 58–100% of patients who were ambulatory upon initial presentation, were ambulatory post-treatment, whereas in those who presented with paraplegia, ambulation post treatment was seen in 0–25% of patients (18,94). Therefore, it is important to identify the signs and symptoms of SCC early and initiate treatment accordingly, in order to optimize neurologic recovery.

There are a few studies on the functional outcome of rehabilitation for patients with SCC. McKinley et al, in 1996, performed a prospective survey of patients diagnosed with SCC and discharged from acute in-patient rehabilitation. FIM scores were utilized to determine functional gains at the time of rehabilitation discharge. Statistically significant functional improvements were noted in self-care and mobility, with 22–72% improvement. Improvement in quality of life was noted up to 3 months after discharge (95).

REFERENCES

1. Constans, JP, de Divitiis, E, Donzelli, R, et al. Spinal metastases with neurological manifestations. *J Neurosurgery* 1983;59:111–118.
2. Black P. Spinal Metastasis: Current Status and Recommended Guidelines for Management. *Neurosurgery* 1979;5(6);726–746.
3. Posner JB. Spinal Metastases. In: Davis,FA, ed. *Neurological Complications of Cancer (Contemporary Neurological Series 45).* Philadelphia, 1995;111–141.
4. Abrahm, JL. Management of Pain and Spinal Cord Compression. In: *Patients with Advanced Cancer* ACP-ASIM End of Life Care Consensus Panel. *Ann Intern Med* 1999;131:37–46.
5. Stark RJ, Henson RA, Evans SJ. Spinal metastases: a retrospective survey from a general hospital. *Brain* 1982;105:189.
6. Bach F, Larsen BH, Rohde K, et al. Metastatic spinal cord compression: occurrence, symptoms, clinical presentations, and prognosis in 398 patients with spinal cord compression. *Acta Neurochir* 1990;107:37-43.
7. Posner JB. Back Pain and Epidural Spinal Cord Compression. *Med. Clin N Am* 1987;71(2):185–204.
8. Byrne TN. Spinal Cord Compression from Epidural Metastases. *N Eng J Med* 1992;327:614–619.
9. Greenberg MS. *Handbook of Neurosurgery, 3rd Ed.* Greenberg Graphics, Florida, 1994.
10. Osborn AG. *Diagnostic Neuroradiology* Mosby, New York, 1994.
11. Levin VA, Leibel SA, Gutin PH. Neoplasms of the Central Nervous System. In: Vincent T. Devita,VT, Jr., Hellman, S, eds. *Cancer: Principles & Practice of Oncology 6th Ed.* Lippincott Williams & Wilkins, Philadelphia, 2001;2100–2160.
12. Arguello F, Baggs RB, Duerst RE, et al. Pathogenesis of Vertebral Metastasis and Epidural Spinal Cord Compression. *Cancer* 1990;65:98–106.
13. Fuller BC, Heiss J, Oldfield EH, Spinal Cord Compression. In: Devita, VT Jr, Hellman, S, Rosenberg, SA, eds. *Cancer Principles & Practice of Oncology, 6th Ed.* Lippincott-Raven, Philadelphia, 2001:2617–2633.
14. Aprin H. Primary Malignant Tumors of the Spine. *Spine: State of the Art Reviews* 1988;2:289–297
15. Merenda JT. Other Primary Benign Tumors and Tumor-like Lesions of the Spine. *Spine: State of the Arts Reviews* 1988;2(2);275–286.
16. American Cancer Society. Cancer Statistics 2000. *CA-a Cancer Journal for Clinicians* 2000;50:6–16
17. Sioutos PJ, Arbit E, Meshulam CF, et al. Spinal Metastases from Solid Tumors. *Cancer* 1995;76:1453–9.
18. Gilbert RW, Kim JH, Posner, JB. Epidural spinal cord compression from metastatic tumor: Diagnosis and Treatment. *Ann Neurol* 1978;3:40–51.
19. Greenberg HS, Kim J, Posner JB. Epidural Spinal Cord Compression from Metastatic Tumor: Results with a New Treatment Protocol. *Ann Neurol* 1980;8:361–366.
20. Rodichok LD, Harper GR, Ruckdeschel JC, et al. Early Diagnosis of Spinal Epidural Metastases. *Am J Med* 1981;70:1181–1188.
21. Hacking HG, Van As HH, Lankhorst GJ. Factors related to the outcome of inpatient rehabilitation in patients with neoplastic epidural spinal cord compression. *Paraplegia* 1993;31:367–374.
22. Thapar K, Laws ER, Jr. Tumors in the CNS in American Cancer Society. In: ACS, eds. *Textbook of Clinical Oncology, 2nd Ed.* Atlanta, Georgia. 1995:378–410.
23. Schwartz TH, McCormick PC. Intramedullary ependymomas: clinical presentation, surgical treatment strategies, and prognosis. *J Neurooncol* 2000;47:211–218.
24. Edelson RN, Deck MD, Posner JB. Intramedullary spinal cord metastases. Clinical and radiographic findings in nine cases. *Neurology* 1972; 22:1222–1231.
25. Murphy KC, Field R, Evans WK. Intramedullary Spinal Cord Metastases from Small Cell Carcinoma of the Lung. *J Clin Onc* 1983;1:99–106.
26. Willis RA. Secondary tumors of bone. In: *The Blood Supply of Bone: An Approach to Bone Biology.* Butterworth, London, 1971:67–91.
27. Coman DR, DeLong RP. The Role of the Vertebral Venous System in the Metastasis of Cancer to the Spinal Column. *Cancer* 1951:610–618.
28. Lam WC, Delikatny EJ, Orr FW, et al. The Chemotactic Response of Tumor Cells. A model of cancer metastasis. *Am J Pathology* 1981; 104:69–76.
29. Ushio Y, Posner R, Posner JB, et al. Experimental Spinal Cord Compression by Epidural Neoplasms. *Neurology* 1977;27:422–429.
30. Siegal T, Siegal T, Shapira Y, et al. Indomethacin and dexamethasone treatment in experimental spinal cord compression. Part l: effect on water content and specific gravity. *Neurosurgery* 1988;22:328–333.
31. Siegel T, Shohami E, Shapira Y, et al. Indomethacin and dexamethasone treatment in experimental spinal cord compression. Part ll.: effect on edema and prostaglandins synthesis. *Neurosurgery* 1988;22: 334–339.
32. Salmon JM, Kilpatrick SE. Pathology of Skeletal Metastases. *Orthopedic Clinics of North Am* 2000;31:537–543.
33. Tarlov IM, Klinger H. Spinal cord compression studies. Time limits

for recovery after acute compression in dogs. *Arch Neurol Psychiatry* 1954;71:271

34. Tarlov IM. Spinal cord compression studies. Time limits for recovery after gradual compression in dogs. *Arch Neurol Psychiatry* 1954;71:588.

35. Nicholas JJ, Christy WC. Spinal pain made worse by recumbency: A clue to spinal cord tumors. *Arch Phys Med Rehabil* 1986;67:598–600.

36. Harrington KD. Current Concepts Review: Metastatic Disease of the Spine. *J Bone Joint Surg* 1968;68:1110–1115.

37. Swenson R. Differential Diagnosis: A Reasonable Clinical Approach in Neuro. *Clin N Am* 1999;17:43-63.

38. NIH Panel, NIH Clinical Practice Guidelines for Acute Low Back Problems in Adults *AHCPR Pub* 1994;95-0642:14.

39. Perrin RG, McBroom RJ, Perrin RG. Metastatic Tumors of the Cervical Spine. In: Congress of Neurological Surgeons, eds. *Clinical Neurosurgery* Williams & Wilkins, Baltimore, 1989:740–755.

40. Bibbo C. Perioperative Considerations in Patients with Metastatic Bone Disease. *Orthop Clin N Am* 2000;31:577–621.

41. Watt I, Cobby, M. Tumors and Tumor-like Conditions of Bone. In: Sutton, D *Textbook of Radiology and Imaging, 6th Ed.* Churchill Livingston, New York, 1998.

42. Gates GF. SPECT bone scanning of the spine. *Seminars in Nuclear Medicine* 1998;28:78–94.

43. McCarthy EF. Histopathologic Correlates of a Positive Bone Scan. *Seminars in Nuclear Medicine* 1997;27:309–320.

44. Li KC, Poon PY. Sensitivity and specificity of MRI in detecting malignant spinal cord compression and in distinguishing malignant from benign compression fractures of vertebrae. *Magn Reson Imaging* 1988;6:547–556.

45. Valk J. GD-DPTA in MR of spinal lesions. *AJNR* 1988;9:345–350.

46. Graus F, Krol G, Foley KM. Early diagnosis of spinal epidural metastases (SEM): Correlation with clinical and radiological findings. *Abstract in Proceedings American Society of Clinical Oncology* 1985;4:269.

47. Rubin P, Constine LS, Williams JP. Late Effects of Cancer Treatment: Radiation and Drug Toxicity. In: Perez, CA; Brady, LW, eds. *Principles and Practice of Radiation Oncology, 3rd.* Lippincott-Raven Publishing, Philadelphia,1997:155–211.

48. John, M J. Radiotherapy and Chemotherapy. In: Legible, SA, Phillips, TL , eds. *Textbook of radiation oncology, 1st Ed.* WB Saunders, Philadelphia; 1998.

49. Caspar W, Pitzen T, Papavero L, Geisler FH, Johnson TA. Anterior cervical plating for the treatment of neoplasms in the cervical vertebrae. *J Neurosurgery (Spine I)* 1999;90:27–34

50. Jackson RJ, Glokaslan ZL, Loh SCA. Metastatic renal cell carcinoma of the spine: Surgical treatment and results. *J Neurosurgery (Spine I)* 2001;94:18–24

51. Fyfe I, Henry A, Mulholland R. Closed vertebral biopsy. *J Bone Joint Surgery [Br]* 1983;65:140–143

52. Dewald RL, Bridwell KH, Prodromas C, et al. Reconstructive spinal surgery as palliation for metastatic malignancies of the spine. *Spine* 1985;10:21–26

53. Sundaresan N, Galicich JH. Treatment of spinal metastases by vertebral body resection. *Cancer Invest* 1984;2:383–397

54. Saunders RL, Pikus HJ, Ball P. Four-level cervical corpectomy. *Spine* 1998;23:2455–2461

55. Sundaresan N, Galicich JH, Lane JM, et al. Treatment of neoplastic epidural cord compression by vertebral body resection and stabilization. *J Neurosurgery* 1985;63:676–684

56. Pelker RR, Friedlaender GE. Biomechanical aspects of bone autografts and allografts. *Orthop Clin North Am* 1987;18:235–239

57. Dunn EJ. The role of methylmethacrylate in the stabilization and replacement of tumors of the cervical spine. *Spine* 1977;2:16–46

58. Miller DJ, Lang FF, Walsh GL, et al. Coaxial double-lumen methylmethacrylate reconstruction in the anterior cervical and upper thoracic spine after tumor resection. *J Neurosurgery (Spine 2)* 2000;92:181–190

59. Caspar W. Anterior Stabilization with the trapezial osteosynthetic plate technique. In: Kehr P, Weidner A, eds. *Cervical Spine I.* Springer Verlag, New York, 1987:198–204

60. Cahill DW, Kumar R. Palliative subtotal vertebrectomy with anterior and posterior reconstruction via a single posterior approach. *J Neurosurgery (Spine I)* 1999;90:42–47

61. Boockvar JA, Philips MF, Telfeian AE, et al. Results and risk factors for anterior cervicothoracic junction surgery. *J Neurosurgery (Spine 1)* 2001;94:12–17

62. Larson SJ, Holst RA, Hemmy DC, et al. Lateral extracavitary approach to traumatic lesions of the thoracic and lumbar spine. *J Neurosurgery* 1976;45:628–637

63. Heary RF, Vaccaro AR, Benevenia J, et al. "En Bloc" vertebrectomy in the mobile lumbar spine. *Surg Neurol* 1998;50:548–556

64. McCormick PC, Post KD, Stein BM. Intradural extramedullary Tumors in Adults. *Neurosurgery Clin North Am* 1990;1:591–608

65. McCormick PC, Stein BM. Intramedullary Tumors in Adults. *Neurosurgery Clin North Am* 1990;1:609–630

66. Hoshmaru M, Koyama T, Hashimoto N, et al. Results of Microsurgical Treatment for Intramedullary Spinal Cord Ependymomas: Analysis of 36 cases. *Neurosurgery* 1999;44:264–269

67. Constantini S, Miller DC, Allen JC, et al. Radical Excision of Intramedullary Spinal Cord Tumors: Surgical Morbidity and Long-term follow-up evaluation in 164 children and young adults. *J. Neurosurgery (Spine 2)* 2000;93:183–193

68. Epstein FJ, Farmer JD, Freed D. Adult Intramedullary Spinal Cord Ependymomas: The result of surgery in 38 patients. *J Neurosurgery* 1993;79:204–209

69. Cooper PR. Outcome after Operative Treatment of Intramedullary Spinal Cord Tumors in Adults: Intermediate and Long-term Results in 51 Patients. *Neurosurgery* 1989;25:855–859

70. Yasuoka S, Peterson HA, McCarthy CS. Incidence of spinal column deformity after multilevel laminectomy in children and adults. *J Neurosurgery* 1982;57:441–445

71. Klekamp J, Samii M. Sugery of spinal nerve sheath tumors with special references to neurofibromatosis. *Neurosurgery* 1998;42:279–290

72. Benzel EC. Spinal Orthotics. In *Biomechanics of Spine Stabilization: Principles & Clinical Practice.* McGraw-Hill; New York, 1995:247–258.

73. Koch R, Nickel V. The halo vest. An evaluation of motion and forces acrosss the neck. *Spine* 1978;3:103–107

74. O'toole DM, Golden AM. Evaluating Cancer Patients for Rehabilitation Potential. *West J Med* 1991;155:384–387.

75. McKenna RJ, Wellisch D, Fawzy FI. Rehabilitation and Supportive Care of the Cancer Patient. In: *American Cancer Society: Textbook of Clinical Oncology; 2nd Ed.* ACS, Atlanta. 1995:639–650.

76. Galasko CSB. Spinal Instability Secondary to Metastatic Cancer. *J Bone Joint Surg* 1991;73-B:104–108.

77. Chad DA, Recht LD. Neuromuscular Complications of Systemic Cancer. *Neurol Clin* 1991;9(4):901-918.

78. Garden FH. Radiation Injury to the Spinal Cord and Peripheral Nerves. In: PM&R: State of the Art Reviews *Rehabilitation.* Hanley & Belfus, Philadelphia, 1994;8(2):405–411.

79. Kelly JJ, Jr, Kyle RA, Miles JM, et al. Spectrum of peripheral neuropathy in myeloma. *Neurology* 1981;31:24–31.

80. Krendel DA, Stahl RL, Chan WC. Lymphomatous polyneuropathy. Biopsy of clinically involved nerve and successful treatment. *Arch Neurol* 1991;48:330–332

81. Lecky BR, Murray NM, Berry RJ. Transient radiation myelopathy: Spinal Somatosensory evoked response following incidental cord exposure during radiotherapy. *J Neurol Neurosurg Psych* 1980;43:747–750.

82. Cascino TL. Radiation Myelopathy. In: Rottenberg, DA, ed. *Neurological Complications of Cancer Treatment.* Butterworth-Heinemann, Boston, 1991:69–78.

83. Glick, JH, Glover, D. Oncologic Emergencies. In: *American Cancer Society: Textbook of Clinical Oncology, 2nd Ed.* ACS, Atlanta, 1995:597–618.

84. Ralston SH, Boyce BF, Cowan RA, et al. Contrasting mechanisms of hypercalcemia in patients with early and advanced humoral hypercalcemia of malignancy. *J Bone Miner Res* 1989;4:103–111.

85. Gucalp R, Theriault R, Gill I, et al. Treatment of cancer-associated hypercalcemia. Double-blind comparison of rapid and slow intravenous infusion regimens of pamidronate disodium and saline alone. *Arch Intern Med* 1994;154:1935–1944.

86. Theologides A. Neoplastic cardiac tamponade. *Semin Oncol* 1978;5:181–192.

87. Consortium for Spinal Cord Medicine. Clinical Practice Guidelines

for Spinal Cord Medicine: Neurogenic Bowel Management in Adults with SCI. *Paralyzed Veterans of America* 1998.

88. Hicks JE. Exercise for Cancer Patients. In: Basmajian, JV, Wolf SL, eds. *Therapeutic Exercise; 5th Ed*. Williams & Wilkins, Baltimore, 1990: 359.

89. Yoshioka H. Rehabilitation for the Terminal Cancer Patient. *Am J Phys Med Rehabil* 1994;7:199–206.

90. Kurtz JC, Given CW. The interaction of age, symptoms, and survival status on physical and mental health of patients with cancer and their families. *Cancer* 1994;74(7 Suppl):2071–2078.

91. Steinberg FU. *The immobilized patient: functional pathology and management*. Plenum, New York, 1980.

92. McKinley WO, Huang ME, Brunsvold KT. et al. Traumatic Spinal Cord Injury: An Outcome Comparison after Inpatient Rehabilitation. *Arch Phys Med Rehabil* 1999;80:1253–1257.

93. Murray PK. Functional Outcome and Survival in Spinal Cord Injury Secondary to Neoplasia. *Cancer* 1985;55:197–201.

94. McKinley WO. Nontraumatic Spinal Cord Injury: Incidence, Epidemiology, and Functional Outcome. *Arch Phys Med Rehabil* 1999;80: 619–623.

95. McKinley WO, Conti-Wyneken AR, Vokac CW, et al. Rehabilitative Functional Outcome of Patients with Neoplastic Spinal Cord Compression. *Arch Phys Med Rehabil* 1996;77:892–895.

INFECTIONS OF THE SPINE AND SPINAL CORD

SUSAN V. GARSTANG

Spinal infections were first noted in the historical record dating back to 400 BC when Hippocrates described the symptoms of tuberculous spondylitis (1). "Pott's paraplegia" was described by Sir Percivall Pott in the eighteenth century. In the early 1900s, surgical techniques for spinal infections were developed. The treatment of spinal infections advanced greatly in the 1940s, with the introduction of antibiotics. However, infections of the spine, spinal canal, and spinal cord remain an important topic due to the potentially high morbidity these infections can cause.

This chapter reviews the topic of infections of the spinal cord, and infections of the spine and surrounding structures that can directly or indirectly cause damage to the spinal cord with subsequent neurologic compromise. The most common etiologies are discussed in depth, and brief mention is made of more-uncommon etiologies.

Infections of the spine can be classified in several ways: pathogenesis, chronicity of infection, extent or type of involvement, and host characteristics. Different types of infections are characterized by certain patterns of involvement, which vary depending on the pathogen, host, and location of infection. The simplest way to unify the topic of spinal infections is to discuss them by anatomic location. Calderone and Larsen proposed the following classification scheme for regions of the spine and spinal canal that can be involved in infections (2). These include infections of the posterior spine, anterior spine, the spinal canal, and the spinal cord (Table 32.1). Infections of the posterior spine are typically an acute or chronic postoperative infection and usually do not lead to myelopathy, so these are not discussed further in this chapter (1).

INFECTIONS OF THE ANTERIOR SPINE

Vertebral Osteomyelitis and Discitis

There are multiple terms in the literature used to describe infections of the vertebral body, including vertebral osteomyelitis, pyogenic vertebral osteomyelitis, adult discitis, septic discitis, and spondylitis. Involvement of the intervertebral disk is common, because of the anatomic relationship between the disk and vertebral body; thus, discitis often coexists with vertebral osteomyelitis. This has led to the term *spondylodiscitis*. Vertebral osteomyelitis accounts for 2% to 4% of all cases of pyogenic osteomyelitis (3).

Infections of the vertebral body and intervertebral disk are typically either hematogenous in nature or secondary to a contiguous focus of infection (4). These infections can be classified based on pathogenesis, chronicity (acute or chronic, with acute infections heralded by recent onset of bone pain and fever, typically occurring after an episode of bacteremia), and host characteristics. Host characteristics include the presence of underlying disease and local factors such as lymphedema, blood supply, venous stasis, and extent of viable tissue (4).

Hematogenous osteomyelitis is usually found in children or the elderly. When found in young adults, hematogenous osteomyelitis is typically caused by intravenous drug use and is found in patients with implanted vascular catheters or sickle cell disease (4). The etiology of discitis in children is thought to relate in part to the relatively preserved vascularity of the disk (compared with adults), allowing increased spread of bacteria (5). Discitis commonly occurs in children because of the immature circulation pattern of the disk. Patients at risk for the development of pyogenic spinal infection include those with advanced age, diabetes, immunocompromising conditions, long-term steroid therapy, and chronic ethanol use (6). In adults, hematogenous vertebral osteomyelitis has been associated with infections of the genitourinary (GU) tract, soft tissue, and respiratory tract. In addition, certain events such as a recent GU procedure, penetrating trauma, or invasive procedures increase the risk of developing spinal infections. Discitis has also been reported after penetrating trauma or invasive spinal procedures including surgery (1,3). In adults, iatrogenic discitis involving adjacent endplates can occur as a postoperative infection after discectomy (2).

Possible sources of osteomyelitis from a contiguous locus of infection include an open fracture, puncture wound or other penetrating trauma, surgical procedure such as a median sternotomy, or extension of a soft tissue, dental, or sinus infection (4).

Etiology

The etiology of vertebral body and disk-space involvement has been studied extensively. Batson paravertebral plexus has been implicated in the spread from pelvic and GU sources; however, Wiley and Trueta (7) showed that the paravertebral venous plexus fills only under pressure and is an unlikely source of

TABLE 32.1. CLASSIFICATION OF INFECTIONS BASED ON REGION INVOLVED

	Anatomic Location	Most Common Etiology
Infections of the posterior spine	The posterior elements and the subcutaneous and subfascial spaces	1. Usually postoperative
Infections of the anterior spine	Vertebral body, intervertebral disk, and the paravertebral space	1. Osteomyelitis and discitis 2. Tuberculosis of the spine
Infections of the spinal canal	Epidural space, meninges, and subdural space	1. Epidural abscess 2. Arachnoiditis
Infections of the spinal cord	The spinal cord itself	1. Intramedullary spinal cord abscess 2. Transverse myelitis 3. Spinal cord involvement in human immunodeficiency virus 4. Human T-cell lymphotrophic virus type 1–associated myelopathy 5. Other infectious etiologies

spread of infection. They also found that there is a rich arterial network supplying the vertebral body metaphysis and the periphery of the disk, filled from the ascending and descending nutrient branches of the posterior spinal arteries (8). Hematogenous spread is thought to occur through this arterial network.

Staphylococcus aureus is the most common pathogen in pyogenic vertebral osteomyelitis, accounting for more than 55% of all reported cases (2,9). *Staphylococcus epidermidis* is also a very common source of vertebral infection (10). Gram-negative bacilli, including *Escherichia coli, Proteus mirabilis,* enterococci, and other bowel flora are common in postoperative and immunocompromised patients and can also be seen from a urinary tract source. *Pseudomonas aeruginosa* infection is more common in users of intravenous drugs.

Clinical Presentation

The clinical presentation of spinal infections varies depending on the virulence of the organism and host characteristics, which determine the chronicity of the disease (1,2). The cardinal presenting feature in adult patients with vertebral osteomyelitis is back pain, seen in 90% of patients (6,11). Fever is not always present and is seen in 50% of patients (4,11). Patients may have tenderness to percussion over the involved vertebrae. If there is extension of infection into the soft tissue, there may be an area of swelling (paraspinal abscess). Delays in diagnosis are common, with reports of patients having symptoms for more than 3 months before the diagnosis is made (11).

Vertebral osteomyelitis occurs in the lumber spine in nearly half of cases. The cervical spine is a common site of involvement in intravenous drug abusers, whereas the thoracic spine is the site of frequent involvement in patients with tuberculous osteomyelitis (3).

Neurologic deficits in patients with vertebral osteomyelitis typically develop as a consequence of a spinal epidural abscess. Most of these purulent collections occur anteriorly, because they originate from the disk space or posterior aspect of the vertebral body. Patients with rheumatoid arthritis, diabetes, advanced age, those on systemic steroids, or those with *S. aureus* infection are at risk for paralysis (3).

Laboratory Findings

Leukocytosis is present in approximately 40% of patients with vertebral osteomyelitis (6,12). An elevated erythrocyte sedimentation rate (ESR) is nonspecific but appears to be the most frequent laboratory abnormality. An elevated C-reactive protein level can also be an accurate indicator of disease (6). The ESR has also been shown to be a good measure of treatment success, with a decrease to two thirds of the original value being indicative of treatment response (11). In patients with an epidural abscess as well as vertebral osteomyelitis, the ESR was elevated in 100%, whereas the leukocyte count was elevated in 90% (12). In postsurgical patients, the ESR typically is elevated, peaking on the fourth to sixth postoperative day and normalizing within the first 2 weeks. In cases of vertebral osteomyelitis or discitis after surgery, the ESR will rise 80% to 90% higher than in normal noninfected postoperative cases (13).

Blood or tissue cultures are useful in establishing a microbiologic diagnosis. Blood cultures are positive in half of all cases of vertebral osteomyelitis (14). Needle biopsy or open surgical biopsy may be necessary to establish the causative organism.

Imaging

Pyogenic infections typically originate in the subchondral bone adjacent to the vertebral endplates and invade the disk from there. By the time the diagnosis is made, typically, there is a loss of disk height and endplate destruction. It can take up to 8 weeks for plain radiographs to detect signs of infection as evidenced by bone destruction (15). Decreased disk height and irregularity of the vertebral endplate are the first abnormalities seen on x-ray. Then there can be widening of the paravertebral space because of the expansion of the inflammatory process outside the disk, causing displacement of the paravertebral line on routine frontal radiographs. Typically, at 8 to 12 weeks, bone regeneration occurs, with visible sclerosis seen on radiographs. Brucellosis has a specific affinity for the anteroinferior vertebral endplate, particularly L4. Localized bone sclerosis, with or without a "parrot's beak" osteophyte, is often seen and should suggest this organism.

Radionuclide imaging study results with technetium-99 compounds will be abnormal in spinal infections well before bone destruction becomes obvious on plain films. An abnormal scan is not specific for infection, because any process involving bone turnover will take up isotope. Gallium or indium scans can be used to assist in difficult diagnoses.

Computed tomography (CT) scanning will reveal areas of bony destruction (endplate erosion) before these are seen on plain film (16). Areas of epidural and paravertebral infection are more easily seen on CT than on plain films.

Magnetic resonance imaging (MRI) with gadolinium is the gold standard in the evaluation of disk-space infection and osteomyelitis of the spine. Early MRI abnormalities are caused when edema and inflammatory cells infiltrate the vertebral body and disk. The marrow will appear dark on T1-weighted images and bright on T2-weighted images. T1-weighted scans with gadolinium contrast agents may show enhancement at the endplate–disk interface fairly early in the course of the infection. Inflammatory tissue and abscess can also be delineated with gadolinium (17). MRI changes seen in degenerative and inflammatory processes (such as rheumatoid arthritis) must be differentiated from infection.

Treatment

Treatment modalities for spondylodiscitis, discitis, and pyogenic facet arthropathy include a combination of antibiotics, percutaneous drainage (if indicated), and surgical intervention. The location of the infection, amount of bony destruction, and presence of neurologic deficits determine the type of treatment indicated. Treatment will usually produce fusion across the disk space, although total vertebral collapse can occur if there is no therapeutic intervention.

Antibiotics, spinal immobilization, and early ambulation have been shown to be effective in approximately three fourths of patients with vertebral osteomyelitis (3). Patients who are younger than 60 years with a healthy immune system and a declining ESR can be expected to do well with medical treatment. Pyogenic vertebral osteomyelitis requires 4 to 6 weeks of treatment with intravenous antibiotics, often followed by a prolonged oral course. Reduction in the ESR can be used to guide the duration of therapy (4). Initial empirical antibiotics must be broad spectrum, with activity against both staphylococci and gram-negative organisms (9). Antibiotic choice is best made based on the results of culture, but if no culture is available, then vancomycin (to cover methicillin-resistant *S. aureus*), along with an aminoglycoside or third-generation cephalosporin, should be used (18).

Surgery is indicated for failure of antibiotic therapy, for resolution of symptomatic spinal cord compression or radicular neurologic deficit, for correction or prevention of deformity, and for management of severe persistent pain (3). Other indications for surgical drainage include extensive destruction of vertebral bodies with sequestra and abscess (4).

Performing a posterior decompression such as a laminectomy is not advised, because this can produce further instability with progression of deformity and possible subsequent neurologic deficit (3). If a posterior epidural abscess is present, posterior debridement may need to be performed, but in a staged manner, with posterior instrumentation and fusion being performed once active infection is resolved (to prevent infection of instrumentation).

Performing anterior decompression has been shown to produce better results when combined with bone grafting (3). In patients receiving a bone graft, fusion occurs sooner and in a higher proportion of patients. The subsequent degree of kyphosis that may develop is lessened if patients undergo bone grafting. If there are concerns of subsequent spinal stability, posterior or anterior instrumentation can be added (although concern about placing hardware in an actively infected region exists) (3).

Outcome

Factors that have been commonly associated with paralysis include increased age, *S. aureus* infection, cervical infection, associated rheumatoid arthritis or diabetes mellitus, and systemic steroids (19). Typically, neurologic deficits are associated with epidural granulation tissue or epidural abscess (primary or secondary) (12). Isolated nerve root deficits have a good prognosis, even without surgery. Patients with spinal cord compression need to undergo surgical decompression before irreversible cord damage occurs to improve outcome (19).

Persistent back pain and instability are common sequelae of spondylodiscitis. Of those treated surgically, 26% had disabling back pain, compared with 64% with back pain who were treated with antibiotics alone. Residual pain in nonsurgically treated patients often was attributable to kyphosis and pseudarthrosis (12). The importance of prompt diagnosis cannot be understated; if diagnosis is delayed, the disease may progress to paralysis.

Tuberculosis of the Spine

Sir Percivall Pott described spinal tuberculosis (TB) in 1779, including the classic pathologic findings and abscess drainage as treatment of the associated paraplegia. However, it was not until the 1940s, with the advent of antimicrobials, that TB could be treated. Pott disease is spinal involvement with TB. Once the spine is involved by TB, the incidence of neurologic involvement (also termed Pott paraplegia) ranges from 10% to 76% (20).

There are approximately 27,000 cases of TB reported annually in the United States. Currently, groups at high risk include those with acquired immunodeficiency syndrome (AIDS), homeless persons, recent immigrants, and drug/Ethanol (ETOH) abusers. The human immunodeficiency virus (HIV) pandemic has coincided with a sharp rise in the incidence of

TB in several developing countries; however, the association has not been clearly proven (21). HIV-positive patients have a higher rate of skeletal TB (60%), compared with HIV-negative patients (3% to 5%).

The skeleton is involved in 3% to 5% of all cases of TB, with 50% of cases of skeletal TB affecting the spine (21,22). The distribution is 5% to 12% cervical, 25% to 40% thoracic, 20% to 40% lumbar and lumbosacral, and 1% to 24% multifocal (21,22). The thoracic spine is typically the most common site of involvement in spinal TB (23–27).

Three patterns of involvement in spinal TB have been described: paradiscal, anterior, and central. The paradiscal lesion is the most common pattern in adults. In this pattern, the vertebral metaphysis is the primary infectious focus. The infection erodes through the endplate and involves the disk. Often two adjacent vertebral bodies will be involved with relative sparing of the disk; this is due to the affinity of *Mycobacterium tuberculosis* for well-oxygenated environments. Anterior lesions develop beneath the anterior longitudinal ligament and spread along several levels. Central lesions involve the entire vertebral body. The disks are only secondarily affected. Narrowing of disks seen on x-ray is due to the herniation through the weakened endplate, rather than due to disk disease (28). The average patient has two to three vertebrae involved, and there can be skip lesions in up to 10% of patients (in which the disk is uninvolved, but the surrounding two vertebrae are involved).

Etiology

TB is caused by *M. tuberculosis*. Typically, spinal TB usually develops via hematogenous spread from a pulmonary focus (21). In most cases, it results form reactivation of resting tubercle bacilli in quiescent lesions. Spinal TB begins with seeding of *M. tuberculosis* in the vertebral body. Abscesses are a common finding in spinal TB. On pathology, there is exudative granulation tissue with abscesses and caseating necrosis.

Clinical Presentation

Patients with spinal TB most commonly present with back pain (90% to 100%), which is often chronic in nature (present for more than 2 weeks) (23,29). However, patients may also present with weight loss (48% to 58%), fever (30% to 58%), kyphosis, and malaise. In those with neurologic involvement (23% to 76%), presenting signs and symptoms can include weakness, sensory loss, and bowel and bladder dysfunction (23). Symptom duration at diagnosis ranges from 2 weeks to several years (21).

Neurologic compromise can be from direct invasion of tissue or from external pressure on the nerves and spinal cord. Paraplegia is present in 11% to 27% of patients (20,21). Factors that have been shown to be associated with the development of paraplegia are a cold abscess or sequestrum in acute TB, and heavy scar tissue or bony deformity impinging on the cord in healed TB (20). Anterior compression of the spinal cord is more common because the vertebral bodies are typically involved. Neurologic involvement is more common in cervical and thoracic lesions (21).

Collapse of anterior spinal elements results in a kyphotic deformity. Lesions in the thoracic spine are more likely to become kyphotic than those in the lumber spine. The loss of a vertebral body may result in up to 35 degrees of kyphosis (30). The potential for collapse and prediction of subsequent deformity can be estimated fairly accurately based on the initial amount of loss of the vertebral body. The loss typically occurs over the first 18 months after treatment.

Direct neural compression from bony deformity is rare, although the term "late" Pott's paraplegia is used when patients with a history of TB present with neurologic decline.

This is often found to be from worsening kyphosis and spinal cord or nerve compression by a bony ridge. Reactivation of disease is an uncommon cause of late neurologic decline.

Laboratory Findings

Typically the ESR is elevated, and the white blood cell (WBC) count is usually within the reference range. Skin testing can be useful, but a negative skin test result does not rule out TB. Skin test results can be negative in up to 14%, and the ESR can be within the reference range in 10% of patients with spinal lesions (31).

Percutaneous needle biopsy (usually CT guided) is the definitive diagnostic test. To confirm the diagnosis of *M. tuberculosis*, one must obtain microbiologic evidence from cultures or histologic sections. However, due to the slow-growing nature of TB, and the fact that few organisms may be present in a spinal lesion, bacteriologic study results are not always positive.

Other laboratory tests such as antigen demonstration, serologic tests, and polymerase chain reaction (PCR) are useful, and PCR can even show discrete genetic mutations that correlate with antibiotic resistance (22).

Imaging

Plain radiographs should be performed but tend to underestimate bony involvement. Radiographic changes seen in TB spondylitis include disk-space narrowing, anterior wedging, and bone destruction (23). These early signs may not be seen for up to 8 weeks (32). CT scan can also be used to evaluate for bony destruction. Abscesses causing soft tissue swelling can sometimes be seen on plain radiographs, and calcium within the region is highly suggestive of TB (21).

Radionuclide study results are often negative but are highly sensitive (89% to 96%) (21). However, even when isotope scans are positive, they are not specific enough to allow a definite diagnosis of TB to be made. Patients with radiographically demonstrable lesions can have a negative bone scan (up to 35% of patients), and there is a high false-negative rate with gallium scans (up to 70%) (25,33).

MRI with gadolinium is the imaging modality of choice, because it can delineate the amount of bony destruction and discriminate abscess from granulation tissue (32). MRI can show early evidence of TB, before plain films are positive. Characteristically, the intervertebral disk is spared. MRI findings include low or intermediate T1 signal intensity, with high T2 signal intensity (21). After gadolinium, involved regions will enhance on T1 images (32). The enhancement with post–gadolinium-diethylenetriamine pentaacetic acid (Gd-DTPA) shows rim enhancement, rather than diffuse enhancement, which would be seen in a pyogenic abscess (28).

The presence of a paravertebral abscess early in the course of the infection is more characteristic of TB than pyogenic infections. CT myelogram or MRI are the imaging procedures of choice if neurologic deficit is present (23). CT myelogram has the advantage of detailing the degree of bone involvement, whereas MRI will better show soft tissue infection and extramedullary lesions.

Treatment

There are two approaches to the treatment of spinal TB: medical (antibiotics and bracing) and surgical. The Medical Research Council (MRC) Working Party on Tuberculosis of the Spine (MRC trials) determined that the mainstay of treatment for spinal TB is drug therapy and that surgery is needed only when there is gross destruction, deformity, or associated neurologic deficit not responding to chemotherapy (28,34–44).

In 1993, guidelines for antituberculous chemotherapy were released by the Centers for Disease Control and Prevention and the American Thoracic Society (45). These guidelines recommend that skeletal TB be treated with a four-drug regimen (isoniazid, rifampin, pyrazinamide, and ethambutol) for 2 months, followed by a two-drug regimen (isoniazid and rifampin) for 4 months. However, short-course medications to treat TB are not considered by all to be long enough in duration. Many other studies support longer treatments of up to 12 months, with at least two antituberculous drugs. The recommended drugs are isoniazid, rifampin, and pyrazinamide for 12 months (46). The addition of a third agent for the initial 2 to 6 months is also advised (23).

Bracing with a conforming orthosis (plaster or molded thermoplastic) has been used in combination with antituberculous drugs as initial treatment. Bracing is continued 3 months after the first radiologic sign of bony fusion. The mean bracing time ranges from 10 to 30 months (47). The MRC trials showed that a favorable outcome could be achieved with chemotherapy alone, without bracing (34–44).

Indications for surgery are acute neurologic deficits, spinal destruction of more than 50%, or unresponsiveness to conservative therapy, progression of disease, intractable pain, and progression of neurologic deficits. Surgical interventions include diagnostic biopsy, drainage of a large paraspinal abscess, decompression of neural elements, debridement of diseased tissue, correction of spinal deformity, or stabilization of the spine (22, 23). Between 10% and 55% of patients have surgical treatment. Significant vertebral body involvement is usually an indication for surgical debridement and stabilization, because patients with this problem who are initially managed nonsurgically may later require fusion procedures for progression of osteomyelitis. When surgery is preformed, it is always combined with antituberculous medications.

Spinal TB affects primarily the anterior column of the spine. One of the main problems to be treated, to prevent deformity and possible neurologic compromise, is the prevention of the development of kyphosis. Both conservative measures, such as

bracing, and surgical techniques have been tried to prevent kyphotic deformity from developing. Focal debridement does not prevent the development of kyphosis (48,49). Decompressive laminectomy is not advised because it destabilizes the spine (22).

There is some discussion in the literature regarding the best surgical approach. The most common technique is to use an anterior strut graft in the defect created by excision of infected vertebral bodies (50). However, when more than two levels are affected, the grafts are more likely to fail or be reabsorbed (51). In those cases, posterior instrumentation can be added to protect the graft, stabilize the segments, and prevent progression of the deformity (23). However, the addition of posterior instrumentation can be associated with increased operating time and increased postoperative morbidity. Therefore, anterior instrumentation alone has been used and has been shown to result in correction of up to 81% of patients, with persistence of the correction in most patients (50).

The following are recommendations for patients with active TB of the thoracic or lumbar spine without paraplegia (51,52):

1. Patients with an initial kyphotic angle of 30 degrees or less should be treated with antituberculous medications, with close monitoring for progression of deformity.
2. Chemotherapy should be with a four-drug regimen for 2 months, followed by isoniazid and rifampin for 4 more months (this regimen is debated, as delineated earlier).
3. Surgery, in addition to medications, is indicated for patients younger than 15 years with a kyphosis of more than 30 degrees. It is also indicated for those who develop kyphosis, for patients with spinal cord compression whose neurologic status deteriorates despite chemotherapy; and for children younger than 10 years, with destruction of vertebral bodies, who have partial or no fusion even during the adolescent growth spurt.
4. Radical excision with anterior strut graft to achieve spinal fusion is the operation of choice. The procedure should be supplemented by posterior fusion, preferably with instrumentation if the graft will span three or more levels.

Outcome

In general, spinal TB is a treatable disease, with more than 90% of patients recovering with appropriate treatment (medical and surgical). Poor prognostic indicators are age older than 70 years and paraplegia (21). Historically, death has resulted from disseminated TB or complications of paraplegia (21).

Recovery of neurologic function in patients with paraplegia is influenced by several factors, including age, general health, severity of damage to the spinal cord, amount of vertebral involvement, severity of spinal deformity, duration and severity of paraplegia, time to initiation of treatment, and type of treatment (22). Duration of paralysis is important, with paralysis of 6 months or more being unlikely to improve. Late paralysis with significant bony deformity is also less responsive to treatment. Lastly, spinal cord atrophy on MRI is a poor prognostic sign.

Spinal deformity and paraplegia are the significant complications of spinal TB, both of which occur more often in cases of delayed diagnosis and management (20). Neurologic recovery for conservatively treated patients can take 2 to 6 months for adults (1 to 4 months in children), and surgically treated patients recover in 2 months (20). In general, in patients with neurologic deficits, prognosis is improved with early anterior surgery (20, 53–55).

Pott paralysis has been divided into early and late forms, also referred to as "paraplegia with active disease" and "paraplegia of healed disease" (56). Early neurologic compromise is typically either from external compression of the cord or from penetration of the dura by infection, as discussed earlier. Late paraplegia, in contrast, is typically caused by cord compression due to a bony ridge or by constriction of the cord by granulation and fibrous tissue (56). Late-onset paraplegia can occur as late as 15 years after the initial infection. The prognosis for neurologic deterioration is worse if the deformity is more proximal or more severe. Spinal cord ischemia and atrophy with gliosis can occur from the mechanical forces of the deformity. Childhood Pott disease carries a higher risk of late neurologic deterioration as growth continues in the posterior part of the spine, despite the lack of growth due to destruction or fusion of the anterior elements (56).

SPINAL CANAL INFECTIONS
Epidural Abscess

The incidence of spinal epidural abscess has been estimated at 0.2 to 1.2 cases per 10,000 hospital admissions (18,57,58). In primary care patients with back pain, the estimated prevalence is 0.000037 (59). The peak age incidence of spinal epidural abscess is in the sixth and seventh decades of life, with the exception of patients with tuberculous abscesses who tend to be young or middle aged (29). Comorbid conditions include diabetes mellitus, intravenous drug abuse, chronic renal failure, alcoholism, and cancer (60,61).

Spinal epidural abscess can be either primary, with hematogenous spread of infection to the epidural space, or secondary from extension into the epidural space from a contiguous process, typically vertebral osteomyelitis or discitis. Hematogenous causes occur in 26% to 50% of cases, 35% to 44% have coexistent vertebral osteomyelitis with direct extension, 16% are from postoperative spread, and blunt trauma accounts for 15% to 35% of all causes of epidural abscesses (9,58,62–64). In 16% to 40% of cases, a source is not identified. Iatrogenic causes include epidural catheters, discography, lumbar puncture, and spinal surgical procedures (65,66). The thoracic spine is involved in 31% to 63% of cases, the lumbar spine in 21% to 44%, and the cervical spine in 14% to 26% (62).

Epidural abscesses caused by hematogenous spread are usually located posteriorly. Those that are a direct extension (from vertebral osteomyelitis or discitis) are typically anterior and can circumferentially surround the thecal sac. Postsurgical cases also surround the thecal sac, because normal anatomic septations are lost during surgery. The average extent of abscess is usually 3 to 6 vertebral segments (29). In epidural abscesses originating from a hematogenous source, there is usually an associated posterior soft tissue abscess, and often these patients have positive blood cultures (3).

Spinal epidural abscesses can also be classified by chronicity as acute or chronic, with the time course varying depending on the virulence of the organism, and host characteristics. An acute abscess has been defined as one in which symptoms have been present for less than 14 days (62). The intraoperative findings have also been used to classify the chronicity of epidural abscesses, with purulent epidural collections thought to be more acute and epidural granulation tissue thought to represent a more chronic infection (63).

Etiology

S. aureus has been isolated in 45% to 73% of patients (58,62). *M. tuberculosis* has been seen in up to 25% of patients in some series. Other less common organisms include *Streptococcus milleri, Haemophilus parainfluenzae, Brucella,* and *Actinomyces. Aspergillus* organisms can cause spinal epidural abscesses in patients with AIDS. *Pseudomonas* has been reported, particularly in those with a history of intravenous drug abuse (61). Most epidural abscesses are from extension, and the bacteria involved are typical of the primary process (see section on vertebral osteomyelitis). One organism is isolated in 51% of patients, two in 16% of patients, and more than two in 8% of patients. Up to 25% of patients have negative cultures (12,58).

The precise pathophysiologic cause of neurologic impairment is not known. Some authors postulate an ischemic mechanism, either from arterial occlusion, venous stasis, or vascular thrombosis. Changes consistent with compression (vacuolization and myelin degeneration with gray-matter preservation) have been shown in animal models. Therefore, compression may be the initial insult, worsened by ischemia.

Clinical Presentation

The most frequent symptom is back pain, which occurs in virtually all patients at some time during the course of the disease (58). Fever is often but not always present (30% to 52% of patients) (18,29,59). Neurologic symptoms such as radicular pain, weakness, numbness, and sphincter dysfunction may be present to varying degrees (67). In cervical epidural abscesses, neck stiffness is common, with weakness involving one to all four limbs (68). The pattern of progression of symptoms is typically from local back pain, to radicular pain, to weakness, and finally paralysis (57). Up to 39% of patients present with paraplegia (18). Patients can also present with septicemia including confusion, which may make detection of subtle neurologic deficits more difficult. Duration of symptoms can range from hours to months, with most patients presenting more acutely (18).

Laboratory Findings

Patients with an epidural abscess will have an elevated WBC count (43% to 50% of cases), and the ESR is almost universally elevated, with mean ESRs of 51 to 94 (18,59). If the ESR is less than 25 mm per hour, spinal infection is unlikely (59). Blood cultures are positive in about 60% of the cases (57).

Diagnosis is typically based on a combination of clinical findings, laboratory tests, and imaging studies. When cerebrospinal fluid (CSF) is obtained, it may range from normal to frank pus. Typical CSF findings include pleocytosis, elevated protein level, and normal glucose level (69). Lumbar puncture to obtain CSF should not routinely be performed, because it may cause spread of the infection to the intrathecal compartment and may cause neurologic deterioration if performed caudal to a spinal block (57).

Imaging

Plain films do not show direct images of an epidural abscess, but nonspecific findings may be seen in 30% to 65% of cases with concurrent vertebral osteomyelitis (57). Osteomyelitis can be seen in 18% to 86% of patients with epidural abscess depending on imaging modality and series (59).

MRI with gadolinium is the radiologic procedure of choice for diagnosing epidural abscess. Abscess fluid is usually higher in signal than CSF on T1 and lower in signal on T2. The membrane of the abscess will usually enhance with Gd-DTPA, although the central portion of the cavity will not enhance. MRI is effective in making the diagnosis but can overestimate bony involvement (18).

If MRI is not available, CT myelography should be performed, although there is the risk of causing acute neurologic deterioration or spreading of the infection. Both MRI and CT myelogram will show a soft tissue mass encroaching on the thecal sac or exiting nerves.

Treatment

Surgical debridement remains the mainstay of treatment for epidural abscess, but there are some studies supporting medical treatment depending on the clinical condition of the patient. Patients who can be considered for medical treatment include those who are poor surgical candidates, those whose abscess involves a significant length of the spinal cord, or those with complete paralysis of more than 3 days (70). In addition, medical treatment can be used in patients with no neurologic deficit, a lumber location of the abscess, and the bacteriologic agent cultured so appropriate antibiotics may be used (57). The length of therapy is typically 8 to 12 weeks of intravenous antibiotics, followed by oral antibiotics, with longer courses needed if vertebral osteomyelitis is present (57).

The duration of antibiotic treatment can be shortened to 4 weeks of appropriate intravenous antibiotics as long as there is no undrained abscess, the patient is clinically doing well, and the ESR has decreased to half of the original pretreatment value (9). Although medical treatment can be successful in carefully chosen cases, sudden neurologic deterioration may occur in patients receiving medical treatment, so close monitoring of clinical status is essential (62).

Surgery is used in cases with rapidly progressive neurologic deficits. As soon as the diagnosis is established, before surgical intervention, empirical antibiotic treatment should be started; it should be delivered intravenously and be continued into the postoperative period, with 4 to 8 week courses of intravenous antibiotics being given (58). Typically, antibiotics are chosen

that are active against *S. aureus,* with further treatment directed by culture.

The surgical approach depends on the location of the abscess, and the presence of concurrent bony infection. An epidural abscess from a hematogenous source is often posterior within the canal (2). These primary epidural abscesses should be evacuated via emergent laminectomy, then stabilized with posterior instrumentation and fusion (12). Some surgeons will advocate a staged procedure, to avoid placing instrumentation into a site of active infection.

Epidural abscesses emanating from extension of an anterior osteomyelitis should be debrided by an anterior surgical approach for better exposure and to avoid further instability from the posterior approach (2,12). This can be supplemented with posterior instrumentation and fusion, with correction of deformity.

A posterior epidural abscess with concurrent spondylodiscitis requires emergent laminectomy, posterior stabilization and fusion, and anterior decompression and fusion (often done as a staged procedure).

Outcome

The outcome of patients with epidural abscess is very dependent on the patient's condition at presentation and the time to definitive treatment. Early surgical treatment consisting of emergency evacuation of the abscess is critical because the outcome of neurologic deficits depends on the time that elapses from onset to surgery (58). Even with appropriate treatment, mortality rates are 5% to 14% (58,67). Delay in diagnosis of more than 3 days is associated with increasing mortality. Those who present with sepsis do poorly (58). Those with deficits for more than 36 hours tend to have minimal neurologic recovery (18). Some have found that the outcome of cervical abscesses is worse than that of thoracic or lumbar abscesses, although others report that thoracic abscesses have the worst outcome. Prompt diagnosis regardless of the region is key to successful treatment.

The severity of the deficit also can be used to predict recovery, with paraparesis associated with a higher incidence of complete recovery than paraplegia. In one study of 13 paraplegics (defined as Frankel grade A, B, or C), 3 had complete recovery, 1 had partial recovery, and 9 had no recovery (12). Patients with root weakness typically recover well (63).

Residual back pain is common (up to 64%) in patients with spinal infections, particularly with vertebral osteomyelitis (12). Despite all of the cautions listed earlier, a good outcome occurs in 60% to 70% (18).

Arachnoiditis

Arachnoiditis is a clinical condition seen in patients who have low back surgery, spinal cord injuries, spinal infections, or invasive spinal procedures. Arachnoiditis results from any injury that causes an inflammatory response of the arachnoid membrane, which leads to fibrosis. This fibrotic process can cause dense adhesions of the nerve roots or the arachnoid to the dura.

Etiology

Infections can cause arachnoiditis, with the most common etiologies being TB and syphilis. Other agents implicated in arachnoiditis include spinal cord injuries, intrathecal hemorrhage, and agents injected into the intrathecal space, including steroids, anesthetics, and radiologic contrast material (particularly hyperosmotic agents). In addition, surgical trauma, retained foreign bodies in the epidural space, or even nucleus pulposus in the epidural space can cause arachnoiditis. It has been estimated that 6% to 16% of patients with persistent low back pain after back surgery have arachnoiditis and that this contributes significantly to failed back surgery syndrome (FBSS) (57).

Clinical Presentation

Patients with arachnoiditis typically present with low back or leg pain, described as burning in nature. Physical examination may reveal signs of nerve root tension and associated neurologic deficits such as motor, sensory, or reflex changes. Multiple nerve root levels bilaterally may be involved. Urinary symptoms can be present in up to 25% of patients (71). Presentation can occur shortly after the causative incident (e.g., surgery or myelography) or can be delayed by several months. Most patients with arachnoiditis will be affected within the first year (71).

Imaging

Historically, myelography has been used to confirm the diagnosis (now with CT imaging rather than plain film myelography). Myelography typically shows a reduction in flow of contrast, ranging from an isolated nerve root filling defect to complete obliteration of the thecal sac (57). There are classification schemes for myelographic appearances in arachnoiditis (72).

MRI is now replacing myelography as the diagnostic procedure of choice. There are three patterns typically seen on MRI (57). In the first pattern, the nerve roots are centrally clumped together, best seen on T1-weighted images. The second pattern shows the roots adherent to the inside of the dura. The third pattern shows increased signal intensity of the intradural compartment on T1-weighted images. There is minimal enhancement on MRI with gadolinium because the collagenous adhesions are minimally vascular.

Arachnoiditis can also be directly visualized during surgery or with a myeloscope. Direct techniques are sensitive for diagnostic purposes but are rarely used because surgery itself is seldom beneficial in arachnoiditis (57).

Treatment

The goals of treatment are to provide relief of symptoms. Arachnoiditis is typically extremely difficult to treat, and although several treatment modalities are available, efficacy is limited (57). Microsurgical lysis of adhesions has been studied, with one study showing up to 75% initial improvement; however, 18% had new neurologic deficits and only 50% maintained good results at 1-year follow-up (57). Many surgeons now advocate against intradural lysis of adhesions, because there is no way to prevent reformation of the scar (72,73).

Spinal cord stimulation has also been tried as treatment of arachnoiditis. The mechanism of pain relief with dorsal spinal cord stimulation is unknown but is thought to involve synaptic inhibition (57). To determine whether the technique will be effective, the patient must undergo a trial of stimulation, with the development of paresthesias over the same region as involved by pain. Long-term follow-up reveals that 52% of patients after 7 years continue to have at least 50% pain reduction, with a 12% unit failure rate and a 5% infection rate (57,74). If the criterion of 50% pain reduction is used as one of the determinants of a good to excellent result, North et al. (74) found that 15% to 88% of patients with FBSS had a good to excellent result. Patients with FBSS with leg pain (rather than back pain) have the best results with spinal cord stimulation.

Neuroablative procedures such as intraspinal, extradural dorsal rhizotomy, or sectioning of the sensory division of involved nerve roots have been attempted with minimal success. Dorsal root ganglionectomy has also been tried in patients with FBSS with poor results. The best results from these procedures appear to be if the pain can be localized to one or two distinct nerve roots. However, in general, these procedures offer little relief.

INFECTIONS OF THE SPINAL CORD
Intramedullary Spinal Cord Abscess

Intramedullary spinal cord abscesses are extremely rare, with approximately 75 cases reported in the literature. These abscesses typically occur in children or the elderly. In the pediatric population, they are commonly associated with lumbosacral dermal sinuses. In older patients, they are often from hematogenous spread from the respiratory tract. However, a primary source is frequently not found (75). Intramedullary spinal cord abscesses may also be associated with epidermoids or ependymomas of the spinal cord (76).

Intramedullary abscesses can be classified by duration of symptoms into acute, subacute, and chronic (77). Patients with acute intramedullary abscess have symptoms that last less than 1 week, those with subacute have symptoms from 1 to 6 weeks, and those with chronic have symptoms lasting more than 6 weeks.

Any region of the spinal cord can be affected, with the thoracic cord affected in most cases in one study, but other studies also show involvement of the cervical cord and conus (78,79). These abscesses typically extend three to six segments. Intramedullary spinal cord abscesses from a primary pulmonary focus have been reported predominantly in the cervical and upper thoracic cord (77,80).

Etiology

The most frequently identified organisms are staphylococci and streptococci. Cases caused by *Haemophilus, Proteus, Listeria monocytogenes, Pseudomonas cepacia, E. Coli, Actinomyces,* and *Pneumococcus* have also been reported (75). There are also case reports of causation by a tapeworm, yeast, and *Toxoplasma* (80). In 36%

of cases, no organism is identified (81). The most common cause of intramedullary abscess is hematogenous spread from another septic focus such as respiratory infection or bacterial endocarditis (80). Meningitis, spinal penetrating trauma such as stab wound or lumbar puncture, and congenital dermal sinus have also been implicated (78,80).

Clinical Presentation

Patients with an acute abscess present with signs of myelopathy including weakness, sensory changes, and sphincter involvement, as well as back pain and fever (57,75). The motor disturbance may be a monoparesis initially that progresses to bilateral deficits. Patients who present with a chronic spinal cord abscess typically are afebrile and may have radicular pain or be pain free. The neurologic deficits are usually slowly progressive.

Laboratory Findings

CSF findings are variable, with normal to high CSF protein levels and variable leukocyte and erythrocyte counts. Typically the CSF is sterile. A sterile abscess is the most common finding when culturing the central pus, but gram-positive and gram-negative organisms as well as multiple organisms have been found (79).

Imaging

CT myelogram can be obtained and will show an expanded cord or complete block to flow of contrast (57). MRI shows enlargement of the cord, consistent with a space-occupying intramedullary lesion. T1-weighted images tend to be hypointense or isointense, whereas T2-weighted images are usually hyperintense (57,75,82). Gadolinium can show peripheral enhancement, similar to an abscess in the brain (79).

Treatment

The treatment of choice is surgical drainage of the abscess, typically performed via laminectomy and midline myelotomy (57). Ultrasound can be used intraoperatively to guide the surgeon to the best site to begin the myelotomy. Parenteral antibiotics should be given for 6 to 8 weeks, guided by culture results. If the culture is sterile, then antibiotics to cover gram-negative rods and anaerobes should be given.

Outcome

Patients with an acute presentation tend to fare poorly and have a high mortality rate (77). Patients with a concurrent brain abscess have a high mortality rate (77,80). Acute meningitis has been associated with the rupture of an intramedullary abscess into the subarachnoid space (81). Neurologic outcome is related to the severity and duration of deficits at presentation. Those with a severe preoperative motor deficit for less than 3 days made a full recovery, whereas three of four patients with a severe motor deficit for 3 or more days did poorly (79). Many patients with a chronic presentation have a good functional outcome with appropriate treatment (81). Even when there is a good outcome, follow-up is essential, because there is a significant rate of recurrence.

Transverse Myelitis

Infections of the spinal cord can be caused by various etiologic agents, including numerous viral and bacterial pathogens. However, neurologic deficits can occur as part of systemic illness, which cannot clearly be linked to an infectious cause. A general term for this process is acute transverse myelitis (ATM). Although 20% to 40% of cases of transverse myelitis are thought to be viral in etiology, often a specific cause cannot be found (83).

ATM is an uncommon neurologic syndrome characterized by intrinsic inflammation of the spinal cord. It is an inflammatory myelopathy in which there is a lesion of the spinal cord, resulting in a horizontal segmental level. The involvement of the cord may be at any region from sacral to cervical. The disease may appear without a history of previous neurologic disease.

ATM can occur in any age group and does not discriminate according to gender (84). The cause of ATM is unknown, although approximately one third of patients with transverse myelitis report flulike illness with fever in close temporal relationship to the onset of neurologic symptoms. The time course typically encompasses days to weeks, and the degree of recovery is variable.

Etiologies

ATM may occur in isolation or in the setting of another illness. Many possible etiologies have been proposed for ATM. Postulated causes include parainfectious, postvaccinal, systemic autoimmune disease, multiple sclerosis, paraneoplastic syndromes, and vascular insufficiency. Infectious agents suspected of causing ATM include herpes simplex virus (HSV), varicella-zoster virus (VZV), cytomegalovirus (CMV), Epstein-Barr virus (EBV), influenza, enteroviruses (poliomyelitis, coxsackievirus, echovirus), *Mycoplasma pneumoniae,* and syphilis (85,86).

Vaccines that have been associated with myelitis include measles, mumps, and rabies vaccine. Measles and mumps vaccine can also cause an acute disseminated encephalomyelitis. Evidence for an autoimmune etiology for ATM includes the fact that individuals suffering from collagen-vascular diseases such as systemic lupus erythematosus often suffer from acute or chronic ATM (87). In the study by Austin et al. (85), the causative agent of ATM could not be determined in one half of the patients. ATM is a diagnosis of exclusion, and treatable causes must be ruled out.

Clinical Presentation

Patients diagnosed with transverse myelitis can exhibit a vast array of symptoms mainly associated with loss of function of spinal cord segments. The initial symptoms of ATM typically are paresthesias, back pain (Ropper and Poskanzer [84] reported the most common location of pain was the dorsal midline at the interscapular), bilateral leg weakness, and urinary retention (88). However, any symptom relating to the spinal cord lesion can be present. The thoracic segments of the spinal cord are most commonly affected (89). The clinical syndrome evolves over several hours to 2 to 3 weeks.

Imaging

Diagnosis of ATM may present as a diagnostic challenge to the clinician. Immediate differential diagnosis must focus on the exclusion of treatable causes of cord compression such as an extramedullary tumor or abscess, as well as exclusion of an intramedullary tumor. MRI has been proven to be the best diagnostic modality for, but does not help in, determining the etiology or prognosis in such cases of ATM (85,90,91). Lesions consist of either cord swelling without abnormal signal or more commonly diffuse increased signal on T2-weighted images within the center of the cord (85,91). Gadolinium has been used to enhance lesions on MRI, and the enhanced lesions show concentration of demyelination in the ventral white matter of the affected spinal cord segments (87).

Treatment

Literature review indicates that the treatment of ATM may include bed rest, analgesics, and corticosteroid therapy. There are controversies in the literature regarding the role of steroids in the treatment of ATM. A pilot study done by Sebire et al. (92) suggests that high-dose methylprednisolone is effective in the treatment of ATM in children. Results of their study showed that the median time of the steroid-treated group to walk independently, compared with that of the historical group, was reduced and the proportion of patients with full recovery within 12 months was significantly higher. A study published the following year by Lahat et al. (93) supported treatment of ATM with high-dose methylprednisolone in the reduction of the median time of motor recovery.

Outcome

Ropper and Poskanzer (84) found that prognosis is predictable on the basis of clinical characteristics. In this study, patients were separated into good, fair, and poor outcome groups. The good outcome group had complete recovery with normal gait and bladder function. The poor outcome group was incontinent and wheelchair bound or bedridden. The remaining patients grouped into the fair category were functional and ambulatory but had a spastic gait, urinary urgency or incontinence, and persistent signs of spinal cord dysfunction. Their study supported back pain as being a predictor of poor outcome. There was no mention of patients receiving any type of acute or long-term rehabilitation that may affect the patients' ultimate mobility outcome.

There is controversy in the literature regarding the risk of development of multiple sclerosis in those with ATM. In patients who show periventricular white-matter lesions, the risk of later development of multiple sclerosis has been speculated to be as high as 90% (94).

Involvement of the Spinal Cord in HIV

Involvement of the spinal cord in patients with HIV occurs both as a direct result of the HIV infection and due to opportunistic infections of the spinal cord. The incidence of myelopathy in patients with AIDS is reported to range from 7% to 20% (95, 96). Often, other neurologic problems such as brain involvement or peripheral neuropathy are superimposed, making detection of the myelopathy less likely. At autopsy, a much higher percentage of patients have spinal cord involvement than is documented clinically. Overall, opportunistic infections involve the spinal cord in 10% of patients as seen by autopsy (96). However, spinal cord involvement is rare in the absence of brain involvement. In addition to infectious causes, vacuolar myelopathy (VM) is seen in up to 55% of patients at autopsy (97,98).

Myelitis in patients with HIV can be from a variety of causes, including the HIV itself, VM, lymphoma, and other infectious etiologies including fungal, viral, and bacterial.

HIV-Related Myelopathy

Patients can develop an acute transverse myelopathy during HIV seroconversion, known as primary acute HIV myelitis (95,99). In addition, an acute or subacute myelitis can develop as an early or late complication of AIDS. HIV myelitis is much less common than HIV encephalitis. When HIV encephalitis extends to the spinal cord, the term encephalomyelitis is used. Spread of HIV encephalitis has been reported in both the white-matter tracts and the gray matter.

Vacuolar Myelopathy

AIDS-associated VM is the most common cause of myelopathy in patients with AIDS (96). The frequency of autopsy-proven VM ranges from 40% to 55% (89,95). VM affects multiple areas of the spinal cord, predominantly the dorsal and lateral columns (89). The typical presentation is a spastic paraparesis, ataxia, a loss of position and vibration sense, urinary complaints, and erectile dysfunction (99). VM is usually seen in patients with a CD4 cell count of less than 200. It is often subclinical, not presenting until the white-matter vacuolization becomes severe. There is no evidence that infection of the spinal cord with HIV is related to the development of VM (100,101).

MRI results are often normal but can show mild atrophy of the thoracic cord or nonspecific areas of increased intensity on T2-weighted images (102). CSF studies can also be normal or may show a mild pleocytosis and a nonspecific increased CSF protein level (99). Somatosensory evoked potentials are often abnormal, even before clinical manifestations are apparent, and can be used to follow the progression of the disease (103).

On pathology, multiple vacuoles are seen, which cause progressive loss of myelin. These contain numerous segmental vacuolar myelin swellings and macrophages residing within vacuoles (16,96). The dorsolateral tracts of the mid-thoracic and low thoracic spinal cord are found to have the most severe vacuolation on pathology (104). These pathologic features are similar to those found in subacute combined degeneration. It has been hypothesized that vitamin B_{12} and folate avitaminosis are possible pathogenic factors, and 7% to 15% of patients with HIV have low serum vitamin B_{12} levels (105). However, the relationship between vitamin B_{12} deficiency and VM has not definitively been proven. Another possible pathogenetic theory is that there are abnormal transmethylation mechanisms induced by HIV and cytokines, which cause the VM (99).

There are currently no treatments for VM, and antiretroviral drugs have not been shown to be effective. Other treatments that have been tried without much effect include vitamin B_{12} and folate supplementation, corticosteroids, and intravenous gamma globulin. Oral L-methionine is currently in clinical trials. A key component of treatment is focused on improving symptoms, including management of gait abnormalities, spasticity, and urologic dysfunction.

Lymphoma

Spinal cord lymphoma is rare, ranging form 2% to 4% in postmortem series. In patients with primary cerebral lymphoma, there is a 25% rate of spread to the spinal cord. Typically, spinal cord lymphoma occurs with a CD4 cell count of less than 100. Lymphoma can affect any part of the spinal cord. Cord edema can be significant and may result in multilevel cord swelling. MRI will reveal increased T2 signal with vigorous contrast enhancement.

Herpes Viruses

Varicella-Zoster Virus
There are few reports of neurologic complications associate with VZV. Presentations of spinal VZV disease in AIDS are encephalomyelitis, mainly involving the gray matter, ependymitis or ventriculitis mimicking CMV infection with secondary meningomyeloradiculitis, and fulminant ascending myeloradiculopathy. VZV myelitis typically involves the posterior horns first because of the spread of the infection from spinal ganglia via the posterior roots (95).

Herpes Simplex Virus Types 1 and 2
HSV myelitis is surprisingly rare in AIDS, although there are cases of ATM due to HSV, which causes a severe necrotizing ascending myelitis (106,107).

Cytomegalovirus

CMV infection of the central nervous system (CNS) is the most common viral disease causing neurologic involvement in patients with AIDS, involving the brain and spinal cord. CMV encephalitis typically occurs in patients with a CD4 cell count of less than 50 (16). CMV causes a necrotizing radiculomyelitis, classically of the cauda equina (96). Clinical presentation is pain, flaccid paraplegia, absence of major sensory deficit, and early sphincter dysfunction (108). The prognosis is often poor, leading to death in a few weeks without treatment.

CMV typically disseminates via the CSF before invading the parenchyma. CMV can cause a rapidly ascending polyradiculoneuropathy similar to the Guillain-Barré syndrome, but with a granulocytic CSF pleocytosis (96,99). The treatment for CMV myelitis and myeloradiculitis is ganciclovir or cidofovir.

Human T Lymphotropic Virus Type 1–Associated Myelopathy in HIV

There are cases of human T-cell lymphotrophic virus-1 (HTLV-1) infection in patients with HIV, particularly in regions in which HTLV-1 is endemic, and in persons who use intravenous drugs (99). A mild to moderate pleocytosis in the CSF may be useful in differentiating HTLV infection from VM.

Fungal Infections

Fungal infections of the spinal cord in patients with HIV include cryptococcosis, aspergillosis, mucormycosis, and candidiasis (96). Cryptococci typically affect the leptomeninges, with involvement of the spinal meninges being less common than the involvement of the basal meninges. *Candida* infection of the CNS is rare in AIDS, given the intact neutrophilic response.

Parasitoses

Toxoplasmosis is by far the most common form of CNS parasitic infestation in patients with AIDS. CNS involvement in AIDS has been reported in 4% to 41% of AIDS autopsy cases (96). CNS toxoplasmosis presents typically as necroses or abscesses, most commonly in the basal ganglia. However, CNS toxoplasmosis may also present as nodular encephalomyelitis. Toxoplasmosis can involve any part of the spinal cord and can cause significant cord edema and multilevel cord swelling extending out from the central portion of the lesion (95).

Bacterial Infections

Bacterial infections are relatively rare in patients with AIDS, due to the intact neutrophilic response in AIDS. The most common pathogen is *M. tuberculosis*. TB is significant among intravenous drug abusers. The clinical presentation can be meningitis, acute abscess formation, or a chronic indolent mass lesion. Spinal meninges may be prominently involved in tuberculous meningitis. Neurosyphilis in AIDS also involves the brain and meninges.

Human T Lymphotropic Virus Type 1–Associated Myelopathy (HTLV-1)

HTLV-1 is a complex type C retrovirus, which has long been known as the causative agent of a highly aggressive T-cell malignancy, adult T-cell lymphoma/leukemia (ATL) (109). However, it was not until the mid-1980s that HTLV-1 was identified as the causative agent in various chronic inflammatory conditions, including a chronic progressive myelopathy. This was referred to as tropical spastic paraparesis (TSP) in the Caribbean and HTLV-1–associated myelopathy (HAM) in Japan (75). The abbreviation TSP/HAM is frequently used to describe the clinical syndrome of a spastic myelopathy in individuals infected with HTLV-1.

There is a closely related virus, HTLV-2, which has only rarely been implicated in myelopathy. The other syndromes associated with HTLV-1 infection include polymyositis, arthropathy, infective dermatitis, and uveitis (109). The mechanism of pathogenesis remains unclear, but it appears to be related to the activation of infected lymphocytes, with the subsequent release of cytokines playing a role (75,109).

Cases of TSP/HAM have been reported in many countries, including the southeastern United States (110). There are endemic foci in the Caribbean, southern Japan, central and South Africa, and South America. The disease is relatively rare in the U.S. population, found chiefly in certain immigrant groups and in intravenous drug users (109). HTLV-1 is unevenly distributed even within endemic areas, with the incidence of seropositivity ranging from 0.1% to 30% (109). The dominant modes of transmission are mother to child in breast milk, sexual transmission, and transmission via infected blood products. In those who are HTLV-1 seropositive, the lifetime risk of developing TSP/HAM is 1% to 2% (109). There are persons who are healthy carriers of HTLV-1, and their risk of progression to TSP/HAM seems to be related to proviral load. There is evidence for HLA-A*02 type being protective against the development of TSP/HAM in those with HTLV-1 (109).

Clinical Presentation

The disease presents with a slowly progressive spastic paraparesis, urinary frequency or incontinence, paresthesias in the legs, autonomic dysfunction, variable sensory loss, and low back pain. The mean age of onset is 40, and women are affected two to three times more commonly than men are. Reports of encephalopathy, involvement of the peripheral nervous system, and inflammatory myopathy in those with HTLV-1 have been made. Physical examination of patients with TSP/HAM typically reveals a spastic gait with hyperreflexia, extensor-plantar responses, and muscle weakness, particularly of the proximal lower limbs.

Laboratory Findings

Testing the serum for antibodies establishes the diagnosis. CSF testing shows a mild pleocytosis, a mild to moderate increase in protein level, and the presence of HTLV-1 antibodies (109). Increased immunoglobulin G synthesis rates in CSF have been noted in 75% of patients (110).

Neuropathologic findings include diffuse demyelinative lesions in the cerebrum and the lower cervical and upper thoracic spinal cord, with a widespread mononuclear cell infiltrate (109). Adhesive arachnoiditis and lesions of vasculitis involving predominantly the spinal cord but also the white matter of the cerebrum, cerebellum, and pons have been described (111).

Imaging

MRI abnormalities include foci of increased T2 signal in the periventricular white matter (110). Evoked potentials can also be abnormal (110).

Treatment

There is no proven successful treatment for TSP/HAM. Medications tried have included corticosteroids, cyclophosphamide, anabolic steroids, zidovudine (AZT), and vitamin C; however, none have showed lasting benefit. Plasmapheresis has also been tried with minimal success. Recently lamivudine (3TC) has been shown to reduce the proviral load of HTLV-1 (112). Management of TSP/HAM centers on treatment of the various symptoms, including medications for spasticity and neurogenic pain, as well as urologic management as would be done in myelopathy from other etiologies.

Outcome

The course of TSP/HAM is variable but typically is progressive over 6 months to 2 years. The disease is not fatal, but life expectancy is usually shortened, with death occurring in about 10 years (109).

Other Infectious Causes

There are various infectious causes of acute myelopathy. Many of the same pathogens that are seen in patients with HIV infection can cause myelopathy in at-risk groups, such as those with advanced age or immunocompromise. Herpesviruses can cause acute myelopathy. The family of herpesviruses includes HSV types 1 and 2, VZV, CMV, EBV, and herpes simiae (monkey B virus), all of which can cause myelopathy (113). Myelopathy after exposure to other herpesviruses is less common but does occur. Myelopathy can be caused by toxoplasmosis, particularly in those with AIDS.

Schistosomiasis can present with spinal cord involvement. The area most typically affected is the lumbar cord, because granuloma form around the conus and roots. Treatment is with praziquantel. Borreliosis (Lyme disease) can cause a spectrum of peripheral and CNS lesions.

REFERENCES

1. Ozuna RM, Delamarter RB. Pyogenic vertebral osteomyelitis and postsurgical disc space infections. *Orthop Clin North Am* 1996;27:87–94.
2. Calderone RR, Larsen JM. Overview and classification of spinal infections. *Orthop Clin North Am* 1996;27:1–8.
3. Khan IA, Vaccaro AR, Zlotolow DA. Management of vertebral diskitis and osteomyelitis. *Orthopedics* 1999;22(8):758–765.
4. Bamberger DM. Osteomyelitis. A commonsense approach to antibiotic and surgical treatment. *Postgrad Med* 1993;94(5):177–184.
5. Glazer PA, Hu SS. Pediatric spinal infections. *Orthop Clin North Am* 1996;27(1):111–123.
6. Rath SA, Neff U, Schneider O, et al. Neurosurgical management of thoracic and lumbar vertebral osteomyelitis and discitis in adults: a review of 43 consecutive surgically treated patients. *Neurosurgery* 1996;38(5):926–933.
7. Wiley AM, Trueta J. The vascular anatomy of the spine and its relationship to pyogenic vertebral osteomyelitis. *J Bone Joint Surg* 1959;41B:796–809.
8. Wood II GW. Anatomic, biologic, and pathophysiologic aspects of spinal infections. *Spine (State-of-the-Art Reviews)* 1989;3:385–396.
9. Sapico FL. Microbiology and antimicrobial therapy of spinal infections. *Orthop Clin North Am* 1996;27(1):9–13.
10. Waldvogel FA, Medoff G, Swartz MN. Osteomyelitis: a review of clinical features, therapeutic considerations, and unusual aspects. *N Engl J Med* 1970;282:198–206.
11. Sapico FL, Montgomerie JZ. Pyogenic vertebral osteomyelitis: report

of nine cases and review of the literature. *Rev Infect Dis* 1979;1(5): 754–776.

12. Hadjipavlou AG, Mader JT, Necessary JT, et al. Hematogenous pyogenic spinal infections and their surgical management. *Spine* 2000; 25(13):1668–1679.

13. Jonsson B, Soderholm R, Stromqvist B. Erythrocyte sedimentation rate after lumbar spine injury. *Spine* 1991;16(9):1049–1050.

14. Patzakis MJ, Rao S, Wilkins J, et al. Analysis of 61 cases of vertebral osteomyelitis. *Clin Orthop* 1991(264):178–183.

15. Rothman SL. The diagnosis of infections of the spine by modern imaging techniques. *Orthop Clin North Am* 1996;27(1):15–31.

16. Simpson DM, Berger JR. Neurologic manifestations of HIV infection. *Med Clin North Am* 1996;80(6):1363–1394.

17. Vaccaro AR, Shah SH, Schweitzer ME, et al. MRI description of vertebral osteomyelitis, neoplasm, and compression fracture. *Orthopedics* 1999;22(1):67–75.

18. Sampath P, Rigamonti D. Spinal epidural abscess: a review of epidemiology, diagnosis, and treatment. *J Spinal Disord* 1999;12(2):89–93.

19. Eismont FJ, Bohlman HH, Soni PL. Pyogenic and fungal vertebral osteomyelitis with paralysis. *J Bone Joint Surg* 1983;65A:19–29.

20. Moon MS, Ha KY, Sun DH, et al. Pott's paraplegia—67 cases. *Clin Orthop* 1996;323:122–128.

21. Pertuiset E, Beaudreuil J, Liote F, et al. Spinal tuberculosis in adults. A study of 103 cases in a developed country, 1980–1994. *Medicine (Baltimore)* 1999;78(5):309–320.

22. Moon MS. Tuberculosis of the spine. Controversies and a new challenge. *Spine* 1997;22(15):1791–1797.

23. Nussbaum ES, Rockswold GL, Bergman TA, et al. Spinal tuberculosis: a diagnostic and management challenge [Comments]. *J Neurosurg* 1995;83(2):243–247.

24. Rezai AR, Lee M, Cooper PR, et al. Modern management of spinal tuberculosis. *Neurosurgery* 1995;36(1):87–98.

25. Weaver P, Lifeso RM. The radiological diagnosis of tuberculosis of the adult spine. *Skeletal Radiol* 1984;12(3):178–186.

26. Colmenero JD, Jimenez-Mejias ME, Sanchez-Lora FJ, et al. Pyogenic, tuberculous, and brucellar vertebral osteomyelitis: a descriptive and comparative study of 219 cases. *Ann Rheum Dis* 1997;56(12): 709–715.

27. Hayes AJ, Choksey M, Barnes N, et al. Spinal tuberculosis in developed countries: difficulties in diagnosis. *J Royal Coll Surg Edinb* 1996; 41(3):192–196.

28. Desai SS. Early diagnosis of spinal tuberculosis by MRI. *J Bone Joint Surg* 1994;76B:863–869.

29. Kaufman DM, Kaplan JG, Litman N. Infectious agents in spinal epidural abscess. *Neurology* 1980;30:844–850.

30. Boachie-Adjei O, Squillante RG. Tuberculosis of the spine. *Orthop Clin North Am* 1996;27(1):95–103.

31. Lifeso RM, Weaver P, Harder EH. Tuberculosis spondylitis in adults. *J Bone Joint Surg Am* 1985;67(9):1405–1413.

32. Ridley N, Shaikh MI, Remedios D, et al. Radiology of skeletal tuberculosis. *Orthopedics* 1998;21(11):1213–1220.

33. Fam AG, Rubenstein J. Another look at spinal tuberculosis [Comments]. *J Rheumatol* 1993;20(10):1731–1740.

34. Medical Research Council Working Party on Tuberculosis of the Spine. A controlled trial of ambulant out-patient treatment and in-patient rest in bed in the management of tuberculosis of the spine in young Korean patients on standard chemotherapy: a study in Masan, Korea. First report of the Medical Research Council Working Party on Tuberculosis of the Spine. *J Bone Joint Surg Br* 1973;55(4):678–697.

35. Medical Research Council Working Party on Tuberculosis of the Spine. Five-year assessments of controlled trials of ambulatory treatment, debridement and anterior spinal fusion in the management of tuberculosis of the spine. Studies in Bulawayo (Rhodesia) and in Hong Kong. Sixth report of the Medical Research Council Working Party on Tuberculosis of the Spine. *J Bone Joint Surg Br* 1978;60-B(2): 163–177.

36. Medical Research Council Working Party on Tuberculosis of the Spine. A controlled trial of anterior spinal fusion and debridement in the surgical management of tuberculosis of the spine in patients on standard chemotherapy: a study in two centers in South Africa.

Seventh Report of the Medical Research Council Working Party on tuberculosis of the spine. *Tubercle* 1978;59(2):79–105.

37. Medical Research Council Working Party on Tuberculosis of the Spine. A 10-year assessment of a controlled trial comparing debridement and anterior spinal fusion in the management of tuberculosis of the spine in patients on standard chemotherapy in Hong Kong. Eight Report of the Medical Research Council Working Party on Tuberculosis of the Spine. *J Bone Joint Surg Br* 1982;64(4):393–398.

38. Medical Research Council Working Party on Tuberculosis of the Spine. A controlled trial of six-month and nine-month regimens of chemotherapy in patients undergoing radical surgery for tuberculosis of the spine in Hong Kong. Tenth report of the Medical Research Council Working Party on Tuberculosis of the Spine. *Tubercle* 1986; 67(4):243–259.

39. Medical Research Council Working Party on Tuberculosis of the Spine. Five-year assessment of controlled trials of short-course chemotherapy regimens of 6, 9, or 18 months' duration for spinal tuberculosis in patients ambulatory from the start or undergoing radical surgery. Fourteenth report of the Medical Research Council Working Party on Tuberculosis of the Spine. *Int Orthop* 1999;23(2):73–81.

40. Medical Research Council Working Party on Tuberculosis of the Spine. A 15-year assessment of controlled trials of the management of tuberculosis of the spine in Korea and Hong Kong. Thirteenth Report of the Medical Research Council Working Party on Tuberculosis of the Spine. *J Bone Joint Surg Br* 1998;80(3):456–462.

41. Medical Research Council Working Party on Tuberculosis of the Spine. A controlled trial of plaster-of-Paris jackets in the management of ambulant outpatient treatment of tuberculosis of the spine in children on standard chemotherapy. A study in Pusan, Korea. Second report of the Medical Research Council Working Party on Tuberculosis of the Spine. *Tubercle* 1997;54(4):261–282.

42. Medical Research Council Working Party on Tuberculosis of the Spine. A 10-year assessment of controlled trials of inpatient and outpatient treatment and of plaster-of-Paris jackets for tuberculosis of the spine in children on standard chemotherapy. Studies in Masan and Pusan, Korea. Ninth report of the Medical Research Council Working Party on Tuberculosis of the Spine. *J Bone Joint Surg Br* 1985;67(1): 103–110.

43. Medical Research Council Working Party on Tuberculosis of the Spine. Controlled trial of short-course regimens of chemotherapy in the ambulatory treatment of spinal tuberculosis. Results at three years of a study in Korea. Twelfth report of the Medical Research Council Working Party on Tuberculosis of the Spine. *J Bone Joint Surg Br* 1993;75(2):240–248.

44. Medical Research Council Working Party on Tuberculosis of the Spine. A five-year assessment of controlled trials of in-patient and out-patient treatment and of plaster-of-Paris jackets for tuberculosis of the spine in children on standard chemotherapy. Studies in Masan and Pusan, Korea. Fifth report of the Medical Research Council Working Party on tuberculosis of the spine. *J Bone Joint Surg Br* 1976; 58-B(4):399–411.

45. Bass JB, Farer LS, Hopewell PC, et al. Treatment of tuberculosis and tuberculosis infection in adults and children. American Thoracic Society and the Centers for Disease Control and Prevention [Comments]. *Am J Respir Crit Care Med* 1994;149(5):1359–1374.

46. Waldvogel FA, Medoff G, Swartz MN. Osteomyelitis: a review of clinical features, therapeutic considerations, and unusual aspects. *N Engl J Med* 1970;282:316–322.

47. Wimmer C, Ogon M, Sterzinger W, et al. Conservative treatment of tuberculous spondylitis: a long-term follow up study. *J Spinal Disord* 1997;10(5):417–419.

48. Chen WJ, Chen CH, Shih CH. Surgical treatment of tuberculous spondylitis. 50 patients followed for 2–8 years [Comments]. *Acta Orthop Scand* 1995;66(2):137–142.

49. Upadhyay SS, Saji MJ, Yau AC. Duration of antituberculosis chemotherapy in conjunction with radical surgery in the management of spinal tuberculosis. *Spine* 1996;21(16):1898–1903.

50. Yilmaz C, Selek HY, Gurkan I, et al. Anterior instrumentation for the treatment of spinal tuberculosis. *J Bone Joint Surg Am* 1999;81(9): 1261–1267.

51. Rajasekaran S, Soundarapandian S. Progression of kyphosis in tuberculosis of the spine treated by anterior arthrodesis. *J Bone Joint Surg Am* 1989;71(9):1314–1323.

52. Parthasarathy R, Sriram K, Santha T, et al. Short-course chemotherapy for tuberculosis of the spine. A comparison between ambulant treatment and radical surgery—ten-year report. *J Bone Joint Surg Br* 1999;81(3):464–471.

53. Bailey HL, Gabriel M, Hodgson AR, et al. Tuberculosis of the spine in children. Operative findings and results in one hundred consecutive patients treated by removal of the lesion and anterior grafting. *J Bone Joint Surg Am* 1972;54(8):1633–1657.

54. Goel MK. Treatment of Pott's paraplegia by operation. *J Bone Joint Surg Br* 1967;49(4):674–681.

55. Hodgson AR, Skinsnes OK, Leong CY. The pathogenesis of Pott's paraplegia. *J Bone Joint Surg Am* 1967;49(6):1147–1156.

56. Bilsel N, Aydingoz O, Hanci M, et al. Late onset Pott's paraplegia. *Spinal Cord* 2000;38(11):669–674.

57. Martin RJ, Yuan HA. Neurosurgical care of spinal epidural, subdural, and intramedullary abscesses and arachnoiditis. *Orthop Clin North Am* 1996;27(1):125–136.

58. Mackenzie AR, Laing RB, Smith CC, et al. Spinal epidural abscess: the importance of early diagnosis and treatment. *J Neurol Neurosurg Psychiatry* 1998;65(2):209–212.

59. Maslen DR, Jones SR, Crisplin MA. Spinal epidural abscess: optimizing patient care. *Arch Intern Med* 1993;153:1713–1721.

60. Broner FA, Garland DE, Zigler JE. Spinal infections in the immunocompromised host. *Orthop Clin North Am* 1996;27(1):37–46.

61. Nussbaum ES, Rigamonti D, Standiford H, et al. Spinal epidural abscess: a report of 40 cases and review. *Surg Neurol* 1992;38:225–231.

62. Wheeler D, Keiser P, Rigamonti D, et al. Medical management of spinal epidural abscesses: case report and review [Comments]. *Clin Infect Dis* 1992;15(1):22–27.

63. Baker AS, Ojemann, Swartz MN. Spinal epidural abscess. *N Engl J Med* 1975;293:463–468.

64. Verner EF, Musher DM. Spinal epidural abscess. Symposium on infections of the central nervous system. *Med Clin North Am* 1985;69:375–384.

65. Ghanayem AJ, Zdeblick TA. Cervical spine infections. *Orthop Clin North Am* 1996;27(1):53–67.

66. Ericsson M, Algers G, Schliamser SE. Spinal epidural abscess in adults: review and report of iatrogenic cases. *Scand J Infect Dis* 1990;22:240–257.

67. Darouiche RO, Hamil RJ, Greenberg SB, et al. Bacterial spinal epidural abscess: review of 43 cases and literature survey. *Medicine* 1992;71:369–385.

68. Lasker RB, Harter DH. Cervical epidural abscess. *Neurology* 1987;37:1747–1753.

69. Hlavin ML, Kaminski HJ, Ross JS, et al. Spinal epidural abscess: a ten-year perspective. *Neurosurgery* 1990;27(2):177–184.

70. Leys D, Lesoin F, Viaud C, et al. Decreased morbidity from acute bacterial spinal epidural abscesses using computed tomography and nonsurgical treatment in selected patients. *Ann Neurol* 1985;17(4):350–355.

71. Benner B, Ehni G. Spinal arachnoiditis. The postoperative variety in particular. *Spine* 1978;3(1):40–44.

72. Roca J, Moreta D, Ubierna MT, et al. The results of surgical treatment of lumbar arachnoiditis. *Int Orthop* 1993;17(2):77–81.

73. Johnston JD, Matheny JB. Microscopic lysis of lumbar adhesive arachnoiditis. *Spine* 1978;3(1):36–39.

74. North RB, Kidd DH, Zahurak M, et al. Spinal cord stimulation for chronic, intractable pain: experience over two decades. *Neurosurgery* 1993;32(3):384–395.

75. Corboy JR, Price RW. Myelitis and toxic, inflammatory, and infectious disorders. *Curr Opin Neurol Neurosurg* 1993;6(4):564–570.

76. Benzil DL, Epstein MH, Knuckey NW. Intramedullary epidermoid associated with an intramedullary spinal abscess secondary to a dermal sinus [Comments]. *Neurosurgery* 1992;30(1):118–121.

77. Menezes AH, Graf CJ, Perret GE. Spinal cord abscess: a review. *Surg Neurol* 1977;8(6):461–467.

78. DiTullio MV Jr. Intramedullary spinal abscess: a case report with a review of 53 previously described cases. *Surg Neurol* 1977;7(6):351–354.

79. Byrne RW, von Roenn KA, Whisler WW. Intramedullary abscess: a report of two cases and a review of the literature. *Neurosurgery* 1994;35(2):321–326.

80. Erlich JH, Rosenfeld JV, Fuller A, et al. Acute intramedullary spinal cord abscess: case report. *Surg Neurol* 1992;38(4):287–290.

81. Miranda ME, Anciones B, Castro A, et al. Intramedullary spinal cord abscess. *J Neurol Neurosurg Psychiatry* 1992;55:225–226.

82. Murphy KJ, Brunberg JA, Quint DJ, et al. Spinal cord infection: myelitis and abscess formation [Comments]. *Am J Neuroradiol* 1998;19(2):341–348.

83. Tyler KL, Gross RA, Cascino GD. Unusual viral causes of transverse myelitis: hepatitis A virus and cytomegalovirus. *Neurology* 1986;36(6):855–858.

84. Ropper AH, Poskanzer DC. The prognosis of acute and subacute transverse myelopathy based on early signs and symptoms. *Ann Neurol* 1978;4(1):51–59.

85. Austin SG, Zee CS, Waters C. The role of magnetic resonance imaging in acute transverse myelitis. *Can J Neurol Sci* 1992;19(4):508–511.

86. Habr F, Wu B. Acute transverse myelitis in systemic lupus erythematosus: a case of rapid diagnosis and complete recovery. *Conn Med* 1998;62(7):387–390.

87. Thomas M, Thomas J Jr. Acute transverse myelitis. *J La State Med Soc* 1997;149(2):75–77.

88. Berger Y, Blaivas JG, Oliver L, et al. Urinary dysfunction in transverse myelitis. *J Urol* 1990;144(1):103–105.

89. Dawson DM, Potts F. Acute nontraumatic myelopathies. *Neurol Clin* 1991;9(3):585–603.

90. Shen WC, Lee SK, Ho YJ, et al. MRI of sequela of transverse myelitis. *Pediatr Radiol* 1992;22(5):382–383.

91. Barakos JA, Mark AS, Dillon WP, et al. MRI imaging of acute transverse myelitis and AIDS myelopathy. *J Comput Assist Tomogr* 1990;14(1):45–50.

92. Sebire G, Hollenberg H, Meyer L, et al. High dose methylprednisolone in severe acute transverse myelopathy. *Arch Dis Child* 1997;76(2):167–168.

93. Lahat E, Pillar G, Ravid S, et al. Rapid recovery from transverse myelopathy in children treated with methylprednisolone. *Pediatr Neurol* 1998;19(4):279–282.

94. Ford B, Tampieri D, Francis G. Long-term follow-up or acute partial transverse myelopathy [Comments]. *Neurology* 1992;42(1):250–252.

95. Quencer RM, Post MJ. Spinal cord lesions in patients with AIDS. *Neuroimaging Clin North Am* 1997;7(2):359–373.

96. Budka H. Neuropathology of myelitis, myelopathy, and spinal infections in AIDS. *Neuroimaging Clin North Am* 1997;7(3):639–650.

97. Artigas J, Grosse G, Niedobitek F. Vacuolar myelopathy in AIDS. A morphological analysis. *Pathol Res Pract* 1990;186(2):228–237.

98. Dal Pan GJ, Glass JD, McArthur JC. Clinicopathologic correlations of HIV-1 associated vacuolar myelopathy: an autopsy-based case-control study. *Neurology* 1994;44(11):2159–2164.

99. Di Rocco A. Diseases of the spinal cord in human immunodeficiency virus infection. *Semin Neurol* 1999;19(2):151–155.

100. Petito CK, Vecchio D, Chen YT. HIV antigen and DNA in AIDS spinal cords correlate with macrophage infiltration but not with vacuolar myelopathy. *J Neuropathol Exp Neurol* 1994;53(1):86–94.

101. Rosenblum M, Scheck AC, Cronin K, et al. Dissociation of AIDS-related vacuolar myelopathy and productive HIV-1 infection of the spinal cord. *Neurology* 1989;39(7):892–896.

102. Sartoretti-Schefer S, Blattler T, Wichmann W. Spinal MRI in vacuolar myelopathy, and correlation with histopathological findings. *Neuroradiology* 1997;39(12):865–869.

103. Pierelli F, Garrubba C, Tilia G, et al. Multimodal evoked potentials in HIV-1–seropositive patients: relationship between the immune impairment and the neurophysiological function. *Acta Neurol Scand* 1996;93(4):266–271.

104. Gonzales MF, Davis RL. Neuropathology of acquired immunodeficiency syndrome. *Neuropathol Appl Neurobiol* 1988;14:345–363.

105. Kieburtz KD, Giang DW, Schiffer RB. Abnormal vitamin B$_{12}$ metabolism in human immunodeficiency virus infection: association with neurological dysfunction. *Arch Neurol* 1991;48:312–314.

106. Levy RM, Beredesen DE, Rosenblum ML. Neurological manifestations of the acquired immunodeficiency syndrome. *J Neurosurg* 1985; 62:475–495.

107. Britton CB, Mesa-Tejada R, Fenoglio CM. A new complication of AIDS: thoracic myelitis caused by herpes simplex virus. *Neurology* 1985;35:1071–1074.

108. Mahieux F, Gray F, Fenelon G. Acute myeloradiculitis due to cytomegalovirus as the initial manifestation of AIDS. *J Neurol Neurosurg Psychiatry* 1989;52:270–274.

109. Bangham CR. HTLV-1 infections. *J Clin Pathol* 2000;53(8): 581–586.

110. Sheremata WA, Berger JR, Harrington WJ, et al. Human T-lymphotrophic virus type I–associated myelopathy. A report of 10 patients born in the United States. *Arch Neurol* 1992;49:1113–1118.

111. Gout O, Gessain A, Bolgert F, et al. Chronic myelopathies associated with human T-lymphotrophic virus type I. A clinical, serologic, and immunovirologic study of ten patients in France. *Arch Neurol* 1989; 46(3):255–260.

112. Taylor GP, Hall SE, Navarette S, et al. Effect of lamivudine on human T-cell leukemia virus type 1 (HTLV-I) DNA copy number, T-cell phenotype, and anti-tax cytotoxic T-cell frequency in patients with HTLV-1–associated myelopathy. *J Virol* 1999;73(12):10289–10295.

113. Pruitt AA. Infections of the nervous system. *Neurol Clin* 1998;16(2): 419–447.

VASCULAR, NUTRITIONAL, AND OTHER DISEASES OF THE SPINAL CORD

STEPHEN S. KAMIN

Although much less prone to vascular disease than the brain, the spinal cord may also be the site of ischemia. This may occur by classical mechanisms of thrombosis or embolism, as well as on a hemodynamic basis. Hemodynamic factors also contribute to the cord damage caused by dural arteriovenous malformations (AVMs). Various other conditions may also lead to spinal cord damage. Nutritional causes of myelopathy, both deficiency states such as subacute combined degeneration (SCD) and exposure to toxins in foodstuffs, as in lathyrism, are discussed in this chapter. Systemic diseases such as lupus erythematosus and Sjögren syndrome may lead to myelopathy. Iatrogenic injury to the cord as a result of radiation therapy also occurs. Finally, many inherited diseases involve the spinal cord. However, only hereditary spastic paraparesis (HSP) presents exclusively or predominantly as a typical myelopathy, and this is the only such disease discussed here.

SPINAL CORD STROKE

The rapid development of paraplegia with complete sensory loss and bowel and bladder dysfunction is a devastating occurrence that may result from ischemia of the spinal cord. Given the frequency of brain infraction, spinal cord stroke is a surprisingly rare phenomenon. The precise mechanism of spinal cord stroke often cannot be determined, but such strokes are frequently seen in the setting of aortic disease or manipulation of the aorta or in the aftermath of profound systemic hypotension. To understand the clinical picture and likely mechanisms of spinal stroke, one must have some knowledge of the vascular anatomy of the spinal cord.

Blood Supply of the Spinal Cord

The blood supply of the spinal cord was first described by Adamkiewicz in 1882 (1). The cord is supplied by a single, midline anterior spinal artery and two posterior spinal arteries (2). All arise from the vertebral arteries in the neck and run the length of the spinal cord. At the level of the conus medullaris, they form an anastomotic network that encircles the cord. They are

contributed to at each segmental level by a small branch of the radicular arteries. Only a few such arteries contribute to the blood supply to a significant extent, 6 to 10 anteriorly and 10 to 23 posteriorly. In the low thoracic and lumbar area, the blood supply is via a single large radicular artery, known as the artery of Adamkiewicz. This usually arises between T9 and L2, most frequently at T11 on the left. It can be distinguished on angiography by the distinctive hairpin turn it makes before entering the thecal sac.

The anterior spinal artery supplies approximately the anterior two thirds of the cord. This includes most of the gray matter of the cord and the anterior and lateral white-matter columns. The posterior spinal arteries supply the remainder, including the tips of the posterior horns and the posterior columns. Paramedian vessels arise from the anterior spinal artery and penetrate the deeper portions of the cord, particularly the gray matter. Anastomotic vessels between the anterior and the posterior spinal arteries give off many small penetrating vessels, which circumferentially supply the white matter. This pattern parallels that seen in the brain stem.

The primary inflow of blood to the spinal arteries is from the vertebral arteries rostrally and the artery of Adamkiewicz caudally. There are minor contributions from other radicular arteries along the remaining length of the spinal cord. This pattern of blood supply leads to a watershed or border-zone area in the upper to mid-thoracic level, which is often reflected in the clinical syndromes of spinal cord ischemia. There is another border-zone region within the gray matter of the cord, because the penetrating arteries are end arteries with limited anastomoses between them.

Spinal Stroke Syndromes

Various patterns of neurologic deficit can be seen in spinal cord ischemia, depending on the specific arteries involved. The most dramatic and devastating picture is that of total transection of the cord. This presents with flaccid paraplegia or quadriplegia, loss of all sensation below the level of the lesion, and bowel and bladder dysfunction. The onset is usually abrupt and progression is rapid. There is often radicular pain at the onset, which may last for hours or rarely days. If the infarct is in the cervical area, there is quadriplegia. Pain is generally interscapular and may radiate to the shoulder. In lower lesions, paraplegia results. Pain may radiate to the abdomen or the anterior thighs. In lesions of the conus medullaris, the pain is referred to the buttocks. The deep tendon reflexes (DTRs) and abdominal reflexes are abolished initially, but hyperreflexia may develop in days or weeks, along with Babinski signs. Sensory loss involves all modalities, and the intensity and level of the sensory loss may change during the course of the stroke. Sphincter dysfunction is generally complete, with urinary retention, constipation, and a lax anal sphincter. Other autonomic disturbances may also occur, including vasodilation with hypotension, bowel pseudoobstruction, loss of thermoregulatory reflexes, and pulmonary edema. The prognosis for functional improvement in this syndrome is poor, and medical complications are frequent.

The "classic" spinal stroke syndrome is the syndrome of the anterior spinal artery (3). This presents with flaccid paraplegia or quadriplegia and dissociated sensory loss below the level of the lesion. Pain and temperature sensations are affected, but vibration and joint position sense are relatively preserved. This reflects the pattern of blood supply to the cord, with the anterior spinal artery supplying only the anterior two thirds. Sphincter disturbance is usually present.

A partial Brown-Séquard syndrome occasionally occurs early in the course of anterior spinal artery infarction (4). This may reflect occlusion of a paramedian penetrating vessel. Other partial syndromes also frequently occur. The anterior horn may be preferentially affected due to the greater susceptibility of gray matter to ischemia, compared with white matter (5). This produces flaccid weakness without sensory or sphincter disturbance, often described as pseudopoliomyelitis. If it occurs in the cervical region, there is isolated arm weakness.

The posterior spinal artery syndrome is rare and difficult to recognize (6). It usually begins with spinal pain and paresthesias in the legs. Examination reveals loss of vibration and joint position sense in the legs and areflexia. There is often variable weakness and sphincter dysfunction due to more anterior extension of the infarction, but the degree of involvement is never as profound as that in the anterior spinal artery syndrome.

Central cord infarctions may result from border-zone ischemia in the central gray matter of the cord. They do not differ clinically from other spinal cord strokes and can only be diagnosed radiographically or pathologically. They often are merely longitudinal extensions of complete transverse infarcts.

Mechanisms of Spinal Cord Infarction

In many cases, the precise mechanism of spinal cord infarction cannot be determined. There are, however, a number of situations that predispose to such infarcts and a specific mechanism may be inferred.

Hypotensive Infarction

Border-zone or watershed infarction of the cord may occur as a result of profound hypotension. As discussed earlier, the vascular supply of the cord makes certain segments, particularly in the mid-thoracic region, more prone to ischemia when the perfusion pressure is reduced. Consequently, in the setting of a marked decrease in blood pressure due to cardiac arrest or massive hemorrhage, infarction may ensue. The usual presentation is acute flaccid paraplegia with sensory loss and areflexia corresponding to the transverse infarction picture discussed earlier. This may be the most common cause of cord infarction. In a review of 11 cases of spinal stroke at the Stokes Mandeville Spinal Injuries Center in Britain, 10 of the cases were due to hypotension and only 1 to aortic occlusion (7). Four additional patients who suffered hypotension during surgery were described later (8). Similar events have also been reported in children (5). The degree and duration of hypotension necessary to produce infarction in humans are unknown. In these series, one patient was in cardiac arrest for 5 minutes and another had a minimum pressure recorded of 47/25, which persisted for 2½ hours. On the other hand, one patient had a lowest recorded pressure of 90/60, but the interoperative records were incomplete. Kobrine et al. (9) found in experimental monkeys that both spinal cord and cerebral blood flow began to decrease when the mean arterial pressure was 50 mm Hg and was unmeasurable at a pressure of 25 mm Hg. They felt that autoregulation was more robust in the brain than the cord, making the cord more sensitive to hypotension. How this information relates to humans with atherosclerosis is uncertain, but it is likely that superimposed arterial narrowing may further compromise the circulation of the cord and increase the risk of ischemia even at higher levels of blood pressure.

Stroke in Association with Aortic Surgery

It has been known for many years that operation on the aorta presents a significant risk of postoperative paraplegia (Fig. 33.1) (10). In experimental dogs, paraplegia can be induced in 50% of animals whose aorta is occluded distal to the left subclavian artery (11). DeBakey et al. (12) reported a 5.5% incidence of paraplegia after resection of aneurysms of the descending aorta. Crawford et al. (13) reported an incidence of 6.8% even with the use of extracorporeal bypass. In correction of coarctation of the aorta, Brewer et al. (14) reported an incidence of paraplegia of 0.41% of 12,532 cases. There was no clear correlation between the risk of paraplegia and the number of intercostal arteries sacrificed or the duration of aortic occlusion. Investigators have generally felt that if the aorta was occluded below the level of the renal arteries, cord infarction would not occur (15). However, even in this situation, paraplegia rarely occurs (16).

It is difficult to determine the precise mechanism of infarction in these cases. Systemic hypotension occurred in some cases. In others, occlusion of radicular arteries by the aortic lesion may lead to infarction, particularly in the setting of relative hypotension. Aortic dissection may result in paraplegia by such a mechanism in the absence of surgical intervention. Coarctation of the aorta may also lead to spontaneous paraplegia. In some cases, the mechanism appeared to be ischemic, whereas in others, it was compressive due to epidural or subarachnoid hemorrhage (17).

Embolism

Fibrocartilaginous material from intervertebral discs is probably the most common source of emboli to the spinal cord. Such

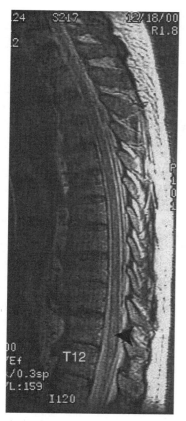

FIGURE 33.1. The patient is a 56-year-old man who underwent an aortic aneurysm repair with postoperative incomplete paraplegia. This T2-weighted magnetic resonance image shows patchy increased intramedullary signal from T9 down through the conus medullaris (*arrowhead*). This finding represents probably spinal cord infarction or ischemia, possibly related to injury to the artery of Adamkiewicz. There is also a less prominent increase in signal extending up to T7.

emboli are hypothesized to originate from Schmorl nodules and to reach the cord via the basivertebral vein of the vertebral body. These emboli most often affect the cervical region. They may be associated with trauma, often of a minor nature, or with pregnancy and the puerperium (18–21). Atheromatous emboli are very rare (17). Cholesterol embolism has also been reported (22).

Venous Infarction

Occlusion of the venous drainage of the cord may also lead to infarction, although reports of such cases are rare. Hughes (23) reported a pathologically proven case that demonstrated hemorrhagic infarction of the central cord from T3 through T6. Clarke and Cumming (24) reported a classic anterior spinal artery syndrome in association with thrombosis of the left common femoral and internal iliac veins. The results of an arteriogram were negative, so infarction was felt to be secondary to the venous lesion. Rao et al. (25) reviewed 15 cases from the literature in 1982. Pain in the back, abdomen, or neck was common at the onset, occurring in ten patients. The infarctions were generally

extensive, six involving the whole cord. Two of these also involved the medulla. The underlying conditions predisposing to venous infarction included chronic infections, polycythemia vera, ulcerative colitis, and pancreatic cancer. In some cases, there was *in situ* venous thrombosis and in others emboli occurred.

Other Causes

Spinal cord infarction has been reported as a consequence of vertebral artery dissection. Crum et al. (26) reported one case and reviewed seven others from the literature. Minor cervical trauma or chiropractic manipulation were reported in some cases. The anterior spinal artery syndrome occurred in two cases and the posterior spinal artery syndrome in three. A combination of spinal cord and medullary infarction was seen in two patients. Unilateral dissection could cause either unilateral or bilateral infarctions, but unilateral infarction always resulted from unilateral dissection.

Vasculitis has rarely been reported to cause spinal cord infarction. In the preantibiotic era, meningovascular syphilis was often presumed to be the cause of spinal stroke, but there are few proven cases (27,28). Other chronic meningitides such as tuberculosis and cryptococcosis can also lead to spinal stroke (29). Two cases of spinal cord infarction due to polyarteritis nodosa were reported by Corbin (30).

SPINAL ARTERIOVENOUS MALFORMATIONS (FOIX-ALAJOUANINE SYNDROME)

In 1926, Foix and Alajouanine (31) described two patients who developed subacute myelopathy leading to death. At autopsy, they discovered necrosis of the spinal cord and numerous thick-walled tortuous vessels lying on the surface of the cord (31). Lhermitte et al. (32) identified these vessels as being associated with an AVM, which usually resides on the dura. It was generally believed that the rapidly progressing myelopathy resulted from thrombosis of these abnormal vessels within the spinal cord (33, 34). Consequently, this process, which came to be known as the Foix-Alajouanine syndrome, was felt to be irreversible and to carry a very poor prognosis. For instance, Aminoff and Logue at Queen Square and Maida Vale analyzed 60 cases (35,36). Within 6 months of onset, 19% of patients required bilateral support to walk or were wheelchair bound. Within 3 years, 50% were at that stage of disability. Only 30% were walking independently at 3 years.

Spinal AVMs are classified into four types (37). Type I AVMs, also called dural arteriovenous fistulas, are the most common type. They generally lie on the dorsal aspect of the lower thoracic cord and conus medullaris. There is usually a single feeding vessel. Type II lesions are intramedullary lesions with a true AVM nidus within the spinal cord. Type III lesions are so-called juvenile malformations and are rare. Type IV AVMs are intradural, extramedullary lesions and are also relatively uncommon. The remainder of this section focuses on type I lesions, and to a lesser extent type II lesions.

The course of the condition is most often gradual, particularly in type I lesions. This was the case in 23 of 27 patients in the series by Rosenblum et al. (38) and 40 of 71 of the patients in the series by Tobin and Layton (39). There may be episodes of stepwise deterioration interspersed with periods of stability or slow progression, as seen in 11 of 71 of the patients in the Mayo Clinic series (39). Acute onset of symptoms is more common in the intramedullary type II lesions (50%, per Rosenblum et al. [38]), probably due to hemorrhage. It may be many years from onset of symptoms before the correct diagnosis is made (38). One third of the patients in the series by Symon et al. (40) had symptoms for 3 years or more before diagnosis.

The most common initial symptoms are sensory disturbance and pain and leg weakness (Table 33.1). Sphincter disturbance is much less common at onset. It is important to realize that the location of pain is not a reliable guide to the site of the vascular malformation (41). By the time of diagnosis, leg weakness, sensory disturbance, and sphincter dysfunction are almost universal. The major physical signs (Table 33.2) include leg weakness, usually of an upper motor neuron type, although Aminoff and Logue (41) found muscle atrophy in two thirds of patients and increased reflexes in only 45% (39). A sensory level is usually found, although radicular sensory loss or the Brown-Séquard syndrome occurs occasionally. None of these signs or symptoms are at all specific for the diagnosis of a spinal AVM. The only pathognomonic finding is a bruit over the spine, and this is not common. It was found in two of eight cases in the Mayo Clinic series in which it was listened for (39,42). A cutaneous angioma may overlie the AVM, and this may be more common than a spinal bruit (43).

Definitive diagnosis of spinal AVMs requires radiographic demonstration of the vascular anomaly. Angiography provides the most detailed information on the vascular anatomy but is technically challenging. Myelography usually demonstrates serpiginous filling defects dorsal to the cord, but small lesions can be missed. It is often necessary to turn the patient onto his or her back to demonstrate the abnormality. Magnetic resonance imaging (MRI) has now nearly replaced myelography in the

TABLE 33.2. FOIX-ALAJOUANINE SYNDROME: NEUROLOGIC SIGNS

Sign	%
Abnormal gait	76
Weakness	75
Reflex abnormality	—
Hyperreflexia	56
Hyporeflexia	14
Both	10
Sensory	—
Radicular	13
Nonradicular	54
Spinal level	55
Sphincter	—
Bladder	52
Bowel	24
Babinski sign	31

From Tobin WD, Layton DD Jr. The diagnosis and natural history of spinal cord arteriovenous malformations. *Mayo Clin Proc* 1976;51:637–646.

initial diagnosis of spinal AVMs, but there are no good studies of the sensitivity of this technique (44).

The pathophysiology of the Foix-Alajouanine syndrome is now felt to be related to increased venous pressure from the AVM, rather than to a primary thrombotic process (45). Even intracranial fistulas may occasionally produce the syndrome by such a mechanism (46). Consequently, the neurologic deficits are potentially reversible with elimination of the fistula. As early as 1979, Logue (36) reported motor improvement from surgical extirpation of dural AVMs in 15 of 24 patients whom he treated at Queen Square. Five of seven chair-bound patients regained some ability to walk. Surgery was relatively ineffective in reversing sphincter disturbance. Only 5 of 23 patients with abnormal bladder function improved and only 2 regained normal bladder function. Eleven of 22 patients had modest improvement in sensation. Eight of 12 patients with pain were pain free postoperatively. Sexual function was unaffected by surgery. Similar or better results were reported by Symon et al. (40). Interestingly, all three patients with intracranial fistulas reported by Wrobel et al. (46) had some improvement with surgery. In addition to surgical obliteration of the fistula, endovascular embolization with polyvinyl alcohol beads or with cyanoacrylate ("superglue") is also effective, although recanalization may occur (47–51). In balancing efficacy and risk, Anson and Spetzler (37) believe that surgery is the preferred treatment in most cases.

NUTRITIONAL MYELOPATHIES

Subacute Combined Degeneration

The association between progressive myelopathy and pernicious anemia has been recognized since the latter part of the nineteenth century (52). This condition was named subacute combined degeneration (SCD) by Russell (53), because of the consistent involvement of both posterior columns and corticospinal tracts (CSTs). The condition was identified quite early to result from

TABLE 33.1. FOIX-ALAJOUANINE SYNDROME: INITIAL SYMPTOMS

Symptom	%
Sensory	97
Radicular	21
Spinal level	37
Leg weakness	56
Pain	49
Radicular	17
Nonradicular	10
Back pain	23
Sphincter disturbance	35
Bladder	25
Bowel	10
Ataxic gait	20

From Tobin WD, Layton DD Jr. The diagnosis and natural history of spinal cord arteriovenous malformations. *Mayo Clin Proc* 1976;51;637–646.

a nutritional deficiency, although the missing factor, vitamin B_{12} was not isolated until 1948 (54). In 1926, Minot and Murphy (55) devised a treatment based on a diet including at least a half a pound of liver per day, for which they won the Nobel Prize. One can imagine the unpalatable nature of this treatment.

The selective deficiency of vitamin B_{12} in pernicious anemia is caused not by a dietary deficiency of B_{12}, but by the absence of intrinsic factor, which is necessary for the absorption of minute amounts of the vitamin in the terminal ileum. SCD also occurs in other settings leading to defects of B_{12} absorption, such as extensive gastric resection, ileal resection, tapeworm infestation and other causes of intestinal malabsorption. Dietary deficiency of B_{12} may also lead to SCD. The condition takes a long time to develop, because normal body stores of B_{12} are approximately 5 mg, and daily loss of the vitamin is only 1 to 2.6 µg per day. Thus, total depletion may take several years to occur (57,58).

The clinical presentation of SCD is quite stereotyped and consistent (57,59). Sensory symptoms, usually numbness or tingling in the legs, are almost always the first complaint. Weakness and unsteadiness of gait occur later. The arms are rarely affected. Sphincter disturbance is uncommon. The earliest neurologic sign is loss of vibration and joint position sense in the legs. Alterations of other sensory modalities occur only in more severe and long-standing cases. Reflex changes are variable early on, but reflexes are invariably diminished in more severe cases. Extensor plantar responses are generally seen in severe cases (9 of 14 cases in reference 57). Lhermitte's sign was seen in 25% of cases seen at the Queen Square Hospital in London (60). Overall, neurologic signs and symptoms are more common in patients with dietary vitamin B_{12} deficiency and pernicious anemia than in those with other causes of B_{12} deficiency (59).

Vitamin B_{12} deficiency has other physiologic effects in addition to SCD. Megaloblastic anemia is common, but it is important to recognize that neurologic involvement may precede the anemia. In the large pathologic series from the Massachusetts General Hospital, all 41 cases had anemia (57). However, SCD without anemia has been well described (61,62). Dementia and affective disorders are also common in B_{12} deficiency. They occurred in 46% of cases in the series by Shorvon et al. (59).

The diagnosis of SCD rests on the determination of vitamin B_{12} levels in a patient with a consistent history and neurologic examination. Borderline-low levels may cause some confusion, and demonstration of elevated homocysteine and methylmalonic acid levels is very useful. These are the main substrates of the enzymes for which B_{12} serves as a cofactor and are therefore typically elevated in B_{12} deficiency. A rather complex algorithm for laboratory evaluation is outlined by Green and Kinsella (63). Electrophysiologic testing may reveal abnormalities. Sensory nerve conduction velocities may be slowed and somatosensory evoked potentials are almost always abnormal. Tibial P37 responses are delayed and median nerve P14 latencies and P9 to P14 and N13 to P14 interpeak latencies are prolonged (64,65). This is consistent with slowed central conduction at the cervical cord level. Central motor conduction times are usually normal. Evoked responses may improve or normalize with treatment in a few patients (64).

MRI findings have now been reported in a number of cases of SCD and correlate very well with the clinical picture. Hyper-intense lesions on T2-weighted scans are typical and are often confined to the posterior columns (64,66–68). Contrast enhancement has been reported (69). High signal has also been seen in the brain stem (66).

The pathologic findings in SCD are very consistent (57). The earliest change is swelling of the myelin sheaths leading to a vacuolated appearance of the white-matter tracts of the cord. Each vacuole represents a single axon. Later, macrophages infiltrate and many lipid-laden macrophages are present. In chronic lesions, there is also a dense fibrillary gliosis. The posterior columns are always affected and may be the only site of degeneration. Lateral and anterior funiculi may also be involved. These findings correlate very well with the clinical presentation of a primarily posterior column type of sensory loss with sensory ataxia. The lower cervical segments are the most severely affected levels in about half of the cases and thoracic segments are comparably affected in most of the rest. Abnormalities of the dorsal root ganglia and peripheral nerves are not prominent. The pathologic changes in experimental animals subjected to a B_{12}-deficient diet are identical (58). It took 3 to 4 years to produce the syndrome in these monkeys, quite similar to the situation in human cases.

It is generally felt that the biochemical basis of SCD is a defect in the synthesis of methionine from homocysteine. However, the enzyme methionine synthase also requires folate as a cofactor, and folate deficiency much less often produces neurologic impairment. Shorvon et al. (59) identified neurologic and psychological abnormalities in 65% of their patients with isolated folate deficiency (compared with 68% of those with B_{12} deficiency), but these were almost exclusively affective disorders and dementia. They identified no cases of SCD due to folate deficiency. However, a number of case reports of SCD induced by folate deficiency have appeared in the literature (70–73). Folate supplementation may reverse the neurologic abnormalities (73).

An interesting iatrogenic cause of SCD is nitrous oxide anesthesia. The first cases actually resulted from nitrous oxide abuse by health care workers, particularly dentists (74–76). Schilling (77) (of the Schilling test fame) reported the first case of SCD induced by nitrous oxide anesthesia in a patient with unrecognized B_{12} deficiency. Other cases have followed (67,78–81).

Treatment of SCD rests on the repletion of the body stores of vitamin B_{12} (63). This is most rapidly accomplished with an intramuscular injection of 100 to 1,000 µg of B_{12} per day for 5 days, followed by 100 to 1,000 µg injected intramuscularly monthly thereafter. Oral therapy is also effective, even for patients with pernicious anemia, because approximately 1% of dietary B_{12} is absorbed by passive diffusion independent of intrinsic factor. Therefore, an oral dose of 1,000 µg of B_{12} per day will provide 10 µg of absorbed B_{12}, an amount greater than daily requirements.

Vitamin E Deficiency

Spinocerebellar degeneration due to vitamin E deficiency is often initially mistaken for SCD. Vitamin E is a fat-soluble vitamin that may be deficient in patients with chronic malabsorption syndromes or liver disease with cholestasis. Its absorption depends on the presence of bile salts, which are reabsorbed in the terminal ileum. Harding et al. (82) published the classic description of patients with spinocerebellar degeneration due to malabsorption. Additional cases have since been reported (83–87). Patients generally present with sensory ataxia due to loss of joint position sense from posterior column involvement. They also typically have leg weakness and absent DTRs. True cerebellar ataxia is present, presumably due to involvement of the spinocerebellar tracts. Dysarthria has also been reported, and one patient had ophthalmoplegia, implicating brain-stem structures as well. Supplementation with vitamin E may lead to substantial improvement in symptoms.

Although pathologic studies are not available in humans, monkeys with experimental vitamin E deficiency show loss of axons and myelin in the dorsal columns (88). There is also marked loss of large myelinated fibers in the sural nerve. This correlates well with the main clinical feature of sensory ataxia in humans. MRI of a human case showed T2 hyperintense lesions in the posterior columns, again correlating well with the clinical picture (87).

A similar condition has been reported in children with chronic liver failure or cystic fibrosis and in experimental animals (89–92). Abetalipoproteinemia, or Bassen-Kornzweig disease, an inherited condition, is also characterized by vitamin E deficiency with acanthocytosis and spinocerebellar ataxia (93). Cases of neuroacanthocytosis without β-lipoprotein deficiency typically present with chorea and self-mutilation, rather than spinocerebellar ataxia (94,95).

Toxic Myelopathy

In addition to the myelopathies caused by the nutritional deficiency states discussed earlier, myelopathies can also be produced by the ingestion of toxins in food. (Here, we are not referring to accidental contaminations, but to naturally occurring toxins in staple foods.) These conditions are not seen in the United States but are not rare in tropical areas where the diet depends nearly exclusively on certain crops.

The best known of these nutritional toxicities is lathyrism (96,97). This term refers to several different syndromes produced by the ingestion of chickpeas of the genus *Lathyrus*. Effects on bones and blood vessels (osteolathyrism and angiolathyrism) are seen only in experimental animals. The human disease, neurolathyrism, is characterized by the subacute onset of weakness in the legs. Pain and paresthesias may also occur. The affected person develops a spastic gait and often needs canes to walk. Sphincter disturbance and erectile dysfunction are common in some series. Sensory loss is less common. In a review of 35 cases from Uttar Pradesh in 1975, 71% of patients presented with motor symptoms (98); 34% had paresthesias; and only 6% had bladder disturbance at onset. The disease developed over less than a week in 3 cases, one to two weeks in 13 cases, and one to six months in 19 cases. The condition is generally permanent. Pathologic studies reveal degeneration of the white matter of the spinal cord, predominantly in the CSTs.

Use of these peas as one third to one half of the diet for 2 months or more is sufficient to produce the syndrome. This generally occurs in conditions of severe disruption of the food supply, as in times of war, flood, or famine. As recently as the 1980s, it was still endemic in parts of India, Bangladesh, and Ethiopia. This condition was recognized by Hippocrates in 46 BC, who wrote, "At Ainos, all men and women who ate peas continuously became impotent in the legs and that state persisted."

Several different compounds present in various *Lathyrus* species have been proposed as causes of lathyrism. These include β-cyano-L-alanine, β-diaminobutyric acid, and N-oxalyl-amino-L-alanine (BOAA) (99–101). This last is generally postulated as the actual species at fault. Feeding BOAA to macaque monkeys does produce a clinically similar upper motor neuron disease, but no pathologic studies have been reported (102). It may exert its effect by neuroexcitatory mechanisms. This compound is closely related to *N*-methylamin-L-alanine, the component in the cycads felt to be the cause of the parkinsonism–amyotrophic lateral sclerosis–dementia complex seen on Guam.

A similar condition known as "konzo" occurs in Africa in populations where the staple food is manioc, or cassava root. This is a plant that contains a number of cyanogens, compounds that release cyanide under acidic conditions. It has been known for centuries by those who use this crop that the roots must be soaked and prepared carefully to extract these compounds before eating. However, during droughts or civil unrest, the people often resort to varieties with higher concentrations of cyanogens and may not prepare the roots as carefully. This has led to outbreaks of konzo in Tanzania, Congo, and elsewhere in Africa. Victims have elevated levels of thiocyanate, the main metabolite of cyanide, in blood and urine (103,104). In one district of Zaire in 1991, Tylleskar et al. (105) found 110 cases in a population of 6,764. In 90% of cases, the disease was full blown in less than 1 day and never progressed over more than 3 days. The gait was always affected, with 25% needing canes and 11% unable to walk. Ninety-seven percent had hyperreflexia, 85% clonus, and 17% Babinski signs. Visual disturbance was also reported by 12% at the onset of the disease. A follow-up of a cohort of patients after 14 years showed no change in their neurologic condition (106). All patients in whom testing has been done had negative titers of human T-cell lymphoma/leukemia virus type 1 (HTLV-1) antibodies (107).

Interestingly, cassava eaters in West African countries such as Nigeria develop a quite different neurologic syndrome dubbed "tropical ataxic neuropathy" (108). This is characterized by sensory ataxia often associated with visual loss and sensorineural deafness. The most common symptoms are numbness and paresthesias (81%), visual loss (71%), ataxic gait (56%), weakness (35%), and hearing disturbance (34%). Neurologic signs include posterior column sensory loss (81%), leg and gait ataxia (67%), a positive Romberg sign (60%), optic atrophy (55%), and deafness (32%). Upper motor neuron signs are much less common (13%). It is not known why the ingestion of the same food causes two such different syndromes in different parts of Africa.

A very similar condition of ataxia and deafness was also reported by Montgomery et al. (109) in Jamaica. Spinal fluid was normal in all 25 cases and poor nutrition was reported in 19 of 21 cases in which this information was available. In contrast, a spastic paraparesis was seen in 181 patients. These latter patients rarely had deafness. Spinal fluid was often abnormal, with up to 49 white cells, and protein was elevated in 35%. There was no apparent association with nutritional status. Autopsies were available only on spastic cases and showed demyelination and perivascular lymphocytic infiltrates. It is my opinion that most of these latter were cases of tropical spastic paraparesis/HTLV-1 associated myelopathy, a condition that was not recognized in 1964.

MYELOPATHY IN COLLAGEN-VASCULAR DISEASE

Systemic Lupus Erythematosus

Neurologic abnormalities are common in systemic lupus erythematosus (SLE). The very first description of the disease by Kaposi (110) in 1872 included two patients with delirium. The classic review of the subject by Johnson and Richardson (111) reported 24 autopsied cases from the Massachusetts General Hospital. Thirteen patients had seizures; ten, cranial nerve disorders; three, hemiparesis; two, peripheral neuropathy; and eight, mental disorders. One patient had paraparesis from spinal cord involvement. They also reviewed 14 other cases of spinal cord disease from the literature.

A more recent review identified 34 cases of myelopathy in the literature and described two more (112). Patients generally presented with paraparesis (67%) and numbness of the legs (53%). Bladder dysfunction was present in 31% and back pain in 31%. The ultimate degree of deficit was generally severe. Fifty-eight percent became paraplegic, and sphincter function was lost in 91%. Loss of reflexes was as common as hyperreflexia. The sensory level was most often thoracic (69%). Outcome was poor overall. On follow-up, 37% of patients had died and 40% had little or no improvement. Only 20% returned to normal.

Although myelopathy is one of the less common neurologic manifestations of SLE, it is not truly rare. In one study from a single center, 3% of the patients had spinal cord disease (113). In five of ten patients, it was the first manifestation of lupus. A prospective study of 500 patients with SLE produced 4 who already had myelopathy and 12 more who developed it during the follow-up (114). Interestingly, 15 of these 16 had anticardiolipin antibodies. The remaining patient had false-positive Venereal Disease Research Laboratories test results and an elevated activated partial thromboplastin time. This obviously suggests a possible mechanism for this rather mysterious condition. In the review by Al-Husaini and Jamal (112), 11 of 17 patients for whom information was available had a false-positive serologic test result for syphilis. On the other hand, Mok et al. (113) found no association with antiphospholipid antibodies.

Cerebrospinal fluid (CSF) is usually abnormal in lupus-associated myelopathy (115). In 20 patients who had lumbar punctures, 16 had elevated protein, generally more than 100 mg/dL. Glucose concentration was reduced in four cases. In contrast, of 21 patients with lupus and neurologic disease other than myelopathy, only one had a low glucose. A leukocytic pleocytosis was seen in 15 of 20 patients, ranging from 7 to 16,100 cells. A significant number of red blood cells were seen in five patients. Even higher proportions of CSF abnormalities were reported in the review by Al-Husaini and Jamal (112), primarily in cases reported after 1973.

Pathologic studies are rare and show various changes. Vascular changes were reported in 11 of 12 cases and 8 of these had myelomalacia, necrosis, or infarction, suggesting a vascular etiology of the myelopathy. In contrast, Johnson and Richardson (111) reported a vacuolar degeneration of all the white-matter tracts with lipid-laden macrophages. Provenzale and Bouldin (116) reported similar findings, which they dubbed "subpial leukomyelopathy," in seven cases; only three cases had cord infarcts.

The most appropriate treatment of lupus-associated myelopathy is unknown. Corticosteroids have been used most often and may be beneficial. Propper and Bucknall (117) reported that of 26 cases, 7 had a partial or full recovery. This included five of eight patients on high-dose steroid treatment and 2 of 18 on low-dose treatment. Berlanga et al. (118) treated one patient with monthly intravenous cyclophosphamide with recovery, after a relapse occurred on tapering the patient's steroid treatment. Slovick (119) employed plasma exchange and reported improvement beginning within 1 day of instituting treatment.

Sjögren Syndrome

The other collagen-vascular disease that has been most frequently associated with myelopathy is Sjögren syndrome. Central nervous system (CNS) disease occurs in up to 20% of all patients with Sjögren syndrome (120,121). Disease is usually multifocal and the spinal cord is often involved. The course of this disease is usually relapsing and remittent. Alexander et al. (122) reported on 20 patients with CNS manifestations of Sjögren syndrome. Out of the 20 patients, 17 had myelopathy; 13 had paraparesis, most often acute or subacute in onset; 10 of the patients had neurogenic bladder, of whom two had no other evidence of spinal cord disease; and two had the Brown-Séquard syndrome. All the patients had evidence of brain disease. Pathology in one case revealed an angiitis of arterioles and venules and necrosis of the cord (123).

The multifocal, relapsing-remitting nature of the manifestations in Sjögren syndrome raises the diagnostic possibility of multiple sclerosis in patients not already diagnosed with Sjögren syndrome. MRI results have been reported in one case of myelopathy, showing increased signal on T2-weighted images and enhancement with gadolinium (124). CSF analysis also resembles the picture of multiple sclerosis. Oligoclonal bands were seen in 89% of patients with Sjögren syndrome (122) and an increased immunoglobulin G (IgG) index is also common. There is often a mild lymphocytic pleocytosis. Of course, the presence of the sicca complex can generally distinguish Sjögren syndrome from multiple sclerosis, and two thirds of patients with Sjögren syndrome have serologic evidence of the disease.

Steroids have generally been employed in the treatment of CNS Sjögren syndrome. This appears to be beneficial, but the occurrence of spontaneous remissions makes this conclusion uncertain. Plasma exchange and chlorambucil have also been used (125,126).

A further complicating issue in the diagnosis of Sjögren syndrome–associated myelopathy is that many patients with HTLV-1 infection also have the sicca syndrome. In two Japanese studies (HTLV-1 is endemic in certain parts of Japan), 12 of 31 and 6 of 10 patients with HTLV-1–associated myelopathy had Sjögren syndrome by standard criteria (127,128).

HEPATIC MYELOPATHY

Liver failure is a well recognized cause of CNS dysfunction. In the presence of spontaneous or surgically produced portosystemic shunts, a reversible syndrome of cognitive dysfunction known as hepatic encephalopathy is common. This syndrome is weakly correlated with hyperammonemia, although it is likely that ammonia is not the actual toxic substance. Protein restriction and treatment with lactulose and nonabsorbable antibiotics such as neomycin generally improve or reverse the encephalopathy. There is also an irreversible hepatocerebral degeneration manifesting as an extrapyramidal syndrome similar to Wilson disease.

Much less well recognized is a generally irreversible myelopathy, which has been named "hepatic myelopathy" or "portosystemic myelopathy." This syndrome, first described by Zieve et al. (129,130) in 1960, is characterized by progressive spastic weakness of the legs. Sensory loss and sphincter disturbance are rare. As of 1999, 50 cases have been reported in the English-language literature (131). Most of the patients had undergone surgical portosystemic shunting, although a few cases have also occurred in patients with spontaneous shunts (132,133). We have seen one case in a patient with no evidence of portosystemic shunting. The mean interval from shunting to onset of paraparesis is 28.7 months, with a range of 4 to 120 months (131). Most (80%) patients have also had episodes of hepatic encephalopathy, often recurrently. The degree of neurologic impairment and its rate of development are variable. Many patients are fairly severely affected, and most require assistance in ambulation.

The diagnosis of hepatic myelopathy is clinical, based on the recognition of myelopathy in the appropriate setting. Other identifiable causes of myelopathy must be excluded. Likely causes in this patient population include vitamin B_{12} or folate deficiency, neurosyphilis, human immunodeficiency virus and HTLV-1 infection, and compressive lesions of the spinal cord. Only a few reports of MRI have been published (131,133–135). None showed any abnormality.

Pathologic information is available in only 15 cases of hepatic myelopathy (see the references in reference 131). This uniformly showed demyelination of the lateral CSTs and occasionally the ventral CSTs and posterior columns. There was variable axonal loss. The lesions are found throughout the length of the spinal cord, becoming more prominent at lower levels.

The pathogenesis of hepatic myelopathy is not well understood. There appear to be no experimental models of the condition. Since portosystemic shunting is almost always present, it is likely to be crucial in the development of myelopathy. It is generally assumed that some toxic substance plays a role, although the exact nature of this substance is unclear (130, 134–139). Hemodynamic factors or nutritional deficiencies are also possibilities (140,141).

Treatment of hepatic myelopathy has generally been unrewarding. The usual interventions for hepatic encephalopathy, including protein restriction, lactulose, and neomycin, usually have no effect on the neurologic deficit. A small number of cases have improved (142–145). Two cases of liver transplantation in patients with hepatic myelopathy have been reported. In one case, the myelopathy improved, and in the other, there was no change (146,147).

PARANEOPLASTIC NECROTIZING MYELOPATHY

When myelopathy occurs in the setting of a systemic malignancy, the cause is almost always extrinsic compression of the spinal cord by metastases to the spine. Rarely, neurologic syndromes may occur in the absence of direct metastatic involvement of the nervous system and without metabolic derangements. These are known as paraneoplastic syndromes, or in the older literature "remote effects of cancer" (148). The mechanism of these syndromes is generally immunologic, with antibodies to tumor cell surface proteins that cross-react with components of normal neural elements. The most common of these are paraneoplastic cerebellar degeneration due to anti–Purkinje cell antibodies or antineuronal nuclear antibodies, and paraneoplastic limbic encephalitis or encephalomyelitis, also due to antineuronal nuclear antibodies. These occur most often in cases of small cell cancer of the lung, ovarian cancer, and lymphomas but have been reported in numerous other malignancies.

A much rarer paraneoplastic syndrome is necrotizing myelopathy. A review by Ojeda (149) in 1984 identified 22 cases in the literature and reported two additional cases. Since then, a handful of further cases have been reported (150–156). This is a fulminant condition characterized by rapidly progressive flaccid paralysis. The patients may be paraplegic or quadriplegic, depending on the site of cord involvement. Reflexes are lost and sensation is diminished to all modalities. Eventually, respiratory function may be compromised and the patient dies either of respiratory failure or of medical complications. The longest reported survival from onset of plegia is 150 days, but the median is 30 days, with a range of 5 to 150 days. The syndrome has been associated with various tumors, with the most common being lymphoma (nine cases), lung (six cases), and breast (four cases). CSF studies have shown increases in protein that can be dramatic (up to 2.7 g/dL), generally normal glucose levels, and small numbers of lymphocytes (2 to 27), neutrophils (2 to 48), and erythrocytes (0 to 800). One case had an increase in CSF IgG and helper T cells (154). Treatment has generally been of no benefit, but one case improved with steroids (151). MRI has been reported in only a few cases and shows T2 hyperintensity with swelling of the cord (155).

Pathologic examination reveals massive hemorrhagic necrosis of the gray and white matter of the spinal cord. There is no predilection for particular tracts or structures. Spinal blood vessels are generally normal, although fibrin thrombi have been reported in venules and arterioles. The longitudinal extent of involvement is variable, ranging from a few segments to the whole cord. Most often, cervical and thoracic levels are involved.

HEREDITARY SPASTIC PARAPARESIS

HSP is a diverse group of inherited disorders characterized by progressive spastic paresis of the legs. The condition has recently been reviewed by McDermott et al. (157). It was first described by Strümpell (158) in 1880 and has acquired the eponym Strümpell-Lorrain syndrome. Over the next 100 years, various authors reported a number of cases that formed a rather heterogeneous group, with variable age of onset, rapidity of progression, and involvement of other neural systems. Harding (159) was the first investigator to impose some order on this rather messy condition in 1981.

Harding divided HSP into "pure" cases with no other significant neurologic findings and "complicated" ones, which had a variety of other neurologic deficits such as amyotrophy, seizures, sensory neuropathy, and dementia. Within the pure group, there also appeared to be a natural division between those with onset before the age of 35 years and slow progression (type I) and those with later onset and more rapid worsening (type II). However, there was still significant overlap between groups and the borders are rather fuzzy. As with the spinocerebellar ataxias, recent information on the genetics of these conditions has shown that there is a good deal of clinical heterogeneity within genetically district groups, as is discussed later (157).

HSP is quite rare, with estimates of 2.0 to 9.6 per 100,000 in various European countries. Patients usually present with difficulty walking. There is often delay in walking in cases with childhood onset. Spasticity and bladder dysfunction are also common. Patients may be asymptomatic and abnormalities are only revealed on examination. The main physical findings are spasticity and hyperreflexia of the legs and less frequently the arms. Weakness is generally much less prominent. Less frequently, there may be sensory abnormalities, usually of vibration sense. Cranial nerve involvement does not occur in pure cases, although complicated cases may have retinal degeneration, optic atrophy, sensorineural hearing loss, or dysarthria.

A review by Durr et al. (160) of 23 index cases of pure autosomal-dominant HSP and 119 other family members revealed 70 cases. Of these, 12 were unaware of their deficits. Insidious onset of stiffness of the legs was the most frequent initial symptom (52 out of 70). Hyperreflexia was present in the legs in all patients and in the arms in 32%. Spasticity in the legs was mild in 14, moderate in 24, and severe in 16. There was proximal muscle weakness in the legs in 66%. Vibration sense was decreased in 65%. Sphincter dysfunction was present in 49%. The mean age at onset was 29 years and the distribution was unimodal. There was a good deal of variation within families.

Results of diagnostic testing are not specific but can be used to exclude alternative diagnoses such as cervical spondylosis or primary progressive multiple sclerosis. There may be cervical cord atrophy on MRI, as seen in 5 of 12 patients reported by Durr et al. (160). Mild brain atrophy occurs occasionally as well (160). CSF is generally normal (157). Electrophysiologic testing has revealed involvement of systems other than motor pathways, even in "pure" cases. Durr et al. (160) found evidence of axonal neuropathy in three members of one family. Visual evoked potentials were abnormal in 2 of 14, brain-stem potentials in 4 of 14, and somatosensory responses in 9 of 14.

There are very few pathologic reports of HSP. Most were published by Schwarz and Liu (161,162). In pure cases, the primary feature is axonal degeneration in CSTs and dorsal columns. The changes are most prominent in the thoracolumbar CST and cervical dorsal columns, particularly in the fasciculus gracilis. Spinocerebellar pathways are affected in about 50% of cases.

The genetics of HSP is very diverse. Cases can be autosomal dominant, autosomal recessive, or X linked. As of 1999, 11 distinct chromosomal loci have been identified for HSP. Many are heterogeneous, both clinically and in terms of the specific mutations involved. In only four is the mutant protein known. One of these is a housekeeping adenosine triphosphatase (ATPase) involved in many cellular functions and one is a mitochondrial protein analogous to yeast ATPases (163,164). Two X-linked forms have the best-characterized mutations. One form affects proteolipid protein and is thus allelic to Pelizaeus-Merzbacher disease (165,166). It causes a complicated form of HSP with cerebellar ataxia and mental retardation. The other X-linked form affects L1CAM, a cell adhesion molecule (167). Other mutations in this gene produce X-linked hydrocephalus, X-linked agenesis of the corpus callosum, and MASA syndrome (i.e., mental retardation, aphasia, shuffling gait, and adducted thumbs). Clearly, much more remains to be learned about these conditions. Further work on HSP will no doubt help shed light on the genetic and cellular basis of various neurodegenerative syndromes. Currently, there is no treatment.

RADIATION MYELOPATHY

Therapeutic radiation of the CNS is a common treatment modality in oncology. The brain or spinal cord may be irradiated as a treatment of primary or metastatic tumor. The nervous system, particularly the spinal cord, may also be an innocent bystander exposed during radiation of nearby malignancies. Although the CNS is generally felt to be relatively resistant to the deleterious effects of radiation because of the low rate of turnover of cells, it is of course not completely immune to injury. Particularly at higher doses, damage to the spinal cord may result from therapeutic radiation.

Two major clinical syndromes occur as a result of irradiation of the spinal cord. Early radiation myelopathy occurs 6 weeks to 6 months after radiation, with a mean of 10 to 16 weeks. The symptoms include numbness and paresthesias of the limbs and the electric-like shock symptom known as Lhermitte's sign. The symptoms may be intermittent. They typically resolved within a few months. The pathology is generally felt to be demyelination of the white-matter tracts, particularly the posterior columns. Such lesions are known to be the basis of Lhermitte's sign in conditions such as multiple sclerosis. An analogous phenomenon occurs after brain irradiation. Somatosensory evoked potentials showed prolongation of the N20 latency 3 months after irradiation of the neck for nasopharyngeal carcinoma. Latencies returned to normal at 9 months (168). In experimental animals, a delayed loss of oligodendrocytes can be observed as a result of radiation (169). There is no clear dose–response effect in this syndrome. Because this is a benign, spontaneously reversible condition, treatment is not indicated.

The more serious, and fortunately much rarer, condition is delayed radiation myelopathy. This generally presents as the gradual development of weakness and sensory loss below the level of irradiation. Sphincter disturbance may also occur. Hyperreflexia and extensor plantar responses are generally present. The condition may progress to a picture of complete cord transection. The onset of the delayed syndrome ranges from 6 months to 4 years from the time of radiation, with an average of 12 to 23 months, depending on the population reported on (170). Rarely, there may be acute onset of symptoms. Survival from onset of symptoms has varied widely in different studies, ranging from an average of 6.4 months to a maximum of 24 months (171).

Schultheiss et al. (171) have proposed three clinical criteria for the diagnosis of radiation myelopathy. First, no other etiology, such as direct involvement by tumor, must be present. Second, the signs and symptoms should be consistent with the picture outlined earlier. Finally, the dose and latency should be consistent with a radiation effect. Onset before 6 months is rare and should raise the question of other etiologies. The dose effects on spinal cord are not fully determined, but the condition is rare with total radiation doses of less than 5,000 cGy. Conventional fractionation with fractions of about 200 cGy yields an estimated incidence of about 0.2% at a total dose of 4,500 cGy. The level at which 5% of patients would develop myelopathy may be between 5,700 and 6,100 cGy. The 50% incidence level is probably between 6,800 and 7,300 cGy. Hyperfractionation, with multiple daily fractions of 40 to 50 cGy, appears to be more dangerous, because cellular repair mechanisms may not be effective with such short intertreatment intervals.

Given these dosage constraints, clinicians are understandably reluctant to reirradiate the spinal cord. This is not of purely theoretical importance, because cord compression due to epidural metastases is frequently a recurrent problem. A review from the Mayo Clinic reports on 54 such patients who were reirradiated (172). Total dosages received over both courses of radiation ranged from 3,650 to 8,089 cGy, with a median of 5,425 cGy. Forty patients were ambulatory at the start of reirradiation and 42 were walking at the end. There was later deterioration in five patients after 6½ to 22½ months. Only one of these patients underwent diagnostic imagining at that time, and he had new epidural metastasis. It is not known whether the other four patients had recurrent metastatic disease or radiation myelopathy. However, these results certainly suggest that reirradiation can generally be done safely if the clinical situation so warrants.

Pathologic studies have demonstrated two main classes of lesions in radiation myelopathy. The most extensive review was presented by Schultheiss et al. (173). In 50 cases, they identified 19 with purely white-matter lesions, 9 with purely vascular lesions, and 22 with a mixture of both. The white-matter lesions were characterized by demyelination, with fat-laden macrophages and sometimes with focal necrosis or axon loss. Vascular lesions included hemorrhage, thrombosis, fibrinoid necrosis, and infarction. A mononuclear cell inflammatory response occurred in approximately half the cases and was seen equally in white-matter and vascular cases. Cases with white-matter lesions had a shorter latency to onset than the vascular cases: 13.6 months in pure white-matter cases, 10.7 months in mixed, and 29.2 months in pure vascular lesions. These data indicate dual mecha-

nisms in the pathogenesis of radiation myelopathy, with both direct injury to oligodendroglia and damage to blood vessels.

The treatment of radiation myelopathy is unsatisfactory. Steroids may offer some transient benefit by decreasing cord edema (174). Prolonged improvement is rare (175,176). Based on the presumed vascular nature of the process, a few investigators have tried anticoagulation, with a few case reports of benefit (177, 178). Interestingly, this approach has also shown some promise in treating radiation necrosis of the brain (179). A French group reported stabilization or improvement of six of nine patients treated with hyperbaric oxygen (180).

DECOMPRESSION MYELOPATHY

With increasing numbers of people participating in sport scuba diving, decompression sickness is a condition that more physicians are likely to see. It has been known for nearly 150 years that rapid return to the surface after underwater activity can lead to serious health effects, often referred to as "the bends." At depth, nitrogen dissolves in the bloodstream and bubbles out of solution as the ambient pressure decreases on surfacing. This condition was first described in 1854 in workers excavating the piers of bridges (181–183). Indeed, Washington Roebling, engineer and builder of the Brooklyn Bridge was himself disabled and ultimately died of what was then called "caisson disease," after the pressurized underwater chambers, or caissons, in which the workers did their jobs.

Neurologic decompression injury is classified as type II decompression sickness. The most common manifestation is myelopathy. A review of 117 cases of neurologic injury reported to the National Diving Accident Network in 1981 and 1982 revealed 70 cases of type II decompression sickness (184). The most common presenting symptoms were progressive paresthesias (24 cases) and numbness of the limbs (39 cases), followed by weakness, nausea, dizziness and vertigo, headache, and ataxia (16, 12, 9, 6 and 4 cases respectively). Both arms and legs can be affected. Symptoms generally began more than half an hour after surfacing, and in 28% at least 6 hours after the dive.

The mechanism of decompression myelopathy has not been fully elucidated. The most widely accepted mechanism is venous congestion (185). Arterial occlusion by air embolus does not seem to be present. Pathologic studies on experimental animals have revealed white-matter hemorrhages and bubbles in the parenchyma of the cord (185,186). One human case of recovered decompression sickness, which came to autopsy, showed degeneration of the fasciculus gracilis from C1 through T4 and of the lateral CSTs from C1 through L4. MRI in 10 cases showed white-matter lesions consistent with the clinical picture (187, 188).

The primary treatment of decompression sickness is recompression therapy, and in mild to moderate cases is generally successful. The U. S. Navy has developed standard protocols for treatment. Hyperbaric oxygen or a 50:50 mixture of helium and oxygen is also effective (189). In the study by Dick and Massey (184), patients with mild symptoms recovered whether they were treated or not. Treatment of cases of intermediate severity was effective, but 4 of 16 such patients had neurologic residua for up to 1 month. Severe cases rarely respond to therapy. Although symptoms may slowly improve, they generally persist for at least 6 months. Residual symptoms included weakness, sensory loss, irritability, and emotional lability (184). In an Israeli review of 68 cases, 22% had persistent neurologic signs and symptoms (189). Even strict adherence to the standard decompression schedules devised by the U. S. Navy does not preclude the development of decompression sickness. In the Israeli study, 41% of the dives were well within the dive-table standards.

REFERENCES

1. Adamkiewicz A. Die blutgefasse des menschlichen ruckenmarkes. II. Die gefasse der ruckenmarksoberflache. Sitzungsberichte der Mathematisch-Naturwissenschaftlichen classe der Kaiserlichen Akademie der Wissenschaften Wien 1882;85:101–130.
2. Turnbull IA. Blood supply of the spinal cord. In: Vinken PJ, Bruyn GW, eds. *Handbook of clinical neurology,* vol 12. Amsterdam: North-Holland Publishing, 1972:478–491.
3. Garcin R, Godlewski S, Rondot P. Etude clinique des medullopathies d'origine vasculaire. *Rev Neurol* 1962;106:558–591.
4. Lapresle J, Decroit JP. Pathologie vasculaire de la moelle (a' l'exception de la pathologie malformative). In: *Encyclopedie Medico-Chirurgicale, Neurologie.* 1984:17067,A10,4.
5. Gilles FH, Nag D. Vulnerability of human spinal cord in transient cardiac arrest. *Neurology* 1971;21:833–839.
6. Gutowski NJ, Murphy RP, Beale DJ. Unilateral upper cervical posterior spinal artery syndrome following sneezing. *J Neurol Neurosurg Psychiatry* 1992;55:841–843.
7. Silver JR, Buxton PH. Spinal stroke. *Brain* 1974;97:539–550.
8. Singh U, Silver JR, Welply NC. Hypotensive infarction of the spinal cord. *Paraplegia* 1994;32:314–322.
9. Kobrine AI, Evans DE, Rizzole HV. Relative vulnerability of the brain and spinal cord to ischemia. *J Neurol Sci* 1980;45:65–72.
10. Ross RT. Spinal cord infarction in disease and surgery of the aorta. *Can J Neurol Sci* 1985;12:289–295.
11. Blalock A, Park EA. Surgical treatment of experimental coarctation (atresia) of aorta. *Ann Surg* 1944;119:445.
12. Debakey ME, Cooley DA, Crawford ES, et al. Aneurysms of the thoracic aorta: analysis of 179 patients treated by resection. *J Thorac Cardiovasc Surg* 1959;36:393.
13. Crawford ES, Fenstermacher JM, Richardson W, et al. Reappraisal of adjuncts to avoid ischemia in the treatment of thoracic aortic aneurysms. *Surgery* 1970;67:182.
14. Brewer LA III, Rosburg RG, Mulder GA, et al. Spinal cord complications following surgery for coarctation. *J Thorac Aortic Aneurysms Surg* 1970;67:182.
15. Adams HD, Van Geertruyden HH. Neurologic complications of aortic surgery. *Ann Surg* 1956;144:574.
16. Askew AR, Wilmshurst CC. Abdominal aortic aneurysm presenting with splenic rupture and subsequent paraplegia. *Vasc Surg* 1973;7:253.
17. Fosburg RG, Brewer LA III. Arterial vascular injury to the spinal cord. In: Vinken PJ, Bruyn GW, eds. *Handbook of clinical neurology.* Amsterdam: North-Holland Publishing, 1976;26:63–79.
18. Strigley JR, Lambert CD, Bilbao JM, et al. Spinal cord infraction secondary to intervertebral disc embolism. *Ann Neurol* 1981;9:296–301.
19. Fergin I, Pyoff N, Adahi M. Fibrocartilaginous venus emboli to the spinal cord with necrotic myelopathy. *J Neuropathol Exp Neurol* 1965;24:63–74.
20. Naina JL, Donohue WL, Pricharch JS. Fatal nucleus pulposus embolism of spinal cord after trauma. *Neurology* 1961;11:83.
21. Jurkovic I, Eiben E. Fatal myelomalacia caused by massive fibrocartilaginous venous emboli from nucleus pulposus. *Acta Neuropathol* 1970;15:284–287.
22. Laguna J, Cravioto H. Spinal cord infarction secondary to occlusion of the anterior spinal artery. *Arch Neurol* 1973;28:134–136.
23. Hughes JT. Venous infarction of the spinal cord. *Neurology* 1971;21:794–800.
24. Clarke CE, Cumming WJ. Subacute myelopathy caused by spinal venous infarction. *Postgrad Med J* 1987;63:669–671.
25. Rao KR, Donnenfeld M, Chusid JD, et al. Acute myelopathy secondary to spinal venous thrombosis. *J Neurol Sci* 1982;56:107–113.
26. Crum B, Mokri B, Fulgham J. Spinal manifestations of vertebral artery dissection. *Neurology* 2000;55:304–306.
27. Williamson RI. Spinal thrombosis and hemorrhage due to syphilitic disease of the vessels. *Lancet* 1894;2:14.
28. Spiller WG. Thrombosis of the cervical anterior median spinal artery: syphilitic acute anterior poliomyelitis. *J Nerv Ment Dis* 1909;36:601.
29. Caplan LR. Case records of the Massachusetts General Hospital: case 5-1991. *N Engl J Med* 1991;324:322–332.
30. Corbin JL. *Anatomie et pathologie arterielle de la moelle.* Paris: Masson, 1961.
31. Foix C, Alajouanine T. La myelite necrotique subaigue. *Rev Neurol* 1926; 2:1–42.
32. Lhermitte J, Fribourg-Blanc A, Kyriaco N. La gliose angeio-hypertrophique de la moelle epiniere (myelitie necrotique de Foix-Alajouanine). *Rev Neurol* 1931;2:37–53.
33. Pia HW, Vogelsang H. Diagnose und therapie spinaler angiome. *Dtsch Z Nervenheilk* 1965;187:74–96.
34. Wirth FP Jr, Post KD, Di Chiro G, et al. Foix-Alajouanine disease. Spontaneous thrombosis of a spinal cord arteriovenous malformation: a case report. *Neurology* 1970;20:1114–1118.
35. Aminoff MJ, Logue V. The prognosis of patients with spinal vascular malformations. *Brain* 1974;97:211–218.
36. Logue V. Angiomas of the spinal cord: review of the pathogenesis, clinical features, and results of surgery. *J Neurol Neurosurg Psychiatry* 1979;42:1–11.
37. Anson JA, Spetzler RF. Classification of spinal arteriovenous malformations and implications for treatment. *BNI Q* 1992;8:2–8.
38. Rosenblum B, Oldfield EH, Doppman JL, et al. Spinal arteriovenous malformations: a comparison of dural arteriovenous fistulas and intradural AVM's in 81 patients. *J Neurosurg* 1987;67:795–802.
39. Tobin WD, Layton DD Jr. The diagnosis and natural history of spinal cord arteriovenous malformations. *Mayo Clinic Proc* 1976;51:637–646.
40. Symon L, Kuyama H, Kendall B. Dural arteriovenous malformations of the spine. Clinical features and surgical results in 55 cases. *J Neurosurg* 1984;60:238–247.
41. Aminoff MJ, Logue V. Clinical features of spinal vascular malformations. *Brain* 1974;97:197–210.
42. Matthews WB. The spinal bruit. *Lancet* 1959;2:1117–1118.
43. Doppman JL, Wirth FP Jr, Di Chiro G, et al. Value of cutaneous angiomas in the arteriographic localization of spinal cord arteriovenous malformations. *N Engl J Med* 1969;281:1440–1444.
44. Minami S, Sagoh T, Nishimura K, et al. Spinal arteriovenous malformation: MR imaging. *Radiology* 1988;169:109–115.
45. Aminoff MJ, Barnard RO, Logue V. The pathophysiology of spinal vascular malformations. *J Neurol Sci* 1974;23:255–263.
46. Wrobel CJ, Oldfield EH, Di Chiro G, et al. Myelopathy due to intracranial dural arteriovenous fistulas draining intrathecally into spinal medullary veins. Report of three cases. *J Neurosurg* 1988;69:934–939.
47. Merland JJ, Reizine D. Treatment of arteriovenous spinal cord malformations. *Semin Intervent Radiol* 1987;4:281–290.
48. Merland JJ, Reizine D. Embolization techniques in the spinal cord. In: Dondelinger RF, Rossi P, Kurdziel JC, et al, eds. *Interventional radiology.* New York: Thieme Medical Publisher, 1990:433–442.
49. Mourier KL, Gelbert F, Rey A, et al. Spinal dural arteriovenous malformations with perimedullary drainage: indications and results of surgery in 30 cases. *Acta Neurochir (Wien)* 1989;100:136–141.
50. Morgan MK, Marsh WR. Management of spinal dural arteriovenous malformations. *J Neurosurg* 1989;70:832–836.
51. Hall WA, Oldfield EH, Doppman JL. Recanalization of spinal arterio-

venous malformations following embolization. *J Neurosurg* 1989;70: 714–720.

52. Lichtheim. Zur kenntniss der perniciosen anamie, verhandl. *D Cong F innere Med* 1887;6:84–99.

53. Russell JSR. The relationship of some forms of combined degenerations of the spinal cord to one another and to anaemia. *Lancet* 1898; 2:5–14.

54. Smith EL. Purification of anti-pernicious anaemia factors from liver. *Nature* 1948;161:638–639.

55. Minot GR, Murphy WP. Treatment of pernicious anemia by special diet. *JAMA* 1926;87:470–476.

56. Adams RD, Victor M. *Principles of neurology*, 4th ed. New York: McGraw-Hill, 1989:833.

57. Pant SS, Asbury AK, Richardson EP Jr. The myelopathy of pernicious anemia. A neuropathological reappraisal. *Acta Neurol Scand* 1968; 44[Suppl 5]:1–36.

58. Agamanolis DP, Victor M, Harris JW, et al. An ultrastructural study of subacute combined degeneration of the spinal cord in vitamin B$_{12}$–deficient rhesus monkeys. *J Neuropathol Exp Neurol* 1978;37: 273–299.

59. Shorvon SD, Carney MWP, Chanarin I, et al. The neuropsychiatry of megaloblastic anaemia. *Br Med J* 1980;281:1036–1038.

60. Gautier-Smith PC. Lhermitte's sign in subacute combined degeneration of the cord. *J Neurol Neurosurg Psychiatry* 1973;36:861–863.

61. Perold JG. Vitamin B$_{12}$ neuropathy in the absence of anaemia. A case report. *S Afr Med J* 1981;59:570.

62. Hensing JA. Subacute combined degeneration, neutrophilic hypersegmentation, and the absence of anemia. A case report. *Ariz Med* 1981; 38:768.

63. Green R, Kinsella LJ. Current concepts in the diagnosis of cobalamin deficiency. *Neurology* 1995;45:1435–1440.

64. Hemmer B, Glocker FX, Schumacher M, et al. Subacute combined degeneration: clinical, electrophysiological, and magnetic resonance imaging findings. *J Neurol Neursurg Psychiatry* 1998;65:822–827.

65. Di Lazzaro V, Restuccia D, Fogli D, et al. Central sensory and motor conduction in vitamin B12 deficiency. *Electroencephalogr Clin Neurophysiol* 1992;84:433–439.

66. Katsaros VK, Glocker FX, Hemmer B, et al. MRI of spinal cord and brain lesions in subacute combined degeneration. *Neuroradiology* 1998;40:716–719.

67. Beltramello A, Puppini G, Cerini R, et al. Subacute combined degeneration of the spinal cord after nitrous oxide anaesthesia: role of magnetic resonance imaging [Letter]. *J Neurol Neurosurg Psychiatry* 1998; 64:563–564.

68. Larner AJ, Zeman AZ, Allen CM, et al. MRI appearances in subacute combined degeneration of the spinal cord due to vitamin B$_{12}$ deficiency [Letter]. *J Neurol Neurosurg Psychiatry* 1997;62:99–100.

69. Kuker W, Thron A. Subacute combined degeneration of the spinal cord: demonstration of contrast enhancement [Letter]. *Neuroradiology* 1999;41:387.

70. Ravakhah K, West BC. Case report: subacute combined degeneration of the spinal cord from folate deficiency. *Am J Med Sci* 1995;310: 214–216.

71. Pincus JH. Folic acid deficiency, a cause of spinal cord system degeneration. In: Botz MI, Reynolds EH, eds. *Folic acid in neurology, psychiatry and internal medicine.* New York: Raven Press, 1979:427–433.

72. Donnelly S, Callaghan N. Subacute combined degeneration of the spinal cord due to folate deficiency in association with a psychotic illness. *Ir Med J* 1990;83:73–74.

73. Lever EG, Elwes RD, Williams A, et al. Subacute combined degeneration of the cord due to folate deficiency: response to methyl folate treatment. *J Neurol Neurosurg Psychiatry* 1986;49:1203–1207.

74. Layzer RB, Fishman RA, Schafer JA. Neuropathy following abuse of nitrous oxide. *Neurology* 1978;28:504–506.

75. Layzer RB. Myeloneuropathy after prolonged exposure to nitrous oxide. *Lancet* 1978;2:1227–1230.

76. Sahenk Z, Mendel JR, Couri D, et al. Polyneuropathy from inhalation of N$_2$O cartridges through a whipped cream dispenser. *Neurology* 1978;28:485–487.

77. Schilling RF. Is nitrous oxide a dangerous anesthetic for vitamin B$_{12}$–deficient subjects? *JAMA* 1986;255:1605–1606.

78. Stacy CB, Di Rocco A, Gould RJ. Methionine in the treatment of nitrous-oxide-induced neuropathy and myeloneuropathy. *J Neurol* 1992;239:401–403.

79. Flippo TS, Holder WD Jr. Neurologic degeneration associated with nitrous oxide anesthesia in patients with vitamin B$_{12}$ deficiency. *Arch Surg* 1993;128:1391–1395.

80. Sesso RM, Iunes Y, Melo AC. Myeloneuropathy following nitrous oxide anesthaesia in a patient with macrocytic anaemia. *Neuroradiology* 1999;41:588–590.

81. Marie RM, Le Biez E, Busson P, et al. Nitrous oxide anesthesia–associated myelopathy. *Arch Neurol* 2000;57:380–382.

82. Harding AE, Muller DP, Thomas PK, et al. Spinocerebellar degeneration secondary to chronic intestinal malabsorption: a vitamin E deficiency syndrome. *Ann Neurol* 1982;12:419–424.

83. Bertoni JM, Abraham FA, Falls HF, et al. Small bowel resection with vitamin E deficiency and progressive spinocerebellar syndrome. *Neurology* 1984;34:1046–1052.

84. Brin MR, Fetell MR, Green PH, et al. Blind loop syndrome, vitamin E malabsorption, and spinocerebellar degeneration. *Neurology* 1985; 35:338–342.

85. Harding AE, Matthews S, Jones S, et al. Spinocerebellar degeneration associated with a selective defect of vitamin E absorption. *N Engl J Med* 1985;313:32–35.

86. Gutmann L, Schockcor W, Gutmann L, et al. Vitamin E–deficient spinocerebellar syndrome due to intestinal lymphangiectasia. *Neurology* 1986;36:554–556.

87. Vorgerd M, Tegenthoff M, Kuhne D, et al. Spinal MRI in progressive myeloneuropathy associated with vitamin E deficiency. *Neuroradiology* 1996;38[Suppl 1]:S111–S113.

88. Nelson JS, Fitch CD, Fischer VW, et al. Progressive neuropathologic lesions in vitamin E–deficient rhesus monkeys. *J Neuropathol Exp Neurol* 1981;40:166–186.

89. Sencer W. Neurological manifestations in malabsorption syndrome. *J Mt Sinai Hosp* 1957;24:331–345.

90. Geller A, Gilles F, Schwachman H. Degeneration of fasciculus gracilis in cystic fibrosis. *Neurology* 1977;27:185–187.

91. Pentschew A, Schwarz K. Systemic axonal dystrophy in vitamin E deficient adult rats: with implication in human neuropathology. *Acta Neuropathol (Berlin)* 1962;1:313–334.

92. Towfighi J. Effects of chronic vitamin E deficiency on the nervous system of the rat. *Acta Neuropathol (Berlin)* 1981;54:261–268.

93. Adam RD, Victor M. *Principles of neurology*, 4th ed. New York: McGraw-Hill, 1989:1059.

94. Herbert PN, Assmann G, Gotto AM, et al. Familial lipoprotein deficiency. In: Stanbury JH, Wyngaarden DS, Fredrickson DS, eds. *The metabolic basis of inherited disease*, 5th ed. McGraw-Hill, New York: 1983:589–621.

95. Miller RJ, Davis CJF, Illingworth DR, et al. The neuropathy of abetalipoproteinemia. *Neurology* 1980;30:1286–1291.

96. Barrow MV, Simpson CF, Miller EJ. Lathyrism: a review. *Q Rev Biol* 1974;49:101–128.

97. Roman GC, Spencer PS, Schoenberg BS. Tropical myeloneuropathy: the hidden endemias. *Neurology* 1985;35:1158–1170.

98. Ludolph AC, Hugon J, Dwivedi MP, et al. Studies on the etiology and pathogenesis of motor neuron disease. I. Lathyrism: clinical findings—established cases. *Brain* 1987;110:149–165.

99. Ressler C. Isolation and identification from the common vetch of the neurotoxin beta-cyano-L-alamine, a possible factor in neurolathyrism. *J Biol Chem* 1962;237:733–735.

100. Ressler C, Redstone PA, Erenburg RH. Isolation and identification of a neuroactive factor from Lathyrus latifolia. *Science* 1961;134: 188–190.

101. Rao SLN, Adiga PR, Sama PS. The isolation and characterization of beta-N-oxalyl alpha, beta-diamino-propionic acid, a neurotoxin from the seeds of Lathyrus sativus. *Biochemistry* 1964;3:432–436.

102. Spencer PS, Roy DN, Ludolph A, et al. Lathyrism: evidence for role of the neuroexcitatory amino acid BOAA. *Lancet* 1986;2:1066–1067.

103. Howlett WP, Brubaker GR, Mlingi N, et al. Konzo, an epidemic

upper motor neuron disease studied in Tanzania. *Brain* 1990;113: 223–235.

104. Tylleskar T, Banea M, Bikangi N, et al. Dietary determinants of a non-progressive spastic paraparesis (konzo): a case-referent study in a high incidence area of Zaire. *J Epidemiol* 1995;24:949–956.

105. Tylleskar T, Banea M, Bikangi N, et al. Epidemiological evidence from Zaire for a dietary etiology of konzo, an upper motor neuron disease. *Bull World Health Organ* 1991;69:581–589.

106. Cliff J, Nicala D. Long-term follow-up of konzo patients. *Trans Royal Soc Trop Med Hyg* 1997;91:447–449.

107. Tylleskar T, Legue FD, Peterson S, et al. Konzo in the Central African Republic. *Neurology* 1994;44:959–961.

108. Osuntokun BO. An ataxic neuropathy in Nigeria. A clinical, biochemical and electrophysiological study. *Brain* 1968;91(2):215–248.

109. Montgomery RD, et al. Clinical and pathological observations in Jamaica. Neuropathy. *Brain* 1964;87:425–462.

110. Kaposi M. Neue beitrage zur kenntnis des lupus erythematosus. *Arch Dermat U Syph* 1872;4:36.

111. Johnson RT, Richardson EP. The neurological manifestations of systemic lupus erythematosus. A clinico-pathological study of 24 cases and review of the literature. *Medicine* 1968;47:337–369.

112. Al-Husaini A, Jamal GA. Myelopathy as the main presenting feature of systemic lupus erythematosus. *Eur Neurol* 1985;24:94–106.

113. Mok CC, Lau CS, Chan EY, et al. Acute transverse myelopathy in systemic lupus erythematosus: clinical presentation, treatment, and outcome. *J Rheumatol* 1998;25:467–473.

114. Lavalle C, Pizarro S, Drenkard C, et al. Transverse myelitis: a manifestation of systemic lupus erythematosus strongly associated with antiphospholipid antibodies. *J Rheumatol* 1993;17:34–51.

115. Andrianakos AA, Duffy J, Suzuki M, et al. Transverse myelopathy in systemic lupus erythematosus. Report of three cases and review of the literature. *Ann Intern Med* 1975;83:616–624.

116. Provenzale J, Bouldin TW. Lupus-related myelopathy: report of three cases and review of the literature. *J Neurol Neurosurg Psychiatry* 1992; 55:830–835.

117. Propper DJ, Bucknall RC. Acute transverse myelopathy complicating systemic lupus erythematosus. *Ann Rheum Dis* 1989;48:5125.

118. Berlanga B, Rubio FR, Moga I, et al. Response to intravenous cyclophosphamide treatment in lupus myelopathy. *Rheumatology* 1992;19: 829–830.

119. Slovick DI. Treatment of acute myelopathy in systemic lupus erythematosus with plasma exchange and immunosuppression [Letter]. *J Neurol Neurosurg Psychiatry* 1986;49:103–105.

120. Molina R, Provost TT, Arnett FC, et al. Primary Sjögren's syndrome in men—clinical, serologic, and immunogenetic features. *Am J Med* 1986;80:23–31.

121. Alexander EL, Arnett FC, Provost TT, et al. Sjögren's syndrome: association of anti-Ro (SS-A) antibodies with vasculitis, hematologic abnormalities, and serologic hyperreactivity. *Ann Intern Med* 1983; 98:155–159.

122. Alexander EL, Malinow K, Lejewski JE, et al. Primary Sjögren's syndrome with central nervous system disease mimicking multiple sclerosis. *Ann Intern Med* 1986;104:323–330.

123. Rutan G, Martinez AJ, Fieshko JT, et al. Primary biliary cirrhosis, Sjögren's syndrome, and transverse myelitis. *Gastroenterology* 1986; 90:206–210.

124. Urban E, Jabbari B, Robles H. Concurrent cerebral venous sinus thrombosis and myeloradiculopathy in Sjögren's syndrome. *Neurology* 1994;44:554–556.

125. Konttinen YT, Kinnunen E, Von Bonsdorff, et al. Acute transverse myelopathy successfully treated with plasmapheresis and prednisone in a patient with primary Sjögren's syndrome. *Arthritis Rheum* 1987; 30:339–344.

126. Wright RA, O'Duffy JD, Rodriguez M. Improvement of myelopathy in Sjögren's syndrome with chlorambucil and prednisone therapy. *Neurology* 1999;52:386–388.

127. Izumi M, Nakamura H, Nakamura T, et al. Sjögren's syndrome (SS) in patients with human T cell leukemia virus I associated myelopathy: paradoxical features of the major salivary glands compared to classical SS. *Rheumatology* 1999;26:2609–2614.

128. Nakamura H, Eguchi K, Nakamura T, et al. High prevalence of Sjögren's syndrome in patients with HTLV-I associated myelopathy. *Rheum Dis* 1997;56:167–172.

129. Zieve L, Mendelson DF, Goepfert M. Shunt encephalomyelopathy. I. Recurrent protein encephalopathy with response to arginine. *Ann Intern Med* 1960;53:33–52.

130. Zieve L, Mendelson DF, Goepfert M. Shunt encephalomyelopathy. II. Occurrence of permanent myelopathy. *Ann Intern Med* 1960;53: 63.

131. Mendoza G, Marti-Fabregas J, Kulisevsky J, et al. Hepatic myelopathy: a rare complication of portacaval shunt. *Eur Neurol* 1994;34: 209–212.

132. Baltzan MA, Olszewski J, Zervas N. Chronic portohepatic encephalopathy. *J Neuropathol Exp Neurol* 1957;16:410–421.

133. Campellone JV, Lacomis D, Giuliani MJ, et al. Hepatic myelopathy. Case report with review of the literature. *Clin Neurol Neurosurg* 1996; 98:242–246.

134. Lebovics E, Dematteo RE, Schaffner F, et al. Portal systemic myelopathy after portacaval shunt surgery. *Arch Intern Med* 1985;145: 1921–1922.

135. Bain VG, Bailey RJ, Jhamandas JH. Postshunt myelopathy. *J Clin Gastroenterol* 1991;13:562–564.

136. Scobie BA, Summerskill WHJ. Permanent paraplegia with cirrhosis. *Arch Intern Med* 1964;113:805–810.

137. Pant SS, Rebeiz JJ, Richardson EP. Spastic paraparesis following portacaval shunts. *Neurology* 1968;18:134–141.

138. Mousseau R, Reynolds T. Hepatic paraplegia. *Am J Gastroenterol* 1976;66:343–348.

139. Sherlock S, Summerskill WHJ, White LP, et al. Portal-systemic encephalopathy: neurological complications of liver disease. *Lancet* 1954;267:453–457.

140. Budillon G, Scala G, Mansi D, et al. Hepatic paraplegia: an uncommon complication of portosystemic shunts. *Acta Neurol (Napoli)* 1979;34:93–100.

141. Giangaspero F, Dondi C, Scarani P, et al. Degeneration of the corticospinal tract following portosystemic shunt associated with spinal cord infarction. *Virchows Arch [A]* 1985;406:475–481.

142. Kissel P, Arnoud G, Tridon P, et al. Sur un cas de myelopathie par shunt portocave. *Rev Neurol (Paris)* 1962;106:782–786.

143. Krake A, Patterson M. Chronic permanent encephalomyelopathy following hepatic shunts. *South Med J* 1964;57:617–621.

144. Liversedge LA, Rawson MD. Myelopathy in hepatic disease and portosystemic venous anastomosis. *Lancet* 1966;1:277–279.

145. Krinashwami V, Radhakrishna T, John BM. Myelopathy in cirrhosis. *J Indian Med Assoc* 1969;53:195–197.

146. Troisi R, Debruyne J, de Hemptinne B. Improvement of hepatic myelopathy after liver transplantation [Letter]. *N Engl J Med* 1999; 340:151.

147. Counsell C, Warlow C. Failure of presumed hepatic myelopathy to improve after liver transplantation [Letter]. *J Neurol Neurosurg Psychiatry* 1996;60:590.

148. Posner JB. Paraneoplastic syndromes. In Posner JB, ed. *Neurologic complications of cancer.* Philadelphia: FA Davis Co, 1995:353–385.

149. Ojeda VT. Necrotizing myelopathy associated with malignancy. A clinicopathologic study of two cases and literature review. *Cancer* 1984;53:1115–1123.

150. Gieron MA, Margraf LR, Korthals JK, et al. Progressive necrotizing myelopathy associated with leukemia: clinical, pathologic, and MRI correlation. *Child Neurol* 1987;2:44–49.

151. Dansey RD, Hammond-Tooke GD, Lai K, et al. Subacute myelopathy: an unusual paraneoplastic complication of Hodgkin's disease. *Med Pediatr Oncol* 1988;16:284–286.

152. Storey E, McKelvie PA. Necrotizing myelopathy associated with multiple myeloma. *Acta Neurol Scand* 1991;84:98–101.

153. Hughes M, Ahern V, Kefford R, et al. Paraneoplastic myelopathy at diagnosis in a patient with pathologic stage 1A Hodgkin disease. *Cancer* 1992;70:1598–1600.

154. Kuroda Y, Miyahara M, Sakemi T, et al. Autopsy report of acute necrotizing opticomyelopathy associated with thyroid cancer. *J Neurol Sci* 1993;120:29–32.

155. Drach LM, Enzensberger W, Fabian T, et al. Paraneoplastic necrotizing myelopathy in a case of AIDS with lymphoma [Letter]. *J Neurol Neurosurg Psychiatry* 1996;60:237.

156. Wilson JWL, Morales A, Sharp D. Necrotizing myelopathy associated with renal cell carcinoma. *Urology* 1983;21:390–392.

157. McDermott CJ, White K, Bushby K, et al. Hereditary spastic paraparesis: a review of new developments. *J Neurol Neurosurg Psychiatry* 2000;69:150–160.

158. Strümpell A. Beitrage zur pathologie des ruckenmarks. *Arch Psychiatrie Nervenkrankheiten* 1880;10:676–717.

159. Harding AE. Hereditary pure spastic paraplegia: a clinical and genetic study of 22 families. *J Neurol Neurosurg Psychiatry* 1981;44:871–883.

160. Durr A, Brice A, Serdaru M, et al. The phenotype of "pure" autosomal dominant spastic paraplegia. *Neurology* 1994;44:1274–1277.

161. Schwarz GA. Hereditary (familial) spastic paraplegia. *Arch Neurol Psychiatry* 1952;68:655–682.

162. Schwarz GA, Liu CN. Hereditary (familial) spastic paraplegia. *Arch Neurol Psychiatry* 1956;75:144–162.

163. Hazan J, Fonknechten N, Mavel D, et al. Spastin, a novel AAA protein, is altered in the most frequent form of autosomal dominant spastic paraplegia. *Nat Genetics* 1999;23:296–303.

164. Banfi S, Bassi MT, Andolfi G, et al. Identification and characterization of AFG3L2, a novel paraplegic-related gene. *Genomics* 1999;59:51–58.

165. Bonneau D, Rozet J-M, Bulteau C, et al. X-linked spastic paraplegia (SPG2): clinical heterogeneity at a single locus. *J Med Genetics* 1993;30:381–384.

166. Johnson AW, McKusick VA. A sex-linked recessive from of spastic paraplegia. *Am J Hum Genetics* 1962;14:83–94.

167. Jouet M, Rosenthal A, Armstrong G, et al. X-linked spastic paraplegia (SPG1), MASA syndrome and X-linked hydrocephalus result from mutations in the L1 gene. *Nat Genetics* 1994;7:402–407.

168. Tang LM, Chen ST, Hsu WC, et al. A longitudinal study of multimodal evoked potentials in patients following radiotherapy for nasopharyngeal carcinoma. *Neurology* 1996;47:521–525.

169. Li Y-Q, Jay V, Wong C. Oligodendrocytes in the adult rat spinal cord undergo radiation induced apoptosis. *Cancer Res* 1996;56:5417–5422.

170. Palmer JJ. Radiation myelopathy. In: Vinken PJ, Bruyn GW, eds. *Handbook of clinical neurology.* Amsterdam: North-Holland Publishing, 1976:81–95.

171. Schultheiss TE, Kun LE, Ang KK, et al. Radiation response of the central nervous system. *J Radiat Oncol Biol Phys* 1995;31:1093–1112.

172. Schiff D, Shaw EG, Cascino TL. Outcome after spinal reirradiation for malignant epidural spinal cord compression. *Ann Neurol* 1995;37:583–589.

173. Schultheiss TE, Stephens LC, Maor MH. Analysis of the histopathology of radiation myelopathy. *J Radiat Oncol Biol* 1988;14:27–32.

174. Schultheiss TE, Stevens LC. Radiation myelopathy. *AJNR* 1992;13:1056–1058.

175. Udaka F, Tsuji T, Shigematsu K, et al. A case of chronic progressive radiation myelopathy successfully treated with corticosteroids. Rinsho Shinkeigaku. *Clin Neurol* 1990;30:439–443.

176. Hirota S, Soejima T, Higashino T, et al. A case of chronic progressive chronic radiation myelopathy treated with long-time corticosteroids administration. *Jpn J Clin Radiol* 1998;43:649–652.

177. Glantz MJ, Burger PC, Friedman AH, et al. Treatment of radiation induced nervous system injury with heparin and warfarin. *Neurology* 1994;44:2020–2027.

178. Koehler PJ, Verbiest H, Jager J, et al. Delayed radiation myelopathy: serial MR-imaging and pathology. *Clin Neurol Neurosurg* 1996;98:197–201.

179. Glantz MJ, Burger PC, Friedman AH, et al. Treatment of radiation-induced nervous system injury with heparin and warfarin. *Neurology* 1994;44:2020–2027.

180. Angibaud G, Ducasse JL, Baille G, et al. Potential value of hyperbaric oxygen in the treatment of post radiation myelopathies. *Rev Neurol* 1995;151:661–666.

181. Pol B, Watelle TSJ. Memoire sur les effets de la compression de l' air. *Ann Hyg Publ (Paris)* 1854;2:241–279.

182. Bert P. La Pression Barometrique. Masson Paris: 1878.

183. Hill L. Caisson sickness and compressed air. *J Royal Soc Arts* 1911;59:400–412.

184. Dick APK, Massey EW. Neurologic presentation of decompression sickness and air embolism in sport divers. *Neurology* 1985;35:667–671.

185. Hallenbeck JM, Bore AA, Elliott DH. Mechanisms underlying spinal cord damage in decompression sickness. *Neurology* 1975;25:308–316.

186. Francis TJ, Griffin JL, Homer LD, et al. Bubble-induced dysfunction in acute spinal cord decompression sickness. *J Appl Physiol* 1990;68:1368–1375.

187. Palmer AC, Calder IM, McCallum RI, et al. Spinal cord degeneration in a case of "recovered" spinal decompression sickness. *Br Med J (Clin Ed)* 1981;283:888.

188. Sparacia G, Banco A, Sparacia B, et al. Magnetic resonance findings in scuba diving-related spinal cord decompression sickness. *Magma* 1997;5:111–115.

189. Aharon-Peretz J, Adir Y, Gordon CR, et al. Spinal cord decompression sickness in sport diving. *Arch Neurol* 1993;50:753–756.

MULTIPLE SCLEROSIS

MARY ANN PICONE
STUART D. COOK

Multiple sclerosis (MS) is a chronic inflammatory disease of the central nervous system (CNS) characterized by focal areas of demyelination and axonal injury. The clinical course can be quite variable, but in most patients, neurologic disability increases incrementally over time. Although its etiology is unknown, MS is generally considered an immune-mediated disorder, occurring preferentially in genetically susceptible individuals, and is probably precipitated by one or more environmental factors, most likely infectious in nature. There is no cure for MS; however, a number of palliative therapies have become available that can modify clinical and magnetic resonance imaging (MRI) disease activity.

HISTORICAL PERSPECTIVE

MS may have occurred as early as the fourteenth century, although the first well-documented case affected Sir Auygustus d'Este, the illegitimate grandson of King George III of England, whose disease course was recorded in his personal diary from 1822 through 1848 (1–3). MS probably existed even earlier but was not recognized as a specific nosologic entity because of the difficulty in differentiating it from other neurologic disorders and diseases of the time. In the 1860s, the great French neurologist Charcot provided the first detailed descriptions of the clinical features of MS, established diagnostic criteria, and correlated clinical manifestations with pathologic findings (4,5). By the late nineteenth century, the clinical and pathologic features of MS were well recognized, leading Guillain to state that "disseminated sclerosis is, after syphilis, the most frequent disease of the nervous system" (6). Although this is obviously not the case today, MS remains a major cause of chronic CNS disease affecting young adults in the Western world.

EPIDEMIOLOGY

MS commonly starts in late adolescence or early adult life, with peak onset occurring at a mean age of about 30 years. Like many other putative autoimmune diseases, MS is more common in women (ratio of 2:1) than in men. However, unlike most other autoimmune disorders, MS has two distinct epidemiologic features: an unusual and as yet unexplained worldwide pattern and

an effect of migration in altering risk for developing the disease. In terms of the former, MS is more likely to occur in white Europeans than in Native Americans, African Americans, Asians, and members of certain ethnic groups (7–10). Prevalence studies indicate a crude North-South gradient in North America, with prevalence rates of 150 to 200 per 100,000 population described in Canada and the northern United States, compared with less than 50 per 100,000 in the American south (7,8,10). In Europe, prevalence rates less predictably relate to latitude, although MS is more common in Scandinavia and Great Britain than in Mediterranean countries (11). In some parts of the Southern Hemisphere, the North-South gradient is reversed, with MS being higher in southern than northern Australia. A relatively low rate of MS has been reported in Asia. Many exceptions to the rate of MS by latitude have been described and remarkable differences in MS prevalence have been documented in populations in close geographic proximity; nevertheless, there seems little doubt about the global pattern of MS, if not the actual prevalence data (10).

In analyzing this unusual geographic distribution, there has been great interest in identifying factors contributing to disease susceptibility. In this regard, a number of variables have been shown to correlate with MS frequency, including white race, higher educational status, urban background, higher socioeconomic status, cold humid weather, meat and dairy food consumption, and human leukocyte antigen DW2 (DR15, DQ6) (11–14). Although it is difficult to dissect out how these variables interact, it seems likely that MS is a complex disorder, whose development requires some combination of hereditary and environmental factors.

Genes appear to play an important role as to who may be affected by MS. Families with at least one member who already has MS are at higher risk to contract the disease than the rest of the general population. Also, the closer the relationship is to an MS affected blood relative, the greater the risk becomes. These factors and the relationship between DW2 and MS risk, lead to the conclusion that there is a genetic factor in the contraction of MS. However, no specific gene has been shown to have a powerful effect in this regard, and it seems likely that multiple, perhaps interacting genes, confer MS susceptibility.

On the other hand, it also seems clear that appropriate environmental triggers are also probably necessary for MS to occur. The most powerful evidence for this comes from migration studies, which indicate that MS risk for individuals or their offspring, often but not invariably, changes upward or downward depending on age of migration and whether migration occurs to or from low to high prevalence areas (7,8,10). The nature of these causative environmental factors is not known, and it is not clear whether a single, a few, or many precipitants are involved. Particular attention has been given to the role of infectious agents because viral-induced models of CNS demyelinating disease, both acute and chronic, are well documented and because serologic and epidemiologic evidence is supportive of this concept (15). Unfortunately, reports of isolation or identification of infectious agents in MS tissue have generally proven nonreproducible or nonspecific. Nevertheless, interest remains in several human (Epstein-Barr virus, human herpesvirus 6, retroviruses, and chlamydial pneumoniae) and animal (canine distemper) viruses as possible candidate agents (16,17).

MECHANISM OF TISSUE INJURY

Regardless of the triggering event, it seems clear that the immune response plays a critical role in causing demyelination. The most impressive evidence for this comes from the effectiveness, at least transiently, of a number of immunomodulating or immunosuppressive agents having markedly different mechanisms of action. Although the precise role of the immune response in causing tissue injury is unknown, it seems clear that macrophages, T cells, and antibodies acting alone or in concert are the major effectors, although it is less clear whether this requires the presence of an infectious agent. A number of alterations in the brain, blood, and cerebrospinal fluid (CSF) T-cell subtypes, cytokines, chemokines, immunoglobulins, and adhesion molecules have been demonstrated consistent with immunologic tissue damage. An animal model of autoimmune CNS demyelination, experimental allergic encephalomyelitis, has many clinical and pathologic features in common with MS.

CLINICAL AND DIAGNOSTIC FEATURES

The diagnosis of MS is based on a thorough history, neurologic examination, and laboratory testing. The key to proper diagnosis is demonstrating multiple lesions in the CNS, occurring at different times, and the exclusion of other disorders with similar features. Early in the course, the diagnosis may not be obvious, but with the passage of time, this becomes less problematic. The predilection for MS lesions to involve motor, sensory, autonomic, and integrative pathways in the brain and spinal cord results in some combination of spastic weakness, impaired sensation, visual loss, internuclear ophthalmoplegia, vertigo, dysarthria, tremor, ataxia, sphincteric problems, impotence, gait disturbance, and cognitive dysfunction. MS deficits can occur in an acute pattern (relapse or exacerbation) or subacutely or may evolve in a more chronically progressive fashion. Symptoms or signs highly suggestive of MS include optic neuritis, internuclear ophthalmoplegia, a Lhermitte sign, and heat sensitivity, whereas generalized areflexia, aphasia, homonymous hemianopsia, diffuse muscle atrophy, multiorgan involvement, or progressive dis-

TABLE 34.1. MOST FREQUENT SYMPTOMS SEEN AT ONSET OF MULTIPLE SCLEROSIS

Sensory symptoms in the arms and legs (usually beginning distally and expanding proximally) (27–40%)
Unilateral visual loss (16–29%)
Motor/gait (19–40%)
Incoordination (9–20%)
Diplopia (due to bilateral intranuclear opthalmoplegia) (7–18%)
Vertigo (4–7%)
Bladder symptoms, bowel or sexual problems (5–10%)
Cognitive (3%)

ease explainable by one lesion in the neuraxis or involving only one neurologic subsystem, should raise a cautionary note about accuracy of diagnosis (18) (Table 34.1).

The differential diagnosis can be quite extensive and considers the temporal presentation, the presence or absence of dissemination of lesions, system involvement, family history, and age at onset. Acute presentations mimicking MS can be seen with infectious disorders (Lyme disease, acute disseminated encephalomyelitis, transverse myelitis, viral infections, and epidural abscess) and vascular disease (vasculitides, arteriovenous malformations [AVMs], and vasculopathy). Focal presentations suggest neoplasms, spondylosis, AVM, human T-cell lymphoma/leukemia virus type 1 (HTLV-1) infection, transverse myelitis, and other structural lesions. If only one system is involved, there is a family history, or onset begins in childhood, one should consider heretidodegenerative disorders such as the spinocerebellar degenerations, leukodystrophies, and mitochondrial disorders. Sjögren syndrome, sarcoidosis, the anticardiolipin syndrome, neurosyphilis, Lyme disease, primary CNS vasculitis, lymphoma, and vitamin B_{12} deficiency should be kept in mind at any stage (19).

Laboratory tests can be of great value to the clinician in supporting the diagnosis of MS and excluding other diseases. Routine blood tests in most patients include a complete blood cell count, SMAC, sedimentation rate, antinuclear antibody, Venereal Disease Research Laboratories test, vitamin B_{12} level, thyroid function tests, anticardiolipin titers, and Lyme serology. Neuroimaging studies (MRI of the brain and often the spinal cord) are generally performed in every patient for diagnostic purposes and to show extent and degree of lesion activity. MRI is also used in assessing prognosis and appropriateness of therapeutic intervention (20,21). If a patient has been on an immunomodulating therapy and continues to have frequent relapses, with repeated MRI showing increased number of lesions with gadolinium enhancement, this would aid in the determination to switch the patient to another immunomodulating agent.

The hallmark of MS on MRI scanning is multiple lesions in the periventricular regions, appearing as areas of increased signal intensity on T2-weighted images. This is a sensitive test for MS, with T2-weighted scans abnormal in 70% to 95% of patients having clinically definite MS and in approximately 50% of patients with an initial presentation of optic neuritis. Lesions often are rounded or ovoid and usually appear homogenous but may possess a rim of altered signal intensity. Similar lesions occur in the white matter of the brain stem and spinal cord. T2 lesions seen on MRI scans reflect increased water content resulting from edema and inflammation or demyelination. These lesions are not specific for MS. Similar lesions can be seen in patients older than 50 years with small vessel ischemic disease, as well as patients with lupus erythematosus, sarcoid, Lyme disease, and other inflammatory disorders. Enhancing lesions on T1-weighted MRI studies after gadolinium administration reflect ongoing or recently active disease.

The detection of new lesions on MRI scanning is a much more sensitive way of assessing disease activity than the patient's history or the physician's neurologic examination. MS traditionally has been characterized based on its clinical features, mainly exacerbation involving different areas of the CNS at different times. Disability progression often occurs over years. However, MRI shows that pathologic changes in MS are more frequent and dynamic than is appreciated by clinical means. When a patient presents with a relapse, MRI shows approximately four to five new lesions. At the time of first presentation with neurologic symptoms referable to MS, MRI will often show evidence of earlier lesions during times when patients have been asymptomatic.

MRI also has prognostic value in predicting the risk of developing MS in certain patients. The optic neuritis study group followed up to 388 patients who did not have a diagnosis of MS but who presented with acute optic neuritis (21). With normal MRI results at presentation, the risk of developing MS after 5 years was 16%, whereas patients with three or more lesions had a 51% risk of developing MS after 5 years.

MRI findings may also correlate with disability (20,21). "Black holes" on T1-weighted imaging, brain or spinal cord atrophy, high lesion load on T2-weighted imaging, and the repeated documentation of many enhancing lesions have been associated with greater disability (22–24).

Evoked potentials, usually auditory and somatosensory, can be of use in difficult cases for demonstrating a second clinically occult lesion. Evoked potentials are used to confirm a pattern of CNS involvement consistent with demyelination, to document lesions disseminated in space, and to provide objective evidence of a subjective complaint such as visual loss. What we are particularly looking at in the evaluation of this test is latency prolongation. This is more helpful than decreased amplitude and wave dispersion because it suggests a demyelinating process. For somatosensory testing, lower extremity somatosensory evoked potentials provide more information than upper extremities because they evaluate the entire spinal cord. With visual evoked potentials, a latency of more than 10 ms between the eyes is abnormal even when the absolute values are within the reference range. However, if patients are drowsy or inattentive or have ocular pathology, the results will be affected. If a patient has positive MRI findings or positive CSF findings consistent with MS, along with the appropriate clinical history and findings on neurologic examination, it is not necessary to perform these tests (25).

CSF analysis is not done as routinely as in the past with the general availability and sensitivity of MRI testing but does play an important role in problematic or atypical cases. Determination of CSF cells, protein, and glucose, as well as testing for

TABLE 34.2. SCHUMACHER CRITERIA FOR MULTIPLE SCLEROSIS

1. Evidence on neurologic examination or by history of involvement of two or more sites in the central nervous system (CNS) (lesions separated in space).
2. Involvement in the CNS in one of the following temporal patterns: two or more distinct patterns of worsening separated by a time period of 1 mo or more, each lasting at least 24 hr; or a slow or stepwise progression over a course of at least 6 mo (lesions separated in time).
3. Objective abnormalities on neurologic examination referable to dysfunction of the CNS.
4. Evidence that CNS disease reflects primarily disease of the white matter.
5. Onset between the ages of 10 and 50 years.
6. A decision that the patient's signs and symptoms cannot be better explained by another diagnosis after a thorough neurologic evaluation.

oligoclonal bands and increased immunoglobulin G (IgG) (IgG index or synthesis rate), is routinely performed when a spinal tap is done. Typically, oligoclonal bands or an increase in CSF IgG is found in the presence of a normal or slightly elevated protein level in about 90% of patients with MS. Oligoclonal bands are generally seen in the CSF, but not in the serum (26).

Criteria often used to make the diagnosis of MS have been the Schumacher criteria for MS (Table 34.2) (25). These criteria can be helpful in diagnosing most patients with MS. However, MS can present before the age of 10 and after the age of 50. Before the advent of MRI, patients were followed for years at times to fulfill the above criteria before making a diagnosis of MS. With the advent of the newer immunologic therapies that should be started as early as possible in the disease course of most patients, this approach is no longer possible. Brain and spine MRI have become the most important diagnostic tests to help confirm lesions separated in space and time. New diagnostic criteria (McDonald criteria) have been developed utilizing MRI more intensively (see appendix at end of chapter).

CLASSIFICATION OF MULTIPLE SCLEROSIS

MS is now classified into four categories based on the temporal profile of clinical disease activity (27). Relapsing-remitting MS is seen in most patients (about 85%) early in the course of their disease. These patients have acute attacks (relapses, exacerbations), followed by periods of stability or improvement, but not slow deterioration between attacks. Secondary progressive MS is seen later in the evolution of the disease in many patients (30%), often after an initial relapsing-remitting phase. Patients in this category show deterioration between attacks. Unfortunately, it is often difficult to assess whether deterioration between attacks represents disease progression or a transient change due to diurnal variation, fatigue, depression, fever, or medications. Primary progressive MS is seen in about 10% of patients who have no obvious relapse or remission, but a progressive course from disease onset. Progressive relapsing MS is even less common, being seen in about 5% of patients and characterized by progression of disease from onset with occasional relapses super-imposed on the progressive course.

This classification is useful for carrying out therapeutic trials to enroll patients with a similar type of clinical disease course. As a result, Food and Drug Administration (FDA) approval of new drugs for MS is based on this classification. However, this classification is not as useful in a practice setting because the distinction between types is not always so clear-cut, particularly between relapsing-remitting and secondary progressive MS. Further, disease type does not necessarily correlate with degree of disability. Theoretically, patients may have relapsing-remitting MS and be more severely disabled than patients with secondary progressive MS with disease of the same duration. Rather than being different entities, it may be that underlying pathogenetic mechanisms are quite similar in these types of MS with clinical phenotype reflective of number, location, and severity of CNS lesions including the degree of axonal damage. This classification is also complicated by the fact that clinical manifestations are much less sensitive than MRI data as to true disease activity.

Poser criteria, published in 1983, are routinely used in research studies. They include definite and probable diagnoses, which are clinically or laboratory supported (Table 34.3). The Poser criteria broadened the definition of relapse to include brief symptoms such as Lhermitte sign, provided they recurred multiple times over a period of days to weeks. Clinical evidence requires documented abnormalities on examination. Paraclinical evidence involves lesions demonstrated by neuroimaging, evoked potential studies, urologic testing, or other modalities. Laboratory-supported diagnosis requires one of two possible immune disturbances in CSF: IgG oligoclonal bands or intrathecal IgG production. In general, a definite diagnosis requires two separate disease attacks to document dissemination in time consistent with multiphasic disease process (25).

The Kurtzke expanded disability status scale (EDSS) is currently considered the gold standard in terms of a rating scale for

TABLE 34.4. KURTZKE EXPANDED DISABILITY STATUS SCALE (SUMMARY)

Score	Explanation
0	Normal neurologic examination
1–1.5	No disability, minimal signs
2–2.5	Impairment, minimal disability
3–3.5	Mild disability
4–5.5	Ambulatory from >500 m to >100 m
6.0	Unilateral assistance for 100 m
6.5	Bilateral assistance for 20 m
7–7.5	Wheelchair bound; <20-m steps
8–8.5	Bedbound; communicates and eats
9.5	Bedbound; cannot communicate or eat
10	Death

measuring disability in clinical trials. This may change, because various composite scales are being investigated, which will evaluate cognitive dysfunction, upper extremity function, and ambulation. The EDSS measures disability on an ordinal 0 (normal) to 10 (death) scale, with 0.5-step increments. This measures a wide disability range: 1 to 3.5 (minimal deficits), 4 to 6.5 (moderate), 7 to 9.5 (severe), and 10 (death) (Table 34.4).

PROGNOSIS

Natural history studies are quite informative about prognosis in patients with MS, although these studies may need to be reevaluated now that effective therapies are available for modifying disease course (27). In these studies, approximately 50% of patients with MS required a cane or other assistive device for ambulation 15 years after disease onset. It is now possible to decrease MS exacerbations, slow the rate of deterioration, and

TABLE 34.3. POSER CRITERIA FOR DIAGNOSIS OF MULTIPLE SCLEROSIS

Clinical Diagnosis

Category		Clinical			Paraclinical Evidence
		Attacks	Evidence		
Definite	1	2	2		—
	2	2	1	and	1
Probable	1	2	1		—
	2	1	2		—
	3	1	1	and	1

Laboratory Supported Diagnosis

Category		Clinical			Paraclinical Evidence	Cerebrospiral Fluid
		Attacks	Evidence			
Definite	1	2	1	or	1	+
	2	1	2		—	+
	3	1	1		—	+
Probable	1	2	—		—	+

TABLE 34.5. CLINICAL FACTORS WITH PROGNOSTIC VALUE IN MULTIPLE SCLEROSIS

Favorable	Unfavorable
Younger age at onset	Older age at onset
Female	Male
Normal MRI at presentation	High lesion load on MRI at presentation
Complete recovery from first relapse	Lack of recovery from first relapse
Low relapse rate	High relapse rate
	Early cerebellar involvement
Long interval to second relapse	Short interval to second relapse
Low disability at 2 and 4 yr	Early development of mild disability
	Insidious motor onset

MRI, magnetic resonance imaging.

diminish MRI lesion formation with appropriate therapy, and it is conceivable that this will translate into a better prognosis, particularly if treatment is started early after the diagnosis is made.

Natural history studies also indicate that MRI findings are a much better barometer of disease activity than clinical evaluations and suggest that MS is neither as intermittent nor as benign as was previously thought. In some studies, frequency type and severity of exacerbations, degree of persistent neurologic deficit, age, sex, symptom profile, and MRI findings may have prognostic value as to future course (29,30) (Table 34.5). Exacerbations of MS are commonly seen in the postpartum period and after viral and possibly bacterial infections. On the other hand, surgery, anesthesia, trauma, and stress have not been clearly shown to aggravate MS, and the 9 months of pregnancy is a time of reduced disease activity.

Unfortunately, some patients with MS may also have a diminished life expectancy. Data from the Danish Multiple Sclerosis Registry indicate that MS may reduce life expectancy by up to 12 years, with premature mortality being seen particularly in patients with the most advanced forms of the disease. These studies will also need to be reevaluated in light of current therapeutic strategies, including the use of drugs to reduce disease activity and disability, the recognition and treatment of depression, and the avoidance of urosepsis, pressure ulcers, and the bedridden state.

TREATMENT

Therapy of MS can be divided into treatments that prevent disease activity, hasten a remission after an exacerbation, relieve symptoms, prevent complications, and improve quality of life. Up until 10 or so years ago, few drugs were proven effective in treating MS. Since that time, a number of treatments have proven useful, albeit palliative, in decreasing clinical and MRI exacerbations or slowing the rate of clinical and MRI deterioration. These include the human proteins or human protein derivatives interferon beta-1a (IFN-β1a) (Avonex, Rebif) and IFN-

β1b (Betaseron), glatiramer acetate (Copaxone), and intravenous gamma globulin, as well as the immunosuppressive drugs including azathioprine, cladribine, cyclophosphamide, methotrexate, and mitoxantrone (31–34). In general, the human proteins are preferable as first-line drugs because of their excellent risk-benefit profile and should generally be administered as soon as the diagnosis of MS is made.

The National Multiple Sclerosis Society published a management consensus statement regarding treatment of relapsing-remitting MS, which stated that patients should be treated as soon as possible after the diagnosis of definite relapsing (active) MS (35). Patients should be treated regardless of relapse rate, age, disability, or most medical conditions. Both interferon treatments and glatiramer acetate can be used for patients on diagnosis of MS. The interferons include IFN-β1a and IFN-β1b. They inhibit synthesis of interferon gamma. They alter the autoimmune cascade in the CNS, manipulate cytokines, reduce relapses, slow progression, and reduce disease burden and activity on MRI.

IFN-β1a is administered as 6 million units intramuscularly on a weekly basis. It has been shown to slow progression as measured by the EDSS. In a recently published study, IFN-β1a administered to patients with a monosymptomatic episode and positive MRI results, showing demyelinating lesions in areas of the CNS other than the presenting neurologic symptom, delayed time to the development of the next neurologic relapse (36).

IFN-β1b is administered subcutaneously as 8 million units every other day. It has been shown to reduce the annual relapse rates by 33%, reduce severity of exacerbations, reduce formation of new lesions on MRI, and in a European study of the drug, was shown to delay progression of disease in patients with secondary progressive MS (35). IFN-β1b has FDA approval in this country for the treatment of relapsing-remitting MS, but not progressive MS.

Glatiramer acetate is the first noninterferon agent for MS. It consists of the acetate salts of synthetic polypeptides containing L-glutamic acid, L-alanine, L-tyrosine, and L-lysine. It was investigated and tested for use in MS because of its strongly suppressive effect on experimental allergic encephalomyelitis. It is given subcutaneously on a daily basis at a dose of 20 mg. Its effects on relapse rate reductions are similar to those of the interferons, and MRI has also shown decreased new lesion formation. There is currently a multicenter placebo-controlled, double-blind study investigating the efficacy of glatiramer acetate in patients with primary progressive MS. The choice of which product to prescribe should be made with the patient, considering lifestyle issues, efficacy, and side-effect profile. Each product has proven efficacy. Making exact comparisons among the agents is difficult because each of the pivotal trials were carried out using dissimilar protocols. In terms of side effects, glatiramer acetate tends to be the best tolerated. Its side effects include mild injection site reaction and a rare systemic reaction with chest pain, dyspnea, and anxiety. There is no direct cardiac effect (32). With the interferons, the main side effects include flulike symptoms, fatigue, increased spasticity, and headaches.

Immunosuppressant drugs have been used for more than 20 years with limited benefit in the treatment of progressive MS. These include azathioprine, methotrexate, cyclophosphamide

(Cytoxan), and cladribine. These can be used in combination with immunomodulators. Mitoxantrone (Novantrone) was recently approved for the treatment of secondary progressive MS. It is an anthracenedione antineoplastic agent that intercalates with DNA and exerts a potent immunomodulating effect that suppresses humoral immunity, reduces T-cell numbers, decreases helper T-cell activity, and enhances suppressor T-cell function. It has been shown to slow worsening of disability. The main limiting factor regarding this drug is a dose-related cardiotoxicity. This limits the length of time that it can be used for the treatment of MS (25).

Corticosteroids are the gold standard for shortening the duration of an exacerbation, although steroids have not been clearly shown to have long-term benefits in MS. We recommend corticosteroid administration for moderate or severe exacerbations, using high-dose oral or intravenous therapy. For acute relapses, the recommended corticosteroid regimen is methylprednisolone (1 g intravenously over 4 hours in 250-mL of D5W). This is given daily for 3 to 5 days, usually 5 days. This is usually followed by an oral prednisone taper, particularly if the patient has not shown complete recovery with the intravenous steroid course. The oral prednisone taper usually consists of a higher dose of 100 mg initially, tapering by 10 mg every 3 days. Patients are usually given an H2-blocking agent concomitantly with medication such as Tylenol or a sleeping aid if insomnia develops due to the steroids.

There are no good data on the duration of steroid therapy, so typically short courses (less than 3 weeks) are preferred to prevent steroid-related complications. Bone density studies should be performed in patients receiving frequent corticosteroid regimens, with prophylactic measures taken to prevent osteoporosis (37).

TREATMENT OF COMMON COMPLICATIONS OF MULTIPLE SCLEROSIS

Symptomatic therapy for weakness, spasticity, tremors, diplopia, paroxysmal attacks (including trigeminal neuralgia), impotence, pain, bladder and bowel dysfunction, depression, fatigue, and pseudobulbar emotional incontinence are available and should be deployed to maximize patient function and comfort (38) (Table 34.6).

Spasticity often responds to treatment with Lioresal, benzodiazepines, and tizanidine. These medications are often combined with a course of physical therapy including a program of daily passive and active range-of-motion stretching exercises. Botulinum toxin has had limited use in MS for localized tremors and spasticity. Patients who do not respond to or cannot tolerate oral antispasticity agents may be candidates for a programmable implantable intrathecal baclofen pump (see chapter 14 for details).

Fatigue is seen in up to 80% of patients and can often interfere with daily activities. Treatment options include medications such as amantadine, methylphenidate, pemoline, modafinil, and selective serotonin reuptake inhibitors. In evaluating patients with fatigue, one should rule out the possibility of drug abuse or a sleep disorder such as sleep apnea. Appropriate use of assistive

TABLE 34.6. MOST COMMON MEDICAL COMPLICATION IN MULTIPLE SCLEROSIS

Symptom	Treatment
Fatigue	Lifestyle management, energy conservation
	Appropriate use of assistive devices
	Pemoline, amantadine, modafinil, selective serotonin reuptake inhibitor
	Treat any sleep disorders
Spasticity	Tizanidine, baclofen (oral and intrathecal)
	Botulinum toxin for appropriate cases
	Physical therapy
	Avoidance of precipitating triggers
Bladder dysfunction (failure to store)	Oxybutinin, tolteridine
Bladder dysfunction (failure to empty)	Intermittent self catheterization
	Urodynamic studies
Constipation	Stool softeners, increased fluid intake
	Bulk forming agents (Metamucil, Citrucel)
Diarrhea	Bowel patterning, dietary management

devices (e.g., scooters, walkers, and wheelchairs) that help to conserve energy expenditure should be discussed with patients (38).

Bladder dysfunction in MS can be broken down into three categories: failure to store, failure to empty, and mixed bladder dysfunction. Patients with failure to store often have symptoms of urgency, frequency, incontinence, nocturia, and a postvoid residua rate of less than 100 mL. An anticholinergic agent, such as oxybutynin, or an antimuscarinic agent, such as tolterodine, can be very helpful. Patients should be instructed to avoid caffeine, aspartate, and alcohol. Behavioral modification and pelvic exercises may also be of value. If the problem is one of failure to empty, patients usually have urgency, hesitancy, double voiding, frequency, incomplete emptying, and a postvoid residual of more than 100 mL. The treatment in this case usually consists of intermittent catheterization or the use of an indwelling catheter. With combined dysfunction, patients note urgency, hesitancy and double voiding, incomplete emptying, and dribbling incontinence. The treatment of choice is intermittent self-catheterization with anticholinergic medication. Sometimes an indwelling catheter is needed (38). Bladder testing including urodynamic studies may be extremely helpful in guiding treatment (see chapter 12 for details).

Constipation, bowel incontinence, diarrhea, flatulence, fecal impaction, and ileus are often seen in patients with MS. Causes for constipation include slow peristalsis, impaired patient mobility, and the use of medications such as anticholinergics. Patients are instructed to drink 1½ to 2 L of water daily, which can be problematic if they have a bladder problem as well, which is usually the case. Stool softeners, oral laxatives, and bulk-forming agents are all recommended. Suppositories or mini-enemas are used as needed.

For loose stools or bowel incontinence, bowel patterning is recommended. Diet is reviewed and anticholinergic medications such as oxybutynin or loperamide (Imodium) are recommended (38). Tremors and incoordination in MS may be helped with medications such as clonazepam, isoniazid, propranolol, and ondansetron or with the use of weighted bracelets and armrests. Unfortunately, tremors are difficult to treat and medication can cause sedation or side effects. For patients with severe tremors, and as a last resort, pallidal stimulation, as used in Parkinson disease, may be useful in improving function.

Paroxysmal motor and sensory attacks frequently occur during the course of MS. If associated with an acute attack of MS, corticosteroids may accelerate their resolution. Symptomatic relief is usually readily achievable using carbamazepine, gabapentin, phenytoin (Dilantin), or Lioresal. Brief courses of these medications may suffice, but long-term therapy is often required (38).

MS can significantly affect sexuality. Sexual excitement and response begin in the brain. Electrical signals from brain areas involved in the sexual response pass to the spinal cord and then exit through nerves at the base of the spinal cord to the genital organs. Demyelination along this pathway can lead to sexual disturbances. The physiology of sexual functioning can be affected by symptoms such as spasticity, fatigue, bowel and bladder problems, and pain. Illness-related neurologic changes such as decreased sensation in the perineal region can affect sexual function. Psychological factors such as anxiety and depression can also interfere with sexual desire. More than 90% of men with MS and more than 70% of women with MS report changes in sexual function. Men most often note decreased libido, inability in achieving and sustaining an erection, decreased force of ejaculation, and impaired genital sensation. Women often report impaired genital sensation, decreased orgasmic response, and loss of sexual desire. Decreased vaginal lubrication also is a common complaint.

It is important to emphasize to patients to feel comfortable with their own bodies and to communicate information about what does and does not feel pleasurable to their partners. To help prevent bowel and bladder problems during intercourse, patients should empty their bladder before sexual intercourse and reduce their intake of fluids approximately 2 hours before sexual activity. Vaginal lubricant such as KY jelly or Astroglide can be used to decrease vaginal dryness. Antispasticity medication can be taken before sexual activity to minimize leg spasms. The use of a vibrator has also been helpful for patients who note decreased vaginal sensation (38).

Options for erectile dysfunction are available (see chapter 22). Recent studies have shown that sildenafil (Viagra) can relieve male impotence, which is frequently seen in patients with spinal forms of MS (39).

Pain can be treated by first identifying its cause. Musculoskeletal pains are common in patients with MS, often due to mechanical imbalances and associated degenerative changes. CNS pain can be treated with analgesics, amitriptyline, carbamazepine, phenytoin, and gabapentin. Muscle spasms can be treated as for spasticity.

Diplopia often resolves spontaneously or with the use of corticosteroids for an acute attack of MS. Persistent diplopia can be treated with eye patching, and severe nystagmus causing oscillopsia may improve with gabapentin or eye prisms.

Depression can be treated with antidepressant drugs, psychotherapy, and avoidance of drugs associated with causing depression whenever possible. Amitriptyline is particularly useful for

pseudobulbar emotional incontinence, and benzodiazepines are of value in treating panic attacks (40).

COGNITIVE FUNCTION

It has only been over the past several years that it has been recognized that MS can cause problems with cognition, planning, and judgment. Approximately one third of patients with MS will have some problems in these areas, particularly in areas of executive functioning. In most patients, these deficits are mild to moderate, with some noticeable impact on everyday activities but not severe enough to prevent functioning at work. However, in about 5% to 10% of patients, cognitive dysfunction may be so severe that the person cannot function without supervision. This can be the case even with mild physical disability. Abstract reasoning and problem solving, verbal fluency, visuospatial skills, speed of information processing, attention and concentration, particularly sustained attention, and memory are the cognitive functions thought to be affected in MS. These changes occur as a result of the cerebral demyelination and axonal damage that occurs in MS. The pattern of deficits noted resembles that seen in subcortical dementias such as seen in patients with Huntington disease. In one study, it was found that 83% of patients with MS with more than 30 cm^2 of total lesion area were cognitively impaired, whereas 22% of those with less than 30 cm^2 of total lesion area met criteria for cognitive impairment (41). Cognitive dysfunction has also been found to be related to enlargement of the ventricles and atrophy of the corpus callosum. Frontal lobe demyelinating lesions have been associated with deficits in executive functions, whereas lesions in the corpus callosum have been associated with deficits in verbal fluency and spatial abilities (42).

Secondary effects of MS can contribute to cognitive dysfunction. Depression, fatigue, and anxiety can affect a patient's attention and ability to concentrate and focus.

To accurately assess cognitive dysfunction, one often must perform full neuropsychological testing. Pharmacologic management of cognitive dysfunction has focused on disease-modifying agents that alter the course of the disease, to slow the neuropathologic changes underlying cognitive deficits. Symptomatic treatments for improving cognition have met with limited success. Donepezil hydrochloride and tacrine hydrochloride, which have been used to treat Alzheimer dementia, have been used to help cognitive problems in MS with mixed results. There is currently a clinical trial in process studying the effects of donepezil hydrochloride in MS. Antifatigue medications such as amantadine and pemoline have helped with attention and fatigue. Cognitive rehabilitation has shown promise in helping patients by using compensatory strategies; such as making lists, or using a computer, and by doing cognitive exercises and drills.

Emotional changes have also been observed in MS. These include depression, suicidal ideation, grieving, emotional lability, euphoria, antisocial behavior, sexual inappropriateness, and psychotic states. Medications used to treat MS such as steroids can produce both depression and hypomanic states. Interferon therapy can also contribute to depression. Patients can be depressed as a reaction to altered life circumstances and increased disease activity. Women often will notice worsening of depression during menses, suggesting a hormonal effect. Assessment of emotional changes in MS is a complex undertaking. Standard treatments such as psychotherapy and pharmacologic management of symptoms such as depression are often helpful (25).

It is important to prevent serious complications such as decubiti, urosepsis, aspiration, and severe depression in patients with MS by identifying those patients at risk and deploying appropriate preventive measures.

DYSPHAGIA AND DYSARTHRIA

Speech impairment has long been recognized as a feature in MS. Scanning speech and dysarthria are often noted. Areas of demyelination, which occur in the periventricular white matter of the brain, brain stem, cerebellum, and spinal cord, can interrupt the transmission of the message between the brain and the muscles in the lips, tongue, soft palate, vocal cords, and diaphragm. Because these muscles control the quality of speech and voice, dysarthria and dysphonia may result. These problems can temporarily worsen with exacerbations and fatigue. Other problems that patients notice include impaired loudness and pitch control, decreased vital capacity, and hypernasality. Spastic dysarthria is due to bilateral lesions of the corticobulbar tracts. Patients with a harsh, strained voice quality often exhibit hypertonicity in facial muscles and palatal muscles. Ataxic dysarthria results from bilateral or generalized lesions of the cerebellum. When vocal tremor is noted, patients also exhibit intention tremor of the head, trunk, arms, and hands. Patients with rapid alternating movements of the tongue and lips often exhibit nystagmus or jerky eye movements. Mixed dysarthrias can be due to a combination of generalized lesions of demyelination in the cerebral white matter and the cerebellum or spinal cord. Patients can then exhibit impaired loudness control, vocal tremor, and impaired articulation and pitch control (25).

To treat dysarthria, medications to help with spasticity, ataxia, tremor, and fatigue, in conjunction with therapy by a speech-language pathologist are recommended. Medications such as baclofen, tizanidine, and diazepam are helpful for spasticity. Spasticity can affect speech and voice in many ways during respiration, phonation, articulation, and resonance. Excess muscle tone can restrict range of motion of the diaphragm, reducing breath support. Excess tone in the vocal cords can result in a harsh, strained voice quality. Choosing the appropriate treatment strategies and objectively monitoring the effects of specific medications on speech and voice are ideally accomplished by a team approach with the physician and speech-language pathologist (25).

REHABILITATION IN MULTIPLE SCLEROSIS

When dealing with an unpredictable, often disabling disease such as MS, one must create an environment in which patients can function as optimally as possible. Occupational therapy can be of great value in enhancing the patient's quality of life through adaptive equipment, home modifications, and hand-control vehicles, as well as in maximizing the use of available motor skills for activities of daily living. Physical therapy can help enhance quality of life and activities of daily living performance with muscle-strengthening programs, Romberg exercises, gait training, bracing, ambulation and transfer training, deployment of safety measures, and use of assistive devices. Speech therapy, as previously mentioned, is often helpful for hypophonation, and dysphaia. Communication devices, cognitive assessment and treatment strategies can also be employed (38).

FUTURE DIRECTIONS

It can be anticipated that as the genetic susceptibility for MS is clarified, as the role of infectious agents in triggering MS is documented, and as the precise pathogenetic mechanisms for immune-mediated tissue injury are defined, more effective and less invasive therapies will emerge. If one exogenous agent is proven to cause most cases of MS, then, like paralytic polio, MS could become a preventable disease through the use of a specific vaccine. If, on the other hand, multiple agents are involved in MS causation, this outcome is unlikely. As the human genome is further defined, it is probable that several genes will prove important in MS susceptibility. Understanding the function of these genes could offer the opportunity to better understand pathogenetic mechanisms and enable research to be focused on the most promising areas. As a result, it may be possible for the pharmaceutical industry to develop better and safer drugs. In the short term, however, it seems likely that early intervention with current drugs and research on the effectiveness of combinations of therapies will be the mainstays of treatment to decrease disease activity while awaiting development of the next generation of treatments.

APPENDIX 34.1

NEW MS DIAGNOSTIC CRITERIA

Clinical (Attacks)	Objective Lesions	Additional Requirements to Make Diagnosis
2 or more	2 or more	• None: clinical evidence will suffice (additional evidence desirable but must be consistent with MS)
2 or more	1	• Dissemination is *space* by MRI[3,4] *or* positive CSF and 2 or more MRI lesions consistent with MS or further clinical attack involving different site
1	2 or more	• Dissemination in *time* by MRI *or* second clinical attack
1 (mono-symptomatic)	1	• Dissemination in *space* by MRI[3,4] *or* positive CSF and 2 or more MRI lesions consistent with MS **AND**
		• Dissemination in *time* by MRI *or* second clinical attack
0 (progression from onset[2])	1	• Positive CSF **AND**
		• Dissemination in *space* by MRI evidence of 9 or more T2 brain lesions *or* 2 or more cord lesions *or* 4–8 brain and 1 cord lesion *or* positive VEP with 4–8 MRI lesions *or* positive VEP with less than 4 brain lesions plus 1 cord lesion **AND**
		• Dissemination in *time* by MRI *or* continued progression for 1 year

From, McDonald et al. Recommended Diagnostic Criteria for MS. *Ann Neurol* 2001;50:121–127 and The National Multiple Sclerosis Society, with permission.

PARACLINICAL EVIDENCE IN MS DIAGNOSIS

What is a Positive MRI?[3,4]
3 out of 4 of the following:
✓ 1 Gd-enhancing lesion **or** 9 T2 hyperintense lesions if no Gd-enhancing lesion
✓ 1 or more infratentorial lesions
✓ 1 or more juxtacortical lesions
✓ 3 or more periventricular lesions
Note: 1 cord lesion can substitute for 1 brain lesion

What Provides MRI Evidence of Dissemination in Time?
✓ A Gd-enhancing lesion demonstrated in a scan done at least 3 months following onset of clinical attack at a site different from attack, **or**
✓ In absence of Gd-enhancing lesions at 3 month scan, follow-up scan after an additional 3 months showing Gd-lesion or new T2 lesion.

What is Positive CSF?
Oligoclonal IgG bands in CSF (and not serum) or elevated IgG index

What is Positive VEP?
Delayed but well-preserved wave form

[2]*Thompson et al.* Diagnostic criteria for primary progressive MS: A position paper. *Ann Neurol* (2000) 47:831–835.
[3]*Barkhof et al.* Comparision of MR imaging criteria at first presentation to predict conversion to clinically definite MS. *Brain* (1997) 120:2059–2069.
[4]*Tintoré et al.* Isolated demyelinating syndromes: comparision of different imaging criteria to predict conversion to clinically definite MS. *Am J Radiology* (2000) 21:702–706.
These new diagnostic criteria were developed through consensus of an International Panel on the Diagnosis of MS. Refer to cited articles for details. Pocket card produced and provided by the National Multiple Sclerosis Society, USA., 7733 Third Avenue, New York, NY.
http://www.nationalmssociety.org: 1-800-FIGHTMS

REFERENCES

1. Medaer R. Does the history of multiple sclerosis go back as far as the 14th century? *Acta Neurol Scand* 1979;60:189–192.
2. Firth D. The case of Auygustus d'Este (1794–1848): the first account of disseminated sclerosis. *Proc Royal Soc Med* 1941; 34:381–384.
3. Fredrikson S, Slavenka K-H. The 150-year anniversary of multiple sclerosis: does its early history give an etiological clue? *Perspect Biol Med* 1989;32:237–243.
4. Charcot J-M. Séance du 14 mars. *C R Seances Soc Biol Fil* 1868;20: 13–14.
5. Cook SD. Multiple sclerosis. *Arch Neurol* 1998;55:421–423.
6. Brain WR. Critical review: disseminating sclerosis. *Q J Med* 1930;23: 343–391.
7. Kurtzke JF. MS epidemiology worldwide. One view of current status. *Acta Neurol Scand Suppl* 1995;161:23–33.
8. Kurtzke JF, Beebe GW, Norman JE. Epidemiology of multiple sclerosis in U.S. veterans: III. Migration and the risk of MS. *Neurology* 1985; 35:672–686.
9. Sadovnick AD, Ebers GC. Epidemiology of multiple sclerosis: a critical overview. *Can J Neurol Sci* 1993;20:17–29.
10. Cook SD. The epidemiology of multiple sclerosis: clues to the etiology of a mysterious disease. *Neuroscientist* 1996;2:172–180.
11. Lauer K. Multiple sclerosis in the old world: the new old map [Editorial]. In: Firnhaber W, Laure L, eds. *Multiple sclerosis in Europe. An epidemiological update.* Darmstadt: LTV Press, 1994:14–27.
12. McLeod JG, Hammond SR, Hallpike JF. Epidemiology of multiple sclerosis in Australia with NSW and SA survey results. *Med J Aust* 1994;160:117–122.
13. Lauer K. Environmental associations with the risk of multiple sclerosis: the contribution of ecological studies. *Acta Neurol Scand Suppl* 1995; 161:77–88.
14. Hillert J. Human leukocyte antigen studies in multiple sclerosis. *Ann Neurol* 1994;36:S15–S17.
15. Cook SD, Rohowsky-Kochan C, Bansil S, et al. Evidence for multiple sclerosis as an infectious disease. *Acta Neurol Scand Suppl* 1995;161: 34–42.
16. Cook SD. Evidence for a viral etiology of multiple sclerosis. In: Cook SD, ed. *The handbook of multiple sclerosis*, 3rd ed. New York: Marcel Dekker Inc, 2001.
17. Cook SD, Rohowsky-Kochan C, Bansil S, et al. Evidence for multiple sclerosis as an infectious disease. *Acta Neurol Scand* 1995;161:34–42.
18. Adams RD, Victor M, Ropper AH. *Principles of neurology.* McGraw-Hill, 1997:909–913.
19. Kesselring J. Differential diagnosis. In: Kesselring J, ed. *Multiple sclerosis.* Cambridge, UK: Cambridge University Press, 1997.
20. O'Riordan JI, Thomson AJ, Kingsley DP, et al. The prognostic value of brain MRI in clinically isolated syndromes of the CNS: a 10 year follow up. *Brain* 1998;121:495–503.
21. Beck RW, Cleary PA, Trobe JD, et al. The effect of corticosteroids for acute optic neuritis on the subsequent development of MS. *N Engl J Med* 1993;329:1764–1769.

22. Stone LA, McFarland HF, Frank JA. Neuroimaging in multiple sclerosis. In: Cook SD, ed. *Handbook of multiple sclerosis,* 2nd ed. New York: Marcel Dekker Inc, 1996.

23. Simon J, Jacobs LD, Campion MK, et al. A longitudinal study of brain atrophy in relapsing multiple sclerosis. *Neurology* 1999;53:139–148.

24. Edwards MK, Bonnin JM. White matter diseases. In: Atlas SW, ed. *Magnetic resonance imaging of the brain and spine.* Baltimore: Williams & Wilkins, 1990:246–450.

25. Burks J, Johnson K. *Multiple sclerosis diagnosis, medical management, and rehabilitation.* Demos Publications, New York, 2000:83–93, 385–391, 405–417.

26. Whitaker JN, Benveniste EN. Cerebrospinal fluid. In: Cook SD, ed. *Handbook of multiple sclerosis,* 2nd ed. New York: Marcel Dekker Inc, 1996.

27. Lublin FD, Reingold SC. Defining the clinical course of multiple sclerosis: results of an international survey. *Neurology* 1996;46:907–911.

28. Weinshenker BG. The natural history of multiple sclerosis. *Neurol Clin* 1995;13:119–146.

29. Filippi M, Horsfield MA, Morrissey SP, et al. Quantitative brain MRI lesion load predicts the course of clinically isolated syndromes suggestive of multiple sclerosis. *Neurology* 1994;44:635–641.

30. Khoury SJ, Guttman CRG, Orav EJ, et al. Longitudinal MRI in multiple sclerosis: correlation between disability and lesion burden. *Neurology* 1994;44:2120–2124.

31. Rudick RA. Disease-modifying drugs for relapsing-remitting multiple sclerosis and future directions for multiple sclerosis therapeutics. *Arch Neurol* 1999;56:1079–1084.

32. Becker CB, Gidal BE, Fleming JO. Immunotherapy of multiple sclerosis, part 2. *Am J Health-Sept Pharm* 1995;52:2105–2120.

33. Wolinsky JS. Copolymer 1: a most reasonable alternative therapy for early relapsing-remitting multiple sclerosis with mild disability. *Neurology* 1995;45:1245–1247.

34. Jacobs LD, Cookfair DL, Rudnick RA, et al. Intramuscular interferon beta 1a for disease progression in relapsing multiple sclerosis. *Ann Neurol* 1996;39:285–294.

35. The IFNB Multiple Sclerosis Study Group. Interferon beta 1b is effective in relapsing-remitting multiple sclerosis. Clinical results of a multicenter, randomized, double-blind, placebo-controlled trial. *Neurology* 1993;43:655–661.

36. Jacobs LD, Beck RW, Simon JH, et al. Intramuscular interferon beta 1a therapy initiated during a first demyelinating event in multiple sclerosis. *N Engl J Med* 2000;343:898–904.

37. Eastell R. Treatment of postmenopausal osteoporosis. *N Engl J Med* 1998;338:736–746.

38. Schapiro RT. *Symptom management in multiple sclerosis,* 3rd ed. Demos Publications, New York, 1998.

39. Litwiller SE. Introduction to neurourology: the treatment of bladder and sexual dysfunction. In: Education program syllabus of the American Academy of Neurology 52nd annual meeting; 4 PC.005-23.

40. Van der Noort S, Holland NJ. *Multiple sclerosis in clinical practice.* Demos Publications, 1999.

41. Rao SM, Leo GJ, Haughton VM, et al. Correlation of magnetic resonance imaging with neuropsychological testing in multiple sclerosis. *Neurology* 1989;39:161–166.

42. Comi G, Filippi M, Martinelli V, et al. Brain magnetic resonance imaging correlates of cognitive impairment in multiple sclerosis. *J Neurol Sci* 1993;115:566–573.

43. McDonald WI, Compston A, Edan G, et al. Recommended diagnostic criteria for multiple sclerosis. *Ann Neurol* 2001;50(1):121–127.

ADULT MOTOR NEURON DISEASE

GREGORY T. CARTER
LISA S. KRIVICKAS

Adult motor neuron disease (MND) is often considered synonymous with amyotrophic lateral sclerosis (ALS). In the United States, the term ALS is frequently used to describe all forms of adult-onset MND. However, it is also used to refer specifically to the most common form of adult MND, which is sporadic, acquired ALS. In the United Kingdom, the converse is true: the generic term for all forms of ALS is MND (1). In reality, adult MND actually encompasses a group of disorders that include ALS, primary lateral sclerosis (PLS), progressive muscular atrophy (PMA), primary bulbar palsy (PBP), adult-onset progressive spinal muscular atrophy (SMA), and X-linked recessive spinobulbar muscular atrophy (SBMA). A presentation with pure upper motor neuron (UMN) signs may be called PLS, whereas pure bulbar presentation may be called PBP and pure lower motor neuron (LMN) presentation may be called PMA. Whether these conditions exist as distinct diseases or represent part of the spectrum of ALS is still debated. This is represented schematically in Fig. 35.1. At least one form of PLS with a benign course and autosomai-dominant inheritance has been reported (2,3). ALS is also referred to as Lou Gehrig disease, after perhaps the most famous person yet afflicted with the disease. SBMA is commonly referred to as Kennedy disease, after the physician who first described this disorder as recently as 1968 (4).

In this chapter, we use the terms ALS, PLS, PMA, PBP, SMA, and SBMA. In the adult population, ALS is far more common than the other disorders. Thus, most of this chapter focuses on ALS, starting with a description of the diseases, including epidemiology and genetics. This is followed by diagnostic workup, including electrodiagnosis, pharmacologic management, and rehabilitation strategies, most of which may be applied to any of the adult MNDs.

OVERVIEW OF THE MAJOR ADULT MOTOR NEURON DISEASES

Amyotrophic Lateral Sclerosis

ALS is a rapidly progressive neuromuscular disease that destroys both UMNs and LMNs, resulting in spasticity and diffuse muscular atrophy and weakness. Most cases of ALS are presumably acquired and occur sporadically. However, approximately 10% of all ALS cases are familial ALS (FALS), usually inherited as an autosomal-dominant trait. About 15% of these cases result from a gene defect on chromosome 21q12.1, which leads to a mutation in the antioxidant enzyme Cu/Zn superoxide dismutase (SOD) (5,6). More than 50 unique SOD mutations have been identified (5–7). Emerging evidence suggests that these mutations result in increased oxidative stress for the motor neurons, leading to cell death, which is believed to be related to free radical toxicity (6,7).

The etiology of sporadic ALS (SALS) and the other 85% of FALS cases is unknown. More data suggest that excessive glutamate activity in the brain and spinal cord may play an important role. Glutamate is one of the main central nervous system (CNS) excitatory neurotransmitters in the brain, and excess levels of this chemical have been demonstrated in the serum, spinal fluid, and brain tissue of patients with ALS (8,9). There appears to be reduced clearance of glutamate from critical motor control areas in ALS, as well as decreased levels of glutamate transport protein (10,11).

Epidemiology of Amyotrophic Lateral Sclerosis

ALS most commonly strikes people between 40 and 60 years of age, with a mean age of onset of 58 years (12–14).

The overall prevalence rate in the worldwide population is somewhere between 5 to 7 per 100,000, making it one of the most common neuromuscular diseases worldwide (15). Further, population studies suggest that the incidence of ALS is increasing, although this is probably due in large part to people living longer and better recognition of the diagnosis (16,17). There appears to be a higher incidence in urban areas, which is believed to be related to environmental factors (17–19). The association of nutrient intake with the risk of ALS was investigated in a population-based case-control study conducted in three counties of western Washington State from 1990 to 1994 (20,21). The authors found that alcohol consumption was not associated with increased risk of ALS. Ever having smoked cigarettes was associated with a twofold increased risk, and a greater than threefold increased risk was observed for current smokers. Significant trends in the risk of ALS were observed with duration of smoking and number of cigarette pack years. Further, dietary fat intake was associated with an increased risk of ALS, whereas dietary fiber intake was associated with a decreased risk. Interestingly, consumption of antioxidant vitamins from diet or supplemental

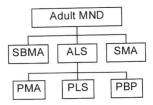

FIGURE 35.1. Schematic representation of adult motor neuron diseases. MND, adult motor neuron disease; SBMA, spinobulbar muscular atrophy; ALS, amyotrophic lateral sclerosis; SMA, spinal muscular atrophy; PMA, progressive muscular atrophy; PLS, primary lateral sclerosis; PBP, primary bulbar palsy.

sources did not alter the risk, but glutamate intake was associated with an increased risk of ALS. The finding that cigarette smoking and glutamate consumption are risk factors for ALS is consistent with current etiologic theories that implicate glutamate excitotoxicity and oxidative stress in the pathogenesis of ALS. The associations with fat and fiber intake warrant further study and biologic explanation.

Considerable clustering has been demonstrated in the western Pacific region of the world (15–17). Other sporadic cluster cases have been reported, but without obvious environmental or causative factors (15). Men appear to be more commonly affected than women, with a male to female ratio of about 1.5:1.0 (12).

Poor prognostic factors include older age at time of onset, bulbar or pulmonary dysfunction early in the clinical course of the disease, short time from symptom onset to diagnosis, and predominance of LMN findings at the time of diagnosis (12–16). More women than men present with bulbar symptoms, and the progression of bulbar palsy appears to be more rapid in women (20,21). Young men with ALS may have a longer life expectancy, but the overall median 50% survival rate is 2½ years postdiagnosis, except in patients with primary bulbar symptoms, in whom the 50% survival rate is only 1 year. Survival rates will obviously vary to a degree depending on the patient's decision to use or not use mechanical ventilation and a feeding tube. Nonetheless, by 5 years postdiagnosis, the overall survival rate is only 28% (12,14,15).

Atypical, "ALS-like," MNDs have been reported infrequently as a remote complication of several malignancies, including lymphoma and small cell carcinoma of the lung (24,25). These likely represent paraneoplastic syndromes and not a true manifestation of ALS (26). Irrespective, patients with atypical MND should be screened for malignancy.

Spinal and Spinobulbar Muscular Atrophy

There are many forms of SMA, all of which involve selective destruction of anterior horn cells (27). The various forms of SMA are clinically dissimilar, with some rare forms affecting distal or bulbar muscles only. The most common forms are often referred to as types I, II, and III (27). These are mostly disorders of childhood and are usually inherited as autosomal-recessive traits. SMA-I, also known as Werdnig-Hoffman disease (WHD) or acute, infantile-onset SMA, is a severe disorder resulting in death before the age of 2. SMA-II, also referred to as early-onset,

intermediate SMA or chronic WHD, is less severe, with signs and symptoms becoming apparent in the first 6 to 18 months of life. SMA-III, also known as Kugelberg-Welander disease, is a chronic, late-onset disorder, associated with significantly less morbidity. Signs and symptoms of SMA-III usually become apparent between the ages of 5 and 15. In prior studies looking at SMA-II and SMA-III over a 10-year period, subjects with SMA-II showed marked weakness and progressive decline of strength (27). Subjects with SMA-III had a relatively static or very slowly progressive course and were far stronger (27). In both SMA-II and SMA-III, proximal weakness was greater than distal weakness. Joint contractures, progressive scoliosis, and restrictive lung disease (RLD) were present in most of the individuals with SMA-II, but these complications were rare in those with SMA-III (27).

There are two forms of SMA that have onset in the adult age-group. One is an adult-onset form of SMA, which may be referred to as SMA-IV, with age of onset of 17 to 55 years with either recessive or dominant forms of inheritance (28,29). The disease clinically appears much like SMA-III, although it may be more progressive. The other form is SBMA, or Kennedy disease. This disorder, which was first described as recently as 1968, is a sex-linked, recessive MND characterized by progressive spinal and bulbar muscular atrophy, gynecomastia, and reduced fertility (4,30). In relation to PMA, adult-onset SMA progresses more slowly. In addition, the bulbar and respiratory muscles are not usually involved in adult SMA but may be involved in PMA.

Patients with adult-onset SMA, SBMA, and SMA-III can have normal lifespans, and many of the rehabilitative modalities discussed in this chapter are applicable to this population. Further, with the rapid advancement of rehabilitation technology, many patients with SMA-II are now living well into adulthood and successful pregnancies have been reported in this disease (31).

Epidemiology and Genetics of Spinal and Spinobulbar Muscular Atrophy

SMA has been mapped to chromosome 5q11.2-13.3. Mutations in exons seven and eight of the telomeric survival motor neuron (SMN) gene are present in more than 98% of patients with autosomal-recessive childhood-onset SMA (28,29,32). Deletions in the neuronal apoptosis inhibitory protein (NAIP) gene are found in approximately 67% of patients with SMA-I, 42% of those with SMA-II, and in some patients with adult-onset SMA, although the percentage is not known (28,29).

SBMA has been mapped to the androgen receptor on the X chromosome (28,30). The mutation, which consists of an expansion of CAG trinucleotide repeats, occurs in the first exon of the gene, producing decreased sensitivity of androgen receptors on motor neurons. The disease has some clinical variability, although phenotypic expression does not correlate with the length of CAG trinucleotide repeats. This is in contrast to myotonic muscular dystrophy and fragile X syndrome, in which an increased number of tandem triplet repeats correlates directly with disease severity (30). Commercially available blood tests (DNA analysis) are now available for SMA and SBMA. SBMA can occur without any family history or gynecomastia, and all men with atypical ALS should be tested for SBMA (30,33,34).

Prevalence rates for types II and III are estimated to range from as high as 40 per million among children to around 12 per million in the general population, with adult-onset SMA and SBMA being far less common (27).

DIAGNOSTIC EVALUATION OF MOTOR NEURON DISEASE

The diagnosis of ALS and other forms of adult MND is primarily a process of exclusion. If based on the history and physical examination, clinical signs and symptoms of MND are detected, one must generate a differential diagnosis and then work to exclude processes mimicking MND. Only in FALS with known SOD1 mutations, Kennedy disease, and the few adult-onset SMA cases in which SMN mutations are detected is a definitive diagnostic test available. For most patients with ALS or its variants (PMA and PLS), electrodiagnostic testing (EDX), laboratory testing, neuroimaging studies, and occasionally a muscle biopsy are used to exclude other diagnoses. The El Escorial criteria, as described later in this chapter, are used to assess the certainty of a diagnosis of ALS once other disease processes have been excluded.

Clinical Presentation

Patients with ALS most often seek evaluation complaining of focal weakness (60%), rarely of generalized weakness or cramps and very rarely of generalized fasciculations or respiratory failure (35). Although fasciculations are a prominent feature in most patients with ALS, patients who complain of fasciculations only and have otherwise normal neurologic examination results usually have benign fasciculation syndrome and are unlikely to develop ALS. Symptom onset may be anywhere within the motor system. A study of 613 patients by Norris et al. (36) identified the following locations of initial symptoms: legs, 41%; arms, 34%; bulbar muscles, 24%; generalized weakness, 1%; and respiratory muscles, 1 of 613 patients.

The evaluation of a patient suspected of having MND begins with a detailed history, general physical examination, and neurologic examination. On neurologic examination, one is looking for evidence of UMN and LMN dysfunction. The mental status, nonmotor cranial nerve function, sensory examination, and cerebellar examination results should be normal.

Patients with UMN pathology often complain of loss of dexterity or a feeling of stiffness in the limbs. They may note weakness, which is caused by spasticity resulting from disinhibition of brain-stem control of the vestibulospinal and reticulospinal tracts. Findings on examination include spasticity and hyperreflexia, indicated by abnormal spread of reflexes and clonus or by the presence of brisk reflexes despite muscle atrophy due to LMN loss. The gold standard used to diagnose UMN pathology is the presence of pathologic reflexes, such as the Babinski sign, the Hoffman sign, and a brisk jaw jerk. If the toe extensors are paralyzed, visualization of contraction of the tensor fascia lata when an attempt is made to elicit a Babinski response has the same significance as great toe extension. Recently, it has been suggested that the corneomandibular reflex may be a more sensitive and specific indicator than the jaw jerk of UMN pathology in the bulbar region (37).

Patients with LMN pathology usually present complaining of muscle weakness. In addition, they may note muscle atrophy, fasciculations, and muscle cramping. Cramping may occur anywhere in the body, including the thighs, arms, and abdomen. Cramping of abdominal or other trunk muscles raises a red flag urging the clinician to consider a diagnosis of ALS. Findings on examination include weakness, atrophy, hypotonia, hyporeflexia, and fasciculations. Head drop is a manifestation of muscle weakness often seen in ALS; although it can be seen in other neuromuscular disorders, ALS and myasthenia gravis are the two most common causes of head drop. Atrophy often appears first in the hand intrinsic muscles. Although fasciculations are not a necessary criterion for the diagnosis of ALS, one should question the diagnosis when none are observed.

Signs and symptoms suggesting bulbar muscle weakness include dysarthria, dysphagia, drooling, and aspiration. These signs and symptoms may be caused by UMN or LMN dysfunction involving the bulbar muscles. Signs of spastic dysarthria, indicating UMN pathology, include a strained and strangled quality of speech, reduced rate, low pitch, imprecise consonant pronunciation, vowel distortion, and breaks in pitch. LMN dysfunction creates a flaccid dysarthria in which speech has a nasal or wet quality; pitch and intensity are monotone, phrases abnormally short, and inspiration audible. Complaints of difficulty chewing and swallowing and nasal regurgitation or coughing when drinking liquids indicate dysphagia. On physical examination, the following tests may be used to assess facial and bulbar muscle function: ability to bury the eyelashes, pocket air in the cheeks, whistle, jaw opening and lip closure strength, and phonation of a variety of syllables such as puh, kuh, tuh, and ah. The tongue should be examined for fasciculations and atrophy, and tongue strength and range of motion should be assessed. The gag reflex and jaw jerk should be assessed to look for UMN dysfunction. Pseudobulbar affect is a symptom of pseudobulbar palsy, which refers to a UMN syndrome caused by motor neuron loss in the corticobulbar tracts, rather than in the medulla or bulb. Patients experience inappropriate laughter or crying that is not concordant with their mood and can be embarrassing. Disinhibition of limbic motor control produces a pseudobulbar affect, sometimes called emotional incontinence.

In patients who present with respiratory failure, the earliest signs are often nocturnal and include poor sleep with frequent awakening, early morning headaches, excessive daytime fatigue and sleepiness, nightmares, and orthopnea. Frequent sighing, a weak cough, and difficulty clearing bronchial or pulmonary secretions are other signs of respiratory muscle weakness. Later signs of respiratory dysfunction are dyspnea with exertion, truncated speech, respiratory paradox, dyspnea when eating, rapid shallow breathing, visible accessory muscle contraction, and flaring of the nasal alae. With advanced, untreated respiratory failure, patients may have an elevated hematocrit level, low serum chloride concentration, respiratory acidosis with a compensatory metabolic alkalosis, hypertension, and cor pulmonale.

Other signs and symptoms frequently associated with ALS are cachexia, fatigue, and musculoskeletal complaints. The term

ALS cachexia refers to a phenomenon experienced by some patients in which weight loss occurs in excess of that caused by muscle atrophy and reduced caloric intake. Both subcutaneous fat and peritoneal fat are lost, presumably because of acceleration of the basal metabolic rate (36,38). In patients with ALS cachexia, more than 20% of body weight is typically lost over a 6-month period. Many patients with ALS feel an overwhelming sense of muscle fatigue, which is probably due to a combination of blocking of neuromuscular transmission in reinnervational nerve terminal sprouts and impairment of excitation–contraction coupling (39). Some patients seek initial medical attention because of fractures or sprains that do not heal. In reality, these patients probably sustained their initial injury because of a fall or other injury (e.g., sprained ankle) that occurred because of underlying muscle weakness; they were then unable to recover to their premorbid level of function because of that weakness. Other common musculoskeletal complaints include neck and back pain, shoulder pain due to a frozen shoulder, elbow flexion and ankle plantar-flexion contractures, and claw hand. Patients may experience osteoporotic fractures or stress fractures because of immobilization-induced bone density loss.

Rare signs and symptoms that usually occur only in advanced ALS include sensory impairment, autonomic dysfunction, bowel and bladder dysfunction, extraocular muscle paralysis, pressure ulcer formation, and dementia. Although ALS is discussed as a pure motor disorder, some patients complain of paresthesias. These may be due to compression or entrapment neuropathies, but subclinical abnormalities in somatosensory evoked potentials and quantitative sensory testing have been reported (40).

Differential Diagnosis

After obtaining a history and examining the patient, the clinician is able to generate a differential diagnosis, which guides further diagnostic testing. The differential diagnosis differs depending on whether the presentation is primarily LMN, UMN, bulbar, or mixed LMN and UMN. Table 35.1 suggests a differential diagnosis for each one of these presentations.

El Escorial Criteria

The El Escorial criteria for diagnosing ALS were developed by a task force of the World Federation of Neurology in 1990 to ensure inclusion of more homogeneous patient populations in ALS clinical trials (41). These criteria have been used to enroll patients in most of the recent clinical trials. The criteria were revised in 1998 to improve the speed and certainty of diagnosis (42). The criteria classify the certainty level of the diagnosis of ALS as falling into one of five categories: definite, probable, probable with laboratory support, possible, and suspected. In brief, the motor system is divided into four regions: bulbar, cervical, thoracic, and lumbosacral. Clinical evidence of UMN and LMN pathology is sought in each region. The certainty level of diagnosis depends on how many regions reveal UMN and LMN pathology. Figure 35.2 summarizes the schema for placing patients in the five diagnostic categories. Clinical weakness, atrophy, and fasciculations are considered evidence of LMN pathology. Pathologic spread of reflexes, clonus, and pseudobulbar features are considered evidence of UMN pathology. Electrophysiologic findings can be used to both confirm LMN dysfunction in clinically affected regions and detect LMN dysfunction in clinically uninvolved regions. Neuroimaging and clinical laboratory studies are used to exclude other conditions that may mimic ALS.

Electrodiagnostic Testing

The various forms of MND, including SMA, Kennedy disease, PMA, SALS, and FALS, share several electrodiagnostic features but differ in some aspects due to varying rates of disease progression. General EDX characteristics of MND include normal sensory nerve conduction study (NCS) results, normal or low motor amplitudes depending on disease stage, and normal distal motor latencies and conduction velocities. However, with profound loss of motor amplitude, conduction velocities may drop as low as 25% lower than the lower limit of normal because of loss of the fastest conducting fibers (43). The needle electrode examina-

TABLE 35.1. DIFFERENTIAL DIAGNOSIS OF SUSPECTED MOTOR NEURON DISEASE BASED ON PRESENTING CLINICAL SIGNS AND SYMPTOMS

LMN Only	UMN Only	Bulbar	UMN and LMN
PMA	PLS	PBP	ALS
SMA	Multiple sclerosis	Myasthenia gravis	Cervical myelopathy with radiculopathy
SBMA	Adrenoleukodystrophy	Multiple sclerosis	Syringomyelia
Polio, post-polio syndrome	Subacute combined	Foramen magnum	Spinal cord tumor or AVM
Benign monomelic amyotrophy	Familial spastic paraparesis	Brainstem glioma	Lyme disease
Hexosaminidase A deficiency	Myelopathy	Stroke	
Polyradiculopathy	Syringomyelia	Syringobulbia	
Multifocal motor neuropathy with conduction block		Syringobulbia	
CIDP			
Motor neuropathy or neuronopathy		Polymyositis	
Lambert–Eaton syndrome		SBMA	
Plexopathy			
Benign fasciculations			

ALS, amyotrophic lateral sclerosis; AVM, arteriovenous malformation; CIDP, chronic inflammatory demyelinating polyneuropathy; LMN, lower motor neuron; PBP, primary bulbar palsy; PLS, primary lateral sclerosis; PMA, progressive muscular atrophy; SBMA, spinobulbar muscular atrophy; SMA, spinal muscular atrophy; UMN, upper motor neuron.

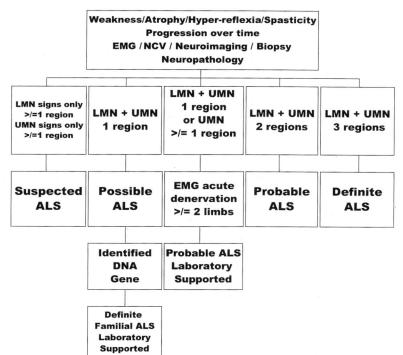

FIGURE 35.2. World Federation of Neurology El Escorial revisited criteria for amyotrophic lateral sclerosis diagnosis. (From Brooks BR. Defining optimal management in ALS: from first symptoms to announcement. *Neurology* 1999;53[Suppl 5]: S1–S3, with permission.)

tion (NEE) reveals a decreased recruitment pattern, either small or large motor-unit action potentials (MUAPs) with or without evidence of remodeling depending on the specific disease process, and spontaneous activity including positive sharp waves (PSWs), fibrillation potentials, fasciculations, and complex repetitive discharges (CRDs). The prominence of the various forms of spontaneous activity varies with the different forms of MND.

Spinal Muscular Atrophies

The EDX features of the autosomal-recessive SMA types I through IV are determined by the rate of anterior horn cell degeneration and the stage in the course of the disease. Sensory NCS results are normal in all forms of SMA. Compound muscle action potentials (CMAPs) are decreased in proportion to the degree of muscle atrophy. Motor velocities are most likely to be abnormally slow in SMA-I because of the extensive loss of motor axons.

The most profound loss of MUAPs is seen in SMA-I. With maximal effort, only a few MUAPs may fire at a rapid rate. Small MUAPs are common because reinnervation cannot compensate for the rapid loss of anterior horn cells. Myopathic-appearing low-amplitude, polyphasic, short-duration units may also be seen because of muscle fiber degeneration. In the other types of SMA, one sees large-amplitude MUAPs (up to 10 or 15 mV), because the number of fibers per motor unit increases as motor-unit remodeling occurs. These large units tend to be polyphasic with increased duration. Satellite potentials appear as remodeling occurs. Myopathic-appearing MUAPs are also seen in some older patients with SMA-III, and their etiology is not well understood.

On NEE in SMA-I, fibrillation potentials and PSWs are diffuse and seen in many muscles, including the paraspinals. Fasciculation potentials are relatively uncommon, but spontaneously firing MUAPs at 5 to 15 Hz, even during sleep, are a unique EDX feature of both SMA-I and SMA-II (44). In the more chronic forms of SMA, fibrillation potentials and PSWs are even more common and increase in frequency as age increases. CRDs are often seen in SMA-II and SMA-III, and fasciculations are more common than in type I (45,46).

Kennedy Disease

Motor NCS abnormalities are similar to those seen in other forms of MND. Although patients generally do not have sensory complaints, absence or reduction of sensory nerve action potentials (SNAPs) is a common finding (47,48). NEE shows large amplitude and long duration MUAPs consistent with the rather indolent disease course. Fibrillation potentials and PSWs may be very prominent and present in all muscles examined. Fasciculation potentials are also abundant in limb, facial, and tongue muscles.

Adult Nonhereditary Motor Neuron Disease

For many years, Lambert's criteria have been the standard for the electromyographic (EMG) diagnosis of ALS (49,50). The following four criteria must be met to make a definite diagnosis of ALS: (a) PSWs or fibrillation potentials in three of five limbs, counting the head as a limb. For a limb to be considered affected, at least two muscles innervated by different peripheral nerves and roots should show active denervation; (b) normal sensory NCS results; (c) normal motor conduction studies; however, if the CMAP amplitude is very low, conduction velocity may drop as low as 70% of the lower limit of normal; and (d) reduced recruitment of MUAPs on needle examination. More recently, Cornblath et al. (51) studied 61 patients with ALS and found that even with low CMAPs, motor distal latencies and F-wave latencies did not exceed 125% of the upper limit of normal, and motor conduction velocities did not fall below 80% of the lower limit of normal. The EDX findings in PMA are identical to those in ALS; the distinction between the two diagnoses is made by the presence or absence of UMN signs on physical examination. By definition, the EDX examination is normal in PLS. In PBP, active denervation is found only in muscles of the head and neck.

The EDX portion of the El Escorial criteria differs somewhat from Lambert's criteria and is generally more liberal. The revised El Escorial criteria allow EDX findings to be used to upgrade the certainty of a diagnosis from clinically possible ALS to probable ALS; this upgrading of the diagnosis is important because it often allows additional patients to participate in clinical trials, which generally require a diagnosis of probable or definite ALS. The El Escorial EDX criteria state that active denervation must be present in two of the four regions (bulbar, cervical, thoracic, and lumbar) to support a diagnosis of ALS. For the cervical or lumbosacral region to be counted, at least two muscles innervated by different nerve roots and peripheral nerves must have EMG changes. In the bulbar and thoracic regions, changes in one muscle are sufficient. Thus, a patient with active denervation in the left arm and thoracic paraspinals would meet the El Escorial criteria for an EDX diagnosis of ALS but not the Lambert criteria because only one limb is involved. On the other hand, a patient with denervation in the tongue and both arms would fulfill Lambert's criteria and the El Escorial criteria for ALS because three limbs and two regions are involved (bulbar and cervical). Early in the progression of ALS, many patients with a suspected clinical diagnosis do not meet EDX criteria for a definite diagnosis. A second study several months later will often fulfill the EDX criteria for diagnosis.

NCS in ALS are characterized primarily by decreased CMAP amplitudes. The mild slowing of motor conduction velocity and the prolongation of F-wave latencies are attributed to loss of the fastest conducting axons. An interesting phenomenon observed in many patients is that of the split hand; CMAP amplitudes are decreased to a greater extent on the radial side of the hand than on the ulnar side. CMAPs obtained from the abductor pollicis brevis and first dorsal interosseous are much lower than those obtained from the abductor digiti minimi. More than two stimulation sites should be used in the evaluation of motor nerves to exclude the presence of conduction block, because multifocal motor neuropathy with conduction block is occasionally misdiagnosed as ALS. The ulnar nerve easily can be stimulated at the wrist, below the elbow, above the elbow, in the axilla, and in the supraclavicular fossa. In limbs with UMN signs, H reflexes may be elicited from muscles in which they cannot normally be obtained. A few patients do have SNAP abnormalities, and the sympathetic skin response is absent in 40%, suggesting subclinical autonomic nervous system involvement (52). Repetitive stimulation studies may show a decrement in CMAP with stimulation at 3 Hz, which is similar to that seen in myasthenia gravis.

A decrement is particularly likely to be detected in patients with rapidly progressing disease and in muscles with an abundance of fasciculations (43).

The NEE is the most important part of the EDX examination in cases of suspected ALS. Fasciculation potentials are seen in most patients with ALS, but they are not necessary to meet diagnostic criteria, and the presence of only fasciculations is inadequate as evidence of LMN involvement of a particular limb or region. The significance of fasciculations depends on the company they keep; they are pathologic only when accompanied by fibrillation potentials, PSWs, or recruitment pattern or MUAP size changes. In patients with advanced ALS, fibrillation potentials and PSWs are prominent in most muscles, but they may be sparse early in the course of the disease. Occasionally, CRDs and doublets or triplets are seen in patients with ALS, but these are not typical EDX findings in ALS. The thoracic paraspinals should be examined with a needle; they are not involved in tandem cervical and lumbar stenosis and can help exclude this as a diagnostic possibility. In addition, when the El Escorial criteria are employed, the finding of denervation in the thoracic and either the cervical or the lumbar region is sufficient for a definite diagnosis, making examination of the tongue or facial muscles (which many patients find unpleasant) unnecessary. Although fasciculations and denervation of the tongue are considered almost pathognomonic for ALS, they are seldom found in patients who do not have clinical evidence of bulbar muscle involvement. The recruitment pattern is decreased in involved muscles. If the disease is progressing relatively slowly, MUAP amplitudes and durations become increased; but if the course is very rapid, denervation outpaces reinnervation, and enlarged MUAPs do not have time to develop. The density and distribution of fasciculations and fibrillations do not correlate with disease course or prognosis, and serial EDX examinations are not useful for monitoring disease progression once a definite diagnosis has been made.

Neurophysiologists have begun to explore the use of transcranial magnetic stimulation as a method of identifying subclinical UMN dysfunction. Results are contradictory with respect to the sensitivity and specificity of various findings as evidence of UMN dysfunction, and these techniques must be considered experimental at present. Abnormalities suggesting UMN pathology include a motor evoked potential (MEP) much lower in amplitude than the CMAP recorded from the same muscle, prolonged central motor conduction time, decreased MEP thresholds and silent periods early in disease, increased MEP thresholds in advanced disease, and decreased cortical representation of individual muscles (53–56).

Neuroimaging

Imaging studies are used to exclude possibilities other than MND from the differential diagnosis. Magnetic resonance imaging (MRI) is the primary imaging modality used in the evaluation of patients with suspected ALS. Almost all patients should have an MRI of the cervical spine to rule out cord compression, a syrinx, or other spinal cord pathology. The location of symptoms will dictate whether other regions of the spinal cord should

TABLE 35.2. SUGGESTED LABORATORY STUDIES

Hematology
  Complete blood count
  Sedimentation rate
Chemistry
  Electrolytes, BUN, creatinine
  Glucose
  Hemoglobin A_{lc}
  Calcium
  Phosphorous
  Magnesium
  Creatine kinase
  Liver function tests
  Serum lead level
  Urine heavy metal screen
  Vitamine B_{12}
  Folate
Endocrine
  T4, thyroid-stimulating hormone
Immunology
  Serum immunoelectrophoresis
  Urine assay for Bence Jones proteins
  Antinuclear antibody
  Rheumatoid factor
  GM1 antibody panel
Microbiology
  Lyme titre
  Venereal Disease Research Laboratories test
Optional
  Human immunodeficiency virus test—if risk factors present
  Anti-Hu antibody—if suspicion of malignancy

be imaged. In patients presenting with the PMA phenotype, an MRI of the involved region of the spinal cord with gadolinium should be considered to look for a metastatic polyradiculopathy. In those presenting with bulbar symptoms, a brain MRI should be performed to rule out stroke, tumor, and syringobulbia.

Although MRI is generally not performed to confirm a diag-

nosis of ALS, a few associated abnormalities have been reported. Rarely, spinal cord and motor cortex atrophy is apparent. Corticospinal tract hyperintensity with T2 imaging has been observed in a few younger patients with a predominance of UMN signs (35).

Laboratory Evaluation and Other Diagnostic Tests

In most neuromuscular clinics, a routine panel of laboratory tests is performed for all patients suspected of having ALS. A suggested set of such tests is provided in Table 35.2. The rationale behind performing this extensive battery of tests is to assess the general health of the patient and to exclude treatable conditions. The differential diagnosis, developed after the history and physical examination, may suggest that more specialized testing be performed. Table 35.3 suggests additional tests that may be warranted when the presentation is with either the PMA, the PLS, or the PBP phenotype. When there is a family history of MND, SOD1 testing should be performed.

PHARMACOLOGIC MANAGEMENT OF MOTOR NEURON DISEASE

Although there is not yet a cure for ALS, significant research advances are being made in an attempt to identify drugs and compounds that will slow disease progression. Although the findings thus far are not overly impressive, offering patients pharmacologic treatment of their disease has psychological benefits that may outweigh the actual slowing of disease progression that currently can be achieved. Offering the patient the opportunity to participate in clinical trials provides hope in the face of a seemingly desperate situation. Riluzole (Rilutek) is the only drug approved by the Food and Drug Administration (FDA) specifically for treatment of ALS. However, many neuromuscular ex-

TABLE 35.3. SPECIALIZED LABORATORY TESTING

Phenotype	Test	Diagnosis Excluded
PMA	DNA test—CAG repeat on X chromosome	SBMA
	DNA test—SMN gene mutation	SMA
	Hexosaminidase A	Hexosaminidase A deficiency (heterozygous Tay-Sachs disease)
	Voltage-gated Ca^{2+} channel antibody test	Lambert-Eaton myasthenic syndrome
	CSF examination	Polyradiculopathy—infectious or neoplastic
PLS	Very-long-chain fatty acids	Adrenoluekodystrophy
	HTLVI antibodies	HTLVI myelopathy (tropical spastic paraparesis)
	Parathyroid hormone	Hyperparathyroid myclopathy
	CSF examination	Multiple sclerosis
PBP	Acetyocholine receptor antibodies	Myasthenia gravis
	DNA test—CAG repeat on X chromosome	SBMA
	CSF examination	Multiple sclerosis

CSF, cerebrospinal fluid; PBP, primary bulbar palsy; PLS, primary lateral sclerosis; PMA, progressive muscular atrophy; SBMA, spinobulbar muscular atrophy; SMA, spinal muscular atrophy; SMN, survival motor neuron gene; HTLV1, human T–cell lymphotrophic viruses.

perts also recommend that their patients take a combination of antioxidant vitamins and creatine.

Riluzole inhibits the presynaptic release of glutamate and reduces neuronal damage in experimental models of ALS. It was approved by the FDA for treatment of ALS in 1995 after the completion of two clinical trials that showed that it slowed disease progression (57,58). Both of these studies showed prolonged tracheostomy-free survival for patients taking riluzole as opposed to placebo, although the benefit was modest. In the larger of the two studies, the relative increased probability of survival at 1 year for patients taking riluzole was 18%, and this benefit diminished after 15 months (58). Median survival benefit was 60 days. Unfortunately, no functional benefit was derived; strength declined at a similar rate in those taking riluzole and placebo.

The recommended dose of riluzole is 50 mg twice daily. It is generally well tolerated with the most common side effects being asthenia, nausea, diarrhea, and gastrointestinal upset. Elevation of hepatic enzymes is a more serious side effect. The alanine aminotransferase (ALT) level should be monitored monthly for the first 3 months and every 3 months thereafter. The drug should be discontinued if the ALT level reaches five times the upper limit of normal. Other serious, but rare, complications are renal tubular impairment and pancreatitis (59,60). The retail cost of riluzole is approximately $700 per month. Because of the marginal survival benefit provided by the drug, if either side effects or the cost has an adverse effect on the patient's quality of life, the drug should be discontinued. A practice advisory published by the American Academy of Neurology recommends that riluzole be prescribed for patients with ALS who are not ventilator dependent (61). There is no evidence of benefit in patients with tracheostomies who are ventilator dependent or in patients with more slowly progressing forms of MND such as SMA or postpolio syndrome.

Because oxidative stress is one of the proposed pathogenic factors in ALS, many physicians recommend a variety of antioxidants. Vitamin E, vitamin C, and coenzyme Q are the most frequently used. Other antioxidants sometimes prescribed are β-carotene and N-acetylcysteine. No double-blind placebo-controlled trials have been undertaken exploring the efficacy of these treatments, but they are generally believed to be nonharmful and are available without prescription. One small study of a cocktail of antioxidant compounds failed to demonstrate either efficacy or harm (62). If these compounds are prescribed, safe recommended daily dose ranges are 1,000 to 3,000 mg of vitamin C, 400 to 800 IU of vitamin E, 60 to 240 mg of coenzyme Q, 10,000 to 25,000 IU of β-carotene, and 100 to 200 mg of N-acetylcysteine.

Another over-the-counter compound taken by many patients with ALS and often recommended by their physicians is creatine. Creatine is an amino acid compound naturally found in skeletal muscle and other tissues. For years, it has been used as an ergogenic aid by athletes. It is part of the cellular energy buffering and transport system supplying adenosine triphosphate to muscle. Two recent studies have generated interest in using creatine to improve strength in patients with neuromuscular diseases. Creatine given to transgenic ALS mice improved motor performance, prolonged survival, and slowed loss of motor neurons (63). In another study that included patients with a variety of

neuropathic (including SMA and postpolio, but not ALS) and myopathic disorders, creatine supplementation improved muscle strength measured both isokinetically and isometrically (64). For patients with ALS who plan to use creatine supplementation on a long-term basis, a dose of 3 g per day will maximize muscle creatine concentration within 1 month and maintain the elevated concentration thereafter (65). The only serious adverse event reported to date is reversible renal dysfunction in an individual with pre-existing renal disease (66). Clinical trials of creatine are currently ongoing.

AMYOTROPHIC LATERAL SCLEROSIS CLINICAL TRIALS

During the last 5 years, the number of clinical drug trials for ALS has increased dramatically. Recent trials have tested a number of growth factors, glutamate antagonists, calcium channel blockers, and amino acids. At present, trials of neurotrophic factors, antioxidants, glutamate antagonists, and creatine are ongoing. In the future, a cocktail approach to slowing disease progression may be the ideal treatment strategy. Such a multidrug regimen might include one or more glutamate antagonists, possibly working on different glutamate receptors, one or more antioxidants, and multiple neurotrophic factors. However, no clinical trials have been performed yet to assess the synergy, or lack of synergy, of different categories of drugs.

Neurotrophic factors are naturally occurring polypeptides that enhance motor neuron survival *in vitro* and in animal models of ALS. Trials of subcutaneous ciliary neurotrophic factor (CNTF), brain-derived neurotrophic factor (BDNF), and intracerebroventricular glial-derived neurotrophic factor have all failed to demonstrate efficacy (67–69). The CNTF and BDNF trials may have failed because too little drug reached the motor neuron. To address this issue, trials of higher dose subcutaneous BDNF and intrathecal BDNF are being performed. The most successful neurotrophic factor tested to date has been insulin-like growth factor-I (IGF-I) (Myotrophin). Two large multicenter clinical trials were conducted, one in Europe and one in the United States. The American trial demonstrated a slightly slower decline in function in patients receiving the drug as opposed to placebo (70). However, the European trial did not demonstrate efficacy (71). Because of the discrepant results of these studies, the FDA has not approved IGF-I. Other neurotrophic compounds that may undergo clinical trials include synthetic compounds that mimic the activity of neurotrophins or stimulate their biosynthesis and a new class of small molecule neurotrophic factors called neuroimmunophilin ligands, which have the advantage of oral administration.

Because glutamate excitotoxicity is believed to play a crucial role in the pathogenesis of ALS, a number of clinical trials have been performed with glutamate antagonists. Riluzole, as discussed previously, reduces glutamate release from presynaptic nerve terminals and has been shown to slow disease progression. Gabapentin, a drug FDA approved for treatment of epilepsy, reduces glutamate activity by an unknown mechanism and has been prescribed to many patients with ALS for the last several years. A phase II trial demonstrated a nearly statistically significant decline in the rate of strength loss, which led many neuromuscular physicians to prescribe gabapentin to their patients because it was available outside of clinical trials (72). Although not yet published, a larger phase III trial was recently completed and failed to demonstrate any slowing of disease progression. Thus, most patients with ALS are now being withdrawn from gabapentin. Dextromethorphan is an *N*-methyl-D-aspartate glutamate receptor antagonist, which failed to slow disease progression in recent clinical trials (73, 74). Topiramate is another FDA-approved antiepileptic drug that reduces glutamate levels in the brain; it is currently undergoing clinical trials for ALS. Because glutamate-induced excitotoxicity produces a rise in the cytosolic calcium concentration, calcium channel blockers have been explored as drugs to slow disease progression. Unfortunately, neither verapamil nor nimodipine demonstrated any efficacy (75,76). Branched-chain amino acids (BCAAs) activate glutamate dehydrogenase, which in turn reduces plasma glutamate levels. This action of BCAAs suggested that they might slow disease progression; however, clinical trials have been negative (77). Other compounds with glutamate antagonist properties are being developed and may soon be available for clinical trials.

Free radical scavengers and antioxidants are candidates for ALS clinical trials because of the suspected role of oxidative stress in disease pathogenesis. Few trials of these compounds have been completed, but a number are in the preclinical investigatory stage. Selegiline, a monoamine oxidase B inhibitor with antioxidant properties, has failed to demonstrate clinical efficacy (78).

Both the Muscular Dystrophy Association (*www.mdausa. org*) and the Amyotrophic Lateral Sclerosis Association (www.al-sa.org) maintain updated websites providing information on drug development and clinical trials. These sites are excellent resources for patients interested in enrolling in a clinical trial. Between the two sites, most active trials and the study sites enrolling patients are listed.

REHABILITATION AND PALLIATIVE CARE

At present, *incurable,* adult MNDs are not completely *untreatable.* The goals of rehabilitation and palliative care for these patients are to maximize functional capacities, prolong or maintain independent function and locomotion, inhibit or prevent physical deformity, and to provide access to full community integration for good quality of life. In ALS, this also includes addressing end of life issues and ensuring that the patient has a comfortable death.

The comprehensive management of all of the varied clinical problems associated with adult MNDs is an arduous task. For this reason, the multidisciplinary approach is much more effective and takes advantage of the expertise of many clinicians, rather than placing the burden on one. Management is best carried out by a team consisting of physicians, physical, occupational and speech therapists, social workers, vocational counselors, and psychologists, among others. Ideally, due to the significant mobility problems associated with these diseases, the physician and all the key clinic personnel should be available at each visit. Tertiary care medical centers in larger urban areas can usually provide this type of service. This may be an independent

clinic or sponsored by one or more of the consumer-driven organizations sponsoring research and clinical care for people with MNDs, including the Muscular Dystrophy Association or the Amyotrophic Lateral Sclerosis Association.

The rehabilitative and palliative care strategies discussed in this section may be applied to any form of adult MND, but the focus of this discussion is primarily on ALS.

Initial Rehabilitation Clinical Evaluation

Initial confirmation of the diagnosis is critical and is a primary responsibility of the consulting neurologist. Due to the ominous prognosis of ALS, a confirmatory second opinion should always be sought. A *physiatrist* is well suited to direct the rehabilitation team and oversee a comprehensive, goal-oriented treatment plan (79,80). Irrespective, a single *primary physician* who coordinates all rehabilitative care should be identified early in the process, either a specialist or the family physician if he or she is willing and knowledgeable of the disease.

At initial evaluation, the patient should be thoroughly educated about the expected outcome and the problems that may be encountered. Enrollment in an experimental drug trial, as discussed previously in this chapter, should be encouraged and facilitated. It not only furthers science but also provides some hope for the patient and ensures frequent follow-up. The physician should then assess the patient's goals and orchestrate a rehabilitative and ultimately a palliative program that matches those goals. In ALS, palliative care should be aimed at maximizing a patient's comfort and quality of life, not necessarily extending their life.

Spectrum of Clinical Problems and Treatment Paradigms

Weakness and Fatigue

Skeletal muscle weakness is the *sine qua non* of all adult MND, including ALS, and is the ultimate cause of most clinical problems associated with these diseases. There have been no well-controlled studies looking at exercise-induced strength gains in this population. However, in slowly progressive neuromuscular diseases, a 12-week moderate-resistance (30% of maximum isometric force) exercise program resulted in strength gains ranging from 4% to 20% without any notable deleterious effects (81). Nonetheless, in the same population, a 12-week high-resistance (training at the maximum weight a subject could lift 12 times) exercise program showed no further added beneficial effect compared with the moderate resistance program and there was evidence of overwork weakness in some of the subjects (82). However, due to the active ongoing muscle degeneration in most cases of ALS, and to a lesser extent in SMA and SBMA, the risk for overwork weakness is great and exercise should be prescribed cautiously and with a common sense approach. Patients should be advised not to exercise to exhaustion, which can produce more muscle damage and dysfunction (83). Patients participating in an exercise program should be cautioned of the warning signs of overwork weakness, which includes feeling weaker rather than stronger within 30 minutes after exercising or excessive muscle soreness 24 to 48 hours after exercising. Other warning signs include severe muscle cramping, heaviness in the extremities, and prolonged shortness of breath (83).

Early intervention with gentle, low-impact aerobic exercise such as walking, swimming/pool exercise, and stationary bicycling will improve cardiovascular performance, increase muscle efficiency, and thus help fight fatigue (84,85). Fatigue in ALS is multifactorial and is due in part to impaired muscular activation (39,86). Other contributing factors include generalized deconditioning from immobility and clinical depression (85). Aerobic exercise not only improves physical functioning but is beneficial in fighting depression and improving pain tolerance.

Restrictive Lung Disease (RLD)

The terminal event in ALS is usually directly related to respiratory failure. RLD usually develops in ALS but may also be present in SMA and SBMA. Although the term RLD is frequently used, this is not *lung disease* per se, but is due to weakness of the diaphragm, chest wall, and abdominal musculature (87). Weakness in the bulbar musculature, which can lead to aspiration, confounds the problem in ALS and SBMA. Patients should be educated early in the disease process so they can make informed decisions down the line (87,88). Routine pulmonary function tests, including forced vital capacity (FVC) and maximal inspiratory and expiratory pressures, should be monitored closely. Dysphagia symptoms closely parallel vital capacity and significantly complicate the clinical course (89,90).

Ultimately, most patients develop hypoventilation, which leads to elevated CO_2 levels (87). Measuring only O_2 saturation levels with pulse oximetry may be inadequate. End-tidal CO_2 levels should be measured periodically, depending on the clinical condition of the patient. Arterial blood gas evaluations are usually not necessary and will not add any needed information. A thorough review of systems will help define any problems. Patients who are hypoventilating will often become hypercapnic and hypoxic at night and complain of a morning headache, restlessness or nightmares, and poor-quality sleep. This may cause daytime somnolence. Insufficient respiration with hypoxia may occur later, particularly if the lungs are damaged by chronic aspiration.

Options for noninvasive interventions include a pneumobelt, which provides diaphragmatic support, or a chest cuirass, which mechanically inflates the lung by creating negative chest wall pressure. Although effective, these devices are cumbersome and may be poorly tolerated (87,88). Bach (89) showed significant success with the use of 24-hour noninvasive positive pressure ventilation (PPV) by mouth. Although it may not prolong survival, this type of ventilation avoids the need for tracheostomy and maintains reasonable quality of life. Noninvasive PPV can be done easily in the home and should be considered the preferred modality of assisted ventilation in ALS. Bimodal positive airway pressure is usually the preferred form of noninvasive PPV in ALS. It can be used via a mouthpiece with or without a lip seal, a nasal mask, or via a full facemask. Patients may benefit initially from using noninvasive PPV mainly at night. In patients who choose to use noninvasive PPV, we recommend starting this when the FVC drops to less than 50%, so they have time to adjust to and accommodate the equipment. In patients with

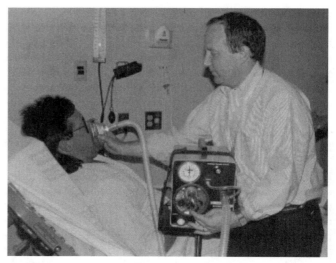

FIGURE 35.3. Photograph demonstrating the use of an In-Exsufflator (JH Emerson Co, Cambridge, MA) to help generate a forceful cough and clear secretions.

severe bulbar dysfunction, noninvasive PPV will not be effective and tracheostomy becomes the only option.

There are various methods of improving respiratory hygiene that may also help the patient with ALS, including devices that produce an artificial cough via a facemask by rapidly going from a positive to a negative airway pressure to bring up secretions (88). This technique has been around since the polio epidemics more than 40 years ago and is now available through several commercial names, including the Cofflator (Respironics, Pittsburgh, PA) or the In-Exsufflator (JH Emerson Co, Cambridge, MA). Figure 35.3 illustrates the use of one of these devices.

If better airway access becomes absolutely necessary and the informed patient wishes more aggressive care, a tracheostomy is then considered. In most centers, only very few patients elect to have a tracheostomy. A laryngeal diversion (laryngotracheal separation) is an alternative procedure wherein the proximal trachea is either oversewn or hooked side on end into the esophagus and the distal trachea is brought out through a stoma in the neck. This procedure has the advantage of completely preventing aspiration, although phonation will no longer be possible (91).

Dysphagia/Dysarthria

Clinical signs and symptoms of dysphagia and dysarthria may closely parallel one another (91). Early signs include changes in voice patterns (voice becoming hoarse) and persistent coughing after swallowing liquids, which can indicate microaspiration. A speech therapist should be consulted early for clinical swallowing evaluations and recommendations on dietary modification such as thickening liquids and preparing food that forms into a bolus easily will help. A modified barium swallow or fiberoptic endoscopic examination of swallowing safety is helpful for accurately determining the presence of aspiration and defining which food textures the patient can safely swallow (92). Cricopharyngeal myotomy may be helpful if dysfunction in this muscle is demonstrated, although this procedure is not likely to be successful if used empirically (85). Placement of a percutaneous endoscopic gastrostomy (PEG) tube may prolong survival and should be strongly considered when the patient loses more than 10% of his or her baseline body weight or is taking longer than 1 hour to eat a meal. It is best to have the PEG tube placed before the patient becomes malnourished or has her FVC drop to less than 50% of the predicted value, because it will be considerably easier for the surgeon to perform the procedure. Patients should be reassured that they will still be able to eat food orally for enjoyment, provided that their caregivers have had some training to manage episodes of choking. Nonetheless, using the PEG tube as the primary route of nutritional intake will ensure adequate fluids and nourishment. Some patients may decline a PEG tube. This choice is left up to the patient, but they must be fully informed that at some point, they may be unable to swallow anything. At that time, PEG placement may be impossible or at the very least technically difficult and involve intubating the patient to facilitate ventilation during the procedure. Thus, it is not really an option to wait until they cannot swallow and then change their mind. Because the gastrointestinal tract generally maintains adequate function in ALS, parenteral hydration and feeding is not necessary and is associated with high nursing needs, cost, and some degree of medical comorbidity. It should not be discussed as a viable option. The patient who can no longer swallow and does not have a feeding tube will eventually die from dehydration and malnutrition. Some patients do elect this route and they can be made comfortable.

Dysarthria in ALS does not respond well to conventional articulation training. However, some adaptive strategies such as maintaining a slow speaking rate with an emphasis on increasing the precision of speech production may be helpful and can be taught by a speech-language pathologist (85,93). As the disease progresses, dysarthria should be approached by prescribing communicative aids, rather than traditional ongoing speech therapy. An alphabet supplementation or word board works well early when patients still have reasonable arm function. After that, developing yes and no or other binary commands with eye-gaze systems may be useful, particularly if the patient is using mechanical ventilation. There have been major recent advancements made in devices such as speech synthesizers or multipurpose, multiaccess, computer-based augmentative communication systems. Although expensive, these devices greatly enhance patients' ability to communicate when they can no longer phonate. These types of devices may often be borrowed or rented from Assistive Technology Centers, which are often found at tertiary care medical centers.

Patients with ALS and bulbar symptoms also usually have difficulty controlling and swallowing the amounts of saliva that are normally present in the oral cavity. Drugs with strong anticholinergic effect, such as benztropine (Cogentin), trihexyphenidyl (Artane), or some of the tricyclic antidepressants (amitriptyline and imipramine), are very effective at drying up secretions. If severe, a transtympanic neurectomy, which blocks the parasympathetic innervation of the salivary glands, or Stenson duct ligation may be tried, but these procedures have met with limited success. Radiation to the salivary glands may also be helpful, although problematic complications are common (85).

Spasticity

Spasticity in ALS is probably induced both at the motor cortex and at the spinal cord level. The γ-aminobutyric acid (GABA) analogue baclofen acts to facilitate motor neuron inhibition at spinal levels and is the agent of choice. Initial doses are 5 to 10 mg twice to three times a day, titrating up to doses of 20 mg four times a day. Occasionally, higher doses (up to 160 mg per day) are more effective but caution is advised. Side effects include weakness, fatigue, and sedation. An intrathecal baclofen pump may be beneficial to some patients with PLS. A new agent tizanidine, an α_2-agonist similar to clonidine, inhibits excitatory interneurons and may also be helpful. Dosing range is 4 to 8 mg three to four times a day, with a similar side effect profile to that of baclofen. Benzodiazepines may also be helpful but can cause respiratory depression and somnolence. Dantrolene, by blocking Ca^{2+} release in the sarcoplasmic reticulum, is effective at reducing muscle tone but will also cause generalized muscle weakness and is not recommended. Slow (30-second sustained), static muscle stretching may be helpful, particularly in the more symptomatic muscle groups such as the gastrocnemius, and may be done in bed. Positional splinting is also a helpful adjunctive modality, but skin must be monitored frequently for pressure areas.

Depression

Reactive clinical depression is expected in ALS (94). Good family, social, and religious support systems, as well as participation in support groups, are all helpful (94–96). Once the diagnosis is confirmed, patients should be counseled with respect to the prognosis. This allows time for grieving, anger, and ultimately acceptance of their fate and is important for the mental well being of the patients and their family (95). Antidepressant medicine should be offered to every patient because it may provide assistance with mood elevation, appetite stimulation, and sleep. As previously mentioned, serotonin mediated tricyclic antidepressants with significant anticholinergic activity will also help dry up oral secretions and minimize drooling. Further, they may help control the symptoms of pseudobulbar affect in ALS. Amitriptyline, starting at a dose of 25 mg 1 hour before bed, is a good choice. Families of patients with ALS with emotional lability should be reassured that the underlying mood state may be normal. Rather, it is their emotional expression that is abnormal. Nonetheless, referral to a psychiatrist or clinical psychologist with experience in treating depression associated with terminal disease may be required. Depression in the spouse, significant other, family, or friends should not be overlooked, and group/family counseling may be helpful.

Pain and Immobility

Although not frequently characterized as a major component of ALS, most of these patients do experience significant pain. The pain is due largely to immobility, which can cause adhesive capsulitis, mechanical back pain, pressure areas on the skin, and more rarely neuropathic pain (85). Frequently, severe weakness in the neck flexors and extensors will cause a "floppy head" associated with severe neck pain and tightness. This may be helped by a hard cervical (Philadelphia type) or a Freeman- or

Headmaster-type collar, which is a wire-frame collar with padding over the pressure points.

Wheelchairs should have adequate lumbar support and good cushioning (gel foam). The chair should be properly fitted to avoid pressure ulcers and inadequate support for the spine. Simply giving the patient a prescription for a wheelchair often ends up with the patient getting a standard manual chair that does not fit properly. A power wheelchair, although expensive, can be justified because it will help prolong independent mobility and thus markedly improve quality of life (96).

A good pressure-relieving mattress (air or dense foam) should be used on the bed at home, along with foam wedges to facilitate proper positioning. This will help prevent pressure ulcers and contractures. Daily passive and active-assisted range of motion is critical. Maintaining mobility and functional independence as long as possible will have positive physical and psychological benefits. Ankle-foot orthoses molded in the neutral position may prolong ambulation and avoid injury if there is unilateral or bilateral footdrop. Wheeled walkers (Gran Tour in particular) or quad (four-point) canes may also help, depending on the pattern of weakness. Other useful equipment includes handheld showers, bathtub benches, grab bars, raised toilet seat, hospital bed, commode chair, aids in activities of daily living (e.g., sock aid and grabbers), and wheelchair ramps. An occupational therapist will help define which, if any, of these devices will be useful to the patient. Other simple suggestions such as moving the patient's bedroom to the first floor, removing any loose rugs, or covering slippery floors are helpful and can be done during an in-home evaluation by the therapist.

Pharmacologic management of pain in ALS includes the use of nonsteroidal antiinflammatory drugs (NSAIDs), particularly if there is evidence of an active inflammatory process such as tenosynovitis or arthritis. Regular dosing of acetaminophen (1,000 mg every 6 hours) may be used along with an NSAID or alone if NSAIDs are not tolerated. Tricyclic antidepressants and antiepileptic drugs such as gabapentin (Neurontin) can sometimes be helpful for pain, particularly if there is a neuropathic component. Gabapentin also has the added benefit of some antispasticity properties. Narcotic medicine should be reserved for refractory pain. Concern for narcotic addiction is pointless in patients with a terminal disease and the medications should be given on a regular dosing schedule and titrated to the point of comfort (97). Concomitant use of the antiemetic, antihistamine hydroxyzine (Vistaril), given along with the narcotic, will enhance the effectiveness (i.e., 30 mg codeine plus 50 mg hydroxyzine every 6 waking hours). Unlike narcotic medications, hydroxyzine is not a cortical depressant but does have direct skeletal muscle relaxant and analgesic properties and is known to potentiate the analgesic effect of narcotic medication, although the exact mechanism is unknown (97). Combination elixirs can be prepared by the pharmacy for ease of administration. Oral or sublingual morphine (Roxanol) (10 to 30 mg every 4 hours) is also effective for comfort care and may also help relieve "air hunger" in the terminal stages of the disease. Another option is taking the total dose of immediate-release morphine required to alleviate pain and giving half of that every 12 hours in a controlled-release preparation such as MS Contin. Intramuscular delivery route should be avoided due to muscle wasting.

Fentanyl or morphine patches may deliver inconsistent dosing, particularly if there is excessive perspiration. A patient-controlled analgesic pump mechanism may not work in advanced stages of ALS due to the inability of the patient to control the delivery. The main problems with narcotic medication in ALS are respiratory depression and constipation. These side effects may be quite acceptable in the final phases of life when respiratory insufficiency or severe pain requires increased doses of morphine and lorazepam. Patients and caregivers should be made aware of these issues.

Autonomic Dysfunction

Although dysautonomia is not generally a predominant feature of ALS, it can cause some unique clinical problems. Patients may complain of feeling quite hot, along with problems of esophageal and gastric motility and cardiac arrhythmias (98). This can cause problems when patients are exercising, particularly if they become overheated and dehydrated. Recommendations include dressing in fabric that wicks away perspiration, such as polypropylene; eating several small meals a day, or if a PEG is being used, switching from bolus feeds to a continuous drip, along with plenty of fluid; and taking care not to exercise to exhaustion.

Incontinence

Although ALS primarily causes denervation of striated skeletal muscle, it may also involve anal and urinary sphincters (99). Despite this, incontinence is usually not a significant clinical problem in ALS. When incontinence is a problem, it is usually due to immobility and difficulty getting to the toilet in time, rather than lack of sphincter control. Patients should avoid drinking large amounts of fluids after dinner to avoid nighttime incontinence. Men may wear a condom catheter at night. Absorbent undergarments may also be used, but skin should be monitored closely for maceration and protected with topically applied moisture-repelling agents. Sympathomimetic agents such as pseudoephedrine (30 to 60 mg up to four times a day) may help increase urinary outlet sphincter tone. However, this may also increase blood pressure and could induce urinary retention, particularly if used in conjunction with anticholinergic agents in men with prostatic enlargement. An indwelling Foley or suprapubic catheter is a reasonable choice later in the course of the disease when mobility problems become significant. Bowels are best regulated by a routine protocol on a time-based regimen (e.g., every morning). Fiber/bulk agents should be given routinely, along with fluids. Suppositories and mini enemas may be used as needed.

Dementia

Dementia is rare in ALS but may be present in later stages of the disease, particularly if there are some overlap symptoms of Parkinsonism. This may cause safety issues requiring 24-hour supervision for the patient.

End of Life Issues

ALS is a disease that poses some unusual ethical and humanitarian considerations. Although it is considered a fatal condition, unlike most cancers or other grave, incurable illnesses, it may take years to die from it, even though the disease continues to debilitate the person in the process. Thus, the patient with ALS has much time to think about the inevitability of the disease and what choices to make in the terminal stages of the disease.

Despite the most aggressive treatment available, ALS will progress. Early in the disease, a social worker should be consulted to help arrange durable power of attorney to a responsible family member, usually the spouse. In most states, this can be done by a paralegal for a nominal fee. A living will should then be drafted, which clearly outlines the patient's wishes regarding extent of medical intervention desired (100). This is particularly important with respect to entering hospice level care. Presumably by the time hospice level care is being considered, patients have had ample time for grieving, anger, and ultimately acceptance of their fate. However, in our experience, many patients with ALS still are hesitant about going into hospice because it implies that the disease has reached *end stage* (101).

The patient should also be referred to a support group. The most prominent consumer-driven organizations facilitating support groups for people with ALS are the Muscular Dystrophy Association and the Amyotrophic Lateral Sclerosis Association. Local branches may be contacted to locate the nearest ALS support group. Support groups are often a great resource, not only for psychological support but also for problem solving and equipment recycling of items such as hospital beds.

Most of this section of this chapter has centered around *comprehensive clinical care* of the patient with adult-onset MND, emphasizing "everything that modern medicine has to offer." The physician must consider that the patient with advanced ALS may not want all of this, which is not necessarily a wrong decision. *Life-sustaining therapy,* defined as any artificial device or intervention that compensates for the failure of an organ system that would normally result in death, is the patient's choice, not the physician's (101–104). The most obvious example of this would be mechanical ventilation, but this also includes artificial hydration and nutrition. Legally and ethically speaking, a mentally competent patient can refuse any prescribed treatment. It is the physician's responsibility to ensure that the patient understands the consequences of this. The physician should always respect and foster the patient's autonomy and self-direction with respect to these types of interventions. This does not extend to the point of physician-assisted suicide, in which the physician takes active steps to end the patient's life. This is an illegal act that carries grievous ethical concerns that are beyond the scope of this chapter. Despite this, a recent study documented that approximately 56% of patients with ALS surveyed in Washington and Oregon states would consider assisted suicide (102). As of October 1997, the Oregon Death with Dignity Act legalizes physician-assisted suicide in that state, although the actual impact of that bill on the care of patients with ALS has not yet been reported. Nonetheless, this stunningly high percentage of patients with ALS who would consider this strongly implies that the quality of care in advanced ALS is inadequate. If the patient is requesting this, then the physician should reassess the situation, making sure that everything has been done to maximize patient comfort and quality of life.

Further, quality of life studies have identified a lack of ade-

quate communication between physician and patient and a poor perception (both positive and negative) on the part of physician of the level of quality of life in these patients (96). It takes a great deal of time to explain all of the *end of life* issues, including the available treatment options and choices. Without this investment of time on the clinician's part, the patient is unaware of the services that may be available to ease his or her suffering.

The most appropriate level of care for patients with ALS may change frequently and these patients should be followed closely. Unfortunately, patients with advanced ALS are often told "there is nothing that can be done," when in fact optimizing in-home care with hospice can maximize quality of life for these patients and provide for a comfortable, painless passing. Krivickas et al. (105) documented that most patients with ALS probably do not receive enough in-home care. Of 98 patients with advanced ALS studied, only 9 received hospice home care, 24 received nonhospice home care, and 7 both hospice and nonhospice home care. The remaining 58 patients received no in-home care at all. Even among those having home care assistance, primary nonmedical ALS primary caregivers spent an average of 11 hours per day caring for patients. Among ALS primary caregivers studied, 42% and 48% felt physically and psychologically unwell, respectively. The authors concluded that home and hospice care received by patients with ALS is inadequate because it starts too late to relieve the burden placed on family caregivers. Because the focus of care in hospice is the family, however defined by the patient, this problem could be easily resolved. Hospice provides an interdisciplinary team of professionals whose mission is to support the patient and the family through their remaining days together. Support is given for physical, psychological, emotional, and spiritual needs of the family unit in the home setting, bypassing the need for laborious trips to clinics.

The National Hospice Organization does have some guidelines for entry of patients with ALS into hospice (Table 35.4), which are somewhat arduous but would allow for early entry into hospice of most patients with ALS in the advanced stages of the disease (106). These guidelines require physicians to make some estimate of life expectancy, which is very difficult to do in ALS and is something for which most physicians are probably ill prepared. Compared with patients with terminal cancer, patients with ALS have a relatively slow progression in respect to the actual dying process, which decreases the clinician's awareness that hospice care may be appropriate. Most clinicians likely perceive that hospice is for "near terminal" patients, which is correct, except that patients with ALS may be in that state for a prolonged period. During this time, hospice care could ease suffering considerably. Lack of physician knowledge of the services provided by hospice is widespread (107). Physicians not familiar with the care of terminal patients may not be comfortable with the aggressive use of opiates and benzodiazepines advocated by hospice clinicians for the control of symptoms in ALS. The physician may find it difficult to give *carte blanche* orders for effective titration of these types of medications, which will ease air hunger and anxiety in the patient with end-stage ALS.

Irrespective, in the final stages of the disease, it is medically appropriate to involve a home hospice team. Regular home visits by hospice nurses will ensure proper medication delivery, pain control, and skin and bowel care, as well as provide the physician

TABLE 35.4. CRITERIA FOR HOSPICE ADMISSION IN AMYOTROPHIC LATERAL SCLEROSIS

Hospice is appropriate when there has been an overall rapid progression of amyotrophic lateral sclerosis (a critical factor), e.g., disability has progressed significantly in the past 12 mo. The patient or family desires no further aggressive treatment or cardiopulmonary recuscitation.

In addition, at least one of the following must also apply:

1. Increased respiratory distress
   a. vital capacity of less than 30% of predicted
   b. significant dyspnea at rest
   c. supplemental oxygen required at rest
   d. patient has refused intubation, tracheostomy, and mechanical ventilation
2. Severely impaired nutrition
   a. tube feeding not elected or discontinued
   b. oral intake insufficient/dysphagia
   c. continued weight loss in spite of tube feedings
   d. dehydration or hypovolemia
3. Life threatening complications
   a. recurrent aspiration pneumonia
   b. decubitus ulcers, multiple, stage 3-4, particularly if infected
   c. upper urinary tract infection, e.g., pyelonephritis
   d. sepsis
   e. fever recurrent after antibiotics

with a progress report without having to bring the patient to the clinic. They can also provide counseling to avoid panic calls to 911 by family members and unnecessary nighttime visits to the emergency department. Most patients wish to die at home, and in most cases with a supportive family and the help of hospice, this is a feasible and worthwhile goal.

An informed patient and family will welcome the comprehensive level of terminal care that hospice offers, consoled with the knowledge that dying with dignity in the serenity and security of one's own home is, in some modest but meaningful way, a measure of victory over this otherwise insufferable illness. Finally, we urge clinicians to attend memorial services because it is a healing and rewarding experience.

ACKNOWLEDGMENT

Supported by Research and Training Center grant no. HB133B980008 from the National Institute on Disability and Rehabilitation Research, Washington, DC, USA.

REFERENCES

1. Rowland LP. What's in a name? Amyotrophic lateral sclerosis, motor neuron disease, and allelic heterogeneity. *Ann Neurol* 1998;43:691–694.
2. Mulder DW. The clinical syndrome of amyotrophic lateral sclerosis. *Proc Staff Meet Mayo Clin* 1957;32:427.
3. Stark FM, Moershc FP. Primary lateral sclerosis: a distinct clinical entity. *J Nerv Ment Dis* 1945;102:332.
4. Kennedy WR, Alter M, Sung JH. Progressive proximal spinal and bulbar muscular atrophy of late onset: and X-linked, recessive trait. *Neurology* 1968;18:671.
5. Siddique T, Deng H. Genetics of amyotrophic lateral sclerosis. *Hum Mol Genetics* 1996;5 Spec No:1465–1470.
6. Lyons TJ, Liu H, Goto JJ, et al. Mutations in copper-zinc superoxide dismutase that cause amyotrophic lateral sclerosis alter the zinc binding site and the redux behavior of the protein. *Proc Natl Acad Sci* 1996;93(22):12240–12244.
7. Hosler BA, Brown RH. Copper/zinc superoxide dismutase mutations and free radical damage in amyotrophic lateral sclerosis. *Adv Neurol* 1995;680:41–46.
8. Plaitakis A, Constantakakis E. Altered metabolism of excitatory amino acids, N-acetyl-aspartate-glutamate in amyotrophic lateral sclerosis. *Brain Res Bull* 1993;30:381–386.
9. Canu W, Billiard M, Baldy-Mouliner M. Fasting plasma and CSF amino acid levels in ALS. *Acta Neurol Scand* 1993;88(1):51–55.
10. Rothstein JD, Martin IJ, Kuncl RW. Decreased glutamate transport by the brain and spinal cord in amyotrophic lateral sclerosis. *N Engl J Med* 1992;326:1464–1468.
11. Rothstein JD, Van Kammen M, Levey AL, et al. Selective loss of glial glutamate transporter GLT-1 in amyotrophic lateral sclerosis. *Ann Neurol* 1995;38:73–84.
12. Norris F, Sheperd R, Denys E, et al. Onset, natural history and outcome in idiopathic adult motor neuron disease. *J Neurol Sci* 1993;118(1):48–55.
13. Pradas J, Finison L, Andres PL, et al. The natural history of amyotrophic lateral sclerosis and the use of natural history controls in therapeutic trials. *Neurology* 1993;43(4):751–755.
14. Ringel SP, Murphy JR, Alderson MK, et al. The natural history of amyotrophic lateral sclerosis. *Neurology* 1993;43(7):1316–1322.
15. Chancellor AM, Warlow CP. Adult onset motor neuron disease: worldwide mortality, incidence, and distribution since 1950. *J Neurol Neurosurg Psychiatry* 1992;55(12):1106–1115.
16. Neilson S, Robinson I, Alperovitch A. Rising amyotrophic lateral sclerosis mortality in France 1968–1990: increased life expectancy and inter-disease competition as an explanation. *J Neurol* 1994;241(7):448–455.
17. Neilson S, Robinson I, Nymoen EH. Longitudinal analysis of amyotrophic lateral sclerosis mortality in Norway, 1966–1989: evidence for a susceptible subpopulation. *J Neurol Sci* 1994;122(2):148–154.
18. Eisen A. Amyotrophic lateral sclerosis is a multifactorial disease. *Muscle Nerve* 1995;18(7):741–752.
19. Eisen A, Schulzer M, MacNeil M, et al. Duration of amyotrophic lateral sclerosis is age dependent. *Muscle Nerve* 1993;16:27–32.
20. Nelson LM, McGuire V, Longstreth WT Jr, et al. Population-based case-control study of amyotrophic lateral sclerosis in western Washington State. I. Cigarette smoking and alcohol consumption. *Am J Epidemiol* 2000;15;151(2):156–163.
21. Nelson LM, Matkin C, Longstreth WT Jr, et al. Population-based case-control study of amyotrophic lateral sclerosis in western Washington State. II. Diet. *Am J Epidemiol* 2000;15;151(2):164–173.
22. Strand EA, Miller RM, Yorkston KM, et al. Management of oral-pharyngeal dysphagia symptoms in amyotrophic lateral sclerosis. *Dysphagia* 1996;11:129–139.
23. Tysnes OB, Vollset SE, Larsen JP, et al. Prognostic factors and survival in amyotrophic lateral sclerosis. *Neuroepidemiology* 1994;13(5):226–235.
24. Stubgen J-P. Neuromuscular disorders in systemic malignancy and its treatment. *Muscle Nerve* 1995;18:636–648.
25. Carter GT, Fritz RC. Pancreatic adenocarcinoma presenting as a monomelic motor neuronopathy. *Muscle Nerve* 1997;20:103–105.
26. Rosenfeld MR, Posner JB. Paraneoplastic motor neuron disease. *Adv Neurol* 1991;56:445–459.
27. Carter GT, Abresch RT, Fowler WM, et al. Profiles of neuromuscular disease: spinal muscular atrophy. *Am J Phys Med Rehabil* 1995;74(5):S150–S159.
28. Fishbeck KH, Ionasecu V, Ritter AW. Localization of the gene for X-linked spinal muscular atrophy. *Neurology* 1986;36:1595
29. MacKenzie AE, Jacob P, Surh L, et al. Genetic heterogeneity in spinal muscular atrophy: a linkage analysis-based assessment. *Neurology* 1994;44:919–924.
30. Amato AA, Prior TW, Barohn RJ, et al. Kennedy's disease: a clinico-

pathologic correlation with mutations in the androgen receptor gene. *Neurology* 1993;43(4):791–794.

31. Carter GT, Bonekat HW, Milio L. Successful pregnancies in the presence of spinal muscular atrophy: two case reports. *Arch Phys Med Rehabil* 1994;75(2):229–231.

32. Moulard B, Salachas F, Chassande B, et al. Association between centromeric deletions of the SMN gene and sporadic adult-onset lower motor neuron disease. *Ann Neurol* 1998;43:640–644.

33. Parboosingh JS, Meininger V, McKenna-Yasek D, et al. Deletions causing spinal muscular atrophy do not predispose to amyotrophic lateral sclerosis. *Arch Neurol* 1999;56:710–712.

34. Parboosingh JS, Figlewicz DA, Krizus A, et al. Spinobulbar muscular atrophy can mimic ALS: the importance of genetic testing in male patients with atypical ALS. *Neurology* 1997;49:568–572.

35. Mitsumoto H, Chad DA, Pioro EP. *Amyotrophic lateral sclerosis.* Philadelphia: FA Davis Co, 1998.

36. Norris F, Shepherd R, Denys E, et al. Onset, natural history, and outcome in idiopathic adult motor neuron disease. *J Neurol Sci* 1993; 118:48–55.

37. Okuda B, Kodama N, Kowabata K, et al. Corneomandibular reflex in ALS. *Neurology* 1999;52: 1699–1701.

38. Kasarskis EJ, Berryman S, Vanderleest JG, et al. Nutritional status of patients with amyotrophic lateral sclerosis: relation to the proximity of death. *Am J Clin Nutri* 1996;63:130–137.

39. Sharma KR, Miller RG. Electrical and mechanical properties of skeletal muscle underlying increased fatigue in patients with amyotrophic lateral sclerosis. *Muscle Nerve* 1996;19:1391–1400.

40. Kothari MJ, Rutkove SB, Logigian EL, et al. Coexistent entrapment neuropathies in patients with amyotrophic lateral sclerosis. *Arch Phys Med Rehabil* 1996;77:1186–1188.

41. Brooks B. El Escorial World Federation of Neurology criteria for the diagnosis of amyotrophic lateral sclerosis. Subcommittee on Motor Neuron Diseases/Amyotrophic Lateral Sclerosis of the World Federation of Neurology Research Group on Neuromuscular Diseases and the El Escorial Clinical Limit of Amyotrophic Lateral Sclerosis Workshop Contributors. *J Neurol Sci* 1994;124:96–107.

42. World Federation of Neurology Research Group on Motor Neuron Diseases. *El Escorial revisited: revised criteria for the diagnosis of amyotrophic lateral sclerosis.* World Federation of Neurology Research Group on Motor Neuron Diseases, 1998.

43. Dumitru D. Central nervous system disorders. In: Dumitru D, ed. *Electrodiagnostic medicine.* Philadelphia: Hanley & Belfus, 1995: 453–462.

44. Hausmanowa-Petrusewicz I, Friedman A, Kowalski J, et al. Spontaneous motor unit firing in spinal muscular atrophy of childhood. *Electromyo Clin Neurophysiol* 1987;27:259–264.

45. Hausmanowa-Petrusewicz I, Karwanska A. Electromyographic findings in different forms of infantile and juvenile proximal spinal muscular atrophy. *Muscle Nerve* 1986;9:37–46.

46. Swift T. Commentary: electrophysiology of progressive spinal muscular atrophy. In: Gamstorp I, Sarnat H, eds. *Progressive spinal muscular atrophies.* New York: Raven Press, 1984:135–139.

47. Ferrante MA, Wilbourn AJ. The characteristic electrodiagnostic features of Kennedy's disease. *Muscle Nerve* 1997;20:323–329.

48. Meriggioli MN, Rowin J, Sanders DB, et al. Distinguishing clinical and electrodiagnostic features of x-linked bulbospinal neuronopathy. *Muscle Nerve* 1999;22:1693–1697.

49. Lambert E. Electromyography in amyotrophic lateral sclerosis. In: Norris F, Kurland L, eds. *Motor neuron disease.* New York: Grune & Stratton, 1969:135–153.

50. Lambert E, Mulder D. Electromyographic studies in amyotrophic lateral sclerosis. *Mayo Clin Proc* 1957;332:441–446.

51. Cornblath DR, Kuncl RW, Mellits ED, et al. Nerve conduction studies in amyotrophic lateral sclerosis. *Muscle Nerve* 1992;15(10): 1111–1115.

52. Dettmers C, Fatepour D, Faust H, et al. Sympathetic skin response abnormalities in amyotrophic lateral sclerosis. *Muscle Nerve* 1993;16: 930–934.

53. Ziemann U, Winter M, Reimers CD, et al. Impaired motor cortex inhibition in patients with amyotrophic lateral sclerosis. Evidence

from paired transcranial magnetic stimulation. *Neurology* 1998;49(5): 1292–1298.

54. de Carvalho MD, Miranda PC, Luis ML, et al. Cortical muscle representation in amyotrophic lateral sclerosis patients: changes with disease evolution. *Muscle Nerve* 1999;22:1684–1692.

55. Schulte-Mattler WJ, Muller T, Zierz S, et al. Transcranial magnetic stimulation compared with upper motor neuron signs in patients with amyotrophic lateral sclerosis. *J Neurol Sci* 1999;170:51–56.

56. Desiato MT, Palmieri MG, Giacomini P, et al. The effect of riluzole in amyotrophic lateral sclerosis: a study with cortical stimulation. *J Neurol Sci* 1999;169:98–107.

57. Bensimon G, Lacomblez L, Meininger V, et al. A controlled trial of riluzole in amyotrophic lateral sclerosis. *N Engl J Med* 1994;330: 585–591.

58. Lacomblez L, Bensimon G, Leigh PN, et al. Dose-ranging study of riluzole in amyotrophic lateral sclerosis. *Lancet* 1996;347:1425–1431.

59. Poloni TE, Alimonti D, Montagna G, et al. Renal tubular impairment during riluzole therapy. *Neurology* 1999;52:670.

60. Drory VE, Sidi I, Korczyn AD, et al. Riluzole-induced pancreatitis. *Neurology* 1999;52:892–893.

61. Practice advisory on the treatment of amyotrophic lateral sclerosis with riluzole. *Neurology* 1997;49:657–659.

62. Vyth A, Timmer JG, Bossuyt PM, et al. Survival in patients with amyotrophic lateral sclerosis treated with an array of antioxidants. *J Neurol Sci* 1996;139[Suppl]:99–103.

63. Klivenyi P, Ferrante RJ, Matthews RT, et al. Neuroprotective effects of creatine in a transgenic animal model of amyotrophic lateral sclerosis. *Nat Med* 1999;5(3):347–350.

64. Tarnopolsky M, Martin J. Creatine monohydrate increases strength in patients with neuromuscular disease. *Neurology* 1999;52:854–857.

65. Hultman E, Soderlund K, Timmons JA, et al. Muscle creatine loading in men. *J Appl Physiol* 1996;81:232–237.

66. Pritchard NR, Kaira PA. Renal dysfunction accompanying oral creatine supplements. *Lancet* 1998;351:1252–1253.

67. ALS CNTF Study Group. A double-blind placebo-controlled clinical trial of subcutaneous recombinant human ciliary neurotrophic factor (rHCNTF) in amyotrophic lateral sclerosis. *Neurology* 1996;46: 1244–1249.

68. BDNF Study Group. A controlled trial of recombinant methionyl human BDNF in ALS. *Neurology* 1999;52:1427–1433.

69. Miller RG, Petajan JH, Bryan WW, et al. A placebo-controlled trial of recombinant human ciliary neurotrophic factor in amyotrophic lateral sclerosis. *Ann Neurol* 1996;39(2):256–260.

70. Lange DJ, Felice KJ, Festoff BW, et al. Recombinant human insulin-like growth factor-I in ALS: description of a double-blind, placebo-controlled study. *Neurology* 1996;47:S93–S95.

71. Borasio GD, Robberecht W, Leigh PN, et al. A placebo-controlled trial of insulin-like growth factor-I in amyotrophic lateral sclerosis. *Neurology* 1998;51:583–586.

72. Miller RG, Moore D, Young LA, et al. Placebo-controlled trial of gabapentin in patients with amyotrophic lateral sclerosis. *Neurology* 1996;47:1383–1388.

73. Gredal O, Werdelin L, Bak S, et al. A clinical trial of dextromethorphan in amyotrophic lateral sclerosis. *Acta Neurol Scand* 1997;96: 8–13.

74. Blin O, Azulay JP, Desnuelle C, et al. A controlled one-year trial of dextromethorphan in amyotrophic lateral sclerosis. *Clin Neuropharm* 1996;19:189–192.

75. Miller RG, Shepherd R, Dao H, et al. A controlled trial of nimodipine in amyotrophic lateral sclerosis. *Neuromusc Dis* 1996;6:101–104.

76. Miller RG, Smith SA, Murphy JR, et al. A clinical trial of verapamil in amyotrophic lateral sclerosis. *Muscle Nerve* 1996;19:511–515.

77. Italian ALS Study Group. Branched-chain amino acids and amyotrophic lateral sclerosis: a treatment failure? *Neurology* 1993;43: 2466–2470.

78. Lange DJ, Murphy PL, Diamond B, et al. Selegiline is ineffective in a collaborative double-blind, placebo-controlled trial for treatment of amyotrophic lateral sclerosis. *Arch Neurol* 1998;55:93–96.

79. Fowler WM, Carter GT, Kraft GH. Role of physiatry in the manage-

ment of neuromuscular disease. In: *Physical medicine and rehabilitation clinics of North America*. Philadelphia: WB Saunders, 1998:1–8.

80. Francis K, Bach JR, DeLisa JA. Evaluation and rehabilitation of patients with adult motor neuron disease. *Arch Phys Med Rehabil* 1999; 80:951–963.

81. Aitkens SG, McCrory MA, Kilmer DD, et al. Moderate resistance exercise program: its effects in slowly progressive neuromuscular disease. *Arch Phys Med Rehabil* 1993;74(7):711–715.

82. Kilmer DD, McCrory MA, Wright NC, et al. The effect of a high resistance exercise program in slowly progressive neuromuscular disease. *Arch Phys Med Rehabil* 1994;75(5):560–563.

83. Kilmer DD. The role of exercise in neuromuscular disease. *Phys Med Rehabil N Am* 1998;9(1):115–125.

84. Carter GT. Rehabilitation management of neuromuscular disease. *J Neurol Rehabil* 1997;11(2):1–12.

85. Carter GT, Miller RG. Comprehensive management of amyotrophic lateral sclerosis. *Phys Med Rehabil N Am* 1998;9(1):271–284.

86. Sharma KR, Kent-Braun JA, Majumdar S, et al. Physiology of fatigue in amyotrophic lateral sclerosis. *Neurology* 1995;45(4):733–740.

87. Krivickas LS. Pulmonary function and respiratory failure. In: Mitsumoto H, Chad DA, Pioro EP, eds. *Amyotrophic lateral sclerosis*. Philadelphia: FA Davis Co, 1998:382–404.

88. Benditt JO. Management of pulmonary complications in neuromuscular disease. In: *Physical medicine and rehabilitation clinics of North America*. Philadelphia: WB Saunders, 1998:167–185.

89. Bach JR. Amyotrophic lateral sclerosis: predictors for prolongation of life by noninvasive respiratory aids. *Arch Phys Med Rehabil* 1995; 76(9):828–832.

90. Bach JR. Amyotrophic lateral sclerosis: communication status and survival with ventilatory support. *Arch Phys Med Rehabil* 1993;72(6): 343–349.

91. Carter GT, Johnson ER, Bonekat HW, et al. Laryngeal diversion in the treatment of intractable aspiration in motor neuron disease. *Arch Phys Med Rehabil* 1992;73(7):680–682.

92. Langmore SE, Schatz MA, Olsen N. Fiberoptic endoscopic examination of swallowing safety: a new procedure. *Dysphagia* 1988;2: 216–219.

93. Miller RG, Rosenberg JA, Gelinas DF, et al. Practice parameter: the care of patients with amyotrophic lateral sclerosis (an evidence-base review). *Muscle Nerve* 1999;22:1104–1118.

94. Hunter MD, Robinson IC, Neilson S. The functional and psychologi-

cal status of patients with amyotrophic lateral sclerosis: some implications for rehabilitation. *Disabil Rehabil* 1993;15(3):119–126.

95. Meininger V. Breaking bad news in amyotrophic lateral sclerosis. *Palliat Med* 1993;7[Suppl 4]:37–40.

96. Abresch RT, Seyden NK, Wineinger MA. Quality of life: issues for persons with neuromuscular diseases. In: *Physical medicine and rehabilitation clinics of North America*. Philadelphia: WB Saunders, 1998: 233–248.

97. Fields HL. Relief of unnecessary suffering. In: Fields HL, Liebeskind JC, eds. *Pharmacologic approaches to the treatment of chronic pain: new concepts and critical issues*, vol 1. Seattle: International Association for the Study of Pain Press, 1994:1–11.

98. Pisano F, Miscio G, Mazzuero G, et al. Decreased heart rate variability in amyotrophic lateral sclerosis. *Muscle Nerve* 1995;18:1225–1231.

99. Carvalho M, Schwartz MS, Swash M. Involvement of the external anal sphincter in amyotrophic lateral sclerosis. *Muscle Nerve* 1995; 18:848–853.

100. Bernat JL. Ethical and legal issues in the management of amyotrophic lateral sclerosis. In: Belsh JM, Schiffman PL, eds. *Amyotrophic lateral sclerosis: diagnosis and management for the clinician*. Armonk, NY: Futura Publishing, 1996:357–372.

101. Carter GT, Butler LM, Abresch RT, et al. Expanding the role of hospice in the care of amyotrophic lateral sclerosis. *Am J Hosp Palliat Care* 1999;16(6):707–710.

102. Ganzini L, Johnston WS, McFarland BH, et al. Attitudes of patients with amyotrophic lateral sclerosis and their caregivers toward assisted suicide. *N Engl J Med* 1998;339(14):967–973.

103. Moore MK. Dying at home: a way of maintaining control for the person with ALS/MND. *Palliat Med* 1993;7[Suppl 4]:65–68.

104. Oppenheimer EA. Decision-making in the respiratory care of amyotrophic lateral sclerosis: should home mechanical ventilation be used? *Palliat Med* 1993;7[Suppl 4]:49–64.

105. Krivickas LS, Shockley L, Mitsumoto H. Home care of patients with amyotrophic lateral sclerosis (ALS). *J Neurol Sci* 1997;152[Suppl 1]: S82–S89.

106. Standards and Accreditation Committee Medical Guidelines Task Force. *Medical guidelines for determining prognosis in selected non-cancer diseases*. The National Hospice Organization, Arlington, Virginia; 1996:24–26.

107. Enck RE. Hospice: the next step. *Am J Hosp Palliat Care* 1999;16(2): 436–437.

108. Brooks BR. Defining optimal management in ALS: from first symptoms to announcement. *Neurology* 1999;53[Suppl 5]:S1–S3.

POSTPOLIO SYNDROME

JAMES C. AGRE
ARTHUR A. RODRIQUEZ

Until the late 1950s, acute paralytic poliomyelitis was a major cause of death, paralysis, and paresis in children and young adults. Although the incidence of acute poliomyelitis dropped precipitously after the development and utilization of vaccines, and the World Health Organization had hoped to eradicate poliomyelitis by the year 2000, cases of acute poliomyelitis still occur. Thus, individuals who survive acute paralytic poliomyelitis will continue to have problems associated with the late effects of polio until late into the twenty-first century.

Although the first reports that cited the development of new problems in polio survivors many years after the acute poliomyelitis illness were published in 1875 (1,2), this problem only became widely recognized by health care professionals in the last two decades. The first descriptions of new weakness occurring years after the initial polio illness were of young men who had poliomyelitis in infancy and who developed new weakness after the performance of physically demanding activity. In 1962, Zilkha (3) described several cases of individuals who developed new weakness and suggested that the new weakness was related to the initial poliomyelitis illness.

Since the initial reports, many reports described finding new problems that were believed to be related to the acute poliomyelitis illness in survivors up to seven decades after the acute illness (4–13). These neurologic changes were commonly diagnosed as a form of progressive muscular atrophy, late progression of poliomyelitis, or a forme fruste amyotrophic lateral sclerosis (5, 6). It was not until the 1980s, three to four decades after the epidemics of the 1940s and 1950s, however, that the late effects of acute paralytic poliomyelitis became widely recognized by health care professionals. This was at the time of the first symposium regarding the late effects of polio, which was held in Warm Springs, Georgia (7).

EPIDEMIOLOGY OF ACUTE PARALYTIC POLIOMYELITIS

During the polio epidemics of the 1940s, the incidence of acute paralytic poliomyelitis was approximately 10 cases per 100,000 people. This incidence increased and peaked during the epidemic of 1952, when 57,800 new cases were reported (an incidence of 15 cases per 100,000 population) (8). After the introduction of the Salk vaccine in 1955 and the Sabin vaccine in 1961, the incidence of acute paralytic poliomyelitis dropped to 0.04 cases per 100,000 in 1963 (8). Paralytic poliomyelitis is now a rare complication of the Sabin (oral, live, attenuated virus) vaccine. The incidence of paralytic poliomyelitis from the Sabin vaccine was reported to be 0.23 cases per 10 million doses in 1989 (8).

Although the number of polio survivors in the United States is unknown, as a result of the National Center for Health Statistics survey in 1987, it has been estimated that there are at least 640,000 survivors of paralytic poliomyelitis in the United States (9). The percentage of polio survivors experiencing new symptoms that may be related to their acute poliomyelitis illness is also unknown, but estimates have ranged from 25% to 60% (10–13). Thus, an estimate of the number of individuals in the United States experiencing the late effects of poliomyelitis is between 160,000 and 380,000. It is most probable that these figures will increase as polio survivors age.

PATHOPHYSIOLOGY OF ACUTE POLIOMYELITIS

Acute paralytic poliomyelitis occurs as a result of a viral infection. The virus is a single-stranded RNA enterovirus belonging to the picornavirus group and has three antigenically distinguishable viruses (14). The wild virus usually enters the body via oral ingestion and then it replicates in the lymphoid tissues of the pharynx and ileum. The virus is extremely infectious, but usually quite benign. Most individuals who are infected with the poliovirus are unaware of any illness (approximately 90% to 95% of cases). Approximately 4% to 8% of cases result in a nonspecific viral illness (fever, myalgia, upper respiratory, or gastrointestinal symptoms). Only 1% to 2% of cases develop paralysis (15). The spread to the central nervous system is thought to be via viremia.

The rate of paralysis varies with the strain of the virus and the age of the individual. Paralysis occurs in approximately 1 of 1,000 infected children, and paralysis occurs in approximately 1 of 75 infected adults (9). The paralysis is usually asymmetric. The lower limbs are usually more severely affected than the upper limbs. Severe bulbar involvement occurs in approximately 10% to 15% of paralytic cases.

The pathologic finding of acute poliomyelitis includes inflammation of the meninges and the motor neurons in the cortex and the spinal cord. Other findings include abnormalities in the cerebellar nuclei, thalamus, hypothalamus, reticular formation, and the dorsal horn (16).

Wallerian degeneration occurs after the death of the motor neurons and the muscle fibers innervated by these neurons become "orphaned." This results in weakness. The amount of recovery of strength and endurance after the acute paralytic illness was determined by four separate factors: (a) the number of motor neurons that recover and resume normal function, (b) the number of orphaned muscle fibers that become reinnervated via terminal motor-unit reorganization, (c) muscle hypertrophy as a result of activity, and (d) improvement in muscle endurance capacity as a result of exercise.

PROPOSED ETIOLOGIES FOR LATE NEUROMUSCULAR DYSFUNCTION

A number of different etiologies—pathophysiologic and functional—have been proposed for late deterioration in survivors of acute paralytic poliomyelitis.

Proposed Pathophysiologic Etiologies

A number of pathophysiologic etiologies have been proposed for late neuromuscular dysfunction in polio survivors. These etiologies include chronic poliovirus infection, death or dysfunction of the surviving motor neurons; loss of muscle fibers from the enlarged motor units; predisposition of motor neuron degeneration due to glial, vascular, and lymphatic changes caused by poliovirus; genetic predisposition of motor neuron degeneration; immune-mediated deterioration; and reduced level of insulin-like growth factor-I (17–19). The most probable of the previously mentioned etiologies are loss of muscle fibers from the enlarged motor units and death of motor neurons associated with the aging process. This process may also lead to dysfunction in patients with spinal cord injury many years after their injury. In particular, at the level of the acute injury, there is often peripheral nerve damage that also results in terminal motor-unit reorganization. Over time, these enlarged motor units may also deteriorate in a similar fashion to those in individuals with postpolio syndrome.

Proposed Functional Etiologies

A number of functional etiologies have also been proposed for late neuromuscular deterioration in polio survivors many years after their acute illness. These factors include chronic muscle weakness, disuse muscle weakness, overuse muscle weakness, and weight gain (9,20). Many years ago, Beasley (21) demonstrated that many polio survivors with apparently "normal" muscle strength (assessed by manual muscle testing) had an average strength of only one half the normal level, when measured quantitatively. Thus, it is possible that many polio survivors with apparently normal muscle strength actually had much less than normal strength after their acute poliomyelitis illness. Over the years, with loss in strength due to the aging process, that deficit

may become much more noticeable. Many polio survivors complain of muscle and joint pain (9,22). This pain can result in a reduced level of activity, which is known to result in disuse muscle weakness (23). Polio survivors are no different from other individuals and will from time to time become ill or require a hospital stay. Both illness and hospitalization may necessitate a period of bed rest, which will result in disuse weakness (23). One clinical study of postpoliomyelitic patients reported that 44% of patients had acknowledged a decline in function that began during a hospital confinement (22). Overuse of muscles can also lead to declining muscular function. Although overuse dysfunction is an old concept, the mechanisms for its effect are not well understood. There are a number of anecdotal reports in the literature citing overuse as the causative factor in declining strength in postpoliomyelitic patients (24–26). Weight gain has also been identified as a risk factor for the development of postpolio syndrome (27). It is well known that individuals tend to become heavier with age. In one study, American postpolio survivors were found to gain 1 kg of body weight per year over a 4-year period (28). During that same time, they were also found to become weaker. The combination of increased body mass (probably related to increased adipose tissue deposition) and reduced strength could certainly make it more difficult to perform usual daily activities.

Combination of Factors Resulting in Declining Function

A number of etiologies, working in combination, have also been hypothesized to result in declining function in poliomyelitis survivors (9). This is the most probable causative factor for declining function in most polio survivors. The most likely pathophysiologic cause for neuromuscular deterioration is a gradual loss of muscle fibers in the enlarged motor units and a gradual loss of motor neurons. The motor units most likely to become dysfunctional or die are those that incorporated the most orphaned muscle fibers during terminal motor-unit reorganization as a part of the natural recovery process after the acute paralytic poliomyelitis illness. The various physiologic and functional etiologies may interact with each other and multiply the effect of any single factor. For instance, a patient with pain due to muscle overuse may reduce his or her level of activity as a result of the overuse problem. This reduction in activity may lead to disuse weakness. The decreasing level of activity may result in weight gain due to excessive (for level of activity) caloric intake. Also, with decreased level of activity, joint contracture may ensue. This will place the patient at a biomechanical disadvantage in performing activities and results in further muscle or joint pain, which can lead to further dysfunction. Treatment of the postpoliomyelitic individual requires an assessment of all possible factors that may be contributing to the patient's dysfunction and intervention whenever possible.

POSTPOLIO CHARACTERISTICS
Clinical Characteristics

Several studies have documented that postpoliomyelitic patients develop similar symptoms regardless of where they may be living

TABLE 36.1. COMMON NEW SYMPTOMS IN PATIENTS POSTPOLIO

Symptom	Halstead and Rossi (29) (n = 132)	Agre et al. (22) (n = 79)	Ramlow et al. (13) (n = 474)	Halstead and Rossi (30) (n = 539)
Fatigue	89%	86%	34%	87%
Joint pain	71%	77%	42%	80%
Muscle pain	71%	86%	38%	79%
New weakness				
Affected muscles	69%	80%	NA	87%
Unaffected muscles	50%	53%	NA	77%
Cold sensitivity	29%	NA	26%	NA

NA, not assessed.

(Table 36.1) (13,22,29,30). The most frequently reported signs and symptoms are listed in Table 36.2. Functional deficits are also commonly acknowledged by postpoliomyelitic patients (Table 36.3) (22,29,30). Although the complaints of postpoliomyelitic patients are varied, the most common complaints are new pain, fatigue, and weakness. Risk factors for the development of postpolio syndrome are listed in Table 36.4.

Pain/Orthopedic Problems

Orthopedic problems resulting in muscle or joint pain are very common in patients seen in postpolio clinics. In one clinical study of 193 postpoliomyelitic patients, 30% had problems with the orthotic devices they were using, with genu recurvatum being a problem in 54 (28%) of 193 patients (31). In 75% of these patients, knee pain was a significant concern. In another clinical study, 61 (77%) of 79 postpoliomyelitic patients complained of joint pain and 55 (70%) of 79 complained of low back pain (22). The most common diagnoses in these patients included degenerative arthritis or arthralgia in 56 (71%) of 79 and muscle overuse or myofascial pain in 56 (71%) of 79 of the patients. In another study of 183 postpoliomyelitic patients, it was found that many patients who could benefit from the use of an assistive device to protect weakened muscles and arthritic joints were not

TABLE 36.2. FREQUENT SIGNS AND SYMPTOMS OF POSTPOLIO SYNDROME

Fatigue
Muscle pain
Joint pain
Muscle weakness
Cold intolerance
Atrophy
Reduced or absent muscle stretch reflexes
Dysphagia (in patients with bulbar involvement initially)
Respiratory dysfunction (in patients with bulbar involvement initially)
Walking difficulty
Stair-climbing difficulty
Difficulty in activities of daily living (particularly those that are instrumental)
Difficulty with use of public transportation

using any such devices (32). Only 14% of the patients were using orthotics or canes at the time of the clinical evaluation, which revealed that 39% of the individuals would benefit from using such devices. In another study of 103 postpoliomyelitic patients, only 18% of the patients were using an orthosis at the time of the clinical appointment (33). As a result of the evaluation, a new orthosis was recommended for 36% of the patients to protect weakened muscles and arthritic joints. In another study, orthopedic problems (including scoliosis, joint pain, or fracture sequelae) were found in 24 (59%) of 41 patients (34).

Fatigue

Fatigue is one of the most common complaints of polio survivors but is a complaint that is impossible to objectively assess. In most of the studies reporting on the prevalence of fatigue in the postpolio population, the term *fatigue* was not defined. It is quite likely that the basis for the complaint of fatigue in postpoliomyelitic patients may vary in different patients (35). Fatigue may be caused by a number of factors including general fatigue, cardiovascular fatigue, local muscle fatigue, or emotional stress. Only after careful evaluation can one properly interpret the complaint of fatigue in a postpoliomyelitic patient and institute appropriate therapeutic measures.

General fatigue can occur in postpoliomyelitic patients. In some postpoliomyelitic patients, this may be a pervasive sense of fatigue that the patient may describe as "hitting the wall" (30). One nationwide survey of polio survivors reported that 43% of respondents acknowledged this problem, and in two thirds of these individuals, it occurred daily (30). This problem most commonly occurred in the mid to late afternoon and in many patients was ameliorated with rest.

Cardiovascular or local muscle factors may also play a role in the fatigue experienced by some postpoliomyelitic patients. One study reported that the average aerobic power of postpoliomyelitic individuals was comparable to that of a non-postpolio individual shortly after an acute myocardial infarction (36). In such individuals, the performance of routine activities of daily living would be performed at close to their maximal capacity, and this could certainly lead to excessive fatigue. In another postpolio study, the most common complaint of patients with postpolio syndrome was decreasing endurance (32). In this

TABLE 36.3. MOST COMMON NEW FUNCTIONAL PROBLEMS IN POSTPOLIO PATIENTS

Functional Problem	Halstead and Rossi (29) (n = 132)	Agre et al. (22) (n = 79)	Halstead and Rossi (30) (n = 539)	Grimby and Einarsson (60) (n = 41)
Walking difficulty	63%	NA	85%	66%
Stair-climbing difficulty	61%	67%	82%	NA
Difficulties with activities of daily living	17%	16%	62%	66%

NA, not assessed.

study, 153 of 154 postpoliomyelitic patients acknowledged this problem. In another clinical report, two thirds of the postpoliomyelitic patients complained of an increasing sense of strength loss in the muscles or a heavy sensation in the muscles while performing daily activities (37). These findings suggest that in at least some postpoliomyelitic patients, fatigue may be caused by cardiovascular or local muscle factors.

It is also well known that depression and significant emotional stress may result in the perception of fatigue. Several studies have reported these factors to play a role in the fatigue experienced by some postpoliomyelitic patients (38–42).

Weakness

Although new weakness is a very common complaint of postpoliomyelitic patients, no studies have conclusively demonstrated that the loss of strength in these individuals is greater than that which could be attributed to the aging process. Two studies, however, have demonstrated an average loss of strength in the quadriceps femoris muscles of 2% per year over 4 years (28,43). This rate of strength loss is twice that expected from the aging process; however, neither study reported on strength change in a control group.

Many postpoliomyelitic patients have difficulty with mobility and ambulation due to significant weakness in their musculature. One study reported that 44% of its patients used orthoses, canes, or crutches at least part time and an additional 18% used a wheelchair at least part time (22). Another study reported that 56% of its patients used a cane or crutch and 20% were wheelchair bound (44).

TABLE 36.4. RISK FACTORS FOR THE DEVELOPMENT OF POSTPOLIO SYNDROME

Present age
Greater time since acute poliomyelitis
Greater severity of acute poliomyelitis illness
Greater functional recovery
Greater level of activity
Muscle or joint pain
Weight gain

Respiratory Dysfunction

Approximately 10% to 20% of patients with acute paralytic poliomyelitis required assisted ventilation during their acute illness (45–47). Most of these individuals could be weaned off ventilators during the convalescent stage after the acute illness (47). The percentage of postpoliomyelitic patients with present respiratory dysfunction is not known. A nationwide survey in 1985 reported that 42% of respondents acknowledged new breathing difficulties (48). Other studies reported lower frequencies of respiratory dysfunction, but in some individuals, these problems were significant (22,30,49). The postpoliomyelitic patients at greatest risk for serious late-onset pulmonary complications are those who had moderate to severe respiratory involvement during their acute poliomyelitis illnesses (9). Respiratory difficulties experienced by polio survivors include both obstructive and restrictive pulmonary disease with chronic hypoventilation, nocturnal rapid eye movement, sleep-induced hypoxemia, and sleep apnea (50,51). Symptoms may include daytime somnolence, morning headache, exertional dyspnea, and generalized fatigue. A number of factors may cause these problems, including weak respiratory musculature, hypoventilation, reduced pulmonary compliance, scoliosis, and the effects of other diseases such as cigarette smoking and asthma.

Swallowing Dysfunction

Approximately 10% to 20% of postpoliomyelitic patients complain of having difficulty with swallowing (52). This results from weakness of the bulbar musculature. One study of 220 postpoliomyelitic patients reported that 18% of the patients acknowledged having dysphagia (53). In another study, 20 postpoliomyelitic patients underwent cinefluorography and 19 were found to have at least some degree of pharyngeal abnormality that was contributing to dysphagia (52). In a random study, 24 of 32 patients with postpolio syndrome acknowledged new swallowing difficulties and 18 had bulbar involvement during their acute paralytic poliomyelitis illness (54). This study suggests that swallowing difficulties may emerge as a late effect of polio even if the bulbar musculature was not apparently involved during the acute illness.

Activities of Daily Living Dysfunction

One study reported that 80% of postpoliomyelitic patients were experiencing difficulties in the performance of personal activities of daily living (such as bathing, dressing, toileting, feeding, and transferring) (44). More difficulties were reported in instrumental activities of daily living (e.g., difficulty with walking several blocks was acknowledged by 90%, difficulties with walking one block or climbing one flight of stairs was acknowledged by 75%, difficulty with performing light housework was acknowledged by 85%, and difficulty with performing vigorous activity was acknowledged by 98%). Use of public transportation was a difficulty for 88% of patients, and 40% were unable to use public transportation because of mobility difficulties. Only 30% of patients were independent in performing household chores, whereas 70% required varied levels of assistance in the performance of these activities.

POSTPOLIO MANAGEMENT

Substantiate Postpolio Diagnosis

It is always important to rule out other medical problems that a postpoliomyelitic patient may have when treating patients with the late effects of polio. The diagnosis of postpolio syndrome is truly one of exclusion of other medical problems that may be causing the patient's problems. The following appear to be reasonable criteria for the diagnosis of postpolio syndrome (9,29):

1. a prior episode of paralytic poliomyelitis confirmed by history and physical examination
2. a period of neurologic recovery followed by an extended interval of neurologic and functional stability preceding the onset of new problems of at least 15 to 20 years
3. a gradual or abrupt onset of new weakness that may or may not be accompanied by other new health problems (such as fatigue, joint or muscle pain, atrophy, and decreased function)
4. exclusion of other medical, orthopedic, or neurologic conditions other than polio-related conditions that might cause the new health problems

The first criterion is documented by history and (whenever possible) by review of the patient's medical records. The history should reveal an acute febrile illness producing motor but not sensory loss. One should also inquire whether other family members, friends, or neighbors also had a similar illness. The physical examination should reveal evidence of a lower motor neuron disease. The weakness and atrophy are usually focal and asymmetric. Muscle stretch reflexes will be reduced. Sensation is intact (unless the patient has a local entrapment neuropathy such as carpal tunnel syndrome or cubital tunnel syndrome).

The second criterion is the characteristic pattern of recovery. Usually the individual achieves a plateau of recovery within a few years of the acute paralytic illness and tends to do well for a few decades thereafter. New problems tend to occur 20 to 30 years or more after the acute paralytic illness in most postpoliomyelitic patients.

The third criterion is the onset of new weakness. This is determined by history obtained from the patient. In many cases, the individual will have difficulty in precisely identifying the onset of new weakness but will often note a gradual onset of

difficulties with ambulation, stair climbing, and so forth. It is imperative that other causes for new weakness are excluded.

The fourth criterion is the exclusion of other medical, orthopedic, and neurologic causes for the complaints of new weakness and the other health-related problems. There is some controversy regarding this criterion, because some clinicians will not make the diagnosis of postpolio syndrome in the presence of such diagnoses as compression neuropathies, arthritis, degenerative disk disease, or obesity. However, these diagnoses are very commonly found in postpoliomyelitic and non-postpoliomyelitic individuals. Additionally, postpoliomyelitic individuals are susceptible to these problems as a result of their chronic weakness; use of biomechanically disadvantaged joints; use of assistive devices such as crutches, canes, and wheelchairs (which can result in compression neuropathies); and reduced level of energy expenditure. In our own practice, we do not use such polio-related diagnoses as exclusionary criteria for the diagnosis of postpolio syndrome.

Electrodiagnostic Assessment

Electrodiagnostic evaluation is not needed in all postpoliomyelitic patients but can be helpful in the evaluation of selected patients based on their complaints and examination. Postpoliomyelitic patients are susceptible to compression neuropathies (such as carpal tunnel syndrome or ulnar neuropathy) from the use of canes, crutches, and wheelchairs. Some patients may develop new neurologic symptoms based on spinal stenosis or radiculopathy due to severe degeneration of the spine from years of activity with poor muscle control in the spine. In such patients, electrodiagnostic testing can be of great help in assessing the patient and determining the best course of therapy for the patient. Electrodiagnostic testing, however, cannot be used to separate postpoliomyelitic patients with new dysfunction from stable postpoliomyelitic patients. Two studies attempted to differentiate postpoliomyelitic patients with new complaints from stable postpoliomyelitic patients with electromyographic (EMG) testing (55,56). Both studies found the two groups to be indistinguishable electrophysiologically using conventional EMG and single-fiber EMG evaluation.

Macro-EMG has also been studied in postpoliomyelitic patients and does demonstrate that postpoliomyelitic individuals do have an increase in the macro-EMG potential (indicating enlarged motor units) (57–59). In one study, using macro-EMG and single-fiber EMG techniques, statistically significant differences were found in macro-EMG amplitude, fiber density, jitter, and blocking when comparing unstable postpoliomyelitic with stable postpoliomyelitic patients (58). However, the authors did not suggest that these methods be used to differentiate stable from unstable postpoliomyelitic patients, because there was a great deal of variance in all the measurements. In another study, single-fiber EMG studies showed a moderate degree of disturbed neuromuscular transmission (increases in jitter and blocking) in postpoliomyelitic patients, which did not appear to significantly change during the 8-year longitudinal study (59). Macro-EMG was found to increase in 20 legs but decreased in 8 legs during this 8-year study. It appeared that the breakpoint was when the macro-EMG amplitude was around 20 times the normal size.

In eight of nine legs with a macro-EMG amplitude more than 20 times the normal value initially, the value had decreased by the time of the 8-year follow-up assessment. This evidence suggests that there is a failing capacity to maintain very large motor units in postpoliomyelitic patients. However, this technique is a very difficult and time-consuming endeavor and is primarily reserved for research purposes. It is doubtful whether this would be useful in the usual clinical evaluation of a postpoliomyelitic patient. Electrodiagnostic testing can be useful in evaluating postpoliomyelitic patients for possible compression neuropathy or as a part of the assessment of a patient with spinal degeneration and stenosis or radiculopathy but cannot be used to differentiate postpoliomyelitic patients with new dysfunction from stable postpoliomyelitic patients.

TREATMENT OF POSTPOLIO PROBLEMS

General Aspects of Treatment

Each and every postpoliomyelitic patient is different. The treatment approach for each patient needs to consider the patient's unique situation. It is important to learn from the patient his or her primary concerns and identify functional problems. The functional sequelae of postpoliomyelitis can be categorized by impairment (on the organic level) and by disability (on the functional level). Management of the patient should focus on reducing impairment whenever possible and avoiding the development of further disability or reducing the level of disability whenever possible. The ultimate goal is to assist each patient in enhancing his or her overall level of function, independence, and sense of well being—that is, to enhance the patient's quality of life (60).

Treatment of Specific Postpolio Problems

Pain

Muscle pain, back pain, and joint pain are very common complaints of postpoliomyelitic patients (22,29,30,48). In many patients, these problems are related to muscle weakness from the initial poliomyelitis illness and the stresses placed on the tissues over the years.

Muscle pain is very common in postpoliomyelitic patients and may be due to overuse of the muscles or to myofascial pain. In one study, 71% of patients had muscle pain related to these two factors (22). Muscle overuse pain can be diagnosed from the patient's history. The patient will complain of muscle pain exacerbated with activity and relieved by rest. Muscle overuse can be caused by overuse of weakened muscles but can also be caused by overuse of relatively strong muscles. It is not uncommon for postpoliomyelitic patients to complain of muscle overuse pain in the lower limb that was not apparently affected by the initial poliomyelitis illness or was only minimally affected. Due to the weakness of the more affected lower limb, excessive stress is placed on the more intact lower limb, leading to muscle overuse pain. Many patients also have poor gait patterns due to weakness and lack of use of an orthosis, which could improve the gait pattern. Also, some postpoliomyelitic patients continue

with their daily activities until the pain is so severe that they simply have to stop the activity. Careful assessment is needed to identify the factors leading to the complaints and implement the appropriate treatment plan to reduce excessive stress on the muscle causing the pain.

Back pain was reported by 70% of postpoliomyelitic patients in one clinical study (22). This pain can be due to a number of factors including scoliosis, biomechanical stress placed on the back during ambulation or transfers, and degenerative joint disease. Back pain can also be caused by a poorly fitted seating system in a patient who primarily uses a wheelchair for mobility.

Joint pain is also commonly found in postpoliomyelitic patients. In one clinical study, 28% of patients were found to have genu recurvatum of the knee (31). This problem was essentially resolved with the fitting of a proper orthosis. Another study reported a significant reduction in lower limb joint pain with the use of a properly fitting orthosis (33). The correct orthosis can reduce pain at multiple sites by altering the lurching type of gait pattern that many postpoliomyelitic patients use without the assistance of an orthosis. Common examples include the forward weight shift to move the center of gravity anterior to the knee joint to assist with knee extension and the side-to-side pattern of weight shift used to circumduct the leg to clear the foot in the patient with footdrop. Shoulder pain is also commonly found in postpoliomyelitic patients. One study reported that 30% of patients complained of shoulder pain (22). This complaint is frequently found in individuals who require the use of canes or crutches for ambulation or in patients who transfer into and out of their wheelchairs. This type of activity can lead to the development of degenerative joint disease of the shoulder, rotator cuff problems, or muscle overuse pain (such as myofascial pain).

Treatment of the specific pain problems requires specific evaluation of the patient to determine the underlying specific causes. The use of nonsteroidal antiinflammatory drugs is helpful for treating joint or muscle pain. Appropriate changes in activities of daily living and use of assistive devices may also be needed. Patients with sleep problems related to their pain may respond to the use of tricyclic antidepressant medications. Compensatory techniques to relieve painful joints are also important. These include education and modifications to transfer techniques to relieve shoulder pain. At times, adaptive equipment such as a mechanical lift or wheelchair for long-distance mobility may be required.

Fatigue

Fatigue is a common complaint of postpoliomyelitic patients. Fatigue may be due to any number of underlying conditions including medical diseases (e.g., thyroid dysfunction, diabetes mellitus, anemia, cardiac disease, and malignancy) and use of some medications (such as β-blockers, sedatives, and antihistamines). Fatigue may also be related to local muscle fatigue, general fatigue, or depression. One needs to carefully assess the postpoliomyelitic patient in an attempt to determine the underlying cause and to design the treatment program based on the assessment. Treatment can include reduction of activity and rest breaks as needed. Some patients "hit the wall" in the mid afternoon and naps can benefit these patients (30).

Pacing (interspersing activity with rest periods) has been quite helpful for many postpoliomyelitic patients with fatigue-related problems. A laboratory study of patients with postpolio syndrome has also shown that interspersing activity with rest breaks not only reduces local muscle fatigue, but also improves strength recovery after activity (61). Lifestyle changes and the implementation of energy conservation techniques can also be very helpful in reducing fatigue in postpoliomyelitic patients. Such changes as using a handicap license plate or use of a motorized scooter for long-distance mobility, when appropriate, can reduce fatigue. Better planning of daily activities, balancing activity with rest, and the use of appropriate assistive devices to reduce energy expenditure during activities can all reduce fatigue in postpoliomyelitic patients.

Weight loss in patients who have gained weight and are overweight can also help decrease fatigue. One clinical study reported an average weight gain in American postpoliomyelitic patients of 1 kilogram per year over 4 years (28). Although not measured, it was presumed that the weight gain was an increase in adipose tissue, because muscle strength declined in that same interval of time. The extra adipose tissue simply increases the energy required to perform activities of daily living. Shedding the extra adipose mass can reduce the energy expended during activities and, thereby, reduce fatigue by reducing the workload.

Disuse and deconditioning can also result in fatigue. Appropriate exercise can be of benefit to patients with this problem (62,63).

Studies have evaluated the effects of various medications (amantadine, prednisone, and pyridostigmine) on fatigue in postpoliomyelitic individuals. Unfortunately, none of the randomized placebo-controlled studies have shown any benefit of these medications on fatigue (64–66).

Disuse Weakness and Deconditioning

The effect of exercise in the postpolio population has been reviewed (62,63). Muscle-strengthening exercise and general conditioning and aerobic conditioning exercises have been found to be helpful in selected postpoliomyelitic patients. Briefly reviewed here are the effects of muscle-strengthening exercise, cardiorespiratory and general conditioning exercises, and aquatic exercise in postpoliomyelitic individuals.

Muscle-Strengthening Exercise

Early reports (before 1970) regarding the effects of exercise in postpoliomyelitic patients yielded conflicting results. Some of the early studies reported that strengthening exercise in postpoliomyelitic individuals was detrimental (24,26,67), whereas others (68–71) reported that it was beneficial. All of the early reports indicating that exercise was detrimental were anecdotal reports, and all indicated that the individuals were excessively active; it was believed that the excessive activity led to the decline (24, 26,67). The three early studies that showed benefit were all experimental studies; two of the studies provided details of the exercise (69,71). In one study, subjects performed two different dynamic exercises (69). Each of the two exercises consisted of three sets of ten repetitions with a 1-minute rest break between each set. Subjects exercised four days per week for up to 4 months. Strength increased by almost 100% on the average. In the second study, subjects performed three 6-second maximal static contractions of the muscle per day for 10 weeks (71). The individual rested for 2 minutes between each of the maximal contractions. Strength increased by 37% on the average.

Four more-recent studies (since the mid-1980s) have all demonstrated an improvement in strength with no apparent deleterious effect (72–75). Each study was different, but the common thread in all four studies was the performance of several sets of dynamic or static muscle contractions with rest breaks between each set to avoid excessive fatigue. All studies only included postpoliomyelitic subjects with greater than antigravity strength in the muscle to be exercised.

In 1987, Einarsson and Grimby (72) reported the effect of a standardized exercise program on quadriceps femoris muscle strength. Twelve postpoliomyelitic patients, nine of whom had postpolio syndrome, participated in this 6-week exercise program. All subjects had grade 3 + or greater strength on manual muscle testing. Subjects exercised three times per week on a special dynamometer in the research laboratory. Each exercise session was comprised of three sets of static and isokinetic muscle-strengthening exercise. Each exercise set consisted of eight 4-second bouts of exercise alternating between isokinetic and static exercise. Each bout was followed by 10 seconds of rest. Subjects rested for 5 minutes between exercise sets. After the exercise program, muscle strength significantly increased by 16% as measured isokinetically and 17% as measured statically. The exercise did not result in muscle damage as determined by muscle biopsy preexercise and postexercise; strength was maintained 5 to 12 months after the exercise (presumably due to increased activity); and 9 of the 12 subjects acknowledged an increased feeling of well-being after the exercise program.

In 1991, Fillyaw et al. (73) reported the effect of long-term nonfatiguing exercise in 17 postpoliomyelitic patients with postpolio syndrome and at least grade 3 + muscle strength of the quadriceps femoris and biceps humerus muscles (73). Subjects exercised the muscles every other day for 1 to 2 years. The exercise consisted of three sets of ten repetitions with 50%, 75%, and 100% of the ten-repetition maximum (RM) (that is, the maximum amount of weight that could be lifted ten times). Subjects rested for 5 minutes between each of the three exercise sets. Every 2 weeks, the ten RM was evaluated and the training resistance adjusted accordingly. After the exercise program, maximum torque significantly increased in the exercised muscles by more than 8% and the ten RM increased in 16 of the 17 subjects, with an average increase in the ten RM of 78%.

In 1996, Spector et al. (74) reported the effect of an exercise program in six patients with postpolio syndrome with at least grade 3 + strength of the knee extensor and elbow extensor muscles. Exercise was performed three times per week on nonconsecutive days for 9 weeks. Exercise was performed on one knee extensor and both elbow extensor muscles. Subjects performed three sets of exercise consisting of 20, 15, and then 10 repetitions of dynamic extension exercise with special exercise machines. The initial resistance was set at approximately 75% of the three RM. Upper and lower limb exercises were alternated to minimize fatigue, with a rest interval of 90 seconds between sets on a particular machine, and 3 minutes between exercises. After the exercise program, the three RM significantly increased for knee extension by 61% and for elbow extension by 71%. Static strength for both muscle groups, however, did not significantly change after the exercise program (this finding is probably related to the specificity of exercise principle). The exercise program did not result in any deleterious effect, because the serum creatine kinase level did not increase during the exercise program (it is known to significantly increase with muscle damage) and muscle biopsies before and after the exercise program demonstrated no significant change.

In 1997, Agre et al. (75) reported on the effect of a supervised 12-week home exercise program on seven patients with postpolio syndrome with at least grade 3+ muscle strength in the knee extensor muscles (75). Subjects exercised at home 4 days per week. On Mondays and Thursdays, subjects performed three sets of four maximal static contractions of the quadriceps femoris muscles held for 5 seconds each. The subjects rested for 10 seconds between each repetition and for 1 minute between each of the three sets. On Tuesdays and Fridays, subjects performed three sets of knee extension exercise in the sitting position with a weight on the ankle. For each set of exercise, the subjects slowly fully extended and then immediately lowered the weight over a 5-second interval with no rest between the 12 repetitions in the set. The subjects rested for 1 minute after the completion of each set. After the completion of the third set, the subjects rated the perception of exertion in the exercised muscle. If this perception was rated at less than a work level of "very, very hard," the ankle weight was increased at the next exercise session. After 12 weeks of exercise, significant improvements were found in a number of variables: the weight lifted increased by 47%, static torque increased by 36%, isokinetic torque increased by 15%, muscular work capacity increased by 18%, and muscular endurance increased by 21%. The exercise program did not appear to result in any deleterious side effect. EMG testing before and after the exercise program demonstrated no significant change in fiber density, jitter, blocking, or macro-EMG amplitude. Also, the serum creatine kinase level did not significantly change from before the start of the exercise program through to the completion of it.

Cardiorespiratory and General Conditioning Exercise

Postpoliomyelitic patients have been reported to be severely deconditioned from a cardiorespiratory standpoint. One study of patients seen in a postpolio clinic reported that the average maximal metabolic capacity of the patients was only 5.6 metabolic equivalents (METs) (1 MET equals the energy expenditure at complete rest) (76). This level of aerobic power is similar to that of individuals shortly after sustaining an acute myocardial infarction (76). Thus, it could be concluded that postpoliomyelitic individuals could be benefited with a general endurance or aerobic conditioning exercise program. Three studies have documented beneficial effects in postpoliomyelitic individuals in such exercise programs (77–79). The results of these three studies are briefly reviewed here.

In 1989, Jones et al. (77) evaluated the response to a 16-week, three times-per-week aerobic exercise program in a group of 37 postpoliomyelitic patients. Sixteen subjects volunteered to be exercise subjects and 21 volunteered to be control subjects. Exercise subjects exercised on bicycle ergometers using lower limb musculature. Exercise was performed at a target heart rate of 70% to 75% of heart rate reserve (i.e., they exercised at a heart rate equivalent to resting heart rate plus 70% to 75% of the difference between resting heart rate and maximal heart rate). Exercise was performed in bouts of 2 to 5 minutes per bout with 1-minute rest breaks between exercise bouts. Patients were instructed to exercise for 15 to 30 minutes of exercise per session. In most subjects, the exercise was initiated at a lower intensity and duration, and over the first few weeks, the exercise intensity and duration were gradually increased. After 16 weeks of exercise, those subjects who exercised had significantly increased their peak oxygen utilization (average increase of 15%) and maximal work power (average increase of 18%), whereas control subjects had no significant change in either of these variables. No subject experienced any untoward effect from participation in the study, and subjects who exercised reported a subjective decrease in fatigue while performing daily activities and an increase in strength in lower limb musculature.

In 1992, Kriz et al. (78) evaluated the response to upper limb aerobic exercise in a group of 20 postpoliomyelitic patients. Subjects were randomly assigned to exercise and control groups, with ten subjects in each group. Exercise was performed with arm ergometers in the subjects who exercised. Exercise was performed at a target heart rate of 70% to 75% of heart rate reserve. Subjects exercised for 20 minutes per session, exercising in bouts of 2 to 5 minutes with 1-minute rest breaks between bouts. Exercise was performed three times per week for 16 weeks. At the conclusion of the study, the subjects who exercised had significant increases in peak oxygen utilization (average increase of 19%) and maximal work power (average increase of 12%), whereas the control subjects had no change in these variables.

In 1996, Ernstoff et al. (79) reported on the effects of endurance training in a gymnasium. Seventeen subjects volunteered for the study. Twelve completed the study, two subjects dropped from the study because they found the exercise program too difficult, one changed jobs, one became ill unrelated to the study, and one was lost to follow-up. Exercise was performed twice per week over a 22-week period, for a total of 40 sessions (group training was discontinued for 2 weeks over Christmas time). Exercise was performed in a gymnasium under the guidance of a physical therapist. Each exercise session lasted for 60 minutes and consisted of 5 minutes of general warm-up exercise, followed by low-resistance, high-repetition exercises for all major muscle groups in the upper and lower extremities and the trunk. After 1 month of training, 5 minutes of exercise on a bicycle ergometer was included at approximately 60% to 80% of maximal heart rate. Each exercise session ended with a 5-minute cool-down period. At the completion of the exercise program, significant increases were found in the strength of some muscle groups. Also, the heart rate at a submaximal workload, on the bicycle ergometer (70 W), was significantly reduced, indicating an improvement in cardiorespiratory fitness. Muscle biopsies, taken both before and after the exercise program, showed no deleterious effects from the exercise. The predominant complaints related to the exercise program were minor musculoskeletal discomfort of the lower limbs in three subjects.

Aquatic Exercise

Two aquatic exercise studies have been performed in postpoliomyelitic patients. Results from these studies are briefly reviewed. In 1994, Prins et al. (80) assessed the effects of aquatic exercise in 16 postpoliomyelitic patients. Subjects were randomly assigned to exercise and control groups. Nine subjects performed exercise and seven served as control subjects; however, complete data were only available on four of the control subjects. Exercise was performed three times per week for 8 weeks in a swimming pool. Exercise sessions ranged from 45 to 70 minutes per session. The exercise regimen for each subject was individually determined before commencement of the program based on the subject's strength and swimming experience. In addition to swimming and isolated use of the legs employing a kickboard, the exercise subjects also performed a series of arm and leg exercises in the water using fins and hand paddles. Each subject's progress was monitored throughout the exercise program and exercise was gradually progressed. After the 8-week exercise program, significant increases were found in muscle strength and range of motion in some of the upper limb muscles and joints in the subjects who exercised, but not in the control subjects. No subject complained of any adverse effects from participating in the study.

In 1999, Willen (81) reported on the effects of dynamic water exercise in 28 postpoliomyelitic patients. A total of 15 subjects volunteered for the exercise program (13 had postpolio syndrome) and 13 (who did not have time to participate in the exercise study) volunteered to be control subjects. Exercise was performed twice a week for 5 months. Exercise was led by a physical therapist and lasted 40 minutes per session. The exercise was designed to train general physical fitness including endurance and resistance activities, balance, stretching, and relaxation. Heart rate was monitored in three individuals chosen at random to obtain information about the intensity of the program. The monitoring indicated that heart rate was, at times, close to peak heart rate, indicating that on some occasions the subjects were exerting themselves at close to peak effort. After the exercise program, heart rate of the subjects who exercised at a submaximal level was significantly reduced, whereas that in the control subjects showed no change. This is an indication of an improvement in cardiorespiratory fitness in the exercise subjects. Muscle strength did not significantly change in the subjects who exercised; they reported a lower level of distress related to pain (using the Nottingham Health Profile), whereas the control subjects reported no change in distress related to pain. Also, after the exercise program, 11 of 15 of the subjects who exercised reported an increased feeling of well being, and 9 of 15 reported an increase in physical fitness.

EXERCISE PRESCRIPTION FOR THE POSTPOLIOMYELITIC PATIENT

To generalize from the previously cited studies, it appears that exercise has its place in the rehabilitation program of many, but not all, postpoliomyelitic patients. You should be reminded that the subjects in these studies were self-selected; they volunteered to participate in the studies, so they were not postpoliomyelitic individuals selected at random. In these individuals, it appears that the different types of exercise were beneficial. For determining an exercise program for an individual postpoliomyelitic patient, it is imperative that the program be designed to match the individual. It must be kept in mind that each patient was affected by the poliomyelitis illness differently. Hence, the late effects experienced by each individual will be unique. In some patients, some of the muscles were essentially spared, whereas others were significantly affected by the acute poliomyelitis illness. In postpoliomyelitic patients, it is unlikely that significantly weakened muscles (those with less than antigravity strength) will be benefited by a strengthening exercise program. Such muscles should be protected from overuse while the individual participates in an exercise program. The effects of strengthening exercise in postpoliomyelitic patients with muscles with less than antigravity strength have not been studied. It should also be kept in mind that joints about significantly weakened muscles may have developed significant degenerative change. The exercise performed by the individual should not aggravate joint pain related to the degenerative change. The exercise program for the patient should be specifically designed for that individual and should avoid excessive fatigue, muscle pain, and joint pain. The term "excessive fatigue" is rather nebulous and has not yet been well studied. Until further research can clarify this issue, a rule of thumb that might reasonably be used clinically is for the individual to fully recover from his or her exercise within an hour or two after its completion. Most certainly, if the patient still feels tired the day after the exercise, or experiences stiffness or soreness as a result of the exercise, the exercise volume or intensity should be lowered and the patient be given more rest and recovery time.

In most patients, a combination of stretching, strengthening, and aerobic conditioning exercise is advised. The program should start with a very low volume of exercise, with plenty of rest interspersed between the intervals of exercise. We recommend that patients start their exercise program with an intensity and duration of exercise that they believe will not cause excessive fatigue, muscle pain, or joint pain. If the performance of exercise at this level does not cause any problem after a week or two, the intensity and duration can be gradually increased and the rest break times gradually reduced. In many patients, it is reasonable to start the exercise program with approximately 15 to 20 minutes of exercise per session, two to three times per week. The exercise should include several minutes of warm-up, including gentle stretching and strengthening exercises. Then several minutes (5 to 10 minutes) of gentle aerobic exercise should follow in intervals of 2 to 3 minutes of activity, with 1 to 2 minutes of rest in between each interval. Finally, several minutes of cooldown activity should be observed at the end of the exercise session. The individual should be allowed those few minutes of rest between each bout of exercise to avoid fatigue and muscle and joint pain. Significantly weakened muscles and the joints near significantly weakened muscles should be protected during the exercise. If the patient cannot tolerate even the most gentle of exercises, he or she may not benefit from the program and careful consideration should be given to discontinue the exercise for that individual. If the person is benefiting from the exercise, the exercise duration and intensity may then be gradually increased, carefully following its effects on the patient, modifying the program as needed. The exercise could be performed either on land or in water or a combination of the two. If the program is carefully designed, monitored, and modified as needed to avoid muscle and joint pain and excessive fatigue, the exercise may be quite beneficial for many postpoliomyelitic patients.

LOCOMOTOR FUNCTION

Many patients seen in postpolio clinics can benefit from the prescription of new assistive devices for mobility. Perry and Fleming (31) reported problems with old orthotic devices in 30% of patients they evaluated, and new devices were needed. Other studies found that many patients seen in a postpolio clinic were not using assistive devices that would be helpful for them. Cosgrove et al. (32) reported that only 14% of patients seen in their postpolio clinic had an orthotic device when seen in the clinic, but they recommended orthoses for 31% of the patients seen. Waring et al. (33) reported similar findings, with only 18% of patients having orthoses when seen in the clinic, and they recommended orthoses for 36% of the patients. Additionally, this later study reported that in follow-up questionnaire, patients using their orthoses found that orthotic use reduced pain, reduced energy expenditure of ambulation, and improved their sense of safety while ambulating. Evaluation for a wheelchair is also important as the distance the patient can safely ambulate decreases. At times, lower limb orthotic devices and assistive devices needed for short-distance ambulation are ordered at the same time as a manual wheelchair for longer distance mobility. If shoulder pain or weakness is present, the prescription for a power wheelchair or motorized scooter may be indicated.

RESPIRATORY DYSFUNCTION

When pulmonary function status is questioned, a screening pulmonary function assessment is advised. Although no standard criteria exist regarding the timing for respiratory intervention, evaluation and management are similar to those used for other neuromuscular diseases. Close monitoring and evaluation are recommended for those individuals with symptoms of hypoventilation and those with vital capacities less than 1.5 liters, or 50% of predicted normal value. Evaluation may include overnight oxyhemoglobin saturation monitoring or polysomnography. Patients with chronic hypoventilation may benefit from inspiratory positive pressure ventilation, which can be delivered by either continuous positive airway pressure or bilevel positive airway pressure, and which can be delivered via an oral, nasal, or oral-nasal interface.

DYSPHAGIA

Patients with dysphagia should undergo videofluoroscopy supervised by a speech and language pathologist to determine the causative factors for the problem and to determine whether compensatory techniques may be helpful for the patient. Compensatory techniques include changing the consistency of the food or liquids; turning or leaning the head to one side so the bolus travels down the patient's stronger side; chin-tuck technique during the swallow; swallowing twice for each bolus; alternating solids and liquids; and not eating or drinking while fatigued (82).

DYSFUNCTION OF ACTIVITIES OF DAILY LIVING

Most postpoliomyelitic patients do not have dependence in the performance of personal activities of daily living; however, many patients have dependence in the performance of some instrumental activities of daily living such as housekeeping, shopping, and using public transportation (44). Each patient has unique needs and this can be assessed with an occupational therapy evaluation (83). The patient's ability to use, and the benefit of using, various assistive devices can be assessed. Modification of activities at home can be made. The patient can also be educated about work simplification and energy conservation techniques.

PSYCHOSOCIAL DISTRESS

Many postpoliomyelitic patients may experience emotional distress. This includes somatization, anxiety, hostility, and phobia for men with depression more frequently seen in women. The emotional responses to the new health problems experienced by polio survivors may cause the individual as much trouble as the physical problems. Some postpoliomyelitic individuals resist making appropriate lifestyle changes or using assistive devices because they had worked so very hard after the acute poliomyelitis illness to overcome their physical limitations. Some have stated that making these changes would be "giving in" to the polio, something they do not wish to consider. Appropriate psychological counseling is helpful for these individuals. It should be kept in mind that very few polio survivors had psychological intervention at the time of their acute illnesses, and they did not have any such counseling thereafter. The new health-related problems that they experience may bring to mind many issues that were not dealt with at the time of the acute illness. In these cases, psychological counseling can be very helpful for the individual. Bruno and Frick (41) recommended psychological and psychosocial evaluation, because the results of such an evaluation can be helpful in the development of a successful treatment program for the patient. Conrady et al. (40) stressed that physical functioning and psychological functioning need to be evaluated and treated in combination, to maximize the benefit to the postpoliomyelitic patient. Postpolio support groups can also be very helpful in providing patients with useful information provided by other individuals with similar problems. Postpolio groups also tend to be aware of the resources within the community, which can be of benefit to the postpoliomyelitic patient.

CONCLUSION

Many polio survivors are experiencing new problems related to their previous acute poliomyelitis illness. A careful assessment of the patient may uncover a number of factors that may be contributing to these problems, many of which may be amenable to treatment. Rehabilitation specialists are in a unique position of being able to assess the patient's functional problems and prescribe a rational treatment program to help the patient achieve the highest level of independence and function.

POSTPOLIO INFORMATION RESOURCE

An excellent resource for postpoliomyelitic patients and their family members, as well as for health care professionals, to contact for further information about postpolio syndrome is Gazette International Networking Institute, at the following address: 4207 Lindell Boulevard, No. 110, Saint Louis, MO 63108-2915 (*www.post-polio.org*).

REFERENCES

1. Raymond M. Paralysie essentielle de l'enfance, atrophie musculaire consecutive. *CR Heb Seances Mem Soc Biol* 1875;27:158–160.
2. Cornil V, Lepine R. Sur un cas de paralysie generale spinale anterieure subaigue, suivi d'autopsie. *Gaz Med Paris* 1875;4:127–129.
3. Zilkha KJ. Discussion on motor neuron disease. *Proc Royal Soc Med* 1962;55:1028–1029.
4. Wiechers DO. Late effects of polio: historical perspectives. *Birth Defects* 1987;23(4):1–11.
5. Kayser-Gatchahan MC. Late muscular atrophy after poliomyelitis. *Eur Neurol* 1973;10:371.
6. Mulder DW, Rosenbaum RA, Layton DD. Late progression of poliomyelitis or forme fruste amyotrophic lateral sclerosis. *Mayo Clin Proc* 1972;47:756–760.
7. Halstead LS, Wiechers DO, eds. *Late effects of poliomyelitis.* Miami: Symposia Foundation, 1985:1–236.
8. Strebel PM, Sutter RW, Cochi SL, et al. Epidemiology of poliomyelitis in the United States one decade after the last reported case of indigenous wild virus associated disease. *Clin Infect Dis* 1992;14:568–579.
9. Gawne AC, Halstead LS. Post-polio syndrome: pathophysiology and clinical management. *Crit Rev Phys Rehabil Med* 1995;7:147–188.
10. Windebank AJ, Lichty WJ, Daube JR. Prospective cohort study of polio survivors in Olmstead County, Minnesota. *Ann N Y Acad Sci* 1995;753:81–86.
11. Codd MB, Mulder DW, Kurland LT, et al. Poliomyelitis in Rochester, MN 1935–1955: epidemiology and long-term sequelae: a preliminary report. In: Halstead LS, Wiechers DO, eds. *Late effects of poliomyelitis.* Miami: Symposia Foundation, 1985:121–134.
12. Speier JL, Owen RR, Knapp M, et al. Occurrence of post-polio sequelae in an epidemic population. *Birth Defects* 1987;23:39–48.
13. Ramlow J, Alexander M, Laporte R, et al. Epidemiology of the post-polio syndrome. *Am J Epidemiol* 1992;136:769–784.
14. Melnick JL, Agol VI, Bachrach HL, et al. Picornaviridae. *Intervirology* 1974;4:303–316.
15. Horstmann DM. Epidemiology of poliomyelitis and allied diseases—1963. *Yale J Biol Med* 1963;36:5–26.
16. Bodian D. Poliomyelitis: pathological anatomy. *Poliomyelitis: papers and discussions presented at the First International Poliomyelitis Conference.* Philadelphia: JB Lippincott Co, 1949.
17. Jubelt B, Cashman NR. Neurological manifestations of the post-polio syndrome. *Crit Rev Clin Neurobiol* 1987;3:199–220.
18. Shetty KR, Matsson DE, Rudman IW, et al. Hyposomatomedin in men with post-poliomyelitis syndrome. *J Am Geriatr Soc* 1991;39:185–191.
19. Rudman D, Shetty KR. Growth hormone and the post-poliomyelitis syndrome. Paper presented at: American Academy of Physical Medicine and Rehabilitation annual meeting; October 30, 1991; Washington.
20. Agre JC, Rodriquez AA, Tafel JA. Late effects of polio: critical review of the literature on neuromuscular function. *Arch Phys Med Rehabil* 1991;72:923–931.
21. Beasley WC. Quantitative muscle testing: principles and applications to research and clinical services. *Arch Phys Med Rehabil* 1961;42:398–425.
22. Agre JC, Rodriquez AA, Sperling KB. Symptoms and clinical impressions of patients seen in a post-polio clinic. *Arch Phys Med Rehabil* 1989;70:367–370.
23. Mueller EA. Influence of training and of inactivity on muscle strength. *Arch Phys Med Rehabil* 1970;51:449–462.
24. Lovett RW. The treatment of infantile paralysis: preliminary report, based on a study of the Vermont epidemic of 1914. *J Am Med Assoc* 1915;64:2118–2123.
25. Bennett RL, Knowlton GC. Overwork weakness in partially denervated skeletal muscle. *Clin Orthop* 1958;12:22–29.
26. Knowlton GC, Bennett RL. Overwork. *Arch Phys Med Rehabil* 1957;38:18–20.
27. Trojan DA, Cashman NR, Shapiro S, et al. Predictive factors for post-poliomyelitis syndrome. *Arch Phys Med Rehabil* 1994;75:770–777.
28. Agre JC, Grimby G, Rodriquez AA, et al. A comparison of symptoms between Swedish and American post-polio individuals and assessment of lower limb strength—a four-year cohort study. *Scand J Rehabil Med* 1995;27:183–192.
29. Halstead LS, Rossi CD. Post-polio syndrome: clinical experience with 132 consecutive outpatients. *Birth Defects* 1987;23(4):13–26.
30. Halstead LS, Rossi CD. Post-polio syndrome: results of a survey of 539 survivors. *Orthopedics* 1985;8:845–850.
31. Perry J, Fleming C. Polio: long-term problems. *Orthopedics* 1985;8:877–881.
32. Cosgrove JL, Alexander MA, Kitts EL, et al. Late effects of poliomyelitis. *Arch Phys Med Rehabil* 1987;68:4–7.
33. Waring WP, Maynard F, Grady W, et al. Influence of appropriate lower extremity orthotic management on ambulation, pain, and fatigue in a post-polio population. *Arch Phys Med Rehabil* 1989;70:371–375.
34. Einarsson G, Broberg C. *Muscle adaptation and disability in late poliomyelitis* [Thesis]. Goteborg, Sweden: University of Goteborg; 1990.
35. Agre JC. Local muscle and total body fatigue. In: Halstead LS, Grimby G, eds. *Post-polio syndrome.* Philadelphia: Hanley & Belfus, 1995:35–67.
36. Owen RR, Jones D. Polio residuals clinic: conditioning exercise program. *Orthopedics* 1985;8:882–883.
37. Berlly MH, Strauser WW, Hall KM. Fatigue in postpolio syndrome. *Arch Phys Med Rehabil* 1991;72:115–118.
38. Frick NM. Post-polio sequelae and psychology of second disability. *Orthopedics* 1985;8:851–853.
39. Kohl SJ. Emotional responses to the late effects of poliomyelitis. *Birth Defects* 1987;23(4):137–145.
40. Conrady LJ, Wish JR, Agre JC, et al. Psychological characteristics of polio survivors: a preliminary report. *Arch Phys Med Rehabil* 1989;70:458–463.
41. Bruno RL, Frick NM. The psychology of polio as prelude to post-polio sequelae: behavior modification and psychotherapy. *Orthopedics* 1991;14:1185–1193.
42. Bruno RL, Frick NM, Cohen J. Polioencephalitis and the etiology of post-polio sequelae. *Orthopedics* 1991;14(11):1269-1276.
43. Grimby G, Hedberg M, Henning G-B. Changes in muscle morphology, strength, and enzymes in a four–five-year follow-up of subjects with poliomyelitis sequelae. *Scand J Rehabil Med* 1994;26:121–130.
44. Einarsson G, Grimby G. Disability and handicap in late poliomyelitis. *Scand J Rehabil Med* 1990;22:113–121.
45. Hodes HL. Treatment of respiratory difficulty in poliomyelitis. *Papers and discussions presented at the Third International Poliomyelitis Conference.* Philadelphia: JB Lippincott, 1955:91–113.
46. Kaufert PL, Kaufert JM. Methodological and conceptual issues in mea-

suring the long term impact of disability: the experience of poliomyelitis patients in Manitoba. *Soc Sci Med* 1984;19:609–618.

47. Lassen HCA. The epidemic of poliomyelitis in Copenhagen, 1952. *Proc Royal Soc Med* 1953;47:6–71.

48. Halstead LS, Wiechers DO, Rossi CD. Late effects of poliomyelitis: a national survey. In: Halstead LS, Wiechers DO, eds. *Late effects of poliomyelitis*. Miami: Symposia Foundation, 1985:11–31.

49. Speier JL, Owen R, Knapp M, et al. Occurrence of post-polio sequelae in an epidemic population. *Birth Defects* 1987;23(4):39–48.

50. Bach JR, Alba AS. Pulmonary dysfunction and sleep disordered breathing as post-polio sequelae: evaluation and management. *Orthopedics* 1991;14:1329–1337.

51. Fisher DA. Poliomyelitis: late respiratory complications and management. *Orthopedics* 1985;8:891–894.

52. Jones B, Buchholz DW, Ravich WJ, et al. Swallowing dysfunction in the post-polio syndrome: a cinefluorographic study. *AJR Am J Roentgenol* 1992;158:283–286.

53. Coelho CA, Ferranti R. Incidence and nature of dysphagia in polio survivors. *Arch Phys Med Rehabil* 1991;72:1071–1075.

54. Sonies BC, Dalakas MC. Dysphagia in patients with the post-polio syndrome. *N Engl J Med* 1991;324:1162–1167.

55. Cashman NR, Maselli R, Wollman RL, et al. Late denervation in patients with antecedent paralytic poliomyelitis. *N Engl J Med* 1987;317:7–12.

56. Ravits J, Hallett M, Baker M, et al. Clinical and electromyographic studies of postpoliomyelitis muscular atrophy. *Muscle Nerve* 1990;13:667–674.

57. Luciano CA, Sivakumar K, Spector SA, et al. Electrophysiologic and histologic studies in clinically unaffected muscles of patients with prior paralytic poliomyelitis. *Muscle Nerve* 1996;19:1413–1420.

58. Rodriquez AA, Agre JC, Franke TM. Electromyographic and neuromuscular variables in unstable postpolio subjects, stable postpolio subjects, and control subjects. *Arch Phys Med Rehabil* 1997;78:986–991.

59. Grimby G, Stalberg E, Sandberg A, et al. An 8-year longitudinal study of muscle strength, muscle fiber size, and dynamic electromyogram in individuals with late polio. *Muscle Nerve* 1998;21:1428–1437.

60. Grimby G, Einarsson G. Post-polio management. *CRC Crit Rev Phys Med Rehabil* 1991;2:189–200.

61. Agre JC, Rodriquez AA. Intermittent isometric activity: its effect on muscle fatigue in postpolio subjects. *Arch Phys Med Rehabil* 1991;72:971–975.

62. Agre JC. The role of exercise on the patient with post-polio syndrome. *Ann N Y Acad Sci* 1995;753:321–334.

63. Agre JC, Rodriquez AA. Muscular function in late polio and the role of exercise in post-polio patients. *Neurorehabilitation* 1997;8:107–118.

64. Stein DP, D'Ambrosia JM, Dalakas MC. A double-blind, placebo-controlled trial of amantadine for the treatment of fatigue in patients with the post-polio syndrome. *Ann N Y Acad Sci* 1995;753:303–313.

65. Dinsmore ST, D'Ambrosia JM, Dalakas MC. A double-blind placebo-controlled trial of high-dose prednisone for the treatment of post-poliomyelitis syndrome. *Ann N Y Acad Sci* 1995;753:285–295.

66. Trojan DA, Collet J-P, Shapiro S, et al. A multi-center, randomized, double-blinded trial of pyridostigmine in post-polio syndrome. *Neurology* 1999;53:1225–1233.

67. Hyman G. Poliomyelitis. *Lancet* 1953;1:852.

68. Mitchell GP. Poliomyelitis and exercise. *Lancet* 1953;2:90–91.

69. DeLorme TL, Schwab RS, Watkins AL. The response of the quadriceps femoris to progressive resistance exercises in polio myelitic patients. *J Bone Joint Surg Am* 1948;30:834–847.

70. Gurewitsch AD. Intensive graduated exercises in early infantile paralysis. *Arch Phys Med* 1950;31:213–218.

71. Mueller EA, Beckmann H. Die trainierbarkeit von kindern mit gelaehmten muskeln durch isometrische kontraktionen. *Z Orthop* 1966;102:139–145.

72. Einarsson G, Grimby G. Strengthening exercise program in post-polio subjects. In: Halstead LS, Wiechers DO, eds. *Research and clinical aspects of the late effects of poliomyelitis*. White Plains, NY: March of Dimes Birth Defects Foundation, 1987:275–283.

73. Fillyaw MJ, Badger GJ, Goodwin GD, et al. The effects of long-term non-fatiguing resistance exercise in subjects with post-polio syndrome. *Orthopedics* 1991;14:1253–1256.

74. Spector SA, Gordon PL, Feuerstein IM, et al. Strength gains without muscle injury after strength training in patients with post-polio muscular atrophy. *Muscle Nerve* 1996;19:1282–1290.

75. Agre JC, Rodriquez AA, Franke TM. Strength, endurance, and work capacity after muscle strengthening exercise in postpolio subjects. *Arch Phys Med Rehabil* 1997;78:681–686.

76. Owen RR, Jones DR. Polio residuals clinic: conditioning exercise program. *Orthopedics* 1985;8:882–883.

77. Jones DR, Speier J, Canine K, et al. Cardiorespiratory responses to aerobic training by patients with post-poliomyelitis sequelae. *JAMA* 1989;261:3255–3258.

78. Kriz JL, Jones DR, Speier J, et al. Cardiorespiratory responses to upper extremity aerobic training by post-polio subjects. *Arch Phys Med Rehabil* 1992;73:49–54.

79. Ernstoff B, Wetterqvist H, Kvist H, et al. Endurance training effect on individuals with postpoliomyelitis. *Arch Phys Med Rehabil* 1996;77:843–848.

80. Prins JH, Hartung H, Merritt DJ, et al. Effect of aquatic exercise training in persons with poliomyelitis disability. *Sports Med Train Rehabil* 1994;5:29–39.

81. Willen C. *Physical performance and the effects of dynamic exercise in water in individuals with late polio* [Dissertation]. Goteborg, Sweden: Goteborg University; 1999.

82. Buckholtz DW, Jones B. Post-polio dysphagia: alarm or caution. *Orthopedics* 1991;14:1303–1304.

83. Young GR. Occupational therapy and the post-polio syndrome. *Am J Occup Ther* 1989;43:97–103.

ACUTE AND CHRONIC INFLAMMATORY DEMYELINATING POLYNEUROPATHIES

JAY M. MEYTHALER

INCIDENCE AND IMPORTANCE

Guillain-Barré syndrome (GBS) is an immunopathy associated with an acute often fulminate evolution of a demyelinating inflammatory polyradiculoneuropathy (1–7). GBS is the most common cause of acute nontraumatic neuromuscular paralysis in developed countries, afflicting 2 to 4 per 100,000 persons annually (1,2,3,6). This translates into 5,000 to 6,000 new cases per year in the United States (1,2,3). With the reduction in worldwide poliomyelitis cases, it is estimated to be the most common cause of acute neuromuscular paralysis in the world. Between 1985 and 1990, the estimated death rate was 628 cases per year (6–8). However, with an approximate 5,000 new cases per year and an expected poor outcome of 20% with regard to mobility or pulmonary function in those who survive, one can conclude this is a significant and understudied cause of disability (1–8). Therefore, GBS is a significant cause of long-term disability for at least 1,000 persons per year in the United States and many more elsewhere (8). However, given the young age at which GBS can occur, it is likely that at least 25,000, and perhaps as many as 50,000 persons, in the United States have residual functional deficits of GBS at this time (8). The resultant economic cost of GBS within the United States is estimated to be $2 to $3 billion annually (6).

Although the disease is primarily demyelinating in nature, a primary axonal variety of GBS has been described (9,10). This variety is linked predominately to *Campylobacter jejuni* infections and is estimated to cause less than one third of the cases of GBS in the United States and the developed world. However, it may account for up to two thirds of cases in less-developed countries.

Chronic demyelinating polyneuropathies have an incidence of at least 1,000 new cases per year within the United States (9). These other inflammatory polyneuropathic syndromes present with many of the same clinical and diagnostic findings of GBS including chronic inflammatory demyelinating polyneuropathy (CIDP), autoimmune neuropathies due to connective tissue diseases, cancer, toxic neuropathies, and hormonal and metabolic neuropathies (10–13). The greatest diagnostic controversy surrounds CIDP and relapsing inflammatory polyneuropa-

thy, which are considered by some to be separable from GBS (9,10,14,15). What is important from a rehabilitation point of view is that the clinical course may vary considerably in these other presentations from those of classically described GBS, so an accurate diagnosis and prognosis is important. Clinically, the major differences between the two entities include the time course, some of the clinical signs, and their response to various treatments (16). CIDP is usually differentiated from the other two most common chronic demyelinating polyneuropathies, multifocal motor neuropathy (MMN) and paraproteinemia (16). The paraproteinemic neuropathies, which include the monoclonal gammopathies, account for approximately 10% of neuropathies of unknown etiology (17).

When all inflammatory polyneuropathies are combined, they have an incidence rate, mortality rate, and direct economic cost similar to those attributed to spinal cord injury (SCI). Yet the amount of attention paid to the disease process of inflammatory polyneuropathies does not even begin to approximate that focused on SCI. Although this chapter focuses predominately on GBS, we do mention other inflammatory polyneuropathies, particularly CIDP, MMN, and paraproteinemic neuropathy.

CLINICAL PRESENTATION

Ascending paralytic illness has been recognized for centuries, but it was Osler (18) who offered the first reasonable clinical description. Years later, Guillain et al. (19) published a report in which the syndrome of a radiculoneuritis associated with elevated protein level in the cerebrospinal fluid (CSF) without a "cellular reaction" was more adequately described. Still, the definition of GBS is based on clinical presentation.

Briefly phrased, GBS is an immunopathy with an acute, often fulminate evolution of a demyelinating inflammatory polyradiculoneuropathy (7). There are three general phases to the disease; a progressive or acute phase, a plateau phase, and a recovery phase. The acute onset is followed by a devastating acute course that may take a person from being absolutely healthy to being bedridden and respirator dependent within 2 or 3 days. The progression usually occurs over 10 to 12 days before a plateau is reached, which is followed by gradual recovery. Some patients

TABLE 37.1. FEATURES REQUIRED FOR THE DIAGNOSIS OF GUILLAIN-BARRÉ SYNDROME

Features Required for Diagnosis	Features Strongly Supportive of the Diagnosis
A. Progressive motor weakness of more than one limb. The degree ranges from minimal weakness of the legs, with or without mild ataxia, to total paralysis of the muscles of all four extremities and the trunk, bulbar and facial paralysis, and external ophthalmoplegia. B. Areflexia (loss of tendon jerks). Universal areflexia is the rule, although distal areflexia with definite hyporeflexia of the biceps and knee jerks will suffice if other features are consistent.	A. Clinical features (ranked in order of importance) 1. Progression; Symptoms and signs of motor weakness develop rapidly but cease to progress by 4 wk into the illness. Approximately 50% will reach the nadir by 2 wk, 80% by 3 wk, and more than 90% by 4 wk. 2. Relative symmetry. Symmetry is seldom absolute, but usually, if one limb is affected, the opposite is as well. 3. Mild sensory symptoms or signs. 4. Cranial nerve involvement. Facial weakness occurs in approximately 50% and is frequently bilateral. Other cranial nerves may be involved, particularly those innervating the tongue and muscles of deglutition and sometimes the extraocular motor nerves. On occasion (less than 5%), the neuropathy may begin in the nerves to the extraocular muscles or other cranial nerves. 5. Recovery. It usually begins 2–4 wk after progression stops. Recovery may be delayed for months. Most patients recover functionally. 6. Autonomic dysfunction. Tachycardia and other arrhythmias, postural hypotension, hypertension, and vasomotor symptoms, when present, support the diagnosis. These findings may fluctuate. Care must be exercised to exclude other bases for these symptoms, such as pulmonary embolism. 7. Absence of fever at the onset of neuritic symptoms. B. Cerebrospinal fluid (CSF) examination features strongly supportive of the diagnosis 1. CSF protein. After the first week of symptoms, CSF protein is elevated or has been shown to rise on serial lumbar punctures. 2. CSF cells. Counts of 10 or fewer mononuclear leukocytes/mm^3 in CSF.

From Asbury AK, Cornblath DL. Assessment of current diagnostic criteria for Guillain-Barré syndrome. *Ann Neurol* 1990;27:521–524, with permission.

may have a stuttering onset, whereas others may present with a rather slow progression that can take place over a few weeks (20). The duration of the illness is usually less than 12 weeks in most patients, with most expected to a have a favorable outcome (generally, this is equated to mean ambulation without assistive devices) (1). There is almost a 2:1 preponderance toward men (1), although this has been questioned (21).

Symptoms usually occur approximately 2 to 4 weeks before the onset of weakness (Table 37.1). About 40% to 60% of the patients have some antecedent infectious process (8,10). Most commonly, patients describe a nonspecific or "flulike" upper respiratory infection (1). Gastrointestinal illnesses, often relatively mild, are reported as the second most common type of illness (1). Viruses that have been most often implicated are cytomegalovirus and Epstein-Barr virus (1,22). Surgical procedures and trauma are predisposing events in a small percentage of patients, certainly less than 2% or 3% (20). Flu vaccines have been implicated in some cases (11,20), and more recently human immunodeficiency virus has been implicated in the development of GBS (22). *C. jejuni* enteritis has recently been recognized as an important preliminary disease (10) and has been linked to the more severe axonal variety (23). Epidural anesthesia and drugs, including thrombolytic agents and heroin, have been associated with a few cases (10). Underlying systemic diseases, such as lupus erythematosus, sarcoidosis, Hodgkin disease, and other neoplasms, have been recognized to cause a small number of "symptomatic" cases of GBS (10,12).

Acute GBS typically begins with fine paresthesias in the toes or fingertips and extends proximally over hours to a few days. This is followed within days by the major clinical manifestation, ascending often symmetric weakness, which evolves over a pe-

riod of several days. Leg weakness may make walking and climbing stairs difficult. In some cases, facial and oropharyngeal weakness may develop (12,24).

Early in the course of illness, there are many clinical features that lead one to suspect the disease. Initially, the patient will demonstrate approximately symmetric limb weakness, absent or greatly diminished tendon reflexes, and minimal loss of sensation despite the paresthesias (10). When sensory loss is present, deep sensibility tends to be more affected than superficial. Pain is common, presenting as either a bilateral sciatica or an aching in large muscles of the upper legs, flanks, or back (25). Weakness of the facial muscles occurs in about one third of all cases (10). In severe cases, the disease progresses to affect respiration and may result in cranial nerve palsies, with associated functional losses in eye movements and deglutition (10). Disturbances of clinical autonomic function develop and can vary from sinus tachycardia, bradycardia, facial flushing, fluctuating hypertension or hypotension, loss of sweating, or episodic profuse diaphoresis. It has been recently reported that cardiac arrhythmias may be a leading cause of death in GBS (10). These disturbances have recently been demonstrated to occur up to several weeks from the initial onset and they often do not manifest until the patient begins to be physiologically stressed in rehabilitative therapies.

The many clinical variants of GBS, which may cause diagnostic difficulty, include Fisher syndrome, which involves ophthalmoplegia, ataxia, and areflexia with little weakness and accounts for approximately 5% of the cases (26,12). Other variants present as weakness without paresthesias or sensory loss (3%); isolated weakness of the arm and oropharynx or the leg (3%);

bilateral weakness of facial muscles with distal paresthesias (1%); severe ataxia and sensory loss (1%); acute dysautonomia, an autonomic polyneuropathy often combined with sensory features (less than 1%); and "axonal" GBS with rapid, almost complete paralysis and electrically inexcitable motor nerves (20%) (9,10, 12,26–29). The effects of these many "subtypes" on the ultimate functional outcome or disability of these afflicted patients are not sufficiently described in the literature. Approximately 10% of patients will have minor relapses, but these relapses do not appear to affect the prognosis (10,21).

In CIDP, cranial nerve involvement, autonomic dysfunction, and antecedent infections are rare (30). In MMN, the CSF protein level is within the reference range and the conduction block is predominately along the distribution of the motor nerves with little involvement of the sensory nerves (15,16). In paraproteinemic neuropathies, there is an immunoglobulin-mediated demyelinating polyneuropathy associated with antimyelin-associated glycoprotein antibodies. Most of the patients present with a prominent sensory ataxia that has a very slow onset and progression, usually over years rather than months (16).

ELECTROMYOGRAPHIC AND LABORATORY FINDINGS

A confirmatory workup should include an examination of CSF, which usually reveals a normal pressure, few or no cells, and a protein concentration of more than 0.55 g/L after the first week of illness in GBS (10). Usually the protein content is within the reference range in the first few days that symptoms are present and then rises, reaching a peak at 4 to 6 weeks. High values have no prognostic significance. In cases of GBS variants, there is a high proportion of persistent reference-ranged protein values. The CSF protein concentration can be elevated in cases of CIDP (31). In contrast, with MMN, the CSF protein concentration is usually within the reference range (16).

Abnormalities of nerve conduction and late responses (f waves and H reflex), reflecting demyelination, are the most sensitive and most specific laboratory findings in inflammatory polyneuropathies. Abnormalities are seen in affected limbs within days of symptomatology. Often enough information can be determined so CSF analysis may not be required. There are proposed diagnostic criteria for the demyelinating versions of the disease (11) (Table 37.2).

Electrodiagnostic and physiologic parameters in GBS associated with a poor outcome include the following:

1. summed motor velocity less than 80% of normal
2. summed proximal motor amplitude less than 20% of normal
3. summed distal motor amplitude less than 20% of normal (20)

A primary axonal variety of GBS has been described (26), which may account for part of the discrepancy between the

TABLE 37.2. ELECTRODIAGNOSTIC STUDIES FOR THE DIAGNOSIS OF CHRONIC INFLAMMATORY DEMYELINATING POLYNEUROPATHY

Mandatory	Supportive
Nerve conduction studies including studies of proximal nerve segments in which the predominant process is demyelination.	1. Reduction in sensory CV <80% of LLN. 2. Absent H reflexes.

Must have three of four of the following:

1. Reduction in conduction velocity (CV) in two or more motor nerves.
   a. <80% of lower limit of normal (LLN) if amplitude >80% of LLN.
   b. <70% of LLN if amplitude <80% of LLN.

2. Partial conduction block or abnormal temporal dispersion in one or more motor nerves: either peroneal nerve between ankle and below fibular head, median nerve between wrist and elbow, or ulnar nerve between wrist and below elbow.

   Criteria suggestive of partial conduction block:
   <15% change in duration between proximal and distal sites and >20% drop in negative-peak area or peak-to-peak (p-p) amplitude between proximal and distal sites.
   Criteria for abnormal temporal dispersion and possible conduction block: >15% change in duration between proximal and distal sites and >20% drop in negative-peak area or p-p amplitude between proximal and distal sites. These criteria are only suggestive of partial conduction block because they are derived from studies on normal individuals. Additional studies, such as stimulation across short segments or recording of individual motor unit potentials, are required for confirmation.

3. Prolonged distal latencies in two or more nerves:
   a. >125% of upper limit of normal (ULN) if amplitude >80% of LLN.
   b. >150% of ULN if amplitude <80% of LLN.

4. Absent F waves or prolonged minimum F-wave latencies (10 to 15 trials) in two or more motor nerves:
   a. >120% of ULN if amplitude >80% of LLN.
   b. >150% of ULN if amplitude <80% of LLN.

From Ad Hoc Subcommittee of the American Academy of Neurology AIDS Task Force. Research criteria for diagnosis of chronic inflammatory demyelinating polyneuropathy (CIDP). *Neurology* 1991;41:617–618, with permission.

clinical diagnostic criteria and the electrodiagnostic criteria. The current proposed electrodiagnostic criteria for GBS are for the demyelinating versions of the disease and do not cover the primary axonal variety (32).

In CIDP, electrophysiologic studies are similar to those initially described for GBS (Table 37.2B) (15,32).

Patients with MMN have no objective sensory abnormalities on nerve conduction studies (NCSs). A subset of MMN has been described that has had demonstrable sensory findings with NCS (31). There usually is a conduction block along the distribution of the motor nerves (16). However, these patients are now thought to have variant of CIDP (31).

DIFFERENTIAL DIAGNOSIS

The separation of CIDP from GBS is based on the clinical time course. In CIDP, the duration of progression should be at least 2 months, whereas the disease nadir for GBS should be reached within 4 weeks (14). This leaves a gap of 4 weeks where there has been some clinical confusion (14). CIDP is similar to GBS in that it is a widespread polyradiculoneuropathy, with similar demyelinating characteristics on electrodiagnostic studies. However, CIDP is more often asymmetric and has a more fluctuating course, a persistent relapsing or slow progression over time.

Other differences include CIDP's responsiveness to steroids and less frequent antecedent infections identified.

CIDP is generally separated from MMN because the latter is usually characterized by asymmetric weakness with motor conduction blocks in the afflicted nerves and a strong association with antibodies against G_{M1} gangliosides (14,16,31).

The clinical features required for diagnosis of inflammatory polyneuropathies are only a progressive motor weakness of more than one limb and areflexia (10). Hence, the clinical course and the pattern of weakness generally determine the differential diagnosis of these similar syndromes and diseases. The most commonly confused diseases or syndromes with inflammatory polyneuropathies include spinal cord compression, transverse myelitis, myasthenia gravis, basilar artery occlusion, neoplastic meningitis, vasculitic neuropathy, polymyositis, metabolic myopathies, and paraneoplastic neuropathy (10). Other diagnoses that can be confused with GBS include hypophosphatemia, heavy-metal intoxication, neurotoxic fish poisoning, botulism, poliomyelitis, and tick paralysis (10).

CLINICAL AND PATHOPHYSIOLOGIC MODELS

Pathologically GBS and CIDP are inflammatory polyradiculoneuropathies that resemble experimental allergic neuritis (EAN)

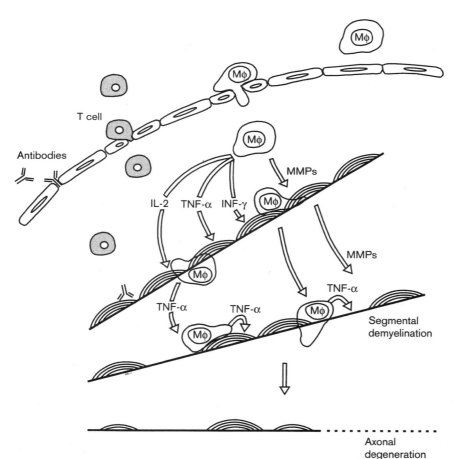

FIGURE 37.1. Diagrammatic scheme of the main cellular elements that seem to play a role in the inflammatory polyneuropathies. (From Dalakas MC. Advances in chronic inflammatory demyelinating polyneuropathy: disease variants and inflammatory response mediators and modifiers. *Curr Opin Neurol* 1999;12:403–409, with permission.)

in animals (14,33). Both EAN and GBS share common histopathologic features characterized by the presence of perivascular mononuclear cell inflammation, demyelination, and edema. Experiments in various animal models have clearly demonstrated that the sensitization of T lymphocytes of the CD4 subclass to proteins in the myelin sheath is necessary for disease induction (33). The principle electrophysiologic finding that accounts for the weakness noted in inflammatory polyneuropathies, at least early in the disease, is the conduction block produced when a portion of the axon fails to transmit impulses in a segment in which myelin has been destroyed or rendered nonfunctional (Fig. 37.1) (34).

Recently, the presence of antiganglioside antibodies, such as antiganglioside G_{M1} antibodies or antiganglioside G_{Q1b} antibodies, has been associated with axonal damage and a poorer outcome (35). G_{M1} gangliosides are used experimentally to promote recovery in SCI and a link has been suggested between the use of gangliosides and GBS but has not been clearly established (36–39). However, a link has been proposed between the presence of immunoglobulin G (IgG) anti-G_{D1a} and anti-G_{M1} antibodies and a more severe presentation of GBS (40,41), so this issue may affect the use of G_{M1} gangliosides.

Cellular and humoral factors have been implicated in CIDP (Table 37.3) similar to those involved with GBS (17). However, there are some differences. It has been demonstrated that patients with CIDP often present with high titers of IgG or immunoglobulin M (IgM) antibodies to acidic glycolipids, but not to sulfated glycolipids (Table 37.4) (16). Antibodies to peripheral myelin protein also have been noted. The role of these antibodies is unclear. However, it is theorized that activated T cells and macrophages release cytokines that upregulate various adhesion

TABLE 37.3. PATHOLOGIC FEATURES OF CHRONIC INFLAMMATORY DEMYELINATING POLYNEUROPATHY

A. Mandatory
  Nerve biopsy showing unequivocal evidence of demyelination and remyelination
  1. Demyelination by either electron microscopy (>5 fibers) or teased fiber studies (>12% of 50 teased fibers, minimum of four internodes each, demonstrating demyelination-remyelination).
B. Supportive
  1. Subperineurial or endoneurial edema.
  2. Mononuclear cell infiltration.
  3. "Onion-bulb" formation.
  4. Prominent variation in the degree of demyelination between fascicles.
C. Exclusion
  1. Vasculitis, neurofilamentous swollen axons, amyloid deposits, or intracytoplasmic inclusions in Schwann cells or macrophages indicating adrenoleukodystrophy, metachromatic, leukodystrophy, globoid cell leukodystrophy, or other evidence of specific pathology.
  Cerebrospinal fluid studies
A. Mandatory
  1. Cell count <10/mm³ if HIV seronegative or <50/mm³ if HIV seropositive.
  2. Negative Venereal Disease Research Laboratories test results.
B. Supportive
  1. Elevated protein level.

HIV, human immunodeficiency virus.

TABLE 37.4. LABORATORY STUDIES ON CHRONIC INFLAMMATORY DEMYELINATING POLYNEUROPATHY

The following studies are suggested: complete blood cell count, erythrocyte sedimentation rate, SMA6/12, creatine kinase, antinuclear antibody, thyroid functions, serum and urine immunoglobulin studies (to include either immunofixation electrophoresis or immunoelectrophoresis), HIV, and hepatitis serology. The list of laboratory studies is not comprehensive. In certain clinical circumstances, other studies may be indicated, such as phytanic acid, long-chain fatty acids, porphyrins, urine heavy metals, α-lipoprotein, β-lipoprotein, glucose tolerance test, imaging studies of the central nervous system, and lymph node or bone marrow biopsy.

Depending on the results of the laboratory tests, patients meeting the criteria can be classified into the groups listed here.
A. Idiopathic CIDP: no concurrent disease
B. Concurrent diseases with CIDP (depending on laboratory studies or other clinical features):
  1. Systemic lupus erythematosus.
  2. HIV infection.
  3. Monoclonal or biclonal gammopathy (macroglobulinemia, POEMS syndrome, osteosclerotic myeloma).
  4. Castleman disease.
  5. Monoclonal gammopathies of undetermined significance.
  6. Diabetes.
  7. Central nervous system demyelinating disease.

CIDP, chronic inflammatory demyelinating polyneuropathy; HIV, human immunodeficiency virus; POEMS syndrome, polyneuropathy, organomegaly, endocrinopathy, monoclonal gammopathy, and skin changes; SMAG/12, serum metabolic assessment.

TABLE 37.5. PROPOSAL FOR CRITERIA FOR DEMYELINATING POLYNEUROPATHY FOR MGUs

A casual relation between demyelinating polyneuropathy and MGUs should be considered in a patient with
  (1) Demyelinating polyneuropathy according to the electrodiagnostic AAN criteria for idopathic CIDP
  (2) Presence of an M protein (IgM, IgG, or IgA), without evidence of malignant plasma cell dyscrasias such as multiple myeloma, lymphoma, Walderstrom macroglobulinemia, or amyloidosis
  (3) Family history negative for neuropathy
  (4) Age >30 yr

The relation is definite when the following is present:
  (1) IgM M protein with anti-MAG antibodies

The relation is probable when at least three of the following are present in a patient without anti-MAG antibodies:
  (1) Time to peak of the neuropathy >2 yr
  (2) Chronic slowly progressive course without relapsing or remitting periods
  (3) Symmetric distal polyneuropathy
  (4) Sensory symptoms and signs predominate over motor features

A casual relation is unlikely when at least three of the following are present in a patient without anti-MAG antibodies:
  (1) Median time to peak of the neuropathy is within 1 yr
  (2) Clinical course is relapsing and remitting or monophasic
  (3) Cranial nerves are involved
  (4) Neuropathy is asymmetric
  (5) Motor symptoms and signs predominate
  (6) History of preceding infection
  (7) Presence of abnormal median SNAP in combination with normal sural SNAP

AAN, American Academy of Neurology; CIDP, chronic inflammatory demyelinating polyneuropathy; MGU, monoclonal gamopathies; SNAP, sensory nerve action potential.

molecules (adhesion molecule-1, E-selectin, vascular cell adhesion molecule-1) on the endothelial walls and initiate breakdown of the blood–nerve barrier (16). The result is theorized to be similar to the models of GBS with a localized increase in putative antibodies, complement, activated T cells, macrophages, and cytokines. Among the cytokines, interferon gamma, interleukin-2, and tumor necrosis factor alpha have been implicated in the final common pathway for GBS, CIDP, MMN, and paraproteinemic neuropathies causing demyelination.

Paraproteinemic neuropathy including monoclonal gammopathy has typically been associated with IgG M proteins and immunoglobulin A (IgA) M proteins, IgM M proteins, often associated with Waldenstrom macroglobulinemia, non-Hodgkin B-cell lymphoma, and chronic B-cell lymphocytic leukemia (17). The rate of malignant transformation in the paraproteinemic neuropathies is estimated to be 2% (Table 37.5) (17).

TREATMENT

It is clear that progress is being made in the treatment of GBS. It has been suggested that improved survival has been related to the use of special care units experienced in handling the complications of the disease (10). Most of these special care units are located in regional medical centers and appear to admit most cases. Many patients with GBS die of avoidable medical complications such as sepsis, adult respiratory distress syndrome, pulmonary emboli (usually secondary to deep venous thrombosis [DVT]), or cardiac arrest that is perhaps related to dysautonomia. It is thought that with appropriate medical supportive care, the rate of mortality could be reduced to less than 5% (10).

Plasmapheresis and intravenous immunoglobulin (IVIg) are now the accepted therapies for GBS (42–44). The North American and French prospective, randomized clinical trials clearly demonstrate that plasmapheresis shortens the time to achieve independent walking and the time a patient stays on a respiratory support. In addition, plasmapheresis is reported to improve functional improvement with regard to mobility at 6 months (42–44). Plasma exchange removes a total of 200 to 250 mL/kg in five to six treatments performed every other day, with replacement of saline and 5% albumin.

Besides plasmapheresis, another alternative treatment is the use of IVIg (45). Infusion of immunoglobulin has been associated with a beneficial outcome in other immunologically mediated diseases (20,34). The usual dosage is 0.4 g/kg daily for 5 consecutive days. Results from a prospective, randomized Dutch trial of 100 patients with GBS treated with IVIg suggest that IVIg is at least as good as, if not better than, plasmapheresis (46). Furthermore, due to the shorter duration of treatment, in general 5 days for IVIg and 10 days for plasmapheresis, it has been favored to reduce the length of time in the acute care setting for those who have not developed ventilatory dependence. However, there have been reports of high incidences of relapse after IVIg (35). Although treatment with plasma exchange and immunoglobulins has decreased the duration of mechanical ventilation by half, GBS still remains the most common cause of acute neuromuscular ventilatory failure (47).

The use of steroids in acute GBS has been controversial (48).

Their use was based on promising trials with EAN in animals (49). In early clinical trials with humans, it was suggested that steroids were useful in decreasing the severity of illness (48). However, in a large randomized prospective study of 242 patients treated with 500 mg of methylprednisolone, it was concluded that steroids were ineffective (2).

CIDP, MMN, and paraproteinemias have also responded to IVIg and plasmapheresis (14,16,17). CIDP has been distinguished by its responsiveness to steroids (9,14). In one controlled study comparing plasma exchange with IVIg, both were found to be beneficial (9). Furthermore, in resistant cases, there has been some success with the use of interferon alpha, cyclosporine, azathioprine, and cyclophosphamide. In contrast, MMN generally has not been responsive to steroids (16). Paraproteinemic neuropathy has been responsive to prednisone in those patients with nonmalignant IgG or IgA monoclonal gammopathies that have been demyelinating. Most other cases of paraproteinemic neuropathies have not been responsive to steroids. Paraproteinemic neuropathies have been responsive to anti–B-cell reagents such as fludarabine, chlorambucil, or cyclophosphamide (Cytoxan), which reduce the M-protein concentration (17).

CLINICAL COURSE

The course of illness may be more prolonged in adults, particularly older adults, than in children (20). Persons who have suffered GBS may continue to improve for up to 2 years after injury (50,51), although there is little information, besides general descriptions about the rate or variability of the neurologic recovery. Prognostic factors with regard to a poor outcome recently identified in a North American study were older age, requirement for respiratory support, rate of progression, abnormal physiologic characteristics of peripheral nerve function, or if no plasmapheresis was performed (20,52). There has been no correlation between recovery from GBS and sex, occupation, the presence of diabetes mellitus, previous steroid usage, or prior immunization (20,53).

The point of maximal neurologic dysfunction is reported as the "disease nadir" (20). The average period from the clinical onset of symptoms to nadir of illness is 8 days (1). The point of time before or at disease nadir has frequently been considered critical with regard to the success of therapeutic interventions using plasmapheresis or IVIg (20), but this has never been established and in one study did not correlate with outcome (54). Yet many institutions will not intervene with plasmapheresis or IVIg if the patient has already begun to obtain neurologic recovery or has not deteriorated neurologically for several days. More work is necessary to delineate whether late intervention after the point of disease nadir is useful. By definition, GBS should reach its maximal nadir within 4 weeks, although most cases will reach nadir within 2 weeks (9,14,15). In contrast, CIDP usually has a duration of progression of more than 2 months (14).

In our experience, patients with GBS who were so severely involved that they required admission to inpatient rehabilitation had an extended period to disease nadir. Clearly, patients with GBS requiring inpatient rehabilitation are the more severely involved cases. The development of relapses may be related to a more extended course of the disease in these patients. Frequent neurologic evaluations will detect the development of relapses, and intervention with plasmapheresis or IVIg may be of therapeutic benefit.

There are multiple medical complications that may develop from inflammatory polyneuropathies. Many of these complications may persist for some time, interfering with rehabilitation or even leading to permanent functional deficits. The course of CIDP, MMN, and paraproteinemic neuropathy has been one of progressive motor weakness. In CIDP and paraproteinemic neuropathy, there can be the development of ataxia as well. Paraproteinemic neuropathy has recently been associated with the eventual development of tremors in most patients (17,55).

Requirement of Ventilatory Support

There has been significant research on the predisposing factors in GBS for the requirement of ventilatory support (21,30). Respiratory failure and pneumonia may be noted in 30% of patients in the acute phases of illness (first 12 weeks), but many will have adequate recovery of their respiratory function (10). Up to 30% of these patients will develop pneumonia (10). Those who do not have full respiratory recovery may have complications leading to long-term morbidity secondary to antecedent chronic obstructive disease, restrictive pulmonary disease from pulmonary scarring secondary to pneumonia, tracheitis from chronic intubation, or respiratory musculature insufficiency (56).

It has been noted that the presence of autonomic dysfunction has a relationship with the requirement of ventilatory support (12,21,24). In epidemiological studies, it is estimated that 10% to 30% of patients will require mechanical ventilation, 5% to 10% will remain seriously disabled, and 3% to 8% will die (8, 21,47). Intubation should be considered when the vital capacity falls to less than 18 mL/kg (10). During the acute phase, the vital capacity should be measured frequently, to monitor for respiratory muscle weakness. The requirement of ventilatory support correlates with outcome as evaluated by ambulatory function and motor functional status (21,24). More recently, the requirement of ventilatory support has been associated with the severity of damage to the peripheral nervous system and has been correlated with longer lengths of stay and increased costs for inpatient rehabilitation (21,53).

In CIDP, MMN, and paraproteinemic neuropathy, there usually is not a problem with patients becoming dependent on ventilators. There are rare cases when this occurs, but this is not frequent (14,57).

Thromboembolic Disorders

DVT is believed to be common in GBS (56); however, the incidence of DVT in GBS has never been systematically studied. Predisposing factors such as the severity of disease or the length of immobilization have not been well delineated (58). In one early study, pulmonary embolus was thought to occur in up to one third of patients who suffered from GBS (58). The prophylactic treatment for DVT is recommended (10,56) based on judgments that immobilization will lead to an increased incidence as predicted by Virchow's triad (59). The incidence of DVT in the other inflammatory polyneuropathies is unknown.

Dysautonomia

Orthostatic hypotension, unstable blood pressure, or abnormal heart rates indicate dysautonomia in GBS. These indications have recently been expanded to include bowel and bladder dysfunction (60). Autonomic dysfunction of the cardiovascular system without bladder and bowel dysfunction has a relationship with the requirement of ventilatory support (12,21,24,61,62). In previous epidemiological studies, dysautonomia has been noted to be present in particularly severe versions of GBS, extending the acute care length of stay (61,62), and is felt to be clinically related to life-threatening cardiac arrhythmias (60). Urologic dysfunction may develop early in the disease process but is felt to resolve in most cases; however, this conclusion appears to be based totally on anecdotal evidence (10,11). Some men will develop residual impotence (10). Dysautonomia has been linked to cardiac arrhythmias, cardiovascular collapse, and death in various case reports of GBS (60). In one case series of 100 patients, 11 developed cardiac arrhythmias sufficient to compromise their circulation and 7 of the 11 died (61). Despite the recent attention to dysautonomia and its relevance to both morbidity and mortality (61), there have been no prospective studies on predicting its onset or evaluating various interventions to limit its impact. One recent report suggests that the incidence of dysautonomia associated with bowel or bladder dysfunction is not statistically related to dysautonomia that involves the cardiovascular system (63). Considering the close statistical interaction between dysautonomia that involves the cardiopulmonary system and the requirement for ventilatory support, the use of beta blockade for prophylaxis in this subgroup should be considered (21,63).

In the other inflammatory polyneuropathies, the incidence of dysautonomia is considered to be much rarer but nevertheless remains a possible complication.

Pain and Sensory Involvement

Most reports of GBS describe pain as a prominent clinical feature of the diagnosis and it has been reported to be the sole initial presenting symptom in some cases (64). The types of pain described include paraesthesia, dysesthesia, axial and radicular pain, meningism, myalgia, joint pain, and visceral discomfort (65). In one small prospective study, pain was reported in 55% of the patients in the acute stages of the illness and in 72% of the patients when evaluated throughout the course of illness (25).

Immobilization

Patients with inflammatory polyneuropathy may be hypotonic or totally immobilized from quadriplegia. They have been reported to develop complications of decubitus ulcers, tendon shortening, joint contractures, and malalignment, as well as peroneal nerve palsies (10). Yet, the treatment approach has been similar to many patients who have an upper motor neuron lesion such as those with SCI or traumatic brain injury (TBI). What is unknown is how these medical complications and functional deficits affect the final disability of these patients. The incidence of immobilization on the development of functional deficits is not well understood in GBS. Can the same treatment milieu be used in this lower motor neuron disease when the predisposing factors and impact of these therapies are not well delineated?

Dysfunction of bone and calcium metabolism can occur in GBS (8). Hypercalcemia of immobilization of such a severe nature that it requires aggressive medical intervention has been noted in a few case reports of GBS (66,67). Rare cases of heterotopic ossification have also been reported in GBS (8,66,68). The incidences of both of these conditions have not been studied in GBS and are thought to be the result of prolonged immobilization (52,69). Treatment for both of these conditions is based on the experience gleaned from case studies and experience with other conditions that cause hypercalcemia of immobilization or heterotopic ossification (66,67).

Anemia

Anemia in persons with GBS with severe involvement requiring inpatient rehabilitation is more common than that found in the corresponding spinal cord population (70,71). The anemia was originally believed to be related to immobilization (21). This assumption was based on studies of the effects of immobilization in healthy male subjects who were confined to bed rest; the studies revealed that the red blood cell count and reticulocyte count declined slowly over 5 weeks (72,73). In a retrospective study, 79% of persons admitted to acute inpatient rehabilitation due to GBS had anemia with hematocrit and hemoglobin levels two standard deviations below the mean (21,70).

In two retrospective studies, patients with a history of undergoing plasmapheresis had higher mean hemoglobin and hematocrit levels (21,70). All these changes reversed with mobilization in one study (21). Plasmapheresis may play a factor, by reducing inflammatory immunoglobulins that may interact with bone marrow precursors (21,70). More recent evidence points to the effects of IVIg, which appears to have some bone marrow suppressive effects (63).

It has been suggested that correcting anemia may aid in the treatment of orthostatic hypotension in persons with GBS (74). However, anemia appears not to relate to rehabilitation outcome or length of stay for those persons with severe involvement requiring inpatient rehabilitation (70).

Cranial Nerve Involvement

Cranial nerve involvement has been described in the more-severe cases of GBS (12,24). The most commonly involved cranial nerve is the facial nerve (cranial nerve VII), with a resultant Bell palsy, but almost every cranial nerve has been implicated (8). Studies have indicated that cranial nerve involvement was associated with an increased total length of hospital stay (acute and rehabilitation combined) for those persons with such severe involvement that they require inpatient rehabilitation (21,53). There has also been an association between cranial nerve involvement and the incidence of dysautonomia that involves the cardiovascular system. In previous studies, cranial nerve involvement was associated with a prolonged duration to reach the plateau phase of illness but did not independently predict future motor deficit (21,24). Cranial nerve involvement may result in dysphagia, bilateral vocal cord paralysis, optic neuritis, and hearing loss (12,24,75–78).

Cranial nerve involvement may develop in CIDP, but it is rare in both MMN and paraproteinemic neuropathy (16,17).

REHABILITATION INVOLVEMENT BEFORE ADMISSION TO THE REHABILITATION UNIT

It must be stressed that rehabilitation of the patient should start before admission to the rehabilitation unit. Many of the problems these patients present with are those listed in the next section of this chapter. However, early attention to cranial nerve involvement is important. Some suggestions include using patches or taping the eyes at night with the use of eyedrops or ointment to prevent dryness; bowel care to prevent constipation; oral hygiene; attention to proper nutrition; skin care with the prescription of frequent turning and a proper mattress; DVT prophylaxis; and orthotic management to prevent contractures. Attention to pain and the proper prescription of medication and therapeutics may relieve considerable psychological and emotional distress.

REHABILITATION

Approximately 40% of the patients who are hospitalized with GBS will require admission to inpatient rehabilitation (8,50, 53). With the recent use of increased plasmapheresis with early transfer to rehabilitation, there are suggestions that the number of patients referred for acute inpatient rehabilitation has increased substantially. Those referred for inpatient rehabilitation are generally considered those that have more severely involved disease. One study describes an incidence of persistent motor weakness in 54% of these patients, ranging from monoplegia to tetraplegia (50). Although it is clear that rehabilitation requires an organized program with defined endpoints, no long-term rehabilitation outcome studies have been performed. The lack of systematic studies on rehabilitation outcome has been noted in the literature (8,10). Consequently, most rehabilitation approaches for measuring functional outcome in GBS have been adopted on the basis of experience with other diseases. The only studies reported are largely descriptive with no well-defined functional outcomes, except for physical findings regarding weakness or alterations in gait (21,50,51,54). Also, there are no detailed studies on the other inflammatory polyneuropathies that evaluate the usefulness of rehabilitation. Consequently, the rest of this chapter focuses generally on GBS, but it is assumed that many of the same general principles apply to other inflammatory polyneuropathies.

There are patients who will suffer a relapse of the disease, and these relapses are believed to be more frequent with the current treatments, particularly IVIg (35). However, IVIg remains the treatment of choice, versus plasmapheresis, due to the ease of delivery and low complication rate (79). Because the course of GBS remains clinically unpredictable at the onset of the disease and patients are, in general, being transferred to rehabilitation more quickly, close supervision of an inpatient rehabilitation service is warranted. This evaluation should include detailed daily physical examinations, documenting motor and sensory test results to evaluate for relapses or complications and measuring vital capacity for patients at risk.

The requirement for ventilatory support has a strong correlation with the functional motor gain and recovery obtained during inpatient rehabilitation as measured by the admit motor and discharge Functional Independence Measure (FIM) Rasch motor converted score (21,53). Those who required ventilatory support were generally more functionally limited and recovered less motor function than those who did not require ventilatory support (21,53). This agrees with other epidemiological studies that generally evaluated outcome in GBS by ambulatory function (4,24).

Poor proprioceptive function has been associated with a longer length of stay on inpatient rehabilitation (53). However, there was no association with proprioceptive changes and functional status as measured by the admit motor and discharge FIM Rasch motor converted score on admission to rehabilitation, so the connection is unclear (53). Also, there appears to be no relationship between the presence of relapses and rehabilitation outcome, except for lower FIM Rasch converted motor discharge scores from inpatient rehabilitation (53). This relationship may be related to the more extended course of the disease in these patients but clearly requires further study.

GBS is a disease that often leads to a functional deficit. At least 20% of the patients will have severe, prolonged residual deficits. As stated, more than 50% will have motor strength changes and up to two thirds may have persistent fatigue or reduced endurance (8,50). It is evident that very little is known about the true incidence of disability in these patients. The absence of deep tendon reflexes in upper or lower extremities, as well as severe distal upper extremity weakness or lower extremity weakness, is indicative of incomplete recovery (54). This may lead to an impairment that is defined as "any loss or abnormality of psychological, physical, or anatomic structure or function" (80). Disability as defined by the World Health Organization exists when an impairment prohibits one from accomplishing a task required for personal independence (80). Assessment of disability in GBS has usually been on a crude 6-point ordinal scale or some modification thereof (2,42–46):

- 0, healthy; 1, minor symptoms or signs
- 2, able to walk 5 m without assistance
- 3, able to walk 5 m with assistance
- 4, chair or bed bound
- 5, requiring assisted ventilation for at least part of the day or night
- 6, dead

One problem with studies using this scale is that the length of time patients were followed varied between 6 months and 12 months, whereas recovery may continue for up to 18 months. Additionally, the usefulness of this scale in relation to the more-traditional scales used to measure outcome in rehabilitation has

yet to be established. More importantly, this scale may not be sensitive enough to detect subtle changes in function with various treatment options.

Another important issue that needs to be addressed by rehabilitation research is how patients with an inflammatory polyneuropathy age with a functional deficit (8). It has been shown that the extent of muscle strength recovery after GBS may be a major determinant of the patient's ultimate functional potential (2,10,40).

Rehabilitation Therapeutics

Motor Recovery and Musculoskeletal Complications

There have been no systematic studies on the efficacy of physical therapy in GBS (8,10). Generally, therapy approaches have been adapted from the experiences with other neuromuscular illnesses and diseases. Patients with GBS may present with such diverse findings as significant involvement with quadriparesis and isolated weakness of the arm, leg, facial muscles, or oropharynx. It has been suggested that overfatiguing the affected motor unit in therapy may impede recovery in patients with GBS (81,82). Clearly, overworking muscle groups in patients with peripheral nerve involvement has been clinically associated with paradoxical weakening (82).

Motor weakness has been associated with muscle shortening and resultant joint contractures. These complications can be prevented with daily range-of-motion exercises (83). Depending on the amount of weakness, exercise can be passive, active assistive, or active. Proper positioning in patients is necessary. Initial exercise, even in the acute phases, can include a program of gentle strengthening involving isometric, isotonic, isokinetic, manual-resistive, and progressive-resistive exercises carefully tailored to the clinical condition of the patient (83). Orthotic devices should be prescribed for proper positioning and optimizing residual motor function (8).

Sensory Dysfunction and Pain

There are patients with significant involvement in vibratory sensation and joint position. Proprioceptive losses cause ataxia and incoordination resulting in functional deficits. In one study, proprioceptive losses were not correlated with long-term functional status or the severity of illness (21). This may be due to the small patient numbers in that study (21). Therapy that uses techniques of sensory reintegration and repetitive exercises to redevelop coordination has been suggested for these patients (8). This will aid in developing motor engrams that are based on the altered sensory perception.

Many patients will relate a history of severe pain in the early stages of recovery from GBS, yet there is a dearth of studies on the nature or duration of this pain. There are no significant studies regarding interventions for deafferent pain syndrome in any of the inflammatory polyneuropathies. Pain in the limbs and axial skeleton has been linked in one report to impaired joint mobility in GBS (84). Patients with GBS with severe pain may have a poor tolerance for activity resulting in longer lengths of stay. Various therapies that use desensitization techniques used in the therapies may be clinically useful. Medical intervention usually starts with tricyclic antidepressants, capsaicin, and transcutaneous nerve stimulation. Second-line agents include the use of anticonvulsants (carbamazepine, gabapentin), that are reported to be effective in neurogenic pain (85,86). Occasionally, in those who have unremitting pain, the use of pain medications such as tramadol or narcotics is indicated for the acute management of pain until the previously cited measures have time to become effective. More recently, it has been suggested that the use of topical capsaicin or transcutaneous electrical stimulation to the specific, well-localized anatomic areas of deafferent pain may be of use (8).

Dysautonomia

Dysautonomia is very prevalent in GBS but is much rarer in the other causes of inflammatory polyneuropathies (14,17,21, 31,55). Most patients who come to inpatient rehabilitation are probably not as threatened by cardiac arrhythmias; however, because these patients are the more severely involved, they may still have problems with postural hypotension, hypertension and excessive sympathetic outflow, or bladder and bowel dysfunction. Recent studies on dysautonomia estimate that between 19% and 50% of all patients with GBS in a hospital setting will have evidence of cardiovascular instability (21,60,63). Patients who have excessive sympathetic outflow and hypertension appear to have extreme sensitivity to vasoactive drugs (60,69). These patients are particularly likely to develop episodes of hypotension or hypertension with suctioning (87). This is of concern, because some patients are prone to cardiac arrhythmias (21,63, 88). Treatment should be directed toward physical modalities such as compression hose, abdominal binders, and proper hydration. There have been suggestions that low-dose beta blockade should be used prophylactically in this patient population (8), particularly with those patients referred for rehabilitation soon after disease nadir and before the cardiovascular system is stressed by therapy.

Bowel and bladder dysfunction is generally of the lower motor neuron variety. Recent evidence does not indicate a link between bowel and bladder dysfunction and dysautonomia that involves the cardiovascular system (63). Urologic dysfunction may develop early in the disease process, in up to 15% of cases, but is believed to resolve in most cases (10,11). Initial management of the bladder should be directed toward avoiding overdistention of the bladder with consequent, bladder wall disruption (8). Furthermore, up to 30% of patients acquire urinary tract infections (10).

Immobilization

The incidence of DVT in the inflammatory polyneuropathies is unknown, because it has never been studied. Predisposing factors for DVT development, such as the severity of disease or the length of immobilization, have not been well delineated (8, 58). Because the most severely involved patients are those referred to inpatient rehabilitation, most rehabilitation physicians use prophylaxis for DVT. Judgments regarding the type and length of prophylaxis are difficult without knowing the inci-

dence or risk factors for DVT development. Early mobilization appears to be beneficial in similar patient groups.

Clearly, prolonged immobilization leads to a reduction of blood volume (72,73) and increased episodes of postural hypotension in the rehabilitation setting (53). In other immobilized patients, use of a tilt table has been a useful therapeutic tool (8).

These patients tend to lose a significant amount of body mass due to immobilization, particularly muscle mass. When this is combined with a significant sensory loss, patients are susceptible to the development of pressure ulcers. Proper bed positioning with frequent postural changes is required to prevent the development of pressure ulcers (8).

The loss of body mass, coupled with an already compromised peripheral nervous system, makes proper positioning a necessity to protect peripheral nerves, which may be compressed between body prominences and the bed (8,83). The nerves that are most frequently involved are the ulnar, peroneal, and the lateral femoral cutaneous sensory nerves.

In the patients noted to have immobilization hypercalcemia, early mobilization even in a therapeutic pool was correlated with a therapeutic drop in the serum calcium level (66). The use of aggressive range of motion may also impede the effects heterotopic ossification may have on joint mobility and function.

No studies have been performed on the nutritional needs of these patients. In our clinical experience, close nutritional monitoring is warranted, because patients tend to lose weight in the acute stage of illness (8). With immobilization and reduced activity, many of those who can eat tend to gain weight after the first few weeks of illness. The consequent weight gain impedes the potential functional gains in transfers and mobility because it may overwhelm any residual motor function.

Psychological-Social Issues

Psychosocial variables have been demonstrated to affect outcome of rehabilitation in many other diagnoses. Symptoms of mild depression long after the initial onset, indicated by persistent mental fatigue, are common, although GBS itself is not believed to result in chronic fatigue syndrome (35). Clearly, an extended period in the intensive care setting, due to ventilatory support, may result in psychological changes. It is expected that patients with severely involved GBS have many of the same psychological and social issues that are suffered by patients with SCI (8). This could then result in the utilization of already established interventions. It is reasonable to consider that a reactive depression may be the result of deafferent pain syndromes that can result from inflammatory neuropathies (8).

Respiratory

Respiratory failure and pneumonia may be noted in 30% of the acute cases in the first 12 weeks (21,54) but are rare in the other causes of inflammatory polyneuropathy (14). Aggressive respiratory therapy with pulmonary toilet is necessary in the early stages of disease, including acute inpatient rehabilitation, as it would be with any patient with a neuromuscular disease affecting pulmonary function. Because this issue appears to be the strongest predictor of hospital length of stay, close monitoring is required (21,53,61,62). Patients with cranial nerve involvement are particularly susceptible to pulmonary infections due to aspiration. Perhaps this is why cranial nerve involvement and dysautonomia have been so closely linked to ventilatory dependence and severity of GBS (21,53,61,62). At our institution, the use of cardiac telemetry has been useful in the quick diagnosis of cardiac arrhythmias induced by therapeutic exercise.

Inflammatory polyneuropathy may lead to restrictive pulmonary function, which may persist for some time after ventilatory assistance is discontinued. Restrictive pulmonary conditions in other diseases have been associated with sleep hypercapnia and hypoxia during rapid eye movement sleep, because within the central nervous system, the centrally mediated ventilatory response to hypoxia and hypercapnia is diminished during sleep (89–92). Many patients may be assessed on the floor by the use of frequent nighttime observations using a pulse oximeter. In those who develop sleep hypoxia or hypercapnia, treatment with bilevel positive airway pressure may be indicated (8). More recently, it has been suggested that theophylline may be of benefit in those patients who present with reduced hypercapnia or hypoxia at night due to central respiratory control mechanisms that accommodate prolonged blood gas alterations (93).

Clearance of secretions, to reduce the work of breathing, is necessary (94). Often this will require the use of resistive inspiratory training. Many of these patients will initially have a tracheostomy; a proper tracheostomy tube capping protocol with frequent rest periods needs to be instituted. One must be careful not to overfatigue the muscles of respiration during the initial period of motor-unit recovery, because this may push the patient into respiratory failure.

OUTPATIENT AND LONG-TERM FOLLOW-UP

The extent and duration of physically disabling sequelae in the inflammatory polyneuropathies, including the incidence of secondary medical complications, have never been adequately described (8). With regard to motor function, poliomyelitis and GBS have many similar clinical issues. Whether the same long-term problems will develop in this population due to a loss in the number of active motor units is unknown. Furthermore, there have been no long-term studies on aging in patients who have suffered GBS (8). These patients will likely suffer a loss of function as they age, similar to postpoliomyelitic patients (95). One can assume that there are outpatient therapy programs that can aid in the maintenance of functional capacity. Until such studies are performed, much of the rehabilitation of GBS will be based on the experience gleaned from similarly presenting neuromuscular conditions.

The incidence of GBS, which may be two thirds that of SCI, is the most prevalent cause of acute nontraumatic neuromuscular paralysis in the world now that polio has been contained. When one adds in all the inflammatory polyneuropathies, there is an incidence close to that of SCI. Undoubtedly, a significant portion of the patients discharged directly to home could benefit from outpatient rehabilitative services. Furthermore, vocational and psychosocial outcomes have not been addressed in any studies. But the services for patients disabled by GBS are as frag-

mented as those originally described two decades ago for TBI and SCI. This led to the creation of Model Systems of care, which developed a comprehensive continuum of care, improving the lives of patients with TBI or SCI. There is a similar need for the development of Model Systems of care in inflammatory polyneuropathies.

REFERENCES

1. Alter M. The epidemiology of Guillain-Barré syndrome. *Ann Neurol* 1990;27:S7–S12.
2. Guillain-Barré Syndrome Steroid Group. Double-blind trial of intravenous methyl-prednisolone in Guillain-Barré syndrome. *Lancet* 1993; 341:586–590.
3. McLean M, Duclos P, Jacob P, et al. Incidence of Guillain-Barré syndrome in Ontario and Quebec, 1983–1989, using hospital service databases. *Epidemiology* 1994;5:443–448.
4. Winer JB, Hughes RAC, Osmond C. A prospective study of acute idiopathic neuropathy: clinical features and their prognostic value. *J Neurol Neurosurg Psychiatry* 1988;51:605–612.
5. Raphael JC, Masson C, Morice V, et al. Le Syndrome de Guillain-Barré: etude retrospective de 233 observations. *Sem Hop Pares* 1984; 60:2543–2546.
6. Prevots D, Sutter R. Assessment of Guillain-Barré syndrome mortality and morbidity in the United States: implications for acute flaccid paralysis surveillance. *J Infect Dis* 1997;175:S151–S155.
7. Asbury AK. Guillain-Barré syndrome: historical aspects. *Ann Neurol* 1990;27:S2–S6.
8. Meythaler JM. Rehabilitation of Guillain-Barré syndrome: a review. *Arch Phys Med Rehabil* 1997;78:872–879.
9. Trojaborg W. Lecture in honour of Professor Emeritus Fritz Buchtal. Acute and chronic demyelinating polyneuropathy: an overview. *Electroencephal Clin Neurophysiol* 1999;50[Suppl]:16S–27S.
10. Ropper AH. The Guillain-Barré syndrome. *N Engl J Med* 1992;326: 1130–1136.
11. Asbury AK, Cornblath DR. Assessment of current diagnostic criteria for Guillain-Barré syndrome. *Ann Neurol* 1990;27:S21–S24.
12. Ropper AH, Wijdicks EFM, Truax BT. *Guillain-Barré syndrome*. Philadelphia: FA Davis Co, 1991.
13. Asbury AK, Arnason BG, Karp HR, et al. Criteria for diagnosis of Guillain-Barré syndrome. *Ann Neurol* 1978;3:565–566.
14. Van der Meche FG, Van Doorn PA. Chronic inflammatory demyelinating polyneuropathy (CIDP). *Electroencephal Clin Neurophysiol* 1999; 50[Suppl]:493S–498S.
15. Ad Hoc Subcommittee of the American Academy of Neurology AIDS Task Force. Research criteria for diagnosis of chronic inflammatory demyelinating polyneuropathy (CIDP). *Neurology* 1991;41:617–618.
16. Dalakas MC. Advances in chronic inflammatory demyelinating polyneuropathy: disease variants and inflammatory response mediators and modifiers. *Curr Opin Neurol* 1999;12:403–409.
17. Latov N. Prognosis of neuropathy with monoclonal gammopathy. *Muscle Nerve* 2000;23:150–152.
18. Osler W. *The principles and practice of medicine*. New York: Appleton Communication, 1892:777–778.
19. Guillain G, Barré JA, Strohl A. Sur un syndrome de radiculonevrite avec hyperalbuminose du liquide cephalorachidien sans reaction cellulaire: remarques sur les caracteres cliniques et graphiques des reflexes tendineurx. *Bull Soc Med Hop Paris* 1916;40:1462–1470.
20. McKhann GM. Guillain-Barré syndrome: clinical and therapeutic observations. *Ann Neurol* 1990;27:S13–S16.
21. Meythaler JM, DeVivo MJ, Braswell WC. Rehabilitation outcomes of patients who have developed Guillain-Barré syndrome. *Am J Phys Med Rehabil* 1997;76:411–419.
22. McFarlin DE. Immunological parameters in Guillain-Barré syndrome. *Ann Neurol* 1990;27:S25–S28.
23. Rees JH, Soudain SE, Gregson NA, et al. Campylobacter jejuni infection and Guillain-Barré syndrome. *N Engl J Med* 1995;333: 1374–1379.

24. Hughes RAC. *Guillain-Barré syndrome.* London: Springer-Verlag, 1990.
25. Ropper AH. Unusual clinical variants and signs of Guillain-Barré syndrome. *Arch Neurol* 1986;43:1150–1152.
26. Fisher M. An unusual variant of acute idiopathic polyneuritis (syndrome of ophthalmoplegia, ataxia, and areflexia). *N Engl J Med* 1956; 255:57–65.
27. Ropper AH, Shahani BT. Pain in Guillain Barré syndrome. *Arch Neurol* 1984;41:511–514.
28. Young RR, Asbury AK, Corbett JL, et al. Pure pan-dysautonomia with recovery: description and discussion of diagnostic criteria. *Brain* 1975; 98:613–636.
29. Feasby TE, Gilbert JJ, Brown WF, et al. An acute axonal form of Guillain-Barré polyneuropathy. *Brain* 1986;109:1115–1126.
30. Melillo EM, Sethi JM, Mohsenin V. Guillain-Barré syndrome: rehabilitation outcome and recent developments. *Yale J Biol Med* 1998;71: 383–389.
31. Saperstein DS, Amato AA, Wolfe GI, et al. Multifocal acquired demyelinating sensory and motor neuropathy: the Lewis-Sumner syndrome. *Muscle Nerve* 1999;22:560–566.
32. Cornblath DR. Electrophysiology in Guillain-Barré syndrome. *Ann Neurol* 1990;27:S17–S20.
33. Brosnan CF, Claudio L, Tansey FA, et al. Mechanisms of autoimmune neuropathies. *Ann Neurol* 1990;27:S75–S79.
34. Soueidan SA, Dalakas MC. Treatment of autoimmune neuromuscular diseases with high-dose intravenous immune globulin. *Pediatr Res* 1993;33:S95–S100.
35. Hughes RA, Rees JH. Guillain-Barré syndrome. *Curr Opin Neurol* 1994;7:386–392.
36. Samson JC, Fiori MG. Gangliosides and Guillain-Barré syndrome: no casual link. *Br Med J* 1994;308:653.
37. Diez-Tejedor E, Gutierez-Rivas E, Gil-Peralta A. Gangliosides and Guillain-Barré syndrome: the Spanish data. *Neuroepidemiology* 1993; 12:251–256.
38. Beghi E. Exposure to exogenous gangliosides and Guillain-Barré syndrome. *Neuroepidemiology* 1995;14:45–48.
39. Grigoletto F. Gangliosides and Guillain-Barré syndrome. Apparent association is a coincidence. *Br Med J* 1994;308:653–654.
40. Yuki N, Yamada M, Sato S, et al. Association of IgG anti-GD1a antibody with severe Guillain-Barré syndrome. *Muscle Nerve* 1993;16: 642–647.
41. Kornberg AJ, Pestronik A. The clinical and diagnostic role of anti-GM1 antibody testing. *Muscle Nerve* 1994;17:100–104.
42. Guillain-Barré Study Group. Plasmapheresis and acute Guillain-Barré syndrome. *Neurology* 1985;35:1096–1104.
43. Plasma Exchange/Sandoglobulin Guillain-Barré Syndrome Trial Group. Randomized trial of plasma exchange, intravenous immunoglobulin, and combined treatments in Guillain-Barré syndrome. *Lancet* 1997;349:1123–1129.
44. French Cooperative Group on Plasma Exchange in Guillain-Barré syndrome. Efficiency of plasma exchange in Guillain-Barré syndrome: role of replacement fluids. *Ann Neurol* 1987;22:753–761.
45. Vermeulen M, van der Meche FGA, Speelman JD, et al. Plasma and gamma-globulin infusion in chronic inflammatory polyneuropathy. *J Neurol Sci* 1985;70:317–326.
46. Van der Meche FGA, Schmitz PIM, A randomized trial comparing intravenal immunoglobulin and plasma exchange in Guillain-Barré system for the Dutch Guillain-Barré Study Group. *N Engl J Med* 1992; 326;1123–1129.
47. Teitbaum JS, Borel CO. Respiratory dysfunction in Guillain-Barré syndrome. *Clin Chest Med* 1994;15:705–714.
48. Feasby TE. Inflammatory-demyelinating polyneuropathies. *Neurol Clin* 1992;10:651–670.
49. Watts PM, Taylor WA, Hughes RAC. High-dose methylprednisolone suppresses experimental allergic neuritis in the Lewis rat. *Exp Neurol* 1989;103:101–104.
50. Zelig G, Ohry A, Shemsesh Y, et al. The rehabilitation of patients with severe Guillain-Barré syndrome. *Paraplegia* 1988;26:250–254.
51. Costa EG. Rehabilitation of patients with Guillain-Barré syndrome. *Rev Neuropsiquiatra* 1970;33:219–232.
52. Mckhann GM, Griffin JW, Cornblath DR, et al. Plasmapheresis and Guillain-Barré syndrome: analysis of prognostic factors and the effect of plasmapheresis. *Ann Neurol* 1988;23:347–353.
53. Meythaler JM, DeVivo MJ, Clausen GC, et al. Prediction of outcome in Guillain-Barré syndrome admitted to rehabilitation. *Arch Phys Med Rehabil* 1994;75:1027A.
54. Eberle E, Brink J, Azen S, et al. Early predictors of incomplete recovery in children with Guillain-Barré polyneuritis. *J Pediatr* 1975;86: 356–359.
55. Ponsford S, Willison H, Veitch J, et al. Long-term clinical and neurophysiological follow-up of patients with peripheral neuropathy associated with benign monoclonal gammopathy. *Muscle Nerve* 2000;23: 164–174.
56. Gareth PJ. *Guillain-Barré syndrome.* New York: Thieme Medical Publisher, 1993.
57. Beydoun SR, Copeland D. Bilateral phrenic neuropathy as a presenting feature of multifocal motor neuropathy with conduction block. *Muscle Nerve* 2000;23:556–559.
58. Raman TK, Blake JA, Harris TM. Pulmonary embolism in Landry-Guillain-Strohl syndrome. *Chest* 1971;60:555–557.
59. Tapson V. Acute venous thromboembolism: diagnostic guidelines. *Am Fam Physician* 2000;62:2226–2231.
60. Zochodne DW. Autonomic involvement in Guillain-Barré syndrome: a review. *Muscle Nerve* 1994;17:1145–1155.
61. Sedano MJ, Calleja J, Canga E, et al. Guillain-Barré syndrome in Cantabria, Spain: an epidemiological and clinical study. *Acta Neurol Scand* 1994;89:287–292.
62. Taly AB, Gupta SK, Vasanth A, et al. Critically ill Guillain Barré syndrome. *J Assoc Physicians India* 1994; 42:871–874.
63. Meythaler JM, DeVivo M, Johnson A, et al. Incidence of leukopenia and anemia in Guillain Barré Syndrome patients admitted to inpatient rehabilitation: effect of IVIG. *Arch Phys Med Rehabil* 1999;80: 1188(abst).
64. Ravn H. The Landry-Guillain-Barré syndrome: a survey and a clinical report on 127 cases. *Acta Neurol Scand* 1967;43[S30]:8–64.
65. Pentland B, Daonald SM. Pain in the Guillain-Barré syndrome: a clinical review. *Pain* 1994;59:159–164.
66. Meythaler JM, Korkor AB, Nanda T, et al. Immobilization hypercalcemia associated with Landry-Guillain-Barré syndrome: successful therapy with combined calcitonin and etidronate sodium. *Arch Intern Med* 1986;146:1567–1571.
67. Evans RA, Bridgeman M, Hills E, et al. Immobilization hypercalcemia. *Miner Electrolyte Metab* 1984;10:244–248.
68. Gitter AJ, Haselkorn JK. Landry-Guillain-Barré syndrome and heterotopic ossification: case report. *Arch Phys Med Rehabil* 1990;71:823.
69. Lichtenfield P. Autonomic dysfunction in the Guillain-Barré syndrome. *Am J Med* 1971;50:772–780.
70. Meythaler JM, DeVivo MJ, Clausen GC, et al. Anemia in Guillain-Barré syndrome patients admitted to rehabilitation. *Arch Phys Med Rehabil* 1994;75:1051A.
71. Hirsch GH, Menard MR, Anton HA. Anemia after traumatic spinal cord injury. *Arch Phys Med Rehabil* 1991;72:195–201.
72. Johnson PC, Fisher CL, Leach C. Hematological implications of hypodynamic states. In: Murray RH, McCally M, eds. *Hypogravic and hypodynamic environments.* Washington: NASA, 1971:27–34.
73. Lancaster MC. Hematologic aspects of bed rest. In: Murray RH, McCally M, eds. *Hypogravic and hypodynamic environments.* Washington: NASA, 1971:299–307.
74. Low PA. Autonomic neuropathies. *Curr Opin Neurol* 1994;7:402–406.
75. Sridharan GV, Tallis RC, Gautman PC. Guillain-Barré syndrome in the elderly. A retrospective comparative study. *Gerontology* 1993;39: 170–175.
76. Panosian MS, Quatela VC. Guillain-Barré syndrome presenting as acute bilateral vocal cord paralysis. *Otolaryngol Head Neck Surg* 1993; 108:171–173.
77. Nadkarni N, Lisak RP. Guillain-Barré syndrome with bilateral optic neuritis and central white matter disease. *Neurology* 1993;43:842–843.
78. Herinckx C, Deggouj N, Gersdorff M, et al. Guillain-Barré syndrome and hypacusia. *Acta Oto-Laryngologica Belgica* 1995;49:63–67.
79. Dalakas MC. Intravenous immunoglobulin in the treatment of autoimmune neuromuscular diseases: present status and practical therapeutic guidelines. *Muscle Nerve* 1999;22:1479–1497.

80. World Health Organization. *International classification of impairments, disabilities, and handicaps: a manual of classification relating to the consequences of disease.* Geneva: World Health Organization, 1980.

81. Bensman A. Strenuous exercise may impair muscle function in Guillain-Barré patients. *JAMA* 1970;214:468–469.

82. Herbison GJ, Jaweed M, Ditunno JF. Exercise therapies in peripheral neuropathies. *Arch Phys Med Rehabil* 1983;64:201–205.

83. Bushbacher L. Rehabilitation of patients with peripheral neuropathies. In: Braddom RL, ed. *Physical medicine and rehabilitation.* Philadelphia: WB Saunders, 1995:972–989.

84. Soryal I, Sinclaire E, Hornby J, et al. Impaired joint mobility in Guillain-Barré syndrome: a primary or a secondary phenomenon? *J Neurol Neurosurg Psychiatry* 1992;55:1014–1017.

85. Calissi PT, Jaber LA. Peripheral diabetic neuropathy: current concepts in treatment. *Ann Pharmacother* 1995;7-8:69–77.

86. Rosner H, Rubin L, Kestenbaum A. Gabapentin adjunctive therapy in neuropathic pain states. *Clin J Pain* 1996;12:56–58.

87. Eiben RM, Gersony WM. Recognition, prognosis and treatment of the Guillain-Barré syndrome (acute idiopathic polyneuritis). *Med Clin North Am* 1963;47:1371–1380.

88. Winer JB, Hughes RAC. Identification of patients at risk of arrhythmia in the Guillain-Barré syndrome. *Q J Med* 1988;68:735–739.

89. Bach JR. Rehabilitation of the patient with respiratory dysfunction. In: DeLisa JA, ed. *Rehabilitation medicine: principles and practice,* 2nd ed. Philadelphia: JB Lippincott Co, 1993:952–972.

90. Redding GJ, Okamoto GA, Guthrie RD, et al. Sleep patterns in nonambulatory boys with Duchenne muscular dystrophy. *Arch Phys Med Rehabil* 1985;66:818–821.

91. Shneerson J. *Disorders of ventilation.* Boston: Blackwell Science, 1988:43.

92. Smith PEM, Edwards RHT, Calverley PMA. Ventilation and breathing pattern during sleep in Duchenne muscular dystrophy. *Chest* 1989;96:1346–1351.

93. Javaheri S, Parker TJ, Wexler L, et al. Effect of theophylline on sleep-disordered breathing in heart failure. *N Engl J Med* 1996;335:562–567.

94. Alba AS. Concepts in pulmonary rehabilitation. In: Braddom RL, ed. *Physical medicine and rehabilitation.* Philadelphia: WB Saunders, 1995:671–685.

95. Trojan DA, Cashman NR, Shapiro S, et al. Predictive factors for postpoliomyelitis syndrome. *Arch Phys Med Rehabil* 1994;75:770–777.

WHEELCHAIRS/ADAPTIVE MOBILITY EQUIPMENT AND SEATING

SANDRA SALERNO
STEVEN KIRSHBLUM

The selection of an appropriate seating and mobility system has become critical for the end user to function at an optimal level. There are many factors that influence the selection of the system, including physical, medical, social, psychological, and environmental. A team approach consisting of the client, family members/caretaker, physician, occupational and physical therapist, assistive technology specialist, driver training specialist, social worker/case manager, and rehabilitation technology supplier (preferred provider) is recommended to address all areas of concern for an appropriate selection.

Due to the rapid growth in technology, seating and mobility types, brands, and components are unlimited, causing the end user to become overwhelmed. The importance of participating in a seating and wheelchair clinic with specialists has become a necessity, particularly because of the funding crisis. It is important for practitioners to be knowledgeable of the basic seating principles and products available. This chapter addresses the types, components, and principles of seating and mobility systems.

GOALS OF SEATING AND WHEELCHAIR SYSTEMS

The client's goals should be discussed with the team to prioritize the importance of each in relation to the client's positional needs, level of function, lifestyle, and environmental barriers. The following goals can assist the practitioner when prescribing and justifying a seating and mobility system (Table 38.1).

TABLE 38.1. GOALS FOR SEATING AND MOBILITY

1. Provide proper positional support to prevent or accommodate postural deformities
2. Maximize function
3. Enhance stability, balance, and physiologic function
4. Reduce the influences of abnormal reflexes and spasticity
5. Ensure skin integrity through an appropriate pressure-relieving system
6. Provide a system to meet the client's lifestyle and environmental factors
7. Aesthetically pleasing

Factors to Consider

Before prescribing a seating and mobility system, the team must assess the client's remaining abilities, function, and potential, in addition to his or her disability, loss of function, and postural deficits. Table 38.2 is a guideline for practitioners to follow when assessing the client, to address all areas of concern.

Frames

Previously, manual wheelchairs were not only limited in style and design but also heavier due to the chrome-folding frame. It was not until the late 1970s when wheelchair-bound athletes began to change the design and frame composition to make lightweight wheelchairs (1). They also set the way for modular

TABLE 38.2. AREAS TO ASSESS BEFORE PRESCRIPTION

Medical history	• Diagnosis (primary/secondary)
	• Cardiac status
	• Respiratory and digestive functions
	• Skin status
	• Prognosis/disorder progression
	• Hypertension
	• Orthostasis
	• Heterotopic ossification
Physical capability	• Active and passive range of motion
	• Strength
	• Sensation
	• Endurance
	• Balance and trunk control
	• Skin integrity
	• Height, weight, and age
Anticipated lifestyle	• Prior Vs anticipated lifestyle
Environment	• Accessibility
	• Transportation
Additional technology	• Environmental control unit
	• Computer access
Transportation concerns	• Car vs. van
	• Driver vs. passenger setup
	• Lock-down system
Insurance/funding	• Coverage
	• Preferred providers (rehab technology supplier)

TABLE 38.3. WHEELCHAIR OPTIONS

Wheelchair Options	Advantages	Disadvantages
1. Frames		
Folding	Easy to transport Absorbs uneven terrain better for smoother ride	Heavier More parts Not as durable Limited width sizes More energy use
Rigid	More energy efficient Fewer parts Lighter weight More durable Smaller turning radius	Difficult to transport Rougher ride LE positioning concerns
2. Armrests		
Full length	Assists with sit-to-stand transfers UE positioning	Obstacle for tabletops
Desk arm	Improved accessibility	Decreased arm support Difficulty with transfers Maintenance
Adjustable height	UE positioning and support Accessibility Assist with transfers	
Fixed height	Less adjustments	Poor UE positioning
Offset	Decreased overall width	Difficulty with mounting back systems
Tubular	Ease of removal Light-weight	Not used for weight-bearing Limited adjustment
Cantilever	Flip back easy Does not require hand function to operate	Do not lock in place Difficulty with mounting back system
3. Footrests		
Swingaway	Ease of removal for transfers Accessibility to countertops	Added weight Maintenance Increases overall length Increases turning radius
Elevating	Positioning for LE limitation Decreases edema Assist with minimizing orthostasis	Added weight Increases overall length Increases turning radius Bulky
Fixed	Fewer parts Increased maneuverability Makes wheelchair lighter and more durable	Transfer concerns Transport issues LE limitations
4. Wheels		
Mag	Decrease maintenance Durable	Heavier
Spoke	Lighter weight	More maintenance to keep tight and true
X-core	Sport look Lighter weight	Expensive Limited type of tires used
Size		
Large (24, 25, 26)	Better UE positioning for propulsion	Increases seat-to-floor height
Small (20, 22)	Decreases seat-to-floor height for ease of foot propulson	Accessibility to tops of tables/desks Assists with sit-to-stand transfers
5. Tires		
Pneumatic-air	Good traction Shock absorption	Maintenance (flats) Resistance due to tread
Airless	Good traction Maintenance free	Harder ride Heavier
Solid	Ease of propulsion on level surfaces Maintenance free	Heavy Slip on wet surfaces
High performance	Ease of propulsion on level surfaces Shock absorption	Maintenance (flats) Slip on wet surfaces Poor performance on rough terrian
Kik	Light tread for better performance than solids Maintenance free	Heavy Poor shock absorption
Knobbie	Good traction on rough terrain	Increased overall width Bulky Not good indoors

(continued)

TABLE 38.3. (continued)

Wheelchair Options	Advantages	Disadvantages
6. **Hand rims**		
Aluminum	Maintenance free	Requires good hand function
Plastic coated	Enhances traction for clients with no grasps	Need to maintain (cracks and cuts)
Projections	Assists with propulsion	Increases overall width
		Uneven placement during propulsion
7. **Casters**		
Large (6–8 in.)	Better performance outdoors and on rough terrain	Increases turning radius
		Not good indoors
		Limits front angle degree
Small (3–5 in.)	Tighter turning radius	Outdoor limitations
	Better maneuverability	Decrease stability
8. **Wheel locks**		
Push/pull	Easy to operate even with limited hand function	Transfer clearance
Scissors	Out of the way during propulsion	Need good balance
		Good hand function needed
High mount	Easy to reach	Transfer clearance
Low mount	Out of the way during propulsion and transfers	Need good balance

LE, lower extremity; UE, upper extremity.

frames and adjustable axle plates for better performance and to address positional needs.

There are two types of frames: folding and rigid (Table 38.3). Folding frames have a cross-brace (X shaped), which connects the side frames, and can be folded by pulling up the center of the seat (Fig. 38.1). Folding frames have more parts, are heavier, and are not as energy efficient as rigid frames because of the cross-brace. They do, however, have better shock-absorption properties, allowing for a smoother ride. Rigid frames are more energy efficient because there is less internal energy needed to propel fewer parts and because of their lighter weight (Fig. 38.2). They can cause difficulty with transportation due to the box frame, although the wheels can be removed and the back can be folded down to be placed in the trunk or back seat for transport (Fig. 38.3).

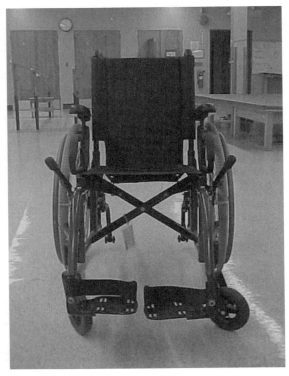

FIGURE 38.1. Folding frame.

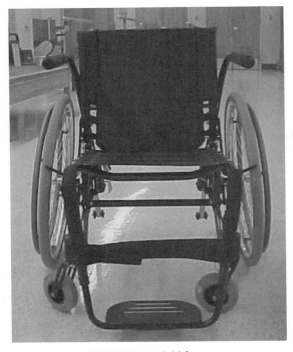

FIGURE 38.2. Rigid frame.

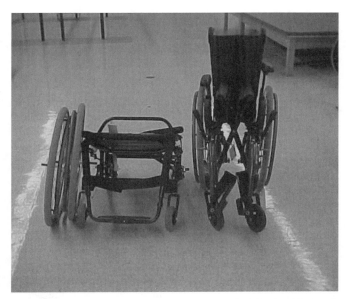

FIGURE 38.3. Rigid **(left)** and folding frame **(right)** wheelchair collapsed.

Performance has become the main issue in selecting a wheelchair to meet the client's lifestyle. The rigid-frame wheelchair is easier to push, has less roll resistance, and is more adjustable to meet the needs of an active user. Due to the benefit of shock absorption in the folding frame, it has led manufactures to construct the option of shocks and suspension system in certain rigid frames. A concern with rigid frames is the front riggings. It is important to evaluate the client's type of transfers to select the degree of angle of the foot riggings. With clients who ambulate, it may be difficult for them to stand with a rigid front, although a flip-up footplate or swing-away footrests can be an option.

Most current wheelchairs are constructed of aluminum, which makes the frames lighter for propulsion and durable for everyday use. Advanced technology has taken a step further by using titanium and carbon fiber to make even lighter frames, although this increases the expense of the system.

TYPES OF WHEELCHAIRS

There are many types of wheelchairs that allow for independent mobility. The material used in constructing them and the ability to adjust for appropriate seating and mobility are used to classify them. Each of these mobility systems differs in features, options, and cost. The major types of wheelchairs include the standard, ultralightweight, heavy-duty, and hemiheight wheelchairs.

Standard or conventional wheelchairs are made of steel and weigh approximately 40 to 65 lb. They are folding-frame wheelchairs with a nonadjustable axle plate, limiting function for the active wheelchair user. The standard wheelchair is usually used for rentals, part-time users, or clients with no positional requirements. The conventional frame wheelchair, made of stainless steel or aluminum, is considered lightweight because it weighs less than 36 lb. They typically do not offer an adjustable axle plate for positioning and are not recommended for the active end user. Due to the lack of adjustability with the rear-wheel placement, the weight, and cross-brace frame, active users will be limited in performance and positioning for stability and wheel placement.

Ultralightweight wheelchairs weigh less than 30 lb and have a semi-axle to full-axle adjustment. These chairs can be constructed of aluminum, titanium, or composite material. This system can be both folding or rigid, depending on the client's positional and lifestyle needs. Semiadjustable wheelchairs refer to the ability to adjust the position of the rear wheels horizontally and vertically in conjunction with the caster assembly. Horizontal adjustment is usually limited in folding frames but is beneficial for improving propulsion, by allowing the rear wheels to be moved forward. Vertical adjustment allows for the ability to lower or raise the rear seat to floor height to address client's with postural trunk instability. Raising the axle plate will in turn lower the rear seat, placing the client in a posterior tilt, or dump, for stability reasons. Better access to the wheels for propulsion, (in conjunction with lowering the casters) for foot propulsion. These reasons are important to state in the letter of justification for an ultralightweight wheelchair. Full-axle adjustment horizontally, wheel alignment, and camber are common for rigid frames.

Some rigid frames offer the ability to adjust the seat-to-back angle for enhancing trunk stability. For the practitioner, these features are great tools for positioning and evaluating a client for an appropriate seating and mobility system. It allows for optimal positioning for the client to be able to maneuver the wheelchair with ease. This feature is beneficial for the first-time user, letting him or her adjust while improving his or her wheelchair skills. Once the client has mastered advanced wheelchair skills and balance has been achieved, the next wheelchair should be a more fixed frame. The weight capacity for this wheelchair is from 250 to 300 lb.

Heavy-duty frame wheelchairs are constructed with a double cross-brace folding frame for clients who weigh more than 250 lb. The wheelchairs weigh approximately 50 to 60 lb and have a strong, durable frame.

Hemiheight wheelchairs vary in seat-to-floor height, allowing for the lower extremities (LEs) to be in a position to reach the floor for clients to propel with their feet. Usually, they are folding frames with swing-away footrests to allow for foot propulsion.

Manual Wheelchair Components

Armrests

Armrests serve many purposes, including support of the upper extremities (UEs), increased postural stability, and a place for the UEs to push up for pressure relief. There are many different styles, which are based on the client's level of function, independence, lifestyle, and seating system (Fig. 38.4).

The two-point armrest can be either fixed or removable depending on the client's transfers. Fixed armrests are durable and inexpensive but are disadvantageous for clients who need to re-

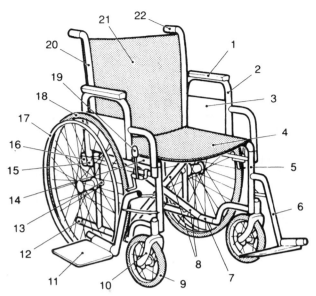

FIGURE 38.4. Components of a typical outdoor sling-seat wheelchair. *1,* arm pad; *2,* desk-style removable arm rest; *3,* clothes guard; *4,* sling seat; *5,* down tube; *6,* foot rest; *7* bottom rail; *8,* cross brace, X bar, or X frame; *9,* caster; *10,* caster fork; *11,* footplate; *12,* tipping lever; *13,* axle; *14,* seat rail; *15,* arm rest bracket or hole for non-wrap-around arm rest; *16,* arm rest bracket or hole for wrap-around arm rest; *17,* handrim; *18,* wheel; *19,* wheel lock, brake lever; *20,* back post; *21,* sling back; *22,* push handle.

move the armrest for lateral or slide-board transfers and for mounting certain seating systems. Two-point armrests have several options: full or desk length, adjustable or fixed height, straight or offset, and flip up. Full-length armrests are beneficial for clients who are able to stand to transfer or ambulate due to the position needed to push up from. However, full-length armrests can become an obstacle for accessibility to tabletops or desks because of their length. Desk-length armrests only extend half of the way improving accessibility, but reducing full arm support to the elbow region.

Height adjustment is a feature that is important when addressing shoulder integrity and position. It allows the armrest to be raised or lowered according to the client's seat-to-elbow height. Some wheelchairs offer an offset option, which decreases the overall width of the wheelchair by wrapping around the back cane eliminating space. They may still be removed for transfer reasons. The ability to flip the armrests back is important for some client's due to limited hand function and strength, and it allows for easier transfers and eliminates misplacing the armrest.

Tubular armrests are for the active enduser who does not rely on the armrest for weightbearing, positioning, or stability. They are not strong enough to provide stability for weight shifts, and it is therefore recommended that the client use the rear tires for this activity. The tubular armrests are used for propping the arms when not propelling and are easy to swing out of the way for transfers.

Cantilever armrests are attached to the back canes on a pivot joint, allowing it to be flipped up out of the way. They can be used for weightbearing, positioning, and transferring. Additional supports, for example, arm troughs, can be added for clients who require more support.

In certain cases in which clients are very active users with good trunk stability, armrests may be omitted. It decreases the weight and eliminates parts from the frame that are not needed.

Footrests/Leg Rests

Manual wheelchairs provide LE support via three different styles: swing-away, elevating, and fixed leg rests. This support is needed for positioning and the prevention of footdrop or other deformities (2). Before selecting the style, one must evaluate the range of motion (ROM) in the LEs, the type of transfer, lifestyle, and function of the client.

Swing-away footrests let users swing the footrest out of the way and remove them for transfers to get closer to the surface being transferred to. They allow for ease of portability to load into a car, which also reduces the weight of the wheelchair when loading. The footrest drop angle comes in certain degrees (60, 70, and 90 degrees), depending on the client's leg length (knee to heel), seat-to-floor height for obstacle clearance, and knee position (ROM). The closer the angle (90 degree), the better the turning radius, access to tables, and transfers, particularly sit-to-stand transfers. The 60-degree front hangers are recommended for clients to accommodate leg length or knee limitations. Heel loops can attach to the footrest for positioning and prevention of the feet from falling off, which would impede propulsion.

Elevating leg rests are used for the client who has limited ROM or edema or to help minimize orthostasis. They are heavier and bulkier than swing-away footrests, and they increase the overall length of the chair. A calf pad or trough comes attached to the center of the leg rest for support.

A fixed footrest does not remove and is mostly seen on rigid-frame wheelchairs. This footrest makes the frame lighter and stronger, although transfers and portability can be difficult.

At times due to client's postural deformities, custom foot boxes are made to accommodate the deformity and maintain skin integrity. Angle-adjustable footplates allow for plantar and dorsiflexion positioning with minimal inversion and eversion adjustment.

Wheels

Wheel type and size affect the performance of the ride. The optimal reach for propelling the wheelchair is determined by the diameter of the wheel size and axle placement in relationship to the client's arm length and function. Wheel size and the seat-to-floor height need to be considered together in making a decision. Wheel sizes vary from 20, 24, to 26 in.

The most common types of wheels available are "mag" and spoke. Mag wheels were previously made of magnesium but now are constructed from plastic. They are more durable and do not require maintenance but are heavier than spoke wheels. Spoke wheels are lighter, but more care is needed to keep them tight and true. Another style that is seen on the more active sports wheelchairs are X-core wheels, which are made of composite material. They are lighter than "mags" and do not require maintenance; however, they are expensive and only accept certain tires.

There are numerous types of tires available (Table 38.3). The most common are the treaded tires with the option of air or airless inserts. They provide good traction on everyday terrain. The airless inserts decrease the maintenance issue, although the ride is harder due to the solid foam insert. Other tire options include (a) high-performance tires, used for indoor mobility and sports, which are air filled with minimal tread, allowing for comfort and low roll resistance; and (b) Kik Tires, which are solid tires with low tread for indoor and outdoor terrain.

Hand Rims

Hand rims are slightly lateral from each wheel and are used to push for propulsion. They can be aluminum for clients with normal hand function or foam and plastic coated for clients with spinal cord injury (SCI) levels between C5 and C7. The option for vertical or oblique projections on the coated rims is available to assist with propulsion, although they are not recommended because they increase the overall width of the chair.

Casters

Casters are the smaller wheels in the front of the wheelchair, which affect the turning performance. They are available in various diameters (3 to 8 in.), widths, and material. The smaller the caster, the tighter the turning radius. However, the smaller casters pose a problem with rougher terrain. The larger and wider casters perform better outdoors and on rougher terrain but increase the turning radius. The material used for casters is similar to that used for tires: pneumatic (air or airless) and solid.

The casters are attached to the wheelchair by stems and forks, which allow the casters to rotate. Suspension forks improve performance and eliminate vibration, which improve the integrity of the wheelchair.

Wheel Locks

Wheel locks, or what some call "brakes," act as a safety feature to stabilize the wheelchair for transfers and prevent the wheelchair from rolling. Wheel locks come in different styles depending on the client's hand function and balance. The two types are either push/pull to lock or scissors. Scissor brakes are for clients who have good hand function and balance. Both styles can be mounted high or low depending on the frame construction. High-mounted brakes are recommended for clients who do not have good balance. Low-mounted braces are appropriate for clients with good balance and they allow for obstacle-free propulsion.

Seat and Back Upholstery

The seat and back of a manual wheelchair usually come standard with sling vinyl upholstery. They are attached to the frame post, allowing the flexibility to easily fold for transport due to the lightweight material. Vinyl material is easy to clean, durable, and inexpensive. The disadvantage is that sling upholstery does not provide much support and over time may cause a hammock effect, which can lead to postural deformities. Cushions with a solid bottom or insert are recommended to prevent this problem.

TABLE 38.4. WHEELCHAIR ACCESSORIES

Type	Purpose
Clothing guards	To prevent clothing or skin from hitting the wheels and impeding function or causing skin breakdown. They can come in plastic or cloth and the option for a "quad hole" for clients with limited hand function is available.
Grade aides	Used to assist clients when propelling up an incline. When flipped down, they will allow the client to propel forward up an incline and prevent the wheelchair from rolling back.
Quick-release wheels	Allows the client to remove the rims from the frame of the chair to disassemble for transport. An option for a quad-release lever for clients who have fine motor deficits is available.
Push handles	They attach to the canes, allowing others to assist with propulsion and negotiating environmental obstacles, such as curbs.
Positional belt	Attaches to the frame of the wheelchair to maintain pelvic position and stability during propulsion.
Ventilator tray	Allows for placement of a ventilator and battery for transport behind or underneath the frame of the wheelchair.
Camber	Angle of the rear wheels. The top part of the wheel angle is inward, whereas the bottom angle is outward, away from the frame of the wheelchair. The advantage of camber is stability, ease of propulsion, and increased performance. The main disadvantage is the increase of overall width of the wheelchair.

Specialty seating can be added and is discussed later in this chapter.

Additional options are listed in Table 38.4.

Positional Wheelchairs

Positional wheelchairs include manual reclining and Tilt-in-Space wheelchairs. These systems are recommended over the standard and lightweight wheelchairs for those who are prone to develop pressure sores due to the inability to perform weight shifts (i.e., those with high-level SCI) and those with postural deformities, balance problems, or orthostasis. A manual positional chair is also usually prescribed as a backup for those with a power wheelchair.

Positional wheelchairs weigh in the range of 50 to 70 lb and are limited in disassembling for transport. The recliner has the ability to fold, but the type of seating system can limit this option, along with the weight of the system. The Tilt-in-Space feature allows for the back canes to fold down to a box-frame construction, although transport requires a van, sports utility vehicle, or station wagon. Certain manufactures will allow for reclining or tilt to be power operated by a switch on a manual frame, to allow the client to perform weight shifts independently. A headrest and high back are recommended for support and stability, particularly when performing weight shifts. Refer to Table 38.5 for the benefits and considerations of both systems.

TABLE 38.5. WHEELCHAIR TYPES AND POWER SEATING FUNCTIONS

Type	Advantages	Disadvantages
1. **Power wheelchairs**		
Power add-on unit	Easy to transport Two chairs in one Lightweight power	Added stress on manual frame Limited performance Warranty issues
Transportable power	Ability to disassemble for transport Direct drive	Heavy parts to transport Limited programming Inability to modify
Conventional power	Ability to integrate specialty controls Programmability	Fixed seat to back angle and seat to floor Decreases durability Inability to modify seating
Modular power	Ability to integrate specialty controls Programmability Ability to add power seating options Ability to modify seating system	Expensive
2. **Recliner**	Passive range of motion Independent seat angle adjustment Improved head control Minimizes orthostasis Easy for catheterization Can help mobilize secretions	Pressure relief/weight shifts Shear May elicit spasms Increases overall length

3. **Tilt-in-space**	Improved head and trunk control
	Minimizes orthostasis
	Diminishes effects of spasticity
	  during positional change
	Tighter turning radius
	Can help mobilize secretions
		Pressure relief/weight shifts (urine back
		  flowing during tilt using a catheter)
		Table clearance
		Lap tray and communication device place
		  ment
		Urologic concerns

4. **Standing**	Weightbearing Urologic benefits Psychological benefits Work/home accessibility	Pressure relief with contractures Limited range of motion Poor bone density Orthostatic problems Not appropriate for clients Clearance issues
5. **Seat elevator**	Assists with transfers Psychological benefits Accessibility	Limited compatibility with other seating functions Tie-down concerns

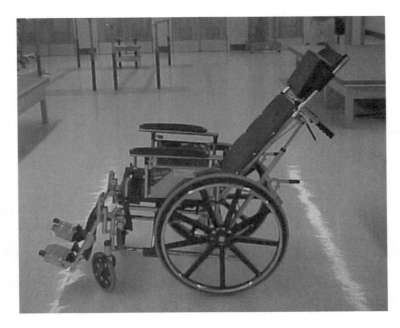

FIGURE 38.5. Recliner wheelchair.

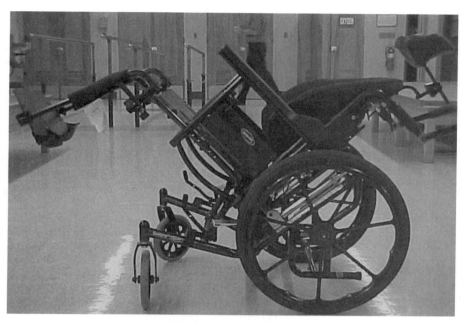

FIGURE 38.6. Tilt-in-space wheelchair.

Recline

A manual reclining wheelchair allows for change at the seat-to-back angle (Fig. 38.5). There are two types of recliners: semi and full. Semireclining wheelchairs allow up to 30 degrees of recline and are approximately 3 in. longer than a standard wheelchair. A full reclining wheelchair allows up to 90 degrees of recline and is approximately 6 in. longer in frame length.

The disadvantages of a reclining wheelchair include the weight, overall length, and bulk of the system. Another factor to consider is shear of skin, which occurs when the forces are parallel to each other such as the force exerted on the tissues in the buttocks when the seat back is reclined (3). Two approaches have been used to reduce this concern: low shear and zero shear. Low-shear systems place the seat-to-back angle hinge a few inches above the seat. By placing the seat-to-back hinge higher, it works in conjunction with the client's rotation point to reduce the movement of the tissue across the seating system. Zero-shear systems attach the back system to sliding mounts that move down as the system is reclined, minimizing the shear force.

Tilt-in-Space

An alternative to the reclining wheelchair is the tilt-in-space system, in which the entire seat and back tilt as a single unit, maintaining all seat angles (seat to back, seat to calf, calf to foot) (Fig. 38.6). The system uses a hydraulic cylinder to assist in the movement. The degree of tilt is at least 45 degrees, but some systems can go to 65 degrees. In a tilt system, the client must tilt at least 45 degrees to obtain an adequate weight shift.

POWER MOBILITY

Power mobility has significantly changed over the decades, with advancement in construction of the bases, electronics, seating

functions, and input devices. There are multiple options to consider: drive-wheel placement, seating systems, and programming features. It is very important for the client to play an active role in the assessment process to make the appropriate selection.

The medical justification for power mobility should be documented for funding issues, which include (a) the inability to propel a manual wheelchair due to limited UE ROM, strength or shoulder integrity concerns (e.g., bursitis or rotator cuff injury); (b) the inability to maintain an upright posture during manual propulsion due to trunk instability; (c) postural deformities; (d) cardiac or respiratory precautions; and (e) community reentry for work, school, or recreation activities.

The client should evaluate various power systems and the appropriate input devices to choose the optimal power system. It is necessary for the client to operate the system first in open terrain and then progress to tighter areas, various terrains, hallways, ramps, van access, and other environmental barriers to select the most appropriate system that will address the client's lifestyle.

Types of Power Mobility

Power Add-on Units

Some clients do not require power mobility full time (Table 38.5). They may be able to propel a manual wheelchair for short distances and on a level surface; however, for distance and rougher terrain, it becomes strenuous for the client's strength, shoulder integrity, or cardiac reserve. A power add-on unit can be added to most folding and rigid-frame wheelchairs, converting the system to power mobility. This system gives the client the advantage of having two chairs in one for funding purposes while offering a transportable lightweight power wheelchair.

An example of this style is the Effix Add-On Unit, which is

a direct-drive unit in which the motors are built into the hubs of the rear wheels. A battery that is removable for transport provides the power source and the system is operated via a joystick. The wheels weigh approximately 20 lb and the battery adds 10 lb to the weight of the wheelchair.

E-motion is another system, which is currently being tested. The system is considered a push-rim–activated power assist. The wheels are replaced with gearless, brushless motors mounted in the hub of each wheel, which weighs approximately 26 lb. The user strokes the push rims, as he would propel a wheelchair. However, the system power assists by increasing the speed at which the wheels rotate, increasing the distance propelled with fewer strokes and limited strength. The system reacts by touch to the rim, not by strength of the stroke. Applying pressure to the push rim, which engages the motor-controlled brakes, reduces downhill descents. The power source is mounted inside the hub of the wheel.

The disadvantages to power add-on units are the extra stress it places on the manual frame; durability compared with a full-power wheelchair, and the limited performance adjustments. It is important to verify the warranty of the wheelchair with the manufacturer before mounting the system, because some companies will void the warranty if the add on requires the frame to be modified.

Scooters

Scooters are very unique compared with power wheelchairs. They are designed for clients who are marginal ambulators and need to conserve energy. It is commonly used for community mobility for individuals with multiple sclerosis and cardiac issues, for example. The construction of the system consists of three or four wheels, a mounted seat, and a tiller steering system.

A three-wheeled scooter is narrower, has a shorter frame, and is available with front- and rear-wheel drive. Front-wheel drive is not as powerful and limits the user to level, smooth terrain. This system is best suited for indoor use due to the smaller dimensions and tighter turning radius. Rear-wheel drive offers better traction due to the center of gravity being directly through the drive wheels.

Four-wheeled scooters are available in both rear- and four-wheel drive, which increases the stability on all terrain. However, they are larger and not as easy to transport. They are better for outdoor use, but all scooters have a tendency to be top heavy and side tipping is a precaution, particularly at high speeds and on uneven surfaces.

The scooter seat is very basic and similar to a bucket seat. There have been improvements made to the seating needs to accommodate specialized seating systems. The seating is typically mounted on a single post, which allows the seat to swivel for transfers. The option for a power seat lift is available for clients to assist with transfers and functional activities.

A tiller steering system is used to operate and drive the scooter. The client requires good UE dexterity and strength to steer the system. The tiller controls steering, and acceleration relies on finger control to operate the lever. The client requires good trunk control and proximal stability to operate the system safely, so it is not appropriate for patients with high-level SCI.

The main advantages of scooters are that they are lightweight and easy to maneuver, they can be disassembled for transport, they are relatively inexpensive, and for some clients, they are aesthetically pleasing and more acceptable than a wheelchair. The disadvantages are that scooters require good UE function and balance, have limited postural support, lack the programming adjustments, and cannot be integrated with specialty controls.

Transportable Power

Power wheelchairs typically are not easy to disassemble and transport via a car. However, there are some manufacturers that construct their frames so users can remove the batteries and fold the frame to be transported. Even with removing the batteries, which weigh approximately 20 lb each, the folded frame weighs about 50 lb or more, due to the motor unit that is attached to the frame.

The advantages of transportable power wheelchairs include a lower cost, household and community mobility, and the ability to transport via a car. The disadvantages are that they are not as compact and lightweight to disassemble and load on a daily basis as a manual wheelchair, they have limited programming and ability to change controls to specialty controls, they cannot be integrated with power-seating functions, and they are less durable.

The advantages of transportable power wheelchairs over add-on units are the stability and durability of the transportable power system. The frames are constructed to handle the power capabilities on various types of terrain, whereas add-on unit is mounted to a manual wheelchair, which can affect the performance, stability, and durability of the frame over time.

The clinician must educate the client and family on the advantages and disadvantages of this type of power system. It is necessary to have the caretaker demonstrate the task of assembling and disassembling the system to see if it is appropriate for the user's lifestyle. This system is not appropriate for clients with progressive diagnoses (e.g., progressive motor neuron disease) due to the inability to modify electronics.

Conventional Power

Conventional power wheelchairs are designed similar to the typical manual cross-frame system, with the power drive system mounted underneath. These systems are belt driven, which acts like a pulley system. Each rear wheel has a large pulley mounted around the rim to rotate the wheels. Conventional power wheelchairs have the large wheels mounted in the rear and they control the steering of the system.

The main advantage of this system versus the transportable power wheelchair is the ability to integrate specialty controls and power seating functions. It comes standard with a proportional joystick and has the ability to be programmed for performance adjustments, such as speed and acceleration. The limitations with conventional frames are the fixed seat-to-back angle and seat-to-floor height, increased overall width due to the seating system sitting between the wheels, and durability due to belt slippage and breaks.

TABLE 38.6. ADVANTAGES AND DISADVANTAGES OF WHEEL PLACEMENT

Type of Wheel Drive	Advantages	Disadvantages
Rear-wheel drive	Greater sense of control Greater speed Stability	Rear tipping is a concern on inclines; need to use antitips Larger turning radius
Mid-wheel/center-wheel drive	Tightest turning radius Maneuverability in tight spaces	Less stable Front tippy, particularly on rougher terrain Concern with clients that lack trunk control
Front-wheel drive	Maneuverability in tight spaces Better getting over rougher terrain	Difficult to track in straight line Takes more skill to operate

Modular Power Bases

To meet the needs of the SCI population, one needs to explore nonfolding power-base wheelchairs. The modular system offers two parts, the power base and seating system on top. The advantage to this system is the separate seating system, which can be modified or adapted without changing the power base. This system is a direct drive, which is directly paired to the wheels through gearboxes. The advantages of direct drive include no slippage, more durability, better performance, and increased speed, torque, and power. The braking system is a dynamic or active brake that provides voltage to stop the motor and prevents rolling. Additional advantages include the ability to adjust the seat-to-back angle and the seat-to-floor height, the advanced programming particularly for specialty controls, and power-seating systems. The modular power bases also have improved outdoor performance for power wheelchairs. The rear wheels are smaller (10 to 14 in.) than those of conventional power wheelchairs (20 in.) with thicker tread width that improves traction on rough terrain.

Due to environmental barriers, manufacturers have started designing the power bases with the drive wheels placed in three different positions on the base: rear-wheel drive, mid-wheel or center-wheel drive, and front-wheel drive (Table 38.6 and Fig. 38.7). The modular bases allow for numerous postural adjustments, growth, and the ability to adapt to meet the client's functional needs.

Before selecting a power base, one must consider the following: compatibility with power-seating systems and specialty controls; transportation, lifts, tie-down system; ground clearance; seat-to-floor heights for table or desk access; battery use; range of travel on a charge; and the seating options and accessories.

Power Wheelchair Components

Power wheelchairs have similar components to those of manual wheelchairs. Technology has advanced to the point that manufactures are constructing interchangeable parts between manual and power wheelchairs.

Armrests

Most power wheelchairs use the two-point height-adjustable and flip-back style to make transfers easier. Additional support may be needed due to the client's level of injury and positional concerns. Arm troughs with hand supports or wide flat armpads are available to prevent subluxation, to distribute pressure equally, and to prevent contractures for those with no or limited UE movement. These contoured supports may increase the overall width or interfere with armrest function to flip back.

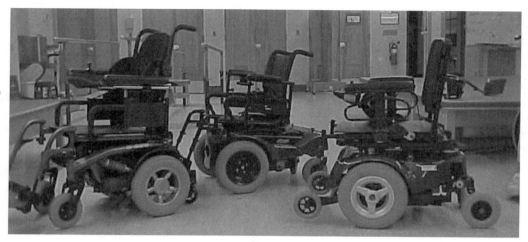

FIGURE 38.7. Positions of power base: rear-wheel, mid-wheel, and front-wheel drive.

Footrest/Leg Rest

Elevating leg rests are available and the option for "smart leg rests" is available. Smart leg rests elevate up and extend outward, keeping the LEs in good position and preventing jamming of the knee and added pressure on the ischial tuberosities. The disadvantage is that they are heavier. Additional support, such as a calf pad or trough, is needed with elevating leg rests to maintain the LE on the leg rest.

Foot supports come in composite plastic with no ankle adjustability and are small and not as durable; extra-large plates that are metal or angle-adjustable plates that accommodate ankle deformities are available. Some power wheelchairs offer a center footrest with a flip-up footplate, which shortens the overall length of the wheelchair and is aesthetically pleasing to the client.

Headrests

There are numerous types of headrests depending on the client's needs. When providing a tilt or recline system, a headrest must be provided to support the cervical region. A custom contoured headrest with lateral and occipital supports can be used to correct or accommodate deformities.

Wheels/Tires

The smaller casters (6 × 2 in.) are more appropriate for indoor or tight environments, whereas 8- and 9-in. diameters are used for outdoor rough or uneven terrain for better performance. The rear wheels used to have a 20-in. diameter; however, to increase performance, manufacturers are producing wheels with 10- to 14-in. diameters by 2- to 4-in. thickness.

The smaller rear wheels have improved turning radius and traction. It is recommended to have a solid insert to prevent flats, which would impede power mobility.

Seat and Back

Most power wheelchairs come with a solid seat pan, with a specialty cushion placed on it. The back system can be either sling upholstery or a specialty solid back. The sling upholstery is not appropriate when using a Tilt-in-Space system, because it is not strong enough to support the client's weight over time. Solid backs come in various styles: flat, curved, contoured, and molded, depending on the client's postural needs.

Power-Seating Functions

Power-seating functions include recline, tilt in space, elevating leg rests, standing and seat elevation (Table 38.5). The importance of these features is to give the client the ability to independently change positions for pressure relief or medical concerns (hypotension), to improve balance and postural alignment, to allow the client to stretch and rest, to provide comfort, and for psychological reasons. The power-seating functions can be used in combination with each other. It is important to consult with the manufacturer to determine the compatibility with the base and the overall dimensions.

Batteries

There are two types of batteries: wet-cell or gel-cell batteries. Wet-cell batteries store more energy, are less expensive, but require more maintenance than gel cell. Gel-cell batteries are required for transport by air. The batteries are charged daily and most power wheelchairs, depending on the terrain, remain charged for up to 12 hours of use.

Additional Accessories

A ventilator tray and battery box are required for clients who require a ventilator. The ventilator is usually mounted to the rear of the wheelchair with the battery mounted underneath. The trays are usually a gimbal style, which has a pivot point to rotate the tray outward during seating functions, or trailer style, which is a flat tray under the seat depending on the frame construction. The gimbal style is used with tilt and recline systems, because it does not impede the function and remains level during tilting and reclining. It is important to keep in mind that the wheelchair may increase in overall length due to how the vent tray is mounted.

Swing-away joystick hardware lets the user retract the joystick out to the side and back, to access tabletops, desks, and a steering wheel.

Lap trays provide support for the UEs and function as a workplace for individuals who cannot access a table. Additional accessories can be mounted to a lap tray, such as book holder, laptop, or communication board, to increase function.

Suspension is a feature to reduce vibration, decrease wear and tear, increase the life of the frame, and improve the performance and ride of the system. Suspension can be within the casters, in the rear, or in the mounting of the seating system to the base.

Integrated controls refer to the ability to plug into the wheelchair's electronics to operate assistive devices. Wheelchair electronics offer the ability to interconnect hardware to control communication devices and environmental control units through the input device that is being used to operate the power base (2).

Types of Input Devices

The input device used to operate the power system is one of the most important decisions to be made. To select the optimal input device, one must address the client's postural needs to allow him or her to accurately operate the input device consistently. The client must operate the power system with the input device on all types of terrain to assess if the input device is consistently and safely activated. Technology has advanced so clients can interchange input devices as their function changes. This is extremely important when addressing medical justification and approval from insurance providers.

Input devices can be categorized into two areas: proportional or nonproportional. Proportional input devices allow the speed and direction of the wheelchair to be directly proportional to the amount of force applied to the input device and in the direction that the force is applied. Proportional input devices allow for greater control over movement of the wheelchair, and speed is infinitely variable from zero to the top speed of the system. These systems are appropriate for clients with fair to good strength with adequate active ROM and coordination. Nonproportional input devices offer the "all or none" signal. Past systems operated the input signal directly into the response or movement of the power system. The result was a less smooth ride and inability to grade movement. Nonproportional input is either on or off; however, advanced electronics with programmability can allow these systems to grade responses to simulate a proportional system to some degree. Nonproportional input devices are used with clients who are limited in strength, ROM, and coordination. It is important to evaluate the cognitive status prior due to the multiple steps needed to scan and select between modes (4).

Joystick (Proportional/Nonproportional)

A joystick-input device is the most commonly used, although considerations need to be addressed in the size, placement, mounting hardware, and accessibility. As already stated, there are two types of joysticks: proportional (continuous) and nonproportional (discrete). A proportional joystick allows for 360-degree directional signal and responds immediately in the direction of the client's movement on the control device. A proportional joystick controls the direction and the rate and speed of movement. A nonproportional joystick (discrete) is for clients who lack the motor control to operate a proportional joystick but have gross motor movement that is consistent. Nonproportional inputs operate in either a four or eight directional. A four-directional joystick will produce movement forward, reverse, left, and right. An eight-directional joystick allows these four directions plus diagonal movements between the standard directions. Nonproportional input devices are either on or off and the amount of response is not proportional to the amount of input. The wheelchair will accelerate at a preset speed and stay at that speed until the switch is no longer closed (activated).

When evaluating for a joystick device, the client must be able to independently place his or her hand on and off the joystick. The joystick can be mounted laterally or medially to the dominant side, or even midline to accommodate for limited active ROM of the UE. Adaptation devices, such as a goal post, can be mounted to the joystick for clients who lack fine motor dexterity to operate the standard knob. If the client has consistent finger movement, a touch pad proportional joystick would be appropriate. The touch pad has a small square control box with a cross outlined on the screen. The client would place the active moving finger in the middle of the cross and slide the finger in the direction she would like to go. It requires minimal movement and is a proportional input, allowing for 360-degree direction.

Joystick input can be at other sites, including the head, chin, elbow, and foot. These sites usually use a remote proportional joystick, which is smaller with no switches for on and off or speed control and is mounted to an interface. A head control joystick is mounted to the back of the headrest on a flexible mount to allow for lateral rotation and flexion-extension of the neck to operate the joystick. Lateral movement will elicit turns and extension will allow the wheelchair to go forward. An addi-

tional switch is needed to allow the forward command to toggle to reverse mode or power-seating functions. This switch can be mounted on the headrest at a site the client can activate. Head control inputs are appropriate for clients with active ROM at the cervical region and no cervical bracing or collars (i.e., those with C4 level SCI).

There is another system that operates with sensors and is a proportional input. The sensors are in a flat or curved headrest and require the client to laterally flex to activate input for right and left, forward flex to go forward, and extension to stop.

The speed is proportional to the amount of forward flexion of the neck away from the headrest. There is a limit switch built into the system; if a client spasms or falls forward, the distance is preset to stop automatically. A visual display is needed to operate drive modes and power-seating functions.

A chin control joystick is mounted in front and directly below the chin. Usually clients (those with C4 level SCI and weak patients with C5 level SCI) who are not able to independently place their hand on a joystick will be appropriate for a head or chin control. A small cup is used to replace the knob for better control and pressure distribution. The input works the same as a proportional hand joystick; the direction the joystick is moved is the direction the wheelchair will go. A foot control joystick is mounted under a footplate on a swivel hinge, which requires plantar flexion, dorsiflexion, inversion, and eversion of the ankle. Most clients who are appropriate for this device have an incomplete SCI (such as central cord syndrome), motor neuron disease, or multiple sclerosis.

Breath Control (Sip and Puff)

Breath control input devices are appropriate for clients who have limited or no use of their arms and legs and weakness in the cervical region (Fig. 38.8). Sip and puff is controlled by a series of breaths: hard and soft sips and puffs through a straw, which is mounted to the wheelchair. The client would have the ability to drive and operate power-seating functions through the breath control. A visual display is needed to see what mode the client is in, which can also give auditory feedback. The client would operate the drive by hard puffing to activate the input to go forward and by hard sipping to stop and reverse the wheelchair. Forward and reverse can be either momentary or latched. Momentary means a response only occurs when the client is interacting with the input device. For example, maintaining a hard puff to go forward and once the breath is stopped, the wheelchair stops. Latched means a cruise control; input is given until the wanted speed or response occurs. Once the desired response is achieved, it will continue until another input is given. For example, one hard puff will allow the wheelchair to go forward and continue to go forward to allow for other breath input, and soft puff and sip turns the wheelchair right or left and is used to maneuver the wheelchair. To stop the wheelchair from latch, the client either gives the opposite command or activates the reset switch. A reset switch is a safety feature, which is a necessity. It is important to place the switch at a site that can be consistently activated in case of emergency to stop the wheelchair. Right and left turns are always momentary.

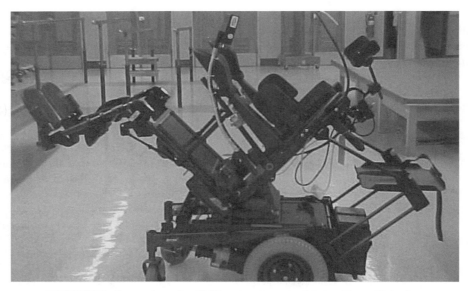

FIGURE 38.8. Power sip and puff tilt and recline wheelchair with ventilator tray.

Head Array

Head array input devices are a type of nonproportional (digital) input (Fig. 38.9). The nonproportional head array input device is a three-piece padded headrest with sensors in each pad. The sensors in the wings control the right and left movement, and the back pad controls forward and reverse. Two sensors can be operated jointly to create veer. Veer is used only with nonproportional input devices. When two switches are closed, which is usually forward or reverse with right or left, it will allow for a controlled turning response. This is similar to a proportional input. It determines how gradual or severe a course correction will be, particularly in a latched mode. The sensors do not require pressure to activate. The client needs to move the head toward the sensor, which can be mounted anywhere in the pad for access to activate the switch.

A reset switch needs to be in place to change forward to reverse and operate seating functions. An electrical switch (beam) or a mechanical (disk) switch can be used. A beam switch would be mounted to the back of the headrest in direct line of the client. The switch would be activated while the client's head is within range and closed when the client moves forward out of range to switch drive modes or operate seating functions. A mechanical switch requires physical contact to activate. It can be a wobble, button, disk, or ribbon switch that can be mounted by a site the client can reach to activate consistently.

Sip and Puff/Head Array

A sip and puff/head array input device is a combination of two types of drive input devices to obtain optimal access. Some clients have great difficulty discriminating between hard and soft commands for breath control. This system allows for any sip

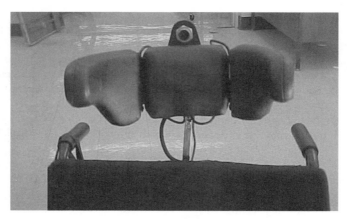

FIGURE 38.9. Head array system.

and puff to operate the reverse and forward drive, and the right and left functions are activated by the sensors in the lateral wings of the headrest. Again a reset switch, either a beam or mechanical switch, must be in place for mode change and safety.

Switches

There are numerous switches on the market to operate power mobility and power-seating functions, such as tilt and recline. Multiple switch input usually consists of four to five switches that are mounted either in a lap tray, on a headrest, or at site of consistent movement to activate. Four of the switches operate the direction of the wheelchair: forward, reverse, right, and left. The fifth switch operates the on and off. If power-seating functions are needed, either add more switches to operate the seating functions or use a mode switch to toggle into seating functions using the drive switches.

Single switch input devices are usually considered the client's "last chance to drive." It is recommended for clients who only have one controlled movement. It requires a visual scanner, which is programmed for speed with four directional arrows that light up on sequence. When the directional arrow is lit up for the desired movement, the client will activate the switch. The switch is an electronic switch that does not require direct physical contact or delayed activation. Single switch input devices can operate power-seating functions also.

A *fiberoptic switch* input device is a red beam of light the size of the head of a straight pin that is activated when covered. This input device is ideal for clients with very limited finger movement. The fiberoptics can be mounted into a lap tray, splint, or armpad to access consistently. It can also be used to activate a single switch scanner for mobility and power-seating functions.

The *tongue touch keypad* input device is a custom dental orthosis that is molded to the roof of the mouth with a number of tiny switches within the orthosis and a radio transmitter that sends radio waves to the wheelchair receiver to operate for mobility. The client must be able to use his or her tongue to operate the switches and be able to tolerate an orthosis in the mouth. This system is recommended for clients who are unable to activate a single switch or who lack head and breath control.

Voice activation input devices have been in the experimental stages over the past few years and will be available soon. A system that is currently being tested is mounted around the neck and activates when the client speaks by sensing the vibration. It requires special programming and training to operate.

SPECIALTY WHEELCHAIRS

Standup Wheelchairs

Standup wheelchairs can be manual or power operated on a manual or power frame (Fig. 38.10A and B). The benefits of a standup wheelchair include weightbearing, which may decrease osteoporosis (4); improved bladder function by improving flow and decreasing residual urine and decreasing the incidence of kidney stones and urinary tract infections (5,6); improved bowel regularity; passive ROM to prevent contractures (7); pressure relief and reduced pressure ulcers (5); decreased effects of spasticity (8); accessibility to reach cabinets, closet shelves, and so on; work and school accessibility; and psychological benefits.

Manual standup wheelchairs are for clients with good upper body strength, to operate the lift mechanism. They are constructed on a manual frame so the client can propel when in a seated position. Some systems are light enough for the client to use as an everyday wheelchair and have the ability to disassemble

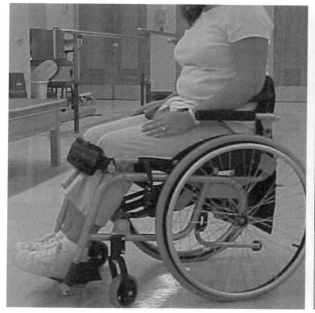
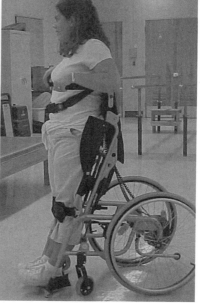

FIGURE 38.10. Stand-up wheelchair: **(A)** seated position, **(B)** standing position.

for car transport. The option to have a power standup on a manual base is for the client who is not able to operate the manual lift mechanism due to limited strength or balance but still has the ability to manually propel the wheelchair. However, the frame will be heavier due to the power lift and battery, which is mounted under the seat.

There are some systems that offer power standup on a power base for the client who is not able to manually propel. Some power bases let the client drive while standing; however, it is recommended to drive only on level surfaces. Usually, top speed is cut in half while operating power mobility while standing due to safety concerns. These systems do not disassemble for car transport; they require van or medical transport.

The actual fitting for a standup wheelchair is very complex and requires detailed measurements for an appropriate fit. It is extremely important to decide if there are any contraindications to standing, such as ROM and risk of fractures. It is recommended that the client be supervised and medically monitored (blood pressure) during the evaluation, and a schedule for standing duration when the system is received.

Sport Wheelchairs

Sport wheelchairs such as those for tennis, basketball, rugby, or racing are specially constructed and adjusted for the specific sport for which it is used (Fig. 38.11). They are not used as the primary wheelchair for the client. The frames are rigid and are constructed of lightweight material such as titanium or carbon fiber. Sport wheelchairs are expensive and require very specific and careful measurements for an appropriate fit. For contact sports such as rugby, the chairs have metal guards at the base to protect the casters and the client from frequent collisions. Racing wheelchairs are very specialized; they require the user to be compressed in a compact shape. The racer chair has two rear wheels with wide camber, to improve stability and minimize tipping, and small-diameter hand rims to maximize arm stroke. The casters are eliminated by a third wheel placed in the front of the system giving the sleek appearance.

Recreational Wheelchairs

Wheelchairs can be for the everyday user who may not be interested in competitive sports but who would like the physical and psychological benefits of exercising. Depending on the client's participation and use, there are lever-drive or arm-crank chairs. The lever drive can be adapted to the current wheelchair wheels so the client can use the lever instead of the push rim to propel. This allows the client an easier push and more rapid speed to travel a longer distance. It acts very similar to a single-speed bicycle.

The arm-crank vehicle is a hand cycle bicycle, which is similar to the mountain bike with gears. The gears allow for the client to choose the efficient gear for the grade of roadway she is traveling. Unlike the lever drive, the client uses this system as a second wheelchair. The limitation to this system is the balance of the client needed to maintain control while operating the system. Steering and drive operation are interconnected. Careful consideration must be paid to the client's required postural and external supports, and it is important that these supports are tried and tested before use (2).

All-Terrain Wheelchairs

Some clients like to experience the rugged outdoors, although their everyday wheelchairs are not equipped to accommodate the extreme rough terrain. The all-terrain wheelchairs appear similar to four-wheeled racers with large front wheels, knobby tires in the rear with a lot of camber, and dual push rims (two per rear wheel). The dual push rims assist the client in accessing the proper gear depending on the terrain. The handlebars and

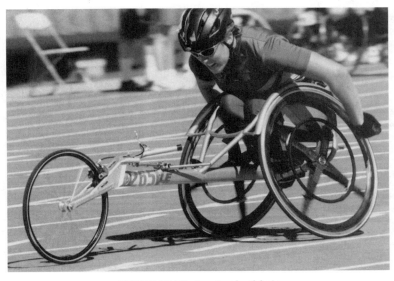

FIGURE 38.11. Sports wheelchair.

brakes, which are mounted in the front, assist with the control declining on rough terrain.

Power all-terrain wheelchairs are more appropriate and efficient for clients who do not have the UE strength and shoulder joint integrity to operate a manual all-terrain wheelchair. The Omega Trac and Permobil Power Base have a wheelchair seating system mounted on top, but the base is powerful enough to climb curbs, hills, and all rough terrain. It is a front-wheel system with suspension and can be operated via joystick and other specialty controls.

Johnson & Johnson is awaiting Food and Drug Administration approval on a new technology wheelchair, the Independence™ IBOT™ 3000 mobility system, which will have the capability to drive on rough unleveled terrain, sand, and curbs, as well as ascend and descend stairs.

Beach Wheelchairs

Beach wheelchairs, which are manually operated, can be used as transport on and off the sand, like lounge chairs, and some can be used in the water. They require a caretaker to assist with propulsion due to the large air-filled tires in the front and rear. They are usually one size fits all and specialized seating is not provided.

TRANSPORTATION CONSIDERATIONS

Transportation of a wheelchair needs to be separated into manual and power systems, as well as car or van versus public transportation. Manual wheelchairs, whether a rigid or folding frame, can easily be disassembled and transported by car. It is important to educate and evaluate the ability of the client and family or caretaker to disassemble and assemble the wheelchair for transport in the vehicle that will most often be used. An option is for a car topper, in which a power mechanical lift can allow the client to load a folding wheelchair on top of the roof in a storage box for transport.

Manual positional chairs can be more cumbersome and may not always fit in a car, particularly with the various seating and accessories. Power add-on systems are similar to manual wheelchairs, except that they have heavier parts such as the battery and power wheels. Most scooters can be disassembled for car transport but can be too heavy, even as parts to lift into a trunk. They do make trunk lifts and rear attachments that can mount to a car to assist with transport.

Power-base wheelchairs are more complex. Even the low-end folding frames, which allow for the batteries to be removed, are still relatively heavy and not easy to load into a car on a regular basis. Transport of a power wheelchair generally requires a van, van lift, or ramp and a specialized tie-down system. Important factors to consider include the overall width, length, and height of the system with the client in it, the setup inside for transport, and the client's ability to drive the vehicle. The type of lockdown system also needs to be assessed.

Public transportation has advanced greatly in many states to allow the client the freedom to explore the world. Buses have specialized lifts and removable seats to accommodate manual and power wheelchairs. Train stations have specific stops desig-

nated for wheelchair users, with elevators to access certain city subways and streets. Airline travel needs special consideration and preparation. Manual wheelchairs, depending on their size, can be taken on board if arrangements are made beforehand. However, power wheelchairs are placed underneath the plane with the baggage, and the batteries must be approved for travel; that is, they must be gel batteries, not lead acid. It is also recommended to remove as many removable parts as possible, particularly the joystick, and box them to prevent damage during travel.

CUSHIONS AND BACKS

The cushion and back are considered the seating system and require special consideration. A wide variety of cushions and backs are available on the market, and they can be divided into several specific classes according to their properties. Factors to consider when selecting a seating system include the patient's motor, sensory, and functional level; skin integrity; degree of spasticity; sitting balance; postural deformities; transfer and weight-shift techniques; bowel and bladder continence; and cognitive status.

Cushions

Cushions can be divided into three support-type surfaces: planar, contoured, and custom contoured (Fig. 38.12). Planar systems are flat surfaces that support the body only where the user makes contact with the system. Planar systems are prescribed for pediatrics because they can "grow" as the child grows. They are appropriate for clients who do not require a lot of support, due to the lack of contour. The main disadvantage is the unequal distribution of pressure that occurs on the bony prominence that it is in contact with.

Commercially or prefabricated contoured surfaces are made in 1-in. increments to fit the client. These systems are adjustable with lateral supports and hip guides to allow for proper position-

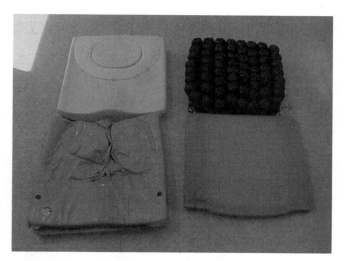

FIGURE 38.12. Cushions: Top left: Invacare Infinity; Top Right: High Profile ROHO; Bottom Left: Jay 2 (Sunrise Medical); Bottom Right: Stimulite Contour.

ing. They also distribute pressure better due to the contour feature, if the client has minimal postural deformities. Growth is limited with this type of system, so it will need to be replaced with a larger-size one.

Custom contour molds can be fabricated on site with the use of simulators to address the client's position and then sent to the shop or manufacturer to be completed. This system provides the greatest amount of contact surface to distribute pressure and support to accommodate or correct the client's posture. The main disadvantages are its cost and the time-consuming process to fit the system. Growth is very limited and will require remolding when changes occur.

Properties

Table 38.7 summarizes the types of cushions, with advantages and disadvantages of each. The properties can be divided into several areas:

1. Resilience: the ability of the material to regain shape after the load has been removed
2. Envelopment: the degree to which the client sinks into the cushion and it conforms around the buttocks; this promotes stability for the client and reduces peak pressures
3. Dampening: the ability of the cushion to soften on impact and absorb shock
4. Temperature: the ability of a cushion to absorb heat and dissipate it to prevent pressure ulcers, as well as the ability to act as an insulator
5. Shear: the forces that act parallel to the surface of the skin and cause tension on the skin and underlying tissue; it is necessary to evaluate the cushion and cover, as well as how the client moves and transfers to see the effects on the skin
6. Suspension: suspension or a cutout in a specific area is seen

to eliminate pressure; this requires specific measurements and trial to ensure that additional problems do not occur
7. Weight: this is important to the client depending on the mobility system; manual users prefer a lighter cushion to be on their lightweight wheelchair, whereas for power mobility, weight is not as much a concern

Foam Cushions

There are various densities and types of foams. They are inexpensive and lightweight. There are two types of cell structures for foam: open cell and closed cell.

Open-cell foam has a membrane that is interconnected with tiny holes to allow for airflow and ventilation. The main problem is absorption into the open cell, which decreases the life of the cushion and makes it difficult to clean. Closed-cell foam has an outside membrane that protects the foam but limits airflow. Examples of foams are polyurethane, latex, Sunmate, or a combination of foams. Life expectancy for foam cushions is about 6 to 12 months.

Gel Cushions

Gel cushions are characterized by viscosity, which is the degree to which fluid molecules move across each other. High-viscosity gel provides a more stable seating surface, although it is limited in shock-absorbing properties and is usually heavy, with fair envelopment and temperature concerns (2). Lower viscosity gels offer greater shock absorption and good envelopment, and temperature is usually not a concern, but resilience is poor.

Air Cushions

Air cushions consist of soft, flexible interconnected air cells that can be ordered in different heights: 2 or 4 in. or a combination

TABLE 38.7. SUMMARY OF TYPES OF CUSHIONS

Type	Advantages	Disadvantages	Examples
Foam	Inexpensive Lightweight Easy to modify Growth	Short lifespan due to light and moisture Loses resilience Limited points of contact depending on the stiffness	T-Foam Polyurethane Sunmate
Gel			
1. High viscosity	Good dampening Stable seating surface Does not change with atmospheric pressure	Poor envelopment Poor resilience Limiting shock absorption Heavy	Royale Action Gel
2. Low viscosity	Good envelopment Good support Better shock absorption	Poor resilience	Jay Fluid Pads
Air	Good pressure relief Good resilience Good envelopment depending on inflation	Maintenance Punctures Air loss depending on temperature and altitude Stability Expensive	Roho Starr
Hybrid	Good pressure relief Good stability and support Good envelopment	Fair resilience Weight Increased thickness Expensive	Jay 2 Varlite

of both sizes to allow airflow and circulation between cells. As the client's body shape changes or shifts, the cushion adjusts and facilitates blood flow for pressure relief and distribution. Air cushions have good resilience and envelopment and are lightweight. The disadvantages include the maintenance required to regulate the pressure to prevent overinflation or underinflation; they are nonpuncture resistant, and they have the possibility of air loss over time, or temperature and altitude change.

Hybrid Cushions

Hybrid cushions are a combination of two types of cushion material mentioned previously. One example, the Jay 2, is a closed-cell foam base with gel placed on top of the contoured base foam. This combination provides good envelopment, good temperature considerations, postural support and stability, and optimal pressure relief. Another example, the Varlite Cushion, combines air and foam, which allows for contouring to the client's seated posture, or can be segmented to adjust for correcting flexible deformities.

Other

The Stimulite cushion is made of a soft, flexible form of aerospace honeycomb, which contours to the body. They are open celled with perforations to allow airflow and moist evaporation. The cells are flexible to reduce shear and provide stabilization. It is extremely lightweight (about 3 lb) and comes in planar and contoured shapes.

Alternating-Pressure Cushions

The cushions previously mentioned are all static cushions, which only redistribute pressure over the seated position and require the client to perform weight shifts. Alternating-pressure cushions were designed on the premise that weightbearing surfaces can tolerate high pressures for a longer period if alternated with periods of no pressure. The alternating-pressure cushions on the market offer an oscillating pump that alternates pressure at specific times. They work off a battery-operated system, which must be mounted to the wheelchair and weigh about 8 lb. If the system goes into fail mode or the battery is not charged, usually the system will remain in a full-air position. Some systems have a 1- to 2-in. foam base. It is important to clinically trial and document the results and failure of static versus dynamic cushions so third-party payers can consider purchase.

Technology

It is difficult to select an appropriate cushion, particularly for clients with a problematic skin history. Pressure mapping, which measures the pressure between the cushion and buttocks, can be used to measure quantitative sitting pressures with various cushions (3).

The most common type of pressure-mapping system used is the multiple-sensor system, which is a very thin map with multiple sensors throughout. It is placed over the entire seating surface and allows measurements simultaneously. The benefit of this system is that it measures at all points and visually illustrates the areas of concern. Pressure mapping is a tool that can confirm a suspected increased pressure area, to compare various cushions, to shorten trial time, and to educate the client on pressure areas and the effectiveness of weight shifts through visual input of the computer screen.

Backs

Back systems are important to consider for the client to maintain an upright position and tolerate that position while participating in everyday activities. Back systems can be divided into high- and low-back support and upholstery, flat or contoured base. A low back extends from the cushion to approximately 2 to 3 in. below the inferior angle of the scapula and is for active users with good trunk stability. It allows for the scapular region to be free to allow for ease of stroke and ability to reach. A high back is needed for clients who lack trunk stability. A high back supports the thoracic and lumbar spine and can range from 2 in. above the inferior angle of the scapula to the shoulder region depending on trunk stability and balance.

The sling upholstery back systems are for active users who have good trunk alignment. Some clients prefer the sling upholstery for ease of folding and because of the lightweight material. Sling upholstery is not recommended on Tilt-in-Space wheelchairs or for clients who are heavy leaners for the fact that the upholstery will bow quickly. Tension-adjustable upholstery is an option. It has straps in the back to reposition and tighten the back to prevent the sling position and improve lumbar support.

A flat solid back allows for additional supports, such as lateral supports and a headrest. It provides a firm surface for clients who require better trunk support. It can vary in height depending on the client's need.

The contoured back systems can be divided into commercial and custom. The commercial backs are the off-the-shelf systems, with the lateral supports symmetrically molded into the base. This is good for the newly injured client or clients with minimal deformities and poor balance. However, if clients require more aggressive contouring or accommodation of their deformities, then a custom-molded system is needed. The custom-molded systems provide the best pressure distribution and points of contact. It is time consuming and expensive and the same considerations as were mentioned with cushions must be considered. Approaches such as the hand-shaped foam, foam in place, and vacuum consolidation methods (Contour U) can be used for custom cushions and back systems.

PRINCIPLES OF SEATING

The seating system is a static system that is used to align and maintain the appropriate posture to improve function. It is vital that clinicians have an understanding of optimal seating specifications and the body's biomechanical alignment to select the appropriate seating system. The clinician should use a systematic approach of proximal to distal support, starting at the pelvis, which is the key to proper posture. A complete description of this approach is beyond the scope of this chapter. However, the optimal seated position achieves the following:

- a level pelvis with a slight anterior tilt
- aligned trunk with normal spinal curves
- the head should be maintained over the pelvis with eyes looking directly ahead and level
- thighs should be slightly abducted
- hips and knees flexed to about 90 degrees
- feet should rest in a slightly dorsiflexed position

If obtaining the optimal seated position cannot be achieved due to postural deformities or inability to function, the clinician needs to accommodate for the client's position to enhance function, mobility, and comfort (Table 38.8). It is important that a mat evaluation (Appendix 38.1) be completed in the supine and seated positions.

The level of the footrests affects the client's position, skin, function, and comfort. If the footrests are too high, added pressure is placed on the ischial tuberosities and there is limited access to tabletops. If the footrests are too low, the client will tend to slide out of the system and increase pressure on the posterior aspect of the thigh by the popliteal fossa.

Seating And Wheelchair Prescription

The proper selection of a seating and mobility system requires careful consideration of the client's needs, posture, function, and community demands. Clients should express their goals and expectations to the team while the team completes a history, a mat assessment, and appropriate systems for trial. The trials should be supervised by a clinician and the client should provide feedback to make an appropriate decision. It is critical during the trials to incorporate the environmental issues, home accessibility, and transportation situations to select the appropriate system.

The Process

A referral is needed by a physician order. Information regarding the client should be ascertained (Table 38.2). It is important to establish the client's goals and expectations before the assessment. The insurance company should be contacted to find out equipment coverage and the preferred provider of the equipment.

A comprehensive mat evaluation (Appendix 38.1) then takes place, with measurements (Table 38.9) and trials of various seating and mobility systems. Once the client and the team have selected an appropriate system, a written prescription is completed. A letter of justification needs to be completed to justify to the funding source the need for the recommended system. This letter should include all the client's background information mentioned earlier, the findings at the mat assessment, the equipment trialed with the reasons certain products did not work and why the recommended system is appropriate. It is extremely helpful to include pictures, particularly when involved seating is required, illustrating how an appropriate seating and mobility system can affect a client's posture and function. Home, work,

TABLE 38.8. SEATING CONSIDERATIONS

Problem	Possible Causes	Possible Solutions
1. Pelvis		
a. Posterior pelvic tilt	TLRP—Flexion	Firm back and seat with correct length and contour
	Extensor thrust	Seat-to-back angle <90 degrees to inhibit hip extensor spasticity
	Tight hamstrings	Add knee block to maintain a neutral pelvic alignment if not fixed
	Limited hip flexion	
Patient sliding out of wheelchair	Seating issues:	
	—seat too long	Use lumbar/sacral pad
	—anterior wedge too high	Adjust foot support
	—footrest too low	Drop seat if a foot propeller
	—seat belt too high	Hip belt 45 degree/Y belt
b. Anterior pelvic tilt	Hip flexion tightness/contracture	Inhibit hip flexor tone through use of flat seat
	Weakness of abdominals	Accommodate hip flexion-contracture via wedging
		Hip belt positioned over ASIS
c. Obliquity	Asymmetry of muscle tone	Solid seat with lateral pelvic blocks for midline orientation
	Scoliosis	
	Sublux-dislocation of the hip	
	—sling upholstery	Build up under buttocks—low side if flexible; high side if fixed
	—seat too narrow	Molded seating to accommodate
		Y hip belt
d. Rotation	ATNR	Midline positioning of the head
	Asymmetry of muscle tone	Y hip belt
	Scoliosis with rotation	Accommodate leg length individually
	Thigh length discrepancy	
	Seating issues:	
	—seat of the chair fitted for longer leg	

(continued)

TABLE 38.8. *(continued)*

Problem	Possible Causes	Possible Solutions
2. Spine		
a. Scoliosis	Hypotonia in trunk and gravity issues	Three points of support with a firm seat
	Asymmetric muscle tone	Power or manual tilt to decrease effect of gravity
	ATNR	Precontoured lateral trunk molding to provide midline feedback
	Pelvic obliquity	
	Fixed spinal deformity	Orthosis
b. Kyphosis	Posterior pelvic tilt	Support pelvis; lumbar/sacral support
	Hypotonia in trunk	Decrease influence of gravity, recline
	Effect of STNR or TLRP	Anterior trunk supporters
	Fixed spinal deformity	Use of arm supports
c. Rotation	Asymmetry of muscle tone	Use of curved trunk support to provide anterior control on rotated side
	Thigh length discrepancy	Chest strap
		Anterior shoulder pads
3. Hips		
a. Extension-flexion	TLRS/primitive tonal patterns	Neutral orientation of the head
	Positive supporting extensor thrust	Seat wedge to decrease extensor tone
		Accommodate hamstrings
		Pelvic support
		Footplate at appropriate height
		Accommodate via wedging
b. Abduction-adduction	Dislocation of hip	Control pelvic rotation
	Surgical adductor release	Pommel
	Seating issues:	Lateral thigh blocks
	—seat depth too short	
	—sling seat	
c. Internal-external rotation	Dislocation of hip	Internal-lateral extension on footplate
		Neutral foot position
4. Knees		
Flexion-extension	Tight hamstrings	Reduce hip flexion angle
	Fixed deformity	Trough the front edge of the cushion to accommodate
5. Ankles		
a. Plantarflexion	Extensor tone/positive supporting reflex	Wedge seat and raise footrest to decrease tone
	Shortening heelcord	Angle adjustable footrests
	Footrest too low	Foot straps at 45 degrees
		Remove footrests
b. Dorsiflexion	Flexor pattern	Angle adjustable footrests
	Hypersensitive plantar surface	Accommodate
6. Scapular		
a. Retraction	Hypertonicity of the trunk (fixings of the shoulder girdle)	Provide trunk and anterior chest support, tray position
		Reposition head in space
	Tone/reflexes	Add protraction wings onto tray
	Tray too high/system tilt too far back	Raise armrest/tray
b. Protraction	Kyphosis	Provide pelvis/lumbar support
		Shoulder harness over lateral aspect of the shoulder
		Raise armrest/tray
7. Head/neck		
a. Forward flexion	Hypotonicity	Support pelvis, trunk, shoulder
	Kyphosis	Alter position in space
		Cervical support
		Anterior head support
b. Hyperextension	Extensor tone	Provide trunk support
	Poor head control	Position headrest below occipital region
		Tilt-in-space to decrease the effect of gravity
c. Rotation	ATNR/rooting reflex tone	Midline head position

TLRP, tonic labyrinthine reflex prone; ASIS, anterior superior iliac spine; ATNR, asymmetric tonic neck reflex; STNR, symmetric tonic neck reflex; TLRS, tonic labyrinthine reflex spine. From Trefler E, Hobson DA, Taylor SJ, et al. Seating and mobility for persons with physical disabilities. Therapy skill builders, University of Tennessee. Tennessee, 1993.

TABLE 38.9. ANATOMIC MEASUREMENTS

Area	Considerations	Concerns
a. Seat width	Measure from trochanter to trochanter and add approximately 1 in. Active users may prefer a tighter fit.	Too wide: promotes scoliosis, back pain, unequal weight distribution, difficulty propelling. Too narrow: difficulty with transfers, promotes pelvic obliquity, pressure on hip region, uncomfortable.
b. Seat depth	Measure from back of the buttocks to the popliteal fossa and minus approximately 2 in. Keep in musculature calf, and if so, measure to the calf muscle.	Too short: increases pressure on ischial tuberosities, may cause tipping, promotes windswept deformity. Too long: pressure on the back of knees, can restrict circulation, promotes sacral sitting.
c. Knee to heel[a]	Measure from the popliteal fossa to the heel. If the client has a plantar contracture, measure the heel and the lowest part of the foot.	Too high: pressure on the ischial area, promotes windswept deformity. Too low: promotes sliding, sacral sitting, pressure on the back of the thighs.
d. Foot length/width	Measure from the toe to heel and across both feet in the position tolerated on the footplate.	Too short: promotes pressure on the dorsal aspect of the foot. Too narrow (rigid front): inability to place feet on footplate, promotes pelvic obliquity. Keep in mind if the client wears braces.
e. Seat to inferior angle of the scapula[a]	Measure from the surface the client is sitting on to the inferior angle of the scapular. Measure both sides. Important for placement of the back system. Active users with good balance minus 2 in. Fair balance to poor, at least 2 in. higher or more.	Too low: trunk instability; may cause spinal deformities. Too high: impedes manual propulsion.
f. Seat to top of shoulder[a]	Measure from the surface the client is sitting on to the top of the shoulder. Measure both sides. Important for clients using a recliner or tilt-in-space wheelchair.	Needed for manual and power tilt-in-space wheelchairs or recliners. If too low, may cause pressure on scapular region; cervical discomfort.
g. Shoulder width	Measure from shoulder to shoulder to have the appropriate width back support.	If too narrow, promotes trunk rotation and pressure. If too wide: promotes scoliosis.
h. Seat to top of head[a]	Measure from the surface the client is sitting on to the top of the head.	Important for van clearance (approx. 2–3 in. of clearance needed inside van).
i. Seat to elbow[a]	Measure from the surface the client is sitting on to the elbow. Measure both sides.	If too high, can cause cervical discomfort, shoulder elevation. If too low, can cause shoulder subluxation; promotes kyphotic posture.
j. Waist width	Measure the client's waist to place lateral supports or to fit between commercial contoured back systems.	If too narrow, promotes trunk rotation and pressure. If too wide, promotes scoliosis.
k. Depth of the chest	Measure the client's thickness to have the appropriate length of a lateral support. Measure both sides and at the placement of the laterals.	If too short, promotes pressure. If too long, impedes functional use of upper extremities.
l. Elbow to tip of finger	Measure from the elbow to tip of the client's fingers on both sides to order proper length armpads.	If too short, lacks support for the wrist and hand. If too long, accessibility issues.
m. Seat to occipital prominence[a]	Measure from the surface the client is sitting on to the occipital prominence to place the headrest in the appropriate position.	If too high, promotes flexion of the head; can cause cervical discomfort. If too low, promotes cervical extension.
n. Seat to floor height	Take the measurement of the knee to the heel minus the cushion thickness and add approximately 2½ in.	If too low, front riggings may get held up. If too high, difficulty with transfers; tabletop accessibility.

Note: These measurements should be performed on a mat and a second time in the recommended seating and mobility system.
[a]Keep in mind the cushion thickness.

and school assessments must be completed before the final prescription and included in the letter of justification.

CONCLUSION

There are unlimited amounts of seating and mobility products on the market. It is very difficult for clinicians to know every product, but it is necessary for clinicians to be knowledgeable of the basic principles of seating and mobility. It is crucial to have specialists in this area to keep abreast of the latest technology in the field.

Seating and mobility systems are a vital part of the client's level of function and postural stability. The client must play an active role in the evaluation process and the clinic team should be advocates for the client to third-party payers for the appropriate system. Prescribing a seating and mobility system takes commitment by the specialists to address all areas of concern without impeding function, posture, mobility, or comfort. A seating and mobility system appropriately selected should enhance the client's function, not overwhelm him or her.

REFERENCES

1. Hasting JD. Seating assessment and planning. *Phys Med Rehabil Clin North Am* 2000;11:183–206.
2. Cooper RA, Trefler E, Hobson DA. Wheelchair and seating: issues and practice. 1996.
3. Cook AM, Hussey SM. *Assistive technologies: principles and practice.* St. Louis, MO: Mosby, 1995.
4. Kaplan PE, Roden W, Gilbert E. Reduction of hypercalciuria in tetraplegic after weight bearing and strengthening exercise. *Arch Phys Med Rehabil* 1982;19:289–293.
5. Dunn RB, Walter JS, Lucero Y, et al. Follow-up assessment of standing mobility device users. *Assistive Technol* 1998;10:84–93.
6. Gould DW, Hsich A, Tinckler L. The effect of posture on bladder pressure. *J Physiol* 1955;129:448–553.
7. Leo LPT. The effects of passive standing. *Paraplegic News* 1985:45–47.
8. Bohannon RW. Tilt table standing for reducing spasticity after spinal cord injury. *Arch Phys Med Rehabil* 1993;74:1121–1122.

APPENDIX 38.1

MAT EVALUATION

SUPINE:

1. Pelvis	Fixed	Flexible
Tilt----Posterior Anterior Neutral	_____	_____
Obliquity----Right Left	_____	_____
Rotation----Right Left	_____	_____

2. Lower extremity R.O.M.	Right	Left
Hip Flexion	_____	_____
Abduction/Adduction	_____	_____
Internal/External rotation	_____	_____
Knee Extension	_____	_____
Ankle Plantar Flexion	_____	_____
Ankle Dorsi-flexion	_____	_____

3. Trunk	Fixed	Flexible
Scoliosis (Apex of the curve_____)	_____	_____
Kyphosis	_____	_____
Lordosis	_____	_____
Rotation (_____ is rotated forward)	_____	_____

4. Upper extremity P.R.O.M.	Right	Left
Scapular Excursion	_____	_____
Shoulder Flexion/Extension	_____	_____
Abduction/Adduction	_____	_____
Internal/External Rotation	_____	_____
Elbow Flexion/Extension	_____	_____
Wrist Flexion/Extension	_____	_____
Supination/Pronation	_____	_____
Fingers	_____	_____

5. Skin Inspection
Clear
History
Current:

Grade_____
Location_____
Size_____

SEATED:

1. Balance:

2. Pelvis
Anterior/Posterior Range
A.S.I.S. Level/Obliquity
Rotation

3. Trunk Alignment:

4. Head Position:

5. Anatomical Measurements:
   (Actual client measurements)
   a. Seat Width_____
   b. Seat Depth Right_____ Left_____
   c. Leg Length (knee to heel) Right_____ Left_____
   D1. Foot Length_____
   D2. Foot Width_____
   e. Seat to Inferior Angle of Scapular Right_____ Left_____
   f. Seat to Top of Shoulder Right_____ Left_____
   g. Shoulder Width_____
   h. Seat to Top of Head_____
   i. Seat to Elbow Right_____ Left_____
   j. Waist Width_____
   k. Depth of Chest_____
   l. Elbow to tip of fingers_____
   n. Seat to Occipital Prominence_____

SPINAL CORD REGENERATION: A REVIEW OF THERAPIES

WISE YOUNG

Published spinal cord injury (SCI) studies often begin with the assertion that the spinal cord cannot regenerate. What is the basis for this frequently repeated assertion? A review of the literature suggests that the notion that the spinal cord cannot regenerate is a relatively recent development. Although pessimism concerning SCI dates back to the beginnings of recorded medical literature, the early pessimism was related to survival from SCI and not the inability of the spinal cord to regenerate (1).

Spinal cord regeneration was a moot issue for much of human history because few people or animals survived long after SCI for regeneration to make a difference (2). It was not until the 1950s, with the advent of modern antibiotics, sterile catheters, and respirators that people began to survive SCI, and rehabilitation of the spinal cord injured became a priority for the first time.

In the beginning, scientists were optimistic that the spinal cord can regenerate (3). For example, Cajal (4,5) emphasized the prolific tendency of spinal axons to sprout. During the 1960s and 1970s, scientists tried many therapies, including peripheral nerve bridges, nerve growth factor (NGF), hormones, and inflammatory mediators to stimulate regeneration.

In the 1980s, however, the mood changed. In the aftermath of a failure to demonstrate regeneration resulting from a controversial enzyme therapy from Russia, many scientists began to search for reasons why the spinal axons do not regenerate.

Scientists attributed the lack of spinal cord regeneration to three obstacles. First, glial scars may prevent axonal growth in injured spinal cords. Second, the spinal cord may contain proteins that block axonal growth. Third, the spinal cord may lack crucial neural growth factors. By 1990, however, it became clear that cell transplants could provide a bridge for growing axons, brain and spinal cord had endogenous neurotrophins (NTs), and proteins from spinal white matter blocked axonal growth.

The decade of the 1990s was one of hope for SCI. Scientists successfully used antibodies to block growth inhibitors, applied growth factors, implanted cells and peripheral nerve bridges, and even used gene therapies to stimulate spinal cord regeneration. This chapter reviews the dogma that the spinal cord cannot regenerate, the evidence that led to the overthrow of the dogma, and the challenges that face us in the coming decade.

EARLY HOPE

Perusal of early neuroscience literature suggests that many scientists were initially optimistic about the possibility of spinal cord regeneration. Cajal (4,5) emphasized the ability of injured spinal axons to grow. In 1955, Windle (3), Galabov (6), and Sasabe and Freeman (7) described a robust growth of spinal axons into peripheral nerve grafts used to bridge the spinal cord. In 1962, McMasters (8) reported that the endotoxin piromen and pituitary hormone adrenocorticotropic hormone stimulated spinal axonal growth. Harvey and Srebnik (9) found that thyroxine increased spinal axon sprouting and locomotor recovery.

Most scientists seemed to believe that the spinal cord could regenerate. Lampert and Cressman (10) and others (11–18) described regrowth of dorsal root axons into injured animal spinal cords and ventral root regrowth. Wolman (19,20) described similar phenomena in injured human spinal cords. Surgeons reinnervated bladder muscles by inserting ventral roots into spinal cord (21–23).

NGF, the original NT, was discovered in the 1960s by Levi-Montalcini (24) and Levi-Montalcini and Angeletti (27). Several scientists described salutary effects of NGF on peripheral and sympathetic axonal growth (28,29). Stenevi et al. (30) injected NGF into the brain to stimulate axonal regrowth. Many scientists expressed optimism in the ability of the brain and spinal cord to regrow (31–38).

Axonal growth and synaptic connections occur in the brain and the spinal cord (39). In the 1970s, Bernstein and Bernstein (40–42) described axonal growth cones and synapse formation in the proximal side of hemisected spinal cord. Björklund et al. (43–46) described regrowth of catecholaminergic fibers in the brain and spinal cord. Other investigators described functional regeneration in premetamorphic lamprey, frog tadpoles, urodeles, lizard, goldfish, and even neonatal mammalian cords.

In the 1970s, Feringa et al. (66–70) reported that the corticospinal tract regenerates in transected rat spinal cords and that immunosuppression with cyclophosphamide enhances the regeneration. They subsequently made rats tolerant of central nervous system (CNS) antigens by inoculating them with myelin and combining the inoculation with immunosuppression, showing that these rats had changes of radioactive transport and electrophysiologic responses suggestive of corticospinal tract regeneration (71). Although later studies raised questions about some of the methodology used to show regeneration, these studies planted the seeds for the current renaissance of regenerative immunotherapies (72,73).

A PERIOD OF PESSIMISM

The notion that the spinal cord cannot regenerate did not become prevalent until the early 1980s. A Russian group had claimed that treating the spinal cord with proteases reduced scarring and promoted axonal regeneration in animals and humans (74). Several laboratories tried but could not confirm these claims (75–78). The Russian results were attributed to incomplete transection of spinal cord. In 1980, Guth et al. (79) proposed that the completely transected spinal cord is required for demonstrating regeneration.

Many scientists subsequently adopted highly critical attitudes toward spinal cord regeneration. Axonal growth was attributed to dorsal root ingrowth, sympathetic sprouting, or simply sprouting (80,81). For example, when Harston et al. (82) found that morphine enhanced axonal growth, they were careful to call the growth "sprouting" and "putative regeneration." Investigators mistrusted behavioral improvements after SCI, because animals can develop locomotor capabilities with treadmill training even after spinal cord transection (83).

Researchers began to ask why axons do not regenerate in mammalian spinal cords. In 1980, Windle (84) proposed that the spinal cord itself inhibits axonal growth. In 1981, David and Aguayo (85) published a seminal paper that showed that spinal axons would grow into peripheral nerve but not back into the spinal cord (86–88). Other investigators proposed that the thin basal lamina that develops at the injury site obstructs axonal growth, leading to efforts to bridge transected spinal cords using peripheral nerves and fetal tissues (89–94).

Scientists searched for growth factors besides NGF. A number of authors hypothesized and identified a brain-derived neurotrophic factor (BDNF) that stimulated neuronal growth and promoted neural survival (95–100). By 1990, several other members of the NT family had been identified, along with their receptors, including NT-3, NT-4, and ciliary neurotrophic factor (CNTF), which stimulate motoneuronal growth and survival (101–103).

In 1988, Caroni et al. (104) found that oligodendroglial cells express a factor that prevents axon growth and fibroblast migration. The inhibitory activity was concentrated in protein fractions with molecular weights of 35 or 250 kd (105). A monoclonal antibody raised against these protein fractions, called IN-1, blocked the inhibitory effects of myelin on axonal growth (106). Myelin extracts prevent axonal growth, effectively collapsing growth cones on contact (107,108). They proposed that a myelin-based protein was responsible for the inability of the spinal cord to regenerate.

THE DISCOVERY OF NOGO

To demonstrate that myelin inhibited axonal growth, Savio and Schwab (109) and Schwegler et al. (110) used x-irradiation to retard myelin formation in newborn rats, showing that the corticospinal tract will regrow many millimeters within 2 to 3 weeks in such irradiated animals. By 1991, Schnell and Schwab (111, 112) reported that implanted hybridomas secreting the antibody IN-1 stimulated corticospinal axonal elongation in injured adult rat spinal cords, to distances of 7 to 11 mm compared with less than 1 mm in untreated control rats. NT-3 enhanced IN-1–induced axonal growth (113). IN-1 also promoted axonal growth across crushed neonatal opossum spinal cords *in vitro* (114). By 1995, Bregman et al. (115) showed that IN-1–treated rats showed better motor recovery than rats treated with a nonspecific antibody.

Schnell and Schwab (111,112) and others (116–121) proposed that myelin-associated growth inhibitors help guide axonal tracts during development and are the primary factors that limit axonal growth and sprouting in mammalian spinal cords. For example, IN-1 strongly stimulates sprouting of remaining pyramidal tract fibers after unilateral pyramidotomies (122). Dantrolene, an inhibitor of calcium release from caffeine-sensitive intracellular calcium, prevented growth cone collapse induced by myelin proteins, suggesting that calcium-dependent intracellular messengers in the growth cone mediate the growth inhibition (123).

IN-1 unfortunately is a mouse immunoglobulin M–kappa antibody and could not be given directly to humans. Direct application of IN-1 to the spinal cord did not facilitate regeneration. IN-1 had to be applied to the spinal cord by implanting an IN-1–secreting hybridoma to the rat brains. It took much of the decade to develop a recombinant human antibody from variable Fab′ regions from IN-1 and to demonstrate that this recombinant humanized antibody blocks myelin-induced inhibition of axonal growth *in vitro* and *in vivo* (124,125).

In 1998, Spillman et al. (126) reported the successful isolation of the bovine neurite growth inhibitor (bNI-220). This led to the recent isolation and identification of the gene for the inhibitor, now called Nogo (127). The Nogo gene encodes for three major protein products, called Nogo-A, Nogo-B, and Nogo-C. Nogo-A is the inhibiting factor recognized by IN-1. It is expressed by oligodendroglia and is a potent inhibitor of neurite growth (128). A member of the reticulon family of proteins, Nogo is reticulon-4A (129). Three other reticulon family members 1, 2, and 3 do not inhibit axonal regeneration. A 66–amino acid sequence on Nogo-A inhibits axonal growth.

OTHER MYELIN-ASSOCIATED INHIBITORS

Nogo, however, may not be the only growth inhibitor in the spinal cord. Nogo should be absent or less effective in the peripheral nerve, in species that can regenerate, or during early development when axons are growing. Phylogenetically, Nogo does appear to be absent or minimally expressed in some fish, reptilian, and amphibian optic nerves (130–132). In the developing opossum, myelin appears 9 days after birth (P9) and IN-1 immunoreactivity appears in the spinal cords by P7, increasing to high levels in the adult opossum spinal cord (133). In the Brazilian opossum, however, the optic nerve shows immunoreactivity to

IN-1 at P26 but does not support axonal growth beyond P14, suggesting that other inhibitors may be present (134).

David et al. (135) found that the peripheral nerve possessed potent inhibitors to axonal growth, but that laminin present on Schwann cells was necessary and sufficient to overcome the inhibition. McKerracher et al. (136) and others (137–139) found that myelin-associated glycoprotein (MAG) promoted growth in dorsal root neurons up to the third postnatal day but strongly inhibited their growth after that period and inhibited growth of neurons from retina, superior cervical ganglia, spinal cord, and hippocampus at all ages tested. Sialidases abolished these effects of MAG (140). However, MAG knockout mice do not show increased regeneration, suggesting that MAG is not the only growth inhibitor (141).

Nogo does not inhibit growth of sensory axons *in vivo* (142). Davies et al. (143,144) showed that adult dorsal root ganglion (DRG) neurons transplanted into injured rat spinal cords will send axons long distances in spinal white matter but invariably will stop at injury sites in the spinal cord. IN-1 does not stimulate corticospinal tract ingrowth into Schwann cell grafts (145). Also, in the presence of astrocytes, oligodendroglia may not inhibit axonal growth, suggesting that a combination of positive and repulsive factors can allow axonal growth (146). IN-1 also stimulates sprouting of surviving axons and such sprouting may account for the functional recovery associated with IN-1 treatment (122,147–149).

Many data argue against the simplistic view that a single growth inhibitor accounts for the failure of regeneration in the spinal cord. Several families of molecules inhibit or facilitate axonal growth in CNS tissues, providing a mixture of positive and negative influences on axonal growth during development and in injured adult spinal cords. Likewise, growing axons may express various receptors to these molecules. The behavior of the axons probably depends on the balance of positive and negative molecules and axonal receptors to these molecules.

EXTRACELLULAR MATRIX MOLECULES

The extracellular matrix contains many molecules that can strongly inhibit axonal growth in the CNS. These include agrin and chondroitin-6 sulfate proteoglycans (CSPG). The last of these represents a large family of glycoproteins that regulate axonal growth, including neurocan, phosphocan, brevican, and versican V2 (150). Agrin is a secreted glycoprotein that clusters cell surface molecules, including acetylcholine (ACh) receptors on muscle cells. An adhesive extracellular glycoprotein and a component of basal lamina, agrin, significantly reduces and may even stop neurite extension but strongly stimulates synaptogenesis (151–155). Agrin plays an essential role in clustering of ACh receptors (156,157). NTs regulate agrin-induced postsynaptic differentiation (158).

In 1993, a number of authors proposed that extracellular matrix proteins are responsible for the failure of DRG axonal growth into spinal cord (159–161). Specifically, they proposed that CSPG suppressed axonal growth in regions of injury and that these molecules are made by reactive astrocytes in the presence of macrophages (162). Davies et al. (143,144) showed that transplanted adult DRG cells sent axons that grew remarkably long distances in adult spinal cord white matter but stopped at wound sites showing CSPG. Both neonatal and adult mouse DRG neurons were capable of such growth, circumventing the argument that embryonic DRG neurons do not express receptors to NI-35/250 (163).

Injury recruits cells that express inhibitory proteoglycans (164). For example, oligodendroglia produce NI-250, MAG, tenascin-R, NG-2, DSE-1/phosphocan, and versican. Astrocytes secrete tenascin, brevican, neurocan, and NG-2. Likewise, meningeal cells produce NG-2 and other proteoglycans. Conditioned media from these cells block axonal growth, and inhibitors of proteoglycan synthesis improve the ability of axons to grow on oligodendroglial cells or astrocytes (165). Injury upregulates CSPG in spinal cord (166) and peripheral nerves (167). Chondroitinase promotes regeneration of CNS axons *in vivo* and *in vitro* (168,169). Proteoglycan synthesis inhibitors stimulate neurite outgrowth (165,170). A metallic metalloproteinase-2 blocks CSPG but not laminin (171). Tenascin is often associated with glial scars but does not seem to prevent axonal growth (159,164,172–174). Chemical removal of collagen "scar" also does not improve corticospinal tract regeneration (175).

CELL ADHESION MOLECULES

Several families of cell adhesion molecules (CAMs) may provide positive trophic influences to counterbalance inhibitory molecules in the spinal cord (176). Growing axons express receptors to many CAMs, including L1, laminin, N-CAM, N-cadherin, ninjurin, and other glial CAMs that may be present in injured spinal cords (177–180).

L1 is essential for long tract formation and myelination (181). A member of the immunoglobulin superfamily of CAMs, L1 binds to L1 and other CAMs. Growing axons express L1 and stimulate each other to fasciculate or grow together in bundles (182,186). L1 is a leading candidate gene for several inherited and congenital neurologic syndromes (187–193). Point mutations in the immunoglobulin and fibronectin domains of L1 lead to blunted, long tract formation and deranged expression of molecules required for myelination, such as ankyrin (194–198). NGF, transforming growth factor -β (TGF-β) and factors that increase intracellular cyclic adenosine monophosphate (cAMP) all upregulate L1 expression, whereas corticosteroids downregulate L1 expression (199–206). In neurons, L1 acts as a receptor that activates various kinases and cytoskeletal enzymes (182,207,208). Glycoproteins such as neurocan and phosphocan tend to co-localize with L1 and may inhibit axonal growth by blocking L1 (209,210). In addition, L1 is a co-stimulus for T-lymphocytic activation (211).

Schwann cells often invade into SCI sites (212). Schwann cells express L1 and laminin, a strong promoter of neurite growth (213–216). Likewise, Schwann cells also express galectin-1, a β-galactoside–binding lectin that stimulates the initial growth of peripheral nerves after axotomy (217). A Schwann cell activation marker, galectin is upregulated during the first 6 days after peripheral nerve injury (218). Oxidized galectin promotes axonal regeneration in DRG explants (219,220). A related compound galectin-3 is upregulated in activated microglia and in wallerian degeneration (218,221). Injury induces interleukin-1 (IL-1) and TGF-β expression in peripheral neurons and spinal cord (222). These cytokines induce expression of leukemia inhibitory factor (LIF) in Schwann cells, a treatment that stimulates spinal axonal growth (223,224). Injured Schwann cells also express ninjurin, a novel L1-like homophilic CAM that promotes axonal growth (177,225,226).

DIFFUSABLE GUIDANCE MOLECULES

During development, several diffusable molecules guide axonal growth, particularly the semaphorins and netrins (176). Semaphorins are a large family of molecules that repel growing axons over long distances (227–234). Semaphorin III (SemaIII) or collapsin turns away or collapses growth cones, increases axoplasmic transport, and are occasionally antirepellents (229, 235–240). Netrins are a family of chemoattractant molecules that usually attract growing axons (241).

Injured adult rat CNS expresses SemaIII that repels axonal growth and inhibits branching of cranial nerve and spinal axons (242–256). In contrast, injury reduces SemaIII in peripheral nerves (257). Injury upregulates SemaIII receptor and the collapsin response mediator proteins (CRMPs), Rac1 and Rho (232,258–268). Activation of cyclic guanosine monophosphate (cGMP) pathways antagonizes SemaIII receptors, whereas NTs reduce responsiveness of growth cones to semaphorins (269, 270). SemaIII induces apoptosis, possibly by antagonizing L1 signaling pathways (271–274). Transgenic SemaIII knockout mice show aberrant axonal projections that correct during development (275–277). Semaphorins may induce cancer susceptibility, possibly by affecting lymphocytes or blood vessels (278–283).

The netrins are secreted laminin-related proteins that strongly attract neuronal migration and axonal elongation and branching, although it may also be a neurorepellent (284–297). Secreted by the basal floor plate of the brain stem, netrin attracts growing axons toward the midline and is responsible for decussation of corticospinal and other central nervous tracts, as well as the development of cranial and peripheral nerves (298–315). Semaphorins and netrins play important opposing roles in the development of motor and sensory axons (293,316–318).

Semaphorins, netrins, and their receptors are phylogenetically old. Netrin, for example, has homologous molecules in worms and insects (288,319–321). The netrin receptor is homologous to DCC in *Caenorhabditis elegans* and the "frazzled" receptor in Drosophila (322–329). Antibodies against DCC block netrin effects (330). Expressed on projecting neurons, netrin receptors activate phospholipase C gamma, require cAMP and calcium, and are regulated by ubiquitin proteosomes (302,331–335). Heparin sulfate proteoglycans bind DCC and block netrin effects (336,337). Without netrin, DCC expression can cause apoptosis (338). In Drosophila, the netrin receptor regulates netrin distribution (339). These mechanisms provide many therapeutic targets for regenerative therapies.

OTHER AXONAL GUIDANCE MOLECULES

Many other molecules are involved in axonal guidance. Several laboratories have identified multiple upregulated and downregulated genes in tissues containing, developing, and regenerating axons (340–343). These include TGF-β, Slit and Robo, nrCAM, engrailed-1, bone morphogenetic proteins (BMPs), LAMP, ephrins, neogenin, Pax, fibroblast growth factor (FGF) tissues, and others (344–358). Many of these molecules share common domains and therefore may serve multiple functions (359–361). Most act synergistically or antagonistically with each other (362,363). Of the guidance molecules, sonic hedgehog (SHH) and ephrins are most likely to influence regeneration.

Named after the video game, SHH is a soluble molecule expressed in spinal cord and is responsible for inducing neuronal and oligodendroglial differentiation, the anteroposterior polarity of the spinal cord, somite development, and neuronal survival (364–376). SHH induces formation of dopaminergic neurons by neural stem cells and motoneuronal differentiation (366,377, 378). SHH also induces expression of netrin (379,380). SHH acts through the G-protein–coupled receptors to promote cyclin and stimulates cell cycling (381,382). BMPs influence the distribution of SHH (383). In the adult rat, SHH signaling components are predominantly located in forebrain structures, although oligodendroglial progenitor cells possess SHH receptors (368,384,385).

Ephrins and Eph receptors have attracted much attention recently (386). Ephrins regulate specificity of synaptic connections, restrict cellular intermingling and communications, and play a major role in dorsal-ventral development as well as segmentation of the spinal cord (387–390). Ephrins are present in adult rodent spinal cords, particularly the substantia gelatinosa and along spinal tracts (391,392). Injury markedly upregulates Ephrin and Eph receptors in the adult rat spinal cords (393). In adult human, Eph5 receptors are highly expressed in the spinal cord (394).

Eph tyrosine receptors stimulate or inhibit neurite outgrowth and collapse, depending on neuronal type, by activating the Rho and Rho kinase (392,395,396). Rho is a guanosine triphosphate (GTP) binding protein that transduces neurite growth and regulates migratory responses of endothelial and epithelial cells (397–399). Rho mediates G protein–coupled receptor activity and neurite responses to NGF (400,401). Inactivation of Rho promotes CNS axon regeneration (402–404). Thus, ephrins are likely to be important players in axonal guidance and cell migration in injured spinal cords.

NEUROTROPHINS

Neurons require growth factors to grow. The first such factor was of course NGF, discovered by Levi-Montalcini (24) and others (27,405–407) and for which a Nobel Prize was awarded. In the 1980s, several additional members of the family now called the NTs were discovered. These include BDNF, NT-3, and NT-4. These molecules turned out to be not only growth factors but also trophic factors that sustained and maintained survival of neurons and are closely related to the cytokines (95, 97,408). BDNF prevents apoptosis in cerebral ischemia (409).

Much evidence suggests that applied neurotrophic factors can facilitate regeneration in spinal cord. NT-3 acts synergistically with IN-1 to promote regeneration of adult rat spinal cord (113, 410). Bregman et al. (411–416) showed that various NTs affected serotoninergic, adrenergic, and corticospinal tract growth into fetal tissues transplanted into rat spinal cords. NT-3 strongly stimulates dorsal root axonal ingrowth into spinal cord, corticospinal growth, and other descending tracts (417–421). NT-3 enhances the effects of IN-1 (113,422).

Direct application of NTs may not be necessary. Injured peripheral nerves and spinal cords express high levels of NT (423). Many conditions stimulate BDNF and NGF expression by neurons, including glutamate exposure, calcium entry, and adenylate cyclase activation with forskolin. These factors increase cAMP, interleukins, and other cytokines (424). IL-1, for example, has been reported to enhance peripheral nerve regeneration and may have beneficial effects on CNS injuries (425–427). LIF induced expression of NT-3, but not the other NTs in the spinal cord; this was associated with robust growth of the corticospinal tract (428). Several cytokines, including LIF, stimulate NT expression (223). LIF is transported by injured axons and may play a role in axonal regeneration (429).

These studies strongly suggest that spinal axons retain sensitivity to neurotrophic factors but that NTs may have synergistic but differential effects on dorsal root afferent and descending spinal tracts (430). Observed improvements in locomotor recovery may be due to regeneration or to other effects of NT on the spinal circuits (431). In contused or hemisected spinal cords, the beneficial effects of NT may be related to sprouting of residual axons and may not be mediated by the regenerated axons.

GENE THERAPY

NTs can be delivered by genetically modified cells (432). Tuszynski et al. (433) and Blesch and Tuszynski (434) found that transplanted fibroblasts modified to secrete NGF induced robust neurite growth of dorsal root afferents. Dorsal root axons invaded into grafts secreting NT-3, NT-4, or basic FGF (bFGF) but not into grafts secreting BDNF; corticospinal axons did not invade the grafts and functional recovery was limited (435,436). Schwann cells secreting NGF also stimulated dorsal root afferent growth in the spinal cord, whereas NT-3–secreting fibroblasts stimulated corticospinal tract regeneration (202,437,438). BDNF-secreting fibroblasts stimulate regeneration of adult rat rubrospinal axons (439). BDNF and NT-3 also may stimulate oligodendroglial proliferation and myelination of regenerating axons (440).

Genetic modification of the cells can be used not only to deliver gene products but also to affect the behavior of grafted cells. For example, Schwann cells transfected to secrete NT-3 tend to survive and grow better after transplantation to the spinal cord (437). It is even possible to introduce genes that inhibit growth of axons. For example, Schwann cells can be modified to express more MAG and such cells inhibit axonal regeneration and branching (138). Finally, nonmodified fibroblasts them-

selves express various growth factors. For example, meningeal fibroblasts implanted into the spinal cord express NGF, NT-3, acidic FGF (aFGF), and bFGF, promoting regeneration of peptidergic axons from dorsal root afferents (441).

NT and other genes can be introduced directly to the spinal cord. Until recently, most investigators have used viral vectors to do so. For example, Romero et al. (442) and others (443, 444) used adenovirus vectors to increase the expression of bFGF, bNGF, NT-3, N-cadherin, or L1 in adult spinal cord. Transgene expression of these factors localized to astrocytes and motoneurons. However, only bNGF stimulates axonal sprouting in the cord. Zhang et al. (419) injected adenoviral vectors containing either the LacZ marker or the NT-3 genes into rat spinal cords, showing strong expression of these gene products in glial cells and neurons and enhanced axonal regeneration into the transfected cords.

OTHER TROPHIC MOLECULES

Many other factors influence neuronal survival and growth. Other neurogenic factors of interest include the BMPs, FGF, and galectin-1 (217,426–446). Several gliagenic factors are also of interest, such as glial growth factor-2 (GGF-2), a neuronal signal that promotes proliferation and survival of oligodendroglia; neuregulin or GGF, which is highly expressed in DRG and spinal cord; and glial-derived neurotrophic factor (GDNF) (447, 48).

FGF stimulates mitogenesis and growth of cells (357). Whereas bFGF promotes survival of sensory neurons, motoneurons, and bulbospinal neurons, aFGF stimulates axonal growth (449–453). In fact, bFGF seems to downregulate injury-induced GAP-43 expression (454). Neurons themselves express aFGF and particularly bFGF, as well as their receptors (455,456). Likewise, microglia express FGF (457). Widely distributed in the CNS, FGF may act synergistically or even mediate some of the actions of NTs or CAMs, as well as antagonize the growth inhibition (145,458). Injury upregulates bFGF expression in DRG and spinal cord (459–464). Many investigators have claimed that aFGF and bFGF play major roles in CNS repair and regeneration (465).

GDNF is a new glial-derived neurotrophic factor (466). For example, two recently discovered homologs of GDNF, neurturin and persephin, increase ACh acetyltransferase activity of postnatal motoneurons, induce neurite outgrowth in the spinal cord, and protect motoneurons against glutamate-induced excitotoxicity. NGF but not GDNF stimulates sensory axonal ingrowth into the spinal cord (467,468). Ramer et al. (469) recently showed that combinations of NGF, NT-3, and BDNF stimulated functional regeneration of dorsal root axons into spinal cord. In general, GDNF seems to work best with other NTs (470).

CNTF prevents degeneration of injured motoneurons. A cytosolic molecule that is expressed by Schwann cells and astrocytes, CNTF remarkably supports the survival of motoneurons (471). In culture, for example, CNTF will permit survival of most motoneurons. However, its effects are synergistic with those of FGF. Combination bFGF and CNTF will result in survival of virtually all motoneurons. In addition, CNTF supports oligodendroglial survival (472).

BRIDGING THE GAP

Injury disrupts the spinal cord, leaving necrotic and cystic areas at the injury site, bereft of many signaling molecules that are normally present in the spinal cord. After a contusion injury, a large cystic structure often develops at the injury site. Many scientists therefore have attempted to bridge the gap by transplanting peripheral nerves or fetal transplants into the injury site.

In 1995, Cheng and Olson (473) reported the first successful bridging of transected rat spinal cords with peripheral nerves. They followed up with a study showing functional recovery in rats that had multiple peripheral nerve implants that routed axonal growth from white to gray matter (474). The axons grew across the peripheral nerve bridges into the spinal cord and continued to grow in gray matter to the distal cord, where they presumably contributed to the functional recovery of adult rats.

More recently, Blits et al. (475) transplanted intercostal nerves transfected to secrete NT-3 with adenovirus vector into dorsally hemisected spinal cords, reporting improved corticospinal tract regeneration and hindlimb function in rats. However, none of the corticospinal axons grew through the grafts, and rats with dorsally hemisected spinal cords tend to recover substantial locomotor function even without therapy. Yick et al. (168) similarly examined the effects of chondroitinases on sensory axonal growth through peripheral nerve grafts in dorsally hemisected cords, with similar results.

A number of authors used Schwann cell–seeded bridges to bridge transected cords (145,476–485). This approach has been useful for demonstrating therapies that encourage axonal growth back into the spinal cord. In particular, a single bolus dose of methylprednisolone improved axonal growth into the distal cord, as well as NT-3 (479,482–486). In some experiments, Schwann cells that were genetically modified to secrete BDNF seemed to be more effective than Schwann cells alone (484). Likewise, FGF seemed to help increase axonal growth, whereas insulin-like growth factor and platelet-derived growth factor improved myelination (145). Xu et al. used fetal cell seeded bridges to bridge hemisected spinal cords (487). Novel bridging biomaterials were developed, including matrigel or neurogel (490–493), poly(α-hydroxy acids), and self-assembling polypeptides (152,480,481,483,486,488–494).

Cell Transplants

Another popular approach to bridging the site has been transplantation of fetal cells and other cells into the injury site (415, 416,497–504). Both central and sensory axons grow into fetal transplants, whereas the fetal cells usually send axons to the host (505,506). Fetal transplants integrate well with spinal cord, often reducing glial responses (507). Serotoninergic neurons cross the fetal cell bridge (508). Fetal transplants also may rescue neurons (509). A number of studies found that careful apposition of transected spinal cord with fetal tissues allowed remarkable functional axonal regeneration (510–515). Demierre et al. (516) and others (517) transplanted embryonic motoneurons into the spinal cords of mice. In general, the cells survived transplantation, but there is little evidence that the motoneurons regenerated axons that innervated muscles. Thomas et al. (518) directly transplanted neurons into denervated muscles, showing the cells innervated the muscles and prevented atrophy.

Olfactory ensheathing glia (OEG) cells are specialized glial cells that reside in the olfactory epithelia and bulb. The olfactory nerve continually regenerates throughout life. OEG cells were thought to be responsible. In 1994, Ramon-Cueto and Nieto-Sampedro (519) reported that OEG cells transplanted to the spinal cord facilitated growth of dorsal root axons into the spinal cord. In 1997, Li et al. (520) reported that OEG transplants allowed the functional regeneration of corticospinal tract in adult rats. Ramon-Cueto et al. (485,521) showed that OEG cells facilitate regrowth of central axons across artificial Schwann cell bridges and allow functional regeneration in transected rat spinal cords. A recent study indicated that OEG cells could be obtained from human olfactory bulb (522).

Schwann cells do not migrate well when transplanted into spinal cord, although they will rapidly myelinate axons in areas where there are few astrocytes (523–527). Schwann cells do not get along with astrocytes (528). However, Schwann cells can integrate well into spinal white matter. Li and Raisman (529) implanted Schwann cells derived from neonatal rat sciatic nerves. Initially positive for p75 NGF receptor, the transplanted Schwann cells organized themselves into rows, forming a precisely arranged mosaic and myelinating axons.

Oligodendroglial cell transplants remyelinate the spinal cord (530). Interestingly, oligodendroglial or O2A precursor cells are more effective in repairing injured tissues than type 1 astrocytes (531). Astrocytic precursor cells filled injured areas better than cultured astrocytes (532). The differentiated oligodendroglia not only may express factors that inhibit growth but may not remyelinate axons (533,534).

PROINFLAMMATORY THERAPIES

Injury produces an intense inflammatory response in the spinal cord, more intense than in the brain (535). Within hours after injury, large rises in messenger RNA expression of cytokines, chemokines, and NTs can be detected (536–541). Inflammation has long been speculated to contribute to secondary injury and reduce recovery by increasing astrogliosis and damaging oligodendrocytes (542,543). Depletion of hematogenous macrophages promotes partial hindlimb recovery in rats (544). Methylprednisolone is a potent antiinflammatory drug. Oudega et al. (545) found that a single bolus dose of methylprednisolone markedly reduced macrophages in the spinal cord, prevented tissue loss at 2, 4, and 8 weeks after injury, and markedly increased axonal growth across the transection site.

However, the evidence for a deleterious effect of the inflammation is weak. Although antiinflammatory therapies, such as the glucocorticoid methylprednisolone and the antiinflammatory IL-10 on injured spinal cords, are neuroprotective, both may be deleterious if continued for more than 24 hours (546).

Klusman et al. (547) found that infusion of the proinflammatory cytokines IL-1, IL-6, and tumor necrosis factor-α reduced tissue damage and improved neurologic recovery in rats after SCI. Frei et al. (548) examined the response of oligodendroglial cells in contused spinal cords. Despite large numbers of macrophages and neutrophils in cord adjacent to the injury site, there was no significant damage to oligodendroglia.

The inflammatory response to injury may be beneficial (549). Macrophages not only remove myelin but also may express molecules that permit long-term growth and persistence of axons (550). Franzen et al. (551) found that transplanted macrophages reduce the expression of MAG in spinal cords associated with neurite growth. The macrophages themselves do not appear to express NTs, including NGF, BDNF, NT-3, aFGF, or bFGF. Prewitt et al. (552) reported that implantation of activated macrophages remarkably enhances dorsal root fiber growth in the spinal cord.

A number of authors proposed that inflammation is essential for repair and showed that peripheral nerve–activated macrophages stimulate regeneration and improve locomotor recovery in rats after spinal cord contusion (553–558). They have further reported that T lymphocytes activated with myelin-based protein are neuroprotective (559). A clinical trial of the activated macrophages is currently underway in Israel.

PURINE NUCLEOTIDES

Most spinal regenerative therapies have aimed at manipulating the environment to make it more permissive for axonal growth. In the last 2 years, a novel therapeutic approach has emerged, aimed at changing the responses of axons to the environment, rather than changing the environment.

In 1995, Schwalb et al. (560) reported the isolation of two factors that strongly stimulated axonal growth in goldfish retina. One of the factors was the common purine nucleotide inosine. Inosine strongly stimulates sprouting in the rat corticospinal tract when applied to the rat sensorimotor cortex (561). In a separate study, Hadlock et al. (562) loaded a slow-release polymer conduit with inosine and showed that it promoted dense peripheral nerve regrowth into the polymer. Benowitz et al. (563) had earlier examined the effects of inosine on retinal ganglion growth and found that exogenously applied inosine and guanosine stimulates axonal growth, acting on an intracellular target that could be blocked by 6-thioguanine (6-TG). The purine analog 6-TG selectively affects a 47-kd protein kinase N that activates an NGF-inducible serine-threonine kinase. Petrausch et al. (564) subsequently compared the mechanisms of inosine and AF-1 stimulation of retinal ganglionic growth in goldfish. Both inosine and AF-1 stimulate axonal growth with concomitant increases of GAP-43 and other growth-related proteins; 6-TG blocked both the inosine and the AF-1 effects.

AIT-082 or neotrofin is a guanosine analog, another purine nucleotide. Unlike inosine, which is only sparingly transported into the brain, AIT-082 passes readily into the brain through a nonsaturable influx mechanism and apparently enhances memory and cognitive performance in people (565). The molecule upregulates synaptophysin expression in PC12 cells, a protein that presumably signifies more synapse formation (566). The purines have long been known to have salutory trophic effects on neurons and glia, including stimulating the synthesis and release of bFGF, NT-3, CNTF, and S-100b proteins (567). In addition, guanosine and GTP also stimulate glial proliferation and axonal growth (568). AIT-082 is now undergoing clinical trial for Alzheimer disease (569).

Both inosine and AIT-082 are likely to go to clinical trials rapidly. Inosine is a natural substance that is ubiquitously present in the body, although it does not pass readily across the blood–brain barrier and must be given directly to the brain or spinal cord. On the other hand, AIT-082 does cross the blood–brain barrier and is already undergoing large clinical trials for Alzheimer disease. In addition, there are likely to be many other analogs of inosine and guanosine that may have better biologic activity.

GROWTH MESSENGERS

The guanosine triphosphatase (GTPase) signaling pathway plays a major role in axonal growth. As pointed out earlier, many of the CAMs, extracellular matrix molecules, and cellular guidance molecules operate through that pathway. Lehmann et al. (402) recently reported that injured axons regrow directly on complex inhibitory substrates when Rho GTPase is inactivated with the C3 enzyme or when the cells are transfected with dominant negative Rho.

Another critical intracellular messenger for axonal growth is cAMP. Qiu et al. (570) reported that intracellular levels of cAMP influence the capacity of mature CNS neurons to initiate and maintain neurite growth. Many drugs affect cAMP. Cai et al. (571) had earlier shown that prior exposure of neurons to mixtures of NTs raised cAMP levels, allowing axons to grow in the presence of axonal growth inhibitors, including MAG. Application of dibutyryl cAMP also overcomes the inhibitory effects of MAG/myelin. Activation of the cGMP and cAMP paths, respectively, converts the SemaIII signal from repulsion to attraction and vice versa (269).

Mann et al. (205) had earlier reported that cholera toxin, a specific inducer of adenyl cyclase, which boosts cAMP, markedly enhances L1 expression by neurons when applied by itself. The cholera toxin acted synergistically with NGF to promote increases in neuritic outgrowth and also increase expression of N-CAM but paradoxically inhibited NGF induction of L1 and Thy1. A similar pattern was seen when FGF was substituted for NGF and forskolin (another adenyl cyclase activator) was used in place of cholera toxin. These data suggest strongly that cAMP differentially modulates the expression of three major CAMs on neurons. Some data suggest that cAMP also regulates the response of glial cells to injury (572).

Finally, An et al. (400) examined the effects of lysophosphatidic acid (LPA) and sphingosine 1-phosphate (S1P) on cAMP levels in cells. These are potent phospholipid messengers that activate multiple G-protein–mediated intracellular signaling pathways. G proteins mediate cAMP, MAP kinases, Rho, and gene transcription pathways. These two phospholipid messengers are released in injured tissues by various inflammatory processes. Similar mechanisms have been described for control of regeneration in aplysia neurons (573). The improved understanding of the signaling pathways involved in axonal growth has opened a world of pharmacologic manipulations of neuronal growth that was never available before.

STEM CELLS, THERAPEUTIC VACCINES, AND IMMUNOTHERAPY

Three novel and promising therapies were reported recently to stimulate regeneration in the spinal cord: stem cell transplants, therapeutic vaccine, and immune demyelination.

Transplanted embryonic stem cells improve locomotor recovery in rats after contusion injury (574). The stem cells had been treated with retinoic acid, which converted most of the cells to oligodendroglial precursors, some astrocytes, and 10% neurons. The transplanted cells were transplanted at 8 days after injury, migrated as far as 8 mm from the implantation site, and apparently myelinated some axons. In a separate study, they transplanted the stem cells into genetically myelin-deficient mice and showed that rapid myelination of axons occurred within 2 weeks (575).

Vaccination of animals with spinal cord homogenates stimulated regeneration and improved locomotor recovery in mice after dorsal spinal cord hemisection (576–577). Based on the hypothesis that spinal cord homogenates will stimulate antibodies against multiple axonal growth inhibitors, the group inoculated the mice for 3 weeks before injury. To quantify the number of cells that regenerated, they labeled the cut axons at the time of injury and then followed by an injection of another dye into distal cord to obtain retrograde labeling of cell bodies in the brain. Double-labeled cells therefore would suggest cells that were cut and then grew into the distal cord. Approximately half the mice showed as many as 75% double labeling of cells in the brain. If confirmed, this would represent an exciting therapeutic vaccination approach to SCI.

Hauben et al. (578,579) recently reported that immunologic demyelination improves neurologic recovery in animals. Dyer et al. (580) had earlier reported that immune demyelination promotes regeneration of brain stem–spinal cord tracts, but Hiebert et al. (581) found that this was not the case for rubrospinal tracts. On the other hand, Keirstead et al. (582) reported that immune demyelination followed by Schwann cell transplants enhanced the number of regenerated axons after dorsal column lesions. Likewise, Baron-Van Evercooren et al. (583) reported that Schwann cell transplants facilitated regeneration after immune demyelination in rats. Ridet et al. (584) found that moderate doses (2 to 20 Gy) of x-radiation improved neurologic recovery. Savio and Schwab (109) had earlier used x-radiation on neonatal rats to produce demyelination and promoted regeneration. The concept of immune-mediated demyelination followed by cell transplant is an important and potentially promising approach.

THERAPEUTIC CHALLENGES

We have a surprising glut of therapies that regenerate the spinal cord of animals. Several are already in clinical trial. For example,

clinical trials have started to assess the safety and feasibility of implanting activated macrophages and porcine neural stem into patients with SCI. Trials involving Schwann cell and OEG transplants are being planned. There is discussion of an IN-1 trial, an inosine trial, and an AIT-082 trial starting in the coming year (2002).

If these treatments prove to be safe and show any promising effects, phase II and III trials will soon be on their way. The onus is now upon the laboratories carrying out regenerative trials to deliver rigorous preclinical data to maximize the success and minimize the risk of the clinical trials. The studies must address several major questions.

First, what is the best dose, duration, and timing of the therapies? Most of the therapies have been tried only in animals shortly after SCI. Dose–response and duration studies have not been systematically performed. Chronic SCI differs considerably from acute SCI. Injury initiates massive increases in cytokines and NTs that may alter the response of the spinal cords to therapy.

Second, what are the effects of combination and sequential therapies? Multiple therapies may be necessary to obtain optimal regeneration. Due to the complexity of interactions between growth regulatory molecules, effects of combination or sequential treatment are unpredictable and must be tested empirically.

Third, how safe are the therapies? Many of the treatments turn on prolonged growth or prevent apoptosis, mechanisms that alter the risk for cancerous growth. Some involve implantation of cells immortalized with genes that may cause cancer, or cells from animals that may pass unknown pathogens to humans.

Finally, we have yet to address one other difficult issue. Recent work suggests that prolonged "nonuse" may lead to neuronal circuits becoming inactive and that intensive forced-use rehabilitation may be necessary to initiate functional recovery (585,586). Thus, even if the therapy were successful, regeneration may not lead to function without appropriate rehabilitation.

REFERENCES

1. Breasted JH. *The Edwin Smith papyrus.* 1930;I.
2. Haynes WG. Acute war wounds of the spinal cord: analysis of 184 cases. *Am J Neurosurg* 1946;3:424–432.
3. Windle WF. *Regeneration in the central nervous system.* 1995.
4. Cajal SR. *Degeneration and regeneration of the nervous system.* 1928.
5. Cajal SR. Notas preventivas sobre la degeneración y regeneración de las vías nerviosas centrales. *Trab Lab Invest Biol Univ Madrid* 1906; 4:295–301.
6. Galabov G. Regeneration of sectioned spinal cord by implantation of a peripheral nerve. *Dokl Bolg Akad Nauk* 1966;19(5):449–452.
7. Sasabe TL, Freeman LW. A chemical potential of proximo-distal nerve implants in experimental spinal cord transection. *Med J Osaka Univ* 1971;21(4):231–240.
8. McMasters RE. Regeneration of the spinal cord in the rat: effects of piromen and ACTH upon the regenerative capacity. *J Comp Neurol* 1962;119:113–125.
9. Harvey JE, Srebnik HH. Locomotor activity and axon regeneration following spinal cord compression in rats treated with L-thyroxine. *J Neuropathol Exp Neurol* 1967;26(4):661–668.
10. Lampert P, Cressman M. Axonal regeneration in the dorsal columns

of the spinal cord of adult rats. An electron microscopic study. *Lab Invest* 1964;13:825–839.

11. Carlsson CA, Thulin CA. Regeneration of feline dorsal roots. *Experientia* 1967;23(2):125–126.

12. Ikeda K, Campbell JB. Dorsal spinal nerve root regeneration verified by injection of leucine-3H into the dorsal root ganglion. *Exp Neurol* 1971;30(3):379–388.

13. Nathaniel EJ, Nathaneil DR. Regeneration of dorsal root fibers into the adult rat spinal cord. *Exp Neurol* 1973;40(2):333–350.

14. Thulin CA, Carlsson CA. Regeneration of transected ventral roots submitted to monomolecular filter tubulation (millipore). An experimental study in cats. *J Neurol Sci* 1969;8(3):485–505.

15. Sjostrand J, Carlsson CA, Thulin CA. Regeneration of ventral roots. A histological study in cats. *Acta Anat* 1969;74(4):532–546.

16. Ochs S, Barnes CD. Regeneration of ventral root fibers into dorsal roots shown by axoplasmic flow. *Brain Res* 1969;15(2):600–603.

17. Carlsson CA, Bolander P, Sjostrand J. Biochemical and histochemical changes in the feline gastrocnemius muscle during regeneration of ventral roots. *J Neurol Sci* 1971;14(1):95–105.

18. Ranish N, Ochs S, Barnes CD. Regeneration of ventral root axons into dorsal roots as shown by increased acetylcholinesterase activity. *J Neurobiol* 1972;3(3):245–257.

19. Wolman L. Axon regeneration after spinal cord injury. *Paraplegia* 1966;4:175–184.

20. Wolman L. Post-traumatic regeneration of nerve fibres in the human spinal cord and its relation to intramedullary neuroma. *J Pathol Bacteriol* 1967;94(1):123–129.

21. Carlsson CA, Sundin T. Reconstruction of efferent pathways to the urinary bladder in a paraplegic child. *Rev Surg* 1967;24(1):73–76.

22. Petrov MA. Transplantations of nerves and roots of the spinal cord. *Reconstr Surg Traumatol* 1971;12(0):250–262.

23. Sundin T, Carlsson CA. Reconstruction of severed dorsal roots innervating the urinary bladder. An experimental study in cats. II. Regeneration studies. *Scand J Urol Nephrol* 1972;6(2):185–196.

24. Levi-Montalcini R. Morphological and metabolic effects of the nerve growth factor. *Arch Biol* 1965;76(2):387–417.

25. Levi-Montalcini R. Growth regulation of sympathetic nerve cells. *Arch Ital Biol* 1965;103(4):832–846.

26. Levi-Montalcini R. The nerve growth factor: its mode of action on sensory and sympathetic nerve cells. *Harvery Lect* 1966;60:217–259.

27. Levi-Montalcini R, Angeletti PU. Nerve growth factor. *Physiol Rev* 1968;48(3):534–569.

28. Liuzzi A, Angeletti PU, Levi-Montalcini R. Metabolic effects of a specific nerve growth factor (NGF) on sensory and sympathetic ganglia: enhancement of lipid biosynthesis. *J Neurochem* 1965;12(8):705–708.

29. Nakazawa T. Study on the nerve growth factor. Effect of a special protein and its antiserum on nerve regeneration. *No To Shinkei* 1966;18(4):344–350.

30. Stenevi U, Bjerre B, Bjorkland A, et al. Effects of localized intracerebral injections of nerve growth factor on the regenerative growth of lesioned central noradrenergic neurones. *Brain Res* 1974;69(2):217–234.

31. Guth L. Axonal regeneration and functional plasticity in the central nervous system. *Exp Neurol* 1974;45(3):606–654.

32. Guth LWW. Physiological, molecular, and genetic aspects of central nervous regeneration. *Exp Neurol* 1973;39(1):3–16.

33. Schneider D. Regenerative phenomena in the central nervous system. A symposium summary. *J Neurosurg* 1972;37(2):129–136.

34. Eccles JC. The plasticity of the mammalian central nervous system with special reference to new growths in response to lesions. *Naturwissenschaften.* 1976;63(1):8–15.

35. Guth L. History of central nervous system regeneration research. *Exp Neurol* 1975;48[Suppl 3, Pt 2]:3–15.

36. The current status of research on growth and regeneration in the central nervous system. Summary of a subcommittee report commissioned by the National Advisory Council of the National Institute of Neurological and Communicative Disorders and Stroke, 1975. *Surg Neurol* 1976;5(3):157–160.

37. Puchala E, Windles WF. The possibility of structural and functional restitution after spinal cord injury. A review. *Exp Neurol* 1977;55(1):1–42.

38. Graftstein B. Cellular mechanisms for recovery from nervous system injury. *Surg Neurol* 1980;13(5):363–365.

39. Marks AF. Regenerative reconstruction of a tract in a rat's brain. *Exp Neurol* 1972;34(3):455–464.

40. Bernstein JJ, Bernstein ME. Axonal regeneration and formation of synapses proximal to the site of lesion following hemisection of the rat spinal cord. *Exp Neurol* 1971;30(2):336–351.

41. Bernstein JJ, Bernstein ME. Neuronal alteration and reinnervation following axonal regeneration and sprouting in mammalian spinal cord. *Brain Behav Evol* 1973;8(1):135–161.

42. Bernstein ME, Bernstein JJ. Dendritic growth cone and filopodia formation as a mechanism of spinal cord regeneration. *Exper Neurol* 1977;57(2):419–425.

43. Björklund A, Baumgarten HG, Lachenmayer L, et al. Recovery of brain noradrenaline after 5,7-dihydroxytryptamine-induced axonal lesions in the rat. *Cell Tissue Res* 1975;161(2):145–155.

44. Björklund A, Katzman R, Stenevi U, et al. Development and growth of axonal sprouts from noradrenaline and 5-hydroxytryptamine neurones in the rat spinal cord. *Brain Res* 1971;31(1):21–33.

45. Björklund A, Lindvall O. Regeneration of normal terminal innervation patterns by central noradrenergic neurons after 5,7-dihydroxytryptamine-induced axotomy in the adult rat. *Brain Res* 1979;171(2):271–293.

46. Björklund A, Nobin A, Stenevi U. Regeneration of central serotonin neurons after axonal degeneration induced by 5,6-dihydroxytryptamine. *Brain Res* 1973;50(1):214–220.

47. Bernstein JJ, Bernstein ME. Effect of glial-ependymal scar and Teflon arrest on the regenerative capacity of goldfish spinal cord. *Exp Neurol* 1967;19(1):25–32.

48. Selzer ME. Mechanisms of functional recovery and regeneration after spinal cord transection in larval sea lamprey. *J Physiol (London)* 1978;277:395–408.

49. Wood MR, Cohen MJ. Synaptic regeneration in identified neurons of the lamprey spinal cords. *Science* 1979;206(4416):344–347.

50. Borgens RB, Roederer E, Cohen MJ. Enhanced spinal cord regeneration in lamprey by applied electric fields. *Science* 1981;213(4508):611–617.

51. Yin HS, Selzer ME. Axonal regeneration in lamprey spinal cord. *J Neurosci* 1983;3(6):1135–1144.

52. Schonheit B. Further studies on the regeneration of the spinal cord in Rana esculenta L. and Rana temporaria L. *Z Mikrosk Anat Forsch* 1968;78(4):557–596.

53. Butler EG, Ward MB. Reconstitution of the spinal cord following ablation in urodele larvae. *J Exp Zool* 1965;160(1):47–65.

54. Schonheit B, Rehmer H. Further studies of the regeneration of the spinal cord of Pleurodeles Waltli Michah (1830). *Z Mikrosk Anat Forsch* 1968;79(2):389–401.

55. Simpson SB Jr. Morphology of the regenerated spinal cord in the lizard, Anolis carolinensis. *J Comp Neurol* 1968;134(2):193–210.

56. Edgar M, Simpson SB, Singer M. The growth and differentiation of the regenerating spinal cord of the lizard, Anolis carolinensis. *J Morphol* 1970;131(2):131–151.

57. Bryant SV, Wozny KJ. Stimulation of limb regeneration in the lizard Xantusia vigilis by means of ependymal implants. *J Exp Zool* 1974;189(3):339–352.

58. Bernstein JJ, Gelderd JB. Regeneration of the long spinal tracts in the goldfish. *Brain Res* 1970;20(1):33–38.

59. Prendergast J, Misantone LJ. Sprouting by tracts descending from the midbrain to the spinal cord: the result of thoracic funiculotomy in the newborn, 21-day-old, and adult rat. *Exp Neurol* 1980;69(3):458–480.

60. Prendergast J, Murray M, Goldberger ME. Sprouting and reflex recovery after spinal nerve lesions in cats. *Exp Neurol* 1981;73(3):732–749.

61. Prendergast J, Stelzner DJ. Changes in the magnocellular portion of the red nucleus following thoracic hemisection in the neonatal and adult rat. *J Comp Neurol* 1976;166(2):163–171.

62. Prendergast J, Stelzner DJ. Increases in collateral axonal growth rostral

to a thoracic hemisection in neonatal and weanling rat. *J Comp Neurol* 1976;166(2):145–161.

63. Gearhart J, Oster-Granite ML, Guth L. Histological changes after transection of the spinal cord of fetal and neonatal mice. *Exp Neurol* 1979;66(1):1–15.

64. Kalil K, Reh T. Regrowth of severed axons in the neonatal central nervous system: establishment of normal connections. *Science* 1979; 205(4411):1158–1161.

65. Kalil K, Reh T. A light and electron microscopic study of regrowing pyramidal tract fibers. *J Comp Neurol* 1982;211(3):265–275.

66. Feringa ER, Gurden GG, Strodel W, et al. Descending spinal motor tract regeneration after spinal cord transection. *Neurology* 1973;23(6):599–608.

67. Feringa ER, Johnson RD, Wendt JS. Spinal cord regeneration in rats after immunosuppressive treatment. Theoretic considerations and histologic results. *Arch Neurol* 1975;32(10):676–683.

68. Feringa ER, Shuer LM, Vahlsing HL, et al. Regeneration of corticospinal axons in the rat. *Ann Neurol* 1977;2(4):315–321.

69. Feringa ER, Wendt JS, Johnson RD. Immunosuppressive treatment to enhance spinal cord regeneration in rats. *Neurology* 1974;24(3):287–293.

70. Feringa ER, Davis SW, Vahlsing HL, et al. Fink-Heimer/Nauta demonstration of regenerating axons in the rat spinal cord. *Arch Neurol* 1978;35(8):522–526.

71. Feringa ER, Nelson KR, Vahlsing HL, et al. Spinal cord regeneration in rats made immunologically unresponsive to CNS antigens. *J Neurol Neurosurg Psychiatry* 1979;42(7):642–648.

72. Feringa ER, Vahlsing HL, Dauser RC. The orthograde flow of tritiated proline in corticospinal neurons at various ages and after spinal cord injury. *J Neurol Neurosurg Psychiatry* 1984;47(9):917–920.

73. Feringa ER, Vahlsing HL, Gilbertie WJ. Failure to promote spinal cord regeneration in rats with immunosuppressive treatment [Letter]. *J Neurol Neurosurg Psychiatry* 1985;48(7):723–735.

74. Matinian LA. Effect of enzyme therapy on the restoration of spinal function after its total resection. *Zh Eksp Klin Med* 1965;5(3):3–13.

75. Kosel KC, Wilkinson JM, Jew J, et al. Enzyme therapy and spinal cord regeneration: a fluorescence microscopic evaluation. *Exp Neurol* 1979;64(2):365–374.

76. Matthews MA, St. Onge MF, Faciane CL, et al. Spinal cord transection: a quantitative analysis of elements of the connective tissue matrix formed within the site of lesion following administration of piromen, Cytoxan or trypsin. *Neuropathol Appl Neurobiol* 1979;5(3):161–180.

77. Kowalski TF, Vahlsing HL, Feringa ER. Lidase treatment of spinal cord transected rats. *Ann Neurol* 1979;6(1):78–79.

78. Guth L, Albuquerque EX, Deshpande SS, et al. Ineffectiveness of enzyme therapy on regeneration in the transected spinal cord of the rat. *J Neurosurg* 1980;52(1):73–86.

79. Guth L, Brewer CR, Collins WF, et al. Criteria for evaluating spinal cord regeneration experiments. *Exp Neurol* 1980;69(1):1–3.

80. Sahgal V, Sahgal S, Subramani V. Morphological and histochemical correlation of recovery after spinal transection in rat. *Paraplegia* 1981; 19(1):1–6.

81. Foerster AP. Spontaneous regeneration of cut axons in adult rat brain. *J Comp Neurol* 1982;210:335–356.

82. Harston CT, Morrow A, Kostrzewa RM. Enhancement of sprouting and putative regeneration of central noradrenergic fibers by morphine. *Brain Res Bull* 1980;5:421–424.

83. Eidelberg E, Story JL, Meyer BL, et al. Stepping by chronic spinal cats. *Exp Brain Res* 1980;40(3):241–246.

84. Windle WF. Inhibition of regeneration of severed axons in the spinal cord. *Exp Neurol* 1980;69(1):209–211.

85. David S, Aguayo AJ. Axonal elongation into peripheral nervous system "bridges" after central nervous system injury in adult rats. *Science* 1981;214(4523):931–933.

86. Benfey M, Aguayo AJ. Extensive elongation of axons from rat brain into peripheral nerve grafts. *Nature* 1982;296:150–152.

87. Aguayo AJ, David S, Bray GM. Influences of the glial environment on the elongation of axons after injury: transplantation studies in adult rodents. *J Exp Biol* 1981;95:231–240.

88. Aguayo AJ, Benfey M, David S. A potential for axonal regeneration in neurons of the adult mammalian nervous system. *Birth Defects* 1983;19(4):327–340.

89. Feringa ER, Kowalski TF, Vahlsing HL. Basal lamina formation at the site of spinal cord transection. *Ann Neurol* 1980;8(2):148–154.

90. Feringa ER, Vahlsing HL, Woodward M. Basal lamina formation at the site of spinal cord transection in the rat: an ultrastructural study. *Neurosci Lett* 1984;51(3):303–308.

91. Feringa ER, Kowalski TF, Vahlsing HL. Basal lamina at the site of spinal cord injury in normal, immunotolerant and immunosuppressed rats. *Neurosci Lett* 1985;54(2-3):225–230.

92. Kao CC. Basic considerations in spinal cord reconstruction. *J Am Paraplegia Soc* 1982;5(1):9–12.

93. Wrathall JR, Rigamonti DD, Braford MR, et al. Reconstruction of the contused cat spinal cord by the delayed nerve graft technique and cultured peripheral non-neuronal cells. *Acta Neuropathol* 1982;57(1):59–69.

94. Wrathall JR, Kapoor V, Kao CC. Observation of culture peripheral non-neuronal cells implanted into the transected spinal cord. *Acta Neuropathol* 1984;64(3):203–212.

95. Lindsay RM, Thoenen H, Barde YA. Placode and neural crest-derived sensory neurons are responsive at early development stages to brain-derived neurotrophic factor. *Dev Biol* 1985;112(2):319–328.

96. Davies AM, Thoenen H, Barde YA. The response of chick sensory neurons to brain-derived neurotrophic factor. *J Neurosci* 1986;6(7):1897–1904.

97. Johnson JE, Barde YA, Schwab M, et al. Brain-derived neurotrophic factor supports the survival of cultured rat retinal ganglion cells. *J Neurosci* 1986;6(10):3031–3038.

98. Kalcheim C, Barde YA, Thoenen H, et al. In vivo effect of brain-derived neurotrophic factor on the survival of developing dorsal root ganglion cells. *Embo J* 1987;6(10):2871–2873.

99. Acheson A, Barde YA, Thoenen H. High K+-mediated survival of spinal sensory neurons depends on developmental stage. *Exp Cell Res* 1987;170(1):56–63.

100. Thoenen H, Barde YA, Davies AM. Neurotrophic factors and neuronal death. *Ciba Found Symp* 1987;126:82–95.

101. Barde YA. The nerve growth factor family. *Prog Growth Factor Res* 1990;2(4):237–248.

102. Hohn A, Leibrock J, Bailey K, et al. Identification and characterization of a novel number of the nerve growth factor/brain-derived neurotrophic factor family. *Nature* 1990;344(6264):339–341.

103. Rodriguez-Tebar A, Dechant G, Barde YA. Neurotrophins: structural relatedness and receptor interactions. *Philos Trans R Soc London B Biol Sci* 1991;331(1261):255–258.

104. Caroni P, Savio T, Schwab ME. Central nervous system regeneration: oligodendrocytes and myelin as non-permissive substances for neurite growth. *Prog Brain Res* 1988;78:363–370.

105. Caroni P, Schwab ME. Two membrane protein fractions from rat central myelin with inhibitory properties for neurite growth and fibroblast spreading. *J Cell Biol* 1988;106(4):1281–1288.

106. Caroni P, Schwab ME. Antibody against myelin-associated inhibitor of neurite growth neutralizes nonpermissive substrate properties of CNS white matter. *Neuron* 1988;1(1):85–96.

107. Bandtlow C, Zachleder T, Schwab ME. Oligodendrocytes arrest neurite growth by contact inhibition. *J Neurosci* 1990;10(2):3837–3848.

108. Bandtlow C, Schmidt MF, Hassinger TD, et al. Role of intracellular calcium in NI-35-evoked collapse of neuronal growth cones. *Science* 1993;259(5091):80–83.

109. Savio T, Schwab ME. Lesioned corticospinal tract axons regenerate in myelin-free rat spinal cord. *Proc Natl Acad Sci U S A* 1990;87(11):4130–4133.

110. Schwegler G, Schwab ME, Kapfhammer JP. Increased collateral sprouting of primary afferents in the myelin-free spinal cord. *J Neurosci* 1995;15(4):2756–2767.

111. Schnell L, Schwab ME. Axonal regeneration in the rat spinal cord produced by an antibody against myelin-associated neurite growth inhibitors. *Nature* 1990;343(6255):269–272.

112. Schnell L, Schwab ME. Sprouting and regeneration of lesioned corticospinal tract fibers in the adult rat spinal cord. *Eur J Neurosci* 1993;5(9):1156–1171.

113. Schnell L, Schneider R, Kolbeck R, et al. Neurotrophin-3 enhances sprouting of corticospinal tract during development and after adult spinal cord [Comments]. *Nature* 1994;367(6459):170–173.

114. Varga ZM, Schwab ME, Nicholls JG. Myelin-associated neurite growth-inhibitory proteins and suppression of regeneration of immature mammalian spinal cord in culture. *Proc Natl Acad Sci U S A* 1995;92(24):10959–10963.

115. Bregman BS, Kunkel-Bagden E, Schnell L, et al. Recovery from spinal cord injury mediated by antibodies to neurite growth inhibitors [Comments]. *Nature* 1995;378(6556):498–501.

116. Schwab ME. Myelin-associated inhibitors of neurite growth and regeneration in the CNS. *Trends Neurosci* 1990;13(11):452–456.

117. Schwab ME. Structural plasticity of the adult CNS. Negative control by neurite growth inhibitory signals. *Int J Dev Neurosci* 1996;14(4):379–385.

118. Kapfhammer JP. Axon sprouting in the spinal cord: growth promoting and growth inhibitory mechanisms. *Anat Embryol (Berlin)* 1997;196(6):417–426.

119. Kapfhammer JP. Restriction of plastic fiber growth after lesions by central nervous system myelin-associated neurite growth inhibitors. *Adv Neurol* 1997;73:7–27.

120. Schwab ME, Brosamle C. Regeneration of lesioned corticospinal tract fibers in the adult rat spinal cord under experimental conditions. *Spinal Cord* 1997;35(7):469–473.

121. Schwab ME. Regeneration of lesioned CNS axons by neutralization of neurite growth inhibitors: a short review. *J Neurotrauma* 1992;9[Suppl 1]:S219–S221.

122. Raineteau O, Z'Gragegn WJ, Thallmair M, et al. Sprouting and regeneration after pyramidotomy and blockade of the myeline-associated neurite growth inhibitors NI 35/250 in adult rats. *Eur J Neurosci* 1999;11(4):1486–1490.

123. Loschinger J, Bandtlow CE, Jung J, et al. Retinal axon growth cone responses to different environmental cues are mediated by different second-messenger systems. *J Neurobiol* 1997;33(6):825–834.

124. Bandtlow C, Schiweck W, Tai HH, et al. The Escherichia coli–derived Fab fragment of the IgM/kappa antibody IN-1 recognizes and neutralizes myelin-associated inhibitors of neurite growth. *Eur J Biochem* 1996;241(2):468–475.

125. Brosmale C, Huber AB, Fiedler M, et al. Regeneration of lesioned corticospinal tract fibers in the adult rat induced by a recombinant, humanized IN-1 antibody fragment. *J Neurosci* 2000;20(21):8061–8068.

126. Spillman AA, Bandtlow CE, Lottspeich F, et al. Identification and characterization of a bovine neurite growth inhibitor (bNI-220). *J Biol Chem* 1998;273(30):19283–19293.

127. Chen MS, Huber AB, van der Haar ME, et al. Nogo-A is a myeline-associated neurite outgrowth inhibitor and an antigen for monoclonal antibody IN-1 [Comments]. *Nature* 2000;403(6768):434–439.

128. Huber AB, Schwab ME. Nogo-A, a potent inhibitor of neurite outgrowth and regeneration. *Biol Chem* 2000;381(5-6):407–419.

129. GrandPre T, Nakamura F, Vartanian T, et al. Identification of the Nogo inhibitor of axon regeneration as a reticulon protein. *Nature* 2000;403(6768):439–444.

130. Wanner M, Lang DM, Bandtlow CE, et al. Reevaluation of the growth-permissive substrate properties of goldfish optic nerve myelin and myelin proteins. *J Neurosci* 1995;14(11):7500–7508.

131. Lang DM, Monzon-Mayor M, Bandtlow CE, et al. Retinal axon regeneration in the lizard Gallotia galloti in the presence of CNS myelin and oligodendrocytes. *Glia* 1998;23(1):61–74.

132. Lang DM, Rubin BP, Schwab ME, et al. CNS myelin and oligodendrocytes of the Xenopus spinal cord—but not optic nerve—are nonpermissive for axon growth. *J Neurosci* 1995;15[Suppl 1, Pt 1]:99–109.

133. Varga ZM, Bandtlow CE, Erulkar SD, et al. The critical period for repair of CNS of neonatal opossum (Monodelphus domestica) in culture: correlation with development of glial cells, myelin and growth-inhibitor molecules. *Eur J Neurosci* 1995;7(10):2119–2129.

134. MacLaren RE. Expression of myelin proteins in the opossum optic nerve: late appearance of inhibitors implicates an earlier non-myelin

135. David S, Braun PE, Jackson DL, et al. Laminin overrides the inhibitory effects of peripheral nervous system and central nervous system myelin-derived inhibitors of neurite growth. *J Neurosci Res* 1995;42(4):594–602.

136. McKerracher L, David S, Jackson DL, et al. Identification of myelin-associated glycoprotein as a major myelin-derived inhibitor of neurite growth. *Neuron* 1994;13(4):805–811.

137. Mukhopadhyay G, Doherty P, Walsh FS, et al. A novel role for myelin-associated glycoprotein as an inhibitor of axonal regeneration. *Neuron* 1994;13(3):757–767.

138. Shen YJ, DeBallard ME, Salzer JL, et al. Myelin-associated glycoprotein in myelin and expressed by Schwann cells inhibits axonal regeneration and branching. *Mol Cell Neurosci* 1998;12(1-2):79–91.

139. DeBallard ME, Tang S, Mukhopadhyay G, et al. Myelin-associated glycoprotein inhibits axonal regeneration from a variety of neurons via interaction with a sialoglycoprotein. *Mol Cell Neurosci* 1996;7(2):89–101.

140. DeBallard ME, Filbin MT. Myelin-associated glycoprotein, MAG, selectively binds several neuronal proteins. *J Neurosci Res* 1999;56(2):213–218.

141. Bartsch U, Bandtlow C, Schnell L, et al. Lack of evidence that myelin-associated glycoprotein is a major inhibitor of axonal regeneration in the CNS. *Neuron* 1995;15(6):1375–1381.

142. Oudega M, Rosano C, Sadi D, et al. Neutralizing antibodies against neurite growth inhibitor NI-35/250 do not promote regeneration of sensory axons in the adult rat spinal cord. *Neuroscience* 2000;100(4):873–883.

143. Davies SJ, Goucher DR, Doller C, et al. Robust regeneration of adult sensory axons in degenerating white matter of the adult rat spinal cord. *J Neurosci* 1999;19(14):5810–5822.

144. Davies SJ, Fitch MT, Memberg SP, et al. Regeneration of adult axons in white matter tracts of the central nervous system. *Nature* 1997;390(6661):680–683.

145. Guest JD, Hesse D, Schnell L, et al. Influence of IN-1 antibody and acidic FGF-fibrin glue on the response of injured corticospinal tract axons to human Schwann cell grafts. *J Neurosci Res* 1997;50(5):888–905.

146. Fawcett JW, Fersht N, Housden L, et al. Axonal growth on astrocytes is not inhibited by oligodendrocytes. *J Cell Sci* 1992;103[Pt 2]:571–579.

147. Buffo A, Zagrebelsky M, Huber AB, et al. Application of neutralizing antibodies against NI-35/250 myelin-associated neurite growth inhibitory proteins to the adult rat cerebellum induces sprouting of uninjured Purkinje cell axons. *J Neurosci* 2000;20(6):2275–2286.

148. Bandtlow CE, Schwab ME. NI-35/250/Nogo-a: a neurite growth inhibitor restricting structural plasticity and regeneration of nerve fibers in the adult vertebrate CNS. *Glia* 2000;29(2):175–181.

149. Wenk CA, Thallmair M, Kartje GL, et al. Increased corticofugal plasticity after unilateral cortical lesions combined with neutralization of the IN-1 antigen in adult rats. *J Comp Neurol* 1999;410(1):143–157.

150. Niederost BP, Zimmermann DR, Schwab ME, et al. Bovine CNS myelin contains neurite growth-inhibitory activity associated with chondroitin sulfate proteoglycans. *J Neurosci* 1999;19(20):8979–8989.

151. Kwiatkowska D, Kwiatkowska-Korczak J. Adhesive glycoproteins of the extracellular matrix. *Postepy Hig Med Dosw* 1999;53(1):55–74.

152. Halfter W, Dong S, Schurer B, et al. Composition, synthesis, and assembly of the embryonic chick retinal basal lamina. *Dev Biol* 2000;220(2):111–128.

153. Chang D, Woo JS, Campanelli J, et al. Agrin inhibits neurite outgrowth but promotes attachment of embryonic motor and sensory neurons. *Dev Biol* 1997;181(1):21–35.

154. Hering H, Kroger S. Synapse formation and agrin expression in stratospheroid cultures from embryonic chick retina. *Dev Biol* 1999;214(2):412–428.

155. Cohen MW, Moody-Corbett F, Godfrey EW. Former neuritic pathways containing endogenous neural agrin have high synaptogenetic activity. *Dev Biol* 1995;167(2):458–468.

156. Gesemann M, Denzer AJ, Ruegg MA. Acetylcholine receptor-aggregating activity of agrin isoforms and mapping of the active site. *J Cell Biol* 1995;128(4):625–636.

157. Saito M, Nguyen J, Kidokoro Y. Inhibition of nerve- and agrin-induced acetylcholine receptor clustering on Xenopus muscle cells in culture. *Dev Brain Res* 1993;71(1):9–17.

158. Wells DG, McKechnie BA, Kelkar S, et al. Neurotrophins regulate agrin-induced postsynaptic differentiation. *Proc Natl Acad Sci U S A* 1999;96(3):1112–1117.

159. Pindzola RR, Doller C, Silver J. Putative inhibitory extracellular matrix molecules at the dorsal root entry zone of the spinal cord during development and after root and sciatic nerve lesions. *Dev Biol* 1993;156(1):34–48.

160. Siegal JD, Kliot M, Smith GM, et al. A comparison of the regeneration of potential dorsal root fibers into gray or white matter of the adult rat spinal cord. *Exp Neurol* 1990;109(1):90–97.

161. Kliot M, Smith GM, Siegal JD, et al. Astrocyte-polymer implants promote regeneration of dorsal root fibers into the adult mammalian spinal cord. *Exp Neurol* 1990;109(1):57–69.

162. Hoke A, Silver J. Heterogeneity among astrocytes in reactive gliosis. *Perspect Dev Neurobiol* 1994;2(3):269–274.

163. Bandtlow CE, Loschinger J. Developmental changes in neuronal responsiveness to the CNS myelin-associated neurite growth inhibitor NI-35/250. *Eur J Neurosci* 1997;9(12):2743–2752.

164. Fawcett JW, Asher RA. The glial scar and central nervous system repair. *Brain Res Bull* 1999;49(6):377–391.

165. Smith-Thomas LC, Stevens J, Folk-Seang J, et al. Increased axon regeneration in astrocytes grown in the presence of proteoglycan synthesis inhibitors. *J Cell Sci* 1995;108[Pt 3]:1307–1315.

166. Lemons ML, Howland DR, Anderson DK. Chondroitin sulfate proteoglycan immunoreactivity increases following spinal cord injury and transplantation. *Exp Neurol* 1999;160(1):51–65.

167. Braunewell KH, Martini R, LeBaron R, et al. Up-regulation of a chondroitin sulphate epitope during regeneration of mouse sciatic nerve; evidence that the immunoreactive molecules are related to the chondroitin sulphate proteoglycans decorin and versican. *Eur J Neurosci* 1995;7(4):792–804.

168. Yick LW, Wu W, So KF, et al. Chondroitinase ABC promotes axonal regeneration of Clarke's neurons after spinal cord injury. *Neuroreport* 2000;11(5):1063–1067.

169. Zuo J, Neubauer D, Dyess K, et al. Degradation of chondroitin sulfate proteoglycan enhances the neurite-promoting potential of spinal cord tissue. *Exp Neurol* 1998;154(2):654–662.

170. Muir E, Du JS, Fok-Seang J, et al. Increased axon growth through astrocyte cell lines transfected with urokinase. *Glia* 1998;23(1):24–34.

171. Zuo J, Ferguson TA, Hernandez YJ, et al. Neuronal matrix metalloproteinase-2 degrades and inactivates a neurite-inhibiting chondroitin sulfate proteoglycan. *J Neurosci* 1998;18(14):5203–5211.

172. Wang X, Messing A, David S. Axonal and nonneuronal cell responses to spinal cord injury in mice lacking glial fibrillary acidic protein. *Exp Neurol* 1997;148(2):568–576.

173. Caubit X, Riou JF, Coulon J, et al. Tenascin expression in developing, adult and regenerating caudal spinal cord in the urodele amphibians. *Int J Dev Biol* 1994;38(4):661–672.

174. Zhang Y, Winterbottom JK, Schachner M, et al. Tenascin-C expression and axonal sprouting following injury to the spinal dorsal columns in the adult rat. *J Neurosci Res* 1997;49(4):433–450.

175. Weidner N, Grill RJ, Tuszynski MH. Elimination of basal lamina and the collagen "scar" after spinal cord injury fails to augment corticospinal tract regeneration. *Exp Neurol* 1999;160(1):40–50.

176. Tessier-Lavigne M. Axon guidance by diffusible repellants and attractants. *Curr Opin Genet Dev* 1994;4(4):596–601.

177. Araki T, Milbrandt J. Ninjurin2, a novel hemophilic adhesion molecule, is expressed in mature sensory and enteric neurons and promotes neurite outgrowth. *J Neurosci* 2000;20(1):187–195.

178. Toyota B, Carbonetto S, David S. A dual laminin/collagen receptor acts in peripheral nerve regeneration. *Proc Natl Acad Sci U S A* 1990;87(4):1319–1322.

179. Chuah MI, David S, Blaschuck O. Differentiation and survival of rat olfactory epithelial neurons in dissociated cell culture. *Dev Brain Res* 1991;60(2):123–132.

180. Ajemian A, Ness R, David S. Tenascin in the injured rat optic nerve and in non-neuronal cells in vitro: potential role in neural repair. *J Comp Neurol* 1994;340(2):233–242.

181. Itoh K, Sakurai Y, Asou H, et al. Differential expression of alternatively spliced neural cell adhesion molecule L1 isoforms during oligodendrocyte maturation. *J Neurosci Res* 2000;60(5):579–586.

182. Crossin KL, Krushel LA. Cellular signaling by neural cell adhesion molecules of the immunoglobulin superfamily. *Dev Dyn* 2000;218(2):260–279.

183. Hall H, Bozic D, Fauser C, et al. Trimerization of cell adhesion molecule L1 mimics clustered L1 expression on the cell surface: influence on L1-ligand interactions and on promotion of neurite outgrowth. *J Neurochem* 2000;75(1):336–346.

184. Aubert I, Ridet JL, Schachner M, et al. Expression of L1 and PSA during sprouting and regeneration in the adult hippocampal formation. *J Comp Neurol* 1998;399(1):1–19.

185. Tran TS, Phelps PE. Axons crossing in the ventral commissure express L1 and GAD65 in the developing rat spinal cord. *Dev Neurosci* 2000;22(3):228–236.

186. Kamiguchi H, Lemmon V. Recycling of the cell adhesion molecule L1 in axonal growth cones. *J Neurosci* 2000;20(10):3676–3686.

187. Higgins JJ, Rosen DR, Loveless JM, et al. A gene for nonsyndromic mental retardation maps to chromosome 3p25-pter [Comments]. *Neurology* 2000;55(3):335–340.

188. Sztriha L, Frossard P, Hofstra RM, et al. Novel missense mutation in the L1 gene in a child with corpus callosum agenesis, retardation, adducted thumbs, spastic paraparesis, and hydrocephalus. *J Child Neurol* 2000;15(4):239–243.

189. Finckh U, Schroder J, Ressler B, et al. Spectrum and detection rate of L1CAM mutations in isolated and familial cases with clinically suspected L1-disease. *Am J Med Genet* 2000;92(1):40–46.

190. Kenwrick S, Watkins A, Angelis ED. Neural cell recognition molecule L1: relating biological complexity to human disease mutations. *Hum Mol Genet* 2000;9(6):879–886.

191. Graf WD, Born DE, Shaw DW, et al. Diffusion-weighted magnetic resonance imaging in boys with neural cell adhesion molecule L1 mutations and congenital hydrocephalus. *Ann Neurol* 2000;47(1):113–117.

192. Ozer E, Sarioglu S, Gure A. Effects of prenatal ethanol exposure on neuronal migration, neuronagenesis and brain myelination in the mice brain. *Clin Neuropathol* 2000;19(1):21–25.

193. Wilkemeyer MF, Sebastian AB, Smith SA, et al. Antagonists of alcoholic inhibition of cell adhesion. *Proc Natl Acad Sci U S A* 2000;97(7):3690–3695.

194. Moulding HD, Martuza RL, Rabkin SD. Clinical mutations in the L1 neural cell adhesion molecule affect cell-surface expression. *J Neurosci* 2000;20(15):5696–5702.

195. Silletti S, Mei F, Sheppard D, et al. Plasmin-sensitive dibasic sequences in the third fibronectin-like domain of L1-cell adhesion molecule (CAM) facilitate homomultimerization and concomitant integrin recruitment. *J Cell Biol* 2000;149(7):1485–1502.

196. Stallcup WB. The third fibronectin type III repeat is required for L1 to serve as an optimal substratum for neurite expression. *J Neurosci Res* 2000;61(1):33–43.

197. Bouley M, Tian MZ, Paisley K, et al. The L1-type cell adhesion molecule neuroglial influences the stability of neural ankyrin in the Drosophila embryo but not its axonal localization. *J Neurosci* 2000;20(12):4515–4523.

198. Garver TD, Ren Q, Tuvia S, et al. Tyrosine phosphorylation at a site highly conserved in the L1 family of cell adhesion molecules abolishes ankyrin binding and increases lateral mobility of neurofascin. *J Cell Biol* 1997;137(3):703–714.

199. Bock E, Richter-Landsberg C, Faissner A, et al. Demonstration of immunochemical identity between the nerve growth factor-inducible large external (NILE) glycoprotein and the cell adhesion molecule L1. *Embo J* 1985;4(11):2767–2768.

200. Seilheimer B, Schachner M. Regulation of neural cell adhesion mole-

cule expression on cultured mouse Schwann cells by nerve growth factor. *Embo J* 1987;6(6):1611–1616.

201. Sajovic P, Ennulat DJ, Shelanksi ML, et al. Isolation of NILE glycoprotein-related cDNA probes. *J Neurochem* 1987;49(3):756–763.

202. Weidner N, Blesch A, Grill RJ, et al. Nerve growth factor-hypersecreting Schwann cell grafts augment and guide spinal cord axonal growth and remyelinate central nervous system axons in a phenotypically appropriate manner that correlates with expression of L1. *J Comp Neurol* 1999;413(4):495–506.

203. Itoh K, Stevens B, Schachner M, et al. Regulated expression of the neural cell adhesion molecule L1 by specific patterns of neural impulses. *Science* 1995;270(5240):1369–1372.

204. Saad B, Constam DB, Ortmann R, et al. Astrocyte-derived TGF-beta 2 and NGF differentially regulate neural recognition molecule expression by cultured astrocytes. *J Cell Biol* 1991;115(2):473–484.

205. Mann DA, Doherty P, Walsh FS. Increased intracellular cyclic AMP differentially modulates nerve growth factor induction of three neuronal recognition molecules involved in neurite outgrowth. *J Neurochem* 1989;53(5):1581–1588.

206. Grant NJ, Claudepierre T, Aunis D, et al. Glucocorticoids and nerve growth factor differentially modulate cell adhesion molecule L1 expression in PC12 cells. *J Neurochem* 1996;66(4):1400–1408.

207. Schmid RS, Pruitt WM, Maness PF. A MAP kinase-signaling pathway mediates neurite outgrowth on L1 and requires Src-dependent endocytosis. *J Neurosci* 2000;20(11):4177–4188.

208. Gutwein P, Oleszewski M, Mechtersheimer S, et al. Role of Src kinases in the ADAM-mediated release of L1 adhesion molecule from human tumor cells. *J Biol Chem* 2000;275(20):15490–15497.

209. Wilson MT, Snow DM. Chondroitin sulfate proteoglycan expression pattern in hippocampal development: potential regulation of axon tract formation. *J Comp Neurol* 2000;424(3):532–546.

210. Oleszewski M, Gutwein P, von Der Lieth W, et al. Characterization of the L1-neurocan-binding site. Implications for L1-L1 Homophilic binding. *J Biol Chem* 2000;275(44):4478–4485.

211. Balaian LB, Moehler T, Montgomery AM. The human neural cell adhesion molecule L1 functions as a costimulatory molecule in T cell activation. *Eur J Immunol* 2000;30(3):938–943.

212. Blight A, Young W. Central axons in injured cat spinal cord recover electrophysiological function following remyelination by Schwann cells. *J Neurol Sci* 1989;91:15–34.

213. Bolin LM, Shooter EM. Characterization of a Schwann cell neurite-promoting activity that directs motoneuron axon outgrowth. *J Neurosci Res* 1994;37(1):23–35.

214. Bignami A, Chi NH, Dahl D. Regenerating dorsal roots and the nerve entry zone: an immunofluorescence study with neurofilament and laminin antisera. *Exp Neurol* 1984;85(2):426–436.

215. Bernstein JJ, Getz R, Jefferson M, et al. Astrocytes secrete basal lamina after hemisection of rat spinal cord. *Brain Res* 1985;327(1-2):135–141.

216. Manthorpe M, Engvall E, Ruoslahti E, et al. Laminin provides neuritic regeneration from cultured peripheral and central neurons. *J Cell Biol* 1983;97(6):1882–1890.

217. Horie H, Inagaki Y, Sohma Y, et al. Galectin-1 regulates initial axonal growth in peripheral nerves after axotomy. *J Neurosci* 1999;19(22):9964–9974.

218. Be'eri H, Reichert F, Saada A, et al. The cytokine network of wallerian degeneration: IL-10 and GM-CSF. *Eur J Neurosci* 1998;10(8):2707–2713.

219. Inagaki Y, Sohma Y, Horie H, et al. Oxidized galectin-1 promotes axonal regeneration in peripheral nerves but does not possess lectin properties. *Eur J Biochem* 2000;267(10):2955–2964.

220. Horie H, Kadoya T. Identification of oxidized galectin-1 as an initial repair regulatory factor after axotomy in peripheral nerves. *Neurosci Res* 2000;38(2):131–137.

221. Walther M, Kuklinski S, Pesheva P, et al. Galectin-3 is upregulated in microglial cells in response to ischemic brain lesions, but not to facial nerve axotomy. *J Neurosci Res* 2000;61(4):430–435.

222. Ryoke K, Ochi M, Iwata A, et al. A conditioning lesion promotes in vivo nerve regeneration in the contralateral sciatic nerve of rats. *Biochem Biophys Res Commun* 2000;267(3):715–718.

223. Matsuoka I, Nakane A, Kurihara K. Induction of LIF-mRNA by TGF-beta 1 in Schwann cells. *Brain Res* 1997;776(1-2):170–180.

224. Kurek JB, Radford AJ, Crump DE, et al. LIF (AM424), a promising growth factor for the treatment of ALS. *J Neurol Sci* 1998;160[Suppl 1]:S106–S113.

225. Araki T, Zimonjic DB, Popescu NC, et al. Mechanism of homophilic binding mediated by ninjurin, a novel widely expressed adhesion molecule. *J Biol Chem* 1997;272(34):1373–1380.

226. Araki T, Milbrandt J. Ninjurin, a novel adhesion molecule, is induced by nerve injury and promotes axonal growth. *Neuron* 1996;17(2):353–361.

227. Kolodkin AL, Matthes DJ, Goodman CS. The semaphorin genes encode a family of transmembrane and secreted growth cone guidance molecules. *Cell* 1993;75(7):1389–1399.

228. Pini A. Axon guidance. Growth cones say no. *Curr Biol* 1994;4(2):131–133.

229. Luo Y, Raible D, Raper JA. Collapsin: a protein in brain that induces the collapse and paralysis of neuronal growth cones. *Cell* 1993;75(2):217–227.

230. Luo Y, Shepherd I, Li J, et al. A family of molecules related to collapse in the embryonic chick nervous system [published correction appears in *Neuron* 1995;15(5):1218]. *Neuron* 1995;14(6):1131–1140.

231. Puschel AW, Adams RH, Betz H. Murine semaphorin D/collapsin is a member of a diverse gene family and creates domains inhibitory for axonal extension. *Neuron* 1995;14(5):941–948.

232. Fukada M, Watakabe I, Yuasa-Kawada J, et al. Molecular characterization of CRMP5, a novel member of the collapsin response mediator protein family. *J Biol Chem* 2000;275(48):37957–37965.

233. Keynes RJ, Cook GM. Repulsive and inhibitory signals. *Curr Opinions Neurobiol* 1995;5(1):75–82.

234. Hu H, Rutishauser U. A septum-derived chemorepulsive factor for migrating olfactory interneuron precursors. *Neuron* 1996;16(5):933–940.

235. Fan J, Raper JA. Localized collapsing cues can steer growth cones without inducing their full collapse. *Neuron* 1995;14(2):263–274.

236. Goshima Y, Kawakami T, Hori H, et al. A novel action of collapsin: collapsin-1 increases antero- and retrograde axoplasmic transport independently of growth cone collapse. *J Neurobiol* 1997;33(3):316–328.

237. Adams RH, Betz H, Puschel AW. A novel class of murine semaphorins with homology to thrombospondin is differentially expressed during early embryogenesis. *Mech Dev* 1996;57(1):33–45.

238. Chen H, He Z, Tessier-Lavigne M, et al. Axon guidance mechanisms: semaphorins as simultaneous repellents and anti-repellents [News; comment]. *Nat Neurosci* 1998;1(6):436–439.

239. Takahashi T, Nakamura F, Jin Z, et al. Semaphorins A and E act as antagonists of neuropilin-1 and agonists of neuropilin-2 receptors [Comments]. *Nat Neurosci* 1998;1(6):487–493.

240. de Castro F, Hu L, Drabkin H, et al. Chemoattraction and chemorepulsion of olfactory bulb axons by different secreted semaphorins. *J Neurosci* 1999;19(11):4428–4436.

241. O'Leary DD. Developmental neurobiology. Attractive guides for axons [News]. *Nature* 1994;371(6492):15–16.

242. Pasterkamp RJ, Giger RJ, Ruitenberg MJ, et al. Expression of the gene encoding the chemorepellent semaphorin III is induced in the fibroblast component of neural scar tissue formed injuries of adult but not neonatal CNS. *Mol Cell Neurosci* 1999;13(2):143–166.

243. Pasterkamp RJ, DeWinter F, Giger, et al. Role for semaphorin III and its receptor neuropilin-1 in neuronal regeneration and scar formation? *Prog Brain Res* 1998;117:151–170.

244. Zou Y, Stoeckli E, Chen H, et al. Squeezing axons out of the gray matter: a role for slit and semaphorin proteins from midline and ventral spinal cord. *Cell* 2000;102(3):363–375.

245. Goshima Y, Sasaki Y, Nakayama T. Functions of semaphorins in axon guidance and neuronal regeneration. *Jpn J Pharmacol* 2000;82(4):273–279.

246. Chen H, Bagri A, Zupicich JA, et al. Neuropilin-2 regulates the development of selective cranial and sensory nerves and hippocampal mossy fiber projections. *Neuron* 2000;25(1):43–56.

247. Pasterkamp RJ, Ruitenberg MJ, Verhaagen J. Semaphorins and their

receptors in olfactory axon guidance. *Cell Mol Biol (Noisy-le-grand)* 1999;45(6):763–779.

248. Pasterkamp RJ, DeWinter F, Holtmaat AJ. Evidence for a role of the chemorepellent semaphorin III and its receptor neuropilin-1 in the regeneration of primary olfactory axons. *J Neurosci* 1998;18(23): 9962–9976.

249. Bagnard D, Thomasset N, Lohrum M, et al. Spatial distributions of guidance molecules regulate chemorepulsion and chemoattraction of growth cones. *J Neurosci* 2000;20(3):1030–1035.

250. Matthes DJ, Sink, H, Kolodkin AL, et al. Semaphorin II can function as a selective inhibitor of specific synaptic arborizations. *Cell* 1995; 81(4):631–639.

251. Kobayashi H, Koppel AM, Luo Y, et al. A role for collapsin-1 in olfactory and cranial sensory axon guidance. *J Neurosci* 1997;17(21): 8339–8352.

252. Messersmieth EK, Leonardo ED, Shatz CJ, et al. Semaphorin III can function as a selective chemorepellent to pattern sensory projections in the spinal cord. *Neuron* 1995;14(5):949–959.

253. Wright DE, White FA, Gerfen RW, et al. The guidance molecule semaphorin III is expressed in regions of spinal cord and periphery avoided by growing sensory axons. *J Comp Neurol* 1995;361(2): 321–333.

254. Puschel AW, Adams RH, Betz H. The sensory intervention of the mouse spinal cord may be patterned by differential expression of and differential responsiveness to semaphorins. *Mol Cell Neurosci* 1996; 7(5):419–431.

255. Shepherd IT, Luo Y, Lefcort F, et al. A sensory axon repellent secreted from ventral spinal cord explants is neutralized by antibodies raised against collapsin-1. *Development* 1997;124(7):1377–1385.

256. Tanelian DL, Barry MA, Johnston SA, et al. Semaphorin III can repulse and inhibit adult sensory afferents in vivo. *Nat Med* 1997; 3(12):1398–1401.

257. Paskterkamp RJ, Giger RJ, Verhaagen J. Regulation of semaphorin III/collapsin-1 gene expression during peripheral nerve regeneration. *Exp Neurol* 1998;153(2):313–327.

258. Tamagnone L, Artigiani S, Chen H, et al. Plexins are a large family of receptors for transmembrane, secreted, and GPI-anchored semaphorins in vertebrates. *Cell* 1999;99(1):71–80.

259. Winberg ML, Noordermeer JN, Tamagnone L, et al. Plexin A is a neuronal semaphorin receptor that controls axon guidance. *Cell* 1998; 95(7):903–916.

260. Goshima Y, Nakamura F, Strittmatter P, et al. Collapsin-induced growth cone collapse mediated by an intracellular protein related to UNC-33. *Nature* 1995;376(6540):509–514.

261. Wang LH, Strittmatter SM. A family of rat CRMP genes is differentially expressed in the nervous system. *J Neurosci* 1996;16(19): 6197–6207.

262. Cohen-Salmon M, Crozet F, Rebillard G, et al. Cloning and characterization of the mouse collapsin response mediator protein-1, Crmp1. *Mamm Genome* 1997;8(5):349–351.

263. Kamata T, Subleski M, Hara Y, et al. Isolation and characterization of a bovine neural specific protein (CRMP-2) cDNA homologous to unc-33, a C. elegans gene implicated in axonal outgrowth and guidance. *Mol Brain Res* 1998;54(2):219–236.

264. Quinn CC, Gray GE, Hockfield S. A family of proteins implicated in axon guidance and outgrowth. *J Neurobiol* 1999;41(1):158–164.

265. Nakamura F, Kalb RG, Strittmatter SM. Molecular basis of semaphorin-mediated axon guidance. *J Neurobiol* 2000;44(2):219–229.

266. Jin Z, Strittmatter SM. Rac 1 mediates collapsin-1 induced growth cone collapse. *J Neurosci* 1997;17(16):6256–6263.

267. Kuhn TB, Brown MD, Wilcox CL, et al. Myelin and collapsin-1 induce motor neuron growth cone collapse through different pathways: inhibition of collapse by opposing mutants of rac1. *J Neurosci* 1999;19(6):1965–1975.

268. Gavazzi I, Stonehouse J, Sandvig A, et al. Peripheral, but not central, axotomy induces neuropilin-1 mRNA expression in adult large diameter primary sensory neurons. *J Comp Neurol* 2000;423(3):492–499.

269. Song H, Ming G, He Z, et al. Conversion of neuronal growth cone responses from repulsion to attraction by cyclic nucleotides [Comments]. *Science* 1998;281(5382):1515–1518.

270. Tuttle R, O'Leary DD. Neurotrophins rapidly modulate growth cone response to the axon guidance molecule, collapsin-1. *Mol Cell Neurosci* 1998;11(1-2):1–8.

271. Gagliardini V, Frankhauser C. Semaphorin III can induce death in sensory neurons. *Mol Cell Neurosci* 1999;14(4-5):301–316.

272. Shirvan A, Shina R, Ziz I, et al. Induction of neuronal apoptosis by semaphorin3A-derived peptide. *Mol Brain Res* 2000;83(1-2):81–93.

273. Castellani V, Chedotal A, Schachner M, et al. Analysis of the L1-deficient mouse phenotype reveals cross-talk between Sema3A and L1 signaling pathways in axonal guidance [Comments]. *Neuron* 2000; 27(2):237–249.

274. He Z. Crossed wires: L1 and neuropilin interactions [Comment]. *Neuron* 2000;27(2):191–193.

275. Taniguchi M, Yuasa S, Fujisawa H, et al. Disruption of semaphorin III/D gene causes severe abnormality in peripheral nerve projection. *Neuron* 1997;19(3):519–530.

276. Catalano SM, Messersmith EK, Goodman CS, et al. Many major CNS axon projections develop normally in the absence of semaphorin III. *Mol Cell Neurosci* 1998;11(4):173–182.

277. White FA, Behar O. The development and subsequent elimination of aberrant peripheral axon projections in semaphorin3A null mutant mice. *Dev Biol* 2000;225(1):79–86.

278. Sekido Y, Bader S, Latif F, et al. Human semaphorins A(V) and IV reside in the 3p21.3 small cell lung cancer deletion region and demonstrate distinct expression patterns. *Proc Natl Acad Sci U S A* 1996;93(9):4120–4125.

279. Xiang RH, Hensel CH, Garcia DK, et al. Isolation of the human semaphorin III/F gene (SEMA3F) at chromosome 3p21, a region deleted in lung cancer. *Genomics* 1996;32(1):39-48.

280. Christensen CR, Klingelhofer J, Tarabykina S, et al. Transcription of a novel mouse semaphorin gene, M-semaH, correlates with the metastatic ability of mouse tumor cell lines. *Cancer Res* 1998;58(6): 1238–1244.

281. Yamada T, Endo R, Gotoh M, et al. Identification of semaphorin E as a non-MDR drug resistance gene of human cancers. *Proc Natl Acad Sci U S A* 1997;94(26):14713–14718.

282. Soker S, Takashima S, Miao HQ, et al. Neuropilin-1 is expressed by endothelial and tumor cells as an isoform-specific receptor for vascular endothelial growth factor. *Cell* 1998;92(6):735–745.

283. Roush W. Receptor links blood vessels, axon [News]. *Science* 1998; 279(5359):2042.

284. Cooper HM, Gad JM, Keeling SL. The deleted in colorectal cancer netrin guidance system: a molecular strategy for neuronal navigation. *Clin Exp Pharmacol Physiol* 1999;26(9):749–751.

285. Blelloch R, Newman C, Kimble J. Control of cell migration during Caenorhabditis elegans development. *Curr Opin Cell Biol* 1999;11(5): 608–613.

286. Yee KT, Simon HH, Tessier-Lavigne M, et al. Extension of long leading processes and neuronal migration in the mammalian brain directed by the chemoattractant netrin-1. *Neuron* 1999;24(3): 607–622.

287. Alcantara S, Ruiz M, DeCastro F, et al. Netrin 1 acts as an attractive or as a repulsive cue for distinct migrating neurons during the development of the cerebellar system. *Development* 2000;127(7):1359–1372.

288. Serafini T, Kennedy TE, Galko MJ, et al. The netrins define a family of axon outgrowth-promoting proteins homologous to C. elegans UNC-6. *Cell* 1994;78(3):409–424.

289. Ren XC, Kim S, Fox E, et al. Role of netrin UNC-6 in patterning the longitudinal nerves of Caenorhabditis elegans. *J Neurobiol* 1999; 39(1):107–118.

290. Kennedy TE, Tessier-Lavigne M. Guidance and induction of branch formation in developing axons by target-derived diffusable factors. *Curr Opin Neurobiol* 1995;5(1):83–90.

291. Lim YS, Mallapur S, Kao G, et al. Netrin UNC-6 and the regulation of branching and extension of motoneuron axons from the ventral nerve cord of Caenorhabditis elegans. *J Neurosci* 1999;19(16): 7048–7056.

292. Colamarino SA, Tessier-Lavigne M. The axonal chemoattractant netrin-1 is also a chemorepellent for trochlear motor axons. *Cell* 1995; 81(4):621–629.

293. Varela-Echavarria A, Tucker A, Puschel AW, et al. Motor axon sub-populations respond differentially to the chemorepellents netrin-1 and semaphorin D. *Neuron* 1997;18(2):193–207.

294. Puschel AW. Divergent properties of mouse netrins. *Mech Dev* 1999; 83(1-2):65–75.

295. Hong K, Hinck L, Nishiyama M, et al. A ligand-gated association between cytoplasmic domains of UNC5 and DCC family receptors converts netrin-induced growth cone attraction to repulsion [Comments]. *Cell* 1999;97(7):927–941.

296. Hopker VH, Shewan D, Tessier-Lavigne M, et al. Growth-cone attraction to netrin-1 is converted to repulsion by laminin-1. *Nature* 1999;401(6748):69–73.

297. Tear G. Molecular cues that guide the development of neural connectivity. *Essays Biochem* 1998;33:1–13.

298. Tessier-Lavigne M, Placzek M, Lumsden AG, et al. Chemotropic guidance of developing axons in the mammalian central nervous system. *Nature* 1988;336(6201):775–778.

299. Kennedy TE, Serafini T, de la Torre JR, et al. Netrins are diffusible chemotropic factors for commissural axons in the embryonic spina cord. *Cell* 1994;78(3):425–435.

300. Tessier-Lavigne M. Axon guidance by molecular gradients. *Curr Opin Neurobiol* 1992;2(1):60–65.

301. Shirasaki R, Mirzayan C, Tessier-Lavigne M, et al. Guidance of circumferentially growing axons by netrin-dependent and -independent floor plate chemotropism in the vertebrate brain. *Neuron* 1996;17(6):1079–1088.

302. Ming G, Song H, Berninger B, et al. Phospholipase C-gamma and phosphoinositide 3-kinase mediate cytoplasmic signaling in nerve growth cone guidance. *Neuron* 1999;23(1):139–148.

303. Placzek M, Tessier-Lavigne M, Jessell T, et al. Orientation of commissural axons in vitro in response to a floor plate-derived chemoattractant. *Development* 1990;110(1):19–30.

304. Placzek M, Tessier-Lavigne M, Yamada T, et al. Guidance of developing axons by diffusible chemoattractants. *Cold Spring Harb Symp Quant Biol* 1990;55:279–289.

305. Colamarino SA, Tessier-Lavigne M. The role of the floor plate in axon guidance. *Annu Rev Neurosci* 1995;18:497–529.

306. Shirasaki R, Katsumata R, Murakami F. Change in chemoattractant responsiveness of developing axons at an intermediate target [Comments]. *Science* 1998;279(5347):105–107.

307. Shirasaki R, Tamada A, Katsumata R, et al. Guidance of cerebellofugal axons in the rat embryo: directed growth toward the floor plate and subsequent elongation along the longitudinal axis. *Neuron* 1995;14(5):961–972.

308. Livesey FJ, Hunt SP. Netrin and netrin receptor expression in the embryonic mammalian nervous system suggests roles in retinal, striatal, nigral, and cerebellar development. *Mol Cell Neurosci* 1997;8(6):417–429.

309. Lauderdale JD, Davis NM, Kuwada JY. Axon tracts correlate with netrin-1a expression in the zebra fish embryo. *Mol Cell Neurosci* 1997;9(4):293–313.

310. Richards LJ, Koester SE, Tuttle R, et al. Directed growth of early cortical axons is influenced by a chemoattractant released from an intermediate target. *J Neurosci* 1997;17(7):2445–2458.

311. Ackerman SL, Kozak LP, Przyborski SA, et al. The mouse rostral cerebellar malformation gene encodes an UNC-5-like protein. *Nature* 1997;386(6627):838–842.

312. Metin C, Deleglise D, Serafini T, et al. A role for netrin-1 in the guidance of cortical efferents. *Development* 1997;124(24):5063–5074.

313. Bloch-Gallego E, Ezan F, Tessier-Lavigne M, et al. Floor plate and netrin-1 are involved in the migration and survival of inferior olivary neurons. *J Neurosci* 1999;19(11):4407–4420.

314. Braisted JE, Catalano SM, Stimac R, et al. Netrin-1 promotes thalamic axon growth and is required for proper development of the thalamocortical projection. *J Neurosci* 2000;20(15):5792–5801.

315. Madison RD, Zomorodi A, Robinson GA. Netrin-1 and peripheral nerve regeneration in the adult rat. *Exp Neurol* 2000;161(2):563–570.

316. Steup A, Lohrum M, Hamscho N, et al. Sema3C and netrin-1 differ-entially affect axon growth in the hippocampal formation. *Mol Cell Neurosci* 2000;15(2):141–155.

317. Culotti JG, Kolodkin AL. Functions of netrins and semaphorins in axon guidance. *Curr Opin Neurobiol* 1996;6(1):81–88.

318. Wang H, Copeland NG, Gilbert DJ, et al. Netrin-3, a mouse homolog of human NTN2L, is highly expressed in sensory ganglia and shows differential binding to netrin receptors. *J Neurosci* 1999;19(2):4938–4947.

319. Wadsworth WG, Bhatt H, Hedgecock EM. Neuroglia and pioneer neurons express UNC-6 to provide global and local netrin cues for guiding migrations in C. elegans. *Neuron* 1996;16(1):35–46.

320. Mitchell KJ, Doyle JL, Serafini T, et al. Genetic analysis of netrin genes in Drosophila: netrins guide CNS commissural axons and peripheral motor axons. *Neuron* 1996;17(2):203–215.

321. Arendt D, Nubler-Jung K. Comparison of early nerve cord development in insects and vertebrates. *Development* 1999;126(11):2309–2325.

322. Keino-Masu K, Masu M, Hinck L, et al. Deleted in colorectal cancer (DCC) encodes a netrin receptor. *Cell* 1996;87(2):175–185.

323. Chan SS, Zheng H, Su MW, et al. UNC-40, a C. elegans homolog of DCC (deleted in colorectal cancer), is required in motile cells responding to UNC-6 netrin cues. *Cell* 1996;87(2):187–195.

324. Fazeli A, Dickinson SL, Hermiston ML, et al. Phenotype of mice lacking functional deleted in colorectal cancer (DCC) gene. *Nature* 1997;386(6627):796–804.

325. Leonardo ED, Hinck L, Masu M, et al. Vertebrate homologues of C. elegans UNC-5 are candidate netrin receptors. *Nature* 1997;386(6627):833–838.

326. Kolodziej PA, Timpe LC, Mitchell KJ, et al. Frazzled encodes a Drosophila member of the DCC immunoglobulin subfamily and is required for CNS and motor axon guidance. *Cell* 1996;87(2):197–204.

327. Kolodziej PA. DCC's function takes shape in the nervous system. *Curr Opin Genet Dev* 1997;7(1):87–92.

328. Guthrie S. Axon guidance: netrin receptors are revealed. *Curr Biol* 1997;7(1):R6–R9.

329. Gong Q, Rangarajan R, Seeger M, et al. The netrin receptor frazzled is required in the target for establishment of retinal projections in the Drosophila visual system. *Development* 1999;126(7):1451–1456.

330. de la Torre JR, Hopker VH, Ming GL, et al. Turning of retinal growth cones in a netrin-1 gradient mediated by the netrin receptor DCC. *Neuron* 1997;19(6):1211–1224.

331. Shu T, Valentino KM, Seaman C, et al. Expression of the netrin-1 receptor, deleted in colorectal cancer (DCC), is largely confined to projecting neurons in the developing forebrain. *J Comp Neurol* 2000;416(2):201–212.

332. Ming GL, Song HJ, Berninger B, et al. cAMP-dependent growth cone guidance by netrin-1. *Neuron* 1997;19(6):1225–1235.

333. Corset V, Nguyen-Ba-Charvet KT, Forcet C, et al. Netrin-1 mediated axon outgrowth and cAMP production requires interaction with adenosine A2b receptor. *Nature* 2000;407(6805):747–750.

334. Hong K, Nishiyama M, Henley J, et al. Calcium signaling in the guidance of nerve growth by netrin-1. *Nature* 2000;403(6765):93–98.

335. Hu G, Zhang S, Vidal M, et al. Mammalian homologs of seven in absentia regulate DCC via the ubiquitin-proteasome pathway. *Genes Dev* 1997;11(20):2701–2714.

336. Bennett KL, Bradshaw J, Youngman T, et al. Deleted in colorectal carcinoma (DCC) binds heparin via its fifth fibronectin type III domain. *J Biol Chem* 1997;272(43):26940–26946.

337. Kappler J, Franken S, Junghans U, et al. Glycosaminoglycan-binding properties and secondary structure of the C-terminus of netrin-1. *Biochem Biophys Res Commun* 2000;271(2):287–291.

338. Mehlen P, Rabizadeh S, Snipas SJ, et al. The DCC gene product induces apoptosis by a mechanism requiring receptor proteolysis. *Nature* 1998;395(6704):801–804.

339. Hiramoto M, Hiromi Y, Giniger E, et al. The Drosophila netrin receptor frazzled guides axons by controlling netrin distribution [Comments]. *Nature* 2000;406(6798):886–889.

340. Livesey FJ, Hunt SP. Differential display cloning of genes induced in regenerating neurons. *Methods* 1998;16(4):386–395.

341. Jacobs JR. The midline glia of Drosophila: a molecular genetic model for the developmental functions of glia. *Prog Neurobiol* 2000;62(5): 475–508.

342. Hotta K, Takahashi H, Asakura T, et al. Characterization of Brachy-urany-downstream notochord genes in the Ciona intestinalis embryo. *Dev Biol* 2000;224(1):69–80.

343. Merz DC, Culotti JG. Genetic analysis of growth cone migrations in Caenorhabditis elegans. *J Neurobiol* 2000;44(2):281–288.

344. Colavita A, Krishna S, Zheng H, et al. Pioneer axon guidance by UNC-129, a C. elegans TGF-beta. *Science* 1998;281(5377): 706–709.

345. Colavita A, Culotti JG. Suppressors of ectopic UNC-5 growth cone steering identify eight genes involved in axon guidance in Caenorhabditis elegans. *Dev Biol* 1998;194(1):72–85.

346. Bashaw GJ, Goodman CS. Chimeric axon guidance receptors: the cytoplasmic domains of slit and netrin receptors specify attraction versus repulsion [Comments]. *Cell* 1999;97(7):917–926.

347. Zallen JA, Kirch SA, Bargmann CI. Genes required for axon pathfinding and extension in the C. elegans nerve ring. *Development* 1999; 126(16):3679–3692.

348. Stoeckli ET, Landmesser LT. Axon guidance at choice points. *Curr Opin Neurobiol* 1998;8(1):73–79.

349. Matise MP, Lustig M, Sakurai T, et al. Ventral midline cells are required for the local control of commissural axon guidance in the mouse spinal cord. *Development* 1999;126(16):3649–3659.

350. Saueressig H, Burrill J, Goulding M. Engrailed-1 and netrin-1 regulate axon pathfinding by association interneurons that project to motor neurons. *Development* 1999;126(19):4201–4212.

351. Augsburger A, Schuchardt A, Hoskins S, et al. BMPs as mediators of roof plate repulsion of commissural neurons. *Neuron* 1999;24(1): 127–141.

352. Zhang B, Levitt P, Murray M. Induction of presynaptic reexpression of an adhesion protein in lamina II after dorsal root deafferentation in adult rat spinal cord. *Exp Neurol* 1998;149(2):468–472.

353. Birgbauer E, Cowan CA, Sretavan DW. Kinase independent function of EphB receptors in retinal axon pathfinding to the optic disc from dorsal but not ventral retina. *Development* 2000;127(6):1231–1241.

354. Mellitzer G, Xu Q, Wilkinson DG. Control of cell behavior by signaling through Eph receptors and ephrins. *Curr Opin Neurobiol* 2000; 10(3):400–408.

355. Gad JM, Keeling SL, Shu T, et al. The spatial and temporal expression patterns of netrin receptors, DCC and neogenin, in the developing mouse retina. *Exp Eye Res* 2000;70(6):711–722.

356. Vitalis T, Cases O, Engelkamp D, et al. Defect of tyrosine hydroxylase-immunoreactive neurons in the brains of mice lacking the transcription factor Pax6. *J Neurosci* 2000;20(17):6501–6516.

357. Eckenstein FP, Shipley GD, Nishi R. Acidic and basic fibroblast growth factors in the nervous system: distribution and differential alteration of levels after injury of central versus peripheral nerve. *J Neurosci* 1991;11(2):412–419.

358. Pirskanen A, Kiefer JC, Hauschka SD. IGFs, insulin, SHH, bFGF, and TGF-beta 1 interact synergistically to promote somite myogenesis in vitro. *Dev Biol* 2000;224(2):189–203.

359. Schultz J, Milpetz F, Bork P, et al. SMART, a simple modular architecture research tool: identification of signaling domains. *Proc Natl Acad Sci U S A* 1998;95(11):5857–5864.

360. Banyai L, Patthy L. The NTR module: domains of netrins, secreted frizzled related proteins, and type I procollagen C-proteinase enhancer protein are homologous with tissue inhibitors of metalloproteases. *Protein Sci* 1999;8(8):1636–1642.

361. Winberg ML, Mitchell KJ, Goodman CS. Genetic analysis of the mechanisms controlling target selection: complementary and combinatorial functions of netrins, semaphorins, and IgCAMs. *Cell* 1998; 93(4):581–591.

362. Galko MJ, Tessier-Lavigne M. Function of an axonal chemoattractant modulated by metalloprotease activity [Comments]. *Science* 2000; 289(5483):1365–1367.

363. Galko MJ, Tessier-Lavigne M. Biochemical characterization of netrin-synergizing activity. *J Biol Chem* 2000;275(11):7832–7838.

364. Rennie J. Super sonic. A gene named for a video game guides development [News]. *Sci Am* 1994;270(4):20.

365. Fietz MJ, Concordet JP, Barbosa R, et al. The hedgehog gene family in Drosophila and vertebrate development. *Dev Suppl* 1994:43–51.

366. Dutton R, Yamada T, Turnley A, et al. Sonic hedgehog promotes neuronal differentiation of murine spinal cord precursors and collaborates with neurotrophin 3 to induce Islet-1. *J Neurosci* 1999;19(7): 2601–2608.

367. Briscoe J, Peirnai A, Jessell TM, et al. A homeodomain protein code specifies progenitor cell identity and neuronal fate in the ventral neural tube. *Cell* 2000;101(4):435–445.

368. Dubois-Dalcq M, Murray K. Why are growth factors important to oligodendrocyte physiology? *Pathol Biol (Paris)* 2000;48(1):80–86.

369. Lu QR, Yuk D, Alberta JA, et al. Sonic hedgehog-regulated oligodendrocyte lineage genes encoding bHLH proteins in the mammalian central nervous system. *Neuron* 2000;25(2):317–329.

370. Echelard Y, Epstein DJ, St-Jacques B, et al. Sonic hedgehog, a member of a family of putative signaling molecules, is implicated in the regulation of CNS polarity. *Cell* 1993;75(7):1417–1430.

371. Johnson RL, Riddle RD, Laufer E, et al. Sonic hedgehog: a key mediator of anterior-posterior patterning of the limb and dorso-ventral patterning of axial embryonic structures. *Biochem Soc Trans* 1994;22(3): 569–574.

372. Fan CM, Tessier-Lavigne M. Patterning of mammalian somites by surface ectoderm and notochord: evidence for sclerotome induction by a hedgehog homolog. *Cell* 1994;79(7):1175–1186.

373. Fan CM, Porter JA, Chiang C, et al. Long-range sclerotome induction by sonic hedgehog: direct role of the amino-terminal cleavage product and modulation by the cyclic AMP signaling pathway. *Cell* 1995; 81(3):457–465.

374. Fan CM, Lee CS, Tessier-Lavigne M. A role for WNT proteins in induction of dermomyotome. *Dev Biol* 1997;191(1):160–165.

375. Oppenheim RW, Homma S, Marti E, et al. Modulation of early but not later stages of programmed cell death in embryonic avian spinal cord by sonic hedgehog. *Mol Cell Neurosci* 1999;13(5):348–361.

376. Britto JM, Tannahill D, Keynes RJ. Life, death, and Sonic hedgehog. *Bioassays.* 2000;22(6):499–502.

377. Hynes M, Porter JA, Chiang C, et al. Induction of midbrain dopaminergic neurons by Sonic hedgehog. *Neuron* 1995;15(1):35–44.

378. Pons S, Marti E. Sonic hedgehog synergizes with the extracellular matrix protein vitronectin to induce spinal motor neuron differentiation. *Development* 2000;127(2):33–42.

379. Strahle U, Fischer N, Blader P. Expression and regulation of a netrin homologue in the zebra fish embryo. *Mech Dev* 1997;62(2):147–160.

380. Lauderdale JD, Pasquali SK, Fazel R, et al. Regulation of netrin-1a expression by hedgehog proteins. *Mol Cell Neurosci* 1998;11(4): 194–205.

381. Kenney AM, Rowitch DH. Sonic hedgehog promotes G(1) cyclin expression and sustained cell cycle progression in mammalian neuronal precursors. *Mol Cell Biol* 2000;20(23):9055–9067.

382. Williams Z, Tse V, Hou L, et al. Sonic hedgehog promotes proliferation and tyrosine hydroxylase induction of postnatal sympathetic cells in vitro. *Neuroreport* 2000;11(15):3315–3319.

383. Liem KF, Jessell TM, Briscoe J. Regulation of the neural patterning activity of sonic hedgehog by secreted BMP inhibitors expressed by notochord and somites. *Development* 2000;127(22):4855–4866.

384. Traiffort E, Charytoniuk D, Watroba L, et al. Discrete localizations of hedgehog signalling components in the developing and adult rat nervous system. *Eur J Neurosci* 1999;11(9):3199–3214.

385. Sussman CR, Dyer KL, Marchionni M, et al. Local control of oligodendrocyte development in isolated dorsal mouse spinal cord. *J Neurosci Res* 2000;59(3):413–420.

386. Wilkinson DG. Eph receptors and ephrins: regulators of guidance and assembly. *Int Rev Cytol* 2000;196:177–244.

387. Feng G, Laskowski MB, Feldheim DA, et al. Roles for ephrins in positionally selective synaptogenesis between motor neurons and muscle fibers. *Neuron* 2000;25(2):295–306.

388. Mellitzer G, Xu Q, Wilkinson DG. Eph receptors and ephrins restrict cell intermingling and communication. *Nature* 1999;400(6739): 77–81.

389. Yue Y, Su J, Cerretti DP, et al. Selective inhibition of spinal cord neurite outgrowth and cell survival by the Eph family ligand ephrin-A5. *J Neurosci* 1999;19(22):10026–10035.

390. Koblar SA, Krull CE, Pasquale EB, et al. Spinal motor axons and neural crest cells use different molecular guides for segmental migration through the rostral half-somite. *J Neurobiol* 2000;42(4): 437–447.

391. Martone ME, Holash JA, Bayardo A, et al. Immunolocalization of the receptor tyrosine kinase EphA4 in the adult rat central nervous system. *Brain Res* 1997;771(2):238–250.

392. Imondi R, Wideman C, Kaprielian Z. Complementary expression of transmembrane ephrins and their receptors in the mouse spinal cord: a possible role in constraining the orientation of longitudinally projecting axons. *Development* 2000;127(7):1397–1410.

393. Miranda JD, White LA, Marcillo AE, et al. Induction of EphB3 after spinal cord injury. *Exp Neurol* 1999;156(1):218–222.

394. Olivieri G, Miescher GC. Immunohistochemical localization of EphA5 in the adult human central nervous system. *J Histochem Cytochem* 1999;47(7):855–861.

395. Gao PP, Sun CH, Zhou XF, et al. Ephrins stimulate or inhibit neurite outgrowth and survival as a function or neuronal cell type. *J Neurosci Res* 2000;60(4):427–436.

396. Wahl S, Barth H, Ciossek T, et al. Ephrin-A5 induces collapse of growth cones by activating Rho and Rho kinase. *J Cell Biol* 2000; 149(2):263–270.

397. Gallo G, Letourneau PC. Axon guidance: GTPases help axons reach their targets. *Curr Biol* 1998;8(3):R80–R82.

398. Aepfelbacher M, Essler M, Huber E, et al. Bacterial toxins block endothelial wound repair. Evidence that Rho GTPases control cytoskeletal rearrangements in migrating endothelial cells. *Arterioscl Thromb Vasc Biol* 1997;17(9):1623–1629.

399. Fenteany G, Janmey PA, Stossel TP. Signaling pathways and cell mechanics involved in wound closure by epithelial cell sheets. *Curr Biol* 2000;10(14):831–838.

400. An S, Goetzl EJ, Lee H. Signaling mechanisms and molecular characteristics of G protein-coupled receptors for lysophosphatidic acid and sphingosine 1-phosphate. *J Cell Biochem Suppl* 1998;31:147–157.

401. Sebok A, Nusser N, Debreczeni B, et al. Different roles for RhoA during neurite initiation, elongation, and regeneration in PC12 cells. *J Neurochem* 1999;73(3):949–960.

402. Lehmann M, Fournier A, Selles-Navarro I, et al. Inactivation of Rho signaling pathway promotes CNS axon regeneration. *J Neurosci* 1999; 19(17)7537–7547.

403. Barth H, Olenik C, Sehr P, et al. Neosynthesis and activation of Rho by Escherichia coli cytotoxic necrotizing factor (CNF1) reverse cytopathic effects of ADP-ribosylated Rho. *J Biol Chem* 1999;274(39): 27407–27414.

404. Tanabe K, Tachibana T, Yamashita T, et al. The small GTP-binding protein TC10 promotes nerve elongation in neuronal cells, and its expression is induced during nerve regeneration in rats. *J Neurosci* 2000;20(11):4138–4144.

405. Levi-Montalcini R. From Turin to Stockholm via St. Louis and Rio de Janeiro. *Science* 2000;287(5454):809.

406. Hamburger V. The history of the discovery of the nerve growth factor. *J Neurobiol* 1993;24(7):893–897.

407. Angeletti P, Calissano P, Chen JS, et al. Multiple molecular forms of the nerve growth factor. *Biochem Biophys Acta* 1967;147(1):180–182.

408. Thoenen H. The changing scene of neurotrophic factors. *Trends Neurosci* 1991;14(5):165–170.

409. Schabitz WR, Sommer C, Zoder W, et al. Intravenous brain-derived neurotrophic factor reduces infarct size and counterregulates Bax and Bcl-2 expression after temporary focal cerebral ischemia. *Stroke* 2000; 31(9):2212–2217.

410. von Meyenburg J, Brosamle C, Metz GA, et al. Regeneration and sprouting of chronically injured corticospinal tract fibers in adult rats promoted by NT-3 and the mAb IN-1, which neutralizes myelin-associated neurite growth inhibitors. *Exp Neurol* 1998;154(2): 583–594.

411. Bregman BS, McAtee M, Dai HN, et al. Neurotrophic factors increase axonal growth after spinal cord injury and transplantation in the adult rat. *Exp Neurol* 1997;148(2):475–494.

412. Bregman BS, Diener PS, McAtee M, et al. Intervention strategies to enhance anatomical plasticity and recovery of function after spinal cord injury. *Adv Neurol* 1997;72:257–275.

413. Broude E, McAtee M, Kelley MS, et al. c-Jun expression in adult rat dorsal root ganglion neurons: differential response after central or peripheral axotomy. *Exp Neurol* 1997;148(1):367–377.

414. Bregman BS. Regeneration in the spinal cord. *Curr Opin Neurobiol* 1998;8(6):800–807.

415. Bregman BS, Broude E, McAtee M, et al. Transplants and neurotrophic factors prevent atrophy of mature CNS neurons after spinal cord injury. *Exp Neurol* 1998;149(1):13–27.

416. Broude E, McAtee M, Kelley MS, et al. Fetal spinal cord transplants and exogenous neurotrophic support enhance c-Jun expression in mature axotomized neurons after spinal cord injury. *Exp Neurol* 1999; 155(1):65–78.

417. Iwaya K, Mizoi K, Tessler A, et al. Neurotrophic agents in fibrin glue mediate adult dorsal root regeneration into spinal cord. *Neurosurgery* 1999;44(3):589–596.

418. Bradbury EJ, Khemani S, Von R, et al. NT-3 promotes growth of lesioned adult rat sensory axons ascending in the dorsal columns of the spinal cord. *Eur J Neurosci* 1999;11(11):3873–3883.

419. Zhang Y, Dijkhuizen PA, Anderson PN, et al. NT-3 delivered by an adenoviral vector induces injured dorsal root axons to regenerate into the spinal cord of adult rats. *J Neurosci Res* 1998;54(4):554–562.

420. Houweling DA, Lankhorst AJ, Gispen WH, et al. Collagen containing neutrophin-3 (NT-3) attracts regrowing injured corticospinal axons in the adult rat spinal cord and promotes partial functional recovery. *Exp Neurol* 1998;153(1):49–59.

421. Ye JH, Houle JD. Treatment of the chronically injured spinal cord with neutrophic factors can promote axonal regeneration from supraspinal neurons. *Exp Neurol* 1997;143(1):70–81.

422. Tatagiba M, Brosamle C, Schwab ME. Regeneration of injured axons in the adult mammalian central nervous system. *Neurosurg* 1997; 40(3):541–546.

423. Meyer M, Matsuoka I, Wetmore C, et al. Enhanced synthesis of brain-derived neurotrophic factor in the lesioned peripheral nerve: different mechanisms are responsible for the regulation of BDNF and NGF mRNA. *J Cell Biol* 1992;119(1):45–54.

424. Zafra F, Lindholm D, Castren E, et al. Regulation of brain-derived neurotrophic factor and nerve growth factor mRNA in primary cultures of hippocampal neurons and astrocytes. *J Neurosci* 1992;12(12): 4793–4799.

425. Wehling P, Wirths J, Evans CH. The effect of cytokines on regeneration results of compressed nerve roots and transected peripheral nerves. *Z Orthop Ihre Grenzgeb* 1993;131(1):83–93.

426. Horie H, Sakai I, Akahori Y, et al. IL-1 beta enhances neurite regeneration from transected-nerve terminals of adult rat DRG. *Neuroreport* 1997;8(8):1955–1959.

427. Streit WJ, Semple-Rowland SL, Hurley SD. Cytokine mRNA profiles in contused spinal cord and axotomized facial nucleus suggest a beneficial role for inflammation and gliosis. *Exp Neurol* 1998;152(1):74–87.

428. Blesch A, Uy HS, Grill RJ, et al. Leukemia inhibitory factor augments neutrophin expression and corticospinal axon growth after adult CNS injury. *J Neurosci* 1999;19(9):3556–3566.

429. Curtis R, Scherer SS, Somogyi R, et al. Retrograde axonal transport of LIF is decreased by peripheral nerve injury: correlation with increased LIF expression in distal nerve. *Neuron* 1994;12(1):191–204.

430. Tuszynski MH, Gabriel K, Gage FH, et al. Nerve growth factor delivery by gene transfer induces differential of sensory, motor, and noradrenergic neurites after adult spinal cord injury. *Exp Neurol* 1996; 137(1):157–173.

431. Tuszynski M, Edgerton R, Dobkin B. Recovery of locomotion after experimental spinal cord injury: axonal regeneration or modulation of intrinsic spinal cord walking circuitry? *J Spinal Cord Med* 1999; 22(2):143.

432. Olson L. Grafts and growth factors in CNS. Basic science with clinical promise. *Stereotact Funct Neurosurg* 1990;55:250–267.

433. Tuszynski MH, Peterson DA, Ray J, et al. Fibroblasts genetically

modified to produce nerve growth factor induce robust neuritic ingrowth after grafting to the spinal cord. *Exp Neurol* 1994;126(1):1–14.

434. Blesch A, Tuszynski MH. Robust growth of chronically injured spinal cord axons induced by grafts of genetically modified NGF-secreting cells. *Exp Neurol* 1997;148(2):444–452.

435. Nakahara Y, Gage FH, Tuszynski MH. Grafts of fibroblasts genetically modified to secrete NGF, BDNF, NT-3, or basic FGF elicit differential responses in the adult spinal cord. *Cell Transplant* 1996;5(2):191–204.

436. Tuszynski MH, Murai K, Blesch A, et al. Functional characterization of NGF-secreting cell grafts to the acutely injured spinal cord. *Cell Transplant* 1997;6(3):361–368.

437. Tuszynski MH, Weidner N, McCormack M, et al. Grafts of genetically modified Schwann cells to the spinal cord: survival, axon growth, and myelination. *Cell Transplant* 1998;7(2):187–196.

438. Grill R, Murai K, Blesch A, et al. Cellular delivery of neutrophin-3 promotes corticospinal axonal growth and partial functional recovery after spinal cord injury. *J Neurosci* 1997;17(14):5560–5572.

439. Liu Y, Kim D, Himes BT, et al. Transplants of fibroblasts genetically modified to express BDNF promote regeneration of adult rat rubrospinal axons and recovery of forelimb function. *J Neurosci* 1999;19(11):4370–4387.

440. McTigue DM, Horner PJ, Stokes BT, et al. Neurotrophin-3 and brain-derived neurotrophic factor induce oligodendrocyte proliferation and myelination of regenerating axons in the contused adult rat spinal cord. *J Neurosci* 1998;18(14):5354–5365.

441. Franzen R, Martin D, Daloze A, et al. Grafts of meningeal fibroblasts in adult rat spinal cord lesion promote axonal regrowth. *Neuroreport* 1999;10(7):1551–1556.

442. Romero MI, Rangappa N, Li L, et al. Extensive sprouting of sensory afferents and hyperalgesia induced by conditional expression of nerve growth factor in the adult spinal cord. *J Neurosci* 2000;20(12):4435–4445.

443. Blits B, Dijkhuizen PA, Carlstedt TP, et al. Adenoviral vector-mediated expression of a foreign gene in peripheral nerve tissue bridges implanted in the injured peripheral and central nervous system. *Exp Neurol* 1999;160(1):256–267.

444. Blits B, Dijkhuizen PA, Hermans WT, et al. The use of adenoviral vectors and ex vivo transduced neurotransplants: towards promotion of neuroregeneration. *Cell Transplant* 2000;9(2):169–178.

445. Cook SD, Rueger DC. Osteogenic protein-1: biology and applications. *Clin Orthop* 1996;(324):29–38.

446. Blottner D, Herdegen T. Neuroprotective fibroblast growth factor type-2 down-regulates the c-Jun transcription factor in axotomized sympathetic preganglionic neurons of adult rat. *Neurosci* 1998;82(1):283–292.

447. Marchionni MA, Cannella B, Hoban C, et al. Neuregulin in neuron/glial interactions in the central nervous system. GGF2 diminishes autoimmune demyelination, promotes oligodendrocyte progenitor expansion, and enhances remyelination. *Adv Exp Med Biol* 1999;468:283–295.

448. Wang L, Marchionni MA, Tassava RA. Cloning and neuronal expression of a type III newt neuregulin and rescue of denervated, nerve-dependent newt limb blastemas by rhGGF2. *J Neurobiol* 2000;43(2):150–158.

449. Malgrange B, Delree P, Rigo JM, et al. Image analysis of neuritic regeneration by adult rat dorsal root ganglion neurons in culture: quantification of the neurotoxicity of anticancer agents and of its prevention by nerve growth factor or basic fibroblast growth factor but not brain-derived neurotrophic factor or neurotrophin-3. *J Neurosci Methods* 1994;53(1):111–122.

450. Hughes RA, Sendtner M, Thoenen H. Members of several gene families influence survival of rat motoneurons in vitro and in vivo. *J Neurosci Res* 1993;36(6):663–671.

451. Pataky DM, Borisoff JF, Fernandes KJ, et al. Fibroblast growth factor treatment produced differential effects on survival and neurite outgrowth from identified bulbospinal neurons in vitro. *Exp Neurol* 2000;163(2):357–372.

452. Archer FR, Doherty P, Collins D, et al. CAMs and FGF cause a local

submembrane calcium signal promoting axon outgrowth without a rise in bulk calcium concentration. *Eur J Neurosci* 1999;11(10):3565–3573.

453. Mohiuddin L, Fernyhough P, Tomlinson DR. Acidic fibroblast growth factor enhances neurite outgrowth and stimulates expression of GAP-43 and T alpha 1 alpha-tubulin in cultured neurons from adult rat dorsal root ganglia. *Neurosci Lett* 1996;215(2):111–114.

454. Piehl F, Hammarberg H, Hokfelt T, et al. Regulatory effects of trophic factors on expression and distribution of CGRP and GAP-43 in rat motoneurons. *J Neurosci Res* 1998;51(1):1–14.

455. Otsuka H, Matsuda S, Fujita H, et al. Localization of basic fibroblast growth factor (bFGF)-like immunoreactivity in neural circuits innervating the gastrocnemius muscle, with reference to the direction of bFGF transport. *Arch Histol Cytol* 1993;56(2):207–215.

456. Grothe C, Meisinger C, Hertenstein A, et al. Expression of fibroblast growth factor-2 and fibroblast growth factor receptor 1 messenger RNAs in spinal ganglia and sciatic nerve: regulation after peripheral nerve lesion. *Neurosci* 1997;76(1):123–135.

457. Liu X, Mashour GA, Webster HF, et al. Basic FGF and FGF receptor 1 are expressed in microglia during experimental autoimmune encephalomyelitis: temporally distinct expression of midkine and pleiotrophin. *Glia* 1998;24(4):390–397.

458. Grothe C, Wewetzer K. Fibroblast growth factor and its implication for developing and regenerating neurons. *Int J Dev Biol* 1996;40(1):403–410.

459. Ji RR, Zhang Q, Zhang X, et al. Prominent expression of bFGF in dorsal root ganglia after axotomy. *Eur J Neurosci* 1995;7(12):2458–2468.

460. Meisinger C, Grothe C. Differential regulation of fibroblast growth factor (FGF)-2 and FGF receptor 1 mRNAs and FGF-2 isoforms in spinal ganglia and sciatic nerve after peripheral nerve lesion. *J Neurochem* 1997;68(3):1150–1158.

461. Follesa P, Wrathall JR, Mocchetti I. Increased basic fibroblast growth factor mRNA following contusive spinal cord injury. *Mol Brain Res* 1994;22(1-4):1–8.

462. Hinks GL, Franklin RJ. Distinctive patterns of PDGF-A, FGF-2, IGF-1, and TGF-beta 1 gene expression during remyelination of experimentally-induced spinal cord demyelination. *Mol Cell Neurosci* 1999;14(2):153–168.

463. Mocchetti I, Wrathall JR. Neurotrophic factors in central nervous system trauma. *Neurotrauma* 1995;12(5):853–870.

464. Mocchetti I, Rabin SJ, Colangelo AM, et al. Increased basic fibroblast growth factor expression following contusive spinal cord injury. *Exp Neurol* 1996;141(1):154–164.

465. Fawcett JW. Spinal cord repair: from experimental models to human application. *Spinal Cord* 1998;36(12):811–817.

466. Trupp M, Ryden M, Jornvall H, et al. Peripheral expression and biological activities of GDNF, a new neurotrophic factor for avian and mammalian peripheral neurons. *J Cell Biol* 1995;130(1):137–148.

467. Bilak MM, Shifrin DA, Corse AM, et al. Neuroprotective utility and neurotrophic action of neurturin in postnatal motor neurons: comparison with GDNF and persephin. *Mol Cell Neurosci* 1999;13(5):326–336.

468. Jones MG, Munson JB, Thompson SW. A role for nerve growth factor in sympathetic sprouting in rat dorsal root ganglia. *Pain* 1999;79(1):21–29.

469. Ramer MS, Priestley JV, McMahon SB. Functional regeneration of sensory axons into the adult spinal cord [Comments]. *Nature* 2000;403(6767):312–316.

470. Terenghi G. Peripheral nerve regeneration and neurotrophic factors. *J Anat* 1999;194[Pt 1]:1–14.

471. Sendtner M, Arakawa Y, Stockli KA, et al. Effect of ciliary neurotrophic factor (CNTF) on motoneuron survival. *J Cell Sci Suppl* 1991;15:103–109.

472. Rosano C, Felipe-Cuervo E, Wood PM. Regenerative potential of adult O1+ oligodendrocytes. *Glia* 1999;27(3):189–202.

473. Cheng H, Olson L. A new surgical technique that allows proximodistal regeneration of 5-HT fibers after complete transection of the rat spinal cord. *Exp Neurol* 1995;136(2):149–161.

474. Cheng H, Cao Y, Olson L. Spinal cord repair in adult paraplegic

rats: partial restoration of hind limb function [Comments]. *Science* 1996;273(5274):510–513.

475. Blits B, Dijkhuizen PA, Boer GJ, et al. Intercostal nerve implants transduced with an adenoviral vector encoding neurotrophin-3 promote regrowth of injured cat corticospinal tract fibers and improve hindlimb function. *Exp Neurol* 2000;164(1):25–37.

476. Paino CL, Bunge MB. Induction of axon growth into Schwann cell implants grafted into lesioned adult rat spinal cord. *Exp Neurol* 1991; 114(2):254–257.

477. Paino CL, Fernandez-Valle C, Bates ML, et al. Regrowth of axons in lesioned adult rat spinal cord: promotion by implants of cultured Schwann cells. *J Neurocytol* 1994;23(7):433–452.

478. Bunge MB. Transplantation of purified populations of Schwann cells into lesioned adult rat spinal cord. *J Neurol* 1994;242[Suppl 1]: S36–S39.

479. Xu XM, Guenard V, Kleitman N, et al. A combination of BDNF and NT-3 promotes supraspinal axonal regeneration into Schwann cell grafts in adult rat thoracic spinal cord. *Exp Neurol* 1995;134(2): 261–272.

480. Xu XM, Guenard V, Kleitman N, et al. Axonal regeneration into Schwann cell-seeded guidance channels grafted into transected adult rat spinal cord. *J Comp Neurol* 1995;351(1):145–160.

481. Xu XM, Chen A, Guenard V, et al. Bridging Schwann cell transplants promote axonal regeneration from both the rostral and caudal stumps of transected adult rat spinal cord. *J Neurocytol* 1997;26(1):1–16.

482. Guest JD, Rao A, Olson L, et al. The ability of human Schwann cell grafts to promote regeneration in the transected nude rat spinal cord. *Exp Neurol* 1997;148(2):502–522.

483. Oudega M, Xu XM, Guenard V, et al. A combination of insulin-like growth factor-I and platelet-derived growth factor enhances myelination but diminishes axonal regeneration into Schwann cell grafts in the adult rat spinal cord. *Glia* 1997;19(3):247–258.

484. Menei P, Montero-Menei C, Whittemore SR, et al. Schwann cells genetically modified to secrete human BDNF promote enhanced axonal regrowth across transected adult rat spinal cord. *Eur J Neurosci* 1998;10(2):607–621.

485. Ramon-Cueto A, Plant GW, Avila J, et al. Long-distance axonal regeneration in the transected adult rat spinal cord is promoted by olfactory ensheathing glia transplants. *J Neurosci* 1998;18(10): 3803–3815.

486. Chen A, Xu XM, Kleitman N, et al. Methylprednisolone administration improves axonal regeneration into Schwann cell grafts in transected adult rat thoracic spinal cord. *Exp Neurol* 1996;138(2): 261–276.

487. Xu XM, Zhang SX, Li H, et al. Regrowth of axons into the distal spinal cord through a Schwann-cell–seeded mini-channel implanted into hemisected adult rat spinal cord. *Eur J Neurosci* 1999;11(5): 1723–1740.

488. Tonge DA, Golding JP, Gordon-Weeks PR. Expression of a developmentally regulated, phosphorylated isoform of microtubule-associated protein 1B in sprouting and regenerating axons in vitro. *Neuroscience* 1996;73(2):541–551.

489. Tonge DA, Golding JP, Edbladh M, et al. Effects of extracellular matrix components on axonal outgrowth from peripheral nerves of adult animals in vitro. *Exp Neurol* 1997;146(1):81–90.

490. Marchand R, Woerly S. Transected spinal cords grafted with in situ self-assembled collagen matrices. *Neuroscience* 1990;36(1):45–60.

491. Marchand R, Woerly S, Bertrand L, et al. Evaluation of two cross-linked collagen gels implanted in the transected spinal cord. *Brain Res Bull* 1993;30(3-4):415–422.

492. Woerly S, Pinet E, De Robertis L, et al. Heterogenous PHPMA hydrogels for tissue repair and axonal regeneration in the injured spinal cord. *J Biomater Sci Polym Ed* 1998;9(7):681–711.

493. Woerly S, Petrov P, Sykova E. Neural tissue formation within porous hydrogels implanted in brain and spinal cord lesions: ultrastructural, immunohistochemical, and diffusion studies. *Tissue Eng* 1999;5(5): 467–488.

494. Gautier SE, Oudega M, Fragoso M, et al. Poly(alpha-hydroxyacids) for application in the spinal cord: resorbability and biocompatibility

with adult rat Schwann cells and spinal cord. *J Biomed Mater Res* 1998;42(4):642–654.

495. Holmes TC, de Lacalle S, Su X, et al. Extensive neurite outgrowth and active synapse formation on self-assembling peptide scaffolds. *Proc Natl Acad Sci U S A* 2000;97(12):6728–6733.

496. Zhang S, Yan L, Altman M, et al. Biological surface engineering: a simple system for cell pattern formation. *Biomaterials* 1999;20(13): 1213–1220.

497. Reier PJ, Perlow MJ, Guth L. Development of embryonic spinal cord transplants in the rat. *Brain Res* 1983;312(2):201–219.

498. Commissiong JW, Toffano G. The effect of GM1 ganglioside on coerulospinal noradrenergic, adult neurons and on fetal monoaminergic neurons transplanted into the transected spinal cord of the adult rat. *Brain Res* 1986;380(2):205–215.

499. Bernstein JJ, Goldberg WJ. Fetal spinal cord homografts ameliorate the severity of lesion-induced hind limb behavioral deficits. *Exp Neurol* 1987;98(3):633–644.

500. Houle JD, Reier PJ. Transplantation of fetal spinal cord tissue into the chronically injured adult rat spinal cord. *J Comp Neurol* 1988; 269(4):535–547.

501. Reier PJ, Anderson DK, Thompson FJ, et la. Neural tissue transplantation and CND trauma: anatomical and functional repair of the injured spinal cord. *J Neurotrauma* 1992;9[Suppl 1]:S223–S248.

502. Reier PJ, Stokes BT, Thompson FJ, et al. Fetal cell grafts into resection and contusion/compression injuries of the rat and cat spinal cord. *Exp Neurol* 1992;115(1):177–188.

503. Itoh Y, Waldeck RF, Tessler A, et al. Regenerated dorsal root fibers from functional synapses in embryonic spinal cord transplants. *J Neurophysiol* 1996;76(2):1236–1245.

504. Connor JR, Bernstein JJ. Vasoactive intestinal polypeptide neurons in fetal cortical homografts to adult rat spinal cord. *Brain Res* 1986; 367(1-2):214–221.

505. Tessler A, Himes BT, Houle J, et al. Regeneration of adult dorsal root axons into transplants of embryonic spinal cord. *J Comp Neurol* 1988;270(4):537–548.

506. Houle JD, Reier PJ. Regrowth of calcitonin gene-related peptide (CGRP) immunoreactive axons from the chronically injured rat spinal cord into fetal spinal cord tissue transplants. *Neurosci Lett* 1989; 103(3):253–258.

507. Eng LF, Reier PJ, Houle JD. Astrocyte activation and fibrous gliosis: glial fibrillary acidic protein immunostaining of astrocytes following intraspinal cord grafting of fetal CNS tissue. *Prog Brain Res* 1987; 71:439–455.

508. Bregman BS. Spinal cord transplants permit the growth of serotonergic axons across the site of neonatal spinal cord transection. *Brain Res* 1987;431(2):265–279.

509. Bregman BS, Reier PJ. Neural tissue transplants rescue axotomized rubrospinal cells from retrograde death. *J Comp Neurol* 1986;244(1): 86–95.

510. Iwashita Y, Kawaguchi S, Murata M, et al. Restoration of function by replacement of spinal cord segments in the rat [Comments]. *Nature* 1994;367(6459):167–170.

511. Kikukawa S, Kawaguchi S, Mizoguchi A, et al. Regeneration of dorsal column axons after spinal cord injury in young rats. *Neurosci Lett* 1998;249(2-3):135–138.

512. Inoue T, Kawaguchi S, Kurisu K. Spontaneous regeneration of the pyramidal tract after transection in young rats. *Neurosci Lett* 1998; 247(2-3):151–154.

513. Asada Y, Nakamura T, Kawaguchi S. Peripheral nerve grafts for neural repair of spinal cord injury in neonatal rat: aiming at functional regeneration. *Transplant Proc* 1998;30(1):147–148.

514. Ito J, Kawaguchi S. Regeneration of the mammalian central vestibular pathway using the rat as animal model. *Eur Arch Otorhinolaryngol* 1999;256(9):442–444.

515. Ito J, Murata M, Kawaguchi S. Regeneration of the lateral vestibulospinal tract in adult rats by transplants of embryonic brain tissue. *Neurosci Lett* 1999;259(2):67–70.

516. Demierre B, Ruiz-Flandes P, Kato AC. Grafting of embryonic motoneurons into spinal cord and striatum of adult mice. *Stereotact Funct Neurosurg* 1990;55:328–336.

517. Nothias F, Horvat JC, Mira JC, et al. Double step neural transplants to replace degenerated motoneurons. *Prog Brain Res* 1990;82: 239–246.

518. Thomas CK, Erb DE, Grumbles RM, et al. Embryonic cord transplants in peripheral nerve restore skeletal muscle function. *J Neurophysiol* 2000;84(1):591–595.

519. Ramon-Cueto A, Nieto-Sampedro M. Regeneration into the spinal cord of transected dorsal root axons is promoted by ensheathing glia transplants. *Exp Neurol* 1994;127(2):232–244.

520. Li Y, Field PM, Raisman G. Repair of adult rat corticospinal tract by transplants of olfactory ensheathing cells [Comments]. *Science* 1997; 277(5334):2000–2002.

521. Ramon-Cueto A, Cordero MI, Santos-Benito FF, et al. Functional recovery of paraplegic rats and motor axon regeneration in their spinal cords by olfactory ensheathing glia. *Neuron* 2000;25(2):425–435.

522. Barnett SC, Alexander CL, Iwashita Y, et al. Identification of a human olfactory ensheathing cell that can effect transplant-mediated remyelination of demyelinated CNS axons. *Brain* 2000;123[Pt 8]: 1581–1588.

523. Blakemore WF. Remyelination by Schwann cells of axons demyelinated by intraspinal injection of 6-aminonicotinamide in the rat. *J Neurocytol* 1975;4(6):745–757.

524. Blakemore WF. Remyelination of CNS axons by Schwann cells transplanted from the sciatic nerve. *Nature* 1977;266(5597):68–69.

525. Blakemore WF. Observations on remyelination in the rabbit spinal cord following demyelination induced by lysolecithin. *Neuropathol Appl Neurobiol* 1978;4(1):47–59.

526. Franklin RJ, Gilson JM, Blakemore WF. Local recruitment of remyelinating cells in the repair of demyelination in the central nervous system. *J Neurosci Res* 1997;50(2):337–344.

527. Shields SA, Blakemore WF, Franklin RJ. Schwann cell remyelination is restricted to astrocyte-deficient areas after transplantation into demyelinated adult rat brain. *J Neurosci Res* 2000;60(5):571–578.

528. Blakemore WF, Crang AJ, Franklin RJ, et al. Glial cell transplants that are subsequently rejected can be used to influence regeneration of glial cell environments in the CNS. *Glia* 1995;13(2):79–91.

529. Li Y, Raisman G. Integration of transplanted cultured Schwann cells into the long myelinated fiber tracts of the adult spinal cord. *Exp Neurol* 1997;145[Suppl 2, Pt 1]:397–411.

530. Franklin RJ, Bayley SA, Milner R, et al. Differentiation of the O-2A progenitor cell line CG-4 into oligodendrocytes and astrocytes following transplantation into glia-deficient areas of CNS white matter. *Glia* 1995;13(1):39–44.

531. Olby NJ, Blakemore WF. Reconstruction of the glial environment of a photochemically induced lesion in the rat spinal cord by transplantation of mixed glial cells. *J Neurocytol* 1996;25(8):481–498.

532. Blakemore WF, Olby NJ, Franklin RJ. The use of transplanted glial cells to reconstruct glial environments in the CNS. *Brain Pathol* 1995; 5(4):443–450.

533. Keirstead HS, Hughes HC, Blakemore WF. A quantifiable model of axonal regeneration in the demyelinated adult rat spinal cord. *Exp Neurol* 1998;151(2):303–313.

534. Keirstead HS, Blakemore WF. The role of oligodendrocytes and oligodendrocyte progenitors in CNS remyelination. *Adv Exp Med Biol* 1999;468:183–197.

535. Schnell L, Fearn S, Klassen H, et al. Acute inflammatory responses to mechanical lesions in the CNS: differences between brain and spinal cord. *Eur J Neurosci* 1999;11(10):3648–3658.

536. Bartholdi D, Schwab ME. Expression of pro-inflammatory cytokine and chemokine mRNA upon experimental spinal cord injury in mouse: an in situ hybridization study. *Eur J Neurosci* 1997;9(7): 1422–1438.

537. Leskovar A, Moriarty LJ, Turek JJ, et al. The macrophage in acute neural injury: changes in cell numbers over time and levels of cytokine production in mammalian central and peripheral nervous systems. *J Exp Biol* 2000;203[Pt 12]:1783–1795.

538. McTigue DM, Popovich PG, Morgan TE, et al. Localization of transforming growth factor-beta1 and receptor mRNA after experimental spinal cord injury. *Exp Neurol* 2000;163(1):220–230.

539. Le YL, Shih K, Bao P, et al. Cytokine chemokine expression in contused rat spinal cord. *Neurochem Int* 2000;36(4-5):417–425.

540. Sugiura S, Lahav R, Han J, et al. Leukaemia inhibitory factor is required for normal inflammatory response to injury in the peripheral and central nervous systems in vivo and is chemotactic for macrophages in vitro. *Eur J Neurosci* 2000;12(2):457–466.

541. Krenz NR, Weaver LC. Nerve growth factor in glia and inflammatory cells of the injured rat spinal cord. *J Neurochem* 2000;74(2):730–739.

542. Fitch MT, Silver J. Activated macrophage and the blood-brain barrier: inflammation after CNS injury leads to increases in putative inhibitory molecules. *Exp Neurol* 1997;148(2):587–603.

543. Fitch MT, Doller C, Combs CK, et al. Cellular and molecular mechanisms of glial scarring and progressive cavitation: in vivo and in vitro analysis of inflammation-induced secondary injury after CNS trauma. *J Neurosci* 1999;19(19):8182–8198.

544. Popovich PG, Guan Z, Wei P, et al. Depletion of hematogenous macrophages promotes partial hindlimb recovery and neuroanatomical repair after experimental spinal cord injury. *Exp Neurol* 1999; 158(2):351–365.

545. Oudega M, Vargas CG, Weber AB, et al. Long-term effects of methylprednisolone following transection of adult rat spinal cord. *Eur J Neurosci* 1999;11(7):2453–2464.

546. Bethea JR, Nagashima H, Acosta MC, et al. Systemically administered interleukin-10 reduces tumor necrosis factor-alpha production and significantly improves functional recovery following traumatic spinal cord injury in rats. *J Neurotrauma* 1999;16(10):851–863.

547. Klusman I, Schwab ME. Effects of pro-inflammatory cytokines in experimental spinal cord injury. *Brain Res* 1997;762(1-2):173–184.

548. Frei E, Klusman I, Schnell ME. Reactions of oligodendrocytes to spinal cord injury: cell survival and myelin repair. *Exp Neurol* 2000; 163(2):373–380.

549. Lazar DA, Ellegala DB, Avellino AM, et al. Modulation of macrophage and microglial responses to axonal injury in the peripheral and central nervous system. *Neurosurg* 1999;45(3):593–600.

550. Frisen J, Haegerstrand A, Fried K, et al. Adhesive/repulsive properties in the injured spinal cord: relation to myelin phagocytosis by invading macrophages. *Exp Neurol* 1994;129(2):183–193.

551. Franzen R, Schoenen J, Leprince P, et al. Effects of macrophage transplantation in the injured adult rat spinal cord: a combined immunocytochemical and biochemical study. *J Neurosci Res* 1998;51(3): 316–327.

552. Prewitt CM, Niesman IR, Kane CJ, et al. Activated macrophage/microglial cells can promote the regeneration of sensory axons into the injured spinal cord. *Exp Neurol* 1997;148(2):433–443.

553. Schwartz M, Moalem G, Leibowitz-Amit R, et al. Innate and adaptive immune responses can be beneficial for CNS repair. *Trends Neurosci* 1999;22(7):295–299.

554. Zeev-Brann AB, Lazarov-Spiegler O, Brenner T, et al. Differential effects of central and peripheral nerves on macrophages and microglia. *Glia* 1998;23(2):181–190.

555. Rapalino O, Lazarov-Spiegler O, Agranov E, et al. Implantation of stimulated homologous macrophages results in partial recovery of paraplegic rats. *Nat Med* 1998;4(7):814–821.

556. Lazarov-Spiegler O, Rapalino O, Agranov G, et al. Restricted inflammatory reaction in the CNS: a key impediment to axonal regeneration? *Mol Med Today* 1998;4(8):337–342.

557. Lazarov-Spiegler O, Solomon AS, Schwartz M. Peripheral nerve-stimulated macrophages stimulate a peripheral nerve-like regenerative response in rat transected optic nerve. *Glia* 1998;24(3):329–337.

558. Schwartz M, Lazarov-Spiegler O, Rapalino O, et al. Potential repair of rat spinal cord injuries using stimulated homologous macrophages. *Neurosurgery* 1999;44(5):1041–1046.

559. Moalem G, Leibowitz-Amit R, Yoles E, et al. Autoimmune T cells protect neurons from secondary degeneration after central nervous system axotomy. *Nat Med* 1999;5(1):49–55.

560. Schwalb JM, Boulis NM, Gu MF, et al. Two factors secreted by the goldfish optic nerve induce retinal ganglion cells to regenerate axons in culture. *J Neurosci* 1995;15(8):5514–5525.

561. Benowitz LI, Goldberg DE, Madsen JR, et al. Inosine stimulates ex-

tensive axon collateral growth in the rat corticospinal tract after injury. *Proc Natl Acad Sci U S A* 1999;96(23):13486–13490.

562. Hadlock T, Sundback C, Koka R, et al. A novel, biodegradable polymer conduit delivers neurotrophins and promotes nerve regeneration. *Laryngoscope* 1999;109(9):1412–1416.

563. Benowitz LI, Jing Y, Tabibiazar R, et al. Axon outgrowth is regulated by an intracellular purine-sensitive mechanism in retinal ganglion cells. *J Biol Chem* 1998;273(45):29626–29634.

564. Petrausch B, Tabibiazar R, Roser T, et al. A purine-sensitive pathway regulates multiple genes involved in axon regeneration in goldfish retinal ganglion cells. *J Neurosci* 2000;20(21):8031–8041.

565. Taylor EM, Yan R, Hauptmann N, et al. AIT-082, a cognitive enhancer, is transported into brain by a nonsaturable influx mechanism and out of brain by a saturable efflux mechanism. *J Pharmacol Exp Ther* 2000;293(3):813–821.

566. Lahiri DK, Ge YW, Farlow MR. Effect of a memory-enhancing drug, AIT-082, on the level of synaptophysin. *Ann N Y Acad Sci* 2000; 903:387–393.

567. Rathbone MP, Middlemiss PJ, Gysbers JW, et al. Trophic effects of purines in neurons and glial cells. *Prog Neurobiol* 1999;59(6): 663–690.

568. Middlemiss PJ, Glasky AJ, Rathbone MP, et al. AIT-082, a unique purine derivative, enhances nerve growth factor mediated neurite outgrowth from PC12 cells. *Neurosci Lett* 1995;199(2):131–134.

569. Grundman M, Corey-Bloom J, Thal LJ. Perspectives in clinical Alzheimer's disease research and the development of antidementia drugs. *J Neural Transm Suppl* 1998;53:255–275.

570. Qui J, Cai D, Filbin MT. Glial inhibition of nerve regeneration in the mature mammalian CNS. *Glia* 2000;29(2):166–174.

571. Cai D, Shen Y, DeBellard M, et al. Prior exposure to neurotrophins blocks inhibition of axonal regeneration by MAG and myelin via a cAMP-dependent mechanism. *Neuron* 1999;22(1):89–101.

572. Scherer SS, Xu YT, Roling D, et al. Expression of growth-associated protein-43 kd in Schwann cells is regulated by axon-Schwann cell interactions and cAMP. *J Neurosci Res* 1994;38(5):575–589.

573. Ambron RT, Walters ET. Priming events and retrograde injury signals. A new perspective on the cellular and molecular biology of nerve regeneration. *Mol Neurobiol* 1996;13(1):61–79.

574. McDonald JW, Liu XZ, Qu Y, et al. Transplanted embryonic stem cells survive, differentiate and promote recovery in injured rat spinal cord [Comments]. *Nat Med* 1999;5(12):1410–1412.

575. Liu S, Qu Y, Stewart TJ, et al. Embryonic stem cells differentiate into oligodendrocytes and myelinate in culture and after spinal cord transplantation. *Proc Natl Acad Sci U S A* 2000;97(11):6126–6131.

576. Huang DW, McKerracher L, Braun PE, et al. A therapeutic vaccine approach to stimulate axon regeneration in the adult mammalian spinal cord. *Neuron* 1999;24(3):639–647.

577. Filbin MT. Axon regeneration: vaccinating against spinal cord injury. *Curr Biol* 2000;10(3):R100–R103.

578. Hauben E, Butovsky O, Nevo U, et al. Passive or active immunization with myelin basic protein promotes recovery from spinal cord contusion. *J Neurosci* 2000;20(17):6421–6430.

579. Hauben E, Nevo U, Yoles E, et al. Autoimmune T cells as potential neuroprotective therapy for spinal cord injury [Letter]. *Lancet* 2000; 355(9200):286–287.

580. Dyer JK, Bourque JA, Steeves JD. Regeneration of brainstem-spinal axons after lesion and immunological disruption of myelin in adult rat. *Exp Neurol* 1998;154(1):12–22.

581. Hiebert GW, Dyer JK, Tetzlaff W, et al. Immunological myelin disruption does not alter expression of regeneration-associated genes in intact or axotomized rubrospinal neurons. *Exp Neurol* 2000;163(1): 149–156.

582. Keirstead HS, Morgan SV, Wilby MJ, et al. Enhanced axonal regeneration following combined demyelination plus Schwann cell transplantation therapy in the injured adult spinal cord. *Exp Neurol* 1999; 159(1):225–236.

583. Baron-Van Evercooren A, Avellana-Adalid V, Lachapelle F, et al. Schwann cell transplantation and myelin repair of the CNS. *Mult Scler* 1997;3(2):157–161.

584. Ridet JL, Pencalet P, Belcram M, et al. Effects of spinal cord x-irradiation on the recovery of paraplegic rats. *Exp Neurol* 2000;161(1): 1–14.

585. Taub E, Uswatte G, Pidikiti R. Constraint-induced movement therapy: a new family of techniques with broad application to physical rehabilitation—a clinical review [Comments]. *J Rehabil Res Dev* 1999; 36(3):237–251.

586. Liepert J, Bauder H, Wolfgang HR, et al. Treatment-induced cortical reorganization after stroke in humans. *Stroke* 2000;31(6):1210–1216.

SUBJECT INDEX

Page numbers followed by f indicate figures; page numbers followed by t indicate tables.

diagnosis of, 188
from endourethral stent, 197
Hydrosyringomyelia, 247, 456, 460–462, 461f
Hydrotherapy, for pressure ulcers, 215
Hyperalgesic border reaction, 394
Hypercalcemia, 169
in children, 444
in Guillain-Barré syndrome, 571, 573
immobilization, 571, 573
Hypercholesterolemia, 128
Hypercoagulability, 128
Hyperextension injuries
cervical, 54–56, 55f
radiography of, 35–37, 36f, 37f
thoracolumbar, 64, 65f
Hyperextension orthoses, 284–285
Hyperflexion injuries
cervical, 54–56, 55f, 57f
thoracolumbar, 62–64, 62f, 63f
Hyperglycemia, 164–167, 165f, 167t
immune function and, 237
Hyperhidrosis, pediatric, 445
Hyperinsulinemia, inactivity and, 166
Hyperlipidemia, 128, 167–169, 168f, 169t, 415
Hypertension, 166–167
in autonomic dysreflexia, 125–127
in children, 444
immediate postinjury, 97, 123
Hyperthermia
exercise-related, 335
pediatric, 445
Hypertonicity. *See also* Spasticity
assessment of, 223, 223t
Hypertriglyceridemia, 168–169, 168f, 169t
Hyperuricemia, 167
Hypoalbuminemia, pressure ulcers in, 212
Hypocapnia, chronic, 151
Hypocortisolism, 171–172
Hypogonadism, 174
Hyponatremia, 172
in head trauma, 270
Hypoosmolar hyponatremia, 172
Hypotension
in neurogenic shock, 97, 123–124
orthostatic, 124–125
spinal infarction in, 514
treatment of, 97, 124
Hypothermia
local, in acute care, 99
in neurogenic shock, 97, 124
pediatric, 445

I

Ibuprofen, 399, 400t
Ice-water test, in voiding dysfunction, 188
Ileal conduit, in urinary diversion, 194
Ileocecal valve, in orthotopic urinary diversion, 194

Ileus, 161
Iliac autograft, in spinal fusion, 101, 102
Imaging studies, 35–40
in acute care, 98, 98t, 100
computed tomography, 37, 98t. *See also* Computed tomography
in dual diagnosis, 254
in head trauma, 254
indications for, 98t
magnetic resonance imaging, 37–40, 38f–40f. *See also* Magnetic resonance imaging
plain-film radiography, 34–37, 35f–37f, 98t. *See also* Radiography, plain-film
in acute care, 97–98, 98t
swimmer's view in, 35
plain-film tomography, 37
in respiratory disorders, 139–140
Imipramine
for depression, 302t
for pain, 401, 402t
for urinary incontinence, 192
Immobility. *See* Inactivity
Immobilization
of pathologic fractures, 242
of spinal fractures. *See* Spine, stabilization of
after tendon transfer, 434
Immune function, 234–238, 235f, 236t
aging and, 238, 414
assessment of, 235
autonomic nervous system in, 236
exercise and, 237–238, 414
Immune system, age-related changes in, 414
Immunization, in spinal cord regeneration, 606
Immunizations, 438
transverse myelitis and, 506
Immunoglobulin, intravenous
for chronic demyelinating polyneuropathies, 569
for Guillain-Barré syndrome, 569
Immunoglobulins, 235
Immunomodulators, for multiple sclerosis, 531–532
Immunosuppressants, for multiple sclerosis, 531–532
Immunosuppression, exercise-related, 335
Immunotherapy, for spinal cord regeneration, 606
Impaired role, 303
Impairment, definition of, 91
Impingement syndromes, shoulder, 243–244
Impotence, 323–324
in multiple sclerosis, 533
Inactivity
body composition changes and, 173–174, 173f
carbohydrate metabolism and, 166

complications of
in Guillain-Barré syndrome, 571
metabolic, 571, 573–574
hypercalcemia of, 571, 573–574
immune function and, 237
osteopenia and, 170
Incentive spirometry, 142
Incidence, 69
age and, 70–71, 70f, 71t, 439
ethnicity and, 71, 71t, 72
gender and, 71, 71t
Incomplete injury, 87
anterior cord syndrome in, 90
Brown-Séquard syndrome in, 89–90
central cord syndrome in, 88–89, 89t
cruciate paralysis in, 89, 89t
posterior cord syndrome in, 90
Incontinence
fecal. *See also* Bowel dysfunction
pediatric, 443, 457
urinary. *See also* Voiding dysfunction
in amyotrophic lateral sclerosis, 547
bladder management for, 280–283
drugs for, 192–193, 200
due to bladder, 191–196, 198–199
due to sphincter, 196
intermittent catheterization for, 191–192
neuroprosthesis for, 374–376
pediatric, 442
posterior rhizotomy for, 374–375
rhizotomy for, 374–375
from sacral lesions, 198–199
supportive treatment for, 195–196
surgery for, 193–195, 199
Independence, age-related decline in, 415–416
Independent living facilities/services, 316–318
Indomethacin, 399, 400t
postoperative, pediatric heterotopic ossification and, 454
Indwelling catheter
bladder cancer and, 202–203
for urinary incontinence, 195–196
for urinary retention, 200
Infants. *See also* Children
myelodysplastic, urodynamic studies in, 191, 456
myelomeningocele in, 455–456. *See also* Myelomeningocele
neural tube defects in, 455–459, 458f
spinal cord injury incidence in, 439
Infarction. *See also* Ischemia
spinal cord, 513–515, 515f
arterial, 513–515, 515f
venous, 515
Infection(s), 234. *See also* Immune function
from artificial urethral sphincters, 199

with extensor carpi radialis longus-to-flexor digitorum profundus, 432

with posterior deltoid-to-triceps, 431–432

with pronator teres-to-flexor digitorum profundus, 432

candidates for, 425, 426t

to flexor digitorum profundus, 432

flexor pollicis longus tenodesis in, passive, 426, 426f, 431

history of, 424

manual muscle test for, 426

neuromuscular electrical stimulation after, 435–436

occupational performance assessment for, 425–426

patient classification for, 427, 427t

physical assessment for, 425–428, 426t, 427t

posterior deltoid-to-triceps, 430, 430f, 432

principles of, 425

procedures for

C5 functional level and, 429–430, 429f, 430f

C6 functional level and, 431–433, 431f, 433f

C7 functional level and, 433

C8 functional level and, 433–434

range of motion assessment for, 427–428

rehabilitation after, 434–435

sensory examination for, 426–427

spasticity and, 428

timing of, 425

Tennis, wheelchair, 341

wheelchairs, 342

Tenodesis, 425–426, 426f, 431

Terazosin, for autonomic dysreflexia, in children, 445

Testis

changes in, 325

structure and function of, 322, 323f

Testosterone

decrease in, 173–175

replacement, 174

Tethered cord, 249

Tetraplegia

classification of, 427, 427t

definition of, 87

renal calculi in, 202

tendon transfers in, 424–436. *See also* Tendon transfers

Thecal sac, 52f

Theophylline, 143

in mechanical ventilation, 148

Therapeutic exercise. *See* Exercise; Exercises

Therapeutic vaccines, in spinal cord regeneration, 606

Thermoregulation

impaired, exercise-related, 335

in neurogenic shock, 97, 124

pediatric, 445

Thiazolidinediones, for diabetes prevention, 167

Thomas collar, 283

Thoracic spinal cord segments, 8

Thoracic spinal surgery, 104–105

Thoracolumbar spine. *See also under* Lumbar; Spine; Thoracic

anatomy of, 27, 28f–32f, 59–61, 60f, 61f

anterior wedge fractures of, 62, 62f

bilateral facet dislocations of, 64, 65f

biomechanics of, 59–61, 60f, 61f

burst fractures of, 62, 63f

Chance fractures of, 64, 64f

degenerative disease of, 61, 61f, 62f

flexion-distraction fractures of, 64, 64f

hyperextension injuries of, 64, 65f

hyperflexion injuries of, 62–64, 62f, 63f

injuries of, 64–65

rotation injuries of, 66

seat-belt fractures of, 64, 64f, 104

shearing injuries of, 66, 66f, 67f

Smith fractures of, 64

surgery of, 104–105

Thoracolumbosacral orthoses, 101, 284–285, 286f

in children, 452–453

Thoracotomy, 104. *See also* Spinal surgery

Three-column model, of spinal stability, 33–34, 34f, 100, 100f

l-Threonine, for spasticity, 227

Thromboembolic disorders, 128–132

etiology of, 128

in Guillain-Barré syndrome, 570–571

in head trauma, 269–270

incidence of, 128–129, 129t

pediatric, 443–444

prevention of, 129–132, 130t, 131t, 382

in cancer, 494

spinal cord infarction and, 514–515

time of onset of, 129

Thyroid function, 171

Thyroxine, 171

Ticket to Work and Work Incentives Improvement Act, 319

Tidal volume, in mechanical ventilation, 145–148, 147t, 148f

Tiedowns, wheelchair, 355, 355f

Tight filum terminale, 455

Tilt-in-Space wheelchair, 211, 583t, 584, 584f

Tiludronate, for osteopenia, 170

Tinzaparin, prophylactic, 131, 131t, 132

Tirilazad mesylate, in immediate postinjury period, 24, 99

Tissue engineering, 118

Tizanidine, for spasticity, 226–227, 226t, 270

in children, 447

TLSO orthosis, 101

in children, 452–453

Tomography

computed, 37, 98t

plain-film, 37, 98t

Tongue touch keypad, 590

Tonic spasticity, 221. *See also* Spasticity

mechanisms of, 222

Topiramate

for amyotrophic lateral sclerosis, 544

for pain, 401, 402t

Toxic myelopathy, 518–519

Toxoplasmosis, 508

Tracheal suctioning, 140

Tracheostomy

in amyotrophic lateral sclerosis, 545

vs. endotracheal intubation, 144

pediatric, 447

Tracheostomy tubes, 143

Trach talk, 140, 143, 149

Traction

in acute care, 98

pin placement for, 98

weight for, 98

Training. *See* Exercise

Tramadol, 399

Transcutaneous electrical nerve stimulation, 399–401

for spasticity, 225

Transfer(s), 281

in acute care, 96–97

neuroprostheses for, 367–370, 367f–370f. *See also* Neuromuscular electrical stimulation

training for, 287–289

transfer board, 288

types of, 287, 288–289

vehicle, 350–351, 353–354, 592

Transfer board, 288, 288f

Transfer board transfer, 288

Transplants

cell, 118–119

fetal spinal cord, 118

Transport, patient, 97

Transurethral sphincterotomy, 197

Transverse atlantal ligament, 40, 41f, 43f, 44

Transverse foramina, cervical, 49, 50f

Transverse myelitis, 474, 506–507

Transverse processes, cervical, 49–51, 50f

Trapezius muscle, 32, 32f, 135

Trapped lung, 138–139

Traumatic brain injury, 261–271

agitation in, 266–268

alertness in, 269

arousal in, 269

behavioral disturbances in, 266–268

cognitive disturbances in, 265–266, 268–269

deep vein thrombosis in, 269–270

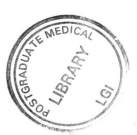